Safe Maternity and Pediatric Nursing Care

THIRD EDITION

Luanne Linnard-Palmer, EdD, MSN, RN, CPN
Professor of Nursing
   Dominican University of California San Rafael, California
RN Clinical Nurse Coordinator
   Pediatric Hematology Oncology
   Stanford Specialty Health Care
   San Francisco, California

Gloria Haile Coats, MSN, RN, FNP
Professor Emeritus of Nursing
   Modesto Junior College
   Modesto, California

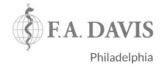

F.A. DAVIS

Philadelphia

F. A. Davis Company
1915 Arch Street
Philadelphia, PA 19103
www.fadavis.com
Copyright © 2025 by F. A. Davis Company

Printed in the United States of America
Last digit indicates print number: 10 9 8 7 6 5 4 3 2 1

Publisher, Nursing: John Goucher
Manager of Project and eProject Management: Catherine H. Carroll
Content Project Manager 2: Sean P. West
Art and Design Manager: Carolyn O'Brien

As new scientific information becomes available through basic and clinical research, recommended treatments and medication therapies undergo changes. The author(s) and publisher have done everything possible to make this book accurate, up to date, and in accord with accepted standards at the time of publication. The author(s), editors, and publisher are not responsible for errors or omissions or for consequences from application of the book, and make no warranty, expressed or implied, in regard to the contents of the book. Any practice described in this book should be applied by the reader in accordance with professional standards of care used in regard to the unique circumstances that may apply in each situation. The reader is advised always to check product information (package inserts) for changes and new information regarding dose and contraindications before administering any medication. Caution is especially urged when using new or infrequently ordered medications.

ISBN 978-1-7196-4884-4

Library of Congress Cataloging-in-Publication Data

Names: Linnard-Palmer, Luanne, author. | Coats, Gloria Haile, author.
Title: Safe maternity and pediatric nursing care / Luanne Linnard-Palmer,
  Gloria Haile Coats.
Description: Third edition. | Philadelphia : F.A. Davis, [2025] | Includes
  bibliographical references and index.
Identifiers: LCCN 2024034067 (print) | LCCN 2024034068 (ebook) | ISBN
  9781719648844 (paperback) | ISBN 9781719654104 (epub) | ISBN
  9781719654111 (pdf)
Subjects: MESH: Maternal-Child Nursing--methods | Pediatric
  Nursing--methods
Classification: LCC RJ245 (print) | LCC RJ245 (ebook) | NLM WY 157.3 |
  DDC 618.92/00231--dc23/eng/20241010
LC record available at https://lccn.loc.gov/2024034067
LC ebook record available at https://lccn.loc.gov/2024034068

About the Authors

Luanne Linnard-Palmer, EdD, MSN, RN, CPN, is a professor of pediatric nursing at Dominican University of California located just north of San Francisco in Marin County. She has been teaching in both undergraduate and graduate nursing programs for over 35 years. She currently practices as a pediatric oncology hematology RN Clinical Nurse Coordinator for Stanford Specialty Health Care in San Francisco. Her passion for teaching and clinical practice spans a 37-year career. She works closely with a diverse clinical team that includes medical assistants, licensed vocational nurses and licensed practical nurses (LVN/LPNs), physicians, medical students and interns, and advanced practice nurses. Her goal in writing this book is to provide a foundation of critical information with a focus on safety based on her clinical practice experiences.

Gloria Haile Coats, MSN, RN, FNP, is a professor emeritus of maternity and pediatric nursing at Modesto Junior College in Modesto, California. She has a diploma from Burge School of Nursing in Springfield, Missouri; a BSN from California State University, Stanislaus; an MSN from California State University, Dominquez Hills; and a Post-Master's Family Nurse Practitioner Certificate from Sonoma State University. She has experience in the development, implementation, and evaluation of nursing education and curriculum. Her expertise in nursing education in both the classroom and clinical setting has enabled her to take difficult concepts of nursing education and make them understandable for nursing students. She understands the time constraints in nursing education, and her goal for this book is to provide the essential need-to-know information for nurses to provide safe and effective maternity and pediatric care.

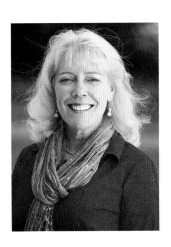

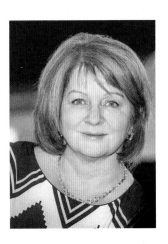

This book is dedicated to my father, Howard Warren Linnard;
my mother, Bernice Elaine Linnard; and my brother, Loren Linnard.

A man whose passion for health, happiness, joy, and love
permeated every aspect of his successful life.

A woman whose strength, creativity, work ethic, and love continue
to influence the well-being of everyone she encounters.

A brother whose creativity flowed endlessly.

Luanne Linnard-Palmer

This book is dedicated to my past and future students:

Thank you for the honor and privilege of being part of your
nursing education.

"Let us never consider ourselves finished nurses . . . we must be
learning all of our lives."

—*Florence Nightingale*

Diana Haile Coats

Preface

This text offers the reader a variety of learning experiences that combine the art of nursing care and practice with the foundations of science. It includes essential nursing content from preconception to conception, pregnancy, delivery, and neonatal care through adolescent care. The book is organized to present principles and concepts of maternity nursing through the principles and concepts of pediatric nursing—health promotion and health restoration. The contents span preconception health through the end of the adolescent developmental stage and across concepts and systems of illness, injury, recovery, and healing.

The authors wish to thank faculty who used previous editions of this book for their generous input into the revision plan for the Third Edition. The feedback informed our decisions to update and improve content and to emphasize critical thinking and clinical judgment. We trust that you and your students will appreciate this approach.

Safety

The concept of safety is presented in this text as the overarching framework. In all aspects of maternity and pediatric nursing, safety remains the ultimate responsibility of the nurse in their role. Safety is incorporated into one's thinking, actions, skills, and caring practice. The safety-related information included in each chapter, including in the boxed features Safety *Stat!* and Safe and Effective Nursing Care, provides guidance about essential safety protocols for maternity and pediatric nursing.

Critical Thinking and Clinical Judgment

Critical thinking is an important and necessary problem-solving process within the profession of nursing, and critical thinking skills are necessary for clinical judgment. Critical thinking is a systematic way of first identifying the key aspects of a problem and then progressing through a process in which solutions are found and are offered to others. Clinical judgment is a means to implement sound interventions and is presented throughout the book as a supportive scaffold for sound decision-making. Within the role of the maternity and pediatric nurse, clinical judgment is a key process across care. Human variation within conception, bearing children, raising children, and providing for their care influences how a maternity or pediatric nurse evaluates families' needs. Providing guidance, education, and care to each unique family is a joy and a challenge. Through the use of critical thinking principles and clinical judgment, you can identify the needs of a family and implement caring practices that provide for each individual within the family.

Students will find critical thinking and clinical judgment features in each of the chapters. It is the intent of the authors to challenge the students in their problem-solving skills by providing exercises that require the student to find resources, solutions to problems, and answers from clinical settings and diverse practice areas, and then work to solve problems as part of a health-care team.

Themes

The unifying principles of excellent and safe nursing care presented throughout this book include the following:

- Family as the unit of care
- Patient- and family-centered care principles
- Safety across all encounters
- Communication
- Culturally sensitive care including how social determinants of health can affect outcomes
- Critical thinking and clinical judgment to help reduce errors and improve outcomes

Features

This text provides extensive chapter features to educate students about various aspects of the chapter topic in patient settings and encounters. Each feature will assist the student in learning more about the chapter content by illuminating important topics and ideas. The following features are included in text chapters:

- *NEW* **Critical Thinking and Clinical Judgment Case Studies:** Case studies with questions open each chapter and appear throughout chapters. Students can use each chapter's case study to challenge themselves to search for answers to the case study questions while reading the chapter. These case studies encourage students to apply nursing knowledge to clinical situations to develop their clinical judgment skills. Suggested answers to the Critical Thinking and Clinical Judgment case study questions are located on fadavis.com.
- **Conceptual Cornerstone:** A concept is an organizing principle, a generalization, a classification, or an idea that is used to understand information. In nursing, concepts categorize relevant information in a way that allows students to apply it to other situations. This type of learning promotes critical thinking because the student is taught to apply a concept and not just memorize facts. Concepts can be applied to understanding disease processes, patient behaviors, family dynamics, and health conditions and to guide professional practice. Each chapter begins with a Conceptual Cornerstone that can be applied to the information in the chapter. This feature is particularly useful in programs that teach conceptually.
- **Phonetic Pronunciations:** These accompany every Key Term to help students to communicate effectively.
- **Word-Building Footnotes:** These appear in most chapters to help students master medical terminology.

- **Evidence-Based Practice:** This boxed content encourages students to think about how they will practice as nurses and how they need to base their practice on the newest and best evidence available.
- **Patient Teaching Guidelines:** These concise guidelines are provided to enable you to answer patient questions and provide or reinforce health-care–related teaching specific to each chapter's topic.
- **Health Promotion:** An important task of nursing is to promote health and empower patients to improve their health and the health of their families. Important health-promotion information is provided in each chapter to assist the student nurse to be knowledgeable about health-promotion behaviors.
- **Labs & Diagnostics:** Laboratory values or diagnostic tests that are pertinent to providing safe maternity and pediatric nursing care are highlighted in this feature.
- **Learn to C.U.S.:** This safety-related feature highlights a method of communication in which you use the format of C: "I am **c**oncerned," U: "I am **u**ncomfortable," and S: "We have a **s**afety issue" to communicate with members of the health-care team.
- **Therapeutic Communication:** Patient- and family-centered care requires you to be adept at therapeutic communication. Examples of therapeutic communication are included to provide the student nurse with a foundation of skills for effective communication with patients and their families.
- **Team Works:** This feature presents you as part of the health-care team who, with other health-care professionals, provides safe patient care.
- **Medication Facts:** Medications that are relevant to the management of patient care are the focus of this feature. It provides basic need-to-know information regarding medications discussed in the chapter, including information related to safe medication administration.
- **Nursing Care Plan:** Nursing care plans are provided to allow students to see how the chapter information can be applied in a nursing care plan. Information may include nursing data collection, diagnoses, interventions, and/or expected patient outcomes.
- **Safety *Stat!:*** The most important safety issues related to safe patient care are highlighted in the Safety *Stat!* features included throughout the chapters.
- **Safe and Effective Nursing Care:** This feature presents nursing practices that support safe care or a patient's physical, emotional, for developmental health and represent the marriage of best practices and patient-centered care.
- **NCLEX®-Style Review Questions:** Each chapter includes NCLEX®-style review questions to assist students with preparing for course and national licensure examinations. Answers are located right after the questions for students' ease of reference. Rationales are located on the Student's Resource page on fadavis.com.
- **Critical Thinking Questions:** Following the review questions, each chapter includes critical thinking questions that can be used in the classroom or completed by the student to apply the chapter information to a critical thinking situation. Answers are located on the Instructor's Resource page on fadavis.com.

Appendices

The appendices support further learning, classroom activities, and application of text material around the evaluation and care of the neonate, child, and adolescent. Appendices include the following:

Appendix A: Best Practices for Medication Administration for Pediatric Patients

Appendix B: Thirty-Five Types of Medical Errors and Tips for Preventing Harm: Quality and Safety Imperatives for Nurses Caring for Patients Across the Developmental Period

Appendix C: Conversion Factors

Appendix D: Common Medication Administration Calculations in Pediatrics

Resources

Study Guide

This essential companion provides the student with a variety of means to demonstrate knowledge, application, analysis, and evaluation of the material provided throughout the text. Each study guide chapter includes exercises that help the learner deepen their understanding and demonstrate mastery of the concepts presented in the book.

The study guide includes exercises that address all of the types of text features, including:

- Multiple choice and other NCLEX®-style review questions
- True or false questions
- Matching exercises
- Short-answer questions
- Fill-in-the-blank questions
- Essay questions
- Crossword puzzle
- Concept maps
- Table completion exercises
- Labeling exercises

Answers to the study guide questions are located on the Instructor's Resource page on fadavis.com. This allows instructors to choose whether students should have the answers before completing the study guide exercises.

Additional Student Resources

Use your unique fadavis.com access code from the inside front cover to access the following resources:

- **Postconference Questions and Activities** that ask the student to consider the specific chapter's content related to relevant aspects of clinical care

- **Suggested Answers to Critical Thinking and Clinical Judgment Case Studies**
- **Printable Care Plans**
- **References**
- **Rationales for In-Text Review Questions**

Instructor Resources
- **ebook**
- **Electronic Test Bank** of NCLEX®-style questions with rationales for correct and incorrect answers and page references, in a learning management system (LMS)-compatible format
- **PowerPoint Presentations** of fully customizable slides
- **Digital Image Collection** includes all of the images from the text
- **Printable Concept Maps**
- **Answers to Critical Thinking Questions, and Postconference Questions and Activities**
- **Answers to Study Guide questions and activities**
- **Skills Checklists**

LPN/LVN Connections

F. A. Davis is pleased to include **LPN/LVN Connections,** a consistent and recognizable approach to design and content that will make it easier for students and instructors to use multiple F. A. Davis textbooks throughout the LPN/LVN curriculum.

We have increased continuity whenever possible without erasing the authors' autonomy or changing legacy content that has been popular in past editions. This makes it easier for instructors and students to move through the textbooks and ancillary products while recognizing shared themes and featured content.

Textbook Design, Style, and Pedagogy
- All textbook chapters include:
  - Numbered Learning Outcomes
  - Key Terms with Phonetic Pronunciations listed on the chapter opener and boldfaced where first defined in the chapter
  - Chapter Concepts
  - Bulleted Key Points
  - NCLEX®-style Review Questions with answers right on the page for ease of reference
  - Chapter References, located online
- A Reading Level Evaluation is performed during the manuscript development to ensure readability.
- Word-Building Footnotes help students build understanding of root terminology.

- A uniform, space-saving internal design features special heads and colors that are shared across titles for features with similar content to increase recognition.
- Consistent and current terminology and laboratory values are used across titles; the authors followed *Davis's Comprehensive Manual of Laboratory & Diagnostic Tests With Nursing Implications* by Van Leeuwen and Bladh for all values.

Standardized Student and Faculty Resources
For Students:

- Davis Advantage online resources for students
- Study Guide with perforated pages so that students can hand in assignments if requested; the Answer Key is provided to instructors online to distribute if desired

For Instructors:

- Davis Advantage online resources for students
- eBook
- NCLEX®-style test bank
- PowerPoint presentations
- Digital image collection

F. A. Davis LPN/LVN Advisory Board

Contributors to the First Edition

Deborah Vance Beaumont, MSN, RN
Mind Body Nutrition RN, Functional Medicine Practitioner
Bend, Oregon
Chapter 37 Child With a Communicable Disease

Olivia Catolico, PhD, MSN, RN, CNL, BC
Professor of Nursing
Dominican University of California
San Rafael, California
Chapter 2 Culture

Leslie Crane, EdD, MSN, RN
Director of the CNA/HHA Program
Santa Rosa Junior College
Santa Rosa, California
Chapter 30 Child With a Respiratory Condition

Catherine E. Cyr-Roy, RN, BSN, MPA/HSA
Manager of Case Management
Kaiser Vallejo
Vallejo, California
Families Experiencing Stressors content

Natalie (Lu) Sweeney, RN, MSN, CNS
Professor of Nursing
Dominican University of California
San Rafael, California
Chapter 31 Child With a Cardiac Condition

Reviewers

Mary Amundson, MSN, RN
Practical Nursing Faculty
Northland Community and Technical College
East Grand Forks, Minnesota

Sandra Barker, BSRN, MS
Master Instructor, Nursing
Tennessee College of Applied Technology at Elizabethton
Elizabethton, Tennessee

Charlene Cowley, MS, RN, CPNP
Pediatric Nursing Instructor LPN Program
Pima Community College
Tucson, Arizona

Carla Crider, MSN, EDDc, RNC, C-EFM
Assistant Professor
Tarrant County College
Fort Worth, Texas

Mary E. Hancock, PhD, RNC-OB
Associate Professor of Nursing
Shepherd University
Shepherdstown, West Virginia

Kathy Johnson, MSN, RN
Practical Nursing Program Coordinator
Greater Lowell Technical School
Tyngsboro, Massachusetts

Rachel Matheson, RN, CAE
Learning Manager in the Practical Nursing Program
Holland College
Charlottetown, Prince Edward Island
Canada

Jane C. Parish, BBA, MSN, PhD, RN, CNE, CPN
Professor of Nursing
Walters State Community College
Morristown, Tennessee

Cheryl Puckett, BSN, MSN, RNC
Associate Professor
Bluegrass Community and Tech College
Danville, Kentucky

Zelda Suzan, EdD, RN, CNE
Associate Professor
Phillips School of Nursing at Mount Sinai Beth Israel
New York, New York

Brief Contents

Contents

CHAPTER 1

Introduction to Maternity and Pediatric Nursing

KEY TERMS

assent (uh-SENT)
autonomy (aw-TAWN-uh-MEE)
beneficence (ben-EFF-ih-senss)
emancipation (ih-MAN-sih-PAY-shun)
empowerment (em-POW-er-ment)
enabling (en-AY-bling)
ethics (ETH-iks)
justice (JUHSS-tiss)
nonmaleficence (NON-mal-EFF-ih-sents)
scope of practice (SKOHP uv PRAK-tiss)
standards of care (STAN-derdz uv KAIR)

CHAPTER CONCEPTS

Family
Growth and Development
Professionalism
Quality Improvement
Safety

LEARNING OUTCOMES

1. Define the key terms.
2. Write a personal definition of *quality health care*.
3. Compare the roles of the licensed practical/vocational nurse (LPN/LVN), registered nurse (RN), nurse practitioner (NP), clinical nurse specialist (CNS), and certified nurse midwife (CNM).
4. Discuss the legalities and ethics of nursing practice including scope of practice, delegation, standards of care, and institutional policies.
5. Explain the ethical principles of autonomy, beneficence, nonmaleficence, and justice as related to maternity and pediatric nursing.
6. Identify possible ethical dilemmas in maternity and pediatric nursing.
7. Analyze the purposes for and essential elements of informed consent, including the concept of assent for school-aged children older than 7 and the emancipated minor.
8. List the children's rights and the family rights in health care.
9. Apply principles of family-centered care to families receiving care in a hospital or home setting.
10. Define evidence-based practice and discuss the importance of evidence-based practice to the nursing profession.
11. Describe the anatomical, physiological, social, and emotional differences between adults and children, emphasizing the critical components that are pertinent to safe, emergent care of children across health-care settings.

CRITICAL THINKING

Lisa, a nursing student, is in her clinical rotation for postpartum care. At the change of shift report, she learns that her assigned patient had a positive drug screen for heroin and that her premature baby is in the neonatal intensive care nursery. Lisa is anxious about providing care for this patient because of her own strong personal beliefs about illicit drug use during pregnancy. Lisa pages her clinical nursing instructor and asks for another assignment. She says to her instructor, "I am uncomfortable with this assignment. It makes me angry to think about what she did to her baby. Can I have another patient instead?"

Questions
1. What do you think the clinical instructor will say?
2. Why would the instructor want Lisa to accept the assignment?

CLINICAL JUDGMENT

Leon, an 11-year-old, is in the pediatric nursing unit. His gastrostomy tube (GT) insertion site requires a surgical revision because acidic gastric contents are spilling out onto the skin of his abdomen, causing redness, irritation, and infection. Leon's cognitive age is approximately that of a 2- to 3-year-old, and he has a minimal vocabulary to express his needs. As you care for Leon during your shift, you experience difficulty communicating with him, which presents challenges with evaluating pain, providing simple instructions, maintaining an intact IV site, and administering medications.

Questions

1. What is your plan to manage Leon's care?
2. What communication strategies will you use?

CONCEPTUAL CORNERSTONE

Safety

During the development period from newborn to adolescence, safety remains one of the most important aspects of care of children. Safety includes providing anticipatory guidance to parents and caregivers as to what they can expect currently and in the future for their child's particular developmental stage. Nurses who care for children role-model safety for parents, caregivers, grandparents, siblings, and visitors.

CONCEPTUAL CORNERSTONE

Quality Improvement

Quality in health care can have many definitions. A nurse manager may view quality as the wise use of resources, a lack of errors in providing care, and positive patient feedback. The nurse at the bedside may view quality as the delivery of safe and effective care. The physician or midwife may view quality as a positive patient response to medications and interventions without complications. The patient may consider health care good only if it meets their own expectations for improvement and recovery. According to the World Health Organization (WHO, 2022), *quality health care* is "the degree to which health services for individuals and populations increase the likelihood of desired health outcomes... it is based on evidence-based professional knowledge and is critical for achieving universal health coverage."

Nurses can improve quality in health care in the following ways:

- Providing safe care to patients by working within the scope of practice, utilizing standards of care built on evidence-based practice, and making sound decisions in providing care

- Delivering family- and patient-centered care with attention to the specific needs, values, and expectations of the patient and family
- Improving patient care by identifying errors and hazards and implementing safety principles
- Collaborating with health-care team members to reduce errors and improve care
- Utilizing hospital resources in a cost-effective manner by not wasting materials and time
- Providing equal care to all patients that does not vary in quality based upon gender, ethnicity, culture, or socioeconomic status (Giddens, 2021)

Welcome to maternity and pediatric nursing! Get ready to build on your nursing foundations knowledge as you learn to care for new patient populations.

Maternity nursing is an exciting field. Welcoming a new life into the world and supporting the family can be two of the most rewarding aspects of health care. Maternity nursing offers a broad range of nursing opportunities that includes providing care from puberty to menopause. Nurses can specialize in prenatal care, labor and delivery, postpartum care, newborn care, neonatal intensive care, women's health, and infertility care.

Nurses caring for children require a unique set of knowledge, skills, and behaviors. Pediatric nursing is considered a specialty practice requiring a body of knowledge acquired through study and experience. Pediatric nursing involves caring for children between birth and 18 years of age, as well as their families, in a variety of clinical settings focusing on normal growth and development; acute, chronic, and critical care issues; and end-of-life and palliative care (Fig. 1.1; Box 1.1).

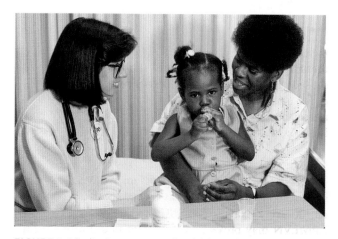

FIGURE 1.1 Pediatric nurses care for children of all ages.

Box 1.1

The Roles of the Pediatric Nurse

- Fostering family-centered care (family unit–based care focusing on partnerships and collaboration)
- Educating families in the prevention of common injuries and accidents across childhood
- Providing health promotion through education, screening, and prevention measures
- Teaching principles of anticipatory guidance and expected behaviors for developmental stages
- Providing for care during acute illnesses or exacerbations of chronic conditions
- Providing community-based nursing care focused on communities and patient groups
- Providing complex care coordination for children with multiple morbidities
- Advocating for the child when families are unable to secure necessary care
- Providing death and dying care and symptom management at the end of life

ROLES IN MATERNAL–CHILD AND PEDIATRIC NURSING

Maternity and pediatric nursing focuses on the care of childbearing women, newborn infants, children, and families. Care may begin before conception with planning for pregnancy or addressing fertility problems. Nursing care continues throughout the pregnancy when you encourage a healthy pregnancy or manage complications of pregnancy. During labor and delivery, you provide labor care until the physician or certified nurse midwife (CNM) arrives for the delivery. After delivery, nurses care for the mother as she recovers and her newborn adjusts to life outside the uterus. Nurses provide patient-centered and family-centered care in a variety of ways as licensed practical/vocational nurses (LPN/LVN), registered nurses (RNs), nurse practitioners (NPs), clinical nurse specialists (CNSs), or CNMs.

Certified Nursing Assistant

The certified nursing assistant (CNA) has a narrow scope of practice that includes assisting with patient care. This care includes supporting the patient's daily needs of nutrition, dressing, and movement, all under direct supervision of a licensed nurse, an advanced practice registered nurse (APRN) or NP, a physician's assistant (PA), or a physician. The CNA assists the nurse with taking the patient's vital signs, collecting specimens, and assisting with transportation.

Licensed Practical/Vocational Nurse

An LPN/LVN has completed a program in a technical school or community college and has passed the National Council Licensure Examination (NCLEX) for LPNs/LVNs. The LPN/LVN may provide nursing care in a doctor's office, clinic, home health-care situation, schools, or hospital under the direction of an RN, NP, physician, or midwife and may assist with preparing patients for pregnancy and delivery.

Registered Nurse

An RN has graduated from an accredited nursing program with either an associate degree in nursing (ADN) or a bachelor's degree in nursing (BSN) and has passed the NCLEX for RNs. The RN can evaluate the patient, plan and provide care, provide teaching, monitor the progression of the pregnancy through delivery, and provide postpartum and newborn care as well as care for pediatric patients across the developmental period.

Nurse Practitioner

An NP is an advanced practice nurse who has graduated from an accredited program with either a master's degree in nursing (MSN) or a doctorate of nursing practice (DNP) degree and has passed a certification examination. An NP provides advanced care and can prescribe medications. The NP may specialize in women's health throughout the life span with emphasis on contraception, fertility problems, prepregnancy care, pregnancy care, postpartum care, lactation problems, newborn care, and menopause care. Pediatric NPs care for children across the developmental period.

Clinical Nurse Specialist

A CNS is an RN who has obtained an advanced degree and clinical preparation at the MSN level with a focus on education, management, and research roles relative to patient care. The CNS often works in clinics and hospitals alongside nurses to educate and support them in providing excellent care to maternity and pediatric patients.

Certified Nurse Midwife

A CNM is an advanced practice nurse with an MSN or a DNP who has passed a certification examination in the area of pregnancy and delivery. The CNM provides care for the woman through pregnancy, labor, delivery, and postpartum. The CNM can prescribe medications and has hospital privileges that allow the CNM to deliver babies in the hospital.

LEGALITIES AND ETHICS

Nurses have guidelines, both legal and ethical, to follow when providing nursing care. This section discusses the legal guidelines that are in place for maternity and pediatric nurses as well as the ethical guidelines that nurses can use when faced with ethical dilemmas.

Legalities

Every licensed nurse, not just maternity and pediatric nurses, must be aware of the laws of the state in which they are licensed regarding the care that they are legally licensed to provide. Nurses who do not meet the standards expected of them may be held legally responsible.

Scope of Practice

The nursing scope of practice is determined by the state in which you are licensed. The **scope of practice** is the legal outline of what you can do according to the laws of that state. For example, an LPN/LVN, an RN, an NP, and a CNM all have different levels of legal authority in providing nursing care to maternity, newborn, and pediatric patients.

Delegation

The act of delegating an activity or task to another caregiver can be tricky. The delegator must know what the scope of practice is for the person being asked to carry out a task for another. In addition, the delegator assumes responsibility for the appropriateness of any activity delegated to another, such as an RN delegating a task to an LVN or LPN. For example, a home health care RN may delegate a dressing change, care of a child's feeding tube and enteral nutrition, or the overnight care of an older infant with an apnea monitor to an LVN. These are general nursing skills that can be safely delegated to an LVN and are within the LVN scope of practice. All boards of nursing in the United States include information on their websites about the state laws and rules that govern nurses' practice in that state. Use the following three steps to determine if a task or action is appropriate for delegation:

1. *Clarify what the specific activity or task is by defining all aspects of the issue:* Look at institutional policies and procedures, check online for information related to your state board of nursing, and then determine whether the person has the documented competency to perform the delegated task.
2. *Review the legal standards of the task:* LVNs/LPNs cannot perform independent assessments and care planning without collaborating with an RN because this is beyond the LVN/LPN scope of practice. Do not jeopardize your nursing license by accepting a delegated task or delegating to another that which is outside of your scope of practice.
3. *Decide whether the preceding elements support or reject the delegated action or task:* If you cannot perform the action legally or safely, then a supervisor should be notified so that a qualified person can be identified to perform the action safely, legally, and proficiently.

Standards of Care

Standards of care are a model of established practice that is accepted as the correct way to provide care for a patient; they are guidelines used to determine what a nurse should do. Standards of care provide a guide to the knowledge, skills, attitude, and judgment needed to practice safe nursing care.

Federal and state laws and professional organizations such as the American Nurses Association (ANA) help define standards of care. For maternity nurses, the Association of Women's Health, Obstetric and Neonatal Nurses (AWHONN) has established standards for the care of women and neonates. For pediatric nursing, the Society of Pediatric Nurses has established standards for care of children and their families.

Institution Policies

Nurses are also held accountable for upholding their agency's or health-care institution's policies. Every hospital has a policy and procedures handbook that clearly outlines how nursing care is to be provided. This handbook might be in paper form, or it could be a document available on the hospital electronic medical record system.

If you are unsure about a policy or a procedure, the policy and procedures handbook will provide specific guidelines. Following the hospital policies and procedures will prevent errors in patient care and promote safe care for the patients.

Ethics

Ethics are defined as moral principles that guide a person's behavior. Ethics are concerned with distinguishing between good and evil and right and wrong. Health-care ethics are concerned with trying to do the right thing while achieving the best possible outcome for every patient.

Nurses do have guidelines for providing ethical care. The ANA Code of Ethics (2018) can be used to guide their nursing practice. Ethical principles that address the issues of fairness, honesty, and respect for human beings are especially important in maternity and pediatric settings:

- *Autonomy:* Patients have the right to have control over their own bodies and make their own decisions. This means that a competent adult can accept or refuse treatment, medications, procedures, diagnostic testing, and surgeries according to their wishes.
- *Beneficence:* This principle refers to acting from a spirit of compassion and kindness to benefit others (Venes, 2021). It also involves balancing the benefits of treatment against the risks and costs involved. Physicians and nurses must view beneficence from the viewpoint of the patient and family. At times, the patient and family may have differing views of the benefits of treatment and disagree with the plan of care.
- *Nonmaleficence:* This principle means to do no harm or to inflict the least possible harm to reach a beneficial outcome. Nurses carefully administer medication and double-check dosages in order to "do no harm" to the patient by making a medication error.
- *Justice:* This ethical principle refers to acting out of fairness such as providing equitable, appropriate medical treatment (Varkey, 2021, para.23). It also refers to the fair allocation of services and resources.

In providing care to maternity and pediatric patients, nurses will encounter challenging ethical problems. No single answer fits every situation and every patient. Hospital ethics committees can provide guidance in clinical situations in which clear-cut answers are not obtainable. Nurses who encounter ethical dilemmas should report through the chain of command to receive assistance. Following are some of the ethical issues you may encounter:

- Abortion
- A mother smoking, drinking alcohol, or using illicit drugs during pregnancy
- A patient who wants a cesarean birth because she does not want to deliver vaginally
- Provision of futile care for an extremely premature newborn
- A young adolescent with no family support leaving the hospital with a newborn
- A mother with substance use disorder and experiencing homelessness who leaves the hospital with her newborn
- Infertility treatment that is expensive and not successful
- A teenager with aggressive cancer who wants to be allowed to die
- A child living in a car with his family being discharged with a new diagnosis of asthma
- A child with type 1 diabetes being cared for by a mother who has dual mental health diagnoses

Nurses are legally and ethically obligated to provide care that meets the standards of practice, regardless of feelings they may have about a patient or a patient's decisions. Nurses must evaluate their own values and beliefs about health care, illness, life, and death and avoid imposing their own values onto the patient.

 ## INFORMED CONSENT

Informed consent means the health-care provider responsible for ordering the procedure is confident that the patient understands the procedure and accepts the risks and benefits. Informed consent applies to individuals 18 years old and older.

- For adults, you have a legal duty to ensure that written consents are signed by a physician or another designated health-care provider in addition to the adult providing consent before the procedure or medical treatment.
- For children, the legal caregiver—namely, the parent or guardian—signs the consent form.

Assent

When a child is 7 years old or older, the health-care team and parents, caregiver, or guardian typically include them in the decision-making process. Feedback from the child is solicited as part of **assent**, or agreement, and the child is asked if they have any questions or concerns about the course of medical treatment. Not all children at age 7 are developmentally ready to participate in assent, but the health-care team should observe the child for their ability to participate in this process.

Emancipated Minor

The **emancipation** of a minor grants basic adult rights to children who are of an age and developmental level to be able to process complex information related to making

Box 1.2

Emancipated Minor Status

The concept of an emancipated minor generally includes one or more of the following criteria:
- Under age 18, usually older than age 14
- Legally married
- On active military service
- Can demonstrate maturity and financial independence; may have to make a legal informed declaration

When emancipated minor status is secured, the following apply:
- Parents are no longer required to pay financial support.
- Minor assumes responsibility for their own medical coverage.
- Minor gives consent for all medical coverage and care without parents' consent, knowledge, or liability.
- Minor can enter into a binding contract and can consent to participate in health-care–related research.

decisions about their health care and medical treatments. A married pregnant teenager is automatically emancipated, but an unmarried pregnant teenager is not automatically emancipated. This teen would need to seek legal assistance to obtain emancipation. The definition of the emancipation of a minor varies among states, and not all states recognize emancipated minor status. Check your state government's website for more information about the legal process and the recognition of the process if the teen was granted this status in another state (Box 1.2).

For example, a 17-year-old boy has a secondary cancer diagnosis of leukemia after treatment for a brain tumor as a child. The boy's parents want to continue chemotherapy treatments even though his prognosis is poor and he has been responding poorly to traditional treatment protocols. The boy wishes to have palliative care only. The profound differences between the parents' and the child's wishes prompt the intervention of a team of social workers, child psychologists, and the legal system. The child is granted emancipation and is then able to make his own treatment decisions.

Children's Rights

Children have the right to provisions, the right to protection, and the right to participation:

1. *Right to provisions:* Children should be provided a standard of living that includes the provisions of safe living; health care; education; clean water; appropriate diets; adequate rest; and sleep, play, and recreation.
2. *Right to protection:* Children should be protected from abuse, exploitation, neglect, and discrimination. Children should be protected from safety risks while at home, school, community areas, and health-care institutions.
3. *Right to participation:* Children should be offered full participation in community activities, art and sports activities, and cultural events according to their individual and family beliefs and practices.

See the UNICEF and Library of Congress websites for more definitions and further discussions on children's rights.

Family Rights

Families are entitled to protected rights within a health-care institution. Family rights include (but are not limited to) the following:

1. Right to full participation in health-care discussions and decision-making concerning the child
2. Right to active participation in cultural beliefs and practices whenever possible, including being allowed to participate in cultural or religious practices at the bedside, providing they are safe (For example, burning incense or candles cannot be permitted because of the fire risk associated with the presence of gases such as oxygen and helium.)
3. Right to visitation and family participation in the treatment and care of the child
4. Right to comfort by having pain and discomfort addressed and treated promptly
5. Right to have interpretation services by a translator when a language barrier exists
6. Right to personal dignity and privacy during assessments, diagnostics, procedures, and treatments
7. Right to receive emergency treatment regardless of the ability to pay
8. Right to be free of restraints or seclusion unless clinically necessary
9. Right to refuse care provided by students
10. Right to decline to participate in research programs or projects

Safety *Stat!*

Secure the use of a certified medical interpreter anytime the health-care team needs to communicate with a family whose primary language is not English. Professional interpreter services provide a valuable service and enhance safety through clear and concise communication.

FAMILY-CENTERED CARE

Definition of Family

A *family* is a biological, legal, and/or emotional relation between two or more persons. There may be a variety of constellations including nuclear, alternative, adoptive, foster, and communal families (Figs. 1.2 and 1.3). See Box 1.3 for a summary of family structures. The most important factor in discussing the structure of a child's family is this: *A family is who they say they are.*

The philosophy of family-centered care recognizes the family as the constant in the child's life and that all members of the family are affected by the illness, injury, or hospitalization that the child is experiencing. Health-care

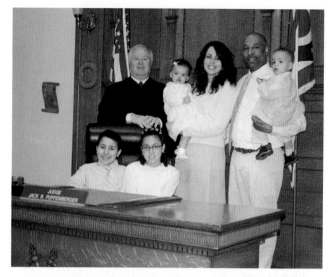

FIGURE 1.2 A family is a biological, legal, and/or emotional relation between two or more persons.

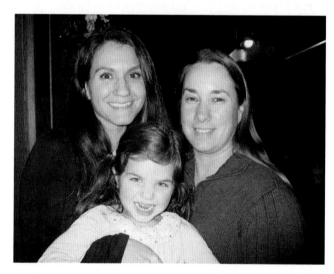

FIGURE 1.3 A family is who they say they are.

institutions across the nation are incorporating the principles of family-centered care into the care team's approach to strengthen the family unit, include all members, and enhance the communication and outcomes of the experience.

Nurses who practice family-centered care provide a safe, child-friendly, and decorative environment, along with the support needed to assist the child and family as a unit. According to one hospital that successfully incorporated family-centered care into its pediatric unit, the provision of hope, love, and engaged care in which the family was supported and strengthened was the basis of a collaborative partnership between the family and health-care providers (Foster et al., 2020).

Two important overarching goals of family-centered care are to empower and enable families:

• *Empowerment:* The interaction between the family and health-care providers is such that the family's sense of

Family Structures

- *Nuclear or conjugal family:* A husband, wife, and children live in the same household.
- *Reconstituted or stepfamily:* Both parents may contribute children from previous relationships or marriages to a new household.
- *Single-parent family:* One parent is responsible for running a household.
- *Same-sex family:* Two members of the same sex are spouses or partners and care for the household.
- *Extended family:* Any constellation of family members lives together in one household.
- *Binuclear family:* A child's time is divided between two households.
- *Foster family:* A family takes care of a child in either a long-term or temporary relationship.
- *Adoptive family:* A family permanently and legally accepts all responsibilities for a child from the biological parents.
- *Communal family:* A group of people who may not be related live together and share responsibilities for the household.

control over their lives continues. Family members are supported so that they can foster their own strengths, abilities, and actions through the caregiving or helping role. The family feels supported, listened to, and competent.

- ***Enabling:*** Professionals provide opportunities for family members to master the child's care. This concept involves the teaching, supporting, and enabling that allows a family to care for their child.

Family-centered care is provided regardless of the practice setting where the encounter takes place. Families need to be encouraged to be present with the child whenever it is safe and possible. If the child is hospitalized, the parents should have access to the child 24 hours a day and should be encouraged to stay with the child throughout the required care. Parents are not always able to stay with their hospitalized child because they must complete work duties and provide for the family's needs. Do not express judgment about this because the functioning of the family may rest on the ability of a parent to provide financial support.

Siblings are another important aspect of family-centered care. Encourage siblings to interact with the hospitalized child while also providing them the opportunity to play and develop. Playrooms should include sibling time and participation. Child life specialists can provide healthy and educative opportunities for siblings while present. If a child is being hospitalized for care of a chronic condition, provide the family with information on sibling support groups and encourage involvement. See Box 1.4 for a list of family-centered care principles.

Family-Centered Care Principles

The philosophy of family-centered care includes the following principles:
- The family is recognized as the constant in the child's life.
- The family is who they say they are.
- The family is treated as one unit because the entire family is affected by the child's illness.
- Health-care providers are acknowledged as providers of collegial support.
- The two core concepts are enabling and empowerment.
- Natural caregiving is supported.
- Decision-making roles within the family structure are supported.
- The unique strengths of the individuals and family unit are built upon.
- Living at home and within the child's greater community is promoted.
- Siblings and extended family members are included in care provisions.
- Diversity among structures is acknowledged, and cultural diversity is promoted.
- Normalization is promoted, and identities are encouraged beyond the illness state.
- A parent–professional partnership is promoted.
- The child is helped to cope with hospitalization.
- The child is helped to cope with separation anxiety that begins at 8 to 10 months and peaks at 16 to 30 months.
- Family goals, dreams, strategies, and activities are supported.
- Support systems, services, education, and information for all members are located and provided to the family.

Therapeutic Communication

Nurses support autonomy by allowing patients to make their own decisions. To assist the patient in decision-making, it may be necessary to help the patient clarify their values as they relate to the health-care situation. Therapeutic communication strategies that might assist you to understand the patient's values and viewpoint are the following:

- "Are you considering another course of action? Tell me about it."
- "How will you discuss this with your family?"
- "Will it be difficult for you to discuss this with your family?"
- "Now that you have made a decision, how do you feel?"
- "What information do you need to make a decision?"
- "How can I help you with this decision?"

EVIDENCE-BASED PRACTICE

Evidence-based practice is nursing care in which all nursing interventions are based on current valid research evidence. Evidence-based practice takes nursing research and puts it into practice at the patient's bedside. Nurses can embrace evidence-based practice by questioning accepted nursing conventions and by being open to changes in nursing care when a scientific study indicates that safe and effective nursing care can be provided in a different way.

SPECIAL CONSIDERATIONS IN PEDIATRIC NURSING

Anatomical and Physiological Differences Between Children and Adults

Children are not simply little adults and cannot be cared for as such. There are 13 important anatomical and physiological differences between children and adults that provide a framework for safety for pediatric health-care team members.

1. Children's airways are anatomically small.
2. Newborns are obligate nose breathers for the first several weeks of life.
3. Children's heads are disproportionately large.
4. Infants have a large posterior head bone (occiput), which makes airway occlusion more likely.
5. Children have poorly developed intercostal chest muscles; fatigue leads to respiratory failure.
6. Children have less tidal volume in their lungs.
7. Young children have a larger body surface area (BSA), which results in greater heat loss and greater insensible water losses.
8. Infants and young children have less total circulating blood volume (80 to 90 mL/kg) than older children and adults.
9. Young children have high glucose needs and poor glycogen stores, which result in a higher metabolic rate.
10. Across childhood, children have relatively healthy cardiovascular systems; primary hypertension and cardiovascular disease are rare.
11. Young children have immature temperature regulation; young infants can rapidly experience hypothermia if not dressed and wrapped appropriately.
12. Young children have immature immune systems and less overall organ maturation (especially kidney function and the concentration of urine).
13. Young children pose challenges in assessment and treatment of the six human symptoms (pain or discomfort, dyspnea, fatigue, sleep disturbances, nausea, and emotional distress); use vital signs and developmentally appropriate pediatric tools to measure symptoms such as pain.

All these anatomical and physiological differences affect the following aspects of the child's status, but by adolescence, differences lessen compared with adults:

• How the child, overall, is affected by trauma and/or injuries

• The presentation of the child's physical illnesses in relation to severity
• A child's rapid rate of decompensation under stress, injury, or trauma
• Blood pressure changes that demonstrate a late sign of shock
• Slower rate of metabolism of medications

Nurses must understand children's patterns of growth and development in order to teach families what to expect at the various developmental levels. Although children grow uniquely and at their own pace, there are consistent patterns that are demonstrated at each stage. Chapters 18 through 22 provide information about the growth, development, and perceptions experienced among the various pediatric populations.

Children's patterns of development follow three progressions:

• *Cephalocaudal:* Development is from head to toe; for example, infants have head control before they are able to crawl, stand, or walk (Fig. 1.4A).
• *Proximal-distal:* Development is from the trunk to the distal extremities; for example, the young infant can move their legs and arms but cannot pick up objects with a finger grasp (Fig. 1.4B).
• *General to specific:* Children master simple tasks before advancing to more complex tasks; for example, the young child will typically master slow crawling behaviors and then fast crawling behaviors and then, progressively, standing, running, and skipping.

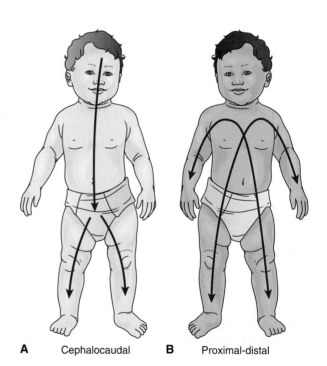

A   Cephalocaudal   **B**   Proximal-distal

FIGURE 1.4 Childhood growth patterns. A, Cephalocaudal. B, Proximal-distal.

CRITICAL THINKING AND CLINICAL JUDGMENT IN MATERNAL CHILD NURSING

Thinking like a nurse first requires you, the student, to obtain a body of knowledge by studying regularly, attending class, and applying the new knowledge in clinical practice. Learning to think critically and make good clinical judgments prepares you for the challenges of clinical practice.

Critical thinking is necessary when providing patient care. It enables you to recognize problems or potential problems, and then helps you decide the best course of action. Nurses spend more time with patients than other health-care providers and are often the first to observe an unexpected problem or complication. Critical thinking involves using what is learned to recognize symptoms and to determine how to provide safe and appropriate patient care.

After collecting data, recalling and understanding what was learned, and knowing that an intervention should occur, you make decisions about changing or implementing care. Clinical judgment is the action or "doing" something for the patient to promote health or to prevent a complication or adverse outcome.

Examples of critical thinking and clinical judgment in maternal–child health include the following:

- You notice that new parents have uncovered the 1-hour-old newborn for 10 minutes. You know (critical thinking) that the newborn is not physically able to maintain a healthy temperature, and this could lead to cold stress. You demonstrate clinical judgment by covering the newborn with a blanket and gently educating the new parents about newborn temperature regulation.

- You are making rounds on your newly assigned patients for the night shift. You observe that the toes of a child in a cast are cold and blue. Using critical thinking, you know that cold blue toes are symptoms of a circulation problem. Using clinical judgment, you report the findings immediately to the charge nurse.

Safety *Stat!*

Some students may not think they need to study the maternity or pediatric content because "I have kids; I've been through this." Having children is not a substitute for the knowledge required by a nursing professional. The student needs to be prepared, complete the assigned reading, and ask the instructor for clarification if their experience differs from what is taught. Patients do not need or want to hear about the student's own labor and birth experience or parenting experiences.

Safety *Stat!*

Even if it is your first day in maternal–child and pediatric nursing, you can still promote patient safety by closely observing possible safety risks whenever you enter a patient's room. For example: Are the side rails up? Is there a spill on the floor? Is the correct IV fluid hanging? Are visitors washing their hands? Is the newborn wrapped warmly and lying in a safe location?

Key Points

- There are many roles available for nurses in providing maternity and pediatric care.
- Health-care ethics provide guidelines for delivering ethical care to patients.
- Autonomy, beneficence, nonmaleficence, and justice are principles that guide medical ethics.
- Applying the principles of family-centered care to families receiving care in a hospital, clinic, or home setting is essential. Two foundational principles are empowering and enabling.

- There are distinct anatomical, physiological, social, and emotional differences between adults and children that emphasize the critical components pertinent to the safe emergent care of children across health-care settings.
- Providing safety in all aspects of care is an important role for the maternity and pediatric nurse.
- Children are at particular risk for being harmed in the hospital environment. Nurses need to employ critical thinking and clinical judgment to ensure their safety.

Review Questions

1. Who or what regulates the nursing scope of practice?
   1. The nurse's employer
   2. State laws
   3. Physicians
   4. Professional organizations

2. To what does the ethical term *justice* refer?
   1. Nurses doing no harm to a patient
   2. Nurses following all the legal requirements of their jobs
   3. Nurses treating a patient with kindness
   4. Nurses being fair in utilizing resources for patients

3. Nurses can contribute to quality health care by doing which of the following? **(Select all that apply.)**
   1. Following standards of care
   2. Delivering patient-centered care
   3. Using aggressive behaviors to get health-care providers to listen
   4. Providing equal care to all patients
   5. Choosing when to follow evidence-based practice

4. You, as a nursing student, are asked by a patient if they can take a medication from home for their headache. You are unsure of the answer. What should you do?
   1. Tell the patient it is all right to take the medication.
   2. Tell the patient to wait and you will find out.
   3. Admit that you do not know.
   4. Act as if you did not hear the patient.

5. While preparing medications for a 3-year-old patient in the pediatric unit, you note that a very large amount of a medication has been ordered. What should be your first step?
   1. Administer the dose and assess the patient's response to the new dose.
   2. Contact the nursing supervisor to discuss options for administration.
   3. Double-check the dose with the original physician's order.
   4. Call the physician to discuss an alternative medication with a similar indication.

6. Although it is the physician's responsibility to explain the purpose, risks, benefits, and alternatives to a medical procedure, there are times when it is appropriate for a nurse to obtain legal informed consent. Which of the following patients may sign for informed consent after you read the consent out loud?
   1. An unconscious patient
   2. A patient who is 14 years of age and alone in the hospital
   3. A patient who has received a sedative medication
   4. A patient who cannot read

7. You have received a child from the pediatric intensive care unit (PICU). The oral report received from the transferring PICU nurse states that the child's vital signs (VS) were stable. Upon observing the child, you note a temperature of 39.8°C (103.6°F). No VS were documented in the patient's chart throughout the night. Which statement accurately summarizes the problem?
   1. The night-shift PICU nurse will be fired for this conduct.
   2. The night-shift PICU nurse needs to be taken off the schedule for an unpaid leave of absence.
   3. The PICU nurse may be found negligent in their care of the child.
   4. The family has a right to sue because of poor documentation of the night shift activities.

ANSWERS 1, 2, 4; 3, 1, 2, 4; 4, 3; 5, 2, 4; 5, 3; 6, 4; 7, 3

CRITICAL THINKING QUESTIONS

1. In your health-care institution, what is the process for obtaining informed consent for an immediate surgical procedure when you have a patient who cannot read, write, or speak English? What steps can you take to assist in this situation?

2. Write about an ethical dilemma you may have observed in a clinical setting.

Resources

For additional resources and information, including Postconference Questions and Activities, Answers, and References, visit www.FADavis.com.

 Student Study Guide

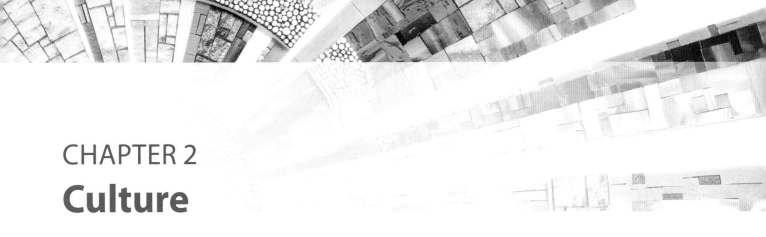

CHAPTER 2
Culture

KEY TERMS

cultural awareness (KUL-chur-uhl uh-WAIR-ness)
cultural competence (KUL-chur-uhl KOM-puh-tents)
cultural sensitivity (KUL-chur-uhl sen-sih-TIV-ih-tee)
culture (KUL-chur)
diversity (dih-VER-sih-tee)
endemic (en-DEM-ik)
ethnicity (eth-NIH-sih-tee)
health literacy (HELLTH LIT-er-ah-see)
National Standards for Culturally and Linguistically Appropriate Services in Health Care (NASH-nuhl STAN-derdz for KUL-chur-uhl-ee and ling-GWIS-tik-uhl-ee uh-PROH-pree-uht SER-viss-uhz in HELLTH KAIR)
race (RAYSS)
social determinants of health (SOH-shuhl DEE-term-i-nants uv HELLTH)
stereotyping (STAIR-ee-oh-tye-ping)
worldview (WERLD-vyoo)

CHAPTER CONCEPTS

Growth and Development
Health Promotion
Safety
Self
Social Determinants of Health

LEARNING OUTCOMES

1. Define the key terms.
2. Discuss the importance of cultural awareness when providing safe and effective nursing care.
3. Examine health-care quality, disparities in care, and social determinants of health (SDOH) across population groups in the community.
4. Examine the factors (social, environmental, economic, and political) that contribute to one's worldview, health beliefs, and health behaviors.
5. Identify and describe cultural assessment tools and their usefulness and limitations in planning care.
6. Demonstrate sensitivity to cultural beliefs, values, and practices when providing care by seeking and giving feedback, listening, and observing.
7. Ensure the use of appropriate and acceptable resources and materials in promoting health teaching and illness prevention with patients and families.
8. Locate community resources that facilitate continuity of care in a culturally sensitive and effective manner for patients and their families.

CRITICAL THINKING & CLINICAL JUDGMENT

Jayden, a 5-year-old, was just admitted to the pediatric unit for dehydration after 4 days of vomiting and diarrhea. Jayden is accompanied by his mother, Kim, who is from Vietnam. Kim gave him a home remedy for diarrhea, but it did not work to stop the symptoms. She brought Jayden to the hospital because he was becoming increasingly lethargic and was continuing to have diarrhea. Jayden and his mother understand conversational English. During the initial assessment and interview, you note that the mother is quiet, does not make eye contact, and nods her head in response to any comment. She does state that she is concerned about the cost of the care and hospitalization, and she is concerned that she does not understand the medical terms being used by the health-care team.

Continued

CRITICAL THINKING & CLINICAL JUDGMENT—cont'd

Questions

1. You found the mother to be quiet and not making eye contact. What concerns do you think the mother has in this situation?
2. What physical and psychosocial evaluations should be conducted to obtain a complete past medical history and summary of the child's current illness from the mother?
3. Using therapeutic communication, how can you maintain cultural sensitivity while inquiring about the home remedy?
4. What teaching needs can you identify for the mother, and what is the best approach for teaching her?

CONCEPTUAL CORNERSTONE
Self

One of the most interesting aspects of being a nurse and caring for families in the fields of maternity and pediatric nursing is the cultural diversity encountered in health-care environments. In health-care settings in the United States, there is a rich diversity of human race, culture, ethnicity, gender identity, sexual orientation, and abilities. Being able to provide safe, effective, and supportive care to diverse families requires skill and knowledge. The terms **cultural awareness** (developing cultural sensitivity) and **cultural sensitivity** (displaying culturally appropriate behaviors) are both used to denote how nurses develop **cultural competence** (ability to function effectively within the cultural context of beliefs, behaviors, and needs of the person or community being served). The term *cultural humility* is also commonly used to denote a genuine attempt to really understand one another in terms of education, socioeconomic status, gender and sexual orientation, race, and ethnicity. According to Miyagawa (2020), one needs both a desire and a commitment to achieve cultural humility; this includes being a lifelong learner, participating in self-reflection, being accountable (personally and institutionally), and mitigating power imbalances so everyone feels respected and heard.

The information in this chapter is intended as a guide to facilitate communication, mutual goal setting, and decision making in the context of **culture**, nursing, and health care; you can find in-depth details in other resource materials.

As you read this chapter, bear in mind some key considerations:

1. Reading about something may enhance your understanding of complex situations and encounters with diverse people, but it is not a substitute for meaningful and productive real-life experiences.

2. Being open to others' perspectives, their life experiences, and the meanings they attribute to conceptions of health and illness is essential to effective communication.
3. Attending to cues, both verbal and nonverbal, allows you to understand cultural needs and communication beyond verbalizations. Tactful and sensitive probing can facilitate effective communication and improve your understanding of the family's process of decision making as well as their underlying beliefs and values.

THE IMPORTANCE OF CULTURAL AWARENESS AND KNOWLEDGE IN NURSING AND HEALTH-CARE DELIVERY

Multiple factors highlight the need for nurses to be skilled in working with and caring for diverse people. *Cultural awareness* is a term used to denote the skills of developing sensitivity to and awareness of the beliefs, values, and behaviors of members of a group different from your own. To be skilled in cultural awareness, you must pay attention to dynamic, changing, and complex factors that include socioeconomics, politics, migration patterns, and personal traits. Statistical and demographic information illustrate the presence of these factors, which have important implications for nursing and health care (Fig. 2.1).

Race

Race is a term used to denote genetic physical characteristics that are similar among members of a group as well as a person's personal identification with one or more social groups. In 2021, this was the racial distribution of the U.S. population: White (59.3%), Black or African American (11.6%), American Indian and Alaskan Native (2.9%), Asian (5.9%), Native Hawaiian and Other Pacific Islander (0.2%), and Hispanic (19%; U.S. Census Bureau, 2021b). Estimates show that almost 3% of people report belonging to two or more races (Kaiser Family Foundation, 2021).

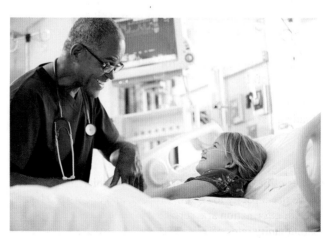

FIGURE 2.1 Cultural diversity in nursing care.

Ethnicity

Ethnicity refers to one's membership in one or more ethnic groups, including commitment to that group's cultural customs and rituals. Ethnicity and race are not synonymous. Ethnic customs can include celebrations and holidays, dress, music, and food preparation, among other things.

Making assumptions about an individual based on the group you think they belong to is **stereotyping**. Stereotyping may result in harmful outcomes, unsafe care, and misunderstanding.

Beyond Race and Ethnicity

Beyond cultural, ethnic, and religious diversity, there are other types of diversity to consider in planning patient-centered care. Nurses providing care for LGBTQ+ (lesbian, gay, bisexual, transgender, queer, + [all other gender identities and sexual orientations not yet defined]) patients must be able to address the unique health concerns of each of these groups. In addition, transgender men and transgender women require sensitive, respectful nursing care for all their health-care needs, not just when they transition. Patients with visual, hearing, or mobility impairments are also diverse patients with unique needs and concerns that you must plan for.

Diversity

Diversity lends enrichment, as well as challenges, to the lives of persons, communities, and environments. **Diversity** means that people of different and diverse backgrounds *are included,* and the term can be further defined as how humans vary according to their religion, culture, sexual orientation, socioeconomic background, and gender (S. Whitman, 2018). Within the context of health-care environments, diversity exists among persons or patients seeking care and among the health professionals providing care (Fig. 2.2).

Quality care includes communicating in a respectful and culturally sensitive manner with patients and their families (Fig. 2.3). Having background knowledge of community demographics and the populations served by the health-care system is vital to this process. This information can be found in internal hospital reports as well as in local and national databases and reports and can be examined to determine differences or similarities across groups. For example, in planning care, the following types of information may be helpful:

- The number of persons who lack health insurance
- Statistics about access to care across the life span
- How many persons have (or lack) a continued and regular source of care
- Languages spoken at home
- Rates of **health literacy** (the degree to which individuals have the capacity to obtain, process, and understand basic health information and services)
- Community rates of acute and chronic disease conditions
- Availability of preventive programs

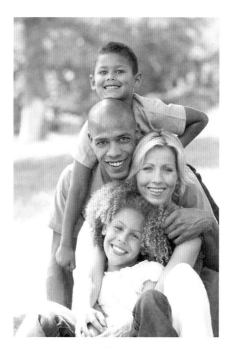

FIGURE 2.2 Culturally diverse families.

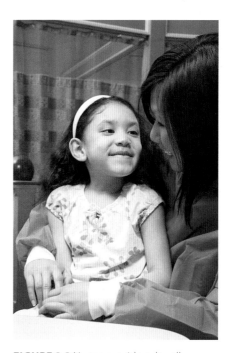

FIGURE 2.3 Nurses provide culturally sensitive care.

Safety *Stat!*

Always use a trained medical interpreter when communicating with a patient who does not speak your language. A child or other family member may not be able to interpret medical information accurately. Moreover, patients may be embarrassed to talk freely about highly sensitive health

Continued

Safety *Stat!*—cont'd

matters in front of family members. Medical interpreters can appear in person; however, depending on geographical location, a phone interpreter or videoconference interpreter may be required. Some institutions are using mobile computer pads that can be rolled into a patient's room to provide remote medical interpreter services in multiple languages. For patients who use sign language, a medical sign language interpreter is essential for effective communication between the patient and health-care personnel.

Health-Care Quality, Disparities, and Social Determinants of Health

Health-care quality can be measured on several dimensions of care: effectiveness, patient safety, timeliness, patient centeredness, care coordination, and access. These quality dimensions of care can then be examined related to their progress and rate of change over time. One aspect of health-care quality relates to **social determinants of health** (SDOH). SDOH are defined as physical conditions and social situations in environments where people are born, live, play, learn, work, worship, and age (*Healthy People 2030,* 2022). A. Whitman and colleagues (2022) describe how SDOH include a family's economic stability, education, access to food, social support systems and integration, housing and neighborhood environments, and health-care coverage including access to health-care providers with cultural competence. These SDOH influence health outcomes including mortality, morbidity, health status, and functional limitations.

Health-care disparity, which is the difference in access or availability of health care and the variation in rates of disease and disabilities among groups within a population, can be further examined. According to Ndugga and Artiga (2021), health disparities are those differences in overall health and differences in the provision of health care between groups. More specifically, disparities are differences in access to and use of quality health care and insurance coverage. Understanding health-care disparities and progress toward *Healthy People 2030* goals among populations served in one's community is important in the planning, implementation, and evaluation of care. For example, national reports indicate that overall health-care quality is slowly improving. However, access to care and health disparities are not improving. Underrepresented groups and people with low incomes receive poorer quality of care and face more barriers in accessing care (Acosta et al., 2021; U.S. Census Bureau, 2021a; Box 2.1). During the early stages of the COVID-19 pandemic in 2020, poverty increased in the United States by 11.4% (U.S. Census Bureau, 2021a).

Disparities were observed in patient and family engagement in making informed decisions and considering treatment options. According to the Agency for Healthcare Research and Quality's *National Healthcare Quality and*

Box 2.1

Health Disparities in the United States

Consider the following data from the Centers for Disease Control and Prevention's (CDC's) seminal report (2021), *Healthy People 2030* (2022), and Acosta and colleagues (2021):

1. Cardiovascular disease remains the leading cause of death among Black (non-Hispanic) Americans, who are 50% more likely to die of stroke or premature heart disease than non-Hispanic Whites.
2. Hispanics have the highest prevalence of diabetes, and the severity of disease is linked to lower income households.
3. Infant mortality rates in the Black population are double the rates in the White population, with the highest rates in the Midwest and South.
4. Noncompletion of high school is directly linked to poorer health.
5. Up to 36.6% of census tracts showed no healthy food retailers; lower income neighborhoods have a higher risk of not having access to nutrient-rich foods, fruits, and vegetables.
6. LGBTQ+ individuals are at higher risk for suicide attempts; have the highest rates of alcohol, tobacco, and other medication use; are more likely to be sexually assaulted and to experience homelessness; and, because of social isolation, have less access to and more barriers to health-care providers.

Disparities Report (2020), having a consistent (or usual) source of health care improved access to health-care services. Racism, both interpersonal and structural, is a major cause of disease and health access and health-care inequities in the United States (Centers for Disease Control and Prevention [CDC], 2021). Compared with Whites, all underrepresented groups reported poor communication with nurses. In addition, when compared with Whites, African Americans, American Indians, Alaska Natives, and patients of more than one race reported poor communication with doctors (U.S. Department of Health and Human Services [USDHHS], 2011b). Patients who spoke Spanish at home reported poor communication with nurses, and patients who spoke some other non-English language at home reported poor communication with both nurses and doctors (USDHHS, 2011b). Compared with all other racial and ethnic groups, Hispanics were the least likely to have health insurance. In the United States, Blacks' life expectancy is 4 years lower than Whites' (CDC, 2021a). Hispanics and African Americans also did not have a specific ongoing source of care (USDHHS, 2011b).

In addition to health-care disparities, disparities in SDOH have an effect on health outcomes. SDOH impact people's health, well-being, and quality of life across the life span and have become very important to the public health community, as they have a strong influence on health and well-being. Separate from traditional medical care, SDOH are those aspects of one's life that highly influence the ability to be safe and feel safe, thrive in school and employment, and live in conditions that promote health (Box 2.2).

Box 2.2

Examples of Social Determinants of Health That Promote Health

- Access to safe housing, reliable transportation, and safe neighborhoods where individuals and families can thrive
- Fair access to job opportunities, income, and education
- Access to nutritious foods including fresh fruits and vegetables
- Access to safe playgrounds and physical activity opportunities
- Access to clean water and air
- Opportunities for developing language and literacy skills

(Healthy People 2030, 2022)

Examples of social conditions that have relevance to this chapter are availability of community resources (education and work opportunities, healthful foods, quality schools, transportation), social support, exposure to crime or violence, public safety, residential segregation, concentrated poverty, mass media, and technology exposure. Examples of physical conditions are the natural and the built environment (buildings, housing, neighborhoods, recreational settings), exposure to toxic substances, and other hazards. *Healthy People 2030* (2022) describes five domains that can assist nurses in planning care for populations:

1. Economic Stability
2. Health Care Access and Quality
3. Education Access and Quality
4. Social and Community Context
5. Neighborhood and Built Environments

WORLDVIEW

To provide quality care to patients, you need effective listening and communication skills, openness and appreciation of differences, and awareness of your own biases that may hinder the process of care. Understanding another's **worldview**, their philosophy or conception of the world, can cultivate these needed nursing abilities and characteristics.

Social Factors Influencing the Worldview

Understanding the patient's or the family's concept of health, wellness, causes of illness, and modalities of treatment lays the groundwork for intercultural communication, informed decision making, and care based on preferences and needs (Fig. 2.4). Social, environmental, economic, and migrational factors influence worldview. Your broad assessment of social factors influencing worldview should include inquiry into the family's cultural beliefs, traditions, and practices or rituals. Specifically, it is helpful to understand the patient's or the family's views on the following:

- What are their cultural ideas of health? What are their cultural ideas of wellness?

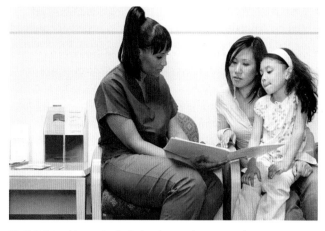

FIGURE 2.4 Nurses include families in decision making.

- What are their health and illness beliefs? How are they different from or similar to medical worldviews of health and illness?
- What self-care treatments, remedies, or interventions, including regional or community ones, are used? What is their perceived effectiveness?
- How do social patterns of family living affect health decision making? How are health decisions made? Are these individualistic or collective decision-making processes? Is assistance sought from others within or outside of the family network?
- How, when, where, and from whom are treatment and care sought? For what reasons?

Environmental Factors Influencing the Worldview

When planning care, it's important to observe the patient's immediate environmental factors, both past and present, and how these affect health status and function. This information also has importance for follow-up and continuity of care, health promotion, and disease-prevention education. To gather information about past and present environmental factors, it can be useful to ask the following:

- What are the availability and accessibility to basic necessities of food and water? What is the quality of food and water?
- What is the average daily air quality?
- What is the availability of residential utilities such as heating, natural gas, fans or air conditioning, electricity, and phone services? What is the availability of high-speed internet?
- Is there exposure to high levels of noise?
- Is there exposure or threat of exposure to toxic waste or hazardous or unsanitary materials?
- Is there exposure or threat of exposure to a disease **endemic**, or native, to a geographical area (Lyme disease, West Nile virus)?

· **WORD · BUILDING ·**
endemic: en–in + dem–people + ic–pertaining to

- What is the quality of immediate living conditions, including sanitation and hygiene? How crowded or cramped are the living spaces? Is there sufficient space for personal privacy needs?
- Do individuals and families feel safe in the neighborhoods where they live?
- Is there access to public recreation areas and playgrounds or nature areas that invite exercise and mobility? Are these areas well-tended and well-lit to prevent accident or injury?

Economic Factors Influencing the Worldview

Economic status also informs a patient's or family's worldview. Does the family have financial resources for day-to-day living? Is payment for health-care services a worry? Information related to both past and present financial resources is useful in determining gaps in health care or deterioration in health status and function that may be attributable to economic factors. For example, it is helpful to know such things as:

- Does health insurance exist in the patient's source culture? If not, who pays for health-care services? What transactions occur?
- Is health care available and affordable there?
- How do individuals and families access health care now? Is access to care feasible?
- Who gets care? Are quality of care and levels of care contingent on ability to pay?
- Who do families go to first when medical attention is needed? How and where do families obtain medical equipment, supplies, and medications, if needed?
- Is care sought out across the life span? Do families have access to comprehensive services including education and support to care for their children (Fig. 2.5)?
- What recourse do individuals or families seek when health-care services are unavailable, unaffordable, or inaccessible?

Political Factors Influencing the Worldview

Information about health care within the political context that people have experienced as they move from one place to another adds another level of understanding in communication and decision making. Questions about political factors and their effect upon worldview of persons would include the following:

- What policies govern (or have governed) the availability of health care to persons?
- Who gets care? Is there fair distribution of health-care resources?
- Is care provided or partially paid for by legislative policies?
- What health-care systems are in place? Are they simple or complex to navigate? Is the health-care system perceived as a benefit or a burden to individuals and families?

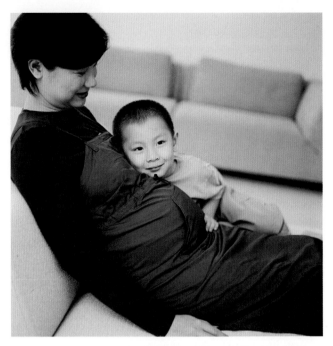

FIGURE 2.5 Families need support and education to care for their children.

- What kinds and levels of health-care coverage are afforded to individuals and families living within a particular political context?
- Are individuals and families able to fully access and benefit from funded community programs? Are these programs long term or short term?

Migrational Factors Influencing the Worldview

For many individuals and families, migration is a significant life event often associated with conflicting emotions, stressors, and both negative and positive experiences. Migration has relevance for understanding the worldview of individuals and families because health status and function could have been compromised during a period of vulnerability. Questions about migrational factors that influence worldview might include the following:

- What were the conditions under which migration occurred?
- Was migration voluntary or involuntary? Planned or unplanned?
- What was the preexisting health status of individuals or family members as compared with the present?
- What were the ages of individual family members at the time of migration?
- How much time was spent in temporary shelters or living arrangements before reaching the final destination? What was the quality of these living conditions?
- Was there exposure or potential exposure to disease, illness, or hazardous or toxic materials?

- Did individuals or family members experience any episodes of illness? How long did they last? Were they recurrent?
- Was health care and treatment provided for illnesses during migration?

CRITICAL THINKING

The concept of intergenerational trauma is used to denote the impact of violence and hardship experienced by parents and elders that is transmitted to their children, even those who may have been born after the trauma took place. Research has shown that children born after parental trauma experience negative consequences of their parents' trauma. This concept demonstrates the impact of the transmission of trauma as a historical event onto the next generation. Consequences of intergenerational trauma include emotional distancing, tumultuous relationships, defensiveness, and denial of the trauma (Ryder & White, 2022; Yehuda & Lehrner, 2018).

While caring for children of parents who experienced trauma, what specifically would you look for as evidence of the impact of intergenerational trauma?

CULTURALLY APPROPRIATE ASSESSMENT

The registered nurse (RN) is responsible for conducting the patient's formal health assessment. However, a knowledgeable licensed practical/vocational nurse (LPN/LVN) or other staff member can share with the RN observations that enhance the quality of that assessment. A culturally appropriate assessment takes into consideration the social, economic, physical, environmental, and political factors that might be relevant to the care of the patient. To elicit the patient's perspectives and preferences requires not just excellent communication skills but also the establishment of a therapeutic relationship based on mutual respect and trust between you and the patient or you and the patient's family.

It is important to recognize that behavioral responses may be influenced by the patient's illness as well as by stress of the patient and family system. Persons of diverse cultural backgrounds may have different conceptions of health and other explanations for signs and symptoms of illness. Their interpretations and experiences of illness, as well as preventive or curative traditions, may be uniquely bound to culture. Nonetheless, all patients and families should be accorded respectful, equitable, and timely care. They should also be given health education and health information in a manner they understand.

The Office of Minority Health in the U.S. DHHS developed 15 national standards on culturally and linguistically appropriate services, **National Standards for Culturally and Linguistically Appropriate Services in Health Care (CLAS)**, for health-care organizations and providers (n.d.). The standards were created to advance health equity by providing structure and a framework to best serve culturally diverse communities. These standards address culturally competent care, language-access services, and organizational supports for cultural competence. The use of a qualified medical interpreter with consideration of preferences for gender is essential in order to provide care that meets the CLAS standards.

Providing effective nursing care to diverse groups of people must take into consideration biocultural variations (such as physical characteristics); illness and disease trajectories; the individual's response to interventions, treatments, and medications; and the socioenvironmental context in which persons live, play, and work.

Do not stereotype a patient based on your beliefs about their culture. Each person is an individual. Environment, psychosocial factors, economics, and health-care status—not just culture—influence the way a person responds to illness.

Therapeutic Communication

Working With a Trained Medical Interpreter
Certified medical interpreters may provide their services in person, via telephone, or through video chat on a tablet computer. Nurses caring for families need to be ready to interact efficiently with interpreters in whatever manner their facility uses. Some tips for working with an interpreter include the following:

- Having a short preconversation to give the interpreter an overview of the discussion planned for the patient
- Speaking directly to the patient, not the interpreter or the screen, if using a tablet computer
- Watching the patient respond to the interpreter or the screen to notice body language
- Using short sentences
- Anticipating that the interpreter may ask you to slow down or repeat complicated words or names of medications
- Encouraging the medical interpreter to ask questions to clarify before interpreting for the patient

Key Points

- It is very important that a nurse develop cultural awareness to provide safe and effective nursing care. Cultural awareness is the development of sensitivity and awareness of the beliefs, values, and experiences of members of a group different from you.
- The term *health disparities* refers to differences in access to or the availability of health-care facilities and services as well as to the variation in rates of disease and disabilities that occurs among different groups within a population. Health disparities for underrepresented groups and people with low incomes are not improving; these groups receive a poorer quality of care and face more barriers in accessing care than do White and/or wealthy people.

- Cultural assessment takes into consideration multiple factors (social, economic, physical, environmental, and political) that affect a person's health status.
- You should demonstrate sensitivity to cultural beliefs, values, and practices when providing care by seeking and giving feedback and by listening and observing.
- The use of a qualified medical interpreter with consideration of preferences for gender can be helpful in communicating effectively with patients and families whose primary language is not English.
- SDOH are defined as physical conditions and social situations in environments where people are born, live, play, learn, work, worship, and age (*Healthy People 2030*, 2022), all of which are very important as they have a strong influence on health and well-being.

Review Questions

1. CLAS standards apply to all of the following except:
   1. Health-care organizations
   2. Individual clinicians and health-care practitioners
   3. Manufacturers of pharmaceutical products
   4. Individual health-care providers

2. Which of the following factors represent a SDOH? **(Select all that apply.)**
   1. Accessibility and availability of healthful foods
   2. Sex, height, weight, and body mass index (BMI)
   3. The number of households per square mile
   4. Prevalence of tuberculosis infections within a geographical location
   5. Availability of health-care providers
   6. Economic status and stability of household

3. When conducting a physical assessment, you recognize that biocultural variation is present in which of the following?
   1. Skin coloring
   2. Oxygen saturation
   3. Socioeconomic status
   4. Education level

4. In evaluating pharmacotherapy interventions, you recognize that which of the following is true?
   1. All patients respond to medication therapy in the same manner.
   2. Dosing and age-specific considerations are minor factors in evaluation.
   3. Environmental, cultural, and genetic factors affect how medications act on an individual.
   4. Pharmacists rely on protocols to determine medication efficacy in individuals.

5. In planning, implementing, and evaluating effective nursing care for diverse patients, which nursing action best illustrates critical thinking?
   1. Refer decisions to a higher-level organizational committee in the health-care system.
   2. Follow organizational policy.
   3. Seek out evidence-based research and practices.
   4. Delegate cultural assessments to charge nurses.

6. A culturally relevant health history considers all *except* which one of the following?
   1. Past and present modalities of self-care and self-treatments
   2. Prevalence of disease conditions among family and relatives
   3. Past and present exposure during migration to illnesses, hazardous conditions, and toxic substances
   4. Presence or absence of health insurance

7. SDOH are described as being:
   1. Conditions that can have an impact on the health and well-being of individuals and families
   2. Laws that provide protection from violence and racism
   3. Personal demographics and sexual identity
   4. Things that influence health-care decision-making for families

ANSWERS 1. 3; 2. 1, 5, 6; 3. 1; 4. 3; 5. 3; 6. 4; 7. 1

CRITICAL THINKING QUESTIONS

1. What are the advantages and disadvantages of a standardized tool (print or electronic) for use in history-taking and health assessment of diverse patients?
2. What are appropriate ways in which you can facilitate high-quality health teaching for patients and families who speak another language?
3. How does your own worldview influence your interactions with patients and their families?
4. Interview someone whose background is different from your own. Use open-ended questions (questions that require more than a "yes" or "no" response) related to foods, childbearing and child-rearing, health-promotion practices, healing practices, and death rituals. Be sensitive to the interviewee's comfort in talking about certain topics. The interviewee's age, race, ethnicity, religion, and gender and your own may influence which topic(s) the interviewee feels comfortable talking about. Discuss in small groups with other students who have also completed this activity how this experience was for you:

- What questions did you ask?
- What responses did you receive?
- How would you have asked the questions differently, if at all?
- What is the most important thing you learned about yourself from this experience? What is the most important thing you learned about the respondent?

Resources

For additional resources and information, including Postconference Questions and Activities, Answers, and References, visit www.FADavis.com.

Student Study Guide

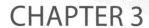

CHAPTER 3
Women's Health Promotion Across the Life Span

KEY TERMS

amenorrhea (AY-men-uh-REE-uh)
contraceptive (KON-tra-SEP-tiv)
cystocele (SISS-to-seel)
dysmenorrhea (DISS-men-uh-REE-uh)
dyspareunia (diss-pa-ROO-nee-uh)
endometrial ablation (en-doh-MEE-tree-uhl a-BLAY-shun)
endometriosis (EN-doh-mee-tree-OH-siss)
fibroids (FYE-broydz)
galactorrhea (ga-LAK-to-REE-uh)
hirsutism (HER-suh-tizm)
hysterosalpingography (hiss-TER-oh-sal-pin-GAW-gruh-fee)
hysteroscopy (hiss-tuh-ROSS-kaw-pee)
hysterosonography (HISS-tuh-roh-son-AWG-ruh-fee)
leiomyoma (LYE-oh-mye-OH-muh)
mittelschmerz (MIT-uhl-shmairts)
myomas (mye-OH-muhz)
osteoporosis (AWSS-tee-oh-puh-ROH-siss)
overflow incontinence (OH-ver-floh in-KON-tih-nents)
prolapse (PROH-laps)
rectocele (REK-tuh-seel)
stress incontinence (STRESS in-KON-tih-nents)
urinary retention (YOOR-ih-nair-ee rih-TEN-shun)
vulvovaginitis (VUL-voh-vaj-ih-NYE-tiss)

CHAPTER CONCEPTS

Health Promotion
Reproduction and Sexuality

LEARNING OUTCOMES

1. Define the key terms.
2. Summarize preventive health screenings suggested for women.
3. Explain the two types of amenorrhea and the possible causes of amenorrhea.
4. Outline medical and nursing interventions for dysmenorrhea.
5. Compare and contrast premenstrual syndrome (PMS) and premenstrual dysphoric disorder (PMDD).
6. Plan nursing interventions for the patient with PMS.
7. Explain endometriosis and list the signs and symptoms.
8. Describe the barrier methods of contraception.
9. Discuss the different types of hormonal contraceptives.
10. Explain permanent contraception options.
11. Define *infertility* and discuss risk factors, causes, and possible treatment options.
12. Define *menopause* and describe physical changes that occur during perimenopause.
13. Plan patient-centered nursing care for a menopausal woman.
14. Summarize treatment options for women who experience severe vasomotor symptoms.
15. Define *uterine fibroids* and list the symptoms of fibroids.
16. Explain how an ovarian cyst forms and list the symptoms of an ovarian cyst.
17. List the characteristics of polycystic ovary syndrome.
18. Discuss the symptoms and treatment for sexually transmitted infections (STIs).
19. Plan nursing interventions for a woman with a vulvovaginal infection.
20. Define the different types of pelvic floor disorders and the treatment options.

CRITICAL THINKING

Scenario #1: **Carina**, aged 46, is your next-door neighbor. Carina is recently divorced and has begun dating again. She knows that you are a nurse and stops by your house for a cup of coffee. She has a few questions. She has been noticing that her periods are becoming irregular and lighter, and sometimes she feels hot during the night. "I'm too young for menopause, right?" Carina asks.

She mentions that she is in a new sexual relationship with a great guy. And she adds, "I didn't have to worry about pregnancy when I was married. My husband had a vasectomy. I'm glad that I'm too old to get pregnant now."

Questions

1. What do you need to think about as you respond to Carina?
2. What are your concerns regarding her comments about her new sexual relationship and becoming pregnant?

CONCEPTUAL CORNERSTONE
Reproduction and Sexuality

To foster sexual health, it is important for nurses to develop a comfort level in evaluating, educating, and providing care related to sexuality. Sexuality across the life span includes physical, emotional, mental, social, and spiritual dimensions that contribute to a state of well-being related to sensuality. It is not just the absence of disease or dysfunction (Giddens, 2021). Nurses are sometimes hesitant to engage patients in discussions related to sexual issues, and patients are often embarrassed to bring up the subject too. Nurses may have difficulty discussing sexual health, but it is important for them to put the patient at ease by using appropriate non-verbal behaviors and by asking open-ended questions to obtain information related to sexual health. Sexuality is a part of a woman's life throughout her life span, and nurses caring for women need to be able to comfortably ask the right questions, encourage the patient to ask questions, and provide education for patients related to the sexuality issues at each stage of life. This chapter has many topics that relate to a woman's sexual health such as **contraceptives** (birth control methods), menstrual disorders, sexually transmitted infections (STIs), infertility, and menopause.

Every woman must have access to knowledge about health issues related to her stage of life. You should be prepared to explain and discuss women's health issues and promote good health by encouraging women to stay on track with screenings and health-care visits. Women and men share many similar health problems, but they have distinct health issues related to sexual health.

PREVENTIVE HEALTH CARE FOR WOMEN

Women tend to put their own health-care needs last. Some women do not obtain routine health maintenance checkups and may go years without a physical examination and preventive screenings. A woman can maintain and improve her health by eating healthy, maintaining a normal weight, exercising daily, practicing safe sex, avoiding tobacco products, limiting alcohol intake, and obtaining preventive care such as pelvic examinations, Papanicolaou (Pap) tests, and mammograms. Table 3.1 outlines timelines for preventive health screenings for women.

Access to health care can pose special challenges for immigrant women. Language and cultural differences between patients and health-care providers can lead to misunderstandings, mistrust, delays, and errors in diagnosis and providing appropriate care. Immigrant women are less likely to receive reproductive services, including cervical cancer screenings, contraception, and comprehensive sex education (Centers for Disease Control and Prevention [CDC], 2022). As a result, they are more likely to experience negative health outcomes, including higher rates of unintended pregnancies and cervical cancer.

Health Promotion
Transgender Patients

- A transgender man or woman will need to continue to see a health-care provider if hormones are prescribed.
- A transgender man who is 21 years old or older, has a cervix, and has had sex with anyone will need to have regular Pap tests to screen for cervical cancer. The Pap tests should be scheduled according to the American Cancer Society (ACS) guidelines.
- A transgender man aged 50 to 69 will need to have mammograms every 2 years to screen for chest cancer, even if the breasts were removed in transitioning (ACS, 2021).

MENSTRUAL DISORDERS

For many women, the monthly menses, or period, occurs regularly and without concerns. However, other women experience a variety of problems related to the menstrual cycle. Nurses must be knowledgeable about problems associated with the menstrual cycle to provide education and supportive counseling. Problems related to the menstrual cycle are discussed in this section.

Table 3.1

Preventive Health Screenings for Women

Screening Test	Purpose	When
Physical examination: including blood pressure screening; cholesterol, diabetes, and thyroid tests; and obesity screening	To maintain health and screen for health problems, discuss lifestyle habits, and keep vaccinations up to date.	Every 1–2 years or more often, depending on general health.
Colorectal cancer screening; stool examination or colonoscopy	To identify and remove cancer and precancerous polyps.	Every 10 years starting at age 45 or every 5 years for high-risk individuals.
Breast self-examination	The American Cancer Society (ACS) no longer recommends breast self-examination for breast cancer screening (ACS, 2022). However, every woman should know how her breasts look and feel normally and report changes to a health-care provider right away.	
Clinical breast examination	According to the ACS, clinical breast examinations are no longer recommended for breast cancer screening (ACS, 2022).	
Mammogram	To detect and diagnose breast cancer.	Women aged 40–44 should have the choice to start screening mammograms. Women aged 45–54 should get mammograms every year. Women aged 55 and older should switch to mammograms every 2 years or can continue yearly screening.
Pelvic examination	To examine the external and internal genitalia for abnormalities.	Yearly starting at age 21.
Papanicolaou (Pap) test	Cells are scraped from the cervix and analyzed under the microscope to identify abnormal cells that could become cancerous.	Women aged 25–65 should get a Pap test every 3 years. Women older than 65 can stop the Pap test if there were normal results in the previous 10 years.
HPV test	To identify the presence of HPV, which can cause cervical cancer.	Every 5 years in women 25–65.
STI tests	Detects and prevents the spread of STIs.	All sexually active women and their partners should be tested before starting sexual activity.
Bone mineral density test	This screening identifies bone loss early before a fracture occurs.	Age 65.

American Cancer Society. (2022). *Prevention and early detection guidelines.* https://www.cancer.org/healthy/find-cancer-early/screening-recommendations-by-age.html#All_ages; United States Department of Health and Human Services. (2022). *Screening tests.* https://health.gov/myhealthfinder/doctor-visits/screening-tests

Amenorrhea

Amenorrhea is the medical term for the absence of menstrual periods. It is classified as:

- *Primary:* The failure of menses to occur by age 16
- *Secondary:* Cessation of menses sometime after the first menstrual period of puberty has occurred, lasting three consecutive cycles or a time period of more than 6 months

The menstrual cycle occurs because of the changing levels of the hormones made and secreted by the ovaries. The ovaries make the hormones because they receive signals from the pituitary gland, which is controlled by the hypothalamus in the brain. Disorders of the ovaries, pituitary, or hypothalamus can interfere with the hormones responsible for the menstrual cycle and cause amenorrhea.

Primary amenorrhea is usually the result of a genetic or anatomical condition. The female reproductive organs either failed to develop normally during fetal development or do not function normally when puberty should begin. Diseases of the pituitary and hypothalamus can prevent stimulation of the reproductive organs, leading to primary amenorrhea.

Pregnancy is the most common cause of amenorrhea, and a pregnancy test is always the first test ordered by the health-care provider. If the test is negative, the health-care provider will order blood tests to check the following hormone levels: prolactin, follicle-stimulating hormone (FSH), estrogen, thyroid-stimulating hormone (TSH), dehydroepiandrosterone (DHEA), and testosterone. If any of these tests is abnormal, the health-care provider will start hormone therapy to restore normal hormone balance and menses.

Imaging studies such as pelvic ultrasound, x-ray, computed tomography (CT) scan, and magnetic resonance imaging (MRI) may be needed to detect anomalies of the reproductive tract. Treatment is based on the findings of the tests and may include surgery to correct anomalies if possible. Counseling should be part of the treatment plan because the young woman may be concerned about future sexual function or fertility.

Secondary amenorrhea may be caused by excessive weight loss, excessive exercise, premature ovary failure, disorders of the pituitary, disorders of the hypothalamus, or emotional stress. Anorexia nervosa, a condition in which a patient restricts food intake to the point of starvation and exercises intensely, typically causes extreme weight loss, amenorrhea, and even infertility. The same diagnostic tests may be ordered to evaluate the cause of secondary amenorrhea. If the cause is excessive weight loss or exercise, nutrition and exercise counseling may be the only treatment required. Estrogen therapy will be instituted for women with premature ovary failure to prevent bone loss (Pitts et al., 2021). In the case of amenorrhea, the patient may require years of treatment to regain hormonal balance, acquire healthy eating patterns, and restore fertility.

- WORD • BUILDING •

amenorrhea: a–without + meno–month + rrhea–flow

Dysmenorrhea

Dysmenorrhea is a medical term for painful menses, referring to menstrual cramps that occur immediately before or during the early part of the menstrual period. The cramping pain is felt in the lower abdomen or back and can be mild or severe. There may be other associated physical symptoms such as malaise, fatigue, nausea, vomiting, lower backache, and headache (Jimenez, 2022). Prostaglandins are responsible for assisting the uterus to contract and shed the lining. High levels of prostaglandins can cause severe cramping. The cramping of the uterine muscle can cause the blood supply to the uterus to be temporarily decreased, and pain results when the muscle does not get enough oxygenated blood.

Severe dysmenorrhea can be caused by the following:

- **Endometriosis** (a condition in which the uterine tissue is growing outside the uterus)
- Infection in the reproductive organs
- Stenosis (narrowing) of the cervix, which slows down the flow of menstrual blood
- **Fibroids** (benign tumors) in the inner wall of the uterus

Medical management of dysmenorrhea includes:

- NSAIDs to block the production of prostaglandins started the day before the menses is due and continued until day two of the menstrual period
- Heating pad or warm bath

For severe dysmenorrhea, the health-care provider may also:

- Complete a thorough history of the menstrual cycle and symptoms.
- Perform a pelvic examination to observe for abnormalities.
- Order an abdominal or transvaginal ultrasound to diagnose reproductive organ abnormalities.
- Prescribe hormonal contraceptives to produce shorter and lighter blood flow periods.
- Perform a laparoscopy to visualize internal organs (Shields & Kho, 2021).

Evidence-Based Practice

A study was conducted on the effects of listening to music while experiencing dysmenorrhea. The findings indicate that a musical composition with no lyrics or percussion at a slow relaxing 60 bpm relieved pain to a greater extent than silence. The participants listened to the music for 30 minutes and reported significantly fewer analgesic treatments.

Martin-Saavedra, J., & Ruiz-Sternberg, A. M. (2020). The effects of music listening on the management of pain in primary dysmenorrhea: A randomized controlled clinical trial. *Nordic Journal of Music Therapy, 29*(5), 398–415. https://doi.org/10.1080/08098131.2020.1761867

- WORD • BUILDING •

dysmenorrhea: dys–bad + meno–month + rrhea–flow

Health Promotion

Relieving Menstrual Cramps

The following suggestions can help to relieve menstrual cramp pain:

- Start ibuprofen at the onset or right before the period starts.
- Exercise regularly. Women who exercise have less menstrual pain.
- Avoid caffeine, salt, and alcohol before the onset of menses.
- Place a heating pad on the lower abdomen (Shields & Kho, 2021).

Dysfunctional Uterine Bleeding

Dysfunctional uterine bleeding is irregular bleeding that occurs in the absence of a pelvic disorder, medical disease, or pregnancy. The bleeding is unpredictable. It can be excessively heavy or very light. It can be prolonged, short, frequent, or random (Harvard Health, 2021). Diagnosis usually begins with testing, such as the following:

- Complete blood count (CBC)
- Thyroid function tests
- Liver function tests
- Hormone panels
- Pap test
- Pelvic examination
- Coagulation tests
- Pelvic ultrasound
- Endometrial biopsy to test for cancer

Abnormal test results will direct the health-care provider to the appropriate therapy. If the testing is all normal, medical management usually begins with hormone therapy. Oral contraceptives suppress endometrial development and reestablish predictable bleeding patterns. **Endometrial ablation**, a procedure that destroys the uterine lining, or hysterectomy may be options for women who are not planning future pregnancies (Bergeron et al., 2020).

Midmenstrual Cycle Pain

Pain that occurs midway through the menstrual cycle is called *mittelschmerz*, which comes from the German words for "middle" and "pain." Ovulation usually occurs 2 weeks before the first day of the menstrual period. Some women notice a slight twinge or more severe pain in the lower abdomen on one side when the egg is released from the ovary. It is usually diagnosed based on the symptoms and the timing of the menstrual cycle. No treatment is needed other than ibuprofen or acetaminophen. If the pain is severe, a pelvic ultrasound or CT scan can be ordered to see if the pain is mittelschmerz or an ovarian cyst.

- WORD • BUILDING •

mittelschmerz: mittel–middle + schmerz–pain

Premenstrual Syndrome

Premenstrual syndrome (PMS) is a recurrent condition associated with the luteal phase of the menstrual cycle in which women experience physical, psychological, and behavioral changes severe enough to interfere with interpersonal relationships and normal activity. The symptoms subside with menses. Symptoms of PMS have been reported to affect as many as 90% of women sometime during their lives (Office on Women's Health, 2021). There are a variety of symptoms and not all women experience the same symptoms. Signs and symptoms associated with PMS include the following:

- Difficulty sleeping
- Irritability
- Crying spells
- Depression
- Weight gain
- Acne
- Dysmenorrhea
- Hot flashes
- Angry feelings
- Tense feelings
- Mood swings
- Headache
- Abdominal bloating
- Breast tenderness
- Swelling of the extremities
- Cravings for sweet or salty food
- General aches and pains

There is no definitive treatment for PMS. Health-care providers suggest the following strategies for managing PMS (Dilbaz & Aksan, 2021):

- Lifestyle changes (Exercise at least 2.5 hours each week at moderate intensity. Eat healthy foods such as vegetables, fruits, and whole grains. Avoid salt, high-sugar foods, and alcohol when feeling the symptoms. Utilize yoga, massage, journaling, and relaxation to manage stress.)
- Medications
- NSAIDs
- Diuretics
- Antidepressants
- Antianxiety medications
- Oral contraceptives (Use of oral contraceptives to treat PMS is controversial. Some studies have shown that they do not improve symptoms [Office on Women's Health, 2021].)

Nutritional supplements are being studied for their effectiveness with relieving PMS symptoms. Some health-care providers may suggest the following:

- Calcium to relieve depression and cravings
- Magnesium to relieve headaches
- Vitamin B_6 to potentially relieve moodiness, anxiety, and bloating (Office on Women's Health, 2021)

Nursing Care Plan for the Patient With Premenstrual Syndrome

Angela, a 19-year-old college student, presents at the campus health center reporting severe menstrual cramps, bloating, and "feeling grouchy and mean." She reports craving pizza and chocolate, but consuming them did not relieve her symptoms. She tried using a heating pad to treat her cramps, but it just made her feel "hot and sweaty."

Nursing Diagnosis: Fluid retention related to cyclic hormonal changes
Expected Outcome: No weight gain before starting menses

Interventions:	Rationale:
Decrease salty foods.	*Excess sodium causes fluid retention.*
Take diuretics as ordered by the health-care provider.	*This medication will eliminate excess fluid.*

Nursing Diagnosis: Anxiety and irritability related to cyclic hormonal changes
Expected Outcome: The patient will verbalize a decrease in irritability and anxiety.

Interventions:	Rationales:
Obtain regular aerobic exercise.	*Release of endorphins is therapeutic for mood stabilization and exercise is an outlet for anxiety.*
Take antianxiety medication as ordered.	*Medications can reduce anxiety.*
Journal feelings and thoughts.	*Journaling can be an outlet for anxiety.*

Nursing Diagnosis: Pain related to breast tenderness
Expected Outcome: The patient will state that the pain is decreased to an acceptable level.

Intervention:	Rationale:
Take NSAIDs as ordered by the health-care provider.	*NSAIDs are effective at managing PMS discomfort.*

Nursing Diagnosis: Ineffective health maintenance related to poor management of PMS symptoms
Expected Outcome: The patient will verbalize that her PMS symptoms are less severe.

Interventions:	Rationales:
Teach the patient to use a calendar to record PMS symptoms and keep track of her menstrual periods.	*She can begin to see a pattern and know when to start managing symptoms.*
Teach lifestyle changes such as a healthy diet and regular exercise.	*Good nutrition and exercise help to decrease the symptoms of PMS.*
Teach stress-reduction techniques such as yoga, journaling, and counseling to reduce stress.	*Reduced stress will make the symptoms of PMS more manageable.*

Premenstrual Dysphoric Disorder

Premenstrual dysphoric disorder (PMDD) is a severe form of PMS in which the woman experiences a severe form of the emotional PMS symptoms such as a labile mood, irritability, anger, and anxiety (Trezza & Krabbe, 2022). PMDD causes more difficulty with interpersonal relationships and a deterioration in functioning at work or school. Additional symptoms experienced with PMDD include the following:

• Decreased interest in usual activities
• Difficulty concentrating
• Marked lack of energy
• **Hypersomnia** or insomnia
• A feeling of being out of control or overwhelmed
• Marked change in appetite with overeating
• Abdominal bloating

Medical management usually begins with ruling out other medical conditions that could cause the symptoms.

• WORD • BUILDING •
hypersomnia: hyper–excessive + somn–sleep + ia–condition

Laboratory studies would include thyroid function tests, CBC, and FSH levels. Treatment for PMDD is similar to the treatment of PMS with more emphasis on medications. Medications indicated for treating PMDD include the following:

- Hormone therapy: drospirenone and estrogen are approved by the United States Food and Drug Administration (FDA)
- Anxiolytics (antianxiety), antidepressants, and mood stabilizers

Nonpharmacological treatment for PMDD includes the following:

- Acupuncture
- Relaxation techniques
- Light therapy
- Cognitive-behavioral therapy (CBT; Dilbaz & Aksan, 2021)

Endometriosis

Endometriosis is common among women in their 30s and 40s. Endometriosis is a condition in which the lining of the uterus, the endometrium, grows outside the uterus. The exact cause of endometriosis is unknown, but it is believed that small pieces of the endometrium travel back through the fallopian tubes into the pelvic cavity and become trapped. These small pieces of tissue begin to grow on the outside of the reproductive organs. Other growth sites for endometriosis have been identified, including the cervix, vagina, vulva, bladder, and rectum (Davila, 2021). This tissue responds to the hormonal influences that cause the menstrual cycle. These abnormal growths of tissue respond similarly to the lining of the uterus. Each month, the tissue builds up, breaks down, and sheds (bleeds), causing pain. Blood from this tissue outside the uterus can cause irritation and scarring.

The signs and symptoms of endometriosis include the following:

- Painful menstrual cramps
- Chronic low back pain
- Pain during or after sexual intercourse
- Painful bowel movements or urination during the menstrual period
- Bleeding or spotting between menstrual periods
- Nausea, vomiting, diarrhea, bloating, or constipation during menstrual periods

Endometriosis is diagnosed by symptoms, pelvic examination, ultrasound, MRI, and abdominal laparoscopy. There is no cure for endometriosis, but medical management may include extended-cycle oral contraceptives to reduce the number of menstrual periods. Surgical management involves removing the patches of endometrial tissue outside the uterus (Davila, 2021).

Nursing Care for Women With Menstrual Disorders

Nurses should encourage patients to seek medical attention for menstrual issues. In addition, nursing care for the woman with a menstrual disorder may include the following:

- Teaching the woman about normal menstrual periods
- Teaching her to keep a record of abnormal bleeding episodes and number of pads or tampons required, to provide accurate information regarding blood loss to the health-care provider
- Discussing avoiding salt, caffeine, and sugary foods, which can contribute to PMS symptoms
- Teaching the importance of adequate nutrition and avoiding excessive exercise (hours per day) to prevent amenorrhea; if exercise and low-calorie intake cause body fat to drop below 16%, she is at risk for amenorrhea (Trezza & Krabbe, 2022).
- Discussing management of menstrual cramps
- Providing information about diagnostic procedures such as pelvic examinations and other tests

 FAMILY PLANNING

The U.S. government has created family-planning goals in *Healthy People 2030* directed at improving pregnancy planning and the prevention of unintended pregnancy. The objective is to reduce the number of unintended pregnancies. The best way to reduce unintended pregnancies is to use an effective contraceptive method, also known as a *birth control method,* consistently and correctly. There are a variety of family planning methods available for use. See Figure 3.1 for the effectiveness of different contraceptive methods. This section discusses contraceptive methods, their correct use, and the advantages and disadvantages of each type.

Natural Family Planning

Natural family planning is one of the most widely used methods of family planning. Women may choose these methods because they are low cost, hormone-free, or more acceptable for people with religious or cultural beliefs against devices or medications for contraception (Casey, 2020). These methods rely on the ability to track ovulation to prevent pregnancy. Examples of natural family planning include the following:

- *Coitus interruptus,* also known as withdrawal, in which when the man withdraws his penis and does not ejaculate into the vagina.
- *Periodic abstinence* from sexual intercourse around the time of ovulation; this is also known as the *calendar method* or *rhythm method* because the woman must keep careful track of her menstrual periods. Ovulation may be estimated by careful monitoring of the menstrual cycle or by monitoring cervical mucus, which becomes more elastic and copious near ovulation.
- *Lactational amenorrhea,* in which a woman is exclusively breastfeeding, which can sometimes prevent her from ovulating. However, breastfeeding is not a reliable method of birth control. A woman who does not menstruate when she is breastfeeding may still ovulate and become pregnant if no other birth control method is used.

Effectiveness of
Birth Control Methods*

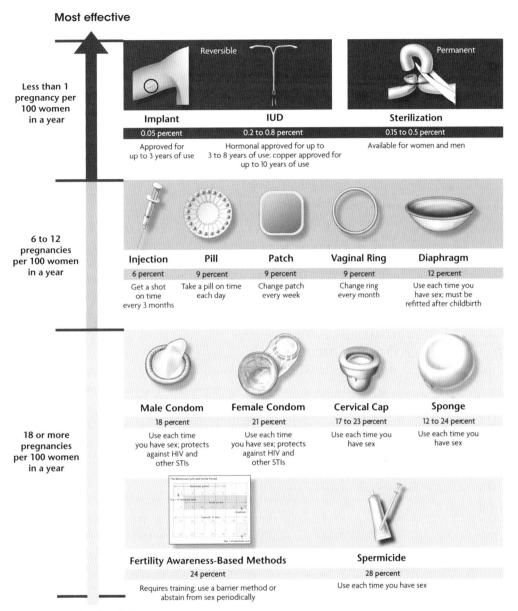

Most effective

Less than 1 pregnancy per 100 women in a year

Implant	IUD		Sterilization
Reversible			Permanent
0.05 percent	0.2 to 0.8 percent		0.15 to 0.5 percent
Approved for up to 3 years of use	Hormonal approved for up to 3 to 8 years of use; copper approved for up to 10 years of use		Available for women and men

6 to 12 pregnancies per 100 women in a year

Injection	Pill	Patch	Vaginal Ring	Diaphragm
6 percent	9 percent	9 percent	9 percent	12 percent
Get a shot on time every 3 months	Take a pill on time each day	Change patch every week	Change ring every month	Use each time you have sex; must be refitted after childbirth

18 or more pregnancies per 100 women in a year

Male Condom	Female Condom	Cervical Cap	Sponge
18 percent	21 percent	17 to 23 percent	12 to 24 percent
Use each time you have sex; protects against HIV and other STIs	Use each time you have sex; protects against HIV and other STIs	Use each time you have sex	Use each time you have sex

Fertility Awareness-Based Methods	Spermicide
24 percent	28 percent
Requires training; use a barrier method or abstain from sex periodically	Use each time you have sex

Least effective

Abbreviations: HIV, human immunodeficiency virus; IUD, intrauterine device; STIs, sexually transmitted infections.

Other methods of birth control

Lactational amenorrhea method: This is a temporary method of birth control that can be used for the first 6 months after giving birth if you are exclusively breastfeeding.
Emergency contraception: Emergency contraceptive pills taken or a copper IUD inserted within 5 days of unprotected sex can reduce the risk of pregnancy.
Withdrawal: The penis is withdrawn from the vagina before ejaculating. 22 out of 100 women using this method will get pregnant in the first year.

*Percentage of women who will get pregnant within the first year of typical use of the method

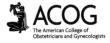

FIGURE 3.1 Effectiveness of contraceptive methods.

• *Cervical mucus monitoring,* in which the woman monitors her cervical mucus daily throughout her menstrual cycle in order to predict fertile days.
• *Body basal-temperature monitoring,* in which the woman monitors her temperature daily before arising from bed to indicate hormonal levels and to predict fertile days.

The advantages of natural family planning methods are that no medications or devices are required. The disadvantages are that these methods are less effective than other types of contraception and the couple must be both motivated and diligent about using their selected method consistently.

Barrier Methods

Barrier methods of contraception prevent the sperm from entering the uterus and traveling to the egg. Some methods are available over the counter (OTC) at a drugstore, and others require a prescription. The barrier methods of contraception are as follows:

• *Male condom:* The condom is placed over the erect penis and prevents sperm from entering the woman's body. The most common types are made from latex and also prevent the transmission of STIs. Each condom can be used only once and should not be combined with oil-based lubricants, which can weaken it.
• *Female condom:* The condom is placed into the vagina up to 8 hours before sexual intercourse and prevents sperm from entering the woman's body (Fig. 3.2).
• *Spermicides:* This method is available in a gel, film, suppository, or tablet. The spermicide is a chemical barrier that inactivates sperm and prevents them from entering the uterus. It is placed in the vagina no more than 1 hour before intercourse and left in place for 6 to 8 hours afterward.
• *Sponge:* The sponge is 2 inches in diameter, made of plastic foam, and inserted into the vagina before intercourse. It releases spermicide and can be left in place for up to 30 hours. It can be purchased in drugstores without a prescription.

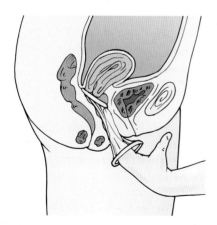

FIGURE 3.2 Female condom insertion.

• WORD • BUILDING •

spermicide: spermi–seed + cide–kill

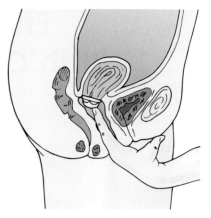

FIGURE 3.3 Cervical cap insertion.

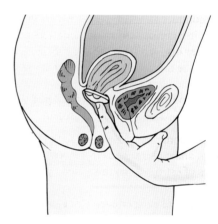

FIGURE 3.4 Diaphragm insertion.

• *Diaphragm or cervical cap:* Each of these methods is placed inside the vagina, where it covers the cervix and prevents sperm from entering the uterus. The cervical cap is clear plastic and thimble-shaped. The diaphragm is shaped similar to a shallow cup. Spermicides must be used with both methods, and both should be left in place for 6 hours after intercourse. Both methods require fitting by a health-care professional (Figs. 3.3 and 3.4).

The advantages of barrier methods are that most are available OTC without a prescription and are inexpensive. The disadvantages are that condoms may decrease the enjoyment of sex, and they can break. Some people are sensitive

Patient Teaching Guidelines

A man may purposely break condoms or remove a condom too early in order to get his partner pregnant. This is controlling behavior seen in abusive relationships and is known as *reproductive coercion.* Women should be made aware of this practice when choosing condoms as a form of birth control (American College of Obstetricians and Gynecologists [ACOG], 2019).

CRITICAL THINKING

Scenario #2: After a woman gives birth, her cervix will not return to its prepregnancy size. Why would it not be advisable to use the same diaphragm or cervical cap she used before her pregnancy?

to spermicides, and their tissues can be irritated with frequent use. Diaphragms and cervical caps require a visit to a health-care provider for a fitting.

Hormonal Contraceptives

Hormonal contraceptives contain progesterone alone or combinations of estrogen and progesterone to prevent ovulation. The contraceptive hormones can be in an oral form, injected, or implanted. Hormonal contraceptives prevent ovulation. They also work by altering the lining of the uterus and changing the mucus at the cervix, which prevents sperm from entering the uterus (Casey, 2020).

Hormonal contraceptives are considered safe for most women, but there some safety concerns:

- The estrogen component can activate the blood-clotting mechanism and cause venous thrombosis.
- High doses of estrogen can raise blood pressure, causing hypertension.
- Women who smoke experience vasoconstriction. The combination of smoking and estrogen leads to an increased risk of blood clots; therefore, women smokers who use hormonal contraception are at higher risk for a cerebral vascular accident (stroke) or a myocardial infarction (heart attack).

Contraindications for hormonal contraceptives are the following:

- A history of deep vein thrombosis (DVT) or pulmonary embolism (PE)
- Untreated hypertension
- Age over 35
- Cigarette smoking
- History of breast cancer

CRITICAL THINKING & CLINICAL JUDGMENT

Your good friend **Susan** recently started taking oral contraceptives. She mentions that she has started having severe headaches. She states that she has only had an occasional headache in the past, and now it is occurring almost daily.

1. What do you think could be a possible cause of the headaches?
2. What should you do?

Combined Oral Contraceptives

The oral contraceptive pill (OCP), also known as "the pill," is taken daily with most formulations having 21 pills with hormones and seven inert pills. Also available is a 91-day OCP that offers the advantage of only four menstrual periods a year. In the United States, there are more than 30 different formulations of estrogen and progesterone. The advantages of the OCP are as follows:

- Highly effective method of birth control
- Easy to use
- Regular and predictable menstrual periods
- Decreased menstrual cramps

The disadvantages of OCPs are:

- No protection from STIs
- Nausea, breast tenderness, and headaches occurring, especially when starting a new cycle
- Breakthrough bleeding (bleeding between periods)
- Failure with inconsistent use

Health Promotion

There are many different dosages of estrogen and progesterone available in oral contraceptives. A woman should be encouraged to return to her health-care provider if she is experiencing uncomfortable side effects such as breast tenderness and nausea. The health-care provider can prescribe a different OCP and work with her to find the right dosage with minimal side effects.

Progestin-Only Pill

Also known as the "minipill," this contraceptive pill contains only one hormone: progestin. The minipill is taken every day of the month at the same time. It is a good option for women who cannot take estrogen. The advantages of the minipill are similar to OCPs, with the addition of safety for breast-feeding mothers. The minipill does not affect milk supply. The disadvantage for the progestin-only pill is that it must be

Patient Teaching Guidelines

A woman may occasionally forget to take an oral contraceptive. If she has forgotten one pill, she should take it as soon as she remembers and then take the next pill at her regular time. No additional contraceptive method is needed. However, if a woman misses two or more pills, she should take the most recent pill missed and continue taking the remainder of the pills at the usual time. She will need to use backup contraception, such as condoms, or abstain from sexual activity until her menstrual period begins and she starts a new pill package.

taken at almost exactly the same time every day to suppress ovulation. Women who take it inconsistently will experience contraceptive failure. The progesterone only pill, the Opill is now available in pharmacies without a prescription.

Implants

This contraceptive is a single thin rod inserted under the skin in the upper arm. The rod contains progestin that is released gradually over 3 years. The advantages of the implant are similar to OCPs; plus it is effective for 3 years and does not require a daily medication. The disadvantages are similar to OCPs with the addition of the following:

- A minor surgical procedure is required for insertion and removal.
- Removal can be difficult.
- Adverse effects include headaches, **hirsutism** (abnormal growth of hair), **galactorrhea** (inappropriate production of milk), and acne.

Transdermal Patch

The transdermal patch is worn on the lower abdomen, buttocks, or upper body but not on the breasts. The patch releases estrogen and progestin into the bloodstream. A new patch is applied weekly for 3 weeks. On the fourth week, no patch is worn so that a menstrual period will start. The advantage of the patch is that there is a decrease in nausea and breast tenderness. The disadvantages are that the patch may irritate the skin or may come off the skin unnoticed.

Vaginal Ring

The vaginal ring is a flexible, colorless ring that contains estrogen and progesterone. The outer diameter of the ring is 54 millimeters. The ring is inserted into the vagina and stays there for 3 weeks.

If properly inserted, the ring will not be noticeable by the woman or her sexual partner. The ring is removed for a week to allow the menstrual period to start, and then a new ring is inserted. The advantages are a decrease in the side effects normally associated with hormonal contraceptives. The disadvantages are that the woman must be comfortable inserting the vaginal ring, the ring may slip out during intercourse, and it may cause vaginal irritation.

Injectable Depot Medroxyprogesterone Acetate

This contraceptive is injected intramuscularly and inhibits ovulation for 3 months. The advantages of this type of contraceptive are that it contains only progesterone and is safe for breastfeeding women or women who cannot take estrogen.

The disadvantages of depot medroxyprogesterone acetate are as follows:

- An appointment at the health-care provider's office is required every 3 months to obtain the injection.

- Missing an appointment may result in a return of fertility and pregnancy.
- Long-term use has been associated with bone density loss (Mayo Clinic, 2021).
- There is a possible delay in fertility after long-term use.
- Acne may develop.
- Weight gain can occur.
- Depression and mood swings can occur.
- It does not protect against STIs.

Medication Facts

The FDA has issued a boxed warning for depot medroxyprogesterone acetate. This medication has been shown to cause bone loss with long-term use of greater than 2 years. It is unknown if use during adolescence and early adulthood will increase future **osteoporosis** (thin, fragile bone) and fracture risk.

Intrauterine Devices

The intrauterine device (IUD) is a T-shaped device implanted into the uterus (Fig. 3.5). Some types of IUDs release progesterone to suppress ovulation. The copper IUD releases a small amount of copper that prevents sperm from fertilizing the egg and usually does not interfere with the menstrual cycle.

The advantages of an IUD include the following:

- It can provide contraception for 3 to 10 years, depending on the type inserted.
- It is more than 99% effective.
- It is not dependent on the woman remembering to use it or affected by her using it incorrectly.
- It is convenient and does not require a trip to the pharmacy or store.

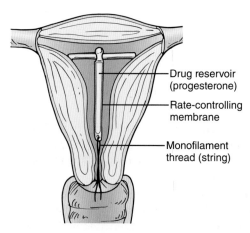

Drug reservoir (progesterone)

Rate-controlling membrane

Monofilament thread (string)

FIGURE 3.5 IUD properly positioned in the uterus.

• WORD • BUILDING •
galactorrhea: galacto–milk + rrhea–flow

• WORD • BUILDING •
osteoporosis: osteo–bone + por–passage + osis–condition

- Hormonal IUDs can reduce menstrual cramps and heavy bleeding during periods.
- Women who prefer to avoid hormones can use the copper IUD.

The disadvantages of an IUD include the following:

- It requires a pelvic examination for insertion and removal.
- To reduce the risk of a pelvic infection, STI screening should be done before insertion of the IUD (Casey, 2020).
- There is a small risk of uterine perforation during insertion.
- Some women experience heavy and painful periods during the first few months after insertion.
- The woman must check every month to see if it is in place.
- The IUD does not protect against STIs.

Emergency Contraception

Emergency contraception is defined as the use of a medication or device to prevent pregnancy after unprotected sex. It is not a form of abortion. Available emergency contraception includes the copper IUD and emergency contraception pills (ECPs).

- Insertion of a copper IUD within 5 days of unprotected sex is the most effective emergency contraception method. It works by making it harder for the sperm to fertilize the egg (World Health Organization, 2021).
- There are three types of ECPs available:
  - Ulipristal acetate 30 mg, taken as soon as possible within 5 days of unprotected sex. This medication works to inhibit or delay ovulation, and it may alter the endometrium to affect implantation.
  - Levonorgestrel 1.5 mg, taken as soon as possible within 3 days of unprotected sex.
  - Combined birth control pills that contain both estrogen and progestin taken in higher-than-normal doses may be prescribed by health-care providers up to 5 days after unprotected intercourse. Doses and number of pills vary depending on the brand of the pill. Two doses are usually given. They work by delaying ovulation.

The major side effects of ECPs are nausea and vomiting because of the high hormone dose.

Permanent Contraception

Sterilization is considered a permanent method of contraception. Although male and female sterilizations can be surgically reversed, the procedures are difficult, and fertility cannot be guaranteed.

The only method of female sterilization available in the United States is the tubal ligation. It may be performed following a cesarean delivery or can be performed surgically by a laparoscopy. The fallopian tubes are closed with clips, rings, sutures, or electrocoagulation.

The advantages of sterilization are that hormone therapy is not required and it is reliable and permanent. The disadvantages are that it requires a surgical procedure, and some women may regret their decision for permanent sterilization.

Vasectomy is permanent sterilization for men. It involves incision of the scrotal sac, cutting of the vas deferens, and closing of the ends by suture. This process prevents the passage of sperm into the seminal fluid. Vasectomy can be performed under local anesthesia in an outpatient setting. The advantages of a vasectomy are that it can be done in an outpatient setting and has minimal risks for complications. The disadvantage is that the man may regret his decision. The patient will not be sterile until after approximately 15 to 20 ejaculations, or 3 months, and therefore another form of birth control must be used until a semen specimen is tested to determine the absence of sperm (Casey, 2020).

Nursing Care Related to Family Planning

Nursing care related to family planning and contraceptives may include the following:

- Providing information to the patient so that she can select a birth control method that is appropriate for her (Fig. 3.6)
- Educating her about the correct administration or use of her chosen method of contraception
- Educating her about the side effects that she may notice
- Educating her about the effectiveness of her chosen method of contraception
- Encouraging her to report side effects to her health-care provider

INFERTILITY CARE

Infertility is the failure to conceive after 1 year of unprotected intercourse. Infertility care is a medical and nursing specialty. Nurses who work in this area develop a special rapport and

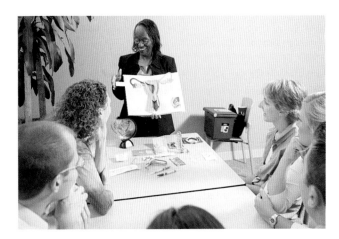

FIGURE 3.6 Teaching about contraception is an essential component of reproductive health care.

close relationship with their patients because they may be working together for months or years to treat the infertility issues. Infertility affects 10% to 15% of reproductive-aged couples (Puscheck, 2020). Risk factors for infertility issues are as follows:

- Maternal age greater than 35 years
- Smoking (can decrease both female fertility and male sperm count)
- Stress (affects the hormones responsible for ovulation)
- Scar tissue (caused by an STI)
- Alcohol use
- Obesity
- Low body mass index (BMI), which means that the patient has a lower level of body fat for estrogen storage, which can interfere with fertility
- Excessive exercise, which causes a release of endorphins that stimulate prolactin and can suppress fertility (Nova IVF Staff, 2022)

Tests and Diagnosis

Testing for infertility can cause anxiety for a couple. For some couples, it can be costly because infertility testing is not covered by all insurance plans. Testing is also time-consuming and can be uncomfortable. Also contributing to the anxiety is the worry about which person will be the one diagnosed with infertility problems and whether the problems can be corrected successfully.

For the woman to be fertile, her ovaries must release healthy eggs regularly, her reproductive tract must allow the egg to enter the fallopian tubes for fertilization, and the egg must travel on to the uterus for implantation. Fertility testing for the female may include the following:

- General physical examination with a pelvic examination and blood tests to evaluate overall health
- Blood tests to evaluate hormone levels and ovulation
- A **hysterosalpingography**: an x-ray with dye to visualize the uterus and fallopian tubes for abnormalities
- Hormone tests: thyroid and pituitary
- Pelvic ultrasound to view the reproductive organs
- Laparoscopy to identify and remove endometriosis (Puscheck, 2020)

For a man to be fertile, he must produce enough sperm to ejaculate into the vagina, and the sperm must be able to travel to the fallopian tube to fertilize the egg. Fertility testing for the male may include the following:

- Semen analysis
- Hormone testing for testosterone levels
- Scrotal ultrasound to visualize the testicles
- Testicular biopsy

• WORD • BUILDING •

hysterosalpingography: hystero–uterus + salpingo–stem or tube + graphy–writing

Causes of Infertility

After testing, the cause of the infertility problem for the couple may be identified. Possible causes of female infertility include the following:

- *Early menopause:* The ovaries have stopped producing hormones for ovulation.
- *Ovulation problems:* The ovaries are not releasing eggs.
- *Reproductive tract abnormalities:* There are fibroids, blocked fallopian tubes, an abnormally shaped uterus, or problems with the cervix or cervical mucus.
- *Endometriosis:* Abnormal tissue growth can alter the function of the uterus, fallopian tubes, or ovaries.
- *Thyroid problems:* Hypothyroidism can influence fertility.
- *Cancer treatment:* Damage to the reproductive tract can occur from earlier cancer treatment.

Possible causes of male infertility are as follows:

- *Inadequate sperm production:* This may be because of undescended testicles, diabetes, or trauma.
- *Problems with delivery of sperm:* There may be damage or anomalies of the reproductive tract.
- *Exposure to toxins:* Pesticides, tobacco smoke, marijuana, excessive alcohol, and steroids can decrease sperm production.
- *Exposure to excessive heat:* Hot tubs, saunas, and tight clothing can increase the temperature of the scrotum, leading to a decrease in sperm production.
- *Cancer treatment:* Damage to the reproductive tract can occur from earlier cancer treatment (Puscheck, 2020).

Treatments

A couple may just need one or two therapies to restore fertility, but it is possible that several treatment approaches may be utilized to restore fertility. Unfortunately, not all treatments for infertility are successful. Possible treatments may include the following:

- Correction of lifestyle issues such as obesity, smoking, hot tub and sauna use, and excessive exercise
- Medications for infections
- Hormones such as thyroid, estrogen, or progesterone
- Surgery to repair reproductive tract disorders
- Stimulating ovulation with medications
- Intrauterine insemination, in which healthy sperm are placed in the uterus at ovulation
- Assisted reproductive technology, which includes using donor eggs or sperm, injecting sperm into an egg, fertilizing eggs in the laboratory, and implanting embryos in the uterus 3 to 5 days after fertilization

General nursing care for couples experiencing infertility begins with referral to a fertility specialist. Nurses can also discuss risk factors that can influence fertility and encourage healthy lifestyle choices for couples desiring to start a family. Couples undergoing fertility testing and treatment will need to realize that even after testing and treatment, fertility may not be instantaneous or successful. Participation in a support group may be beneficial for them, as it may allow them to work through their fears and frustrations with infertility.

 ## MENOPAUSE

Menopause is defined as cessation of menstrual activity and is confirmed when the woman has missed her period for 12 consecutive months. Most women experience menopause between the ages of 40 and 58, and the average age is 51 (The North American Menopause Society [NAMS], 2022). The transition phase from regular periods to menopause is called *perimenopause,* and it may last for 4 to 10 years.

Some women experience no physical changes during perimenopause except irregular menstrual periods. Other women may experience any or all of the following:

- Hot flashes, which are sudden waves of heat that may be accompanied by sweating; tachycardia; and reddening of the face, neck, and chest. Hot flashes are caused by a decrease in estrogen that signals the hypothalamus in the brain to dilate blood vessels in the skin to cause the heat to disperse (Coney, 2021).
- Night sweats (heavy sweating from hot flashes at night) that interfere with sleep.
- Vaginal atrophy, which is a thinning and drying of the vaginal walls because of the drop in estrogen. Vaginal atrophy makes sexual intercourse uncomfortable or painful, a condition known as **dyspareunia.**
- Dry skin because of a reduction in collagen and decrease in oil production.
- Difficulty sleeping, ranging from insomnia to waking frequently during the night.
- Mental fogginess and forgetfulness because of a decrease in estrogen.
- Vaginal changes, including decreased lubrication, dryness, and a loss of normal vaginal flora, which is replaced with diverse flora that can cause urinary tract infections (UTIs) and vaginal infections.
- A general loss of pelvic muscle tone.
- *Osteoporosis,* a condition in which the bones become thinner and fragile; bone loss accelerates at menopause and continues for the first few years after menopause (Banks, 2021).

Psychologically, at menopause, some women experience a feeling of relief that they do not have to worry about birth control or menstrual periods. For other women, the hormone fluctuations can affect the neurotransmitters in the brain and lead to mood swings, irritability, sadness, and depression.

• WORD • BUILDING •

dyspareunia: dys–painful + pareun–lying beside + ia–condition

Medication Facts

Medications and supplements can prevent or slow bone loss among postmenopausal women. These include the following:

Calcium: 1,000 to 1,500 mg daily
Vitamin D: 1,000 IU daily
Estrogen: 0.025 mg daily
Bisphosphonates (alendronate, risedronate, ibandronate): weekly or monthly

(NAMS, 2022)

Treatment for menopausal symptoms depends on the woman and the severity of the symptoms. Some women do not want medications and prefer to try natural approaches to dealing with the symptoms. Women with severe hot flashes and night sweats often prefer to use medications. Medical management for menopausal symptoms may include the following:

- Low-dose hormone replacement therapy (HRT) with estrogen. Many health-care providers begin with a low-dose estradiol 0.05 mg patch. Estrogen is also available in oral preparations, creams, gels, sprays, and vaginal rings. Menopausal women with a uterus must be given progestin 2.5 mg daily to prevent the uterine lining from overgrowing (Coney, 2021).

Labs & Diagnostics

Bone density scanning, also called dual-energy x-ray absorptiometry (DEXA scan), is used to measure bone loss. A DEXA scan is a low-dose x-ray performed on the lower spine and hips that measures bone loss and can predict fracture risk for postmenopausal women.

- Selective serotonin reuptake inhibitors (SSRIs) such as venlafaxine, paroxetine, and fluoxetine are used to treat depression and can be effective in controlling hot flashes for some women.
- Clonidine is used for blood pressure control but can control hot flashes for some women.
- Gabapentin, a medication that is used to control seizures, is moderately effective in controlling hot flashes (Caporuscio, 2022).
- Intravaginal DHEA can be prescribed to manage moderate-to-severe dyspareunia. DHEA is an inactive steroid that is converted into estrogens. Estradiol vaginal inserts were approved by the FDA in May 2018 for treatment of dyspareunia of menopause (Coney, 2021).

Nursing care of the menopausal woman includes the following:

- Teaching her about perimenopause and menopause
- Instructing her that pregnancy is a possibility during perimenopause and that she should continue to practice birth control until she has gone 1 year without a menstrual period
- Providing information about HRT and encouraging her to discuss it with her health-care provider
- Instructing her to manage heat intolerance by layering clothing
- Instructing her to talk to her health-care provider about any depression symptoms
- Suggesting vaginal lubricants to improve vaginal moisture and relieve discomfort during sexual intercourse
- Encouraging a calcium-rich diet to support bone health
- Encouraging weight-bearing exercise to maintain bone strength
- Providing emotional support

FEMALE REPRODUCTIVE TRACT DISORDERS

The most common female reproductive tract disorders are uterine fibroids and ovarian cysts. Women with these conditions may experience a range of symptoms from none to so severe that they can interfere with work and lifestyle.

Uterine Fibroids

Uterine fibroids are the most common benign tumor found in women and can cause health problems such as abnormal menstrual bleeding and infertility. Fibroids are also known as **myomas** and **leiomyomas**, and they develop from the smooth muscular tissue of the myometrium. The cause of fibroids is unknown. A single cell divides uncontrollably and produces a firm, rubbery mass. The size of a fibroid can range from pea-sized to as large as a melon. A fibroid can grow suddenly or slowly. It can shrink, or it may remain the same size for years. Fibroids usually shrink during menopause. Multiple fibroids can distort and enlarge the uterus. Risk factors associated with the development of fibroids include the following:

- *Heredity:* Fibroids tend to run in families.
- *Race:* Black women are more likely to develop fibroids than other ethnic groups (Nutan, 2021).
- *Lifestyle:* A diet high in red meat and alcohol and low in vegetables can encourage fibroid development.

Symptoms of fibroids are as follows:

- Heavy menstrual bleeding
- Severe menstrual cramping
- Passing of large clots during menses

- Prolonged menstrual periods
- Pelvic pressure or pain
- Infertility

Diagnostic tests may include the following:

- Pelvic examination
- Ultrasound
- **Hysterosonography** (a saline-infusion ultrasound) to view the uterus
- Hysterosalpingography, a test that uses dye to visualize the fallopian tubes and uterus
- **Hysteroscopy**, in which a lighted scope is placed through the cervix into the uterus to visualize the uterine cavity

Many women with uterine fibroids do not have any signs or symptoms, or the symptoms are mild. In these cases, medical management usually consists of watching and waiting to see if the fibroids grow large enough to cause problems or shrink on their own as the woman enters menopause. If the fibroids are large, the health-care provider may recommend the following actions:

- Prescribing medications that inhibit estrogen and progesterone in order to shrink the fibroids
- Prescribing oral contraceptives or GnRH agonist medications to decrease menstrual bleeding and shrink the fibroids (University of California San Francisco [UCSF], 2022)
- Performing uterine artery embolization, in which small particles are injected into the arteries of the uterus, cutting off blood supply to the fibroids and causing them to shrink and die
- Performing surgery to remove the fibroids from the uterus or a hysterectomy to remove the uterus itself (Milton, 2021)

Nursing care for a woman with uterine fibroids may include the following:

- Explaining uterine fibroids
- Explaining diagnostic tests
- Preparing the patient for diagnostic tests
- Encouraging her to ask questions
- Providing emotional support

Ovarian Cysts

Ovarian cysts are fluid-filled sacs in the ovary. There are two types of ovarian cysts related to when they originate in the menstrual cycle. During a normal cycle, the ovary releases an egg, and the egg grows inside a follicle. When the egg is mature, the follicle breaks open to release the egg. A follicle cyst forms when the follicle does not break open to release the egg and instead keeps on growing. This type of cyst is usually not painful and ruptures in 1 to 3 months. A second

• WORD • BUILDING •

leiomyoma: leio–smooth + my–muscle + oma–tumor

• WORD • BUILDING •

hysterosonography: hysteron–uterus + sono–sound + graphy–writing

hysteroscopy: hysteron–uterus + scopy–look at

type of cyst can occur after the follicle ruptures. After the egg is gone, the empty follicle is supposed to shrink into a mass of cells called the corpus luteum. The corpus luteum makes hormones to prepare for the next egg, but a cyst can occur if the follicle sac does not shrink down. Instead, the sac reseals and begins to fill with fluid. It may disappear in a few weeks, or it may grow large, twist the ovary, and cause pain.

The most common causes of ovarian cysts are hormonal imbalances and endometriosis. Some women produce many small cysts on their ovaries and have a condition known as polycystic ovary syndrome (PCOS).

If a large cyst ruptures, it will cause sudden severe pain in the lower abdomen on one side. If the cyst is twisting the ovary, it will cause abdominal pain along with nausea and vomiting. Other symptoms of an ovarian cyst may include the following:

- Pressure or swelling in the abdomen
- Problems emptying the bladder or bowels
- Dull aching in the lower back
- Pain during sexual intercourse
- Painful menstrual periods
- Abnormal bleeding

Diagnosis of an ovarian cyst is made by symptoms and by a pelvic or transvaginal ultrasound. Medical management may include waiting to see if it resolves on its own or performing surgery to remove the cyst. Women who get frequent painful cysts may benefit from oral contraceptive medication to prevent ovulation and therefore prevent cyst formation (Amesse, 2019; Mayo Clinic, 2022).

Nursing care for a woman with an ovarian cyst may include the following:

- Determining the level of pain and administering pain medications as ordered by the health-care provider
- Explaining the disorder
- Explaining diagnostic tests
- Providing emotional support

Polycystic Ovary Syndrome

PCOS is caused by different factors working together in the body. It affects the entire body, not just the reproductive tract. The typical characteristics of this syndrome are increased levels of androgens, insulin resistance, and irregular menstrual periods.

A hormonal imbalance causing higher levels of androgens in a woman's body prevents the ovaries from releasing eggs. The ovaries may have small cysts inside. Androgens affect the endometrial layer, causing it to thicken, which increases the risk of endometrial cancer. The androgens also cause unwanted hair growth on the face (hirsutism) and acne. Insulin resistance increases the woman's risk of diabetes, metabolic syndrome, and cardiovascular disease (Lucidi, 2021).

Symptoms of PCOS are as follows:

- Irregular or absent menstrual periods
- Extra hair growth on the face
- Acne that is difficult to resolve

- Weight gain and difficulty losing weight
- Patches of dark, velvety brown skin on the neck and other areas, such as under the arms and in the groin area

Medical management of polycystic syndrome includes the following:

- Performing ultrasound imaging of the ovaries
- Obtaining hormone levels for a baseline for correction
- Obtaining fasting blood glucose, HbA1c, and lipid levels to determine if metabolic syndrome is occurring
- Prescribing hormonal therapy in the form of oral contraceptives, the vaginal ring, or the transdermal patch
- Prescribing metformin if the patient has high levels of blood glucose
- Prescribing spironolactone to lessen hair growth
- Encouraging the patient to lose weight if she is overweight or obese
- Encouraging lifestyle changes of increasing exercise and consuming a heart healthy diet
- Screening for anxiety and depression (Boivin et al., 2020)

Nursing care for the patient with PCOS includes the following:

- Educating the patient about her diagnosis and managing the medications prescribed by the health-care provider
- Encouraging the patient in making lifestyle changes that will improve her health such as increasing exercise and eating a healthier diet
- Directing the patient to community resources such as support groups or internet resources about PCOS

INFECTIOUS DISORDERS OF THE REPRODUCTIVE TRACT

Infections of the reproductive tract can affect the vagina, cervix, fallopian tubes, or ovaries. Some infections are sexually transmitted. All women should seek medical care for an infection of the reproductive tract to prevent possible complications such as infertility, ectopic pregnancy, and cancer.

Therapeutic Communication

A patient may feel very anxious and embarrassed about a possible exposure to an STI. You should remember to be therapeutic in discussing it with the patient. Avoid judgmental or shaming attitudes. Be matter-of-fact and encourage the patient to verbalize her fears and discuss her symptoms. Establish rapport with kindness and empathy and use the encounter as an opportunity to teach the patient.

Sexually Transmitted Infections

Anyone who has oral, anal, or vaginal sex, or genital touching, can acquire an STI, formerly known as a sexually transmitted disease. Every woman should know for sure that her partner does not have an STI or should insist on condoms for every sexual encounter. Some STIs have no or only subtle signs, particularly in women, and a woman can pass the infection along to a partner without realizing she is infected. See Table 3.2 for information about the signs, symptoms, diagnosis, and treatment of STIs.

Table 3.2
Sexually Transmitted Infections

Infection	Signs and Symptoms	Diagnosis	Treatment
Trichomonas vaginalis: caused by a parasite	Symptoms appear within 5–28 days of exposure: Thin green vaginal discharge, erythema, edema, and itching of the vulva Strong vaginal odor Dysuria	Wet mount slide under a microscope to identify the organism Culture DNA and polymerase chain reaction (PCR) testing from a swab sample	Metronidazole 2 g orally in a single dose
Chlamydia: bacterial infection of the genital tract	Symptoms start 1–3 weeks after exposure. Early-stage infections may not cause symptoms, which delays treatment. Late stage: Vaginal discharge Pain during intercourse Dysuria Bleeding between periods Lower abdominal pain	Vaginal or endocervical swab for culture Urine	Azithromycin 1 g orally as a single dose, or doxycycline 100 g orally twice a day for 7 days
Gonorrhea: bacterial infection of the vagina, penis, mouth, throat, eyes, or anus	Symptoms may start within 10 days of exposure or longer: Thick, cloudy vaginal discharge Heavy menstrual bleeding	Vaginal, urethral, anal, or pharyngeal swab for culture Blood tests: venereal disease research laboratory test (VDRL) or rapid plasma reagent (RPR)	Ceftriaxone 500 mg IM once; if patient >150 kg, the dose is increased to 1,000 mg once
Syphilis: bacterial infection that can affect the genitals; skin; mucous membranes; and, in later stages, the brain and heart	Primary: Symptoms occur within 10 days–3 months Small painless sore (chancre) wherever the bacteria were transmitted Secondary: Symptoms occur 3–6 weeks after the chancre appears Red or brownish red rash Fever Enlarged lymph nodes Fatigue Tertiary: without treatment, it progresses to affect internal organs Lack of coordination Numbness Paralysis Blindness Dementia Headache	Microscopy of swab from lesion Blood: enzyme immunoassay (EIA), *Treponema pallidum* particle agglutination (TPPA), VDRL	Benzathine penicillin G 2.4 million units IM in a single dose

Table 3.2

Sexually Transmitted Infections—cont'd

Infection	Signs and Symptoms	Diagnosis	Treatment
Pelvic inflammatory disease (PID): caused by *Chlamydia trachomatis* and *Neisseria gonorrhoeae* Infection travels from the vagina to the fallopian tubes; can cause permanent damage to the fallopian tubes	Abdominal pain Green or yellow vaginal discharge Dysuria Fever Chills Nausea Vomiting Painful intercourse	Vaginal swab for culture Blood tests: VDRL or RPR	Depends on severity; broad spectrum antibiotics such as azithromycin and cephalosporins may be used
HPV: viral infection that puts a woman at high risk for cervical cancer; genital warts is one type	Small flesh-colored papules Warts close together take on a cauliflower shape Itching Bleeding with intercourse	Physical examination and signs and symptoms Biopsy of warts	Podofilox topical 0.5% applied to affected areas twice daily for 3 days followed by 4 days of no treatment; may repeat for 4 cycles to treat the warts, not the underlying HPV infection
Herpes simplex virus (HSV): virus that enters the body through small breaks in the skin or mucous membranes	Some people never have symptoms Small clusters of vesicles and ulcers in the genital and anal areas Pain Itching Dysuria Headache Muscle weakness Swollen lymph nodes in the groin	Physical examination and signs and symptoms Confirmed by viral culture antibody or DNA-based rapid test	There is no cure; antivirals can reduce symptoms and suppress outbreaks Acyclovir 200 mg every 4 hours while awake for 10 days Valtrex 1,000 mg by mouth every 12 hours for 10 days
HIV: viral infection that can cause AIDS	Early signs: Fever Headache Sore throat Swollen lymph glands Rash Fatigue Late signs: Swollen lymph glands Weight loss Fever Diarrhea Night sweats Opportunistic infections	Saliva test for HIV Blood: HIV enzyme-linked immunosorbent assay (ELISA), HIV rapid test, Western blot, deoxyribonucleic acid (DNA) Polymerase chain reaction (PCR), CD4 cell count, viral load	There is no cure; patients should be referred to an infectious disease specialist to begin antiviral treatment to reduce viral load and slow down or prevent progression of the disease

Source: Centers for Disease Control and Prevention. (2021). *Sexually transmitted infection treatment guidelines 2021.* https://www.cdc.gov/std/treatment-guidelines/toc.htm

Health Promotion

A vaccine, human papillomavirus 9-valent vaccine recombinant, is available to prevent nine strains of human papillomavirus (HPV). The vaccine is effective against oropharyngeal, cervical, vulvar, vaginal, and anal cancers and genital warts. Vaccination against HPV is recommended for girls and boys from ages 9 to 26 years old. The vaccine is most effective if given before exposure to the virus.

Health Promotion

Avoiding a Sexually Transmitted Infection
There are several ways to avoid contracting an STI:

- Abstain from sex.
- Avoid oral, vaginal, or anal intercourse with new partners until you both have been tested for STIs.
- Get the HPV vaccination before you are sexually active.
- Use condoms correctly and every time you have sex.
- Stay in a monogamous relationship.
- Do not drink excessive alcohol or use illicit drugs because you may be more likely to take sexual risks.

Vulvovaginitis

Vulvovaginitis is a term used to describe many types of vaginal infections that involve the vagina and vulva. The most common vaginal infections are vulvovaginal candidiasis, atrophic vaginitis, and contact dermatitis. See Table 3.3 for more information about these infections.

Toxic Shock Syndrome

Toxic shock syndrome (TSS) is a rare but life-threatening illness usually caused by infection from *Staphylococcus aureus* or group A *Streptococcus*. Toxins produced by these bacteria cause the symptoms. Men, women, and children can develop TSS, but at least 50% of patients with TSS are menstruating women (Venkataraman, 2020). TSS has been associated with the use of superabsorbent tampons, and it usually develops within 5 days after the onset of menstruation.

Symptoms can be diverse and may include the following:

- High fever and chills
- Influenza-like symptoms
- Hypotension
- Vomiting and diarrhea
- Muscle aches
- Change in mental status
- Headaches
- Redness of the eyes, mouth, and throat

- Petechiae (tiny purple-brown spots under the skin caused by bleeding)
- Signs of soft tissue infection
- Rash that resembles a sunburn on the palms and soles that eventually peels off

Patients become severely hypotensive quickly and do not respond to IV fluid administration, leading to renal dysfunction. Other organs, such as the liver and lungs, become infected and the multiorgan dysfunction can eventually lead to death. Respiratory distress syndrome occurs in 55% of patients (Venkataraman, 2020). Successful treatment requires early recognition, transfer to an intensive care unit, antibiotic treatment, IV fluids, and dialysis if the kidneys are severely infected. The mortality rate can be as high as 30% to 70% (Venkataraman, 2020).

Nursing care for women who are experiencing an infection of the reproductive tract may include the following:

- Administering antibiotics and pain medication as ordered
- Monitoring vital signs and reporting abnormal findings
- Educating the patient about self-care to avoid contracting reproductive tract infections
- Encouraging the patient to practice safe sex and use condoms
- Encouraging open communication by avoiding judgmental attitudes

Safety *Stat!*
To prevent TSS, a woman should be educated to change her tampons every 4 to 6 hours, wear a pad at night, and wear minipads rather than tampons when her menstrual flow is light.

PELVIC FLOOR DISORDERS

Pelvic floor disorders involve a **prolapse** (dropping down) of the bladder, urethra, small intestine, rectum, vaginal wall, or uterus because of a weakness or injury to the ligaments, connective tissue, and muscles of the pelvis. The following factors may contribute to the development of pelvic floor disorders:

- Childbirth
- Obesity
- Hysterectomy
- Aging
- Engaging in activities that increase pressure in the abdomen, such as heavy lifting or straining during bowel movements

The different types of pelvic floor disorders are as follows:

- *Cystocele:* The bladder drops down and protrudes through the vagina, causing **stress incontinence** (leaking of urine

• WORD • BUILDING •
vulvovaginitis: vulvo–womb + vagin–sheath + itis–inflammation

• WORD • BUILDING •
cystocele: cysto–bladder + cele–swelling

Table 3.3
Vulvovaginitis

Type	Cause	Symptoms	Treatment
Vulvovaginal candidiasis	*Candida* is a naturally occurring organism in the vagina. Its growth is kept under control by *Lactobacillus* bacteria. If an imbalance occurs because of medications, heat, or restrictive clothing, the *Candida* can overgrow, causing symptoms.	• Thick, white, curd-like discharge • Vulvar and vaginal itching • Erythema and edema of the labia major and minora	• Fluconazole 150 mg in a single dose or • Terconazole 0.8% cream 5 g intravaginally for 3 days or • Over-the-counter products available without a prescription such as miconazole 2% cream intravaginally for 7 days
Atrophic vaginitis	Extremely low levels of estrogen can lead to atrophy of the vagina wall, causing thinning of the tissue. This affects the glycogen in the tissues, leading to a decrease in lactic acid and increase in vaginal pH, which allows other bacterial flora to cause infections.	• Vaginal soreness • Dyspareunia (painful sexual intercourse) • Burning, white discharge	• Topical vaginal estrogen • Vaginal lubricants during sexual intercourse
Bacterial vaginitis	The exact cause is unknown, but it is thought to be caused by multiple bacteria that accumulate because of the reduction of natural flora in the vagina.	• Thin white or gray vaginal discharge • Fishlike odor after having sexual intercourse • Itching and burning in the vagina	• Metronidazole 500 mg twice a day for 7 days, or • Metronidazole gel 0.75% 5 g intravaginally daily for 5 days
Contact dermatitis	This infection is irritant- or allergy-induced. Possible causes are: spermicides, vaginal discharge, latex, cosmetics, douching, fragrances, underwear, and cleansing products.	• Red swollen skin • Ulceration of skin	• Remove irritant • Triamcinolone ointment 0.1% applied twice a day • Hydrocortisone cream 0.5%–1% applied twice a day

Sources: Davis, S. (2020). Bacterial vaginosis and *Candida* vulvovaginitis. *Professional Nursing Today, 24*(3), 17–20; Leclair, C., & Stenson, A. (2022). Common causes of vaginitis. *American Medical Association, 327*(22), 2238–2239. https://doi.org/doi:10.1001/jama.2022.6375; Walter, K. (2022). Premenopausal vaginitis. *American Medical Association, 327*(22), 2255–2256. https://doi.org/10.1001/jama.2022.9256

when coughing or laughing), **overflow incontinence** (passing urine when the bladder is too full), or **urinary retention** (the bladder cannot empty completely).

• *Rectocele:* The rectum drops down and protrudes into the back wall of the vagina, making it difficult to have a bowel movement.

• *Prolapse of the uterus:* The uterus drops down into the vagina because of weakening of the connective tissue and ligaments. It can cause pain in the lower back or pain with walking, and it can make urination difficult (Fig. 3.7).

• *Prolapse of the vagina:* The upper part of the vagina drops into the lower part, causing the vagina to turn inside out. This causes pain while sitting and walking. It may also make it difficult to urinate or defecate.

The health-care provider can diagnose pelvic floor disorders with a pelvic examination.

Treatment for pelvic floor disorders may include the following:

• Exercises, such as Kegel exercises, to strengthen the muscles and ligaments
• Pessaries, devices shaped similar to a diaphragm, cube, or doughnut, inserted into the vagina to support the prolapsed organ
• Surgical repair (Diokno, 2021; Scott et al., 2022)

• WORD • BUILDING •
rectocele: recto–rectum + cele–swelling

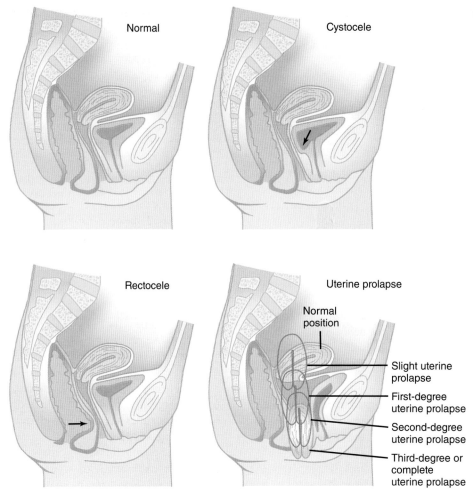

FIGURE 3.7 Cystocele, rectocele, and uterine prolapse.

Nursing care for the patient with a pelvic floor disorder may include the following:

- Teaching the patient Kegel exercises
- Encouraging her to drink plenty of fluids to avoid a UTI
- Providing information about how to insert a pessary if ordered by the health-care provider
- Providing emotional support and reporting signs of depression, which is common in women with pelvic floor disorders (Scott et al., 2022)

Key Points

- Nurses need to develop their therapeutic communication skills so that they are comfortable discussing issues related to sexual health.
- The most common cause of amenorrhea is pregnancy. Amenorrhea can also be caused by hormonal dysfunction or reproductive organs that did not develop properly or are not functioning correctly.
- Dysmenorrhea can be caused by endometriosis, infection, stenosis of the cervix, or fibroids and, for most women, can be treated effectively with ibuprofen.
- PMS is a condition in which women experience physical, psychological, and behavioral problems during the luteal phase of the menstrual cycle.
- PMDD is a severe form of PMS.
- Endometriosis is a condition in which the uterine tissue is living outside the uterus. It can cause pain and infertility.
- Natural family planning methods include coitus interruptus, periodic abstinence, and lactational amenorrhea.
- Barrier methods of birth control prevent sperm from entering the uterus.
- There are a variety of hormonal methods of contraception available, including pills, vaginal rings, injections, implants, and patches.
- IUDs, injections, and implants provide long-term contraception without the patient needing to remember a daily medication.

- Emergency contraception is most effective if started within 48 hours of unprotected sex.
- Permanent contraceptive methods include tubal ligation and vasectomy.
- Infertility is defined as failure to conceive after 1 year of unprotected sex.
- Infertility treatment may include hormones, surgery, lifestyle changes, or assisted reproductive technology.
- A woman is in menopause if she has not had a menstrual period for 1 year.
- Menopause causes physical changes such as vasomotor symptoms, vaginal thinning, and osteoporosis.
- Fibroids are benign tumors that grow in the uterine muscle. They can cause pain, bleeding, and infertility issues.

- Ovarian cysts can cause severe abdominal pain if they rupture. The most common causes of these cysts are hormonal imbalances.
- PCOS affects the entire body and requires hormone adjustments and metformin to manage the symptoms and prevent infertility.
- STIs are easy to transmit to another person. To avoid complications, a patient should seek medical care as soon as possible if they have been exposed to an STI or if they exhibit symptoms of an STI.
- TSS is a life-threatening infection that is associated with tampon use.
- Pelvic floor disorders involve a prolapse of the bladder, uterus, small intestine, rectum, vagina wall, or uterus. These disorders can cause pain and may need treatment with surgery.

Review Questions

1. A breastfeeding woman is requesting to be prescribed the minipill. You will include which statement in the patient teaching session?
   1. "The pills are taken for 3 weeks and then off a week."
   2. "The pills can cause nausea."
   3. "The pills must be taken at the same time every day."
   4. "The pills cannot be taken if you continue to breastfeed."

2. A woman is planning to undergo a tubal ligation. You will include which statement in the patient teaching session?
   1. "Your menstrual period will stop after the procedure."
   2. "The procedure requires anesthesia."
   3. "You will need to use a spermicide for 3 months."
   4. "The procedure is easily reversible."

3. A 30-year-old woman indicates understanding about health screening for women when she states:
   1. "I should get a Pap test every 3 years."
   2. "I should perform self-breast examination at least twice a year."
   3. "I should have a mammogram every 5 years."
   4. "A colonoscopy is only needed if there is a family history of colon cancer."

4. Which of the following statements about vaginal changes during menopause is accurate?
   1. The vaginal wall becomes moister.
   2. Vaginal lubrication during sex is increased.
   3. There is a decreased risk of vaginal infections.
   4. Normal vaginal flora are replaced by diverse flora.

5. Usual treatment for PMS includes which of the following? **(Select all that apply.)**
   1. Avoiding sugar and salt during the entire menstrual cycle
   2. Obtaining regular exercise
   3. Taking calcium and magnesium
   4. Taking antipsychotic medications
   5. Taking NSAIDs

6. A patient calls the clinic because she thinks she may have an STI. The *best* responses by you are which of the following? **(Select all that apply.)**
   1. "Can you come in for an appointment today?"
   2. "We will need a list of all your sexual contacts as soon as possible."
   3. "Abstain from sex until your appointment."
   4. "It sounds like you had unprotected sex. What were you thinking?"
   5. "We don't have any open appointments until next month."

7. The most common cause of amenorrhea is:
   1. A pituitary disorder
   2. Early ovarian failure
   3. A thyroid disorder
   4. Pregnancy

8. Pelvic floor disorders may be treated by which of the following? **(Select all that apply.)**
   1. Pessaries
   2. Medications
   3. Pelvic exercises
   4. Surgical procedures
   5. Nutrition counseling

9. A patient at the gynecology clinic is interested in using oral contraceptives for birth control. Which statement indicates that the patient understands oral contraceptives?
   1. "Oral contraceptives are not as effective as barrier methods of birth control."
   2. "I shouldn't smoke when using oral contraceptives."
   3. "I may have painful menstrual cramps when taking the pill."
   4. "Now I have increased protection from pregnancy and STIs."

10. A patient is receiving teaching about her newly diagnosed ovarian cysts. Which statement by the patient indicates that she needs clarification?
    1. "Ovarian cysts can cause abdominal pain and pressure."
    2. "Ovarian cysts are always treated by surgical removal."
    3. "Ovarian cysts are diagnosed by symptoms and an ultrasound examination."
    4. "Oral contraceptives are sometimes prescribed to prevent cyst formation."

ANSWERS 1. 3; 2. 2; 3. 1; 4. 4; 5. 2, 3; 6. 1; 7. 4; 8. 1; 9. 2; 10. 2

CRITICAL THINKING QUESTIONS

1. What are some nonpharmacological treatments for dysmenorrhea?
2. A friend has confided to you that she thinks she has an STI and that she has no money for an appointment with her health-care provider. What should you think about before giving advice to her?

Resources

For additional resources and information, including Postconference Questions and Activities, Answers, and References, visit www.FADavis.com.

 Student Study Guide

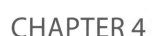

CHAPTER 4

Human Reproduction and Fetal Development

KEY TERMS

amniotic fluid (am-nee-OT-ik floo-id)
amniotic membrane (am-nee-OT-ik MEM-brayn)
blastocyst (BLAST-oh-sist)
cervix (SER-viks)
chorion (KOR-ee-on)
colostrum (ko-LOSS-truhm)
corpus luteum (KOR-puhss loo-TEE-uhm)
dizygotic twins (dye-zye-GOT-ik TWINZ)
ductus arteriosus (DUHK-tuhss ar-TEER-ee-OH-suhss)
ductus venosus (DUHK-tuhss vee-NOH-suhss)
embryo (EM-bree-oh)
endometrium (en-doh-MEET-ree-uhm)
epimetrium (ep-ih-MEET-ree-uhm)
estrogen (ESS-troh-jen)
follicle-stimulating hormone (FSH) (FOLL-ih-kuhl STIM-yoo-lay-ting HOR-mohn)
foramen ovale (fo-RAY-men oh-VAL-ee)
human chorionic gonadotropin (hCG) (HYOO-muhn kor-ee-AWN-ik goh-NAD-oh-TROH-pihn)
human placental lactogen (HYOO-muhn pla-SEN-tuhl LAK-toh-jen)
luteinizing hormone (LH) (LOO-tee-in-EYE-zing HOR-mohn)
microencephaly (MYE-kroh-en-SEF-uh-lee)
monozygotic twins (MON-oh-zye-GOT-ik TWINZ)
multiple pregnancy (MUL-tih-puhl PREG-nuhn-see)
myometrium (MYE-oh-MEE-tree-uhm)
placenta (pla-SEN-tuh)
progesterone (proh-JES-ter-ohn)
relaxin (rih-LAK-sin)
teratogen (ter-RAT-oh-jen)
testosterone (tes-TOSS-ter-ohn)
umbilical cord (um-BILL-ih-kuhl KORD)
villi (VIL-ee)
Wharton jelly (WOR-tuhn JEL-ee)

CHAPTER CONCEPTS

Reproduction and Sexuality
Safety

LEARNING OUTCOMES

1. Define the key terms.
2. Identify the structures and functions of the female reproductive system.
3. Identify the structures and functions of the male reproductive system.
4. Summarize the actions of the hormones that affect reproductive functioning.
5. Discuss the female and male reproductive cycles.
6. Describe the fertilization process.
7. Discuss the stages of embryonic development.
8. Describe fetal circulation.
9. Identify significant developmental changes of the fetus at various gestations.
10. Describe the functions of the placenta, umbilical cord, amniotic membranes, and amniotic fluid.
11. Contrast the differences between monozygotic twins and dizygotic twins.
12. Discuss TORCH infections and risks to the mother and fetus.
13. Discuss possible risks to safe fetal development caused by possible teratogens in medications, street drugs, foods, and the environment.

CRITICAL THINKING & CLINICAL JUDGMENT

Layla

Layla, aged 28, just confirmed with a home pregnancy test that she is pregnant with her first baby. She is employed at a plant and floral nursery in a rural agricultural area. Layla has an active job that provides physical exercise. She is of average weight, eats healthy food, and takes her lunch to work daily. At her first visit to the obstetrician's office, she is curious about fetal development and is concerned about having a healthy pregnancy and baby.

Continued

CRITICAL THINKING &
CLINICAL JUDGMENT—cont'd

Questions

1. What information can you provide Layla about the development of the fetus in the early weeks of pregnancy?
2. How might Layla's job impact the health of her pregnancy and baby?
3. What dietary advice regarding safe food choices should you give Layla?

CONCEPTUAL CORNERSTONE
Reproduction and Sexuality

The concept of reproduction is a foundational concept in the biological sciences. This chapter begins the discussion of human reproduction. Pregnancy is usually an expected event for couples who engage in sex without contraceptive measures. Unplanned pregnancies occur when couples lack education regarding contraception, do not choose to use contraception, experience nonconsensual intercourse (rape), or use contraceptives that fail.

You must be familiar with the structures and functions that make conception and childbearing possible. This chapter presents a brief summary of the male and female reproductive cycles, organs, and functions. The process of fertilization, embryonic development, and fetal development are discussed along with possible risks to the developing fetus.

FEMALE REPRODUCTIVE SYSTEM

The female reproductive system consists of external organs, internal organs, the female pelvis, breasts, and the female reproductive cycle.

External Organs

The external genital organs in women are the mons pubis, the labia majora and minora, the clitoris, the vestibule of the vagina, and the Bartholin glands (Fig. 4.1).

- The mons pubis is a pad of fat that lies over the symphysis pubis. After puberty, the mons is covered with hair. The labia majora, two folds of tissue that extend from the mons pubis to either side of the vulva, develop during puberty and are also covered with hair. After menopause, hormonal decline causes some atrophy of the labia.
- The labia minora are two smaller folds of tissue that form a hoodlike structure, called the prepuce, which surrounds the clitoris. The labia minora have sweat and sebaceous glands to lubricate the surface.
- The clitoris, a small sensitive organ containing erectile tissue, lies in front of the vulva and below the mons pubis.
- The vestibule of the vagina is the area between the labia minora and where the urethra and vagina open.

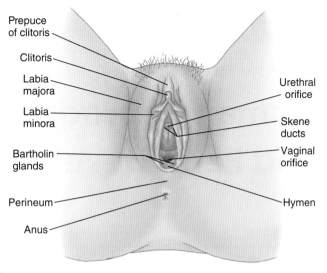

FIGURE 4.1 Female external genitalia.

- The Bartholin glands are located on either side of the vagina under the labia majora. Their ducts open to secrete lubricating fluids to moisten the vulva and to facilitate sexual intercourse.
- In addition, the perineum is the skin from the vaginal opening to the anus; it lies over muscles and fibrous tissue that separate the vagina and rectum.

Internal Organs

The internal organs of reproduction are the ovaries, the fallopian tubes, the uterus, and the vagina (Fig. 4.2). The ovaries are two small glands located on either side of the uterus slightly behind and below the fallopian tubes. The ovaries are attached to the broad ligament, a suspensory ligament, and the ends of the fallopian tubes. The ovaries are about the size and shape of almonds, and they store approximately one-half million eggs. The ovaries also secrete the hormones estrogen and progesterone during each reproductive cycle.

The fallopian tubes are attached to the uterus at one end; at the opposite end, they curve over the ovaries with fringelike projection. The function of the fallopian tubes is to provide a channel for the sperm to travel to the egg and to transport the fertilized egg into the uterus.

The uterus, a muscular triangle-shaped organ located between the rectum and bladder, provides the environment for the growth of a fetus (Fig. 4.3). The top portion of the uterus is called the fundus, whereas the lower portion that projects into the vagina is called the **cervix**. It provides a protective entrance to the uterus. This portion of the cervix is surrounded and supported by the uterosacral ligaments, the transverse ligaments, and the pubocervical ligaments. The cervix is very elastic and has the ability to stretch to allow for childbirth. The elasticity is caused by the high fibrous and collagenous content of the supportive tissue and the large number of folds in the cervical lining. The cervical canal contains mucus-secreting glands. The functions of

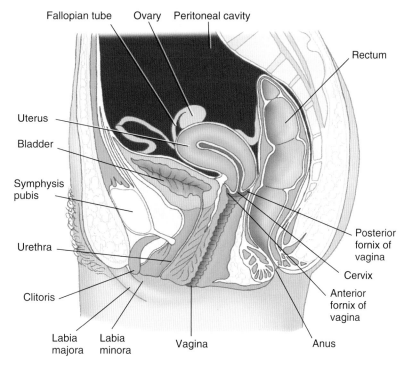

FIGURE 4.2 Internal female genitalia and cross section of the rectum.

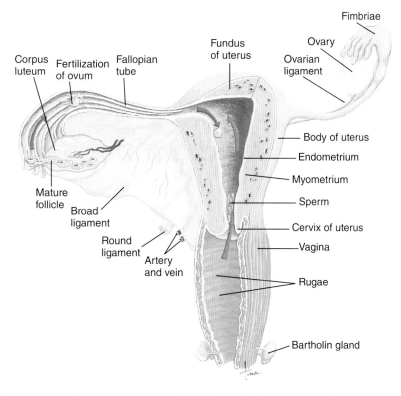

FIGURE 4.3 Female reproductive system shown in anterior view. The left ovary has been sectioned to show the developing follicles. The left fallopian tube has been sectioned to show fertilization. The uterus and vagina have been sectioned to show internal structures. Arrows indicate the movement of the ovum toward the uterus and the movement of sperm from the vagina toward the fallopian tube.

the cervical mucus are to prevent the growth of bacteria, to lubricate the vaginal canal, and to provide an alkaline environment to protect sperm from the acidic vaginal secretions.

The uterus has two coats: a muscular coat with longitudinal and circular fibers and an inner mucous membrane, which is in folds, also known as rugae. The uterus has three layers:

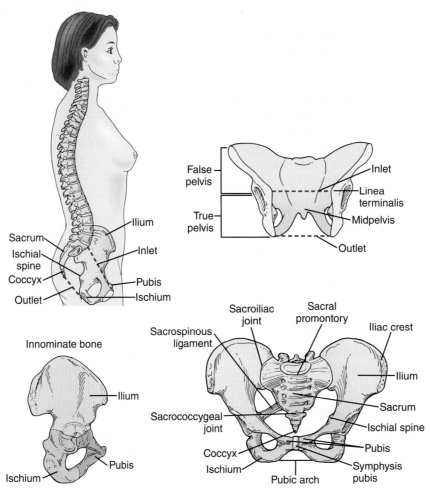

FIGURE 4.4 Female bony pelvis.

- The **endometrium**, a mucous membrane that lines the cavity of the uterus, is the site where the embryo implants after arriving in the uterus.
- The **myometrium** is the middle layer of smooth muscle that contracts and expels the fetus and placenta during childbirth.
- The **epimetrium** is a smooth, transparent membrane that lines most of the external surface.

The uterus is held in place by several ligaments. These ligaments provide support and stabilize the reproductive organs:

- The broad ligament, which keeps the uterus centrally placed and provides stability, is located on each side of the uterus and attaches to the pelvic sidewall (see Fig. 4.3).
- The round ligaments are situated between the broad ligaments, anterior and inferior to the fallopian tubes.

- WORD · BUILDING ·

endometrium: endo–inside + metrium–uterus
myometrium: myo–muscle + metrium–uterus
epimetrium: epi–on or at + metrium–uterus

- The cardinal ligaments arise superiorly and laterally from the uterus and inferiorly from the vagina to provide the primary support for the uterus.
- The uterosacral ligaments attach the uterus to the sacrum.

The vagina is a 4- to 6-inch elastic muscular tube that extends from the cervix to the external vaginal opening. Vaginal tissue is composed of smooth muscle and elastic connective tissue and is lined with stratified squamous epithelium, which is similar to skin. The vagina lies behind the bladder and urethra and in front of the rectum. The vagina begins at the vulva and ends at the cervix, and its two main functions are for sexual intercourse and childbirth.

Female Pelvis

The bones of the female pelvis are formed posteriorly by the sacrum and coccyx and on the sides and front by the hip bones. The hip bones consist of three sections: the ilium, the ischium, and the pubis. The female pelvis is shorter, wider, and more circular than the male pelvis, which makes the female pelvis the right shape for childbearing. The ischial spines are the narrowest diameter the fetus must pass through during childbirth (Fig. 4.4).

Breasts

The breasts are two glands that secrete milk. In the center of the surface is the nipple, which projects outward beyond the skin level. The nipple is a light color until pregnancy, and then it becomes darker because of hormonal changes. Inside the breasts are ducts that lead to the nipple. The tissue of the gland is similar to a sebaceous gland but is more highly developed to produce milk instead of sebum. The gland is divided into lobes by fibrous tissue, and the lobes are further subdivided into lobules. The breasts begin to develop during puberty, and further development occurs during pregnancy because of the effects of hormones from the pituitary and ovaries. **Colostrum**, a fluid rich with antibodies, may be secreted in small amounts during pregnancy and before milk production. Milk production typically begins 2 to 3 days after childbirth (Fig. 4.5).

Female Reproductive Cycle

The menstrual cycle begins on the first day of menstrual bleeding and ends on the first day that menstrual bleeding begins again (Fig. 4.6). **Follicle-stimulating hormone (FSH)**, **luteinizing hormone (LH)**, estrogen, and progesterone are involved in the female reproductive cycle.

Follicular Phase

During the follicular phase, the anterior lobe of the pituitary secretes FSH, which stimulates the development of a follicle in the ovary. The follicle consists of cells that surround an egg. As the egg follicle matures, it begins to secrete **estrogen**, which causes the endometrium in the uterus to thicken and prepare for the fertilized egg to implant. When the level of estrogen increases, it prevents FSH from further secretion. The pituitary gland responds to the decrease in FSH and begins to release LH.

Luteal Phase

The luteal phase begins on the day the egg is released. The levels of LH peak approximately day 14 of the cycle, causing

ovulation or the release of the egg from the follicle. After the follicle on the ovary releases an egg, LH converts the ruptured follicle into the **corpus luteum**, which secretes the hormone progesterone. **Progesterone** completes the development of the uterine lining in preparation for a fertilized egg. If the egg is not fertilized, the corpus luteum begins to degenerate, causing the levels of progesterone and estrogen to decrease, which leads to the shedding of the uterine lining (menstruation). The menstrual cycle then begins again. If fertilization and implantation occur, the endometrium does not degenerate, and the woman is pregnant (see Fig. 4.6).

Health Promotion

Preconception Health

Couples who desire to become pregnant should prepare ahead of time. Important things a couple can do for preconception health are the following:

- Stop smoking and drinking alcohol.
- The woman should take 400 mcg of folic acid each day along with eating foods with folate from a varied diet to lower the risk of fetal defects of the brain and spine (Centers for Disease Control and Prevention [CDC], 2022).
- Obtain an optimal weight.
- Continue to exercise.
- If the woman has a medical condition, such as diabetes, epilepsy, or asthma, she should make an appointment to discuss her pregnancy with her health-care provider.
- Avoid contact with toxic substances at home or work.
- Discuss the use of over-the-counter (OTC) and prescription medications with her health-care provider.
- The male should be aware that fever; exposure to excessive heat, such as hot tubs, saunas, or tight clothing; cigarette smoking; and heavy alcohol use may reduce the number of sperm.
- Make sure vaccinations are up to date.

MALE REPRODUCTIVE SYSTEM

The male reproductive system consists of the scrotum, penis, and testicles in which the sperm are produced.

External Organs

The external male reproductive organs are the scrotum and the penis. The scrotum is made of two sacs separated by a septum, or wall of tissue. Within each sac are a testicle, the epididymis, and the beginning of a spermatic cord.

The penis contains cavernous tissue. During arousal, spaces in this tissue fill with blood, and the arteries that supply blood to this region become dilated and filled with blood, which produces an erection. Semen is expelled, or ejaculated, through the end of the penis when a male reaches sexual climax (Fig. 4.7).

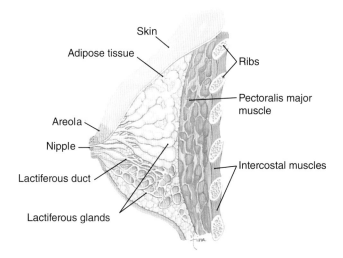

FIGURE 4.5 Mammary gland shown in a midsagittal section.

Labels: Skin, Adipose tissue, Ribs, Pectoralis major muscle, Areola, Nipple, Lactiferous duct, Intercostal muscles, Lactiferous glands

• WORD • BUILDING •
estrogen: estro–desire + gen–produce

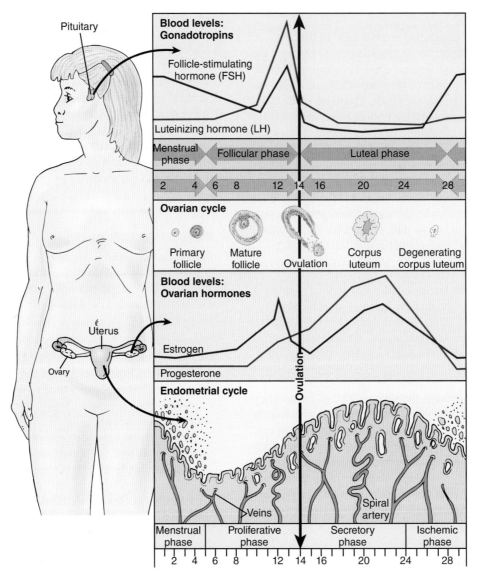

FIGURE 4.6 The female reproductive cycle. Levels of the hormones secreted from the anterior pituitary are shown relative to one another and throughout the cycle. Changes in the ovarian follicle are depicted. The relative thickness of the endometrium is also shown.

Internal Organs

The testicles, the reproductive glands of the male, are located in the scrotum and are suspended there by the spermatic cords. Each testicle consists of 200 to 300 lobules, each of which contains tiny tubules called the *convoluted seminiferous tubules.* The lining of the tubular walls contains cells that develop into spermatozoa. The tubules are supported by loose connective tissue containing groups of interstitial cells, which secrete the hormone testosterone. **Testosterone** promotes the development of male reproductive organs and the secondary male characteristics, such as body hair growth and the deeper voice that occur during puberty.

The seminiferous tubules open into the epididymis, a tightly coiled tube attached to the back of each testis. The epididymis transports sperm and brings the sperm to maturity, because they are immature when they leave the testis.

The sperm gain motility (the ability to move) in the epididymis after 18 to 24 hours. During sexual arousal, contractions force the mature sperm from the epididymis into the vas deferens, where they are stored until ejaculation. The vas deferens is a continuation of the duct of the epididymis; it passes through the inguinal canal and runs between the base of the bladder and the rectum to the prostate gland. At the prostate gland, located below the bladder and in front of the rectum, the vas deferens is joined by the duct of the seminal vesicle. The urethra runs through the center of the prostate, which provides additional fluid to support the sperm.

The seminal vesicles are two pouchlike sacs that create a sugar-rich fluid that provides energy to the sperm, and they attach to the vas deferens near the bladder. The fluid from the seminal vesicles composes most of the volume of the ejaculate. Ejaculatory ducts are formed by the fusion of the vas

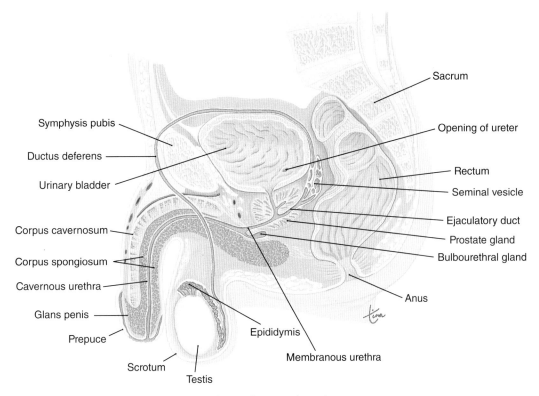

FIGURE 4.7 The male reproductive system shown in a midsagittal section through the pelvic cavity.

deferens (transporting mature sperm) and the seminal vesicles (producing seminal fluid). The ejaculatory ducts empty into the urethra.

The urethra carries urine out of the body and also carries sperm when the male reaches climax. When the penis is erect, the flow of urine from the bladder is blocked, and only semen is ejaculated.

The Male Reproductive Cycle

The hormones FSH and LH are responsible for regulating the production of sperm in the male. Both hormones are released from the anterior pituitary gland, with FSH stimulating sperm production in the testes and LH stimulating the production of testosterone. Testosterone allows immature spermatozoa to develop and become mature sperm cells during a 72-day process.

FERTILIZATION

For fertilization to occur, a sperm and egg must be in the same place at the same time. Typically, this occurs after sexual intercourse has taken place. The sperm and the egg, called gametes, meet in the fallopian tubes, where fertilization usually occurs. Of 14 million sperm deposited into the vagina during ejaculation, only 1 to 10 sperm reach the fallopian tube. One sperm will penetrate the egg's outer layer and fertilize the ovum. Typically, each gamete shares one

set of 23 single chromosomes. When fused, the total of 46 chromosomes produces a cell called the zygote (Fig. 4.8).

The sex of the embryo is determined at fertilization. The female shares only an X sex chromosome, and the male contributes either an X or a Y. At the moment of fertilization, if the zygote has an X chromosome from the mother and an X chromosome from the father, it is genetically female (XX); if the zygote has an X chromosome from the mother and a Y chromosome from the father, it is genetically male (XY).

If fertilization occurs, the lining of the uterus does not begin to degenerate and instead provides a place for the zygote to implant. Estrogen and progesterone levels remain high. An additional hormone, **human chorionic gonadotropin (hCG)**, is produced to support the development of the embryo. This hormone is made by the cells that will form the placenta. Elevated levels of hCG can be first detected by a blood test about 11 days after conception and in urine tests about 12 to 14 days after conception.

Labs & Diagnostics

Women who want to become pregnant can monitor their hormone levels at home with an OTC ovulation test that detects the changes in estrogen and in LH that trigger ovulation. The home test indicates the peak fertility days in a woman's menstrual cycle.

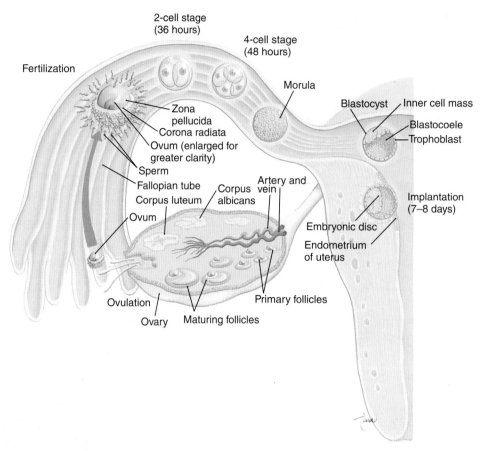

FIGURE 4.8 Ovulation, fertilization, and early embryonic development.

The zygote begins to divide immediately by mitosis. During mitosis, the cell replicates each of the chromosomes and then separates the chromosomes in the cell nucleus into two identical sets of chromosomes, each with a new nucleus that produces two complete cells. Then the zygote continues to grow from two cells to four cells to eight cells to 16 cells and to 32 cells to produce an **embryo**. An embryo is the stage of development between the fertilized ovum and the fetus. A **blastocyst** is a maturing embryo in which some cell differentiation has occurred. In the blastocyst stage, the embryo will implant 7 to 10 days after fertilization into the thickened, vascular uterine endometrium.

The placenta develops at the site of implantation. The placenta is an organ that provides the fetus with oxygen and nourishment from the maternal blood during intrauterine life, also known as the gestation period.

STAGES OF FETAL DEVELOPMENT

The embryo changes from a hollow ball of cells through two processes: morphogenesis and cell differentiation. During morphogenesis, the cells are moving and maturing to

complete a human form. Cell differentiation means that the cells specialize into different kinds of cells needed to build a human body, such as nerve cells, muscle cells, skin cells, and so on. The circulatory system for the fetus develops differently than normal human circulation because of the unique way that blood travels between the placenta and fetus during pregnancy.

Fetal Circulation

While in the uterus, the fetus does not need as much blood to circulate through the liver or lungs; the mother's body provides oxygenation and filtration as well as nutrition.

Oxygen from the mother's blood crosses the placenta, enters the fetus's blood, and passes through the umbilical vein. The oxygenated blood bypasses the liver through the **ductus venosus** and combines with deoxygenated blood in the inferior vena cava. Blood then rejoins deoxygenated blood from the superior vena cava and empties into the right atrium. Pressure is greater in the right atrium than the left atrium, so most blood will move through the **foramen ovale**. A small amount of blood does travel from the right atrium to the right ventricle into the pulmonary system, but most bypasses the pulmonary arteries and moves directly into the aorta through the **ductus arteriosus** and out to the rest of the body. Deoxygenated blood returns to the placenta through the umbilical arteries (Fig. 4.9).

· WORD · BUILDING ·

blastocyst: blasto–germ or sprout + cyst–bladder

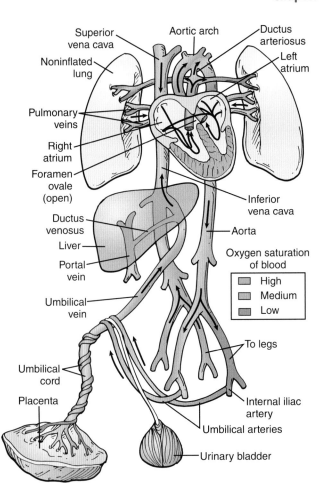

FIGURE 4.9 Fetal circulation.

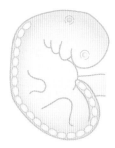

FIGURE 4.10 Embryo at 4 weeks' gestation (28 postovulatory days). All four limb buds are present. Source: Smith, B. (2013). *The multidimensional human embryo, Carnegie Stages.* http://embryo.soad.umich.edu/carnStages/carnStages.html

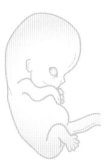

FIGURE 4.11 The embryo at 8 weeks (56 to 57 postovulatory days) has a human appearance. Source: Smith, B. (2013). *The multidimensional human embryo, Carnegie Stages.* http://embryo.soad.umich.edu/carnStages/carnStages.html

Significant events that occur during fetal development are noted next by trimester.

Learn to C.U.S.

You are working in the emergency department and providing care to Anna, a 16-year-old patient. Anna is being treated for pyelonephritis. The health-care provider has ordered trimethoprim/sulfamethoxazole 80 mg/400 mg every 12 hours. As you prepare to administer the first dose of the medication, the patient confides that she may be pregnant. Her menstrual period is approximately 2 weeks late. You call the health-care provider and uses the C.U.S. communication strategy.

C: "Hello, doctor. I am *concerned* about administering this medication to Anna.

U: I am *uncomfortable* about it because she has confided that she may be pregnant.

S: There may be a *safety* issue for the fetus. Can I have an order for a pregnancy test before administering the medication?"

First Trimester (Week 1–Week 12)

Even before a woman is aware that she is pregnant, the first trimester is a critical time of rapid changes to the fertilized cell and the development of major organs and structures. Morphogenesis and cell differentiation establish three germ layers in the embryo within 2 weeks after fertilization. These three layers are the foundation for the tissues and organs of the body (Figs. 4.10 and 4.11).

* *Ectoderm:* The cells of the ectoderm, or outer layer, become the nervous system, the epidermis of the skin, tooth enamel, and the lens and cornea of the eye.
* *Mesoderm:* The middle layer, the mesoderm, becomes the connective tissue, skeleton, skeletal muscles, the circulatory system, kidney cortex, and the dermis of the skin.
* *Endoderm:* The inner layer, the endoderm, becomes the digestive tract and accessory organs, the respiratory tract, the bladder, and endocrine glands.

Table 4.1 notes significant events that occur during the development of the embryo through the third month.

Second Trimester (Week 13–Week 28)

During the second trimester, the organs and structures continue to develop as a woman becomes more aware of her growing fetus. Table 4.2 notes significant events that occur during the development of the embryo in months 4 through 6.

Table 4.1

Fetal Growth and Development in the First Trimester

Gestational Age	Developmental Milestones
Week 3	• 2 mm length, crown to rump (C-R). • A fluid-filled membrane called the *amnion* surrounds the embryo. • The placenta begins to develop.
Week 4	• 4–6 mm length C-R, 0.4 g weight. • The heart beats and is pumping blood. • The limb buds are formed. • The placenta is developed and working.
Week 6	• 12 mm length C-R, 0.8 g weight. • The limb buds develop digits. • A skeleton of cartilage forms. • The liver is functioning.
Week 8	• 2.5–3 cm length C-R, 2 g weight. • All internal organs are produced. • Heart development is complete. • The embryo has a humanlike appearance.
Week 10	• 5–6 cm length C-R, 14 g weight. • Fingers and toes begin nail growth. • The eyelids are fused. • Fingerprints are apparent in the skin.
Month 3	• 8 cm length C-R, 45 g weight. • Large head. • Two distinct eyes. • The sex can be determined by examining the external organs. • Bone tissue is replacing cartilage.

Table 4.2

Fetal Growth and Development in the Second Trimester

Gestational Age	Developmental Milestones
Month 4	• 13.5 mm length crown to heel (C-H), 200 g weight. • The skeleton is established. • The appearance of scalp hair and lanugo (body hair) begins. • The skeletal muscles contract and produce body movement.
Month 5	• 19 cm length C-H, 435 g weight. • The internal organs continue to develop. • The fetus reacts to loud noises. • Brown fat and vernix begin to form. • The fetus actively sucks and swallows amniotic fluid.
Month 6	• 23 cm length C-H, 780 g weight. • Fused eyelids begin to open. • Hand grip and startle reflex have developed. • Respiratory movements occur. • Alveoli appear in lungs.

Table 4.3
Fetal Growth and Development in the Third Trimester

Gestational Age	Developmental Milestones
Month 7	• 27 cm length C-H, 1,200 g weight. • Internal organs are maturing. • Body fat increases. • The fetus uses the senses of vision and hearing. • Hiccups may occur.
Month 8	• 31–35 cm length C-H, 2,000–2,700 g weight. • Active periods are more noticeable by the mother. • A few sole creases form on the bottom of the feet. • Earlobes are soft, with little cartilage. • A layer of fat begins to be stored for insulation and nourishment.
Month 9	• 48–52 cm length C-H, 3,200+ g weight. • The fetus matures and becomes prepared for birth. • The fetus has smooth, pink skin with vernix present in skin folds. • Lanugo is present in small amounts on the fetus's shoulders and upper back. • The fetus's earlobes are firmer because of increased cartilage.

Source: Landon, M. B., Galan, H. L., Jauniaux, E. R., Driscoll, D. A., Berghella, V., Grobman, W. A., Gabbe, S. G., Niebyl, J. R., & Simpson, J. L. (2019). *Gabbe's obstetrics essentials.* Elsevier.

Third Trimester (Week 29–Week 40)

The third trimester is a time for the fetus to gain weight, mature, and prepare for life outside the uterus. Table 4.3 notes significant events that occur during the development of the embryo in months 7 through 9.

Patient Teaching Guidelines

Reducing the Risk of Birth Defects

- Avoid all medications, even OTC medications, unless directed by your health-care provider.
- Avoid alcohol, tobacco products, and street drugs.
- Notify any dentist or health-care provider that you are pregnant.
- Eat a variety of healthy foods from all food groups.
- Follow safe food-handling practices.
- Avoid exposure to environmental substances that can have a harmful effect on the fetus.
- Avoid cat feces and changing a cat litter box to decrease the risk of contracting toxoplasmosis.

ACCESSORY STRUCTURES OF PREGNANCY

The accessory structures of pregnancy include the placenta, the umbilical cord, placental membranes, and amniotic fluid.

Placenta

The **placenta** provides the fetus with oxygen and nourishment. It begins to grow when cells from the fetus, called *trophoblasts,* attach to the uterine wall and then grow deep into the tissues of the uterus. The cells of the placenta connect indirectly with the mother's blood vessels. At the same time, the fetal circulatory system is developing as the fetal blood vessels form in the placental villi. These vessels connect back to the fetus through the umbilical cord, which attaches the fetus to the placenta. As the placenta continues to grow, **villi**, fingerlike projections that are surrounded by the mother's blood, form. The mother's blood enters the space around the villi in the placenta through arteries that form out of the uterine arteries and flows around the villi. Gas, nutrient, and antibody exchange as well as waste removal take place across the villi walls. The walls also keep the fetus's blood from mixing with the mother's blood. The placenta, which is 15 to 20 cm in diameter and weighs approximately 1 pound, provides for all fetal oxygenation and nutritional needs while in the uterus (Fig. 4.12).

The placenta also functions as an endocrine organ because it produces hormones that support the pregnancy. The hormones produced include the following:

- *Progesterone*
  - Supports the endometrium to support the developing embryo
  - Calms and quiets the uterine muscle

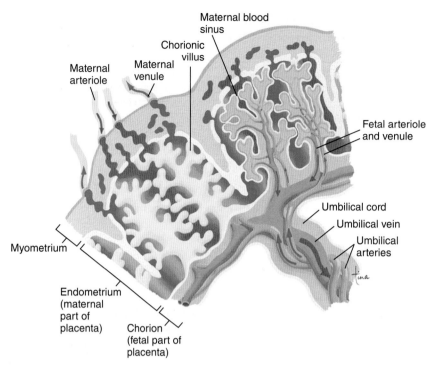

FIGURE 4.12 Placenta and umbilical cord.

- *Estrogen*
  - Stimulates growth of the myometrium and improves blood flow to the placenta and fetus
  - Stimulates breast development to prepare for breastfeeding
- *Human chorionic gonadotropin*
  - Stimulates the corpus luteum to produce estrogen and progesterone during the first 10 weeks after conception
  - Is used to determine pregnancy either by urine or blood test
  - Is used to help indicate if there is a viable pregnancy or if pregnancy loss has occurred based on levels
- *Human placental lactogen*
  - Assists with milk preparation
  - Increases the mother's metabolism during pregnancy
- *Relaxin*
  - Works with progesterone to maintain the pregnancy
  - Causes relaxation of pelvic ligaments to aid in birthing (acts as a source for hormone information)

After the delivery of the baby, the placenta is delivered. Often, the placenta is referred to as the *afterbirth.*

Umbilical Cord

The **umbilical cord**, which is formed by the fifth week of gestation, joins the fetus to the placenta. The umbilical cord is composed of two arteries and one vein. The vein carries oxygenated, nutrient-rich blood from the placenta to the fetus. The two arteries carry deoxygenated, nutrient-depleted blood from the fetus to the placenta. The vessels

are surrounded by Wharton jelly. **Wharton jelly** is a gelatinous substance that provides support and protection for the vessels inside the cord. The average umbilical cord at full-term is about 55 cm long and 1 to 2 cm in diameter (Stewart, 2022). After delivery of the placenta, the umbilical cord is clamped and cut. The site where the umbilical cord was attached to the fetus is commonly known as the *umbilicus, navel,* or *belly button.*

Placental Membranes and Amniotic Fluid

The chorionic membrane supports the embryo as it grows. The **chorion** is a thick membrane that develops from the trophoblast and becomes part of the placental villi. The chorionic villi can be used for genetic testing at 8 to 11 weeks' gestation. After 12 weeks, the chorion degenerates except for the portion that has become part of the placental villi.

The **amniotic membrane** is a thin membrane formed from the ectoderm layer. It contains the **amniotic fluid**, also known as the *bag of waters* (BOW), and the growing fetus. The functions of the amniotic fluid are as follows:

- Cushioning the fetus
- Providing buoyancy, which allows movement, symmetrical growth, and muscle development
- Preventing the amniotic membrane from adhering to the fetus
- Preventing compression of the umbilical cord
- Protecting the fetus from bacteria from the vagina
- Providing fluid for the analysis of fetal health and maturity

Nursing Care Plan for the Pregnant Patient

Kym, age 17, visits the community health clinic because of persistent nausea and vomiting of 1 week's duration. She reports having unprotected sex with her boyfriend, so the nurse runs a test to rule out pregnancy. The test is positive. Kym is surprised, but not unhappy, to be pregnant. She says that she wants to keep the baby, but she also admits that she knows almost nothing about pregnancy and fetal development.

Nursing Diagnosis: Insufficient knowledge of fetal development
Expected Outcome: The patient will verbalize general understanding of fetal development.

Interventions:	Rationale:
Provide a month-by-month guide to fetal development.	
Provide a website to explore fetal development photographs.	*The patient will have a reference for fetal development and know the important milestones in fetal development.*

Nursing Diagnosis: Insufficient knowledge of environmental teratogens
Expected Outcome: The patient will avoid environmental teratogens during her pregnancy.

Interventions:	Rationale:
Discuss potential teratogens and provide written material to review at home.	
Provide a website that includes information pertaining to teratogens.	*The patient will have an up-to-date reference for potential teratogens.*

Nursing Diagnosis: Anxiety because of concerns about possible birth defects
Expected Outcome: The patient will state that her anxiety is reduced because of her knowledge of healthy lifestyle choices that she will make during her pregnancy to reduce the risk of birth defects.

Interventions:	Rationale:
Encourage a healthy lifestyle with a nutritious diet and avoidance of possible teratogens.	*Lifestyle, nutrition, and teratogen education will promote a healthy pregnancy and fetus and therefore reduce anxiety.*
Allow the pregnant woman to verbalize her fears and provide appropriate reassurance.	*Talking about anxiety and fears reduces anxiety as the patient verbalizes her fears and receives appropriate reassurance.*

The average volume of amniotic fluid is 700 to 800 mL. Variations in the amount of fluid can indicate potential health problems of the fetus.

MULTIPLE PREGNANCY

A **multiple pregnancy** means that a woman has two or more embryos in her uterus. These embryos can come from the same egg or different eggs. Babies born from the same egg are termed *identical*, whereas babies born from two or more eggs are termed *fraternal*.

In the case of twins, **monozygotic twins** form when a single fertilized egg splits. The split occurs most often in the blastocyst stage, and each embryo will have its own amniotic sac but will share a placenta. Both embryos implant in the uterus, and they are always the same sex.

When two eggs are fertilized by two separate sperm, **dizygotic twins** result. Each zygote develops separately and implants into the uterus. Each embryo will have its own amniotic sac and placenta. There will be genetic similarities because the twins are siblings, but they will not have the exact same genetic material (Fig. 4.13).

A woman is more likely to have a multiple pregnancy if she falls in any of the following categories:

- Older than age 35
- Black
- Family history of twins
- Undergone fertility treatment to become pregnant
- Given birth to multiples previously

· WORD · BUILDING ·
monozygotic: mono–one + zygot–yoked + ic–pertaining to

· WORD · BUILDING ·
dizygotic: di–two + zygot–yoked + ic–pertaining to

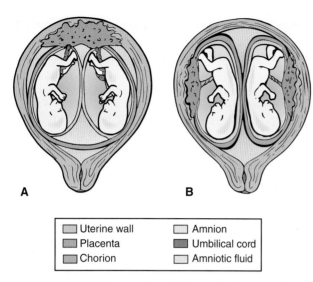

▢ Uterine wall	▢ Amnion
▢ Placenta	▢ Umbilical cord
▢ Chorion	▢ Amniotic fluid

FIGURE 4.13 Multiple gestations. A, Monozygotic twins with one placenta, one chorion, and two amnions. B, Dizygotic twins with two placentas, two chorions, and two amnions.

EFFECTS OF TERATOGENS ON FETAL DEVELOPMENT

Many substances can present a risk for the developing fetus, so the safest approach regarding medications in pregnancy is to use as little as possible. A **teratogen** is any substance that may cause a birth defect. Most substances have the ability to cross the placenta from the mother to the fetus and possibly cause abnormalities. The fetal susceptibility depends on the period of development. For example, the brain and

Safety *Stat!*

The fetus is very vulnerable to the effects of medications during the first trimester. Before administering any medication to a woman of child-bearing age, you should verify that the date of her last menstrual period is in the woman's health record. If you have any concern that the patient may be pregnant, you should report the concern to the charge nurse or health-care provider.

Medication Facts

If a woman currently taking medication for depression, asthma, diabetes, seizures, HIV, or other health problems becomes pregnant, she should talk to her health-care provider right away. Abruptly stopping such medications may be more harmful for her than her fetus. She needs to discuss the benefits and risks of the medications during pregnancy with her health-care provider.

· WORD · BUILDING ·

teratogen: terato–monster + gen–that which produces

skeleton are at risk for damage by teratogens from the third week of gestation to the end of the pregnancy. The heart is most susceptible to injury during the third and fourth weeks of gestation. The genitalia are more sensitive to injury during the eighth and ninth weeks (Maudlin, 2022).

Medications

The Food and Drug Administration (FDA) has discontinued the Pregnancy Category System for medication use in pregnancy. The FDA does not believe that the A, B, C, D, and X categorization appropriately addresses the risk that a medication may have during pregnancy and lactation. Pregnancy categories are being removed from medication prescribing information and replaced with a summary that describes the potential risks of using the medication during pregnancy and lactation. Information is also included for women and men of the need for contraceptives, pregnancy testing, and infertility related to use of the medication (Vallerand & Sanoski, 2023).

Safety *Stat!*

A pregnant woman should be cautioned that OTC medications may not be safe in pregnancy. She should always check with her health-care provider before taking any medications, even OTC ones.

Tobacco

Smoking is one of the most important modifiable causes of poor pregnancy outcomes (CDC, 2020). Inhaling e-cigarettes, also known as vaping, is not considered safe in pregnancy because many e-cigarettes contain nicotine, which affects the fetus in the same way as smoking tobacco does (CDC, 2020). Smoking or vaping causes vasoconstriction, which leads to a smaller placenta. A smaller placenta decreases the nourishment and oxygenation that the fetus receives. This can lead to a small baby with delayed development. The adverse effects of smoking in pregnancy and excessive exposure to secondhand smoke are as follows:

• Low birth weight
• Premature rupture of membranes
• Placenta previa
• Placenta abruption
• Preterm labor
• Ectopic pregnancy
• Increased risk of cleft lip or palate in the fetus

The American College of Obstetricians and Gynecologists (ACOG, 2020b) suggests that nurses use the Five *As* Model to address smoking in pregnancy:

1. Ask about tobacco use.
2. Advise the woman to quit.
3. Assess willingness to make an attempt to quit.
4. Assist in a quit attempt.
5. Arrange for follow-up.

Smoking interventions may provide a tool to assist the pregnant woman to stop smoking and promote a healthy pregnancy and fetus.

Safety *Stat!*

A pregnant woman who does not smoke but breathes secondhand smoke is more likely to have lower birth-weight babies than women who are not exposed to secondhand smoke. After birth, babies who are around secondhand smoke have more ear infections, asthma, and respiratory infections and are more likely to die from sudden infant death syndrome (SIDS; CDC, 2020).

Alcohol

ACOG (2023) recommends that the pregnant woman should avoid alcohol throughout the pregnancy to prevent lifelong problems for the child. Children born with fetal alcohol spectrum disorders (FASDs) may exhibit the following symptoms:

- Small for gestational age at birth
- Vision and hearing problems
- Facial abnormalities, such as a small head, flat face, and narrow eye openings
- Trouble with concentration and learning in school
- Trouble controlling behavior

Caffeine

High usage of caffeine during pregnancy has been linked with miscarriage and preterm birth. However, the ACOG (2020a) states that light and moderate use of caffeine (less than 200 mg per day) are not likely to cause miscarriage or preterm birth.

Marijuana

Marijuana is the substance most widely used by pregnant women. Marijuana usage in early pregnancy alters the trophoblast cells as they are implanting into the uterine wall, which affects placental development and implantation. Therefore, the placenta may not nourish the fetus effectively, leading to increased risk for low birth weight, smaller head circumference, and preterm labor. Research has also shown that intrauterine exposure to tetrahydrocannabinol (THC), the chemical responsible for most of marijuana's psychological effects, can affect the neurological development of the newborn in ways that will be evident as the child grows and develops (Splete, 2022).

Cocaine

Cocaine use has been studied for many years with the conclusions that use during pregnancy leads to growth retardation and microencephaly. *Microencephaly* is the term for a small brain and head. Depending upon when cocaine use occurs during pregnancy, the fetus's genitals, kidneys, or brain may have

abnormalities. Cocaine use during pregnancy has been associated with increased risk of placental abruption and neurobehavioral abnormalities that are exhibited after birth (Villa, 2022).

Opioids

Untreated opioid addiction can interfere with the function of the placenta and expose the fetus to periods of withdrawal (CDC, 2021). Opioids cross the placenta and can lead to neonatal addiction and withdrawal symptoms after birth. Opioid addiction during pregnancy is often associated with a lack of prenatal care and can lead to adverse outcomes including:

- Increased risk of premature birth
- Low birth weight
- Hypoglycemia
- Intracranial hemorrhage in the uterus
- Neonatal abstinence syndrome (NAS; see Chapter 17)

Methamphetamines

Any use of methamphetamines during pregnancy is of concern. Research is limited, but methamphetamine use in pregnancy has been associated with elevation in the heart rate of the mother and fetus, increased risk of preterm labor, and increased risk of placental abruption (Wang, 2020).

Therapeutic Communication

Nurses play an important role in providing support and education during pregnancy. Authenticity and truthfulness are essential for developing a therapeutic relationship with a pregnant woman and her partner. Nurses need to be open and honest with women and their partners as they discuss sensitive lifestyle issues, such as tobacco, drug, and alcohol use, which could cause birth defects. Techniques that encourage communication include using nonjudgmental open-ended questions, conveying acceptance, and focusing on patient concerns.

Evidence-Based Practice

A study investigated the association between the COVID-19 pandemic and congenital birth anomalies. A population of infants born before the pandemic was compared with a similar group born during the COVID-19 pandemic. In the COVID-19 group, the authors found statistical evidence of an increase in central nervous system and genitourinary anomalies. The authors concluded that there were several factors that could have contributed to the increase in congenital anomalies including viral infection, maternal fever during the first trimester, chronic maternal stress, decrease in quality and quantity of prenatal care, and poverty created by the pandemic.

Heidarzadeh, M., Taheri, M., Mazaheri, Z., & Abbasi-Khameneh, F. (2022). The incidence of congenital anomalies in newborns before and during the COVID-19 pandemic. *Italian Journal of Pediatrics, 48,* 174. https://doi.org/10.1186/s13052-022-01368-6

· WORD · BUILDING ·

microencephaly: micro–small + encephaly–brain

Environmental Toxins

Exposure to substances in the home or outdoor environment can have harmful effects on pregnancy. The pregnant woman will want to be aware of the following potential hazards:

- To prevent exposure to chemicals, cleaning products, or heavy metals, follow safety guidelines at work.
- Avoid exposure to lead. It is toxic to the brain and nervous system of the fetus. Lead is found in some toys, costume jewelry, pottery, and folk remedies.
- Avoid exposure to mercury by not consuming fish that contain high levels of mercury. Mercury affects brain development in the fetus. Fish that contain high levels of mercury are marlin, sea bass, orange roughy, swordfish, and tuna.
- Avoid foods that may harbor listeria, a type of bacteria found in water and soil. Listeria has been found in uncooked meats, uncooked vegetables, unpasteurized milk, and food made from unpasteurized milk. Deli meats have the potential to be contaminated with listeria after cooking and before packaging.
- Avoid exposure to paint. It is a mix of chemicals that can lead to birth defects and developmental disabilities.
- Avoid exposure to pesticides used to control weeds, insects, and cockroaches (Organization of Teratology Information Specialists [OTIS], 2021).
- To reduce the risk of potential problems for the developing fetus, the pregnant woman should look for bisphenol A (BPA)-free plastic products. According to the *National Report on Human Exposure to Environmental Chemicals* (2024) by the CDC, the BPA in plastic bottles was shown to have hormonelike effects on the developing reproductive system and to cause neurobehavioral changes in the offspring in animal testing.
- Avoid hot tubs and saunas. Maternal hyperthermia has been linked to possible central nervous system defects in the fetus (Millard, 2022).
- Avoid infections known as the TORCH infections. The acronym TORCH stands for toxoplasmosis, other organisms (parvovirus, HIV, Epstein-Barr virus, herpes, varicella, syphilis, West Nile, Zika), rubella, cytomegalovirus (CMV), and hepatitis. See Chapter 7.

Team Works

Some women become pregnant while they are struggling with alcohol or drug addiction. Women who have these problems and want to deliver a healthy baby will require a team approach to assist them with living drug- and alcohol-free lives during the pregnancy. The team approach to assisting these women includes nurses, obstetricians or midwives, mental health workers, social workers, self-help groups such as Alcoholics Anonymous (AA) and Narcotics Anonymous (NA), and the patient's family or significant other.

Key Points

- The female external reproductive organs include the mons pubis, the labia minora, the labia majora, the clitoris, the vestibule of the vagina, and the Bartholin glands.
- The female internal organs of reproduction are the ovaries, the fallopian tubes, the uterus, and the vagina.
- The female pelvis is shorter, wider, and more circular than a male pelvis, which makes it the right shape for childbearing.
- The menstrual cycle, which occurs because of the influence of the hormones estrogen and progesterone, prepares the uterus for a fertilized egg to implant. If fertilization does not occur, menses begin.
- The male reproductive system is composed of the scrotum, penis, and testicles.
- Testosterone promotes the development of male reproductive organs and secondary male characteristics.
- Fertilization takes place in the outer third portion of the fallopian tube, leading to the formation of a zygote that begins dividing and traveling down the fallopian tube to implant in the uterus.
- There are three embryonic layers of cells that differentiate. The ectoderm layer becomes the central nervous system, skin, and glands. The mesoderm layer becomes the musculoskeletal, urinary, reproductive, and circulatory systems. The endoderm layer develops into the respiratory system, liver, digestive system, and pancreas.
- The placenta provides oxygen and nutrition and removes waste products for the fetus. It also produces hormones: progesterone, estrogen, hCG, human placental lactogen, and relaxin, all of which support the pregnancy.
- The amniotic fluid surrounds the fetus to provide buoyancy and protection. The fluid allows for fetal movement and can be studied to monitor fetal health.
- Fetal circulation transports blood to the heart and brain and shunts it away from the lungs and liver. The mother's body carries out the functions of the fetus's lungs and liver.
- The first trimester is the most critical time for organ development in the fetus when the cells are differentiating and forming the foundation for the tissues and organs of the body.
- Pregnant women should avoid medications unless directed by their health-care provider.
- Teratogenic substances such as lead, mercury, pesticides, bacteria, and street drugs can adversely affect the growth and development of the fetus.

Review Questions

1. Which hormones do the ovaries secrete during the menstrual cycle? **(Select all that apply.)**
   1. Estrogen
   2. Testosterone
   3. Thyroxine
   4. Progesterone
   5. Oxytocin
   6. FSH

2. In which structure does fertilization usually occur?
   1. Uterus
   2. Vagina
   3. Fallopian tube
   4. Ovary

3. After an ovum is fertilized, where does it usually implant?
   1. Endometrium of the uterus
   2. Upper portion of the fallopian tube
   3. Inside the cervix
   4. Near the ovary

4. The hormone first detected by a blood test about 11 days after conception and in urine tests about 12 to 14 days after conception is:
   1. Estrogen
   2. hCG
   3. Progesterone
   4. Placental lactogen

5. Which structure produces the major male hormone of reproduction, testosterone?
   1. Pituitary
   2. Thyroid
   3. Adrenal glands
   4. Testicles

6. Which of the following are functions of the placenta? **(Select all that apply.)**
   1. Supply oxygen to the fetus
   2. Supply nourishment to the fetus
   3. Produce hormones
   4. Provide protection from infection
   5. Provide cushioning protection for the fetus

7. _____ is the substance that provides support and protection for the vessels inside the umbilical cord.

8. Which of the following adverse outcomes are associated with opioid use during pregnancy? **(Select all that apply.)**
   1. Neonatal withdrawal
   2. Increased risk of premature birth
   3. Low birth weight
   4. Hypoglycemia
   5. Increased risk of placental abruption

9. Twins who share the same placenta in the uterus are called _____ twins.

ANSWERS 1. 1, 4, 6; 2. 3; 3. 1; 4. 2; 5. 4; 6. 1, 2, 3, 4; 7. Wharton jelly; 8. 1, 2, 3, 4; 9. Monozygotic

CRITICAL THINKING QUESTIONS

1. At birth, you notice that the umbilical cord has one vein and one artery. Which body system of the fetus is at risk for a congenital anomaly?

2. Is it safe for a pregnant patient to use a nicotine patch to stop smoking?

3. If the pregnant patient has a low level of amniotic fluid, what problems could occur for the fetus?

Resources

For additional resources and information, including Postconference Questions and Activities, Answers, and References, visit www.FADavis.com.

 Student Study Guide

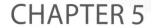

CHAPTER 5
Physical and Psychological Changes of Pregnancy

KEY TERMS

anemia (an-NEE-mee-uh)
ballottement (bal-ot-MAWN)
Chadwick sign (TSHAD-wik SINE)
Couvade syndrome (koo-VAHD SIN-drohm)
dysuria (dis-YOO-ree-uh)
Goodell sign (GUD-uhl SINE)
Hegar sign (HAY-gar SINE)
hemorrhoids (HEM-uh-roydz)
Kegel exercise (KAY-guhl EK-ser-size)
linea nigra (LIN-ee-uh NYE-gruh)
melasma (meh-LAZ-muh)
pruritic urticarial papules and plaque of pregnancy (PUPPP) (proo-RIT-ik er-tih-KAIR-ee-uhl PAP-yoolz and PLAK uv PREG-nuhn-see)
quickening (KWIK-uh-ning)
striae gravidarum (STRY-ee gra-vih-DA-ruhm)
varicose veins (VA-rih-kohz VAYNZ)
vena caval syndrome (VEE-nuh KA-vuhl SIN-drohm)

CHAPTER CONCEPTS

Health Promotion
Reproduction and Sexuality
Self

LEARNING OUTCOMES

1. Define the key terms.
2. Differentiate presumptive, probable, and positive signs of pregnancy.
3. Describe the physiological changes in each body system occurring during pregnancy.
4. Plan safe and effective nursing interventions that address the common physiological discomforts of pregnancy.
5. Identify physiological discomfort symptoms that should be reported to the health-care provider.
6. Identify normal laboratory values for the pregnant woman.
7. Discuss Reva Rubin's four maternal tasks that the woman accomplishes during pregnancy.
8. Discuss the psychosocial changes occurring during pregnancy for the woman, her partner, and her family.
9. Identify psychosocial issues of the pregnant adolescent.

CRITICAL THINKING & CLINICAL JUDGMENT

Scenario #1: **Lisa**, aged 23, is pregnant with her first baby and is 32 weeks' gestation. She has had an uncomplicated pregnancy and is eagerly awaiting her due date. Today she is at the office of her health-care provider for her routine prenatal checkup. She reports that she is experiencing heartburn almost every day and especially when she lays down at night to go to bed. She asks you, "Can I take antacids that I bought at the store?"

Questions

1. What physiological change of pregnancy is causing the heartburn?
2. What would you suggest the patient do to safely manage the heartburn?

CONCEPTUAL CORNERSTONE

Health Promotion

Some pregnant women are curious about pregnancy changes. They read pregnancy literature, surf the internet, and attend classes. Other pregnant women rely on the advice of family, friends, and health-care providers for pregnancy concerns. Nurses encounter a variety of patients who have diverse learning needs. Patient-centered teaching involves assessing the educational needs of the patient and then planning personalized teaching appropriate for that patient. It is important to keep in mind some principles of adult learning. Adults learn best when the learning is related to an immediate need and is person-centered and problem-centered (Bloomberg, 2022). Education empowers the pregnant patient to make changes in her life to improve her health and to promote a safe pregnancy and healthy fetal outcome.

Pregnancy is a state that causes considerable physical and psychological changes in the woman. In addition to the obvious changes in the reproductive system, virtually every body system is affected, and changes occur to adapt to the pregnancy and the growing fetus. Even before the woman suspects she is pregnant, changes are occurring.

DIAGNOSIS OF PREGNANCY

Every woman is different and pregnancy symptoms can vary from one woman to the next and from pregnancy to pregnancy in the same woman. The signs and symptoms of pregnancy are generally grouped into three categories: presumptive, probable, and positive.

Presumptive Signs of Pregnancy

Presumptive signs of pregnancy are the subjective signs that a woman notices occurring in her body. These signs are the least reliable because they can sometimes be caused by health conditions not related to pregnancy. Many of the early signs are caused by the rapid rise in hormone levels that begins at implantation of the trophoblast. The first sign many women notice is amenorrhea, the absence of a menstrual period. Usually within 2 weeks after missing a period, the woman will begin to experience some of these other presumptive signs:

- Nausea and vomiting
- Fatigue
- Urinary frequency
- Breast enlargement and tenderness

Most women notice fetal movement by 20 weeks. With a first pregnancy it may be between 18 and 21 weeks; in subsequent pregnancies, the mother may feel **quickening**, or fetal movement as early as 15 to 17 weeks (Rigby, 2020).

Probable Signs of Pregnancy

Probable signs of pregnancy are objective signs that indicate the woman is likely to be pregnant. These signs can be detected by a health-care provider during a physical examination or can be evaluated by a laboratory test or an in-home pregnancy test.

- *Goodell sign:* softening of the cervix
- *Chadwick sign:* a bluish-purple coloration of the vaginal mucosa and cervix
- *Hegar sign:* softening of the lower uterine segment
- *Ballottement:* a technique in which the health-care provider pushes against the woman's cervix and then can feel the fetus floating away from the cervix
- *Positive pregnancy test:* a test in which human chorionic gonadotropin (hCG) is detectable in more than 98% of patients by day 11 of gestation (Shields, 2022)

Positive Signs of Pregnancy

Positive signs of pregnancy can be attributed only to the presence of a fetus. An experienced health-care provider can confirm that a fetus is growing inside the uterus.

- Fetal heart auscultation by Doppler
- Fetal movement felt by an experienced practitioner
- Ultrasound: a means of testing used to verify an embryo or a fetus

After a pregnancy has been confirmed, the health-care provider will arrange a schedule of visits with the pregnant woman to provide prenatal care to ensure the health of the mother and baby and to prepare for the upcoming birth.

NORMAL PHYSIOLOGICAL CHANGES IN PREGNANCY

Maternal physiology undergoes many changes throughout gestation. Most changes occur as the result of the effects of progesterone and estrogen and the increasing demands of the growing fetus. You can provide teaching and anticipatory guidance to the pregnant patient and her family on how to manage the physiological changes of pregnancy.

The normal physiological changes in pregnancy are presented in seven body-system tables. Each table notes the types of changes experienced by patient observations and the nursing implications for care.

Reproductive System Changes

The types of reproductive system changes in pregnancy, what the patient observes, and the related nursing care implications are found in Table 5.1. See also Figure 5.1.

Table 5.1

Reproductive System Changes in Pregnancy

Types of Changes	Patient Observations	Nursing Implications
Uterus: • Length from 6.5–32 cm • Width from 2.5–24 cm • Depth from 2.5–22 cm • Weight from 50–1,000 g • Wall thickness from 1–0.5 cm	• The uterus expands to accommodate the fetus, placenta, umbilical cord, 50–100 mL of amniotic fluid, and fetal membranes.	• Growth occurs at a predictable pace. • At 12 weeks' gestation, the uterus can be palpated above the symphysis pubis. • At 20 weeks' gestation it is located at the umbilicus (Fig. 5.1).
Cervix: • Estrogen causes the cervix to become congested with blood, causing a bluish purple color to the cervix, vagina, and labia (*Chadwick sign*). • Softening occurs of the lower uterine segment (*Hegar sign*). • Estrogen and progesterone cause cervical softening by decreasing collagen fibers, increasing vascularity, and causing edema (*Goodell sign*). The soft cervix is preparing for dilation during labor and childbirth. • Cervical mucus forms a plug in the cervical canal. The closed cervix with the mucous plug prevents bacteria from entering the uterus.	• "Bloody show" may be evident during early labor as the congested cervix starts to dilate and the mucous plug is released.	• Loss of the mucous plug and "bloody show" are early signs of labor.
Vagina and Vulva: • Increased vascularity causes the vagina and vulva to appear bluish. • Vaginal mucosa thickens, and the vaginal folds become more noticeable. A softening of the collagen fibers occurs because of hormonal influences. • Increased levels of glycogen are present in vaginal cells. An acidic vaginal environment develops because of the effect of *Lactobacillus acidophilus* on glycogen in the vaginal cells. • Softening of the connective tissue allows the vagina to distend during childbirth. This causes rapid sloughing of cells and an increase in vaginal discharge. • The acidic environment prevents growth of bacteria normally found in the vagina. • The glycogen-rich environment favors the growth of *Candida albicans*.	• Increased vaginal discharge is noted by the patient. • Increased vascular congestion of the vulva and decreased venous blood return from the lower extremities will cause edema of the vulva. • Yeast infections are common in pregnant women.	• Reassure the patient that the increased vaginal discharge is normal and may increase as the due date approaches. • Discuss vulvar hygiene through gentle external cleansing with nonscented soap and water. • Teach the patient to avoid douching and to wear breathable underwear, such as cotton. • Instruct the patient to avoid petroleum-based lubricants during sex. • Teach the patient the signs and symptoms of vaginal yeast infection, such as increased vaginal discharge that is white and thick (similar to cottage cheese) and vaginal itching. These symptoms should be reported to the health-care provider.
Ovaries: • After ovulation, luteinizing hormone stimulates the corpus luteum, which produces progesterone for 6–7 weeks. The corpus luteum continues to increase in size during this period, and sometimes the cyst can rupture.	• The corpus luteum may rupture and cause pain and vaginal bleeding in some women.	• Advise the woman to contact her health-care provider if pain or bleeding occurs.

Table 5.1
Reproductive System Changes in Pregnancy—cont'd

Types of Changes	*Patient Observations*	*Nursing Implications*
Breasts: • There is increased blood volume in the breast tissue. Estrogen and progesterone cause breast enlargement, tingling, and increased sensitivity. During the second trimester, colostrum develops from the acini cells in the milk glands.	• Breasts feel engorged with a feeling of heat and tingling. • Breasts become tender and enlarge. Colostrum may leak from the nipples.	• Reassure the woman that leaking colostrum is a normal process of the breasts preparing for lactation. • To promote comfort, advise the woman to wear a supportive bra.
Sexual Activity: • During pregnancy, there is an increase in vaginal lubrication and an increase in blood flow to the genital area.	• Many pregnant women feel that during the first trimester the libido decreases because of nausea, fatigue, sore breasts, and anxieties about miscarriage. • During the second trimester, women generally feel more energetic and have an increase in libido. • By the third trimester, physical discomfort can make traditional sexual acts more difficult and less frequent. Fatigue is a major predictor to sexual frequency during pregnancy.	• Reassure the woman and her partner that sexual intercourse will not harm the fetus. • Sexual needs can be met in a variety of ways. Positions such as side by side, woman on top, and hands and knees can be used during pregnancy. • The literature does not support an association between sexual intercourse and increased risk of preterm labor and delivery (Goodfellow et al., 2021).

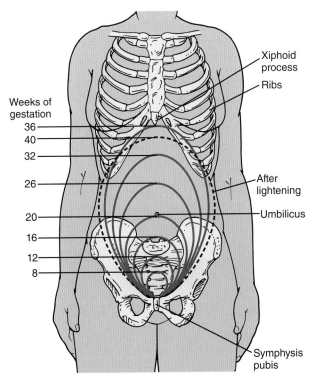

Weeks of gestation
36
40
32
26
20
16
12
8

Xiphoid process
Ribs
After lightening
Umbilicus
Symphysis pubis

FIGURE 5.1 Pattern of uterine growth during pregnancy.

Patient Teaching Guidelines

Kegel Exercises
Kegel exercises will help the patient to strengthen her perineal muscles.
Instructions:
• With an empty bladder, contract the muscles of the perineum and vagina and hold for 10 seconds.
• Relax for 20 seconds.
• Repeat the routine.
• The number of repetitions should be increased gradually to between 50 and 150 per day.

Respiratory System Changes

The types of respiratory system changes in pregnancy, what the patient observes, and the related nursing care implications are found in Table 5.2.

Cardiovascular System Changes

The types of cardiovascular system changes in pregnancy, what the patient observes, and the related nursing care implications are found in Table 5.3. See also Figure 5.2.

Table 5.2

Respiratory System Changes in Pregnancy

Types of Changes	Patient Observations	Nursing Implications
• The respiratory rate increases to 18–20 respirations per minute (RPM). • Oxygen consumption increases by 20%, and the tidal volume (amount of air breathed in each minute) increases. This provides for the extra oxygen demands of the uterus, placenta, and fetus.	• Pregnant women may feel short of breath easily when lying down and with mild exertion.	• To reduce the feeling of shortness of breath, encourage the woman to elevate her head on an extra pillow at night and to walk up stairs more slowly.
• Estrogen causes hypertrophy and increased vascularity of nasal and lung tissue, whereas progesterone causes relaxation of the smooth muscle of the bronchi, bronchioles, and alveoli. These hormonal changes cause an increase in oxygen consumption. The effects of the hormones also cause increased mucus production (Medcrine, 2020).	• A pregnant woman breathes faster and more deeply. The increased vascularity causes a feeling of nasal and lung congestion (Rigby, 2020). • Rhinitis and nosebleeds can occur.	• The pregnant woman needs education regarding these normal changes and reassurance. • The woman should use gentle nose-blowing, use a cool mist humidifier, drink fluids, and avoid overuse of nasal spray decongestants because of the rebound effect of prolonged use. • If frequent nosebleeds occur, she should notify her health-care provider.
• The enlarging uterus causes upward pressure and elevation of the diaphragm. • Cartilage and muscles relax and the chest broadens to allow room for the enlarging uterus.	• Chest circumference may increase by as much as 6 cm.	• Educate the pregnant woman of this normal physiological change of pregnancy.

Table 5.3

Cardiovascular System Changes in Pregnancy

Types of Changes	Patient Observations	Nursing Implications
General Cardiovascular System Changes: • An increase in circulatory blood volume begins by week 6 and will reach 50% more than the prepregnancy volume. • 500 mL of blood is needed to provide for increased oxygen consumption of the growing fetus, the enlarging uterus, and the breasts. • Increased blood volume helps balance blood loss at delivery (Pascual & Langaker, 2022). • Heart rate increases 10–20 beats/minute greater than prepregnancy levels. • Increased blood volume causes veins to enlarge. • Increase in blood volume correlates with the increase in fetal weight.	• Pregnant women have warm hands and feet. • Nasal blood flow is increased, causing nasal congestion. • The weight of the uterus obstructs blood return from the veins in the legs. This may result in varicose veins of the legs, vulva, and rectum (hemorrhoids). • **Varicose veins** are swollen veins raised above the surface of the skin. They may be twisted or bulging and are dark purple or blue in color. They are located most often on the backs of the calves or on the inside of the leg.	• On assessment, slight cardiac hypertrophy may be identified as well as an asymptomatic systolic murmur. • Inform the pregnant woman that she should avoid the supine position. Lying on her back can cause feelings of lightheadedness and cause her blood pressure to drop. This is called supine hypotension or **vena caval syndrome**. Side-lying provides for better brain and placental profusion (Fig. 5.2).

Table 5.3
Cardiovascular System Changes in Pregnancy—cont'd

Types of Changes	*Patient Observations*	*Nursing Implications*
• 30% more blood circulates through the kidneys to remove waste from the mother and fetus. • Cardiac output increases up to 50% during the first half of pregnancy. • Blood pressure remains stable even though there is an increase in blood volume. There may be a slight decrease in systolic pressure and increase in diastolic pressure.	• When the pregnant woman is supine, the weight of the uterus may cause hypotension when the uterus partially occludes the vena cava and aorta.	
Blood Components: • Red blood cell mass increases by 40%. This provides increased oxygen-carrying capacity to the mother and growing fetus. • More red blood cells also give the mother some protection from hemorrhage in childbirth. • Hemodilution occurs because of increased volume causing physiological anemia of pregnancy. **Anemia** is a reduction of red blood cells. • Leukocytes increase during pregnancy, ranging from 5,000–15,000 mcL. The cause is unknown but may be because of the physical stress of pregnancy and hormonal changes. • Fibrinogen levels rise by 50%. • Increased risk for thrombophlebitis and thrombus formation (Pascual & Langaker, 2022).	• The anemic pregnant woman may experience fatigue, hair loss, or pica. • *Pica* is an abnormal craving for a nonfood substance, such as ice, dirt, paint, or clay. • If a venous thrombus occurs, the woman may notice erythema (hot or warm skin), pain on the leg, and swelling of the surrounding area of the calf.	• An iron supplement is usually prescribed to pregnant women by the second trimester to prevent anemia. • The woman should be instructed to include iron-rich foods in her diet, such as red meat, spinach, kale, broccoli, and raisins. • It may be difficult to determine whether infection is occurring during the pregnancy. Any possible signs of infection should be reported to the health-care provider. • Inform the woman that if she develops signs of a venous thrombus, such as warmth, redness, or swelling of her calf, she should notify her health-care provider. • Instruct the pregnant woman to avoid standing or sitting for prolonged periods to prevent venous stasis.

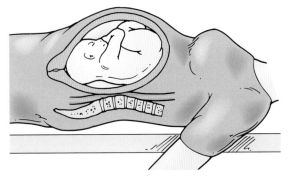

FIGURE 5.2 Supine hypotension, or vena caval syndrome, may occur if the pregnant woman lies on her back. The weight of the uterus causes compression of the vena cava.

· WORD · BUILDING ·
anemia: an–without + em–blood + ia–condition

CRITICAL THINKING & CLINICAL JUDGMENT

Scenario #2: **Della** is waiting for the nurse midwife to come into the room for her 36-week appointment. She is lying on her back on the examination table and begins to feel lightheaded, a little nauseous, and reports a rapid heart rate to you.

1. Why is Della experiencing these symptoms?
2. What should you do before asking the nurse midwife to hurry into the room?

Gastrointestinal System Changes

The types of gastrointestinal (GI) system changes in pregnancy, what the patient observes, and the related nursing care implications are found in Table 5.4.

Table 5.4

Gastrointestinal System Changes in Pregnancy

Types of Changes	Patient Observations	Nursing Implications
• Advancing maternal age; high levels of hCG, estrogen, and prostaglandin; reduced tone of the GI system; and reduced stomach acidity are all thought to contribute to nausea and vomiting, also known as morning sickness (Smith et al., 2021).	• Usually occurs between 6 and 12 weeks' gestation. • Nausea may occur in the mornings or may occur because of strong aromas.	Instruct the patient to: • Eat several small meals instead of three large meals to keep her stomach from being empty. • Eat dry toast, saltines, or dry cereals before getting out of bed in the morning. • Sip on water, weak tea, or clear soft drinks. • Avoid smells that upset her stomach.
• Progesterone causes smooth muscle relaxation, which affects the esophageal sphincter and allows gastric contents to reflux into the esophagus, causing heartburn.	• The woman may experience heartburn or epigastric discomfort after eating a large meal or if she lies down right after eating.	• If experiencing heartburn, eat bland foods that are low in fat and easy to digest, such as cereal, rice, and bananas. • Avoid lying down after a meal. • Avoid overeating. • Eating smaller frequent meals may eliminate heartburn.
• The increased levels of hormones slow down digestion and relax the smooth muscles in the intestines, causing constipation for many women. • In addition, the pressure of the expanding uterus on the intestinal tract can contribute to constipation.	• Signs of constipation include having hard, dry stools; less than three bowel movements per week; and painful bowel movements.	Educate the patient to: • Drink 8–10 glasses of water daily. • Eat fiber-rich foods, such as fresh or dried fruit, raw vegetables, and whole-grain cereals. • Increase mild physical activity, such as walking. • Avoid straining for a bowel movement. • Notify health-care provider if constipation is severe.
• The gallbladder becomes hypotonic because of the effects of progesterone on smooth muscle. • This causes a delay in emptying, which can predispose the patient to the development of gallstones.	• The woman may develop upper right quadrant pain after a fatty meal.	• Instruct the woman to notify her health-care provider of any abdominal pain.
• Up to 50% of pregnant women get hemorrhoids (Rigby, 2020). • Hemorrhoids are common for many reasons. The increase in blood volume causes veins to enlarge. • The expanding uterus also puts pressure on the veins in the rectum. • Constipation can worsen hemorrhoids if the woman strains to have a bowel movement.	• **Hemorrhoids** are swollen and bulging veins in the rectum. They can cause itching, pain, and bleeding.	• Educate the woman to notify her health-care provider if the hemorrhoids are painful and/or bleeding. • Increase fiber and fluid intake to avoid straining for a bowel movement. • Reassure the woman that hemorrhoids usually improve after delivery.

• **WORD • BUILDING** •

hemorrhoid: hemo–blood + rrhoid–flow

Labs & Diagnostics
Common Laboratory Blood Values

Common Laboratory Blood Values	Nonpregnant Woman	Pregnant Woman
Hemoglobin (HGB)	11.7–15.5 g/dL	11.5–13 g/dL
Hematocrit (HCT)	33%–45%	31.5%–41%
Red blood cells (RBCs)	3.91–5.11 cells/mcL	No change
White blood cells (WBCs)	4.5–11.1	5.9–14
Serum creatinine	0.51–1.1 mg/dL	0.49–0.9 mg/dL
Serum blood urea nitrogen (BUN)	8–21 mg/dL	8–10 mg/dL
Serum uric acid	2.5–7 mg/dL	2–5.8 mg/dL
Urine creatinine clearance	75–115 mL/min	150–200 mL/min
Urine uric acid	250–750 mg/24 hr	Increases
Serum glucose	<100 mg/dL	Gradual decrease of 10%
Alanine transaminase (ALT)	7–35 units/L	Unchanged
Aspartate aminotransferase (AST)	15–30 units/L	Unchanged
Alkaline phosphatase (ALP)	25–125 units/L	Up to two to four times because of placental tissue and fetal bone growth
Lactate dihydrogenase (LDH)	100–330 units/L	Upper end of normal to 700 units/L
Fibrinogen (factor I)	200–400 mg/dL	Progressive increase of 1–2 g/L
Platelets	150,000–450,000 per mm^3	Less than 150,000 per mm^3
Fibrin split products (FSPs); also known as fibrin degradation products (FDPs)	Less than 10 mcg/mL	Increased greater than 10 mcg/mL
D-dimer	0–0.5 mcg/mL	Greater than 0.5 mcg/mL

Van Leeuwen, A. M., & Bladh, M. L. (2021). *Davis's comprehensive manual of laboratory and diagnostic tests with nursing implications* (8th ed.). F. A. Davis.

Learn to C.U.S.

Marta is 14 weeks' pregnant and arrives for her prenatal visit. She has gained only 1 pound since her last visit, which was 1 month ago. She states that she is still experiencing nausea and vomiting "practically all day." "I mentioned it to my doctor last month, and he said it would stop when I entered my second trimester. I really feel like he thought I was overly concerned about it and acting like a baby over a little nausea. I don't feel like he was listening to me." Concerned, you discuss the issue with the physician using the C.U.S. method of communication.

C: "I am *concerned* about Marta.

U: I am *uncomfortable* with this situation because she is still experiencing nausea and vomiting and is not gaining adequate weight.

S: We have a *safety* issue regarding her health and the health of the fetus."

Patient Teaching Guidelines
Foods High in Fiber

Pregnant patients who increase fiber intake can reduce or avoid the discomforts of constipation and hemorrhoids. Foods high in fiber include the following:

- Prunes (dried plums)
- Pears
- Mangoes
- Apples
- Whole-grain breads and cereals
- Beans
- Lentils
- Nuts
- Broccoli
- Cabbage

Medication Facts

Iron Supplements

Iron supplements may be prescribed to prevent
or treat iron-deficiency anemia in the pregnant patient.
    Nursing implications:

- For best absorption, the patient should take the medication 1 hour before or 2 hours after a meal.
- Absorption is improved if iron is taken with orange juice.
- If gastric irritation occurs, iron can be taken with meals.
- Advise the patient that the stool may become dark green or black.
- Constipation is the major side effect, so encourage the patient to drink adequate amounts of water (Vallerand, 2023).

Urinary System

The types of urinary system changes in pregnancy, what the patient observes, and the related nursing care implications are found in Table 5.5. See also Figure 5.3.

Integumentary System

The types of integumentary system changes in pregnancy, what the patient observes, and the related nursing care implications are found in Table 5.6. See also Figure 5.4.

Musculoskeletal System

The types of musculoskeletal system changes in pregnancy, what the patient observes, and the related nursing care implications are found in Table 5.7.

Table 5.5
Urinary System Changes in Pregnancy

Types of Changes	Patient Observations	Nursing Implications
• Kidney workload increases because of increased blood volume and cardiac output. • The increase in blood flow is necessary to remove metabolic wastes from the mother and fetus. • The glomerular filtration rate increases, but the ability of the renal tubules to reabsorb glucose does not increase; therefore, mild glycosuria is common in pregnancy. • Mild proteinuria is also common. • The effect of progesterone on the renal pelvis causes dilation, and the distention can lead to urinary stasis and possible UTI (Pascual & Langaker, 2022).	• If the patient develops a urinary tract infection (UTI), she may experience urinary urgency, frequency, and dysuria. **Dysuria** is painful urination.	• You should monitor the kidney function tests, creatinine, BUN, and so on, for abnormalities and report them to the health-care provider. • The woman has an increased risk of UTIs and should be educated on the signs and symptoms. Signs and symptoms of a UTI are urinary urgency, frequency, and dysuria.
• Temporary bladder control problems are common in pregnancy. The enlarged uterus and fetus push down on the bladder, urethra, and pelvic floor muscles (Fig. 5.3).	• Increased pressure on the bladder can lead to a more frequent need to urinate as well as leaking of urine when sneezing, coughing, or laughing.	Educate the woman to: • Take frequent bathroom breaks. • Increase consumption of fluids to avoid dehydration. • Instruct the patient on performing Kegel exercises. See Patient Teaching Guidelines for Kegel exercises. Inform the woman that if she experiences burning along with frequency of urination, it may be an infection and she should notify her health-care provider.

• WORD • BUILDING •

dysuria: dys–abnormal + ur–urine + ia–condition

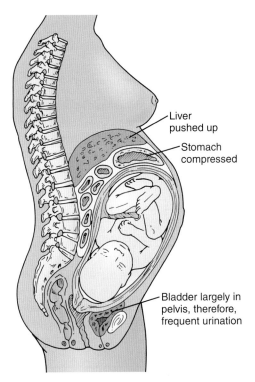

FIGURE 5.3 Compression of the bladder results from the growing uterus.

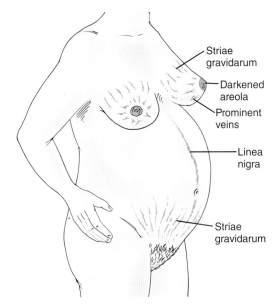

FIGURE 5.4 Integumentary system changes include darkening of the areolae, appearance of the linea nigra, and striae gravidarum.

Table 5.6
Integumentary System Changes in Pregnancy

Types of Changes	Patient Observations	Nursing Implications
• Hyperpigmentation occurs because of elevated levels of estrogen, progesterone, and melanocyte-stimulating hormone (Rigby, 2020).	• **Melasma**, also called the *mask of pregnancy,* is indicated by brownish patches on the forehead, cheeks, and nose. • **Linea nigra**, a hyperpigmented line, may extend from the symphysis pubis to the fundus. • On the breasts, the areola may darken.	• Educate the pregnant woman that melasma increases with exposure to the sun. Sunscreen may reduce the severity. • Reassure the woman that the hyperpigmentation usually disappears after childbirth.
• **Striae gravidarum**, also known as *stretch marks,* occur because of separation of collagen fibers of the connective tissue as the skin expands. See Figure 5.4 for skin changes in pregnancy.	• Striae gravidarum occur on the abdomen, hips, thighs, and breasts. They may be red and itchy.	• There is no documented proof that creams prevent striae; however, creams may soothe the itchiness.
• **Pruritic urticarial papules and plaque of pregnancy (PUPPP)** describe the most common pregnancy-specific dermatosis, occurring in 1 of 130 to 300 pregnancies. The disorder is more common with first pregnancies and multiple gestations, and familial occurrences have been reported (Pierson, 2020).	• The rash appears on the abdomen and occasionally involves extremities. The face usually is not affected. • PUPPP are itchy plaques and papules with erythematous patches of papules and vesicles.	• Usually develops in the third trimester. • Oral antihistamines and topical corticosteroids may be administered for pruritus. For extreme symptoms, oral corticosteroids may be prescribed. • Reassure the woman that the rash will disappear after childbirth.

Table 5.7
Musculoskeletal System Changes in Pregnancy

Types of Changes	Patient Observations	Nursing Implications
• Postural changes: The upper spine extends to support the enlarging uterus. This gives the pregnant woman a "swayback" appearance and leads to backache. • Her center of gravity shifts forward, placing more strain on the lower back.	• Increased backache as the uterus enlarges and the woman gains weight.	• Teach the woman to practice good posture; wear low-heeled shoes; sleep on her side; and try heat, cold, or massage to manage backache.
• Loose joints: The effects of relaxin, a pregnancy-related hormone, affect the sacroiliac joints and the symphysis pubis, causing them to soften and stretch to allow more room in the pelvis to make birth easier. • Carpal tunnel syndrome can occur when weight gain and edema compress the median nerve (Daneau et al., 2021).	• She may feel clumsy and may experience "waddling" because of the laxity of her joints. • She may feel tingling, numbness, and pain in the thumb, index finger, middle finger, and the radial side of the ring finger.	• Teach her to lift with good body mechanics and to wear low-heeled shoes and exercise caution when walking on unlevel surfaces. • Splinting of the wrists to maintain a neutral position will decrease pain. • Warn the patient that the syndrome can persist for years postpartum and recur in future pregnancies (Danuea et al., 2021).

Evidence-Based Practice

This study utilized data from the National Electronic Injury Surveillance System for emergency department visits for pregnant women aged 12 years and older who sustained stair-related falls. Falls are the leading cause of trauma during pregnancy and lead to serious complications and concerns for maternal and fetal well-being. The physiological changes of pregnancy combined with hazards of water and ice greatly increase the risk of falling. Nurses and health-care providers who have multiple opportunities for patient education during pregnancy can provide anticipatory and safety guidance for pregnant women to prevent falls.

Wallberg, C. D., Smart, D. M., Mackelprang, J. L., & Graves, J. M. (2021). Stair-related injuries among pregnant women treated in the United States emergency departments. *Maternal and Child Health Journal, 25,* 892–899. https://doi.org/10.1007/s10995-021-03141-3

Health Promotion

Skin Care During Pregnancy
To promote skin health during pregnancy, encourage the patient as follows:

• Wear sunscreen every day and avoid prolonged exposure to the sun. This will prevent or minimize the appearance of melasma on the face.
• Use moisturizing lotion to decrease dry skin and minimize itching of the abdominal skin.
• Use gentle face wash and scrubs to control acne.
• Read package labels carefully and avoid skin products containing retinoids, benzoyl peroxide, or salicylic acid.

PSYCHOLOGICAL ADAPTATION TO PREGNANCY

Pregnancy and childbirth are considered life transitions, also known as *maturational crises.* Even a woman and her partner who planned and wanted a pregnancy may experience ambivalent feelings and worries about the pregnancy, impending parenthood, and integrating a child into the family. You should keep in mind that there are many factors that influence how a pregnant woman, her partner, her other children, and her extended family react to the news of a new baby entering their lives. Factors that may cause ambivalence include limited access to health care, financial issues, lack of family support, lack of available day care, transportation problems, and previous negative experiences with childbirth and child rearing. The nurse who observes problems with adaptation to pregnancy can make appropriate referrals and provide assistance to ensure that the adaptation to this maturational crisis is as smooth as possible.

The Maternal Role

The psychological journey to the role of motherhood is described by Rubin (1984) and Mercer (2004) in their classic theories of maternal role attainment.

According to Rubin, four maternal tasks that the woman accomplishes during pregnancy lead to maternal identity:

1. Seeking safe passage for herself and her fetus
2. Securing acceptance of herself as a mother and for her fetus
3. Learning to give up self and to accept herself as mother to the infant
4. Committing herself to the child as she progresses through pregnancy

Seeking Safe Passage for Herself and the Fetus

During the first trimester, the woman expresses concern for her own health and her pregnancy symptoms. Even women profoundly happy about the pregnancy are surprised to experience emotions that rapidly change from tears to irritability to joy without provocation, all because of the hormonal shifts that are occurring physically. A woman typically seeks information by observing mothers with their children or other pregnant women; she may also read books or websites about pregnancy and childbirth.

Some women experience ambivalence about pregnancy but still seek competent prenatal care and engage in healthy self-care, such as avoiding alcohol consumption and eating healthy foods. The reality of pregnancy often causes introspection during the first trimester as the woman adapts to her own physical changes and to the changes in her life and lifestyle.

Seeking Acceptance of the Child by Others

In this task, support and acceptance of the pregnancy by the woman's partner and family are most important. The woman also desires their acceptance of her developing maternal identity. If there are other children in the family, the woman works to build acceptance of the new baby. This may involve adjustments of psychological, social, and physical space within the family to make a place for the coming child.

Mercer (1995) states that a pregnant woman's relationship with her own mother is significant in adapting to pregnancy. Ideally, her mother's positive reaction to the pregnancy indicates acceptance of the grandchild. As the pregnant woman's mother reminisces about her pregnancy and her daughter's early childhood, it helps the daughter to anticipate and prepare for pregnancy, labor, and motherhood.

Bonding With the Infant

During the developmental task of pregnancy, most mothers begin to develop bonds of attachment and feelings of love for the infant. They feel fetal movement and feel an intimate connection with the unborn fetus. A woman may fantasize about the ideal child. This strong emotional "binding-in" process motivates the woman to be a good mother. The woman observes women mothering their children and reflects on her own style of mothering.

The woman's own mother was identified by Rubin as the strongest model of mothering behavior. If the pregnant woman's mother was perceived as a good mother, the woman takes on her mothering style. If the woman's own mother was a poor role model, the pregnant woman adjusts her thinking to prepare herself to be a better mother.

Committing Herself to the Child Through Pregnancy

Next, the woman begins to develop the ability for self-denial and learns to meet the needs of another being before herself. She begins to prepare for the baby by creating a nursery and accumulating clothing and baby-care items. At this time, some women begin reading books on newborn care and parenting and attending childbirth classes.

According to Rubin and Mercer, the pregnant woman undergoes psychosocial changes throughout the pregnancy. Unsuccessful resolution of these changes has been associated with difficulties in pregnancy and delivery and, later, child abuse and neglect.

The Pregnant Adolescent

The pregnant adolescent has many psychosocial issues to manage. She is completing the developmental tasks of adolescence as well as the developmental tasks of becoming a mother. Priorities typical for her age are the importance of appearance, the importance of the peer group, and a focus on her own needs.

Most teens do not plan on becoming pregnant and may keep the pregnancy a secret as long as possible. Denial of the pregnancy until late in gestation is common. The young woman may experience anxiety related to informing her parents, the baby's father, and her friends about her pregnancy. Ambivalence, resistance, and inconsistency can be expected with the pregnant adolescent. You will need to evaluate the young woman's developmental level and her support system when planning physical and psychological care for this patient.

Therapeutic Communication

Elizabeth, aged 17, is in her second trimester of her pregnancy. She is visibly upset as she arrives for her prenatal appointment. As the nurse, you can use therapeutic communication to inquire about Elizabeth's mood.

You: "Elizabeth, you seem upset." (Technique: making an observation.)

Elizabeth: "I am so mad at my mother. I hope I am not like her with my child."

You: "What's the problem?" (Technique: clarifying.)

Elizabeth: "She is just so bossy."

You: "You feel like she tells you what to do too much?" (Technique: reflecting.)

The Partner

The most important person to the pregnant woman is usually her spouse or partner. The mother has a need for the partner to accept their child. The partner's role is important in the couple's and the family's adjustment to the new baby. Some spouses or partners of pregnant women do experience physical changes called **Couvade syndrome**, which is a sympathetic response to the pregnancy. Some may gain weight and even experience nausea.

The partner may not exhibit many physical changes, but they do undergo psychological changes throughout the pregnancy. The partner experiences psychological changes during each trimester, just as the woman experiences psychological adjustments. In the first trimester, the partner may feel ambivalence about becoming a parent or have strong protective feelings of nurturing and protecting the woman. As the pregnancy progresses, some may be concerned about their ability to be a good parent and may examine their own family relationship to determine the type of parent to be.

If the pregnancy is unplanned or unwanted, some partners may not readily accept changes in lifestyles or life plans. The parent-to-be may feel left out and unsure of their position in the relationship after the baby is born. Many eventually adjust to the unwanted pregnancy and begin to look forward to parenthood. However, some male partners or spouses express their disappointment and frustration with violence. Some women are battered by their partner for the first time during a pregnancy. Domestic violence has become an issue during pregnancy, and the American College of Obstetricians and Gynecologists (ACOG, 2021) suggests that screening for domestic violence should be done at each prenatal visit.

Partners may also be concerned about their ability to be an emotional support during childbirth. Parents-to-be may not discuss their fears and worries but often cope with their uncertainties by finding concrete tasks to do, such as preparing the baby's room, painting furniture, shopping for baby furniture, assembling car seats, and attending childbirth classes. Toward the end of the pregnancy, most partners or spouses are preparing for parenthood with thoughtful contemplation of being a loving, nurturing, supportive parent.

Siblings

For the woman's other children, a new baby is a major crisis. Each sibling's response is influenced by the child's age, the parents' attitudes, and how well prepared the child is for the upcoming birth. Parents can prepare siblings by encouraging their participation in preparing the baby's room, taking them on a tour of the hospital, reading books on babies, visiting friends with infants, and promoting a positive attitude about the coming addition to the family.

Toddlers may notice physical changes in the mother and may sense that there are changes coming, which often leads them to be clingy and irritable. Older children take an interest in the physical changes occurring in the mother and may ask questions about conception, pregnancy, and childbirth. Older children and teenagers may feel embarrassed by the sexuality of their parents and may express embarrassment about the pregnancy but be pleased about the arrival of a new sibling.

The parents need to introduce the news that a new baby is coming at an appropriate time for the child. For an older sibling, it is best to give them the news earlier rather than later. A toddler who has a limited concept of time will begin to think that a new baby is only a "story" and not a reality if informed too early of the new baby's arrival. Toddlers have difficulty sharing the parent with another child. The preschool child may feel a sense of loss, a feeling of being "replaced," or may feel jealous of the baby. Older school-aged children will contemplate and plan for ways to be helpful with a new baby in the home.

Nursing Care Plan: Body Image in Pregnancy

Nadia is 28 years old and pregnant with her first baby. She is in the 28th week of her uncomplicated pregnancy. Nadia has been an athlete and very active physically for her entire life. She ran a marathon when she was 4 weeks pregnant and has continued to run until the last 2 weeks. At that time, it became too uncomfortable to continue running. She states that she feels "slow and fat. I hate the way I look." She is at her health-care provider's office for a routine prenatal visit.

Nursing Diagnosis: Dissatisfied body image
Expected Outcome: By the next prenatal visit, Nadia will express acceptance of her body size.

Interventions:	Rationale:
Acknowledge her feelings. Listen to her concerns empathetically.	*The nurse needs to establish rapport and avoid minimizing the patient's feelings.*
Explore other methods of moderate exercise that are safe during pregnancy, such as swimming and walking.	*The patient has always been active. Continuing moderate safe exercise will help her manage her feelings of being "fat."*
Encourage healthy nutritional intake to decrease excessive weight gain.	
Educate Nadia on the expected weight gain pattern during pregnancy to promote a safe pregnancy and healthy fetus.	*Educating the patient on a healthy diet and expected weight gain will help her to be active in promoting a healthy pregnancy.*

Grandparents

With the news of the impending arrival of a grandchild, most expectant grandparents are pleased with the possibility of a new baby in the family. The news of a new baby causes them to remember their own experiences of pregnancy and raising children. They begin to recall the "firsts" of their child, such as the first steps or first words. These memories are shared in the family, and the grandparents use them as a way of providing a link between the generations. The grandparents' support and presence strengthen the family and provide nurturing for the parents-to-be as they attain their parenting roles.

However, expectant grandparents have to face the reality of aging when they realize that their child will become a parent. They may react negatively to the news and state they "are too young to be grandparents." Nonsupport of the pregnancy adds stress and decreases the self-esteem of the parents-to-be.

Key Points

- This chapter has outlined the physiological, anatomical, and psychological changes that develop during the course of pregnancy.
- There are presumptive, probable, and positive signs of pregnancy.
- Early physical changes are caused by the increasing levels of estrogen and progesterone, which rise in response to the demands brought on by the fetus, placenta, and uterus.
- Physiological changes that occur later in the pregnancy are more anatomical and are caused by the expanding uterus.

- When a woman becomes pregnant, she expects to see an expanding abdomen but does not often expect the other changes occurring in her body in response to the growing fetus.
- There are major psychosocial changes that occur as the woman makes the transition to motherhood.
- The mother's partner and the grandparents will also have psychosocial issues to address.
- The pregnant adolescent has special needs during the pregnancy.

Review Questions

1. You are discussing pregnancy care with a woman who just had her pregnancy confirmed by her health-care provider. The woman is 8 weeks' pregnant. Which of the following topics should be discussed with the pregnant woman at this time? **(Select all that apply.)**
   1. Nutrition for a healthy pregnancy
   2. Her feelings about being pregnant
   3. Managing nausea
   4. Her birth plan
   5. Managing back pain

2. A woman states that she is feeling a "little confused or uncertain about being pregnant." A therapeutic response by the nurse would be:
   1. "Don't worry. Everything will be all right."
   2. "There are plenty of women who would be happy to be pregnant."
   3. "It's not unusual to have ambivalent feelings about pregnancy."
   4. "As long as you take care of yourself, you will be just fine."

3. A pregnant woman at 37 weeks' gestation is lying on her back. She is experiencing lightheadedness and states, "I feel like I'm going to faint." You should:
   1. Reassure her that she is OK.
   2. Turn her to her left side immediately.
   3. Administer oxygen at 4 L/min.
   4. Call the health-care provider immediately.

4. A woman at 36 weeks' gestation states that she does not understand why her ankles are swelling by the end of the day. The best response by the nurse is:
   1. "You may need to pay more attention to your dietary intake of salt."
   2. "Your circulation in your legs is compromised by the weight of the uterus."
   3. "You may be developing a complication; you should contact your health-care provider."
   4. "Every pregnant woman experiences swollen ankles."

5. A woman states that she "thinks she is pregnant." Which of the following presumptive signs of pregnancy may she be experiencing? **(Select all that apply.)**
   1. Absence of menstruation
   2. Fetal heart heard by Doppler
   3. Nausea
   4. Sore, tender breasts
   5. Positive pregnancy test

6. A pregnant patient at 9 weeks' gestation arrives at the clinic for a routine pregnancy visit. She comments on the morning sickness that she experiences "every day." You know that morning sickness is caused by which of the following? **(Select all that apply.)**
   1. High levels of hCG, estrogen, and prostaglandin
   2. Reduced tone of the GI system
   3. Reduced stomach acidity
   4. Overeating at meals
   5. The enlarging uterus pressing on the stomach

7. During early pregnancy, the cervix and vagina become congested with blood, causing a bluish hue to the skin. This sign is called:
   1. Goodell sign
   2. Hegar sign
   3. Chadwick sign
   4. McMurry sign

8. A patient says that her friend warned her about the risk of vaginal yeast infections during pregnancy. She wants to know how to prevent a vaginal yeast infection. What do you tell her to do? **(Select all that apply.)**
   1. Soak in a hot tub every night.
   2. Use a gentle unscented soap to clean her perineal area.
   3. Douche the vagina once a week.
   4. Wear breathable underwear, such as cotton.
   5. Avoid petroleum-based lubricants during sexual activity.

9. A pregnant patient in her third trimester is experiencing heartburn daily. What information can you provide to the patient to reduce her heartburn? **(Select all that apply.)**
   1. Eat only three meals a day.
   2. Lie down after eating.
   3. Select foods that are easy to digest.
   4. Avoid overeating.
   5. Increase her consumption of over-the-counter antacids.

10. A woman experiencing constipation in pregnancy should be educated to:
    1. Limit fluids to 3 to 4 cups daily.
    2. Limit activity such as walking.
    3. Purchase an over-the-counter laxative.
    4. Increase her intake of fiber-rich foods.

ANSWERS 1. 1, 2, 3; 2. 3, 3; 3. 4; 4. 5; 5. 1, 3, 4; 6. 1, 3; 7. 3; 8. 2, 4, 5; 9. 3, 4; 10. 4

CRITICAL THINKING QUESTIONS

1. A woman who is 8 weeks' pregnant reports that she is so nauseated in the morning she can't really eat breakfast. How would you explain the nausea of pregnancy? What nursing interventions could you offer this patient?

2. What strategies can you suggest to a pregnant woman to assist her to prepare her other children, ages 2 and 8, for the new addition to the family?

Resources

For additional resources and information, including Postconference Questions and Activities, Answers, and References, visit www.FADavis.com.

Student Study Guide

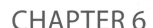

CHAPTER 6
Nursing Care During Pregnancy

KEY TERMS

amniocentesis (AM-nee-oh-sen-TEE-siss)
antepartum (an-tee-PAR-tuhm)
bimanual examination (bye-MAN-yoo-uhl
  eks-AM)
diagonal conjugate (dye-AG-on-uhl
  KON-joo-gayt)
gravida (GRA-vih-duh)
ischial tuberosity diameter (ISS-kee-uhl
  too-ber-ROSS-ih-tee dye-AM-uh-ter)
lithotomy position (lih-THAW-tuh-mee
  po-ZIH-shun)
Naegele's rule (NAY-gel-eez ROOL)
obstetric conjugate (ob-STET-rik KON-joo-gayt)
papanicolaou (Pap) test (PAP-uh-NEE-ka-low
  TEST)
para (PA-ruh)
viability (vye-uh-BIH-lih-tee)

CHAPTER CONCEPTS

Health Promotion
Professionalism
Reproduction and Sexuality
Violence and Neglect

LEARNING OUTCOMES

1. Define the key terms.
2. Discuss diagnostic testing to confirm pregnancy.
3. Explain the GTPAL system.
4. Explain scopes of practice and roles of the family practice physician, the obstetrician, and the certified nurse midwife on the health-care team.
5. Determine the estimated date of delivery (EDD) using Naegele's rule.
6. Describe how patient-centered care is dependent on a thorough past medical history, cultural history, social history, and pregnancy history.
7. Explain the purpose and procedure of the complete physical examination and pelvic examination.
8. Define the common laboratory tests utilized during pregnancy.
9. Explain the commonly used screening tests and diagnostic tests for fetal health.
10. List the usual pattern of prenatal visits to the health-care provider.
11. Discuss nursing care provided during subsequent visits to the health-care provider.
12. Communicate effectively with the patient regarding intimate partner violence (IPV).
13. Discuss the monitoring of fetal growth and development.

CRITICAL THINKING

Jean is 40 years old. She arrives for her first prenatal visit with the obstetrician. This is her sixth pregnancy, and Jean thinks she is at 6 weeks' gestation. Her past medical history reveals that she had a therapeutic abortion at age 15 and one spontaneous abortion at 22 years old. Jean has three living children aged 15, 12, and 8 at home. Her last child was born at 32 weeks' gestation and spent 2 weeks in the hospital neonatal intensive care unit.

Questions

1. What is Jean's GTPAL?
2. Considering Jean's medical history, what would be the frequency of prenatal visits for Jean?
3. Review Jean's medical history in the scenario. What screening tests for fetal health would be recommended for Jean?

For a pregnant woman, the **antepartum** period begins with conception and ends with the onset of labor. As she begins her prenatal care, the nurse frequently answers questions and provides support to the pregnant woman. The nurse should have an understanding of the elements of antepartum assessment and the usual plan of care to promote a healthy pregnancy. Assessment involves history, examination, and diagnostic testing. This chapter discusses the selection of a health-care provider, the initial prenatal interview and examination with the health-care provider, and subsequent prenatal care. Commonly used laboratory tests and screening tests for health of the mother and fetus are also covered.

INITIAL PRENATAL ASSESSMENT

The initial prenatal assessment begins with the woman's suspicions of pregnancy, such as a missed menstrual period and other physical signs. This section discusses the diagnosis of pregnancy, the selection of a health-care provider, terminology specific to pregnancy, and the components of a prenatal history.

Diagnosis of Pregnancy
The diagnosis of pregnancy can be made by several methods. Amenorrhea, which is the absence of a menstrual period, is usually the first sign that a woman notices. Amenorrhea can be caused by other medical reasons such as thyroid abnormalities, poor nutrition, hormonal imbalances, anorexia, obesity, fad diets, stress, medications, and viral infections.

• *Pregnancy testing of human chorionic gonadotropin (hCG) levels:* The hCG hormone is produced by the trophoblast after conception and is the first hormone to rise with pregnancy. There are at least 25 home pregnancy tests marketed in the United States. The test is generally used in the week after the missed menstrual period. Urine

· WORD · BUILDING ·
antepartum: ante–before + partum–giving birth

hCG is variable at that time but can be detected with a home test (Shields, 2022).
• *Abdominal ultrasonography:* This procedure can be done to confirm pregnancy at 6 to 8 weeks' gestation. It can also be done at 18 to 20 weeks and again later in the pregnancy to confirm the age of the fetus and to monitor for any problems with the internal organs and body systems. Ultrasound waves create a picture of the fetus on a monitor. The mother needs to have a full bladder and must be able to lie still for several minutes for the examination.
• *Transvaginal ultrasonography (TVUS):* This method can detect a pregnancy at 4 to 5 weeks' gestation, which is 1 week sooner than traditional abdominal ultrasonography. With TVUS, the patient is not required to have a full bladder or endure uncomfortable abdominal pressure on the abdominal wall (Shields, 2022). However, some women may object to insertion of the vaginal probe.

Pregnancy Terminology
The terms *gravida* and *para* are used to describe pregnancies, not the number of fetuses. **Gravida** refers to the number of times a woman has been pregnant. For example, a woman pregnant for the second time is a gravida 2. **Para** refers to

a woman who has produced a viable infant, regardless of whether the fetus was alive at birth. ***Viability*** is defined as the point in a pregnancy that the fetus could theoretically survive outside its mother's womb. The lower limits of viability are a fetal weight of 500 g or a gestation greater than 20 weeks.

A multiple birth is considered to be a single parous experience (Venes, 2021). The gravida and para system does not provide enough detail regarding the pregnancy and childbirth experience. Most health-care providers use the GTPAL acronym to give data that are more comprehensive in order to provide appropriate care:

- G: the number of pregnancies regardless of the outcome or number of fetuses (G represents *gravida*)
- T: the number of *term* births born at 37 weeks' gestation and beyond
- P: the number of *preterm* births born after 20 weeks' gestation and before 37 weeks' gestation
- A: the number of pregnancies that ended in a spontaneous or therapeutic *abortion* (included as gravida if before 20 weeks' gestation)
- L: the number of *living* children

For example, Maria is pregnant for the third time, and she had a spontaneous abortion 2 years ago. She has a 5-year-old daughter who was born at 39 weeks' gestation. Maria's GTPAL is G3, T1, P0, A1, and L1.

Selection of a Health-Care Provider

There are options available for the pregnant woman as she selects a health-care provider to give medical care during her pregnancy and birth.

- *Family physicians:* They provide health care for the complete life span. Their medical education qualifies family physicians to manage most uncomplicated pregnancies, including minor surgical procedures for vaginal delivery. Some family physicians perform cesarean sections but may need to refer a patient to an obstetrician for that procedure.
- *Obstetrician-gynecologists* (*OB-GYNs*): They provide health care for all phases of pregnancy, from preconception planning to postpartum recovery. Women with preexisting medical conditions or at risk to develop complications, such as diabetes or preeclampsia, should select an OB-GYN.
- *Certified nurse midwives* (*CNMs*): They provide preconception, maternity, and postpartum care for women at low risk of complications during pregnancy. Midwives generally offer a low-technology approach to the birthing process. Midwives cannot perform cesarean sections and will need to transfer care to an OB-GYN if complications occur.

Determining the Estimated Date of Delivery

Most women do not deliver on their due date. However, the establishment of a due date or the estimated date of delivery (EDD) is important. It allows the health-care provider to monitor the growth and progress of the pregnancy. The method for determining the EDD is based on **Naegele's rule**. The formula is to subtract 3 months from the first day of the last menstrual period (LMP) and then add 7 days, which will indicate the approximate date of delivery (Venes, 2021).

For example, if the first day of the woman's LMP was January 1, subtracting 3 months is equal to October 1. Next, add 7 days. The EDD would be October 8.

A pregnancy wheel, which is based on Naegele's rule, can also be used to determine the estimated due date or date of delivery. The pregnancy wheel works by adding 40 weeks to the date of the LMP. It provides the approximate conception date, gestation week, and due date (Fig. 6.1).

Initial Patient History

To provide patient-centered care, thorough past medical history, family history, cultural preferences, and gynecological and obstetrical histories are very important to obtain. The information in Box 6.1 should be obtained by the health-care provider.

Health Promotion

As soon as a pregnancy is confirmed, the nurse can reinforce health promotion with the woman to ensure a healthy pregnancy. Health promotion and maintenance in early pregnancy include:

- Encourage the woman to schedule the first prenatal visit as soon as she confirms pregnancy.
- Obtain a thorough past medical history and current health history to detect any potential problems.
- Encourage the woman to ask questions.
- Answer all questions honestly.
- Encourage the patient to obtain all laboratory tests ordered by the health-care provider.
- Stress the importance of subsequent prenatal visits and care throughout the pregnancy.

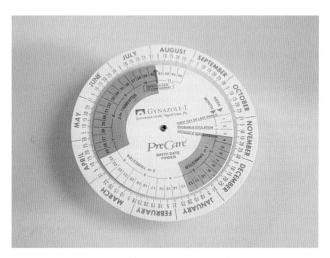

FIGURE 6.1 A gestation wheel is a handy tool for determining the gestational age. The arrow labeled "first day of LMP" is placed on the date of the LMP. The date at the arrow labeled "expected delivery" is then noted.

Box 6.1

Initial Patient History

Personal Information
- Age
- Relationship status
- Support systems
- Race or ethnic background
- Occupation
- Economic level
- Educational level
- Any history of emotional or physical abuse in her current relationship (Does the patient feel safe in her current living situation?)

Patient Medical History*
- Surgical procedures
- Hospitalizations
- Childhood diseases

Family Medical History
- Occurrence of multiple births
- History of birth defects
- History of chromosomal abnormalities, such as Down syndrome
- History of diabetes; hypertension; cardiovascular issues; bleeding disorders; and/or thyroid, respiratory, or kidney diseases
- Causes of death of deceased parents or siblings
- History of genetic disorders, such as CF or sickle cell disease

Cultural, Religious, and Spiritual History
- Any religious or spiritual beliefs that may influence the acceptance of medical treatment or care
- Any attitudes the patient or family may have regarding their attitudes about the sex of the fetus
- Cultural preferences that may influence obstetric care and the childbirth experience
- Does the patient want a religious preference noted on the medical record?

Gynecological and Obstetric History
- Age of menses onset
- Menstrual cycle: frequency and duration of menstrual flow
- History of dysmenorrhea
- History of infertility and any fertility treatment
- Previous STIs
- Date of last Pap test
- Contraception history
- Number of past pregnancies
- Number of spontaneous or elective abortions
- Number of living children
- Loss of a child (SIDS, accident, disease, relinquishment)
- Complications with previous pregnancy or childbirth
- Prenatal education

Partner's History*
- Age
- Use of alcohol, tobacco, and/or illicit drugs
- Occupation
- Blood type and Rh
- Thoughts and feelings about the pregnancy
- Does the father know of any genetic diseases in his family?

Current Medical Status
- Height, weight, and current body mass index (BMI)
- Blood type and Rh, if known
- Current medications
- Allergies to foods or medications
- Chronic diseases such as diabetes; hypertension; cardiovascular issues; bleeding disorders; and/or thyroid, respiratory, or kidney disease
- Illicit drug use
- Tobacco use
- Alcohol use
- Immunization record, especially rubella
- History of mental health problems, such as depression and anxiety

Current Pregnancy
- First day of LMP
- Planned or unplanned pregnancy?
- Results of pregnancy tests, if completed
- Thoughts and feelings about the pregnancy
- Any pregnancy discomforts noted
- Any personal preferences regarding the birth
- Any educational needs regarding pregnancy and childbirth

*History-taking is a little different if a patient has used assisted reproductive technology to become pregnant. Questions about chromosomal abnormalities and family medical history relate to the donor who provided the egg and/or sperm. Questions about current medical status refer to the woman who is carrying the pregnancy and her partner.

Therapeutic Communication

When interviewing a patient for her prenatal visits, remember these points for effective communication:

- Avoid the initial discussion of the patient's gravida or para status in front of her partner or family.
- Maintain sensitivity in discussions with the patient seeking a therapeutic abortion or choosing to put her baby up for adoption. Avoid any tone or body language that might imply a judgmental attitude. (See Chapter 12 for information on caring for the woman placing her newborn for adoption.)
- Always provide privacy. The patient may not feel comfortable discussing health issues with her family, friends, or spouse or partner present.
- Avoid judgmental comments or behaviors when the patient shares past medical history and obstetrical history.
- Be an active listener in order to recognize patient concerns and educational needs.

PRENATAL ASSESSMENT AND CARE

Ideally, a woman should schedule her first prenatal visit as soon as she knows she is pregnant. The first prenatal visit is important as it is a time for the health-care provider to determine a baseline of the woman's overall health and identify any potential problems that may influence the course of the pregnancy. Laboratory and diagnostic tests will be ordered to obtain a baseline and identify health problems. The woman will also be advised of the need for subsequent visits to monitor her pregnancy for potential complications and to monitor the health of the fetus until labor begins.

Medication Facts

When interviewing the patient for past and current medical history, it is important to develop a list of medications that she is currently taking. Some medications pose a hazard to the fetus and should be reported to the health-care provider as soon as possible. The woman should be provided with a list of safe or acceptable over-the-counter medications during pregnancy.

Initial Prenatal Assessment

After a detailed health history is obtained, the health-care provider will proceed to do a thorough physical examination. During the physical examination, the woman should be provided with privacy and should be made comfortable, both physically and psychologically. Rapport should be established that allows her to ask questions and verbalize any concerns during the examination.

Physical Examination

The health-care provider should perform a head-to-toe physical examination that covers all major systems. The examination will provide the health-care provider with information regarding the woman's current overall health.

In addition to the complete physical examination, a pelvic examination is performed. The patient is draped and placed in the **lithotomy position**. In this position, the patient lies on her back with hips and knees flexed and the legs spread and raised above the hips. The feet are placed in stirrups attached to the examination table. This position allows the health-care provider with a clear view of the external and internal genitalia.

The external genitalia are examined to detect lesions or discharge. A culture for sexually transmitted infections (STIs) is generally done at this time.

Examination of the internal genitalia is done with a vaginal speculum to observe the cervix for the signs of pregnancy (Fig. 6.2). A **papanicolaou (Pap) test**, which is used

· WORD · BUILDING ·
lithotomy: litho–stone + tomy–cutting

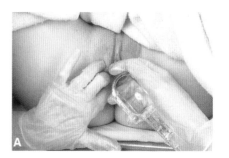
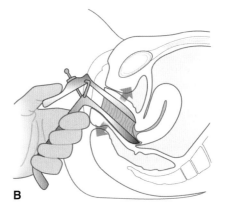
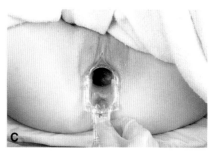
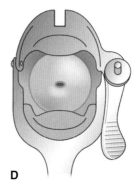

FIGURE 6.2 Pelvic examination. A, Inserting the speculum. B, Proper position of speculum in the vagina. C, Opening the speculum. D, View through the speculum.

to detect cervical cancer, is obtained. After the speculum is removed, the examiner will perform a **bimanual examination** of the uterus to determine its size. During the bimanual examination, the health-care provider places the gloved middle and index fingers into the vagina to identify the cervix. Then the examiner places the other hand midway between

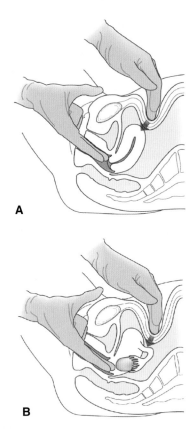

FIGURE 6.3 Bimanual examination for determining uterine size, position, tenderness, and consistency. A, Palpating the uterus. B, Palpating the ovaries.

the umbilicus and the symphysis pubis and presses downward toward the pelvic hand. Using the fingers, the examiner palpates for the uterine fundus to determine its size, position, tenderness, and consistency. The ovaries are also palpated for size, position, and tenderness (Fig. 6.3).

The pelvic bones are assessed to determine their size and adequacy for a vaginal birth. The examiner obtains information on pelvic size to be aware of the potential for cephalopelvic disproportion, a mismatch between the size of the fetus's head and the mother's pelvis. (See Chapter 10.) The pelvic assessment measurements are featured in Figure 6.4.

- **Diagonal conjugate:** This is the distance from the lower posterior border of the symphysis pubis to the sacral promontory.
- **Obstetric conjugate:** This diameter extends from the sacral promontory to the upper inner border of the symphysis pubis and measures approximately 11 cm. It is the most important of the pelvic measurements because it is the first bony strait through which the fetus has to pass during the birth process.
- **Ischial tuberosity diameter:** This is the smallest dimension of the pelvis. It should be at least 10 cm to allow the fetus's head to pass through the pelvis. The examiner will note whether the ischial spines are blunt or prominent (Fig. 6.4).

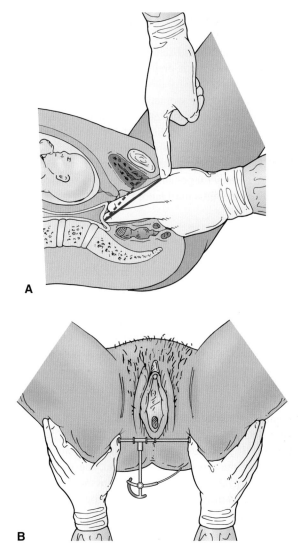

FIGURE 6.4 Pelvic measurements to determine adequacy for vaginal delivery. A, The diagonal conjugate and the true conjugate (conjugate vera). B, Use of a pelvimeter to measure the ischial tuberosity diameter.

Laboratory Tests

The American College of Obstetricians and Gynecologists (ACOG, 2021b) recommends the following laboratory testing for all pregnant women to be done early in the pregnancy:

- *Complete blood count (CBC)* to determine overall health and to detect anemias
- *Antibody screen* to determine whether the mother has been exposed to fetal blood
- *Blood typing and Rh* to identify the mother's blood type (A, B, AB, or O) and Rh status (+ or −)
- *Rubella titer* to determine whether the patient has immunity or will need the immunization after giving birth
- *Varicella titer* to determine immunity to varicella or need to vaccinate after childbirth
- *Hepatitis B and C* to determine presence of the antigen and to detect infection

- *HIV and STI screen* to detect HIV status and any STIs that may require treatment
- *Pap test* for detecting cervical cancer
- *Urinalysis* to detect bacteria, ketones, glucose, and protein in the urine
- *Tuberculosis* testing

Laboratory testing done later in the pregnancy should include the following:

- A repeat *CBC* may be performed.
- A *glucose challenge test* is used to screen for gestational diabetes. It is usually done between 24 and 28 weeks' gestation unless the mother is at high risk for diabetes. If she is high risk, the test is usually ordered by the health-care provider to be done after the initial prenatal visit. For the 1-hour test, the patient is given 50 g of oral glucose. After 1 hour, the blood glucose level is checked. Normal is less than 140 mg/dL. If greater than 140, a 3-hour screening test is done (Moore, 2022).
- A *group B streptococci test (GBS)* can be performed. GBS are bacteria that live in the vagina and rectum, and

---

Safety *Stat!*

Pregnant women are tested for rubella immunity with a rubella titer early in the pregnancy. Rubella is a virus that can cause congenital defects of the heart, hearing, and vision, especially if a pregnant woman contracts the virus during the first trimester. If the pregnant woman is not immune to rubella, she cannot have the vaccine during pregnancy. Rubella outbreaks have been documented in many countries around the world. A pregnant woman who is not immune should be careful about foreign travel, especially during the first trimester, when the fetus is at the highest risk for problems associated with the virus.

Labs & Diagnostics

An antibody screen is a test done to find antibodies that attack red blood cells. The most common problems with antibodies are related to the Rhesus (Rh) factor. For example, if an Rh-negative woman is pregnant and the fetus has Rh-positive blood, any amount of fetal blood that enters the mother's circulation causes her body to make antibodies. This is called Rh sensitization. There are other rare blood factors that can cause problems for the fetus if the mother is sensitized and begins making antibodies. Regardless of the cause, the mother begins making antibodies that destroy red blood cells during future pregnancies. The antibody screen is usually repeated at 28 and 36 weeks' gestation. Typically, the medication RhoGAM is used to treat Rh-negative women exposed to Rh-positive blood (see Chapter 11).

most women have no symptoms. They can be passed to the fetus during birth and cause health problems for the newborn. A swab is used to collect samples from the vagina and rectum (ACOG, 2021b).
- The *Rh antibody* test may be repeated.

Screening and Diagnostic Tests for Fetal Health

Screening tests are recommended by ACOG (2021b) as a routine part of prenatal care to find conditions that may increase the risk of complications for the mother and fetus. Additional diagnostic tests may be required to confirm the diagnosis.

FIRST TRIMESTER
- Along with hCG testing, another maternal blood test called pregnancy-associated plasma protein-A (PAPP-A) is done at 11 to 13 weeks to help detect the fetal genetic abnormalities trisomy 18 and trisomy 21, better known as Down syndrome (Springer, 2022).
- Fetal ultrasonography is a reliable method of determining fetal age.
- Nuchal translucency testing (NTT) is performed between 11 and 13 weeks' gestation to screen for chromosomal abnormalities. An ultrasound examination is used to measure the translucent area on the back of the fetal neck. Fetuses with genetic disorders often have excessive accumulation of fluid in this area that can be seen by the end of the first trimester (Springer, 2022).
- Chorionic villus sampling (CVS) is also done between 11 and 13 weeks' gestation. With ultrasound guidance, a thin tube is inserted into the chorionic villi via the cervix or abdomen. Cells are obtained for karyotyping for genetic disorders (Fig. 6.5). Possible complications following CVS are spontaneous abortion and infection.
- Preimplantation genetic testing is performed in cases where a fetus has a high risk of inheriting a genetic disorder and in cases where a woman has experienced repeated miscarriages because of a fetal chromosomal abnormality. After in vitro fertilization (IVF), a technician removes and analyzes a single cell from an embryo at the eight-cell stage of development. Based on the results of the test, only genetically healthy embryos are transferred into the uterus (Springer, 2022).

SECOND TRIMESTER
- Quadruple screen (Quad screen) is performed on the mother's serum between 15 and 20 weeks' gestation to detect levels of specific serum markers:
  - *Alpha-fetoprotein (AFP):* High levels may indicate fetal neural-tube defect; lower levels could indicate risk for Down syndrome (trisomy 21) or trisomy 18.
  - *hCG:* High levels indicate risk for Down syndrome.
  - *Unconjugated estriol (UE):* Low levels indicate a risk for Down syndrome.
  - *Inhibin-A:* High levels indicate a risk for Down syndrome.

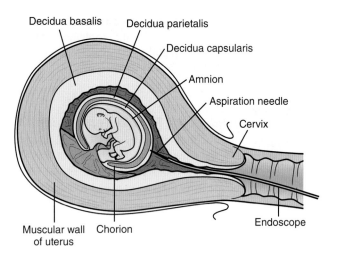

FIGURE 6.5 Chorionic villi sampling (CVS) test done for genetic disorders.

Labels: Decidua basalis, Decidua parietalis, Decidua capsularis, Amnion, Aspiration needle, Cervix, Endoscope, Chorion, Muscular wall of uterus

- **Amniocentesis** may be performed to diagnose Down syndrome, cystic fibrosis (CF), spina bifida, and other genetic disorders. Under ultrasound guidance, a thin needle is used to remove amniotic fluid and cells from the amniotic sac surrounding the fetus. Possible complications after amniocentesis are as follows:
  - Spontaneous abortion
  - Infection
  - Needle injury to the fetus
  - Leaking of amniotic fluid
  - Rh sensitization
  - Infection transmission; if the mother is HIV+ or has hepatitis C or toxoplasmosis (Fig. 6.6)
- Percutaneous umbilical cord sampling (PUBS), or cordocentesis, is a test of cells obtained directly from the umbilical cord. A 20- to 22-gauge needle is inserted transabdominally to obtain cells from the umbilical cord.

Nursing Care Plan for Prenatal Care

Samantha, age 21, presents at the community health clinic for her first prenatal examination at 12 weeks' gestation. She has never had a gynecological examination before and doesn't know what to expect. Unaware that she was pregnant, Samantha occasionally drank alcohol and smoked marijuana during the first trimester. She is concerned about the effects of her actions on her unborn baby.

Nursing Diagnosis: Insufficient knowledge of the pelvic examination and first prenatal visit
Expected Outcome: The patient will verbalize understanding of the need for the pelvic examination and importance of prenatal care.

Interventions:	Rationales:
Provide positive feedback to the patient for scheduling the prenatal appointment with the health-care provider.	*Positive reinforcement helps to change behavior.*
Explain the importance of prenatal visits.	*Patients are more likely to be compliant if the reasons are explained.*
Explain the reason for the pelvic examination and what to expect during the procedure.	*The patient will understand that the pelvic examination will provide the health-care provider with information and allow the health-care provider to plan appropriate care.*
Provide for privacy to answer questions.	*Providing privacy will promote trust between the nurse, patient, and health-care provider.*
Offer to stay with the patient during the procedure.	*Staying with the patient can help to allay anxiety.*

Nursing Diagnosis: Anxiety caused by fear of chromosomal abnormalities and birth defects
Expected Outcome: The patient will verbalize that her anxiety is decreased because she has information regarding testing options.

Interventions:	Rationales:
Acknowledge her fear and allow her to verbalize concerns.	*Fear is real to the patient. By allowing the patient to talk without criticism, her fears and anxieties will become more manageable for her.*
Provide information regarding diagnostic tests that can be completed during early pregnancy, such as chorionic villi sampling, NTT, quadruple screen blood test, and amniocentesis.	*Educating the patient on options will help to reduce her fears and anxieties.*

· **WORD** · **BUILDING** ·

amniocentesis: amnio–amniotic sac + centesis–puncture

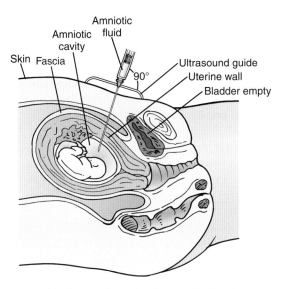

FIGURE 6.6 Amniocentesis testing for genetic disorders.

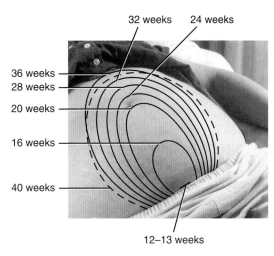

FIGURE 6.7 Fundal height measurements as the pregnancy progresses. Fundal measurement should approximately equal the number of weeks of gestation.

Safety *Stat!*

Following an amniocentesis, the woman should not leak fluid from the abdominal puncture site. The amniotic sac should seal over after the needle is removed. Instruct the patient to immediately call her health-care provider if she notices any leaking of fluid from the abdominal puncture site. Leaking fluid could lead to infection of the uterus.

This test can be used to conduct DNA studies, to diagnose hematological problems or infections in the fetus, and to evaluate fetal oxygenation (Springer, 2022).

Subsequent Prenatal Visits

The pregnant woman will usually visit her health-care provider according to the following schedule:

- Monthly for the first 28 weeks' gestation
- Every 2 weeks until 36 weeks' gestation
- Weekly after 36 weeks until childbirth

Care During Subsequent Prenatal Visits

It is important for the pregnant woman to obtain regular care during her pregnancy in order for the health-care provider to identify complications early and implement appropriate care. During each visit, the patient can expect the health-care provider and nurse to do the following:

- Evaluate any physical or psychological patient concerns and answer questions. Be especially sensitive to the patient who has a history of sexual assault or abuse. Routine care may trigger posttraumatic stress disorder (PTSD) for these women. Be patient, explain everything that will be done, ask permission to touch them, and don't rush these patients (O'Laughlin et al., 2021).

- Weigh the patient to monitor for appropriate weight gain.
- Monitor vital signs for increasing blood pressure.
- Perform urinalysis to monitor for:
  - Glucose, which may indicate gestational diabetes
  - Ketones, which are produced when the body is breaking down fat for energy
  - Protein, which may be a sign of preeclampsia, kidney damage, or urinary infection
  - Nitrates, which indicate urinary tract infection
- Measure fundal height:
  - The fundal height is the distance between the top of the pubic bone and the top of the uterus.
  - The fundus reaches the level of the umbilicus at approximately 20 weeks and measures approximately 20 cm (Fig. 6.7).
  - Each subsequent visit to the health-care provider should indicate growth of the uterus.

Safety *Stat!*

During prenatal visits, the fundal height is measured to determine appropriate fetal growth. The pregnant patient should not be placed flat on her back any longer than necessary to complete an accurate measurement. In the supine position, the large uterus can compress the vena cava and cause a drop in blood pressure and cardiac output. This causes the patient to feel faint and dizzy. She should be encouraged to lie on her side to prevent supine hypotensive syndrome.

- Monitor fetal heart rate (FHR).
  - A handheld device called a Doppler is used to listen to the FHR. Heart tones may be heard as early as 8 weeks but more commonly at 10 to 12 weeks.

- Perform a psychological assessment.
  - Warning signs:
    - Increasing anxiety about the pregnancy
    - Inappropriate responses to or preoccupations about the pregnancy
    - Failure to acknowledge quickening
    - Signs of substance use disorder
    - Inability to cope with stress
    - Failure to prepare for the baby, such as preparing clothing and selecting a feeding method

Evidence-Based Practice

Evidence in previous studies indicates that 13% to 21% of prenatal persons experience anxiety. A study investigated prenatal persons' internet discussion concerning their experiences with anxiety. Blogs are an accessible resource for people to anonymously discuss anxiety symptoms and management of anxiety. The bloggers commonly discussed emotional, cognitive, physical, and behavioral symptoms. The researchers followed and analyzed the blogs, determining that three main themes were evident throughout the blogs. The first theme was that people were concerned about the cause of the anxiety, such as previous pregnancy loss. The second theme was triggers for anxiety, such as the mother's health and baby's health. The third theme was concern about the symptoms of anxiety, such as loss of joy and poor sleeping. The study concluded that one way to address prenatal anxiety is for nurses and other health-care professionals to make credible information on anxiety in pregnancy easily accessible through online mediums, such as blogs.

Pierce, S. K., Reynolds, K. A., Hardman, M. P., & Furer, P. (2022). How do prenatal people describe their experiences with anxiety? A qualitative analysis of blog content. *BMC Pregnancy and Childbirth, 22*, 398. https//doi.org/10.1186/s12884-022-04697-w

Learn to C.U.S.

During a prenatal visit with Lauren, she acknowledges that she has not prepared any clothes or a crib for her newborn. Lauren "can't decide" whether she wants to bottle feed or breastfeed. You are concerned because this is Lauren's first baby, and she is at 37 weeks' gestation. You discuss her concerns with the obstetrician using the C.U.S. method of communication.

C: "I am *concerned* about Lauren.
U: I am *uncomfortable* because she has not started preparing for the birth of her newborn and she is at 37 weeks' gestation.
S: We have a possible *safety* issue and a warning sign that she is not coping well with the pregnancy."

- Provide education.
  - Address topics appropriate to gestational age.
  - Include signs that should be reported to the health-care provider and could indicate potential complications such as preeclampsia and placenta problems (see Chapter 8) such as:
    - Vaginal bleeding
    - Severe headache
    - Unusual or severe abdominal pain
    - Leaking fluid from the vagina
    - Blurry or impaired vision
    - Excessive vomiting and or diarrhea
    - Swelling of the feet, hands, and face
- Screen for intimate partner violence (IPV). Pregnancy often triggers IPV or exacerbates the problem (ACOG, 2021a).
  - Screening questions:
    - "Do you feel safe at home?"
    - "Do you and your partner fight?"
    - "Does the fighting become physical?"
    - "Have you ever been hit or hurt by your partner?"

Assessment of Fetal Development

The assessment of fetal development most commonly includes FHR and quickening.

- *FHR:* The ultrasound Doppler is used in the prenatal setting to evaluate the FHR. The normal FHR is 110 to 160 bpm. If unable to hear the FHR by 12 weeks' gestation, an ultrasound examination may be completed to evaluate fetal development.
- *Quickening (the mother's sensation of fetal movement):* This is expected between 16 and 22 weeks' gestation. A **primigravida** woman usually notices quickening later than a woman who has been pregnant before.

Safety *Stat!*
Warning Signs of Intimate Partner Violence
- Late or absent for prenatal appointments
- Injuries to the face, head, neck, chest, or abdomen
- Vaginal bleeding
- Genitourinary infections
- Signs of anxiety, depression, and self-harm
- Signs of alcohol or substance use disorder
- The partner demands to attend all clinic visits.
- The partner answers all the questions for the woman.

Document all information and report using the established agency policy.

· WORD · BUILDING ·
primigravida: primi–first + gravida–pregnant

Key Points

- Family practice physicians, obstetricians-gynecologists, and certified nurse midwives can provide prenatal and delivery care for the patient.
- A complete medical history, family history, spiritual history, cultural history, gynecological history, and pregnancy history are required to provide patient-centered care.
- A complete head-to-toe assessment with a pelvic examination is required to evaluate the overall health of the mother and the adequacy of the pelvis for childbirth.
- Laboratory tests, including a CBC, rubella screen, varicella screen, antibody screen, HIV test, STI panel, Pap test, urinalysis, Rh test, and blood type test, provide baseline information about the patient's health status.

- Prenatal visits are planned throughout the pregnancy to continually monitor maternal and fetal health.
- The GTPAL system is used to provide data on pregnancy and childbirth history.
- Screening tests, such as CVS, NTT, and quadruple screen, are performed for early diagnosis of genetic abnormalities.
- IPV often begins or gets worse during pregnancy. Screening questions should be asked at each prenatal visit.
- FHR and quickening are two early assessments of fetal development.

Review Questions

1. Typically, when does a pregnant woman notice quickening for the first time?
   1. Between 8 and 11 weeks' gestation
   2. Between 12 and 15 weeks' gestation
   3. Between 16 and 20 weeks' gestation
   4. Between 21 and 24 weeks' gestation

2. A pregnant patient asks why the quadruple screen test is done. You answer that the test is performed:
   1. To detect Rh sensitization
   2. To detect cardiac and renal abnormalities
   3. To detect central nervous system abnormalities
   4. To detect Down syndrome, trisomy 18, and neural tube defects

3. A pregnant patient at 8 weeks' gestation is at her first prenatal visit. Most likely, if no complications have developed, her next visit would be scheduled in _____ weeks.

4. A urinalysis is performed at each prenatal visit to screen for which of the following? (**Select all that apply.**)
   1. Ketones
   2. Glucose
   3. Bacteria
   4. Protein
   5. Drugs
   6. Anemia

5. Mary, aged 24, is pregnant with her second baby. She is at 20 weeks' gestation. You are concerned that Mary may be experiencing psychological stress. Which of the following is a sign that she may be experiencing psychological stress?
   1. She has not started preparing the baby's room.
   2. She is excited about her upcoming baby shower.
   3. She frequently misses her prenatal appointments.
   4. She has not selected a name for the baby.

6. You are concerned that a pregnant patient may be the victim of IPV. Signs of IPV include which of the following? (**Select all that apply.**)
   1. Lateness to or absence from prenatal appointments
   2. Signs of injuries to the face, neck, chest, or abdomen
   3. Reports of backache after working all day
   4. Shortness of breath when climbing stairs
   5. Signs of anxiety and self-harm
   6. Vaginal bleeding

7. Why is the height of the uterine fundus measured?
   1. To determine appropriate fetal growth
   2. To estimate the weight of the fetus
   3. To monitor abdominal weight of the mother
   4. To estimate the date of delivery

8. What is the frequency of prenatal visits for a pregnant woman at 38 weeks' gestation?
   1. Daily
   2. Weekly
   3. Every 2 weeks
   4. Every 3 weeks

9. The health-care provider would be very concerned if an FHR were not detected with a Doppler at how many weeks' gestation?
   1. 14 to 16 weeks
   2. 6 to 8 weeks
   3. 18 to 20 weeks
   4. 10 to 12 weeks

10. Emily is 36 years old and is currently pregnant with twins. She has a 10-year-old daughter born at 30 weeks' gestation and a 16-year-old son born at 40 weeks' gestation. Eighteen years ago, she had a miscarriage at 8 weeks' gestation. Emily's GTPAL is _____.

ANSWERS 1. 3; 2. 4; 3. Four (4); 4. 1, 2, 3, 4; 5. 3; 6. 1, 2, 5, 6; 7. 1; 8. 2; 9. 4; 10. G4, T1, P1, A1, L2

CRITICAL THINKING QUESTIONS

1. Martha is 39 years old and pregnant for the first time. She has type 1 diabetes, takes medication for hypertension, and is very concerned about delivering a healthy baby. Which type of health-care professional would be the best choice to provide prenatal and delivery care for Martha?

2. Jennie, aged 45, is at 8 weeks' gestation. She is concerned about potential genetic problems of the fetus because of her age. Which screening tests is the health-care provider likely to recommend?

3. Estelle, aged 36, is 32 weeks' pregnant with her third child. She works as a hairdresser and stands for long periods during her workday. What questions should you or the health-care provider ask Estelle about her occupational history to assist her with maintaining a healthy pregnancy?

Resources

For additional resources and information, including Postconference Questions and Activities, Answers, and References, visit www.FADavis.com.

Student Study Guide

CHAPTER 7
Promoting a Healthy Pregnancy

KEY TERMS

chorioretinitis (KOH-ree-oh-RET-in-EYE-tiss)
hydrocephalus (HYE-droh-SEF-uh-luhss)
hyperthermia (HYE-per-THER-mee-uh)
leukorrhea (loo-ko-REE-uh)
morbidity (mor-BID-ih-tee)
mortality (mor-TAL-ih-tee)
neural tube defects (NOO-ruhl TOOB DEE-fekts)
nocturia (nok-TOO-ree-uh)
oligohydramnios (OL-ih-goh-hye-DRAM-nee-ohss)
pica (PYE-kuh)
pneumonitis (NOO-moh-NYE-tiss)
polyhydramnios (POL-ee-hye-DRAM-nee-oss)
thrombosis (throm-BOH-siss)

CHAPTER CONCEPTS

Health Promotion
Infection
Nutrition
Safety

LEARNING OUTCOMES

1. Define the key terms.
2. Provide guidance to the pregnant patient on managing the common discomforts of pregnancy.
3. Promote safe and effective self-care practices during pregnancy.
4. Discuss the nutritional needs of the pregnant patient.
5. Define *pica* and its dangers for the pregnant patient.
6. Discuss the dangers and prevention of viral infections in pregnancy.
7. Teach the pregnant patient about the recommended weight gain in pregnancy.
8. Plan appropriate prenatal care for the pregnant adolescent.
9. Discuss the additional nutritional needs of the pregnant adolescent.
10. Discuss culturally competent care of the LGBTQ+ couple.
11. Identify risks for the pregnant patient over the age of 35.
12. Explain the tests used to monitor fetal well-being during the pregnancy.
13. Compare and contrast the Bradley method and Lamaze method of childbirth education.
14. Discuss the components of a birth plan.

CRITICAL THINKING & CLINICAL JUDGMENT

Ruby is 25 years old at 34 weeks' gestation of her first pregnancy. She has experienced no complications with her pregnancy and is in good health. Her prepregnancy body mass index (BMI) was 19, and she has gained 15 pounds during the pregnancy. She is taking her prenatal vitamins and an additional iron tablet daily. She states, "I am very constipated because of the iron supplements ordered by my nurse midwife. I have never had this problem before."

Questions

1. Based on Ruby's BMI of 19, has she gained enough weight in the pregnancy?
2. What questions could you ask about her constipation?
3. What suggestions could you make for managing the constipation?
4. You ask Ruby what she is doing to manage the constipation and Ruby says, "I'm taking a walk every day." Exercise is usually effective, but what are other strategies for managing constipation you can suggest?

CONCEPTUAL CORNERSTONE
Health Promotion

The concept of health promotion can be defined as the improvement of health and the prevention of disease. The focus of health promotion includes nutrition, exercise, hygiene, vaccinations, protection from environmental hazards, avoidance of harmful substances, protection from accidents, and stress reduction. Health promotion usually requires people to change behaviors, and change is not easy. However, pregnant women are typically very motivated to change behaviors to improve their health and to promote a healthy fetus and pregnancy. When providing care, a nurse has many opportunities to teach and support the pregnant patient in health promotion.

The focus of this chapter is on promoting a healthy pregnancy and providing nursing care during pregnancy. The patient will undergo profound changes to her body and will experience discomforts that are a natural part of pregnancy.

Nurses caring for pregnant patients need a clear understanding of care that will promote a healthy and safe pregnancy and that will prepare the woman for her eventual delivery.

FOCUS ON THE PATIENT

Nearly every body system is affected in pregnancy. As hormones change and the fetus grows, the pregnant woman will experience changes in her body that produce physical discomforts. As the pregnancy progresses, she will have questions about maintaining her health, managing the discomforts of pregnancy, providing self-care, and ensuring safety for herself and her fetus.

Relief of Common Discomforts of Pregnancy

The common discomforts of pregnancy are caused by hormonal and physiological changes. You can provide anticipatory guidance and teach strategies for managing the common discomforts (Table 7.1).

Table 7.1
Relieving the Common Discomforts of Pregnancy

Discomfort	Methods of Relief
Nausea and vomiting	• Eat crackers first thing when arising. • Avoid foods with strong odors. • Consume peppermint candies. • Use relaxation techniques with slow breathing to decrease nausea. • Eat small, frequent meals. • Avoid spicy foods.
Nasal stuffiness, discharge, and obstruction	• Increase fluid intake. • Use nasal saline drops. • Use a humidifier in the home.
Urinary frequency, urgency, and **nocturia** (urination during the night)	• Perform Kegel exercises to improve the muscle tone of the perineum. • Maintain adequate hydration during the day but decrease fluids 2 hours before bedtime.
Increased **leukorrhea** (vaginal discharge)	• Avoid tight-fitting clothing. • Wear cotton underwear. • Wear a pad or panty liner to absorb moisture. • Perform daily perineal hygiene to prevent infection.
Increased fatigue	• Schedule rest periods throughout the day. • Maintain a regular, consistent bedtime with adequate sleep.
Heartburn	• Avoid overeating and eat small, frequent meals. • Do not eat less than 3 hours before bedtime. • Avoid spicy and greasy foods. • Elevate the head with an extra pillow at night. • Consume milk products.

· WORD · BUILDING ·

nocturia: noct–night + ur–urine + ia–condition
leukorrhea: leuko–white + rrhea–flow

Table 7.1

Relieving the Common Discomforts of Pregnancy—cont'd

Discomfort	*Methods of Relief*
Constipation	• Increase fluid intake. • Increase fiber intake to 35 g per day. • Exercise daily. • Use only bulk-forming laxatives or mineral oil (*not* stimulant laxatives) and only after increasing fluids, fiber, and exercise.
Hemorrhoids	• Avoid straining at defecation. • Increase fluid intake. • Increase fiber intake. • Avoid standing for long periods.
Backache	• Maintain good posture. • Use correct body mechanics when lifting; bend at the knees, not the waist. • Wear low-heeled shoes. • Support the uterus with a pillow underneath when lying on the side to sleep.
Leg cramps	• Avoid constrictive clothing. • Elevate the legs periodically. • Dorsiflex the foot to stop the cramp. • Include adequate amounts of dietary calcium and magnesium. Consult with a health-care provider before adding a magnesium supplement (Marnch, 2021).
Shortness of breath	• Avoid constrictive clothing. • Sleep with an extra pillow to elevate the head. • Allow extra time for stair climbing and walking.
Ankle edema	• Elevate the legs periodically to increase venous return. • Rest in a side-lying position to promote placental circulation and to increase venous return.
Round ligament pain	• Support the uterus with a pillow or pregnancy support garment. • Take a warm bath. • Apply warmth to the ligament area. • Avoid standing for long periods.

CRITICAL THINKING

Marta is 36 weeks' gestation and mentions jokingly that "I think I'm addicted to my nasal decongestant spray. I have to use it at least twice a day to keep my nose open and breathe easier. I've been using it for weeks."

1. What is causing Marta's nasal congestion?
2. Should you be concerned about the use of the nasal decongestant?
3. Are there other ways to manage nasal congestion without a decongestant spray?

PROMOTION OF SELF-CARE DURING PREGNANCY

Self-care is personal, medical care performed voluntarily by the patient. Most pregnant women are motivated to learn about self-care by reading books and conducting internet searches. Although some of the information they find may be helpful, some may be inaccurate. You can support the pregnant woman's self-care by providing her with accurate information. Self-care during pregnancy empowers the woman to make healthy lifestyle choices in order to maintain or improve her health and the health of her fetus.

Personal Hygiene

An increase in vaginal discharge and perspiration during pregnancy makes personal hygiene very important. Showers are safe throughout pregnancy. Tub baths are also permitted throughout pregnancy except after the amniotic membranes rupture. The pregnant woman should avoid excessively hot showers and baths because of the detrimental effects of **hyperthermia**. Hyperthermia is elevated body heat caused by fever or by hot tubs, saunas, or sunshine. Maternal hyperthermia has been linked to neural tube defects in the fetus. **Neural tube defects** affect the spinal cord or brain.

Safety *Stat!*

Women should be cautioned about tub baths during the last trimester of pregnancy. The pregnant woman is at risk for falling and should ask for help when exiting the tub.

Breast Care

A daily shower or bath usually provides for breast cleanliness. During late pregnancy, colostrum may crust on the nipples. Colostrum, rich in antibodies and minerals, is a yellowish fluid secreted by the breasts during late pregnancy that precedes the production of milk. It can be removed with a washcloth and warm water; however, the pregnant woman should avoid using strong soap on the nipples because of its drying effect.

During pregnancy, breast support helps to prevent back strain and retain breast shape. Whether a woman plans to breastfeed or bottle feed, support from a well-fitting bra will enhance comfort. Tips for bra selection include the following:

- The breast tissue should fit entirely inside the cup.
- The straps should be wide and not too tight.
- The bra should have sufficient hooks to allow it to expand as needed.

Clothing

Maternity clothing has changed over the years from large, loose smocks that hid the pregnant abdomen to stylish, more fitted garments. Because maternity clothes can be expensive and are worn for only a short time, many women improvise a maternity wardrobe using their prepregnancy clothes supplemented with a few essential items. The most important points to remember about choosing maternity clothes are comfort and safety. The clothes need to be loose enough to allow for movement and circulation. High-heeled shoes are not recommended because of the potential for falls as the abdomen expands and the pregnant woman's center of gravity shifts.

Exercise

An exercise regimen is safe and beneficial to continue during pregnancy. Women who did not exercise before pregnancy can begin moderate exercise during the pregnancy. Benefits of exercise include preventing excess maternal weight gain, promoting normal fetal growth, preventing gestational

diabetes, and decreasing the risk of preeclampsia (ACOG, 2022a; Fig. 7.1). Table 7.2 provides information about the benefits of exercise, forms of safe exercise, forms of exercise that are not appropriate during pregnancy, and safety tips for exercising during pregnancy.

Patient Teaching Guidelines

Patient Exercise

Teach patients to stop exercising and see their health-care provider if they experience any of the following symptoms:

- Dizziness or feeling faint
- Fluid leaking from the vagina
- Vaginal bleeding
- Chest pain
- Headache
- Increased shortness of breath
- Decreased fetal movement

Safety *Stat!*

Many health clubs offer prenatal yoga classes. Yoga can be continued throughout the pregnancy with some modifications to promote a safe pregnancy. Pregnant women who practice yoga should note the following guidelines:

- Increased body heat is never recommended during pregnancy. Avoid "hot yoga" classes.
- Avoid yoga poses that involve lying flat on the abdomen or back.
- Avoid poses that involve twisting, hopping, and jumping.
- Maintain adequate hydration during exercise.

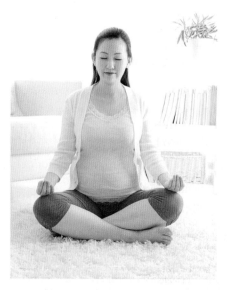

FIGURE 7.1 Exercise during pregnancy has many benefits and enhances the woman's sense of well-being.

• **WORD** • **BUILDING** •

hyperthermia: hyper–excessive + therm–heat + ia–condition

Table 7.2
Exercising During Pregnancy

Benefits of exercise	• Reduction of backaches and constipation • Potential prevention of gestational diabetes • Improved muscle tone, strength, and endurance • Improvement in sleep
Forms of safe exercise	• Walking • Swimming • Cycling • Aerobics • Running, if the pregnant woman was a runner before pregnancy
Forms of exercise not appropriate during pregnancy	• Skiing, gymnastics, and other sports that include a risk of falling • Contact sports such as hockey, basketball, and soccer • Scuba diving because decompression sickness can affect the fetus
Safety tips for exercising during pregnancy	• Maintain adequate hydration. • Avoid overheating. • Wear a supportive bra and well-fitting shoes. • After the first trimester, avoid exercising on the back; the supine position restricts blood flow, causing vena caval syndrome.

Evidence-Based Practice

Exercise is considered safe for the pregnant woman and her fetus. A study published in *BMC Pregnancy and Childbirth* examined the level of physical activity and sedentary time in relationship to pregnancy weight gain and complications during pregnancy and childbirth in a sample of pregnant individuals. The main findings indicate that only 27% of the participants exercised 30 minutes or more per day. The largest group of participants were sedentary for 4 to 6 hours per day. The study concluded that the group with a higher level of daily physical activity had a reduced risk of emergency cesarean section, lower pregnancy weight gain, and self-rated their overall health during pregnancy higher than the sedentary group. Encouraging women to increase their physical activity during pregnancy can reduce excessive weight gain, reduce the risk of emergency cesarean section, and improve overall health.

Meander, L., Lindqvist, M., Mogren, I., Sandlund, J., West, C. E., & Domellof, M. (2021). Physical activity and sedentary time during pregnancy and associations with maternal and fetal health outcomes: An epidemiological study. *BMC Pregnancy and Childbirth, 21,* 166. https://doi.org/10.1186/s12884-021-03627-6

Sleep and Rest

Pregnant women typically experience fatigue and will need more rest; fatigue increases as the fetus gets larger. The woman should incorporate rest periods into her day to decrease fatigue and should allow for 8 hours of sleep at night. At times, sleep may be difficult because of backaches and the growing fetus. The woman may need to use additional pillows to support her uterus and take the strain off the lower back when lying down.

Employment

Pregnant women without complications can continue to work throughout the pregnancy. However, hazards to fetal well-being need to be considered at the job site as well as in the home. Even prolonged standing may increase maternal fatigue. In addition, heavy lifting can pose a risk of musculoskeletal injury and low back pain. A woman who must lift heavy loads for long periods at work should consult with her health-care provider for guidance or to obtain modified work accommodations. The pregnant woman should contact her industry nurse for information about environmental hazards at the job site and research environmental hazards related to her employment (Marcin, 2021).

Seatbelts

Seatbelts should be worn to protect both the mother and the fetus. The belt should be placed low, across the abdomen and across the hipbones. The shoulder strap should be placed between the breasts and over the clavicle (Fig. 7.2). Pregnant women should try to keep the abdomen 10 inches from the air bag (DelCastillo, 2021).

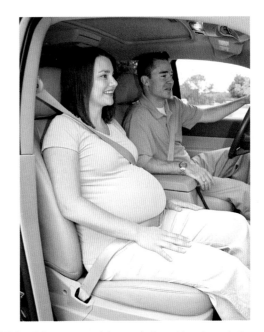

FIGURE 7.2 Proper use of the seatbelt and headrest during pregnancy.

Travel Restrictions

The second trimester is considered to be the safest time for the pregnant woman to travel. Prolonged sitting during pregnancy increases the risk of venous stasis, which leads to thrombosis. **Thrombosis** is a blood clot, usually in the lower extremities, which restricts blood flow. Adequate hydration and ambulation every 2 hours will help to decrease the risk of developing a venous thrombus.

Air travel can cause dehydration because of low oxygen tension, low humidity, and recirculated air. Drinking water and avoiding caffeine are important to prevent dehydration when traveling.

Dental Care

Overall, good health includes dental care. During pregnancy, the gums are commonly edematous and may bleed easily because of the effects of hormones and increased blood supply. If treatment for cavities or infection is required, the dentist should be informed of the pregnancy. X-rays should be done only if necessary and with appropriate abdominal shielding utilized to protect the fetus.

Sexual Activity

Sexual intercourse during pregnancy is safe unless the amniotic membrane has ruptured or vaginal bleeding is occurring.

Therapeutic Communication

A patient may feel uncomfortable asking questions about sexual activity during pregnancy. However, the pregnant couple usually has concerns and needs education regarding safe sex in pregnancy. You need to initiate the conversation with open-ended questions and use a matter-of-fact approach such as, "Your body is going through many changes right now. Some of the changes can affect your sexual activity. What questions do you have about that?"

Patient Teaching Guidelines

Signs That Something May Be Wrong

These warning signs in a pregnant patient must be reported to the health-care provider:

- Abdominal pain
- Vaginal bleeding
- Infection
- Severe headaches
- Swelling of the hands and face
- Premature rupture of membranes
- Preterm labor
- Absence of fetal movement

• WORD • BUILDING •

thrombosis: thromb–blood clot + osis–condition

ACOG (2021b) states that sexual activity during pregnancy is safe for most women unless there is a specific contraindication. The woman should limit or avoid sex if she has preterm labor; has had more than one miscarriage; has placenta previa, an infection, or bleeding; or has ruptured amniotic membranes. ACOG recommends that the couple try different positions for comfort as the pregnancy advances.

Health Promotion

Prevention of infections in pregnancy is important. Some general instructions for the pregnant woman to prevent infections include the following:

- Practice good hand-washing techniques, especially after changing diapers or wiping children's noses.
- Avoid young children with colds and infections.
- Avoid raw or undercooked meat.
- Avoid cleaning the cat litter box.
- Avoid yard work that may cause exposure to cat feces.
- Avoid sharing drinks and eating utensils with small children.
- Make sure vaccinations are current before becoming pregnant again.
- Get a yearly flu vaccine.

 AVOIDING INFECTIONS

Infections in pregnancy are major causes of maternal and fetal morbidity and mortality. The medical definition of **morbidity** is a disease state, and **mortality** refers to death (Venes, 2021). The usual way that a fetus acquires an infection is by transmission through the placenta. Infections known to cause congenital defects (defects present at birth) can be remembered with the acronym TORCH (toxoplasma, others, rubella, cytomegalovirus [CMV], and herpes). "Other" infectious agents include parvovirus B19, HIV, measles, hepatitis, varicella-zoster virus (VZV), syphilis, West Nile virus, and Zika virus. Physical signs and symptoms of disease may be apparent in the newborn at birth or may not be evident until years later.

T = Toxoplasmosis

Toxoplasmosis can be acquired by eating raw or undercooked meat or through exposure to cat feces. The symptoms are vague and the pregnant woman may experience body aches, headache, fatigue, enlarged lymph nodes, and a sore throat. When the woman becomes infected, the parasite invades the placenta and the fetus is infected for life (Cleveland Clinic, 2022). The disease is transmitted more frequently during the third trimester. The signs of infection may not be present at birth, but those infected may develop clinical illness by young adulthood (Health Resources & Services Administration [HRSA], 2022). Infected infants develop **chorioretinitis**, inflammation of the choroid and retina of the eye that can lead to blindness; obstructive hydrocephalus; mental retardation; seizures; motor delays; and developmental delays (Cleveland Clinic, 2022).

O = Others

Parvovirus B19

Parvovirus B19 (B19V) is the virus that causes erythema infectiosum, also known as fifth disease. Fifth disease is a childhood disease characterized by the "slapped face" rash that appears along with a fever. It is transmitted by the respiratory route, through blood products, and by placenta transmission during pregnancy. Approximately 40% of pregnant women do not have antibodies for this virus and are at risk for infection (Marino, 2021). If the pregnant woman acquires the virus, it is often asymptomatic for the woman, but can affect the fetus and cause fetal death. This is a disease that causes the fetus to have anemia and be unable to manage fluid. The fluid builds up in the fetal lungs or heart. The neonate may be born with liver swelling, heart failure, jaundice, and edema of the body (Riley & Caraciolo, 2022).

Varicella-Zoster Virus

Primary varicella infection, also known as *chickenpox,* is considered a medical emergency during pregnancy. VZV, which is transmitted as an airborne virus, causes fever, anorexia, and itchy vesicles. The person is contagious until the last vesicle crusts over. **Pneumonitis**, which is inflammation of the lungs, is a complication that is likely to occur with the adult pregnant patient (Centers for Disease Control and Prevention [CDC], 2019). The risk for life-threatening respiratory complications is significant if the fetus acquires the virus. It can result in spontaneous abortion, chorioretinitis, cataracts, limb malformations, and brain dysfunctions (Riley, 2021b).

Patient Teaching

- Avoid any person known to have the disease.
- Follow vaccination guidelines for children in the home.

Measles Virus

Measles, also known as *rubeola,* can have severe consequences for the pregnant woman. It is transmitted by the airborne route of coughing and sneezing. The symptoms are fever, cough, conjunctivitis, and rash. Pregnant women are also at risk to develop pneumonitis with this disease. Most pregnant women have been vaccinated. However, measles is not eradicated worldwide. Travel outside of North America can also increase the risk of exposure to measles. Rubeola is not known to cause specific birth defects but has been associated with spontaneous abortion, premature labor, and low birth weight (Marino, 2021).

Patient Teaching

- When planning travel during pregnancy, be aware that measles is present in Europe, Asia, Africa, the Pacific Islands, and even some areas within the United States.
- Avoid any person known to have the disease.
- Follow vaccination guidelines for children.

HIV

Congenital HIV infection is a major cause of infant and child mortality worldwide. HIV has been responsible for an estimated 40 million deaths worldwide since the start of the HIV pandemic in the 1980s (UNAIDS, 2022). Most countries have placed an emphasis on prenatal treatment to prevent mother-to-fetus transmission.

Approximately 25% of women in the United States are not tested for HIV during pregnancy (CDC, 2022c). The CDC recommends routine third trimester screening for women with high-risk behaviors or who have symptoms of the disease.

Before becoming pregnant, women diagnosed with HIV should be counseled about decreasing the risk of mother-to-fetus transmission with highly active antiretroviral therapy (HAART). The risk of transmission to the fetus is linked to the mother's viral load, also known as the amount of active virus in her bloodstream. Zidovudine (ZVD) is the most common medication used to reduce viral load. This medication also crosses the placenta and provides protection against HIV to the fetus. Antiretroviral therapy has not been shown to cause any negative effects on pregnancy. It should be started as early as possible during the pregnancy to reduce the risk of disease transmission to the fetus (Choudrary, 2022).

Patient Teaching

- Notify the health-care provider if HIV+.
- If HIV status is unknown, get tested for HIV.
- Take all antiretroviral medications as prescribed.
- Avoid a high-risk lifestyle, such as IV drug use, and practice safe sex with untested partners.

Syphilis

Syphilis is a sexually transmitted infection (STI) that can cause miscarriage, premature birth, and stillbirth when acquired during pregnancy (CDC, 2021).

• WORD • BUILDING •

chorioretinitis: chorio–choroid + retin–retina + itis–inflammation

pneumonitis: pneumon–lung + itis–inflammation

Patient Teaching

- Avoid unprotected sex with a new partner.
- Maintain a monogamous relationship.
- Notify the health-care provider of any painless lesions on the genitals, mouth, or rectum after unprotected sex.

West Nile Virus

West Nile virus is transmitted by mosquitoes. The risk is low, but a few cases of transmission of the virus to the fetus have been documented (MotherToBaby, 2021). Symptoms include high fever, headache, neck stiffness, tremors, seizures, and coma.

Patient Teaching

- Prevent infection by using insect repellent and wearing long-sleeved shirts and pants.
- Control mosquitoes around the home.

Hepatitis

Hepatitis B can be transmitted to the fetus at the time of delivery. Hepatitis C can be transmitted to the fetus during the pregnancy, especially if there is a codiagnosis of HIV (ACOG, 2021a).

Patient Teaching

- Avoid exposure to blood and body fluids.
- Obtain the hepatitis B vaccination.

Zika Virus

Zika virus is spread through mosquitoes, sexual contact, and perinatal transmission to the fetus during pregnancy. It can cause severe congenital abnormalities including

Patient Teaching

- Pregnant women or women desiring to become pregnant should avoid travel to countries with active Zika virus transmission such as the Americas, the Caribbean, and the Pacific Islands (Marino, 2021).
- Wear long sleeves and pants in high-risk areas.
- Wear insect repellent for prevention. For 3 weeks after travel to a country with high incidence of Zika, wear insect repellent to prevent passing the virus to mosquitoes that could infect other people locally.
- Zika virus can be transmitted through sex. After travel to a high-risk area, condoms should be used for sexual activity for 3 months (Marino, 2021).

microencephaly, hearing loss, glaucoma, retinal dysplasia, optic nerve abnormalities, and nystagmus (CDC, 2022a).

R = Rubella

Rubella (German measles) is spread by contact with respiratory secretions and is very dangerous to the developing fetus. Signs and symptoms of maternal infection include a rash starting on the face or neck, enlarged lymph nodes, joint pain, fever, and cough. The fetus is infected through placental transmission, and the most dangerous time for the fetus is the first 12 weeks of the pregnancy. Rubella can cause miscarriage and stillbirth. Congenital rubella syndrome is associated with four common abnormalities: deafness, central nervous system abnormalities, eye defects, and cardiac malformations (Riley, 2021a).

Patient Teaching

- Avoid exposure to young children, especially during the first trimester.
- Report any rash or illness to the health-care provider.

C = Cytomegalovirus

CMV is a herpes virus that is acquired through contact with saliva, urine, and other body fluids. It can be acquired through sexual contact, organ transplantation, transmission through the placenta, and breast milk. Maternal CMV infection may cause no symptoms or may be noticeable by fever, mild depression, and muscle aches. Infection of the fetus can cause intrauterine growth retardation (IUGR), hearing loss, seizures, rash, vision loss, microencephaly (small brain), **hydrocephalus** (increased fluid in the brain), and delayed motor development. The most important risk factor for CMV infection for the pregnant woman is exposure to young children. Approximately 20% of young children shed CMV in their saliva or urine even if they never had symptoms (Cedeno-Mendoza, 2021).

H = Herpes Simplex Virus

Herpes simplex virus (HSV) is one of the most common STIs. Symptoms of herpes typically appear as a blister or as multiple blisters on or around affected areas such as the mouth, genitals, or rectum. The greatest risk to the fetus occurs if the mother becomes initially infected with HSV during the third trimester. Neonatal herpes infection occurs more frequently in babies from mothers who acquired HSV during the pregnancy (Grove, 2020). Most neonatal infections result from exposure to genital HSV during the delivery. Most obstetricians will schedule a cesarean birth if the woman has a history of frequent outbreaks of herpes or

· WORD · BUILDING ·

hydrocephalus: hydro–water + cephalus–head

an active case at the due date. The newborn infected with HSV may have skin, eye, or mouth lesions; encephalitis; or dysfunctions of the liver, lungs, central nervous system, and brain (Grove, 2020).

Patient Teaching

- Inform the health-care provider of any past history of herpes outbreaks.
- Inform the health-care provider of any new herpes outbreaks during the pregnancy so that antiviral therapy can be started.
- Practice safe sex with a new partner by using condoms and avoiding sexual contact with anyone with an open sore on the genitals.

Labs & Diagnostics

Types of HIV Tests

- Antibody tests look for HIV antibodies in the patient's blood:
  - Enzyme immunoassay (EIA) tests use blood, saliva, or urine to detect HIV antibodies. Results can take up to 2 weeks.
  - Rapid HIV antibody tests also use blood, saliva, or urine to detect HIV antibodies. These results take 10 to 20 minutes. Rapid HIV self-tests can be obtained at a pharmacy or ordered online for home delivery.
  - A positive result from either test requires a follow-up test called a Western blot to confirm the result.
- Antigen tests require a blood sample and detect HIV earlier than an antibody test. Antigens are foreign substances, such as chemicals, bacteria, viruses, or pollen, that cause the activation of the immune response.
- The polymerase chain reaction (PCR) test detects the genetic material of the HIV and identifies HIV in the blood within 2 to 3 weeks of infection. Babies born to HIV-infected mothers are tested using this method because the baby may have HIV antibodies from the mother for several months and would test positive on a standard antibody test. Another test, the nucleic acid test (NAT), looks for HIV in the blood, not the antibodies (HIV.gov, 2022).

COVID-19

COVID-19 (SARS-CoV-2) is a potentially severe respiratory syndrome that was identified as a pandemic by the World Health Organization in March of 2020 (CDC, 2022b). The virus spreads through close person-to-person contact by inhaling airborne droplets or direct contact with respiratory secretions on a contaminated surface. Symptoms include fever, cough, headache, sore throat, chills, difficulty breathing, fatigue, congestion, nausea, vomiting, diarrhea, body aches, and loss of taste or smell. Because of physiological and immunological changes of pregnancy, the COVID-19 virus is more likely to cause severe illness in pregnant individuals (Rosenberger et al., 2023). Knowledge of this virus and its variations are continually evolving. Refer to the CDC for the most up-to-date information on the virus and for providing patient care.

Patient Teaching

- Avoid sick individuals.
- Wash hands frequently.
- Wear a mask in crowded conditions or around sick individuals.
- The COVID-19 vaccination is recommended for pregnant persons (CDC, 2022b).
- Report any possible COVID symptoms to the health-care provider.

 ## NUTRITION IN PREGNANCY

Healthy eating in pregnancy enables optimal weight gain for the fetus and reduces complications. The requirement for many nutrients is increased; the mother should take a multivitamin with iron during the pregnancy. During pregnancy, the basic principles of healthy eating remain the same. There are a few nutrients in pregnancy that the woman may want to pay special attention to when choosing foods. General guidelines for nutrition include the following:

- The pregnant woman should avoid empty calories such as soft drinks, desserts, and fried foods.
- Limit caffeine to less than 200 mg daily, which is about equal to two 6-ounce cups of coffee (ACOG, 2022b).
- Folate (folic acid) is a B vitamin that helps prevent neural tube defects in the developing fetus. A lack of folic acid in the diet during pregnancy can also increase the risk of low birth weight and preterm delivery. Foods high in folic acid include cereal grains, beans, spinach, kale, broccoli, romaine lettuce, asparagus, and peanuts. The recommended daily allowance of folic acid is 600 mcg per day (ACOG, 2022b).
- Calcium and vitamin D are needed by the mother for healthy bones and teeth. The fetus needs calcium for developing a healthy heart, nerves, muscles, and blood clotting abilities. Dairy products are the best sources of these nutrients. Good calcium sources for the vegan patient would include cabbage, turnip greens, tofu, and almonds. The recommended daily allowance of calcium is 1,000 mg/day and vitamin D is 15 mcg/day.
- Protein is important for fetal growth, especially during the second and third trimesters. Good sources of protein are lean meat, poultry, eggs, dried beans, tofu, dairy products, and peanut butter. It is recommended that pregnant

women consume 75 to 100 grams of protein daily. In some cultures, protein might be restricted. A culturally competent nurse and health-care provider should evaluate the pregnant woman's diet to determine whether she is obtaining adequate protein to promote fetal growth and development (Hussain et al., 2021).

- Iron needs are increased in pregnancy as the woman's blood volume expands to meet the needs of the fetus. Iron is also needed to make hemoglobin, which carries oxygen to the tissues. Good sources of iron include lean red meat, poultry, iron-fortified cereals, green leafy vegetables, and dried fruits.
- Most women pregnant with a single fetus need 340 more calories a day during the last 6 months of pregnancy (ACOG, 2022b).

Recommended Weight Gain

ACOG has developed guidelines for weight gain in pregnancy. Excessive weight gain is associated with an increased risk for gestational diabetes, pregnancy-associated hypertension, and the delivery of infants who are large for their gestational age (ACOG, 2021d). The guidelines for weight gain for a woman pregnant with one fetus are as follows:

- BMI less than 18.5 is considered underweight, and she should gain 28 to 40 pounds.
- BMI between 18.5 and 24.9 is considered normal weight, and she should gain 25 to 35 pounds.
- BMI between 25 and 29.9 is considered overweight, and she should gain 15 to 25 pounds.
- BMI greater than 30 is considered obese, and she should gain 11 to 20 pounds.

Nutritional Needs of the Obese Patient

Obesity during pregnancy increases the risk of spontaneous abortion, gestational diabetes, preeclampsia, sleep apnea, a large-for-gestational-age (LGA) fetus, and a longer labor. Obese patients should be referred to a nutrition counselor for education on selecting a healthy diet. Exercise is recommended to assist with weight control. The goal should be 30 minutes of activity most days of the week.

The weight gained in pregnancy is caused by changes in the mother's body and the growth of the uterus and fetus. The breakdown for weight gain is as follows:

- Breasts: 1 to 2 pounds
- Blood volume: 3 to 4 pounds
- Fat: 6 to 9 pounds
- Body fluid: 2 to 3 pounds
- Uterus growth: 2 to 3 pounds
- Placenta: 2 to 3 pounds
- Amniotic fluid: 2 to 3 pounds

Pica

Pica is an eating disorder that can occur with pregnant women. **Pica** is the practice of eating nonnutritive foods or nonfood substances. It involves intensely craving, then ingesting, these substances. There are three common forms of pica:

- *Geophagy:* the ingestion of soil, clay, or similar substances
- *Amylophagy:* the ingestion of raw starch or similar substances
- *Pagophagy:* the ingestion of ice or freezer frost

The cause of pica is not known, but several theories have been proposed to explain it: nutritional deficiencies, cultural and familial factors, stress, low socioeconomic status, learned behavior, or underlying chemical disorder (Burke, 2021).

Common substances craved during pregnancy are dirt, clay, laundry starch, charcoal, ice, toothpaste, coffee grounds, baking soda, and cigarette ashes. If the mother eats nonfood substances instead of a healthy diet, she may not supply the nutritional needs of herself or her fetus. It is also possible that the nonfood substances could be toxic or contain parasites.

Management of Pica

The nurse or health-care provider should question the woman in a nonjudgmental way about pica practices. She may be embarrassed to admit that she is eating nonnutritive substances. The management of pica practices can include the following:

- Encouraging her to eat a balanced diet with sufficient vitamins and minerals
- Recommending that she select a close friend, family member, or spouse to be her support person who can assist her with avoiding harmful substances
- Limiting her access to the nonnutritive substances that she is craving
- Substituting chewing gum or healthy, low-calorie snacks for the substance that she is craving
- Using distraction, such as taking a walk, calling a friend, or reading a book, until the craving disappears

CARE OF THE PREGNANT ADOLESCENT

Adolescence is a period of transition between childhood and adulthood. Developmental issues need to be considered when planning care for the pregnant adolescent. When you are working with a pregnant adolescent, you must keep in mind that the developmental tasks can impact care and compliance with planned prenatal care. Normal adolescent development has implications for the ways in which teens experience pregnancy and prenatal care.

The emerging ability to think abstractly may enable the teen to see the relationship between her behavior and the health of the fetus. You should use direct, concrete communication with the adolescent and provide information about the positive effects of healthy behaviors and fetal health. The adolescent may need more frequent prenatal visits or follow-up phone calls to encourage compliance with physician visits and nutrition guidelines.

Body image is a major issue for the adolescent. She may resist gaining weight, which could lead to complications of the pregnancy. You should stress the relationship between healthy nutrition and exercise and good physical appearance.

Adolescents experience egocentric thinking in which they think everyone else is focused on their behavior or that their feelings, fears, and experiences are unique. The pregnant teen may think that normal pregnancy discomforts are unique to her situation. Addressing discomforts of pregnancy in a group-teaching session may help her to see that pregnancy discomforts are normal and common among pregnant women.

You should remember that the adolescent is establishing emotional independence from her parents and is becoming more emotionally reliant on friends. Peer groups are an important part of her identity. Peers may supply support for her pregnancy needs. She may also view the pregnancy as a way to strengthen her relationship with the father of the baby. Parents and other family members should be encouraged to allow the pregnant adolescent to take responsibility for her own pregnancy-related care, yet give her time to be a "regular teenager."

Experimentation with risk-taking behaviors is common in adolescents. The pregnant adolescent may experiment with alcohol or smoking during the pregnancy. The health-care provider and nurse need to be clear on the dangers of risk-taking behaviors and pregnancy.

Legal Issues for Pregnant Teens

The pregnant teen's parents cannot force the teen to make a decision regarding abortion, adoption, or raising the baby. Some states require parental permission for an abortion if the teen is under the age of 18, and some states require parental permission for placing the baby for adoption if the teen is under the age of 17.

Emancipation is a legal process that allows a teen under the age of 18 to be independent of her parents. A married pregnant teenager is automatically emancipated, but an unmarried pregnant teenager is not. This teen would need to seek legal assistance to obtain emancipation. The definition of the emancipation of a minor varies among states, and not all states recognize emancipated minor status. The pregnant teen should check with a local pregnancy center or government website to obtain information on teen rights and emancipation.

Nutritional Needs of the Pregnant Adolescent

Adolescents often do not have good eating habits. They enjoy convenience foods that are high in fat, salt, and sugar and low in nutritional value. The lifestyle of adolescents contributes to their poor nutritional status. They often do not want to get up early enough for a healthy breakfast before school, and they may have jobs or extracurricular activities and prefer to hang out with friends after school and on the weekends. This type of schedule does not leave time for healthy family meals.

Most adolescents who desire to maintain their pregnancy want to have a healthy baby. This goal can be used to assist the adolescent to make healthier food choices.

Weight gain can be a major issue for the pregnant adolescent. She may not want to see the changes in her body and may resist gaining weight. This is detrimental to her own physical growth that is occurring during pregnancy and has a negative impact on the development of the fetus.

Inadequate consumption of calcium is a problem for many pregnant adolescents. Their own bones are still growing, and they need additional calcium for the bones of the fetus during the third trimester.

Poor nutrition choices may cause the pregnant adolescent to consume a diet low in iron. This can make her fatigued, short of breath, and unable to concentrate.

The combination of inadequate weight gain and poor nutritional choices can lead to delivery of a small-for-gestational-age (SGA) newborn.

Suggestions to improve adolescent nutrition include the following:

- Encouraging her to consume an additional 300 calories per day during the last 6 months of pregnancy, choosing foods from all food groups (American Pregnancy Association, 2021)
- Keeping a daily food diary to record protein, vegetables, dairy products, and fruit consumed
- Replacing soft drinks and juices with milk or yogurt
- Taking 1,300 mg of a calcium supplement with food to increase absorption (American Pregnancy Association, 2021)
- Taking iron supplements with water or orange juice between meals to increase absorption
- Avoiding anemia by eating meat; beans; and dark, leafy green vegetables
- Avoiding eating too much convenience or fast food
- Choosing healthy food options at fast-food restaurants
- Providing positive reinforcement for healthy food choices
- Providing a referral to a dietitian if needed

 ## CARE OF LGBTQ+ PATIENTS

The number of alternative family structures has risen in the last 40 years. Approximately 5.6% of Americans identify as lesbian, gay, bisexual, or transgender (Jones, 2021). Gestational parents and their partners have the same physical and educational needs as heterosexual women and their partners but have additional needs of acceptance and acknowledgment as a couple.

Assisted reproductive technology (ART) has opened up the possibility of pregnancy and motherhood to LGBTQ+ (lesbian, gay, bisexual, transgender, queer, + [all other gender identities and sexual orientations not yet defined]) couples by making available three main ways to get pregnant: through donor insemination, in vitro fertilization (IVF), or intrauterine insemination (IUI). Another option is known as reciprocal IVF. In reciprocal IVF, one partner's eggs are harvested and fertilized by an anonymous or known sperm donor, and then the embryo is placed into the hormonally prepared uterus of their partner. Although the baby will not share genetic material with both partners, egg sharing is a way for both partners to participate in the pregnancy (Villines, 2021).

Lesbians have historically faced obstacles to obtaining health care as well as stigma once they are in the health-care system (McCann et al., 2021). LGBTQ+ patients who have experienced discrimination may be fearful that communication with doctors, midwives, and nurses will be uncomfortable after revealing their sexual orientation. Even today, lesbians may be denied care and fertility assistance because of some health-care providers' personal beliefs (Scheitle & Platt, 2020).

Challenges faced by LGBTQ+ patients during pregnancy include the following:

- They may not receive the same education and assistance as other pregnant patients because caregivers are uncomfortable with providing physical care and emotional support.
- Caregivers may exclude or ignore the patient's partner during teaching sessions and examinations.
- Medical forms often only have spaces for "mother" and "father," not any other type of coparent or partner.
- Health-care providers may ask overly inquisitive questions regarding sexuality that are not related to caregiving (Scheitle & Platt, 2020).

You can provide culturally competent care for these patients and their partners by doing the following:

- Demonstrating an open-minded accepting attitude toward the couple
- Providing respectful care to the patient and their partner
- Using gender-neutral terms such as *parent* (instead of *mother*) and *partner* (instead of *spouse*). Even better is to ask the couple what terms they prefer you to use.
- Avoiding insensitive questions such as: "Where is the father?"; "Where did you get the sperm?"; "Won't it be confusing for your child to have two mothers?"
- Advocating for a change in the clinic and hospital forms for inclusivity of all individuals

CARE OF THE EXPECTANT WOMAN OLDER THAN AGE 35

Advanced maternal age for child bearing has been traditionally set at 35 years old, although the average age for a first pregnancy in the United States has been increasing in recent years (ACOG, 2022c). Some of the reasons women delay pregnancy are that they want to be in a stable relationship, they have fertility problems, or they want to be established in their careers. Advanced maternal age for child bearing is correlated with poorer outcomes in pregnancy. This may be because of a higher incidence of chronic medical conditions among older women (ACOG, 2022c).

Risks for Pregnancy in Patients Older Than Age 35

Women older than age 35 have an increased risk for pregnancy complications. These include the following:

- It may take longer for the woman older than age 35 to conceive. An older woman may not ovulate each month even if she is still having regular menstrual periods.
- Men older than age 45 have an increased risk of fathering children with neural tube defects, autism spectrum disorders, schizophrenia, and bipolar disorder (Carroll, 2021).
- The chance of having twins increases with age. ARTs such as IVF or fertility medications contribute to the risk of a multiple pregnancy.
- The risk of chromosome abnormalities is higher because of the aging of the eggs (ACOG, 2022c).
- There is an increased risk of miscarriage. This may be because of the higher likelihood of fetal chromosomal abnormalities.
- There is a higher risk for complications of pregnancy such as gestational diabetes, placenta previa, and high blood pressure.
- There is an increased risk for developing labor complications that may lead to a cesarean birth.

Despite the risks noted previously, women older than age 35 can and do have healthy pregnancies. You should be sensitive to the feelings and experiences of the older patient to meet her health-care educational needs and to provide emotional support. To improve pregnancy outcomes, a patient at an advanced maternal age should plan to do the following:

- Meet with a health-care provider for preconception counseling, especially if the mother-to-be has chronic health problems.
- Obtain early prenatal care and regular prenatal follow-up care.
- Receive education regarding testing for chromosomal abnormalities.
- Follow all prenatal care recommendations regarding nutrition, medications, and self-care as with any younger pregnant patient.

FOCUS ON THE FETUS

During pregnancy visits to the health-care provider, maternal and fetal well-being are monitored. Sometimes simple noninvasive tests are conducted to determine fetal well-being. If complications arise, more invasive tests may be ordered by the health-care provider to evaluate the health of the fetus. Table 7.3 provides information about tests that may be performed to determine fetal well-being.

Table 7.3

Tests Performed to Determine Fetal Well-Being

Fetal Measure	Procedure	Explanation	Nursing Care	Patient Teaching
Fundal height measurement	A tape measure is used to measure the distance from the symphysis pubis to the top of the fundus at each prenatal visit.	• Growth is expected at each visit to determine normal fetal growth.	N/A	When the fetus is growing appropriately, there will be an increase in fundal height at each prenatal visit.
Fetal kick counts	This count is done to monitor fetal well-being. The mother lies on her side and counts distinct fetal movements daily. After counting 10 movements, the count is discontinued.	• Ten fetal movements in 2 hours are considered reassuring for fetal well-being. • If fetal movements are decreased, the pregnant woman should eat, rest, and refocus on fetal movement. • Fewer than 10 movements in 2 hours should be reported to the health-care provider.	• Teach the pregnant woman how to do a fetal kick count. • Teach her when to report her findings to the health-care provider.	• The mother is to palpate and note fetal movement daily for 1 hour.
Amniocentesis	A thin needle is used to remove amniotic fluid and cells from the amniotic sac surrounding the fetus (see Fig. 6.6). Amniocentesis later in pregnancy can indicate fetal well-being, and the amniotic fluid will indicate whether the fetus is mature enough for delivery.	• Bilirubin levels can be obtained to determine whether the fetus is experiencing hemolytic disease. • Fluid can be cultured to determine whether infection is present. • Fetal lung maturity can be determined by testing the lecithin/sphingomyelin (L/S) ratio, phosphatidyl glycerol (PG), and lamellar body count (LBC). • L/S ratio greater than 2:1 indicates mature fetal lungs. • L/S ratio less than 2:1 indicates immature fetal lungs and risk for respiratory distress at birth. • Positive PG indicates mature fetal lungs. • Lamellar bodies present indicate fetal lung maturity.	• Explain the procedure to the woman. • Explain that the fetus will be monitored, and ultrasound guidance is used for needle placement. • Provide comfort and emotional support. • Label specimens and send to the laboratory for analysis. • Administer Rh-immune globulin (RhoGAM) to Rh-negative women after the procedure to decrease the risk of antibody formation.	• Report any decrease in fetal movement, bleeding, cramping, leaking of fluid, or fever to the health-care provider.
Nonstress test (NST)	This test is performed after 28 weeks to monitor for fetal distress. A fetal monitor is attached to the mother's abdomen, and the fetus is monitored for several minutes.	• For a fetus at greater than 32 weeks' gestation, the NST is considered reactive when the FHR increases 15 beats above baseline for 15 seconds twice in 20 minutes.	• Apply the fetal monitor. • Interpret the FHR and accelerations, and report to the health-care provider. • Provide comfort and emotional support.	• Explain the procedure. • Explain the interpretation and the need for follow-up tests if indicated.

Continued

Table 7.3

Tests Performed to Determine Fetal Well-Being—cont'd

Fetal Measure	Procedure	Explanation	Nursing Care	Patient Teaching
	Every time the woman perceives fetal movement, it is noted on the fetal monitor. A healthy fetal response is a rise in the heart rate with fetal movement.	• For a fetus at less than 32 weeks' gestation, accelerations of at least 10 beats per minute and lasting 10 seconds are considered reactive. • A nonreactive NST is a test without sufficient accelerations of heart rate with movement in 40 minutes of testing (ACOG, 2021c).		
Contraction stress test (CST)	The purpose is to evaluate the well-being of a fetus by observing the fetal response to the stress of contractions. An external fetal monitor is applied and IV oxytocin is administered until there are three uterine contractions in 10–20 minutes lasting 40 seconds or longer.	• The CST is considered negative or normal when there are no late or variable decelerations of FHR noted on the fetal monitor. A negative CST is associated with good fetal outcomes. • The CST is considered positive if there are late or variable decelerations of FHR with 50% of the contractions. Further testing with a biophysical profile is recommended.	• Apply the fetal monitor. • Start the IV access and safely administer the oxytocin. • Provide comfort and emotional support. • Monitor the patient throughout the procedure. • Report interpretation of the test to the healthcare provider.	• Explain the procedure. • Explain that the uterine contractions will not be severe and should stop when the test is over and the oxytocin is discontinued. • Teach the patient to report any increase in contractions or decrease in fetal movement after she returns home.
Amniotic fluid index (AFI)	Ultrasound is used to measure the depth of the pockets of amniotic fluid in four quadrants of the uterus. Amniotic fluid amount is based on fetal urine production, which depends upon fetal renal function. If the fetus is not obtaining enough oxygenation through the placenta, blood is shunted from the kidneys to other vital organs and, therefore, fetal urine is decreased.	• The average measurement of amniotic fluid pockets is greater than 2 cm and less than 8 cm per pocket (Lord et al., 2022). • Abnormal AFI is less than 5 cm total measurement and is called **oligohydramnios**, which is the state of low amniotic fluid. • Oligohydramnios is associated with poor fetal outcomes. • If the AFI is greater than 24 cm total measurements, it is considered to be **polyhydramnios**, which is excessive amniotic fluid. This condition is associated with congenital anomalies, such as neural tube defects and gastrointestinal defects.	• Explain the procedure to the patient. • Provide comfort and emotional support.	• This test is non-invasive and requires only that the patient lie quietly. • There are no needles involved and no risk to the fetus.

Table 7.3

Tests Performed to Determine Fetal Well-Being—cont'd

Fetal Measure	Procedure	Explanation	Nursing Care	Patient Teaching
		(See Chapter 10 for more about oligohydramnios and polyhydramnios.)		
Biophysical profile (BPP)	This test is done in the third trimester to monitor the overall health of the fetus. This test involves an abdominal ultrasound along with a stress test. The BPP monitors the fetal movement, breathing movements, heart rate, and the amount of amniotic fluid. The BPP test consists of an NST with an additional 30 minutes of ultrasound observation. A score of 0 (absent) to 2 (present) is given to each component of the test.	• One or more episodes of fetal breathing movements of 30 seconds or more within the 30 minutes of observation are expected. • Three or more body limb movements are expected in 30 minutes. • One or more fetal extremity extension with return to fetal flexion or an opening and closing of the hand is expected. • An amniotic fluid depth of 2 cm or more in two pockets of fluid perpendicular (at a 90° angle) is expected. • An overall score of 8–10 is reassuring of fetal well-being. • A score of 6 may indicate a need to deliver the fetus early, depending upon the gestational age. • Special training is required to interpret the results.	• Explain the procedure. • Apply the external fetal monitor.	• Explain any required follow-up and assist the patient to understand the results.
Group B streptococcus screen	This test is done at 36–37 weeks to screen for group B streptococcus, which can be a danger to the fetus. Group B streptococcus, also known as *group B strep,* is a common bacterium carried in the genital tract and intestines. It does not usually cause problems for adults, but a fetus could pick up the bacterium during delivery and become ill. The health-care provider swabs the mother's vagina and rectum during the third trimester and sends the samples to the laboratory.	• If the test is negative, no action is needed. • A positive strep B test requires antibiotics to be given during labor to decrease the risk of transmitting group B strep disease in the newborn.	• Administer IV antibiotics as ordered during labor if necessary.	• Explain the need for antibiotics to prevent disease in the newborn.

Nursing Care Plan for Health Promotion in Pregnancy

Cadence is 12 weeks pregnant with her first baby and arrives for her second prenatal appointment at the clinic. Cadence is concerned about gestational diabetes because she is slightly overweight with a BMI of 26 and reports that her mother and sister both had gestational diabetes when they were pregnant. Cadence admits that she does not exercise except for walking around at her job as a teacher and that she eats "whatever I want." Cadence is concerned about preventing gestational diabetes during her pregnancy.

Nursing Diagnosis: Insufficient knowledge of risk factors for gestational diabetes
Expected Outcome: Cadence will state an understanding of risk factors.

Intervention:	Rationale:
Teach Cadence that two major risk factors are excessive weight gain and inactivity.	*These are two risk factors that Cadence can control, and teaching will increase her awareness.*

Nursing Diagnosis: Sedentary lifestyle
Expected Outcome: Cadence will begin exercising at least four times a week for 30 minutes.

Interventions:	Rationale:
Assist Cadence to select a safe exercise for pregnancy, such as walking or swimming, that she would enjoy.	*She needs to participate in planning exercise so that she will want to follow through on the plan.*
Assist Cadence to look at her weekly schedule and schedule specific times to exercise for 30 minutes a day at least four times a week.	*She will be more likely to exercise if it is scheduled as part of her daily routine.*

Nursing Diagnosis: Inadequate nutrition
Expected Outcome: Cadence will select foods that are healthy for pregnancy.

Interventions:	Rationale:
Review with Cadence healthy pregnancy nutrition.	*Face-to-face teaching will enable Cadence to ask questions.*
Provide written instructions for nutrition for a healthy pregnancy.	*Patients need written materials to refer to after they leave the clinic.*
Ask the health-care provider about a referral to a dietitian for Cadence.	*A dietitian can help Cadence plan a healthy diet to promote fetal growth and to avoid excess weight gain, which is a risk factor for gestational diabetes.*

Learn to C.U.S.

You are preparing a woman for a nonstress test (NST) in the labor and delivery unit. The patient is at 36 weeks' gestation. The woman states, "The baby doesn't move around as much as he did a week or so ago." During the NST, you note that the fetal heart rate (FHR) only accelerates for 10 seconds, and there is minimal fetal movement. You call the health-care provider using the C.U.S. method of communication.

C.: Hello, doctor. I am *concerned* about the patient's NST today.

U.: I am *uncomfortable* because it was not entirely normal.

S: I wanted to notify you as soon as possible because I feel that we have a patient *safety* issue.

Labs & Diagnostics

The CDC recommends that all pregnant women be screened for group B streptococcus (GBS) at 35 to 37 weeks' gestation. Rapid GBS test kits can provide results within minutes on vaginal or rectal fluid swab specimens submitted in a sterile redtop tube. Optimally, a specimen should be sent for culture *before* any antibiotics are started (Van Leeuwen & Bladh, 2021).

 FOCUS ON THE GROWING FAMILY

In the months leading up to the birth, many couples prepare by attending childbirth classes and by developing a birth plan. There are a variety of childbirth classes available and many options for childbirth that the woman and her partner can consider.

This section highlights common childbirth preparation methods and choices available when planning a birth. The patient should be encouraged to discuss her birth plan with her family, health-care providers, and the nurses providing labor care.

Childbirth Preparation

Many first-time parents prepare for the upcoming birth by attending childbirth preparation classes. Most of these classes begin at approximately 30 to 32 weeks' gestation, and a variety of classes are available. The two most popular are Lamaze techniques and the Bradley method of childbirth preparation. Childbirth educators should be certified by a national organization such as Lamaze International, Childbirth Educator Certification Program (offered by the International Childbirth Education Association [ICEA]), or the Bradley method certification through American Academy of Husband-Coached Childbirth (AAHCC). The classes are usually taken with a partner, friend, or relative to be the birth coach and assist the woman throughout her labor (Fig. 7.3).

Lamaze

Lamaze classes are the most widely used childbirth preparation classes in the United States. This method is named after the French obstetrician Fernand Lamaze and was introduced in the United States in the 1950s. The method provides women with techniques to assist them with coping with the pain of labor. It centers on breathing patterns with a focal point and relaxation techniques that conserve energy for the pushing stage of labor. The Lamaze method does not support or discourage medications in labor but views medications as an option if needed. Lamaze classes educate the mother-to-be and her partner on the birth process and options available for managing the pain and making decisions during the labor and delivery process.

The Bradley Method

The Bradley method was developed by obstetrician Dr. Robert Bradley and popularized by his book *Husband-Coached Childbirth*, published in 1965. The Bradley method prepares the woman to deliver without medications or unnecessary medical interventions. It also prepares the husband to coach his wife through the birth experience. The Bradley method

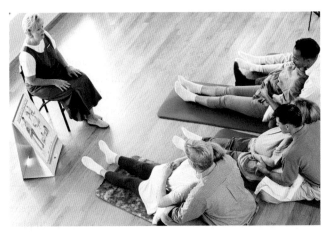

FIGURE 7.3 Childbirth education classes help to prepare the expectant couple for many aspects of the childbearing year.

does not emphasize breathing techniques; instead, its focus is on muscle control. Muscle tension increases the pain of labor, and active relaxation during labor reduces pain.

Childbirth Class Topics

Topics typically covered in childbirth classes include the following:

- Normal labor, birth, and postpartum care
- Relaxation techniques
- Breathing techniques
- Comfort measures during labor
- Medical procedures that may become necessary during labor and/or delivery
- Breastfeeding
- Tour of the hospital labor and delivery unit
- Developing a birth plan

Birth Plan

Some women choose to develop a birth plan to communicate their desires for the labor and delivery with their health-care provider and the labor and delivery nurses. A birth plan may be very detailed, or it may be brief. Some topics typically included in a birth plan are provided in Table 7.4.

Table 7.4
Birth Planning

Topics Related to Birth Planning	Items to Consider in Birth Planning
Before labor or early labor	• Induction preferences • Laboring at home • Hospital admittance
Induction of labor	• Timing of the induction • Choice of induction techniques
Environment during labor	• Birthing bed or chair • Music and television • Shower and birthing tub • Comfort measures
Medical interventions	• Fetal monitoring • Epidural • IV access and/or fluids • Vaginal examinations
Second stage of labor	• Pushing positions • Pushing methods
Delivery	• Inclusion of family and friends • Episiotomy • Cord cutting • Placenta delivery
The newborn	• Medications • Initiating breastfeeding • Separation from the mother

Key Points

- A nurse can provide anticipatory guidance for managing physical discomforts because of the hormonal and physiological changes of pregnancy.
- The patient should be educated on self-care during pregnancy to promote a safe, healthy pregnancy.
- Infections are major causes of morbidity and mortality in pregnancy. You should be aware of common infections and teach the patient methods to avoid the infectious agents.
- Healthy nutrition and appropriate weight gain in pregnancy promote optimal health for the fetus and mother-to-be.
- Pregnant adolescents have additional nutritional needs because of their own growth and development.

- The developmental needs of the pregnant adolescent must be considered when planning care during pregnancy.
- Nurses need to demonstrate culturally competent, patient-centered care for their LGBTQ+ patients and their partners.
- There are pregnancy risks for women older than age 35, but a healthy pregnancy and fetus are possible.
- There are many tests outlined in the chapter that are available to monitor fetal well-being during pregnancy.
- The Bradley method and Lamaze method are two childbirth education programs that assist pregnant couples to prepare for childbirth.
- Some women prepare a birth plan to communicate their desires for labor and delivery.

Review Questions

1. The pregnant patient states that she has a low iron level. Which foods can you suggest to increase patient dietary intake of iron? (**Select all that apply.**)
   1. Milk
   2. Spinach
   3. Beef steak
   4. Carrots
   5. Kale
   6. White bread

2. Which statement made by the patient indicates understanding of the amniocentesis procedure?
   1. "I will need to avoid food and water for 8 hours before the procedure."
   2. "The test is only done in the third trimester."
   3. "A long needle is placed through my abdomen to obtain amniotic fluid."
   4. "The procedure requires 48 hours of bedrest afterward."

3. Which statement made by a pregnant adolescent indicates that more teaching is needed regarding her understanding of pregnancy nutrition?
   1. "I should eat at least 300 additional calories a day and eat from all food groups."
   2. "I can drink diet soft drinks because they have no calories."
   3. "I can make healthy food choices at a fast-food restaurant."
   4. "I need extra calcium for my bones and for fetal development."

4. Which risks of pregnancy do women face over the age of 35? (**Select all that apply.**)
   1. Miscarriage
   2. Twins
   3. Leg cramps
   4. Anemia
   5. Gestational diabetes
   6. Cesarean birth

5. Which conditions does a biophysical profile of the fetus evaluate? (**Select all that apply.**)
   1. Fetal movement
   2. Fetal position
   3. Placenta location
   4. FHR
   5. Fetal breathing movements
   6. Amount of amniotic fluid
   7. Cervical changes

6. You are preparing to teach a class of pregnant women about seatbelt use during pregnancy. You should include which statement in the discussion?
   1. "The shoulder belt is not safe; just use the lap belt."
   2. "Place the lap portion of the belt low across the abdomen and hipbones."
   3. "The abdomen should be 5 inches from the steering wheel."
   4. "Loosen the seatbelt so that it will not be too tight."

7. To prevent venous thrombosis formation during travel, which precaution should the pregnant woman take? **(Select all that apply.)**
1. Change position frequently.
2. Walk around every 2 hours.
3. Restrict fluid intake.
4. Take aspirin daily.
5. Elevate the legs whenever possible.

8. What patient teaching should be given to decrease the risk of a pregnant woman developing hemorrhoids?
1. Use a laxative daily.
2. Increase fiber intake.
3. Decrease fluid intake.
4. Decrease exercise.

ANSWERS 1. 2, 3, 5; 2. 3; 3. 2, 4; 4. 1, 2, 5, 6; 5. 1, 4, 5, 6; 6. 2; 7. 1, 2, 5; 8. 2

CRITICAL THINKING QUESTION

1. Allison is 15 years old and pregnant with her first baby. She is 8 weeks' pregnant and voicing concern about gaining too much weight in the pregnancy. What approach can you use to educate Allison about nutrition and weight gain in pregnancy?

Resources

For additional resources and information, including Postconference Questions and Activities, Answers, and References, visit www.FADavis.com.

 Student Study Guide

CHAPTER 8

Nursing Care of the Woman With Complications During Pregnancy

KEY TERMS

abortion (uh-BOR-shun)

cerclage (ser-KLAZH)

cervical incompetence (SER-vih-kuhl in-KOM-puh-tents)

choriocarcinoma (KOH-ree-oh-KAR-sih-NOH-muh)

dilation and curettage (D&C) (dye-LAY-shun and koo-ruh-TAZH)

eclampsia (ek-LAMP-see-uh)

ectopic pregnancy (ek-TOP-ik PREG-nuhn-see)

elective abortion (uh-LEK-tuhv uh-BOR-shun)

hydatidiform mole (HYE-duh-TID-uh-FORM MOHL)

hyperemesis gravidarum (HYE-per-EM-uh-siss gra-vih-DA-ruhm)

hypofibrinogenemia (HYE-poh-fye-BRIN-oh-juh-NEE-mee-uh)

hysterectomy (HISS-teh-REK-to-mee)

insulin resistance (IN-suh-lin rih-ZISS-tents)

isoimmunization (EYE-so-IM-yoo-nih-ZAY-shun)

ketones (KEE-tohnz)

perfusion (per-FYOO-zhun)

placenta abruptio (pla-SEN-tuh ab-RUP-shee-oh)

placenta accreta (pla-SEN-tuh ak-REE-tuh)

placenta previa (pla-SEN-tuh PREE-vee-uh)

preeclampsia (PRE-ek-LAMP-see-uh)

salpingectomy (sal-pin-JEK-tuh-mee)

salpingostomy (sal-ping-OSS-toh-mee)

threatened abortions (THRET-uhnd uh-BOR-shun)

viable (VYE-uh-buhl)

CHAPTER CONCEPTS

Communication
Grief and Loss
Health Promotion
Perfusion
Self-Care

LEARNING OUTCOMES

1. Define the key terms.
2. Discuss the nursing care of a patient experiencing hyperemesis gravidarum.
3. Identify bleeding complications of early and late pregnancy.
4. Recognize signs of complications following a spontaneous abortion.
5. Discuss the nursing care for the patient following a ruptured ectopic pregnancy.
6. Compare and contrast the abnormalities of placenta abruptio, placenta accreta, and placenta previa.
7. Define *hydatidiform mole* and explain usual medical treatment and nursing care.
8. Provide safe and effective nursing care for patients experiencing a placental abnormality such as placenta abruptio, placenta accreta, or placenta previa.
9. Identify signs of hypovolemic shock caused by blood loss from bleeding complications of pregnancy.
10. Discuss the medical interventions and nursing care for the patient with an incompetent cervix.
11. Summarize the management of patients with Rh incompatibility.
12. Develop a plan of care for women with multiple gestation pregnancy.
13. Develop a plan of care for a patient experiencing pregnancy-related hypertensive disorders.
14. Outline the nurse's role in assessment, managing care, and patient teaching for a patient with gestational diabetes.

CRITICAL THINKING & CLINICAL JUDGMENT

Scenario #1: **Tonya** is a 30-year-old patient, pregnant with her first baby. She is in gestational week 41 and has had no previous complications during her pregnancy. Tonya arrives in the labor and delivery unit experiencing severe abdominal pain and vaginal bleeding. As you assist her into bed, Tonya says: "I used cocaine this afternoon. I haven't used drugs my entire pregnancy, but because it was my birthday and I was overdue, I used the cocaine. I thought the only risk to using drugs was during the first trimester. Did I cause this bleeding? Is my baby in danger?"

Continued

CRITICAL THINKING & CLINICAL JUDGMENT—cont'd

Questions

1. Why is Tonya having severe abdominal pain and bleeding?
2. What nursing interventions are appropriate for this situation?
3. How would you answer Tonya's questions of "Did I cause this bleeding? Is my baby in danger?"

CONCEPTUAL CORNERSTONE
Self-Care

An aspect of self-care is *adherence,* which can be defined as the extent to which a patient follows the health-care provider's instructions for prescribed treatments to promote health or to manage a condition (Giddens, 2021). Nurses have an opportunity to work with patients undergoing life-changing events such as pregnancy. When working with a pregnant patient, you have the chance to educate the patient about preventive health-care measures to promote a safe and healthy pregnancy.

When a patient experiences pregnancy complications such as the conditions discussed in this chapter, you can reinforce the treatment plan of the health-care provider and suggest actions to improve the chance of a good outcome for the patient and her fetus. Nurses play a major role in assisting patients to accept and maintain needed changes during a crisis such as a complicated pregnancy. While planning patient-centered care, nurses should recognize that the patient's willingness and ability to adhere to a treatment plan is influenced by the patient's own personal experiences, attitudes, motivation, and culture.

Complications can occur during pregnancy that threaten the fetus and the expectant mother. This chapter discusses the care of the woman with complications of hyperemesis gravidarum, bleeding disorders of early and late pregnancy, maternal-fetal blood incompatibility, hypertensive disorders of pregnancy, and gestational diabetes.

CARE OF THE WOMAN WITH HYPEREMESIS GRAVIDARUM

Nausea and vomiting, also known as *morning sickness,* are common during the first trimester of pregnancy for many women. **Hyperemesis gravidarum**, however, is a more severe form of morning sickness that persists past 20 weeks' gestation. It is characterized by severe nausea and vomiting along with ketosis and weight loss (greater than 5% of prepregnancy weight). This condition may cause dehydration, electrolyte and acid-base imbalances, nutritional deficiencies, and even death.

Incidence and Risk Factors

Hyperemesis gravidarum occurs in 0.3% to 2% of all pregnancies (Ogunyemi, 2022). The cause is unknown, but there are several theories as to why some women experience this condition. Women who experience hyperemesis often have high human chorionic gonadotropin (hCG) levels that cause short-lived hyperthyroidism. The hormone hCG can physiologically stimulate the thyroid gland's thyroid-stimulating hormone (TSH) receptor. There is a positive correlation between the serum hCG elevation level and free T4 levels. The severity of nausea appears to be related to the degree of thyroid stimulation. The hormone hCG may not independently be the cause of hyperemesis gravidarum but may be indirectly involved by its ability to stimulate the thyroid (Ogunyemi, 2022).

Some studies link high estradiol levels to the severity of nausea and vomiting in pregnant patients. Previous intolerance to oral contraceptives is associated with nausea and vomiting in pregnancy. Also believed to contribute to this condition is the hormone progesterone. Progesterone peaks in the first trimester, which can cause the relaxation of smooth muscle, resulting in delayed gastric emptying (Ogunyemi, 2022).

Hyperemesis can cause problems for both the mother and fetus. Women with hyperemesis gravidarum in the second trimester have an increased risk for preterm labor, preeclampsia (an increase in blood pressure, protein in the urine, and edema), and placental abruption. For the fetus, the dehydration that occurs may lead to poor placental perfusion and inadequate oxygenation. Fetal growth can be compromised, leading to an infant who is small for gestational age (Smith, 2022).

Signs and Symptoms

Signs and symptoms of hyperemesis gravidarum include the following (Rosenberger et al., 2023):

- Vomiting multiple times throughout the day
- Poor appetite
- Weight loss (greater than 5% of prepregnancy weight)
- Dehydration
  - Dry mouth and skin
  - Poor skin turgor
  - Concentrated urine
  - Decreased urine output
  - Elevated heart rate
  - Alkalosis from loss of hydrochloric acid

Medical Care

Most care may be provided at home, but some women will require outpatient treatment or hospitalization for IV fluid

---

· WORD · BUILDING ·

hyperemesis gravidarum: hyper–excessive + emesis–vomiting + gravidarum–of pregnancy

administration and antiemetics. Research studies have determined that acupuncture and acupressure are effective for some women as modes of treatment to avoid the use of medications in the critical first trimester of pregnancy. Initial management is usually conservative and may include the following:

- Vitamin B_6 10 to 25 mg three times daily
- Doxylamine 12.5 mg three to four times daily
- Ginger capsules 250 mg four times daily

If the nausea and vomiting are severe, the following medications may be prescribed next:

- Metoclopramide 5 to 10 mg every 8 hours
- Promethazine 12.5 mg oral or rectal every 4 hours
- Dimenhydrinate 50 to100 mg every 4 to 6 hours
- Ondansetron 4 to 8 mg orally or IV every 8 hours (Smith, 2022)

In severe cases, the health-care provider will also investigate other possible causes of nausea and vomiting, such as gastroenteritis, pancreatitis, hepatitis, ulcers, and kidney disorders.

　The health-care provider may order the following laboratory studies to monitor the patient's health status:

- Complete blood cell count (CBC) to monitor for signs of infection and dehydration
- Electrolytes to monitor for imbalances caused by dehydration
- **Ketones** to monitor the use of fat stores to provide energy to the mother and her fetus
- Liver enzymes to monitor liver inflammation

Nursing Care

Nursing care of the patient with hyperemesis gravidarum includes the following:

- Administering IV fluids and antiemetics
- Monitoring laboratory results and reporting any abnormalities to the health-care provider
- Monitoring for weight loss
- Providing for psychosocial needs by referral to appropriate resources and by allowing time to therapeutically listen to the patient's concerns

Patient Teaching

Teach patients with hyperemesis gravidarum to do the following:

- Eat small, frequent meals.
- Avoid spicy and fatty foods.
- Identify and avoid odors or foods that may trigger nausea.
- Maintain fluid intake by sipping throughout the day to avoid dehydration.

- Monitor for signs of dehydration. Teach the patient these signs if she does not already know them.
- Notify her health-care provider if she notices any of the following warning signs:
  - Dark urine
  - Bloody vomitus
  - Abdominal pain
  - Dehydration
  - Lack of urine output for 8 hours
  - Inability to keep food down for 24 hours
  - Ketones in the urine (Instruct the patient on use of urine dipsticks to monitor for ketones at home.)

Therapeutic Communication

Nonadherence

Margarita is a primigravida patient who had her initial prenatal appointment with the nurse midwife at 8 weeks of gestation but has missed her appointments since that time. Now, she is at 22 weeks of gestation, and the nurse midwife calls to discuss the missed prenatal appointments. In this situation, the communication approach by the nurse midwife should not shame or scold Margarita for missing her prenatal visits.

Nurse Midwife: "Hello, Margarita, we would like to schedule a prenatal appointment with you. We haven't seen you for a while."

Margarita: "Well, I didn't really need an appointment. I have been feeling fine."

Nurse Midwife: "Sometimes pregnant women have questions that we can answer during your appointment."

Margarita: "My grandmother has answered my questions. I am really doing fine."

Nurse Midwife: "Could we make an appointment just to check that everything is progressing well with the pregnancy and your baby? We can also talk about future appointments at that time."

Margarita: "Sure, let me check my work schedule."

 CARE OF THE WOMAN WITH BLEEDING DISORDERS OF EARLY PREGNANCY

Bleeding during pregnancy is always abnormal and, especially in the first trimester, threatens the viability of the pregnancy. Bleeding disorders of early pregnancy include spontaneous abortion, ectopic pregnancy, and gestational trophoblastic disease (GTD).

Abortion

The term *abortion* is used to describe a pregnancy loss or termination before the fetus is viable. The term *viable* describes a fetus that is able to live outside the uterus. Medically, *fetus viability* is defined as attaining an age greater than

20 weeks of gestation or a fetal weight greater than 500 g (Venes, 2021). See Chapter 10 for more information about pregnancy loss.

Incidence and Risk Factors

Spontaneous abortion, also known as *miscarriage,* is the most common type of pregnancy loss. It occurs in up to 20% of all clinically recognized pregnancies (Rosenberger et al., 2023). A spontaneous abortion can be caused by chromosomal abnormalities of the fetus, uncontrolled diabetes, hypothyroidism, maternal infection, reproductive abnormalities, moderate to high alcohol consumption, cocaine use, or maternal injury. Spontaneous abortions are classified according to symptoms and the outcome (Rosenberger et al., 2023):

- **Threatened abortions** are diagnosed when vaginal bleeding occurs, possibly accompanied by abdominal cramping. The woman may or may not lose the fetus.
- Inevitable abortions happen when the cervix dilates and the amniotic membranes rupture. The fetus and placenta are expelled unless a health-care provider intervenes.
- Incomplete abortions occur when some of the uterine contents of pregnancy are expelled but not all. This retention of products of conception leads to uterine bleeding and cramping.
- Complete abortions occur when all uterine contents are expelled. When this occurs, uterine cramping and bleeding stops without interventions.
- Missed abortions occur when the fetus dies during the first half of the pregnancy. The fetus is not expelled, and the woman carries the fetus until spontaneous abortion occurs or the products of conception are removed by the health-care provider.

Signs and Symptoms

The signs and symptoms of a spontaneous abortion include lower abdominal cramping and vaginal bleeding. These symptoms can also occur with other early pregnancy complications; therefore, a thorough history, physical examination, ultrasonography, and serum hCG testing should be completed before treatment begins.

Medical Care

A complete spontaneous abortion usually needs no additional treatment, medically or surgically. If the woman suspects that she has had a spontaneous abortion, she should contact her health-care provider. After an examination, the patient can return home unless there are concerns about excessive bleeding or infection. If bleeding does not stop after a spontaneous abortion, a **dilation and curettage (D&C)** may be necessary. A D&C is a surgical procedure in which the cervix is dilated and the physician gently scrapes the lining of the uterus to remove the products of conception. Another common procedure is vacuum extraction, in which a cannula is attached to a suction device to remove the products of conception. These procedures will usually stop the bleeding. Some patients may require medications such as oxytocin or methylergonovine to control bleeding. These medications cause uterine contraction and therefore slow uterine bleeding.

If the patient has a missed, incomplete, or inevitable abortion present before 13 weeks' gestation, the standard therapy has traditionally been vacuum D&C. The advantage of a suction D&C is that the procedure is scheduled and occurs at a known time. The risks of a D&C include bleeding, infection, and possible perforation of the uterus.

Medical management can be considered in women without infection, hemorrhage, severe anemia, or bleeding disorders (Alves & Rapp, 2022). Therapy with misoprostol and mifepristone is an acceptable alternative to D&C for most women. The advantage of medical therapy is that no surgical procedures are needed if it is successful.

A dose of mifepristone (200 mg orally) is given to the woman 24 hours before treatment with misoprostol. Then, an initial dose of misoprostol 800 mcg (4 tab 200 mcg placed vaginally) is given. Prescriptions for pain medication should be provided to the patient. The patient is reevaluated on day three. If expulsion of the products of conception has not occurred, then a second dose of 800 mcg of misoprostol is placed vaginally. Passage of tissue should happen within a few days of receiving medical therapy. If it is not successful, then a surgical approach may follow. The risks for medical therapy include bleeding, infection, possible incomplete abortion, and possible failure of the medication to work (Alves & Rapp, 2022).

Nursing Care

Nursing care of the patient who has experienced a fetal loss in the first half of pregnancy may include the following:

- Monitoring vital signs, intake and output, oxygen saturation, and laboratory test results
- Recognizing the signs of hypovolemic shock, which include decreased blood pressure, increased heart rate, clammy skin, lightheadedness, and confusion
- Anticipating the need for IV fluids and oxygen therapy
- Administering medications, such as oxytocin or methylergonovine, ordered by the health-care provider to control bleeding
- Possibly alerting the laboratory to blood type; crossmatching the patient for a possible blood transfusion
- Administering Rho(D) immune globulin (RhoGAM) to an Rh-negative woman within 72 hours to prevent isoimmunization
- Assisting the patient to discuss her feelings of loss; some patients have feelings of guilt and need an opportunity to ask questions and talk about the experience

Patient Teaching

Teach the patient who has had a planned, a spontaneous, or an elective (Box 8.1) abortion the following information:

- Warning signs of complications after a D&C or administration of misoprostol. The following warning signs should be reported to the health-care provider:
  - Heavy, bright-red bleeding
  - Foul-smelling vaginal discharge

Elective Abortion

An **elective abortion** is performed when a woman chooses to terminate a pregnancy. In early pregnancy, elective abortions are accomplished by a medical approach with a combination of mifepristone and misoprostol or prostaglandin administered vaginally or orally. A surgical approach may be required if the medical approach is not successful or the pregnancy is more advanced (Casey, 2022). Medical care, nursing care, and patient teaching will all be similar to those presented previously.

- Fever
- Pelvic pain
- Do not resume sexual activity or use of tampons or douches for at least 2 weeks or until advised by the health-care provider (Rosenberger et al., 2023).
- If there was significant blood loss, take iron supplements with orange juice between meals for maximum absorption.
- Add liver, green leafy vegetables, and eggs to the diet to increase dietary iron.
- It is normal to go through a grieving process that may last 6 to 12 months.
- The body needs to rest and recover before attempting another pregnancy. Customary advice is to wait for two to three menstrual cycles. Have the woman discuss when to attempt another pregnancy with her health-care provider (Rosenberger et al., 2023).

Ectopic Pregnancy

An **ectopic pregnancy** occurs when the fertilized ovum implants outside the uterus. Most ectopic pregnancies occur in the fallopian tubes, but they can occur anywhere outside the uterus (Fig. 8.1).

Incidence and Risk Factors

Ectopic pregnancies occur in 1 out of 40 pregnancies (Sepilian, 2022). Risk factors for ectopic pregnancies include scarring of the fallopian tubes or blocks in the tubes, which can slow down the movement of the fertilized ovum; advanced maternal age; reproductive anomalies; a history of fallopian tube surgery; a history of pelvic inflammatory disease (PID); repeated induced abortions; repeated sexually transmitted infections (STIs); use of intrauterine devices (IUD); a history of assisted reproductive technology (ART); regular douching; and smoking (Sepilian, 2022).

Signs and Symptoms

Signs and symptoms of ectopic pregnancy include vaginal bleeding and abdominal pain.

If the fallopian tube ruptures, the following additional symptoms may occur:

- Severe abdominal pain
- Shoulder or neck pain from blood leaking out of the fallopian tube into the abdomen and irritating the diaphragm
- Weakness
- Dizziness
- Decreased blood pressure
- Increased heart rate

Medication Facts

Methotrexate

If methotrexate is used to treat an ectopic pregnancy, the patient should avoid foods high in folic acid, such as leafy green vegetables, orange juice, beans, enriched bread or pasta, and vitamins with folic acid. Also, the patient should not consume alcohol. These can all decrease the effectiveness of methotrexate.

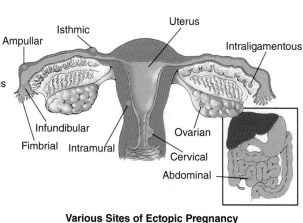

Actual Ectopic Pregnancy

Various Sites of Ectopic Pregnancy

FIGURE 8.1 Various sites of ectopic pregnancy implantation.

• **WORD** · **BUILDING** ·

ectopic: ec–out of + top–place + ic–pertaining to

Medical Care

If the fallopian tube has not ruptured, methotrexate may be administered. Methotrexate is an **antineoplastic** medication, as well as a folic acid antagonist that interferes with DNA synthesis. Methotrexate interferes with cell division. It causes the embryo to stop growing and reduces the chance of fallopian tube rupture. Certain criteria must exist to use this medication: The fetus must be fewer than 3.5 cm long and lack cardiac activity, and the patient must be stable hemodynamically. That means that her blood pressure and pulse rate are stable, indicating that no active bleeding is occurring, and she does not have anemia, thrombocytopenia, or leukopenia (Sepilian, 2022).

If the fallopian tube has ruptured, laparoscopic surgery is performed to save the tube. A **salpingostomy** is a small linear incision made into the fallopian tube to remove the products of conception. The tube is allowed to heal without suture to prevent scarring (Jazayeri, 2021). If the fallopian tube cannot be saved or the patient does not desire a future pregnancy, the tube may be removed by a laparoscopic salpingectomy. A **salpingectomy** is surgical removal of the fallopian tube.

Nursing Care

Nursing care of the patient who has an ectopic pregnancy includes the following:

- Administering methotrexate if ordered
- Monitoring the patient for signs of hypovolemic shock caused by hemorrhage:
  - Decreased blood pressure
  - Increased heart rate
  - Restlessness
  - Confusion
- If the patient undergoes a salpingostomy or salpingectomy, monitoring postoperative vital signs, oxygen saturation, intake and output, and vaginal bleeding according to institutional policies
- Assessing and controlling pain
- Administering RhoGAM to Rh-negative women within 72 hours to prevent isoimmunization
- Assisting the patient with emotions such as anger, sadness, or guilt, which are a part of coping with pregnancy loss

Patient Teaching

Teach the patient who has had an ectopic pregnancy the following:

- Notify the health-care provider if fever, chills, or significant bleeding occurs.
- If methotrexate was administered, anticipate nausea and vomiting, which are common.

- Grieving after a pregnancy loss is normal and may last for 6 to 12 months.
- Have the woman discuss the timing of another pregnancy attempt with her health-care provider.

Gestational Trophoblastic Disease

GTD includes several disease processes involving rare tumors that begin in the uterus during placental development. Hydatidiform mole is the most common of the GTDs and occurs at the extremes of the reproductive years. That is, women in their early teens and women in perimenopause are at most risk. A **hydatidiform mole** or molar pregnancy is a rare type of tumor that occurs during very early placental attachment and embryonic development. The trophoblast cells, which would normally attach the embryo to the uterine wall, develop abnormally. The abnormal development causes the placenta, but not the fetus, to grow and develop. The chorionic villi of the placenta swell, forming fluid-filled sacs. The sacs resemble tiny clusters of grapes inside the uterus. The fluid-filled villi may grow large enough to fill the uterus to the size of an advanced pregnancy (Fig. 8.2).

The molar pregnancy is classified as complete or partial. A complete molar pregnancy completely fills the uterus. A complete hydatidiform mole most commonly develops when two sperm fertilize an egg cell that has no DNA. Therefore, all the genetic material comes from the sperm, so no fetus can develop. In a partial molar pregnancy, two sperm fertilize a normal egg, and some fetal tissue develops. An amniotic sac is present along with the fluid-filled sacs of the hydatidiform mole, but no viable fetus exists (Ghassemzadeh et al., 2022).

Incidence and Risk Factors

Hydatidiform pregnancies occur in 1 out of 1,200 pregnancies in the United States and Europe (Moore, 2021). Women of Asian descent, of advanced maternal age, or who have had a previous molar pregnancy are at an increased risk of having a molar pregnancy.

Signs and Symptoms

Signs and symptoms of hydatidiform mole are as follows:

- Light-to-heavy bleeding with blood that may be brown or bright red

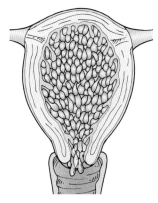

FIGURE 8.2 Hydatidiform mole, in which the chorionic villi break down into fluid-filled clusters inside the uterus.

• WORD • BUILDING •

antineoplastic: anti–against + neo–new + plastic–growth
salpingostomy: salping–stem or tube + ostomy–surgical opening
salpingectomy: salping–stem or tube + ectomy–surgical excision

- Uterine growth that is larger than expected for gestational age
- Absent fetal heart tones and movement
- Serum hCG levels that may be as high as 100,000 mIU/mL, which indicates extremely rapid trophoblastic growth (Moore, 2021)
- Hyperemesis caused by high levels of hCG
- Gestational hypertension

Medical Care

The preferred method of treating or removing the molar pregnancy is suction evacuation and curettage. The abnormal tissues are removed by vacuum aspiration or by surgical curettage to entirely empty the uterus. Hemorrhage is a frequent complication after the evacuation of a molar pregnancy (Moore, 2021). IV oxytocin is then administered after the procedure to contract the uterus and prevent hemorrhage.

A possible complication of a molar pregnancy is a **choriocarcinoma**, a fast-growing cancer that can develop in the uterus following a molar pregnancy. This type of cancer develops from germ cells, which are cells that ordinarily turn into sperm or eggs. Choriocarcinomas resemble the cells that surround an embryo in the uterus. Upon diagnosis of a hydatidiform mole, a chest x-ray should be ordered to establish a baseline for future monitoring because the lungs are the primary site of metastases of choriocarcinoma (Ghassemzadeh et al., 2022). To monitor for malignancies, the patient will need follow-up care with serially monitored hCG levels for 9 to 12 months and must avoid pregnancy during this time. Gestational trophoblastic malignancies are almost 100% curable; however, pregnancy makes it difficult to monitor for abnormalities.

Nursing Care

Nursing care of the patient who has had a hydatidiform mole includes the following:

- Monitoring for signs and symptoms of shock:
  - Decreased blood pressure
  - Increased heart rate
  - Restlessness
  - Confusion
- Ensuring preoperative patient preparation:
  - CBC
  - Blood type and crossmatching
- Administering RhoGAM to Rh-negative women to prevent isoimmunization
- Monitoring postoperative vital signs, oxygen saturation, intake and output, and vaginal bleeding according to institutional policies
- Supporting the patient in her reaction to grief and loss
- Emphasizing the importance of consistent follow-up; there is a small, but real, risk of developing malignant disease (Moore, 2021)

- WORD · BUILDING ·

choriocarcinoma: chorio–chorion + carcin–cancer + oma–tumor

Patient Teaching

Teach the patient who has had a hydatidiform mole the following:

- Report to her health-care provider if she experiences any of the following signs and symptoms of complications:
  - Excessive bleeding
  - Foul-smelling vaginal discharge
  - Fever
- Avoid tampons, douches, and sexual activity until the health-care provider indicates that it is safe to resume these activities.
- Regular follow-up appointments are essential to monitor serum hCG levels because of the risk of choriocarcinoma.
- Delay another pregnancy for at least 6 months to monitor the hCG levels without the interference of hCG from pregnancy (Moore, 2021).
- It is normal to go through a grieving process that may last 6 to 12 months.
- Ensure that future pregnancies are monitored by early sonographic evaluation because of the increased risk of the recurrence of hydatidiform mole.

CONCEPTUAL CORNERSTONE
Perfusion

Concepts integrate thinking and assist with transferring knowledge from one patient problem to another patient with a similar condition. The concept of perfusion is applicable in this chapter because of the complications of pregnancy that may result in blood loss. **Perfusion** is blood circulating through the body and oxygenating the tissues. Impaired central perfusion occurs in conditions that decrease cardiac output or cause shock. If adequately oxygenated blood cannot freely travel to all parts of the body, a state of inadequate tissue perfusion exists. The bleeding disorders of pregnancy all relate to the concept of perfusion. Regardless of the cause of poor perfusion, whether it is caused by blood loss from a spontaneous abortion, placenta previa, or placental abruption, the basic nursing care is similar. Immediate nursing interventions include monitoring vital signs, noting capillary refill time, noting peripheral pulses, inspecting perineal pads, noting the color and amount of blood, and administering IV fluids and blood products as ordered by the health-care provider.

 ### CARE OF THE WOMAN WITH BLEEDING DISORDERS OF LATE PREGNANCY

Bleeding in late pregnancy can be a potential emergency because it usually indicates placenta attachment problems, which cause the fetus not to receive sufficient oxygen or nourishment. Bleeding disorders of late pregnancy include placenta previa, placenta abruptio, and placenta accreta.

Placenta Previa

Placenta previa is a placenta that is implanted near the opening of the cervix. As the pregnancy nears term and the cervix begins to dilate, bleeding occurs because the placenta is becoming detached from the uterus. This bleeding puts the fetus at risk because the placenta supplies oxygen to it until the baby begins to breathe.

There are different forms of placenta previa (Fig. 8.3):

1. *Marginal:* The placenta is next to the cervix but does not cover the opening.
2. *Partial:* The placenta covers part of the cervical opening.
3. *Complete:* The placenta covers all of the cervical opening.

Incidence and Risk Factors

Placenta previa occurs in 0.5% of all pregnancies. The risks increase 1.5 to 5 times with a history of cesarean birth (Anderson-Bagga & Sze, 2022). There are several risk factors for placenta previa:

- Previous cesarean delivery
- Cocaine use
- Previous placenta previa
- Uterine scarring from endometriosis
- Previous spontaneous abortion
- Short pregnancy interval
- Previous uterine surgery
- Previous or recurrent abortions

- NonWhite ethnicity
- Smoking
  (Lockwood & Russo-Stieglitz, 2022)

Signs and Symptoms

The characteristic symptom of placenta previa is painless, bright-red bleeding. Spotting may occur throughout the second and third trimesters. Painless hemorrhaging may occur in late pregnancy or when labor begins.

Medical Care

Placenta previa can be diagnosed by transabdominal ultrasound or a vaginal ultrasound. Vaginal cervical examination must be avoided if a patient has painless bleeding. A vaginal cervical examination may result in hemorrhage if the healthcare provider further disrupts the implantation of the placenta.

Medical management will depend on the type of placenta previa, the gestational age of the fetus, the amount of bleeding, and fetal status. Bedrest may be required to reduce the pressure of the uterus and fetus on the cervix and placenta. The patient will also be advised to avoid exercise, sexual intercourse, and douching. Nonstress tests (NSTs) may be done during bleeding episodes to evaluate fetal status.

A cesarean delivery is necessary for a complete placenta previa. It may also be necessary for the other types as well, depending on the exact location of the placenta previa and the amount of blood loss occurring during labor. A trial of labor may be allowed if the placenta edge is greater than 2 cm from the cervical os or opening (Lockwood & Russo-Stieglitz, 2022). Bleeding is monitored, the fetal heart rate is monitored closely, and any signs of fetal distress will indicate the need for an emergency cesarean birth.

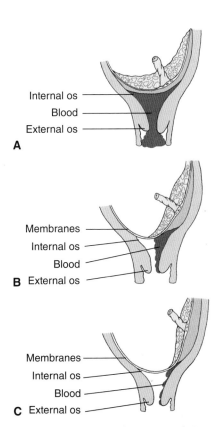

FIGURE 8.3 Placenta previa: A, complete; B, partial; C, marginal.

Safety *Stat!*

Possible Placenta Previa

If a laboring patient is experiencing vaginal bleeding, the examiner should not perform a vaginal cervical examination. The bleeding could indicate a placenta previa. The examiner could inadvertently puncture the placenta during the examination and cause additional separation of the placenta and hemorrhage. This could lead to a life-threatening event for the mother and fetus.

Nursing Care

Nursing care of the patient with placenta previa includes the following:

- Instructing the patient to avoid vaginal cervical examinations to prevent perforation of the cervix
- Monitoring fetal heart tones with external monitoring; reporting nonreassuring or abnormal heart rate patterns to the health-care provider immediately
- Monitoring fetal heart rate and movement

- Obtaining venous access for the prompt administration of fluids or blood products that may be ordered by the health-care provider
- Instituting medical orders for blood typing and cross-matching to prepare for possible blood transfusion

Patient Teaching

Teaching for the patient with placenta previa includes the following:

- If ordered by the health-care provider, reinforcing the importance of maintaining bedrest to reduce pressure on the placenta and cervix
- Abstaining from sexual intercourse or douching
- Notifying the health-care provider of any increase in vaginal bleeding
- Performing a daily fetal kick count and reporting to her health-care provider if fewer than 10 kicks are counted in a period up to 2 hours (Anderson-Bagga & Sze, 2022)

Placenta Abruptio

Placenta abruptio is the premature separation of the placenta from the wall of the uterus. Bleeding occurs between the uterine wall and the placenta. An abruption can be partial or complete. An abruption is partial if the margins of the placenta remain attached and a section detaches from the uterine wall (Fig. 8.4). With a complete abruption, the entire placenta separates from the uterine wall. Placenta abruptio is a life-threatening event for the fetus and the patient. A patient experiencing an abruption is at risk for severe hemorrhaging, resulting in hypovolemic shock, disseminated intravascular coagulation (DIC), and death (Schmidt et al., 2022). The placenta provides oxygenation to the fetus, so an abruption of the placenta can lead to fetal hypoxia and death.

Incidence and Risk Factors

Placental abruption occurs in 1 out of 100 to 120 deliveries (Schmidt et al., 2022). Risk factors for placenta abruptio include the following:

- Hypertension (44% of all cases; Rosenberger et al., 2023)
- Abdominal trauma (1.5%–9.4% of all cases; Rosenberger et al., 2023)

- Cocaine use
- Alcohol abuse
- Cigarette smoking
- Multiple pregnancy
- Short umbilical cord
- Advanced maternal age
- History of placental abruption
- Sudden decompression of the uterus (premature rupture of membranes, delivery of the first twin)
- Prolonged rupture of membranes

Classification and Signs and Symptoms

Placental abruptions are classified based on the extent and the location of separation.

- *Class 0* is asymptomatic and is diagnosed after delivery of the placenta.
- *Class 1* is mild and the patient will have no or mild vaginal bleeding, slightly tender uterus, normal heart rate and blood pressure, and no fetal distress.
- *Class 2* is moderate and the patient will have no vaginal bleeding to moderate bleeding, moderate to severe uterine tenderness, possible boardlike firmness of the abdominal wall, possible severe contractions, maternal bradycardia and orthostatic blood pressure changes, fetal distress, and **hypofibrinogenemia** (lack of fibrin in the blood, which decreases clotting time).
- *Class 3* is severe and the patient will have no vaginal bleeding to severe bleeding, very painful uterus, boardlike firmness of the abdominal wall, signs of maternal shock, hypofibrinogenemia, poor blood clotting, and possible fetal death (Rosenberger et al., 2023)

Medical Care

The diagnosis of placental abruption is made based on the symptoms and abdominal ultrasound. Treatment is determined by the severity of the abruption. The patient will need to be hemodynamically stabilized as much as possible, and then an emergency cesarean section may be required to save the fetus. A vaginal delivery may be attempted if the abruption is small and the mother and fetus are stable. Delivery is usually rapid because of increased uterine tone and contractions (Schmidt et al., 2022).

Nursing Care

Nursing care of the pregnant patient with placenta abruptio should include monitoring the status of the patient and the fetus.

- Frequently check vital signs and fetal heart tones, reporting abnormal results to the health-care provider immediately.

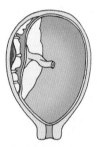 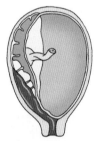 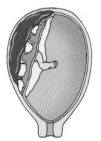

Partial separation (concealed hemorrhage)   Partial separation (apparent hemorrhage)   Complete separation (concealed hemorrhage)

FIGURE 8.4 Placenta abruptio.

• **WORD** • **BUILDING** •

hypofibrinogenemia: hypo–deficient + fibrinogen–fibrinogen + em–blood + ia–condition

- Notify the health-care provider and document any nonreassuring fetal heart patterns.
- Monitor for blood loss, and weigh pads and sheets for accurate measurement of blood loss.
- Administer IV fluids per physician's order.
- Administer oxygen per physician's order.
- Alert the laboratory for emergency type and crossmatch of blood per physician's order.
- Evaluate and document the patient's pain levels.
- Inform the patient of the status of the fetus.
- Provide emotional support to the patient and her family.

Patient Teaching

Patient teaching for the patient with a placenta abruptio includes the following:

- Report any bleeding or abdominal pain to her health-care provider.
- A cesarean birth may be required.
- Answer any questions the patient or family may have about the condition.

Placenta Accreta

Placenta accreta, also known as placenta accreta spectrum, occurs when the placenta villi are attached too deeply into the wall of the uterus, causing complications with removal. After childbirth, the placenta normally releases easily from the uterine wall. However, a patient with placenta accreta encounters a difficult removal with possible complications of hemorrhage and hysterectomy (National Accreta Foundation, 2020).

Incidence and Risk Factors

There are three types of placenta accreta:

- *Placenta accreta:* The placenta attaches directly to the myometrium, the middle layer of the uterine wall.
- *Placenta increta:* The placental villi invade into, but not through, the myometrium.
- *Placenta percreta:* The placental villi invade through the full thickness of the myometrium and may cause uterine rupture (American College of Obstetricians and Gynecologists [ACOG], 2021a).

The incidence of placenta accreta is 1 in 200 pregnancies. There has been an increase in placenta accreta corresponding to the increased number of cesarean births (ACOG, 2021a). Risk factors include the following:

- Abnormalities of the uterine wall, such as scarring after a cesarean delivery or uterine surgery
- Low implanted placenta
- Maternal age greater than 35 years old
- Previous cesarean delivery (risk increases with each cesarean delivery)
- Risk increases with each pregnancy
- Previous placenta accreta

- Previous endometrial ablation
- Pelvic irradiation
- Previous D&C
  (National Accreta Foundation, 2020)

Signs and Symptoms

Placenta accreta is undiagnosed before delivery in one-half to two-thirds of cases (ACOG, 2021a). There may be no signs and symptoms of placenta accreta until delivery except for third trimester vaginal bleeding. A placenta accreta may be identified on an ultrasound examination.

Medical Care

An extensive placenta accreta that is diagnosed before or during labor may require a cesarean birth. If diagnosed at the time of delivery, the patient may be taken to the operating room for general anesthesia. The physician will then attempt to remove the placenta and preserve the uterus if possible. If the placenta cannot be removed, a hysterectomy will be performed. A **hysterectomy** is a surgical procedure to remove the uterus. This procedure prevents severe hemorrhage, which could be life-threatening.

Nursing Care

Nursing care of the patient with placenta accreta includes the following:

- Preparing the patient for a cesarean birth
- Preparing the patient for the operating room
- Monitoring for signs of hypovolemic shock, such as low blood pressure
- Providing emotional support for the patient who is coping with an unexpected complication and a possible hysterectomy at a young age

Evidence-Based Practice

In vitro fertilization (IVF) is becoming increasingly popular as a method of managing infertility. There has been emerging evidence that IVP is associated with placental abnormalities. A large retrospective study was conducted with 17 million deliveries between 2013 and 2018 in China. This study concluded that IVF-conceived pregnancies had a higher risk of placental-related adverse outcomes than non-IVF pregnancies, including placenta previa, placental abruption, and placenta accreta.

Kong, F., Fu, Y., Shi, H., Li, R., Zhao, Y., Wang, Y., & Qiao, J. (2022). Placental abnormalities and placental-related complications following in-vitro fertilization: Based on national hospitalized data in China. *Frontiers in Endocrinology, 13,* 924070. http://doi.org/10.3389/fendo.2022.924070

• WORD • BUILDING •

hysterectomy: hyster–uterus + ectomy–surgical excision

Patient Teaching

Teach the patient who has placenta accreta the following:

- There is nothing she could have done to prevent placenta accreta.
- A cesarean birth may be scheduled for as early as 35 weeks of gestation to avoid an unscheduled delivery (Shepherd & Mahdy, 2022).
- Have the patient discuss surgical options with her physician.
- Explain to the patient that, after the hysterectomy, she will no longer have menstrual periods or be able to become pregnant again.

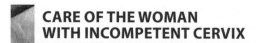

CARE OF THE WOMAN WITH INCOMPETENT CERVIX

Cervical insufficiency, also known as **cervical incompetence**, is defined by the ACOG as the inability of the uterine cervix to retain a pregnancy in the second trimester in the absence of uterine contractions. The diagnosis is based on a history of a previous second trimester loss with the absence of uterine contractions, preterm premature rupture of membranes (PPROM), painless dilation of the cervix, and a rapid delivery of the fetus (Norwitz, 2021).

Nursing Care Plan for Bleeding in Pregnancy

At 12 weeks' gestation, Ashley, age 25, is brought to the emergency department by her boyfriend. Ashley states that she noticed some slight vaginal bleeding yesterday while taking a shower, but the bleeding has increased today. The couple are worried about their baby, and Ashley feels guilty for not having called her health-care provider right away.

Nursing Diagnosis: Knowledge deficit regarding effects of bleeding in pregnancy
Expected Outcome: The patient will verbalize understanding the effects of bleeding during pregnancy for herself and her fetus.

Interventions:	Rationale:
Inform the patient and her partner of the effect bleeding can have on the mother, the course of the pregnancy, and the fetus.	*Patients who are knowledgeable about their condition are more likely to be cooperative with the treatment plan and understand the consequences of their condition.*
Teach the patient the signs and symptoms of bleeding.	*Patients will understand that vaginal bleeding or abdominal pain in the presence of a positive pregnancy test requires evaluation. Bleeding with or without abdominal pain or cramping should be reported to the health-care provider.*
Explain that a spontaneous abortion (miscarriage) can rarely be prevented.	*Understanding that spontaneous abortion cannot be prevented may alleviate some feelings of anguish or guilt.*
Educate the patient about any medications that may be prescribed, including the name, purpose, possible side effects, and correct administration.	*A knowledgeable patient is more likely to be compliant with the planned care. Also, the patient will understand correct administration and side effects of medications, optimizing a positive outcome for the pregnancy.*

Nursing Diagnosis: Anticipatory grieving related to the potential loss of pregnancy
Expected Outcome: The patient will verbalize that she feels emotional support from the nurses and her partner.

Interventions:	Rationale:
Encourage the patient and her partner to verbalize their concerns, feelings, and fears regarding the potential loss.	*This will assure the patient that grief is a normal reaction to the potential loss.*
Observe the patient's behavioral response.	*Responses such as guilt, anger, denial, and depression are normal reactions to grief.*
Clarify any misconceptions about possible fetal loss caused by vaginal bleeding.	*Vaginal bleeding does not always result in fetal loss. You can educate the patient and family about factual information without providing false hope.*
Collaborate with social services in the care of the patient.	*The social worker can evaluate the patient for concerns that can be addressed through social services and support groups.*

Causes and Symptoms

Cervical insufficiency may occur because of anatomical abnormality of the uterus or from obstetric trauma such as a cervical laceration from a previous delivery. Treatment for cervical dysplasia and cancer has been associated with cervical incompetence as well as multiple pregnancy terminations. For many women with cervical insufficiency, the cause is unknown (Norwitz, 2021).

Most patients have no obvious symptoms of cervical insufficiency, but pelvic pressure, back pain, increased vaginal discharge, and mild cramping may be noticed. Women with a previous history of cervical incompetency should be screened with a diagnostic ultrasound and physical examination during the late first trimester.

Medical Interventions

Medical intervention for an incompetent cervix is surgical cerclage. **Cerclage** is the use of sutures around the cervix to prevent the opening of the cervix (Fig. 8.5). It is usually performed at 12 to 14 weeks' gestation and removed after 37 weeks' gestation or the onset of labor.

Cerclage is usually performed as an outpatient procedure and the patient will return home a few hours after the procedure. Nursing care for the patient after cerclage is performed includes:

- Monitoring for signs of infection
- Monitoring for signs of ruptured membranes
- Monitoring for signs of bleeding
- Monitoring for signs of uterine activity
- Teaching the patient signs of ruptured membranes, signs of infection, and signs of preterm labor.
- Providing emotional support to the patient and her family

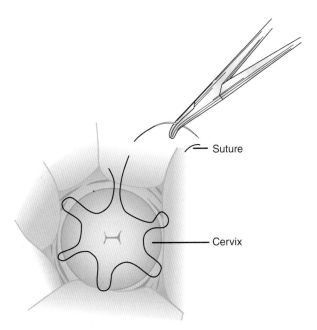

FIGURE 8.5 Cerclage.

CARE OF THE WOMAN WITH RH INCOMPATIBILITY BETWEEN MATERNAL AND FETAL BLOOD

Rh incompatibility can occur during pregnancy if the woman who is Rh-negative has been exposed to fetal blood cells that are Rh-positive. Rh factor is a surface antigen on a red blood cell. An antigen is any substance that causes the immune system to produce antibodies against it. Rh incompatibility occurs when a woman who does not have the surface antigen (Rh–) is exposed to blood that has the antigen (Rh+). When the Rh-negative woman is exposed to Rh-positive blood, her immune system produces antibodies against the Rh factor. This is called *isoimmunization*. The antibodies will attack any Rh-positive blood cells. This will not cause a problem for the mother. However, the antibodies can pass to the developing baby and destroy some of the baby's blood cells.

Exposure to the Rh-positive blood may occur during a spontaneous abortion, trauma, invasive obstetric procedures, or normal childbirth (Salem, 2022). In 90% of cases, sensitization occurs at delivery (Salem, 2022). Blood from an Rh-positive fetus may enter in small amounts during any of these events and sensitize the woman, causing her to produce antibodies. The fetus during the first pregnancy is rarely affected and not at risk. However, when a subsequent pregnancy occurs, the sensitized woman's immune system produces Rh antibodies that cross from the placenta into the fetal circulation. Once in the fetus's circulation, these antibodies form antigen-antibody complexes with the fetal red blood cells. These complexes destroy the red blood cells, causing the fetus to have a condition known as *alloimmune-induced hemolytic anemia* (Fig. 8.6).

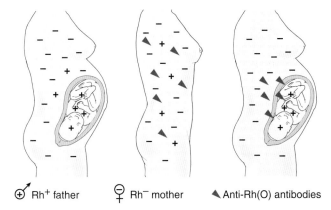

⊕ Rh⁺ father   ♀ Rh⁻ mother   ◀ Anti-Rh(O) antibodies

FIGURE 8.6 Isoimmunization occurring with an Rh+ father and Rh– mother. The fetus is Rh+; at childbirth, a small amount of fetal blood enters the mother's bloodstream. The mother's immune system produces antibodies against the Rh+ blood. In subsequent pregnancies, if the fetus is Rh+, the mother's immune system sends the antibodies through the placenta to attack the fetal red blood cells.

· WORD · BUILDING ·
isoimmunization: iso–equal + immuniz–safe + ation–action

Incidence and Risk Factors

The incidence of Rh-negative blood type is 15% to 20% for Whites and 5% to 10% for Blacks. For individuals of Asian and American Indian descent, the incidence of Rh-negative blood type is less than 5% (Salem, 2022).

Signs and Symptoms

The woman will not notice any signs or symptoms of Rh incompatibility. The disorder is only detected by a routine prenatal laboratory test, the indirect Coombs test, ordered by the health-care provider.

Medical Care

All pregnant women should have a blood test to determine Rh and blood type. Rh-negative women should have an antibody titer test (indirect Coombs test) to determine if they are sensitized and have developed antibodies against Rh-positive blood. If the indirect Coombs test is negative, the health-care provider will repeat the test at 28 weeks of gestation. A negative indirect Coombs test indicates that the fetus is not at risk of developing hemolytic disease.

If the woman has a positive indirect Coombs test, she will be evaluated at intervals to determine the level of antibodies and to monitor the condition of the fetus. To prevent hemolytic disease in the Rh-positive fetus, RhoGAM is administered at 28 weeks of gestation. RhoGAM prevents the formation of antibodies against Rh-positive blood and helps to prevent the fetus from developing complications of hemolytic anemia. If antibodies do attack the Rh-positive fetal blood cells, the fetus compensates by producing extra red blood cells. Amniocentesis may be performed to evaluate the amount of bilirubin from the destroyed red blood cells that is in the amniotic fluid. Amniocentesis is a procedure in which amniotic fluid is taken from the uterus and the cells are analyzed to provide information on the health of the fetus. A rise in the bilirubin in the amniotic fluid indicates that the fetus is losing too many red blood cells. The health of the fetus may be in danger.

Nursing Care

Nursing care of the woman with Rh incompatibility with her fetus includes the following:

- Encouraging the Rh-negative mother to be compliant with all requests by the health-care provider for blood tests to determine antibody titers
- Providing emotional support for the Rh-negative woman with a positive antibody titer as she undergoes testing throughout the remainder of the pregnancy
- Administering RhoGAM after spontaneous abortion, chorionic villus sampling, amniocentesis, abdominal trauma, or at 28 weeks of gestation unless there is laboratory documentation that the father of the baby is Rh-negative
- Sending umbilical cord blood to the laboratory at the time of birth to determine the baby's blood type, Rh, and antibody titer (direct Coombs test); RhoGAM should be administered to the mother within 72 hours of childbirth if the baby is Rh-positive

Patient Teaching

Teach the patient who has Rh incompatibility with her fetus the following:

- Rh incompatibility is a potentially serious condition. The antibodies the patient's body makes do not harm her but are a potential problem for the fetus.
- If RhoGAM is not administered, antibodies may develop that can cross the placenta and destroy the red blood cells of the fetus.
- It is important to receive RhoGAM at 28 weeks of gestation and possibly within 72 hours of childbirth.

CARE OF THE WOMAN WITH A MULTIPLE GESTATION PREGNANCY

Multiple gestation pregnancy is becoming more common as women with fertility issues are receiving treatment. These women are monitored closely, and multiples are detected early. In the past, multiple gestation pregnancies were often a surprise. Nowadays, women who receive adequate prenatal care are rarely surprised at the time of birth by twins, triplets, or other multiple births.

Incidence and Risk Factors

According to the Centers for Disease Control and Prevention (CDC, 2020), the U.S. twin birth rate is 31.1 per 1,000 live births. The triplet or higher birth rate for the United States is 79.6 per 100,000 live births (CDC, 2020). There is an increased risk for twins if the mother used fertility medications, is older, is obese, has a family history of multiples, or used assisted reproductive technologies to become pregnant (Heard, 2021).

Signs and Symptoms

Possible signs that may indicate a multiple pregnancy are as follows:

- Rapid weight gain and excessive hunger in the first trimester
- Severe nausea and vomiting because of higher-than-usual hormone levels
- Extreme breast tenderness because of higher-than-usual hormone levels
- Simultaneous fetal movements in different areas
- Larger-than-expected uterine size
- Higher-than-usual levels of hCG and alpha-fetoprotein
- Multiple fetal heartbeats
  (Heard, 2021)

Medical Management

Management of multiple gestation pregnancies is focused on maintaining the pregnancy as long as possible so that the fetuses will be viable and at less risk of preterm complications. Medical management may include the following:

- *Increased calories and well-balanced nutrition:* It is recommended that women carrying twins gain at least 35 to 45 pounds. Mothers of multiples need more calories, protein, and other nutrients, including iron. Consumption of calories should be around 3,000 Kcal per day (March of Dimes, 2021).
- *Frequent prenatal visits:* Multiple pregnancy increases the risk for complications. Frequent visits to the health-care provider may help detect complications early enough for effective management.
- *Increased rest:* Some women may need increased rest or even bedrest if complications develop. Multiple pregnancies often require bedrest beginning in the middle of the second trimester.
- *Referrals:* Referral to a perinatologist or maternal-fetal medicine specialist for special testing and evaluations and to coordinate care of complications may be necessary.
- *Maternal and fetal testing:* Testing may be needed to monitor the health of the fetuses, especially if there are pregnancy complications. Ultrasound biophysical profiles (BPP) may be required to monitor the health of the fetuses.
- Monitoring for complications:
  - Incompetent cervix
  - Preterm labor
  - Preeclampsia
  - Gestational diabetes
  - Placental abruption
  - Infants small for gestational age
  - Spontaneous abortion
  - Malpresentation of the fetus complicating delivery
  - Increased risk for cesarean birth
    (Doshi, 2022)

Nursing Care

Nursing care of the patient with multiple gestations includes the following:

- Prenatally, providing information about nutrition, an increased need for rest, and signs and symptoms of complications
- Encouraging the patient to verbalize her fears and ask questions
- During labor, monitoring fetal heart rates continually
- Preparing the woman for a possible cesarean birth
- Ensuring that extra nurses and physicians are available at the birth for any newborn complications

Patient Teaching

Teach the patient who has multiple gestations the following:

- Eat a healthy pregnancy diet with extra calories for the multiple fetuses.
- Watch for signs of preterm labor:
  - Contractions
  - Cramping
  - Low backache
  - Increase in vaginal discharge
  - Loss of mucous plug
  - Pelvic pressure
- Keep all office visits to monitor for pregnancy complications.
- Schedule rest periods daily.
- Report any increase in edema, headaches, and visual disturbances to her health-care provider. These could be signs of hypertension.
- Report any vaginal bleeding to her health-care provider.

Patient Teaching Guidelines

Urinalysis

During each prenatal visit, the patient is asked to give a clean-catch urine specimen for analysis. This analysis provides early information about possible complications of pregnancy. This urinalysis checks for high levels of sugars, proteins, ketones, white blood cells, bacteria, leukocytes, and nitrates related to the following conditions:

- Bladder or kidney infections
- Diabetes
- Dehydration
- Preeclampsia

Protein: Higher levels of protein may indicate a possible urinary tract infection or kidney disease. Preeclampsia may be a concern if high levels of protein are found later in pregnancy, combined with high blood pressure.

Sugar: During pregnancy, it is normal for the kidneys to leak some sugar from the blood into the urine. However, high levels of sugar could indicate gestational diabetes.

Ketones: When the body is breaking down fats instead of carbohydrates for energy, ketones are found in the urine. High levels of ketones indicate that the patient is not getting enough to eat or may be dehydrated.

Bacteria, leukocytes, and nitrites: The presence of these items indicates that there may be a urinary tract infection.

 ## CARE OF THE WOMAN WITH HYPERTENSIVE DISORDERS

The following hypertensive disorders can complicate pregnancy:

- Chronic/preexisting hypertension
- Gestational hypertension
- Chronic hypertension with superimposed preeclampsia
- Preeclampsia
- Eclampsia
- HELLP syndrome

These disorders are discussed next with information regarding medical management, nursing care, and patient teaching found in Table 8.1.

Table 8.1
Hypertensive Disorders of Pregnancy

Disorder	Medical Management	Nursing Care	Patient Teaching
Chronic/Preexisting Hypertension Blood pressure (BP) of 140/90 mm Hg or greater before pregnancy or occurring before 20 weeks' gestation	• Increase frequency of prenatal checkups. • Periods of rest to improve placental perfusion and promote diuresis to decrease blood pressure. • Administration of antihypertensive medications is not recommended unless the BP is consistently above 160/100 mm Hg to decrease likelihood of fetal growth restriction (Carson, 2022). Appropriate antihypertensive medications are labetolol and nifedipine (Carson, 2022). Ultrasonography to evaluate fetal growth.	• Monitor BP and report elevations to the health-care provider. • Administer antihypertensive medication and monitor for side effects.	• Rest on left side to increase placenta blood flow and promote diuresis. • Drink eight glasses of water a day to prevent dehydration. • Eat a low-sodium diet: do not add table salt, avoid canned foods, read labels carefully. • Consume daily diet of high-protein and high-fiber foods. • Correctly administer antihypertensive medications if ordered and recognize any possible side effects. • Schedule regular prenatal checkups with health-care provider. • Take and record daily BP and check urine for protein. • Perform daily fetal kick counts. • Record weight daily.
Gestational Hypertension BP of 140/90 mm Hg or greater for first time during pregnancy • BP returns to normal less than 12 weeks postpartum. • No proteinuria.	Same management as chronic hypertension.	Same nursing care as chronic hypertension.	Same patient teaching as chronic hypertension.
Preeclampsia and Chronic Hypertension With Superimposed Preeclampsia Preeclampsia *without severe features*: BP greater than or equal to 140/90 mm Hg on two occasions at least 4 hours apart Preeclampsia with severe features • Systolic BP of 160 mm Hg or higher, or diastolic BP of 110 mm Hg or higher, on two occasions at least 4 hours apart	• Prescribe home bedrest for mild preeclampsia symptoms. • Order diagnostic tests: CBC, liver function tests (LFTs), and platelet levels. • Hospitalize patient. • Conduct daily urinalysis to detect protein in urine. • Prescribe antihypertensive medications. Hydralazine and labetolol are recommended as first-line treatment.	• Monitor BP at least every 2 hours. • Monitor urine output hourly and check for protein. • Measure weight daily. • Administer antihypertensive medications. • Check patient's level of consciousness (LOC) and vision and report any changes.	Same patient teaching as for chronic hypertension with some additions. Instruct patient to report to health-care provider immediately if any of these signs occur: • Increase in BP • Excessive heartburn • Sudden weight increase • Frontal headache • Decrease in fetal movement

Signs and Symptoms	Management	Nursing Interventions	Patient Teaching
Oliguria of less than 500 mL/24 h • Proteinuria of more than 0.3 g in a 24-hour collection OR more than 3+ on two random samples collected at least 4 hours apart • Pulmonary edema or cyanosis • Serum creatinine greater than 1.1 mg/dL • Persistent headaches • Epigastric or right upper quadrant pain • Impaired liver function • Thrombocytopenia • Visual disturbances (e.g., blurred vision, dark spots in the visual field) • Peripheral edema	• Induction of labor if after 37 weeks' gestation. • Daily retinal examination to monitor for retinal spasm. • NST and BPP to monitor fetal health. • Magnesium sulfate given IV via an infusion pump in an initial loading dose of 4 to 5 g diluted in NS/D5W given over 4–5 hours (Vallerand & Sanoski, 2023) if BP consistently above 160/100. • Prostaglandin gel may be given to prepare cervix for labor. • Oxytocin may be given to induce labor. Vaginal delivery preferred to reduce risks associated with surgical births. Corticosteroid treatment to help fetus's lungs mature faster.	• Monitor for nervous system irritability by testing for ankle clonus. Record number of beats noted and report to health-care provider. • Monitor laboratory results for signs of liver impairment. • Auscultate lungs for signs of pulmonary edema, such as crackles and dyspnea. • Monitor fetus for well-being. • Provide a quiet environment for patient. • Administer magnesium sulfate as ordered and monitor for signs of toxicity: hyporeflexia and depressed respirations. • Check brachial, radial, and patellar reflexes (DTRs) for hyperreflexia, indicating brain irritability. • Provide emotional support for patient and family. • Postpartum management: • Continue to monitor BP, hyperreflexia, urine output, and proteinuria for 48 hours after delivery.	Severe nausea and vomiting • Abdominal pain • Vision changes Instruct patient about importance of magnesium sulfate administration and possible side effects.
Eclampsia Same symptoms as preeclampsia with the addition of one or more seizures	• Magnesium sulfate 4–6 grams over 15–30 minutes. If seizures continue, midazolam or lorazepam may be prescribed (Ross, 2022) • Plan either vaginal or cesarean birth after seizures are controlled and patient is stable.	Same nursing care as preeclampsia with some additions. During seizure, clear airway, administer oxygen, and provide for patient safety. • Document description of seizure, its duration, and nursing care provided. • Following seizure, reorient patient. • Provide emotional support for patient and family. Postpartum management: • Continue to monitor BP, hyperreflexia, urine output, and proteinuria for 48 hours after delivery.	Same patient teaching as for the other disorders of hypertension in pregnancy with some additions. Explain importance of preventing another seizure. • Explain that the main treatment for eclampsia is delivery. After delivery, patient's BP will return to normal and seizures will discontinue. • Reassure patient that she will never be alone during a seizure.

Continued

Table 8.1

Hypertensive Disorders of Pregnancy—cont'd

Disorder	Medical Management	Nursing Care	Patient Teaching
HELLP Symptoms of preeclampsia and/or eclampsia with the following additional signs and symptoms: • Elevated lactate dehydrogenase (LDH), AST, ALT, BUN, and bilirubin level caused by liver damage • Elevated uric acid level and creatinine caused by kidney damage • Low platelet count • Fluid retention • Pain in upper right quadrant of abdomen • Blurry vision • Nosebleeds or other bleeding that is difficult to stop • Jaundice (Rosenberger et al., 2023)	Deliver baby as soon as possible. • Provide corticosteroid treatment to help fetus's lungs mature faster. • Provide blood transfusions if required. • Provide antihypertensive medications. • Provide magnesium sulfate to prevent seizures (Khan, 2022).	Monitor BP at least every 2 hours. • Monitor urine output hourly and check for protein. • Administer medications such as antihypertensive medications, corticosteroids, and magnesium sulfate. • Monitor for signs of bleeding. • Administer platelets or packed red blood cells (PRBCs). • Check and report any changes in the patient's LOC and vision. • Monitor for nervous system irritability by testing for ankle clonus. • Monitor laboratory results, as well as LFTs, for signs of liver impairment. • Auscultate the lungs for signs of pulmonary edema, such as crackles and dyspnea. • Monitor fetus for well-being. • Provide a quiet environment for patient. • Check DTRs for hyperreflexia, indicating brain irritability. • Monitor for signs of magnesium toxicity; hyporeflexia and depressed respirations. • Provide emotional support for patient and family.	Teach patient what her medications are and possible side effects to report. • Immediately report bleeding from gums, nose, or venipuncture site, and any unusual bruising. • Need to deliver fetus to stop progression of HELLP syndrome.

Chronic Hypertension

Chronic hypertension refers to patients who are hypertensive before pregnancy or who become hypertensive during early pregnancy. Frequently, hypertension is related to obesity or to a strong family history of hypertension. Many young women do not receive routine health care until they become pregnant and so may be diagnosed with hypertension at the first prenatal visit.

Gestational Hypertension

Gestational hypertension is a condition of elevated blood pressure that begins in pregnancy and can lead to preeclampsia if not treated. Typically, the blood pressure returns to normal after delivery.

Preeclampsia

Preeclampsia is defined as hypertension and proteinuria after 20 weeks of gestation. Edema is commonly present also but not necessary for a diagnosis of preeclampsia.

Incidence and Risk Factors

The incidence of preeclampsia is estimated to range from 2% to 6% in healthy **nulliparous** women (Carson, 2022).

Risk factors for preeclampsia include the following:

- Primigravida
- Maternal age more than 35 years or younger than 18
- Previous history of preeclampsia
- Chronic hypertension
- Multiple gestations
- Chronic kidney disease
- Chronic hypertension
- Obesity
- Hydatidiform mole
- Egg donation or donor insemination
- Urinary tract infection
- Family history of preeclampsia
- Interpregnancy interval less than 2 years
  (Carson, 2022)

Eclampsia

Preeclampsia becomes **eclampsia** with the onset of a seizure. Most cases of eclampsia occur in the third trimester through the first 48 hours of the postpartum period. Although early detection of preeclampsia is possible, there are no tests that can indicate that preeclampsia will progress to eclampsia (Ross, 2022).

Incidence and Risk Factors

Eclampsia occurs in about 1 in 2,000 pregnancies. The risk factors for eclampsia are as follows:

- Primigravida
- Family history of preeclampsia

· **WORD** · **BUILDING** ·

nulliparous: nulli–none + parous–bearing children

eclampsia: eclamps–a sudden development + ia–condition

- Multifetal gestations
- Chronic hypertension
- Gestational diabetes
- Obesity
- Lower socioeconomic status
- Vascular and connective tissue disorders
  (Ross, 2022)

HELLP Syndrome

HELLP syndrome is considered by most health-care providers to be a variant of preeclampsia and eclampsia that can be life-threatening. HELLP is named for the three main features of the disease: hemolysis, elevated liver enzyme levels, and low platelet counts:

H = hemolysis of red blood cells
EL = elevated liver enzymes
LP = low platelet count

The breakdown of red blood cells (hemolysis) can cause oxygenation and perfusion problems for the woman and her fetus. Inflammation in the liver, manifested by the elevated liver enzymes, can cause right upper quadrant abdominal pain. The inflamed liver is unable to detoxify the blood as usual, and the low platelet count will cause bleeding and clotting problems for the patient. The symptoms of HELLP are sometimes mistaken for gastritis, gallbladder disease, hepatitis, or the flu. The mortality rate for women diagnosed with HELLP syndrome is about 25%. The cause of HELLP syndrome is unknown, and there is no preventive management (Khan, 2022).

Incidence and Risk Factors

HELLP syndrome occurs in 10% to 20% of pregnant women with severe preeclampsia and eclampsia. It occurs most often before 37 weeks of gestation or after the baby is born (Khan, 2022).

Risk factors for HELLP syndrome include the following:

- White race or European descent
- Maternal age greater than 34 years
- History of hypertension
- Previous history of HELLP syndrome

Pathophysiology of Pregnancy-Induced Hypertension

Gestational hypertension, preeclampsia, eclampsia, and HELLP syndrome are all examples of pregnancy-induced hypertension (PIH). These disorders are multisystem diseases that are specific to the second half of pregnancy. A pregnant patient can experience any hypertensive disorder alone, but PIH is thought to be an evolving manifestation of a single pathological process and share a common origin.

The exact cause of preeclampsia, eclampsia, and HELLP syndrome remains unknown, despite much research. Yet these are the most serious disorders of hypertension in pregnancy.

The following discussion examines current understanding of the causes and effects of PIH.

The Placenta

Current thinking is that the primary pathophysiology of PIH disorders is related to the placenta. Preeclampsia occurs both in women who have an intrauterine pregnancy and also in those with a hydatidiform mole, indicating that the placenta is playing a role in the pathophysiology (Carson, 2022). The problem has been identified as abnormal trophoblastic implantation, which causes reduced placental perfusion. During implantation, the tiny villi in the placenta that eventually form arteries do not develop, and the placenta does not receive the blood supply that it should. The restriction of placental blood flow leads to hypoxia of the placental environment, which causes a release of factors called *antiangiogenic proteins* that enter the mother's circulation and act on endothelial cells, causing injury to the cells and producing vasospasm (Rosenberger et al., 2023). Decreased blood flow to the placenta can also cause infarctions of the placenta tissue that lead to increased risk for placenta abruptio, chronic fetal hypoxia, and a fetus with intrauterine growth retardation.

The Cardiovascular System

Hypertension in preeclampsia is caused by vasoconstriction. Also, if the placenta does not develop normally, the increased blood supply that should be going from the mother to the placenta does not occur, causing hypertension and edema.

Endothelial cell damage, which causes arteriolar vasospasm, may contribute to an increased capillary permeability. This increases edema and further decreases intravascular volume, predisposing the woman with preeclampsia to pulmonary edema. Women with preeclampsia also exhibit a hyperresponse to angiotensin-II and epinephrine, both of which elevate the blood pressure (Carson, 2022).

Genetic Factors

Over 100 maternal and paternal genes have been studied for their relationship with preeclampsia, including those genes known to play a role in diabetes, blood pressure regulation, and immune system functions. Preeclampsia tends to run in families. A study showed that 20% to 40% of daughters and 11% to 37% of sisters of women with preeclampsia also developed the disease (Carson, 2022).

The Kidney

Endothelial cell injury, which results in vasospasm, causes poor renal perfusion. This leads to a loss of protein, which reduces the colloid osmotic pressure (Ross, 2022). This will cause the woman with preeclampsia to have protein in her urine. Poor renal perfusion allows fluid to shift to interstitial spaces, resulting in edema. There is also a rise in blood urea nitrogen (BUN), creatinine, and uric acid levels.

The Liver

Vasospasm in the liver impairs liver function. This causes hepatic edema and bleeding, which leads to necrosis of liver tissue. The necrosis causes an elevation in liver enzymes. A report of epigastric pain by the patient may indicate liver

---

Labs & Diagnostics

Liver Enzymes

The liver performs many biochemical functions such as eliminating toxins; managing the breakdown of red blood cells; and detoxifying drugs, alcohol, and environmental toxins. Liver enzymes help the liver to do its job. They are substances that speed the rate of chemical or metabolic reactions. Enzymes utilized by the liver primarily exist in the cells of the liver. Under normal circumstances, these enzymes are also present in the bloodstream in low concentrations. However, when the liver is not working as it should, either because of inflammation or injury, these enzymes spill over into the bloodstream. In obstetrics, liver enzyme tests are used to determine liver disease that may occur with PIH:

- *Alanine aminotransferase (ALT):* Normal range 24 to 36 units/L; found in liver cells and in muscle and kidney cells; released with tissue damage
- *Aspartate aminotransferase (AST):* Normal range 15 to 30 units/L; found in liver cells and in muscle and kidney cells; released with tissue damage
- *Alkaline phosphatase:* Normal range 25 to 125 units/L; if found, it will be in the liver, biliary tract, bone, intestine, and placenta (Van Leeuwen & Bladh, 2021)

---

damage. Liver damage also activates the coagulation cascade with thrombocytopenia. The thrombocytes are increased in activation and size but have a shorter life span (Ross, 2022). When HELLP syndrome develops, the hemolysis that occurs produces red blood cell fragments that leave fibrin in the blood vessels. The fibrin causes decreased blood flow to the liver and leads to liver impairment.

The Immune System

Immunologic factors may play a role in the development of preeclampsia. The presence of a foreign protein, for example, in the placenta or fetus, may be identified by the mother's immune system as an antigen. This may then trigger an abnormal response by the immune system (Carson, 2022). This theory is supported by the increased incidence of preeclampsia or eclampsia in first-time mothers or to multiparous women pregnant by new partners (August & Silbai, 2022). Preeclampsia may be an immune disease in which the maternal antibody system is overwhelmed by excessive fetal antigens in the maternal circulation.

The Brain and Central Nervous System

Cerebral edema, vasoconstriction from vasospasm, and damage to capillary linings may lead to seizures or hemorrhage. Cerebral vasospasm in the pregnant woman may be observed as a throbbing frontal headache. The woman may also experience vision symptoms associated with central nervous system irritation, an indication of cerebral edema. Vision changes include a temporary loss of vision, flashing lights, auras, light sensitivity, and blurry vision or spots.

Learn to C.U.S.

Lucille, aged 17, has arrived late for her scheduled prenatal appointment with her health-care provider and is reporting a severe headache and seeing dark spots in front of her eyes. She admits that she missed her last prenatal visit because she had "a test at school." She is at 36 weeks of gestation. On physical assessment, you note that Lucille has a blood pressure of 160/94 mm Hg, she has swollen feet and hands, and the fetal heart rate is 160 bpm. The office is very busy; there are several patients to be seen before Lucille. You locate the health-care provider and use the C.U.S. method of communication.

C: "I am *concerned* about Lucille. She is 17 years old and at 36 weeks of gestation.

U: I am *uncomfortable* because she is reporting a severe headache and vision disturbance, and I noted swelling of her hands and feet. Her blood pressure is 160/94 mm Hg.

S: We have a *safety* issue because she may get worse before you have a chance to evaluate her and provide orders for her care."

Medication Facts

Magnesium Sulfate Therapy

Pharmacological effects: Magnesium sulfate blocks neuromuscular transmission. Effects include a minor-to-moderate neurological depression manifested by diminished reflexes and somnolence (drowsiness). *Indications:* It is prescribed to depress the central nervous system to prevent seizures. *Dose:* An initial loading dose of 4 to 5 g diluted in NS/D5W given IV over 4 to 5 hours followed by a maintenance dose of 1 to 2 g/h IV as a continuous infusion. Calcium gluconate is the antidote for magnesium sulfate toxicity.
  (Vallerand & Sanoski, 2023)

Nursing Implications

- Before administering this medication, inspect the patient for a respiratory rate of at least 12 breaths per minute, an oxygen saturation of 95% or higher, urine output of at least 30 mL/hour, and the presence of deep tendon reflexes (DTRs).
- Monitor reflexes; if a response is absent, no additional doses should be given.
- Administer on time and with the correct dosage.
- Have a second practitioner independently double-check the original order, dose calculations, and infusion pump settings. Accidental overdose can result in serious harm to the patient.
- Monitor for signs of toxicity, such as hypotension, depressed DTRs, flushing, drowsiness, and decreased respirations.

Labs & Diagnostics

Assessing Deep Tendon Reflexes

- *Brachial reflex:* Support the woman's arm by laying it on your forearm. Instruct her to relax and let her arm go limp. Place your thumb over the tendon. Strike your thumb with the small end of the reflex hammer. A normal response is a slight flexion of the forearm.
- *Patellar reflex:* Dangle the patient's legs over the side of the bed. Place your hand on the patient's thigh and strike the distal patellar tendon just below the kneecap. If the patient is supine, flex each leg to a 45-degree angle and place your dominant hand behind her knee to support it. The normal response is contraction of the quadriceps muscle with extension of the knee.

The reflexes are graded on the following DTR rating scale:

- Reflex absent = 0
- Hypoactive reflex = +1
- Normal reflex = +2
- Slightly above average reflex = +3
- Hyperactive reflex = +4

1. Report and document 0, +3, and +4 reflexes.
2. Evaluate for clonus (involuntary muscle contractions). Support the patient's lower leg with your hand. The foot is dorsiflexed to stretch the Achilles tendon. Hold the flexion. If clonus is present, you will observe a rapid tapping motion of the foot. This indicates hyperreflexia.
3. Report and document hyperreflexia.

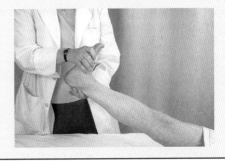

CARE OF THE WOMAN WITH GESTATIONAL DIABETES

Gestational diabetes is defined as a condition in which the blood glucose level is elevated during pregnancy in a woman not previously diagnosed as diabetic. Similar to other types of diabetes, gestational diabetes affects how cells use glucose.

When a pregnant woman eats a meal, a series of hormonal actions begin. Glucose is absorbed into the bloodstream, which elevates blood glucose levels. This rise in glucose stimulates the secretion of insulin from the beta cells of the pancreas. Insulin binds to cell receptors and facilitates the entry of glucose into the cell, which uses the glucose for energy. The increased insulin secretion from the pancreas and the subsequent cellular utilization of glucose results in lower blood glucose levels. Lower glucose levels then result in decreased insulin secretion.

If insulin production and secretion are altered by disease, blood glucose is affected. If insulin production is decreased, glucose entry into cells is inhibited, resulting in hyperglycemia. The same effect will be seen if insulin is secreted from the pancreas but is not used properly by target cells. If insulin secretion is increased, blood glucose levels may become very low (hypoglycemia) as large amounts of glucose enter tissue cells and little remains in the bloodstream. Pregnant women tend to develop hypoglycemia between meals and during sleep because the fetus continues to draw glucose across the placenta from the maternal bloodstream.

The placenta provides the growing fetus with nutrients and produces hormones to maintain the pregnancy. The hormones of pregnancy produced by the placenta include estrogen, cortisol, and human placental lactogen, all of which can have a blocking effect on insulin. Unlike other types of diabetes, gestational diabetes is not caused by a lack of insulin, but by the blocking effects of other hormones on the insulin that is produced. This condition is referred to as *insulin resistance*, a condition in which the body produces insulin but does not use it effectively. When people have insulin resistance, glucose builds up in the blood instead of being absorbed by the cells and used by the body. As the placenta grows, more of these hormones are produced, and insulin resistance becomes greater. Normally, the pancreas is able to make additional insulin to overcome insulin resistance, but when the production of insulin is not enough to overcome the effect of the placental hormones, gestational diabetes results. Gestational diabetes usually starts halfway through the pregnancy at about 20 to 24 gestational weeks.

Incidence and Risk Factors

Gestational diabetes occurs in 3% to 10% of all pregnancies (Moore, 2022). Risk factors for a woman to develop gestational diabetes include the following:

- Age greater than 25 years
- Physical inactivity
- Being obese with a body mass index (BMI) of 30 or higher
- Gestational diabetes with a previous pregnancy
- Previous birth of a baby weighing more than 9 pounds
- Unexplained stillbirth
- Black, Native American, Hispanic, or Asian individual
- Having prediabetes, a condition in which blood glucose is higher than normal but is not high enough for a diagnosis of diabetes
- Having a parent or sibling with type 2 diabetes
- History of polycystic ovary syndrome (PCOS). (For more information on PCOS, see Chapter 3.)
- Current use of steroids
- Hypertension
  (Rosenberger et al., 2023)

Signs and Symptoms

Some women will have no noticeable symptoms. Of those who do, signs and symptoms of gestational diabetes are as follows:

- Increased thirst
- Feeling hungrier and eating more than usual
- Increased urination
- Fatigue
- Frequent infections of the bladder, vagina, and skin
- Blurred vision

Medical Management

When planning medical care, the obstetrician will need to distinguish between pregestational diabetes and gestational diabetes. Pregestational diabetics have a higher risk than gestational diabetics for pregnancy and fetal complications. Gestational diabetes can also be divided into two subclasses. A1GM is non-insulin dependent–diet controlled gestational diabetes and A2GM is insulin dependent gestational diabetes. Care will be individualized based upon the subtype of gestational diabetes. Current recommendations by the American Diabetes Association are that high-risk women should be identified at the first prenatal visit and screened at that time with a two-step glucose tolerance test (GTT). All pregnant women should receive an oral GTT between the 24th and 28th weeks of pregnancy to screen for the condition, regardless of whether they tested nondiabetic at a previous screening (Rosenberger et al., 2023).

The woman with gestational diabetes requires careful medical management, which may include weekly or biweekly appointments, and nursing care to prevent complications for her and her fetus. In addition to routine pregnancy laboratory tests, the following tests are needed to monitor for possible complications related to diabetes: hemoglobin A1c (HbA1c), BUN, serum creatinine, thyrotropin (TSH), free thyroxine (FT4), and capillary blood sugar levels two to four times daily (Moore, 2022).

The woman will also need to be monitored for ketoacidosis. Diabetic ketoacidosis (DKA) is an accumulation of ketones in the blood because of high glucose levels. In pregnancy, there is a state of accelerated starvation, especially in the second and third trimesters. The fetus and the placenta use large amounts of maternal glucose as a source of energy, which leads to decreased maternal fasting glucose. This increased use of glucose, along with insulin deficiency, leads to an increase in free fatty acids, which are then converted to ketones in the liver. In gestational diabetes, DKA can occur at blood sugar levels of 200 mg/dL as compared with 350 mg/dL with nonpregnant diabetics (Moore, 2022). This condition requires immediate management to prevent complications for the mother such as coma and possible death of the fetus.

Signs and symptoms of DKA are as follows:

- Increased urine production
- Increased thirst
- Nausea
- Vomiting
- Abdominal pain

- Weakness
- Weight loss
- Hyperventilation
- Ketone breath (sweet-smelling breath)
- Tachycardia
- Hypotension
- Dry mucous membranes
- Disorientation
- Coma

Complications

Complications of diabetes for the mother include diabetic retinopathy, which is damage to the retina and vision related to elevated glucose levels. In addition, hypertension complicates 10% of diabetic pregnancies (Rosenberger et al., 2023). Hypertension can lead to preeclampsia and stroke.

The fetus can experience accelerated growth and become large for gestational age (LGA). The large fetus develops a condition called *macrosomia,* or overgrowth, and deposits fat in the abdomen and shoulder areas. If the mother gains excessive weight during the pregnancy, it increases the chance for preterm delivery, an LGA baby, and a cesarean birth. Birth injuries are more common in infants of diabetic mothers because of the infants' size. Injuries that can occur are brachial plexus injury, facial nerve injury, and **cephalohematoma**. After birth, the infant is at risk for hypoglycemia, which can lead to neonatal seizures, coma, and brain damage. Infants of diabetic mothers also have an increased risk for respiratory distress syndrome. Medical studies have determined that there is a positive relationship between levels of maternal average blood glucose levels and perinatal morbidity and mortality. The stillbirth rate is four to six times higher and neonatal mortality is two to four times higher in diabetic than in nondiabetic pregnancies (Riskin & Garcia-Prats, 2022).

PREVENTING FETAL COMPLICATIONS. Throughout the pregnancy, the goal is to prevent diabetic complications. Periodic testing for fetal well-being is part of the management of care. The recommended tests are as follows:
- Fetal movement counting performed every night from 28 weeks of gestation until birth
  - A reassuring result is 10 movements in fewer than 2 hours.
- NSTs to begin at 28 to 34 weeks for insulin-dependent diabetic women and at 36 weeks for diet-controlled diabetic women
  - Reassuring results are two heart rate accelerations in 20 minutes.
- Contraction stress test done weekly, beginning at 28 to 34 weeks for insulin-dependent diabetic women and at 36 weeks for diet-controlled diabetic women
  - Reassuring results are no heart rate decelerations in response to three contractions in 10 minutes.
- Ultrasonic BPP starting at 34 weeks of gestation
  - A reassuring result is a score of 8 in 30 minutes (ACOG, 2021b).

· **WORD** · **BUILDING** ·

cephalohematoma: cephalo–head + hema–blood + toma–tumor

Team Works

Care of the Patient With Gestational Diabetes
A woman with gestational diabetes can have a healthy fetus and avoid complications. Often, to provide optimal care, a team approach is used. The patient may be referred to the following health-care professionals:

- Dietitian to educate her about calories, carbohydrates, and selecting healthy meals
- Diabetic educator nurse to teach her how to administer her medications
- Endocrinologist to provide medical management of her diabetes
- Neonatologist if complications have occurred during the pregnancy
- Obstetric nurse to educate her about how to perform fetal kick counts and explain normal pregnancy discomforts as well as warning signs to report to the health-care provider

---

Recommended Therapies

The woman should check and record her blood sugar with a finger stick on the schedule suggested by her health-care provider and bring the log to each visit. As the pregnancy progresses there will be increased fetal demand for glucose, which can cause the woman to experience episodes of hypoglycemia. Also, as she progresses into each trimester, insulin resistance rises. The increase in insulin resistance prevents its proper use at the cellular level. Glucose cannot enter cells and accumulates in the bloodstream, resulting in hyperglycemia.

Dietary therapy is the first line of treatment for women with gestational diabetes. Guidelines include:

- Eating six meals per day, with three major meals and three snacks
- Including plenty of complex carbohydrates with cellulose, such as whole grains and legumes
- Ensuring that carbohydrates make up 50% or less of each meal

Insulin may be prescribed to achieve optimal glucose levels if diet alone cannot keep the glucose levels acceptable. The goal of insulin therapy is to achieve glucose profiles similar to the nondiabetic woman. The blood sugar range for the nondiabetic woman is 70 to 120 mg/dL. See Table 8.2 for target blood glucose ranges for the woman with gestational diabetes. Obtaining these blood sugar levels will require the woman and her health-care provider to pay meticulous attention to her care. Lispro, aspart, regular (also known as *Humulin R*) and NPH insulins (neutral protamine Hagedorn, also known as *Humulin N* and *Novolin N*) are well-studied in pregnancy and are considered safe. An insulin regimen for patients with gestational diabetes requires frequent adjustments in the amount, type, and timing of insulin injections. Some patients would benefit from an insulin pump (Rosenberger et al., 2023).

Table 8.2

Target Blood Glucose Levels for Women With Gestational Diabetes

Time of Day	*Target*
When patient awakens and before meals	95 mg/dL
1 hour after a meal	140 mg/dL or lower
2 hours after a meal	120 mg/dL or lower

CRITICAL THINKING & CLINICAL JUDGMENT

Scenario #2: **Josephina**, 32 weeks' gestation, has gestational diabetes. She had an office visit with her obstetrician yesterday and her insulin dose was adjusted based upon her fingerstick blood sugar readings of the past 2 weeks. She called the office and reported to you that she increased her dose of insulin this morning and now she "doesn't feel well."

1. What could be causing Josephina to feel unwell?
2. What questions should you ask Josephina?
3. What should you tell Josephina to do?

Nursing Care

Nursing care of the woman with gestational diabetes includes the following:

- Determining the patient's understanding of gestational diabetes and providing additional teaching and reference materials
- Referring the patient to a registered dietitian and reinforcing the dietary plan
- Monitoring blood sugar levels and adjusting care based on orders from the health-care provider
- Administering insulin or oral hypoglycemic medications as prescribed by the health-care provider
- Teaching the patient how to perform a capillary finger stick for glucose monitoring
- Monitoring for signs of hyperglycemia and DKA
- Monitoring fetal growth and well-being by performing NSTs as ordered by the health-care provider

Patient Teaching

Discuss the following with the patient with gestational diabetes:

- Teach the patient the capillary finger stick blood glucose procedure for home glucose monitoring. Encourage the patient to perform a return demonstration to monitor for understanding.

Health Promotion

How to Prevent Health Problems Related to Gestational Diabetes

A woman with gestational diabetes can prevent problems or complications during her pregnancy and have a healthy newborn. Guidelines she should follow are these:

- Keep all prenatal appointments. She may need to see her health-care provider more often than someone without gestational diabetes.
- Check her blood sugar on schedule and keep a log to take to her prenatal appointments.
- If medications are prescribed, take them as directed and on time.
- Follow a healthy diet, choosing foods from all food groups.
- Get regular daily exercise to use the excess sugar in the bloodstream.
- Know the symptoms of low blood sugar: sleepiness, perspiration, tremors, rapid heart rate, cool clammy skin, blurred vision, and confusion.
- Treat low blood sugar quickly. Keep glucose tablets or gel nearby at all times.
- Notify the health-care provider if she is not able to maintain her blood sugars within the parameters that are expected by her health-care provider.

- Explain the health-care provider's preferred schedule for monitoring blood sugars at home.
- Teach how to administer insulin. Encourage the patient to perform a return demonstration.
- Identify the signs of hyperglycemia and hypoglycemia
- Engage in at least 30 minutes of exercise daily.
- Monitor fetal well-being with daily kick counts beginning at 28 weeks of gestation.
- Keep a daily log of blood sugar levels, diet, and exercise to monitor her progress and to provide information to her health-care provider at her visits.

Key Points

- Pregnancy is usually a natural process that ends with a healthy baby and mother. However, there are many possible complications that threaten the positive outcome. The nurse is essential in assisting the health-care provider to manage the care of women with complications of pregnancy.
- Hyperemesis gravidarum can cause complications for the mother and fetus, such as fluid and electrolyte disturbances and preterm labor.
- Spontaneous abortion (miscarriage) is a pregnancy loss before the fetus is a viable size. There are several types of spontaneous abortions: threatened, inevitable, incomplete, and complete. All have the potential for excessive blood loss and infection.
- An ectopic pregnancy occurs when a fertilized ovum implants outside the uterus. This condition can be life-threatening to the woman and may require surgical treatment.
- Hydatidiform mole is abnormal growth of the placenta without fetal growth occurring. This condition requires aggressive treatment and follow-up for 1 year to monitor for cancer.

- Bleeding disorders of late pregnancy include placenta previa, placenta abruptio, and placenta accreta. They all have the potential to cause maternal hemorrhage and possible fetal loss if not identified and managed appropriately when diagnosed.
- The Rh-negative woman requires monitoring throughout pregnancy and after delivery to prevent isoimmunization.
- Multiple gestations are becoming more common, and women pregnant with multiples require careful monitoring throughout pregnancy to prevent complications and preterm delivery.
- There is a range of hypertensive disorders of pregnancy that can complicate a pregnancy. Women with hypertensive disorders such as chronic hypertension, gestational hypertension, preeclampsia, eclampsia, and HELLP syndrome require close monitoring to prevent adverse outcomes for the mother and fetus.
- Women with gestational diabetes may require a team approach to manage the condition and prevent complications such as an infant who is LGA, requiring a cesarean birth.

Review Questions

1. A 30-year-old pregnant woman, gravida 1, para 0 is 30 weeks' pregnant. She reports at her regularly scheduled office visit that she is experiencing vaginal bleeding that began "about 3 days ago." She also states, "I didn't call because I am not having any pain, and I can feel the baby moving." Which of the following would be the appropriate diagnostic procedure for her?
   1. A vaginal cervical examination
   2. A contraction stress test
   3. Abdominal ultrasound
   4. Internal fetal monitoring

2. A nurse is caring for a patient who just experienced a first trimester spontaneous abortion. Which comment by the nurse is considered appropriate? (**Select all that apply.**)
   1. "It must have been God's will."
   2. "You can try getting pregnant again soon."
   3. "If you have any questions, I am available to talk."
   4. "At least you weren't very far along."
   5. "There must have been something wrong with the fetus."
   6. "Is there anyone I could call for you—a friend, pastor, or rabbi?"

3. Which of the following is a priority nursing intervention for a patient with a ruptured ectopic pregnancy?
   1. Obtain IV access and begin infusing IV fluids.
   2. Reassure the patient that everything will be okay.
   3. Provide pain medication.
   4. Infuse IV antibiotics.

4. The purpose of administering RhoGAM is to _____ _____ the mother from developing Rh antibodies.

5. A woman at 38 weeks of gestation was involved in a car accident. She has numerous abrasions but no broken bones or head injury. The emergency department nurse knows that the most common complication that may occur for this woman is:
   1. HELLP syndrome
   2. Placenta previa
   3. Placenta abruptio
   4. Preeclampsia

6. Which of the following is a major risk factor for gestational diabetes?
   1. Anemia
   2. Hypertension
   3. Obesity
   4. Asthma

7. The most serious complication of a hydatidiform mole pregnancy is the development of:
   1. Cancer
   2. Diabetes
   3. Infertility
   4. Hypertension

8. Patient teaching for the patient with preeclampsia should include which of the following?
   1. Continue normal activities, including daily exercise.
   2. Monitor blood pressure twice daily.
   3. Limit fluid intake to 320 mL per day.
   4. Monitor weight monthly.

9. Why is magnesium sulfate administered to the pregnant patient with preeclampsia?
   1. Prevent nausea and vomiting.
   2. Decrease the pain of labor contractions.
   3. Reduce central nervous system irritability to prevent seizures.
   4. Replace magnesium in a patient with a low magnesium level.

10. Immediately after birth, the infant born to a mother with gestational diabetes should be monitored for which of the following?
    1. Seizures
    2. Hypoglycemia
    3. Respiratory distress
    4. Jaundice

ANSWERS 1. 3; 2. 3, 6; 3. 1; 4. Prevent; 5. 3; 6. 3; 7. 1; 8. 2; 9. 3; 10. 2

CRITICAL THINKING QUESTIONS

1. A patient diagnosed with preeclampsia has been on bedrest for a week. The home health nurse visits the patient. What signs would indicate to the nurse that the bedrest is effective in treating the patient's preeclampsia?
2. At her regularly scheduled clinic visit, a pregnant teenager states, "Several of my friends smoke, and I have a cigarette occasionally. My older sister is a nurse, and she said that it can cause placenta problems if I smoke. Is that true?" What explanation should you give the teenager?

Resources

For additional resources and information, including Postconference Questions and Activities, Answers, and References, visit www.FADavis.com.

 Student Study Guide

CHAPTER 9

Nursing Care During Labor and Childbirth

KEY TERMS

acceleration (ak-SELL-uh-RAY-shun)
acme (AK-mee)
amnioinfusion (AM-nee-oh-in-FYOO-zhun)
amniotomy (AM-nee-OT-uh-mee)
Apgar score (AP-gar SKOR)
atony (AT-on-ee)
attitude (AT-ih-TOOD)
Braxton Hicks contractions (BRAK-ston HIKS kon-TRAK-shunz)
deceleration (dee-SELL-uh-RAY-shun)
decrement (DEK-ruh-ment)
dilation (dye-LAY-shun)
doula (DOO-luh)
early decelerations (ER-lee dee-SELL-uh-RAY-shunz)
effacement (eh-FAYSS-ment)
epidural (EP-ih-DOO-ruhl)
episiotomy (ih-PIZ-ee-OT-uh-mee)
episodic decelerations (ep-ih-SOD-ik dee-SELL-uh-RAY-shunz)
estriol (ESS-tree-ol)
fetal lie (FEE-tuhl LYE)
fetal presentation (FEE-tuhl pree-zen-TAY-shun)
fetal station (FEE-tuhl STAY-shun)
increment (IN-kre-ment)
intrathecal space (IN-truh-THEE-kuhl SPAYSS)
intrauterine pressure catheter (IUPC) (IN-truh-YOO-tuh-rin PRESH-uhr KATH-uh-ter)
late decelerations (LAYT dee-SELL-uh-RAY-shunz)
Leopold maneuvers (LEE-oh-pold mah-NOO-verz)
lightening (lite-n-iNG)
meconium (mee-KOH-nee-uhm)
ophthalmia neonatorum (off-THAL-mee-uh NEE-uh-na-TOR-uhm)
oxytocin (ok-sih-TOH-sin)
periodic decelerations (pee-ree-OD-ik dee-SELL-uh-RAY-shunz)
prostaglandins (PROS-tuh-GLAN-dinz)
pudendal block (pyoo-DEN-duhl BLOK)
somatic pain (soh-MAT-ik PAYN)
spinal anesthesia (SPYE-nuhl AN-ess-THEE-zha)
tocolytic medications (toh-koh-LIT-ik MED-ih-KAY-shunz)
variability (VAIR-ee-uh-BILL-ih-tee)
variable decelerations (VAIR-ee-uh-buhl dee-SELL-uh-RAY-shunz)
visceral pain (VISS-er-uhl PAYN)

CHAPTER CONCEPTS

Collaboration
Comfort
Communication
Leadership and Management

Oxygenation
Reproduction and Sexuality
Stress and Coping

LEARNING OUTCOMES

1. Define the key terms.
2. Discuss the theories related to the factors that cause the onset of labor.
3. List the signs of labor.
4. Describe the process of effacement and dilation that occurs in the cervix during labor.
5. Distinguish between true and false labor.
6. List and describe the "Seven Ps" of labor.
7. Distinguish between fetal lie, presentation, and position.
8. Teach a patient how to time uterine contractions.
9. Recognize the characteristics of a normal labor so as to provide knowledgeable care to the laboring patient.
10. Outline the stages and phases of labor.
11. Compare and contrast the advantages and disadvantages of a hospital birth, birthing center birth, and home birth.
12. Review the initial maternal care in the labor and delivery unit.
13. Describe the process of a cervical examination and discuss the information obtained during the cervical examination.
14. Demonstrate Leopold maneuvers and discuss the purpose of the maneuvers.
15. Explain medical interventions that may occur during each stage of labor.
16. Plan safe and effective patient-centered nursing care for each stage of labor.
17. Identify nursing responsibilities and safety issues that may arise when the patient receives analgesic and anesthetic medications for pain control in labor.
18. Analyze a fetal-monitor strip.
19. Identify unsafe or nonreassuring fetal heart decelerations and choose appropriate nursing interventions for nonreassuring fetal heart patterns.
20. Complete an Apgar score on a newborn.
21. Explain the immediate needs and goals of care for the newborn.
22. Discuss immediate postdelivery care for the woman.

CRITICAL THINKING & CLINICAL JUDGMENT

Nadia is pregnant with her first baby. She is in her 37th week of gestation and has noticed an occasional episode of a few mild uterine contractions. They seem to stop after a few minutes and are not really painful. Nadia calls her obstetrician's office. She has questions about labor contractions. "Are these mild contractions, and am I having preterm labor? How do I know if I am having true labor contractions?"

Questions

1. What are your concerns about contractions at 37 weeks' gestation?
2. Do you think Nadia is in labor? Why?
3. How would you teach Nadia about labor contractions?

CONCEPTUAL CORNERSTONE
Comfort

Labor and childbirth involve acute pain that is short-lived and diminishes with healing. Every woman has a different pain tolerance and response to pain. You should conduct a thorough pain assessment and should avoid making assumptions about the patient's pain experience. A complete pain assessment requires questioning the patient about the location, intensity, quality, onset, and duration of the pain. The nurse in labor and delivery has a key role in managing the patient's pain. The patient should be educated about safe, pharmacological strategies available for pain management as well as nonpharmacological strategies. Nonpharmacological techniques may be effective alone for mild to moderate pain and give comfort to the patient (Giddens, 2021). Unrelieved pain can interfere with the patient's ability to relax and participate in her birth experience.

You can be instrumental in assisting the woman in coping with the pain of labor and promoting self-esteem and positive memories about her childbirth experience.

In the hospital setting, nurses provide most of the care during labor. The nurse caring for a patient in labor has the responsibility of carefully monitoring the mother and fetus. Topics discussed in this chapter include the physiology of labor, signs of labor, true versus false labor, critical factors that influence labor, the stages of labor, maternal systemic response to labor, fetal response to labor, medical management of labor, and nursing care. Fetal monitoring and pain management are important parts of the care provided for the laboring woman. Fetal monitoring is a crucial part of the assessment of the health of the fetus; and this chapter includes information about examining a fetal monitoring strip and nursing interventions for nonreassuring fetal heart patterns. The chapter concludes with discussion of a birth and immediate nursing care afterward for the mother and baby.

THE PHYSIOLOGY OF LABOR

Labor is a physiological process during which the fetus, umbilical cord, placenta, and amniotic membranes are expelled from the uterus. This process of expelling the uterine contents is accomplished through uterine contractions and cervical effacement and dilation. This section discusses the theories of the causes of labor, the uterine and pelvic musculature, changes in the cervix during labor, and signs of labor.

Therapeutic Communication

Lenora, aged 17, is pregnant with her first baby. The nurse discusses childbirth education classes with Lenora using therapeutic communication.

Nurse: "Are you signed up for a childbirth class?"
Lenora: "No."
Nurse: "The classes fill up quickly; you don't want to miss it."
Lenora: "I don't think I'll go to one."
Nurse: "What are your concerns about it?"
Lenora: "I don't have the money, and they aren't at the right time."
Nurse: "Let's work together to find one that works for you. We have several options available in this area."

Possible Causes of Labor Onset

Labor usually begins between 38 and 42 weeks of gestation. The exact cause of labor onset is not clearly understood, but several theories have been proposed. It is believed that a combination of factors leads to the onset of labor:

- Increased levels of **oxytocin**, a pituitary hormone that is secreted into the bloodstream and stimulates the uterine muscle. Oxytocin is also produced in uterine tissues in late pregnancy with concentrations increasing at the onset of labor. Oxytocin receptors in the uterus also increase at the end of pregnancy. This leads to an increased sensitivity of the uterine tissues to oxytocin and subsequent myometrial (uterine muscle) activity.
- Oxytocin also helps in stimulating increased prostaglandin production through receptors in the decidua (the lining of the uterus). **Prostaglandins** are hormonelike substances with a variety of effects on tissues, including contraction and relaxation of smooth muscle. Prostaglandins produce cervical softening and increase uterine muscle sensitivity. Oxytocin and prostaglandins are thought to be the most important biochemical factors in stimulating contractions (Walter et al., 2021).

- During pregnancy, progesterone is produced by the placenta. Progesterone relaxes uterine smooth muscle by hindering the conduction of impulses from one cell to the next. Toward the end of pregnancy, progesterone levels decline, which allows estrogen to stimulate contractions.
- The *corticotropin-releasing hormone hypothesis* is based on the fact that the maturing fetus produces cortisol from the adrenal glands. The cortisol is detected in the fetal blood, and then the placenta converts the hormone into estriol. **Estriol** is one of three types of estrogens that occur naturally in the body. The rising level of estriol produces an imbalance with estradiol, another estrogen, which triggers labor.
- The *uterine stretch theory* is that the large, hollow organ becomes overstretched, leading to a natural expulsion of the contents.

Uterine Muscle

The musculature of the pregnant uterus is arranged in three layers (Fig. 9.1).

- An external layer arches over the fundus and extends to the ligaments that support the uterus.
- An internal layer has fibers that act as sphincters around the openings of the fallopian tubes and internal opening of the cervix.
- Between the external layer and internal layer is a middle layer that is composed of a dense network of fibers perforated by blood vessels. This network of muscle fibers and blood vessels contracts after placenta delivery to control blood loss (Ameer et al., 2022).

Musculature Changes in the Pelvic Floor

The muscles of the pelvic floor—the levator ani muscle and the fascia—pull the vagina and rectum upward and forward with each contraction. The pressure of the fetal head progressing through the birth canal causes these muscles to thin from approximately 5 cm to 1 cm at the time of birth (Ameer et al., 2022).

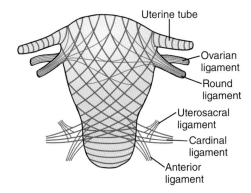

FIGURE 9.1 Arrangement of the direction of the smooth muscles of the myometrium and ligaments.

Labels: Uterine tube · Ovarian ligament · Round ligament · Uterosacral ligament · Cardinal ligament · Anterior ligament

Signs of Labor

Although every woman's experience is unique, most women experience the following signs of the onset of labor.

Bloody Show

Bloody show is evident when the mucus from inside the cervix is released. This blood-tinged mucus is sometimes referred to as the *mucous plug* and may be noted any time before or during labor.

Burst of Energy

Some women experience a burst of energy, which is also called *nesting,* about 24 to 48 hours before labor begins. The woman may experience the desire to complete many projects before her baby arrives.

Spontaneous Rupture of Membranes

Spontaneous rupture of membranes (SROM) is also referred to as the *water breaking.* The rupture of the membranes surrounding the fetus and amniotic fluid often signals that labor is beginning. The membranes can rupture any time during labor. The fluid should be clear with no offensive odor. The rupture can manifest as a large gush or a small trickle of fluid.

Safety Stat!

Amniotic fluid that is not clear, but rather yellow or green, should be reported immediately to the health-care provider. It could indicate an unhealthy fetus.

Lightening

Lightening is usually noticed by the mother after the 38th week of pregnancy as the fetus descends or drops into the pelvis. The mother notices the drop of the fetus because she has more room in her upper abdomen and finds breathing easier. After lightening takes place, she will notice that she has to urinate more often because of pressure of the fetal head on her urinary bladder, and she may experience an increase in leg cramps from the increased pressure on the nerves and blood vessels in her pelvis and legs.

Contractions

During pregnancy, women often experience contractions.

- **Braxton Hicks contractions** are irregular, mild contractions that begin during the second trimester and do not produce cervical effacement and dilation. Braxton Hicks contractions are described by women as feeling similar to menstrual cramps.
- Uterine contractions that occur regularly and become more intense as time passes indicate true labor. Contractions are sometimes described as pressure or aching in

the lower back or pelvis that then spreads around to the abdomen. The contraction starts mildly, gets stronger, progresses to a peak, and then fades away.

Cervical Changes

During most of pregnancy, the cervix is approximately 3 to 4 cm thick and closed. Toward the end of the pregnancy, the cervix starts to soften and begins to open. During labor, the cervix continues to dilate to 10 cm or large enough to accommodate the fetal head.

Effacement is the cervix-thinning process that may begin toward the end of pregnancy. Each uterine contraction causes the muscles of the upper uterine segment to shorten and cause a longitudinal traction on the cervix, causing this thinning effect. Effacement is measured in percentages. A thick, uneffaced cervix is defined as 0% effaced, and a fully thinned or effaced cervix is 100% effaced. This measurement is subjective, depending upon the skill and opinion of the practitioner performing the cervical examination. The cervix of the primipara woman effaces slowly before significant dilation occurs. With the multipara woman, effacement and dilation usually occur simultaneously.

Dilation is the opening of the closed cervix to approximately 10 cm or large enough to accommodate the fetal head.

CRITICAL THINKING

Scenario #1: Your neighbor, **Gabby**, is pregnant with her fourth child.

Question

1. What are your concerns regarding labor onset?

Differences Between True and False Labor

When labor begins, it may not be easy for you or the patient to determine if it is real or false labor. There are some points to remember when evaluating a patient for signs of true labor:

- True labor contractions:
  - Come at regular intervals
  - Become increasingly more intense as labor progresses
  - Increase in duration over time
  - Include discomfort that usually begins in the back and radiates to the front
  - Cause effacement and dilation to occur
  - May intensify with walking
  - Do not diminish with a warm shower or rest
- False labor contractions:
  - Are irregular
  - Do not increase in duration
  - Do not cause cervical effacement and dilation to occur
  - May cease with rest or a warm shower
  - Do not intensify with a walk

CRITICAL FACTORS IN LABOR

Traditionally, educators and health-care providers have used the acronym of "Ps" to describe the significant factors in the process of labor: The "Seven Ps" of labor are *passage, passenger, powers, position, psyche, pain management,* and *patience.*

> ### Safety *Stat!*
> The hormone relaxin affects all joints of the body. A term pregnant patient is at risk of falling because of the loosening of her pelvic joints, knees, and ankles.

Passage

The passage is the route through which the fetus must pass to be delivered vaginally. The passage consists of the pelvis and the soft tissues. The soft tissues yield to the pressure of the fetal presenting part, which is usually the head. The pelvis is most important to the outcome of labor because bones and joints do not yield easily to the fetal head. The pelvis is usually measured by the health-care provider at the first prenatal visit to determine if the woman's pelvis is adequately sized for a vaginal delivery.

During late pregnancy, concentration of the hormone relaxin increases, causing a softening of the cartilage that connects the pelvic bones. This softening of cartilage allows the pelvis to stretch somewhat to allow for passage of the fetus through the pelvis.

Passenger

The passenger is the fetus with the placenta. When providing labor care, the health-care provider and the nurses determine the fetal lie, presentation, position, attitude, and station and continue to monitor fetal changes as labor progresses.

Fetal Head

The structure of the fetal head accommodates labor and birth. The frontal, parietal, and occipital bones are not fused in the fetus. These bones are soft and pliable with gaps between them known as *suture lines.* This allows the bones to overlap as the head progresses through the pelvis from the force of the uterine contractions. This overlapping process causes an elongation shape of the skull and is called *molding.*

The diameter of the fetal skull affects the ease or difficulty of the labor process. The optimal position for the fetal head at birth is fully flexed with the chin on the chest, which produces the smallest fetal head dimension.

Fetal Lie

Fetal lie is the position of the fetus in the uterus. It refers to how the fetal spine lines up with the mother's spine. Determining the fetal lie helps to anticipate problems that may

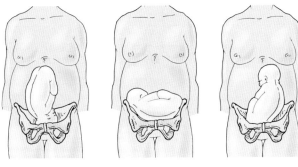

FIGURE 9.2 The fetal lie refers to the relationship of the long axis of the woman to the long axis of the fetus. A, Longitudinal lie. B, Transverse lie. C, Oblique lie.

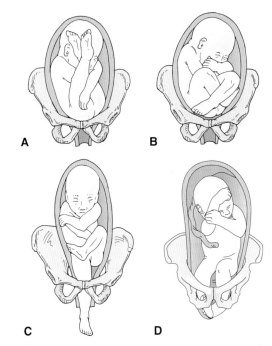

FIGURE 9.3 Breech presentation. A, Frank. B, Complete or full. C, Footling (single). D, Footling (double).

arise during labor and birth. The longitudinal lie, when the maternal and fetal spines are parallel and the fetal head is down toward the cervix, is the most common position and the easiest to deliver.

- *Longitudinal lie* refers to a fetus that is lying parallel with the mother.
- *Transverse lie* refers to a fetus that is lying perpendicular to the mother's body.
- *Oblique lie* refers to a fetus that is lying at an angle between the transverse lie and the longitudinal lie (Fig. 9.2).

Fetal Presentation

Fetal presentation refers to the part of the fetus that is first to enter the pelvis. A cephalic presentation is the most common and the easiest to deliver. In this presentation, the fetus with the head extended toward the neck can enter the pelvis in a face presentation, or a partially flexed head may create a brow presentation. Most brow presentations convert spontaneously by flexion to a true cephalic presentation (Murray & Huelsmann, 2021). A shoulder presentation will require a cesarean delivery. A breech presentation may also require a cesarean delivery; however, a footling breech presentation will require one.

- *Cephalic presentation:* The head is the presenting part.
- *Breech presentation:* The buttocks are the presenting part (Fig. 9.3A and B).
- *Shoulder presentation:* The shoulder is the presenting part.
- *Footling breech presentation:* The feet are the presenting part (Fig. 9.3C and D).

Fetal Position

Fetal position refers to the relationship of a given point on the fetus's presenting part with the mother's pelvis. The landmark for the head or cephalic presenting part is the occipital bone (indicated by the letter *O*). For a breech presentation, the landmark is the sacrum (indicated by the letter *S*). The maternal pelvis is divided into four quadrants: left anterior, right anterior, left posterior, and right posterior. The fetal position is determined by noting the presenting part and the

maternal pelvis quadrant that the fetus is facing. The position is indicated by a three-letter abbreviation:

- The first letter indicates whether the presenting part is tilted toward the left (*L*) or right (*R*) of the maternal pelvis.
- The second letter indicates the presenting part of the fetus (*O* for occipital or *S* for sacrum).
- The third letter indicates the location of the presenting part in relationship to the anterior (A), transverse (T), or posterior (P) part of the maternal pelvis.

The most common fetal position in labor is *LOA* (left occiput anterior), which means that the fetus's occipital bone (the back of the head) is facing the left anterior quadrant of the mother's pelvis (Fig. 9.4). An anterior presentation is the optimal position for the fetus to move through the birth canal.

Fetal Attitude

The fetal **attitude** refers to the positioning of the fetus's body parts. The most common fetal attitude and the most successful for a vaginal delivery is when the fetus is in a fully flexed position with the chin on the chest, the back rounded, the thighs flexed on the abdomen, and the legs flexed at the knees. A fetus that is not fully flexed exhibits changes in the presenting part diameter as passage through the pelvis occurs, leading to birthing difficulty (Fig. 9.5).

Fetal Station

Fetal station is the measurement in centimeters of the fetal head in relationship to the maternal ischial spines in the

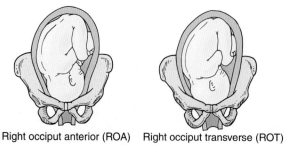
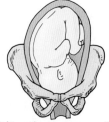
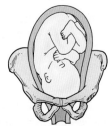

Right occiput anterior (ROA)   Right occiput transverse (ROT)   Right occiput posterior (ROP)

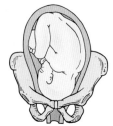
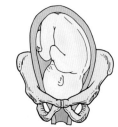
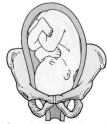
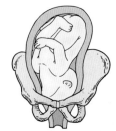

Left occiput anterior (LOA)   Left occiput transverse (LOT)   Left occiput posterior (LOP)   Right mentum anterior (RMA)

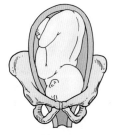
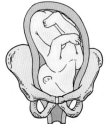
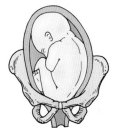
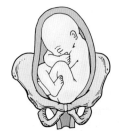

Right mentum posterior (RMP)   Left mentum anterior (LMA)   Left sacrum anterior (LSA)   Left sacrum posterior (LSP)

FIGURE 9.4 Fetal presentations and positions. The position refers to how the presenting fetal part is positioned in relationship to the maternal pelvis: front (anterior), back (posterior), or side (transverse).

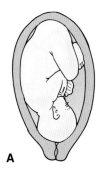
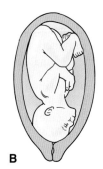
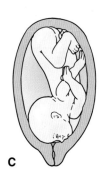

A   **B**   **C**

FIGURE 9.5 The fetal attitude describes the relationship of the fetal body parts to one another. A, Flexion (cephalic or vertex). B, Moderate flexion. C, Extension.

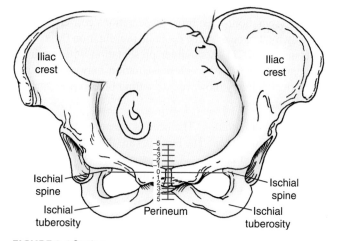

FIGURE 9.6 Station.

pelvis. Station measurements provide information on the descent of the fetus through the birth canal.

- The measurement ranges from –5 cm to +5 cm.
- When the head is above the ischial spines, a negative number is applied. For example, when the head is 1 cm above the ischial spines, the measurement is –1.
- When the fetal head is at the level of the ischial spines, it is measured as 0 station.
- When the head is 1 cm through the ischial spines, it is termed +1 station (Fig. 9.6).

Powers

During labor, the power of the uterine contractions and the woman's ability to push are critical factors. At the onset of labor, the patient and her support person will be timing contractions at home. After arrival at the hospital, the health-care provider and labor and delivery nurses will time and evaluate contractions with the use of the fetal monitor or manually by palpating contractions. Uterine contractions in labor occur in a regular, rhythmic fashion. Each contraction has three phases:

1. The **increment**, which is the onset and build-up of intensity of the contraction
2. The **acme**, which is the peak of the contraction
3. The **decrement**, which is the subsiding of the contraction (Fig. 9.7)

To describe contractions, the following terms are used:

- *Onset:* The exact time that a contraction begins
- *Duration:* The actual time that a contraction lasts from beginning to end
- *Frequency:* The time between contractions, which is measured from the beginning of one contraction to the beginning of the next contraction
- *Intensity:* The strength of the contraction at its peak, or acme; intensity can be measured by palpation by an experienced practitioner and by internal fetal monitoring

At the peak of a strong contraction, uteroplacental blood flow is decreased, and the fetus receives no fresh oxygenated blood supply until the contraction passes. Between each contraction is a period of relaxation.

During the second stage of labor, the woman pushes along with contractions to continue to move the fetus through the birth canal. Her pushing efforts can prevent interventions such as forceps or vacuum extraction assistance during the birthing process.

Position

Maternal position changes can influence the length of the labor. Upright positions, such as standing, sitting, kneeling,

Patient Teaching Guidelines

How to Time Uterine Contractions

An informed woman who knows how to time contractions will have valid information to provide the health-care provider if she thinks she is starting labor. Such knowledge will also help the patient to distinguish between true and false labor. The steps for timing contractions are as follows:

- Note the exact time that a contraction begins. This is the *onset* of the contraction.
- Note the exact time that the contraction stops. From the onset to this point is the *duration*, or length, of the contraction.
- Note the exact time that the next contraction begins. From the first onset to this point is the *frequency* of the contractions.

Teach your patient that contraction frequency is the time from the beginning of one contraction to the beginning of the next. Duration of the contraction is the actual length of time the contraction was noticeable. For example, a patient's contractions have occurred at 0400, 0404, 0409, 0413, 0418, 0423, 0428, 0432, and 0437. Each contraction lasts from 40 to 60 seconds. You would report that the patient is having contractions 4 to 5 minutes apart with a duration of 40 to 60 seconds.

or walking, have been shown to reduce the length of labor by approximately 1 hour and are associated with less epidural anesthesia (Murray & Huelsmann, 2021). Women should be encouraged to choose a position that is comfortable for

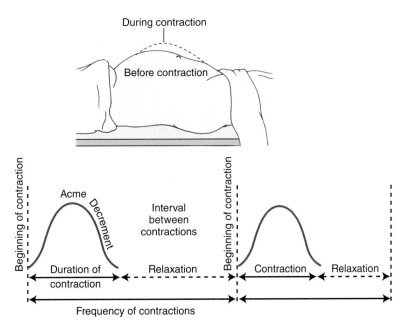

FIGURE 9.7 Counting contractions. Contraction frequency is the time from the beginning of one contraction to the beginning of the next. Contraction duration is the time from the beginning to the end of the same contraction.

them; an exception is the supine position, which can produce blood-flow problems for the woman and the placenta.

Studies have shown that an upright, lateral, or squatting position during the second stage for pushing and delivery reduces the need for assisted delivery. These positions have been shown to reduce reports of severe pain during this stage and to reduce abnormal fetal heart rate (FHR) patterns (American College of Obstetricians and Gynecologists [ACOG], 2019). Women without an epidural should be encouraged to deliver in an upright position.

Psyche

Physical and mental preparation for labor and delivery are very important aspects of managing the labor process. It is generally noticed by nurses in the labor and delivery unit that women who lack confidence in their ability to manage and cope with labor seem to have longer labors with more interventions and a higher rate of cesarean births. The woman's state of mind (psyche) before and during the birthing process is important to create a positive outcome for her and her family. Factors that contribute to a positive birth experience include the following:

- Childbirth education, which prepares the woman for labor and delivery; patients with childbirth education tend to arrive at the labor and delivery unit in active labor and are confident of their ability to manage labor (Berghella & Di Mascio, 2020)
- Trust in the health-care provider and the staff who care for her
- Nurses who integrate the patient's birth philosophy, cultural beliefs, and religious values and beliefs into the plan of care
- Information updates provided about labor progress
- Clear, concise information given on necessary procedures during the labor and birth process
- Nurses, the health-care provider, and the support person giving reassurance and praise for managing labor and offering advice regarding coping techniques
- Continuous one-on-one support throughout labor and birth by someone who can advocate for the woman's desires or birth plan
- Assisting the laboring woman to maintain her sense of control of herself and the labor situation

Pain Management

Labor and delivery are normal physiological processes, but they are painful. Every woman perceives and reacts to pain differently. Women who are anxious during labor have high levels of the stress hormone epinephrine in the blood, which can lead to abnormal FHR patterns, decreased uterine contractility, and a longer active labor phase (Berghella & Di Mascio, 2020). The challenge of the birthing team (woman, support person, nurse, anesthesiologist, and health-care provider) is to find the right combination of pain management methods to promote a positive experience for the woman in labor as well as a safe delivery for the fetus.

Pain management methods used by women during childbirth include both nonpharmacological measures, such as massage, warm baths, and relaxation techniques, and pharmacological methods.

Patience

The process of labor takes time. Many obstetric interventions that are widely used, such as the induction of labor, the augmentation of labor with oxytocin, and regional anesthesia (epidural), influence the length of the labor process. Delaying these types of interventions and allowing labor to progress naturally may decrease medical interventions and decrease the cesarean birth rate. *Healthy People 2030* has two goals related to cesarean birth in the United States:

1. Reduce the rate of cesarean birth among low-risk women.
2. Reduce the rate of cesarean births among women who have had a prior cesarean birth.

To achieve these goals, patience during labor is required. Methods to increase patience include:

- Educate the woman and her family that every labor is different and it is difficult to predict how long a labor will last.
- Avoid interventions such as epidural anesthesia that reduce the woman's ability to push and her participation in delivery of the fetus (Olsen, 2022).
- Avoid induction of labor when the cervix has not softened sufficiently to make it receptive to induction methods.
- Avoid the induction of labor for nonmedical reasons. Women induced have a significantly longer time in labor (Olsen, 2022).
- Provide reassurance to the mother of fetal well-being during the labor process.
- Provide nonpharmacological pain interventions as well as pharmacological support for pain during labor.
- If the fetal monitor indicates that the fetus is tolerating labor well, do not place pressure on the obstetrician or midwife to rush the birth. Allow a longer pushing phase. Longer pushing has not been associated with poor outcomes.

 ## MATERNAL SYSTEMIC RESPONSE TO LABOR

The most significant response during labor occurs in the reproductive system. However, the mother's cardiovascular, respiratory, renal, gastrointestinal, and hematopoietic systems are also affected during labor.

Cardiovascular System

At the peak of a contraction, blood flow to the placenta from the mother is decreased. This decrease of blood to the placenta causes the woman's blood volume to increase. An increase in blood volume will cause a rise in blood pressure and a decrease in the pulse rate. Supine hypotension may occur if the woman is allowed to lie on her back during labor. The mother should be encouraged to labor in a side position or slightly upright to avoid hypotension.

Respiratory System

Anxiety and pain will cause an increase in the rate and depth of respirations. If the woman is allowed to breathe too deeply and too fast, hyperventilation can occur because she exhales too much carbon dioxide.

Renal System

The position of the fetus in the uterus places pressure on the urinary bladder. The woman adjusts physically to the constant feeling of pelvic pressure and may not notice a full bladder. A full bladder can impede the labor process and fetal descent; therefore, the patient should be encouraged to empty her bladder at regular intervals. A woman with an epidural during labor will have a catheter inserted to keep the bladder from becoming too full.

Gastrointestinal System

During labor, gastric motility slows down. Nausea and vomiting can occur, so large quantities of food and liquids are usually not advisable. It is common for the woman to experience thirst and dry mouth from the increased respiratory rate.

Hematopoietic System

Expected blood loss for a vaginal delivery is 500 mL. Because of the increased blood volume during pregnancy, most women have no adverse effects from this amount of blood loss. A hemoglobin of 11 g/dL and a hematocrit of 33% or higher further indicates that the woman can handle the blood loss without problems (Van Leeuwen & Bladh, 2021). The leukocyte count for a pregnant woman at term is usually higher than that of a nonpregnant woman, averaging 14,000 to 16,000 per mm^3. Fibrinogen is elevated throughout pregnancy and continues to remain elevated during labor. Although there is an increase in clotting factors, fibrinolysis (clot breakdown) actually slows down, which promotes coagulation when the placenta separates from the uterus.

FETAL RESPONSE TO LABOR

The fetus experiences labor along with the mother. If the fetus is healthy, the stress of labor does not produce adverse effects for the fetus. Fetal responses to labor include the following:

- The heart rate accelerates with fetal movement and decelerates with head compression as the fetus moves through the birth canal
- Decreased circulation and perfusion during the peak of a contraction
- An increase in arterial carbon dioxide pressure (Pco_2)

- A decrease in fetal oxygen pressure (Po_2)
- A decrease in fetal breathing movements (Funai & Norowitz, 2022)

> **Team Works**
>
> Women with an understanding of the normal labor and delivery process will experience less stress during labor (Berghella & Di Mascio, 2020). A team approach to educating the woman and her partner about the labor experience would include the following team members:
>
> - The office nurse during prenatal visits
> - The childbirth educator who provides childbirth education classes
> - The nurse in labor and delivery who determines the immediate learning needs of the patient
> - The doula, if one is present, providing labor support
> - The nurse midwife or obstetrician providing care and delivering the fetus

STAGES OF LABOR AND BIRTH

Labor is divided into four stages that occur in a continuous progression. The first stage is usually the longest. During this stage of labor, fetal monitoring and pain management are usually part of the labor experience. The second stage of labor involves pushing the fetus through the birth canal and delivery. The third stage of labor is the delivery of the placenta, and the fourth stage is recovery.

Labor Stage 1:

The first stage of labor begins with regular uterine contractions and ends with complete cervical dilation at 10 cm. The first stage is divided into early and active phases (ACOG, 2021b; Olsen, 2022). Medical management and nursing care are outlined in Table 9.1 for each phase of stage 1 of labor.

Early Phase

The early phase of labor can be unpredictable from woman to woman and from labor to labor. Typically for the **primiparous** woman, the early phase may last close to 20 hours. For a **multiparous** woman, it is usually around 10 to 12 hours. The amniotic membranes may spontaneously rupture in the early-to-midportion of the first stage of labor. If they rupture, the labor process usually speeds up because the presenting part is able to apply pressure to the cervix during contractions.

· WORD · BUILDING ·
primiparous: primi–first + parous–bearing
multiparous: multi–many + parous–bearing

Table 9.1

Stage 1 of Labor

Stages of Labor	Characteristics	Medical Management	Nursing Care
Stage 1: Early Phase	• Uterine contractions are mild and may be erratic. The contractions may range from 5–20 minutes apart and last 20–40 seconds. • Most of the cervical effacement occurs. • Cervical dilation increases to 6 cm (ACOG, 2021b) • The woman and her partner may feel excited and relieved that labor has started but anxious about the birth process. • The woman usually can cope with the pain of contractions by using relaxation and breathing techniques. • For the primiparous woman, this stage may last close to 20 hours; for multiparous women, it varies but is generally 10–12 hours.	• Admit to hospital • CBC, blood type, Rh, GBS screen, and urinalysis • STI screen, depending on state laws • Order IV infusion of lactated Ringer's solution or normal saline to prevent dehydration in labor • Intermittent or continual fetal monitoring	• Orientation of the patient and her support person to the labor room • Establishing a therapeutic relationship • Inquiring about concerns or questions • Reassuring the support person that the nurse will be assisting with providing comfort measures and support for both of them during labor • Reinforcing relaxation techniques or teaching simple relaxation techniques • Inserting the IV or saline lock for fluid maintenance or medication administration • Reviewing laboratory results and notifying the physician, if necessary • Administering penicillin G IV, if indicated, for GBS • Encouraging fluid intake with clear fluid and ice chips • Explaining the fetal monitor and applying it for intermittent or continual monitoring • Ongoing monitoring of the vital signs, cervical dilation and effacement, FHR, and contractions
Stage 1: Active Phase	• Uterine contractions are 2–3 minutes apart. The duration is around 60–90 seconds and increasingly painful. • The rate of dilation increases until fully dilated. • Fetal descent is progressing. • The woman becomes labor-focused and may require more assistance to cope with the increasing intensity of the uterine contractions. • The woman may feel pelvic or rectal pressure caused by fetal descent into the pelvis. • She may have a strong desire to push the fetus down and out. • She may have more trouble with concentration and coping and may become irritable. • Nausea and vomiting are common.	• Performing an **amniotomy**, which is the artificial rupture of the membranes (AROM) with an amniohook • Orders for pain medication or **epidural** anesthesia • Evaluation of the maternal condition and progression of labor • Evaluation of the fetal condition • Pain medication if safe, depending upon the labor progress • The health-care provider will be monitoring fetal descent and preparing to deliver the fetus	• Pain assessment, including the description, location, radiation, and degree of discomfort • Performing vaginal examinations to monitor cervical dilation, fetal position, and descent • Providing the woman and her support person frequent updates on progress • Providing emotional support in the form of praise, reassurance, listening, and physical presence • Assisting the woman's support person to provide comfort and encouraging the support person to take a break as needed • Encouraging clear liquids • Monitoring vital signs every 30 minutes • Monitoring the FHR and contractions every 15–30 minutes, adjusting the transducers as needed

• **WORD** • **BUILDING** •

amniotomy: amnio–amniotic sac + tomy–incision
epidural: epi–on or over + dural–relating to dura mater

Table 9.1

Stage 1 of Labor—cont'd

Stages of Labor	Characteristics	Medical Management	Nursing Care
	• For the primiparous woman, this stage can last 3.5 hours; for multiparous women, it varies but is generally shorter.		• Providing nonpharmacological pain relief and comfort measures (See the Nonpharmacological Pain Management section later in this chapter.) • Administering pain medication as ordered and per patient requests Evaluating the effectiveness of pharmacological and nonpharmacological pain relief • Changing the disposable pad underneath the patient as she continues to leak fluid and mucus from the vagina • Encouraging position changes; encouraging walking if her membranes are intact • Assisting with elimination to prevent a full bladder, which can slow down the descent of the fetus into the pelvis • Reviewing and reinforcing relaxation and breathing techniques using a calm, soothing voice and touch • Communicating labor progress to the healthcare provider • Assisting with breathing techniques, particularly if she loses focus or has a strong desire to push • Preparing the patient and the room for delivery • Remaining in the room with the patient and family • Providing encouragement to the woman and her support person

The uterine contractions are generally mild and erratic before becoming regular and stronger, and they may range from 5 to 20 minutes apart and last 20 to 40 seconds. For a primiparous woman, most of the cervical effacement occurs in this phase and cervical dilation increases to 6 cm (ACOG, 2021b). The woman and her partner may feel excited and relieved that labor has started but anxious about the birth process. The woman can usually cope with the pain of contractions by using relaxation and breathing techniques. The woman and her support person and/or family may arrive at the hospital or birthing center during this phase. If they are planning a home birth, they should alert their midwife that labor has begun.

Active Labor

The next part of the first stage of labor is the active phase. Active labor begins when the rate of cervical change increases at 6 cm and faster dilation occurs. For the primiparous woman, this stage can last 3.5 hours; for multiparous women, it varies but is generally shorter. Commonly, the contractions are 2 to 3 minutes apart with a duration of at least 60 seconds;

toward the end of the active phase the contractions may be as long as 90 seconds. As the rate of dilation increases, fetal descent progresses and causes feelings of pelvic pressure. Toward the end of active labor, the woman may feel pelvic or rectal pressure because of fetal descent into the pelvis. She may have more trouble with concentration and coping and may become irritable. Nausea and vomiting commonly accompany this phase of labor.

During this phase she may have the urge to push. The patient and the support person should be taught by the nurse to call the nurse immediately if the patient begins to push or bear down. A nurse should check the patient to determine if she is fully dilated. Pushing too early can cause the cervix to swell and slow dilation of the cervix.

The patient is no longer talkative or interested in conversation. She becomes labor focused and may require more assistance to cope with the increasing intensity of the uterine contractions. Pain management and comfort measures become more important during this phase. The woman may change positions frequently to find one that feels right to her (Fig. 9.8).

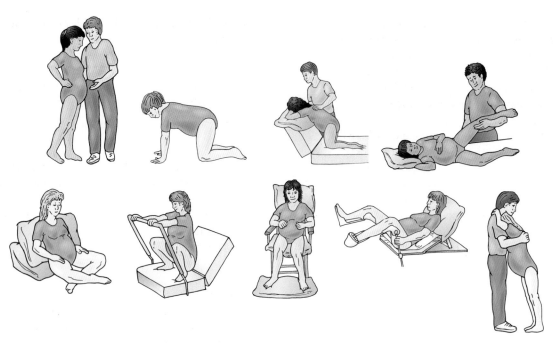

FIGURE 9.8 Various positions for labor and birth.

Safe and Effective Nursing Care

Hyperventilation can occur if the woman breathes too fast and too deeply in response to pain in labor. Hyperventilation causes a decrease in carbon dioxide in the blood. Signs of hyperventilation include feelings of anxiety, a feeling that she cannot get enough air, an elevated heart rate, lightheadedness or vertigo, numbness or tingling of the fingers, and chest tightness. To manage hyperventilation, encourage the patient to do one of the following: (a) slow down breathing and breathe through pursed lips, as if blowing out a candle; (b) close her mouth and one nostril and breathe through one nostril only; or (c) cover her nose and mouth with a paper bag and breathe in and out into the bag for a few breaths only or for about 15 seconds. These interventions will raise the level of carbon dioxide in the blood and decrease symptoms.

Team Works

Assisting a patient in labor requires teamwork. The health-care provider, labor and delivery nurse, support person or coach, doula, and friends can all work together to provide positive support and comfort measures for the laboring woman. Continuous support has a more beneficial effect for reducing anxiety and pain than intermittent support (Murray & Huelsmann, 2021).

Safe and Effective Nursing Care

If the patient becomes nauseated, you need to assist her to a safe position, such as sitting up or elevating her head, to prevent aspiration if she vomits. The health-care provider may order antinausea medication if the nausea is severe.

Patient Teaching During Labor

During labor, the patient will need ongoing teaching regarding the process of labor and reassurance that labor is progressing appropriately.

- Inform her that the contractions are mild at the beginning of labor but will get progressively stronger and last longer.
- Encourage her to relax by listening to music, receiving a massage, or engaging in a distraction such as television or conversation.
- Encourage her to change position and walk to promote labor progress.
- Remind her to urinate every 2 hours to prevent distension of her bladder, which could slow down the descent of the fetus.
- Invite her to sip clear liquids to avoid dehydration. If the health-care provider consents, she can eat light, easily digested food.
- Instruct her to notify you if her water breaks or any bleeding is noted.
- Instruct the patient that if she notices strong pressure in her lower back and rectum or feels a desire to push, she should notify you. Pushing too early can cause the cervix to become edematous (swollen) and slow down dilation of the cervix.

- Instruct her to use pant-blow breathing to prevent early pushing and assist her in this breathing technique. Pant-blow breathing is quick breathing in and out of the mouth. After every 3 to 5 quick breaths (panting), the patient should do a longer exhale (blowing).
- Caution her that nausea and vomiting may occur, and she should call you for assistance.
- Mention that she may notice more blood-tinged vaginal mucus as the capillaries in the cervix rupture.
- Reassure her that it may become more difficult to maintain focus and concentration, but you will be available to assist her. It is normal for her to feel impatient, overwhelmed, and irritable at some points in labor.
- Instruct the patient to report the following signs to you: nausea, vomiting, leg shakiness, and alternating chills and sweats.

SETTINGS FOR CHILDBIRTH

Pregnancy and childbirth are normal life events for most women and their newborns. For women with uncomplicated pregnancies, there are a variety of settings that may be utilized for childbirth: the hospital, the birthing center, and the home.

Hospital

In the United States, most births occur in hospitals. Table 9.2 notes the advantages and disadvantages of giving birth in a hospital.

Birthing Center

A birthing center is a homelike setting where certified nurse midwives (CNMs) provide family-centered care. Birthing centers are typically located in large urban areas; therefore, many women may not have access to a birthing center. Table 9.3 notes the advantages and disadvantages of giving birth in a birthing center.

Home

According to the ACOG (2020b), 0.9% of births in the United States occur outside a hospital. Home births may be attended by a licensed CNM or by lay midwives who have varying degrees of formal education. The American Academy of Pediatrics (AAP) supports a woman's right to make a medically informed decision about delivery and has published

Table 9.2
Advantages and Disadvantages of a Hospital Birth

Advantages of a Hospital Birth	*Disadvantages of a Hospital Birth*
• It is the safest environment for high-risk patients. • Emergency equipment and personnel are available at all times. • The pediatrician can be present for the delivery if a problem is anticipated. • It is the only option if a cesarean delivery is required. • Until discharge, the woman has 24-hour support from nurses.	• Many women giving birth for the first time have never been in a hospital and find the environment intimidating. • The woman's partner may be less actively involved with the process. • The birth is managed by experts who may not agree with the mother's birth plan. • Hospitals can be noisy, and the new mother may not receive much rest.

Table 9.3
Advantages and Disadvantages of a Birthing Center Birth

Advantages of a Birthing Center Birth	*Disadvantages of a Birthing Center Birth*
• The facility is dedicated to providing labor and delivery care only. • The woman is encouraged to make her own decisions regarding comfort measures, eating, and moving during labor. • The woman can give birth in any position she prefers. • The woman can invite family and friends to participate in the birth process. • A birthing center is usually affiliated with a hospital in the event that an emergency occurs and the woman needs to be transported.	• Most centers have rigid screening criteria, and high-risk mothers are not allowed to use the center for labor and birth. • Discharge is usually within 24 hours. • Transfer to a hospital may be required if a complication occurs. • There are no pediatricians present at the birth.

Table 9.4

Advantages and Disadvantages of a Home Birth

Advantages of Having a Home Birth	*Disadvantages of a Having a Home Birth*
• The mother is able to relax in her home environment and have more privacy. • Continuous one-on-one care is given. • The caregivers are invited into the home and will not leave because their shifts are over or another patient needs care. • Labor is allowed to progress normally, without interventions. • The cost of a home birth is less than a birthing center or hospital. • Bonding is enhanced because the mother and baby are not separated.	• The patient has to accept the consequences of medical and health decisions made during labor and birth. • Medication for pain is usually not available. • The laboring woman must be moved to the hospital in the event of an emergency. • Home deliveries are 10 times more likely to result in an Apgar score of 0 than hospital deliveries (Ratini, 2022).

Patient Teaching Guidelines

When to Go to the Hospital or Birthing Center

The obstetrician or nurse midwife may give the patient specific guidance on monitoring early labor at home. However, some general guidelines for when to arrive at the hospital or birthing center include the following:

• The amniotic membranes rupture (water breaks).
• The contractions are 5 minutes apart for an hour and increasing in intensity and duration.
• Her previous labor was rapid; she should come in if contractions are 7 to 10 minutes apart.
• Any vaginal bleeding occurs, even if it is painless.
• She feels any urge to push or bear down during contractions.

a position paper informing mothers-to-be about standards of care for a newborn. The AAP recommends that there be a person dedicated to the care of the newborn at every home delivery. This person would provide resuscitation and warmth and would assign Apgar scores at 1 and 5 minutes. Table 9.4 notes the advantages and disadvantages of giving birth at home.

ADMISSION TO THE HOSPITAL OR BIRTHING CENTER

Patients can often complete hospital or birthing center paperwork and supply medical insurance and payment information before arriving in labor. This will streamline the admissions process when the woman arrives in labor and may be unable to focus on completing hospital forms.

On arrival, the hospital will ask the patient to sign consent for admission and medical and nursing care. This process places the patient information into the hospital computer system and allows the ordering of laboratory tests and medications. The patient is then transported to the labor and delivery unit.

Upon arrival in the unit, the patient and her support person should be greeted by a registered nurse who reviews the patient's admission data. Most health-care providers forward prenatal care records to the hospital before the patient's due date. You have two patients to evaluate: the woman and her fetus.

Admission Data Collection

You should review the records to identify any potential problems and high-risk patients. A medication history should be obtained, including information about current medications, vitamins, supplements, or alternative therapies.

Maternal Care

Every patient who comes under the care of a nurse must be evaluated to obtain a baseline of the patient's condition. In the labor and delivery unit, this baseline provides information that will assist you in monitoring the progress of labor and noticing early signs of potential problems and possible safety issues for the patient and fetus. You should prioritize the admission assessment in the event that the labor is progressing quickly. You may need to check the contractions, cervical dilation, and fetus immediately to notify the obstetrician or nurse midwife of an impending delivery. A complete admission assessment usually includes the following:

• Vital signs (temperature, respiratory rate, pulse, and blood pressure)
• Documentation of allergies to food and medications
• Documentation of the last food intake
• A complete head-to-toe assessment
• Skin assessment
• Falls risk assessment
• Pain assessment
• Cultural needs assessment

- Documentation of the time labor began, including the frequency and duration of contractions
- The presence or absence of bloody show
- Cervical examination

Cervical Examination

You will perform a cervical examination to determine the patient's cervical dilation, effacement, and fetal position. The cervical examination provides the woman with a progress report and gives you needed data for anticipating the birth and reporting progress to the health-care provider. Vaginal examinations can be uncomfortable for the woman, so you must be gentle. The steps to perform a vaginal cervical examination are as follows:

1. You should perform hand hygiene and provide for privacy.
2. You will position the woman onto her back with her knees flexed.
3. You will apply sterile gloves and place a drop of lubricant on the dominant hand.
4. With the nondominant hand, while gently opening the labia, you should inspect the labia and note any blood or fluid leaking from the vagina. You will also note any ulcerated lesions or vesicles that should be reported to the health-care provider.
5. With the dominant hand, you will introduce the index and middle fingers into the vagina toward the posterior vaginal wall.
6. You will touch the cervix and note the position and the amount of effacement and dilation present. At the same time, you will confirm the presenting part and rate the station in the pelvis. As dilation increases, you can determine fetal position by palpating the posterior fontanelle.
7. You will withdraw your hand and remove lubricant from the labia by wiping from front to back to avoid rectal contamination in the vaginal area.
8. You will assist the woman to sit up or lie on her side.
9. You will document findings and report progress, if needed, to the health-care provider (Fig. 9.9).

Vaginal cervical examinations are performed periodically. There are no rules about timing for the vaginal examinations. The patient is usually eager for labor progress updates, but you need to educate the patient that frequent cervical examinations can lead to an increased risk for infection. The experienced nurse takes into consideration the woman's parity, past labor length, contraction pattern, and response to labor

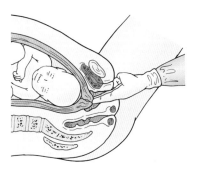

FIGURE 9.9 Vaginal examination to determine cervical dilation.

to determine the frequency of the vaginal cervical examinations. The information about dilation, effacement, and station provide the woman and her family with a progress report on the labor process.

Assessment of Amniotic Membranes

If the amniotic membranes have ruptured before admission, you should obtain the time of rupture and characteristics of the fluid (color, odor, amount) from the patient. The membranes can rupture as a gush or a slow leak. The amniotic fluid should be clear.

Yellow-stained fluid can indicate a blood incompatibility between the mother and fetus. The breakdown of red blood cells that occurs because of the incompatibility produces the yellow tint.

Greenish amniotic fluid can indicate fetal distress, which causes the fetus to pass meconium into the fluid. **Meconium** is usually the newborn's first bowel movement. If the fetus experiences stress or hypoxia (decreased oxygen), it expels meconium while still in the uterus. Any abnormal color of amniotic fluid should be reported to the health-care provider immediately.

Amniotic fluid is alkaline and can be tested with nitrazine paper. You take a small piece of nitrazine paper and touch it to any fluid around the perineum. If amniotic fluid is present, the alkaline fluid will produce a deep blue color on the nitrazine paper.

The amniotic membranes may rupture spontaneously or the health-care provider may use an amniohook to break the bag of fluids. An amniohook is a sterile, long, thin plastic hook that slides through the cervix to rupture the amniotic sac. After rupture, you should inspect the fluid for color, odor, and amount.

Safety Stat!

A vaginal cervical examination must never be attempted if the woman is bleeding from the vagina. The bleeding may be caused by placenta previa, and you could puncture the placenta and cause hemorrhage.

Safe and Effective Nursing Care

The FHR must be determined immediately when the amniotic membranes are ruptured in case the umbilical cord becomes compressed with the sudden loss of the cushioning amniotic fluid. You should listen to the FHR with a Doppler as soon as possible after rupture of the amniotic membranes. The health-care provider must be immediately notified of any drop in FHR.

CRITICAL THINKING

Scenario #2: Sherri arrives for her weekly visit with her nurse midwife. She comments, "I think my water broke."

Question

1. What question should you ask Sherri?

Laboratory Tests

Admission laboratory tests are completed to evaluate the health of the woman. Although protocol varies among hospitals and health-care providers, the following laboratory tests are commonly ordered on admission:

- *Complete blood cell count (CBC):* This test evaluates the red blood cells, white blood cells, and platelets. The results provide diagnostic information regarding the general health of the patient.
- *Blood type and screen:* This test evaluates the blood type and Rh in the event of a need for a blood transfusion. Generally, the health-care provider will ask the laboratory to hold the specimen for 72 hours in the event a blood transfusion is required.
- *Urinalysis:* This test screens for infection, glucose, bilirubin, nitrates, and proteins and provides information about the overall health of the patient.
- *Group B streptococcus (GBS) screen:* This test determines if the organism is present.

Obstetricians screen patients for GBS at 37 weeks of gestation. If no screening has occurred, a rapid GBS test kit can provide results in minutes on a vaginal or rectal fluid swab. Women who have a positive screen usually do not have symptoms. However, the fetus can be exposed to the organism during the birth process, and it can cause pneumonia and sepsis in the newborn (Centers for Disease Control and Prevention [CDC], 2022).

Labs & Diagnostics

Because of the blood loss of delivery, it is important to know if the laboring patient has a low hemoglobin and hematocrit before giving birth. Often the woman is screened for anemia at the initial prenatal appointment and then again at 24 to 28 weeks of gestation. Screening at admission will provide important information for planning care in the event that she has become anemic during the last weeks of pregnancy.

Additional Assessment Data

The nurse who wants to provide patient-centered care will also collect information regarding the patient's desires and needs for support in labor. Additional information that should be collected includes the following:

- *Birth plan:* If the woman arrives with a birth plan, the nurse should review it with the patient and make sincere efforts to follow the plan as long as it does not interfere with a safe birth. (For more about birth plans, see Chapter 7.)
- *Support person:* The nurse should determine who the main support person is and reassure that person that the labor and delivery staff will also provide any needed support during labor.
- *Childbirth classes:* If the patient attended Lamaze or Bradley childbirth classes (see Chapter 7), the nurse should be prepared to support and assist with breathing and relaxation techniques. If not, the nurse should be prepared to teach relaxation and breathing techniques as labor progresses.

Therapeutic Communication

Many patients arrive in labor and delivery with a birth plan. The woman and her support person may be anxious and fearful that you will not listen to or implement her birth plan. You should use open-ended questions and, with an open mind, gently explore options that may be agreeable to the patient, you, and the health-care provider if the team cannot safely adhere to the complete birth plan.

Fetal Assessment

On admission, you should perform **Leopold maneuvers**, a series of palpations, to determine fetal position and presentation. This provides information about possible complications in labor and makes it easier to position electronic fetal monitoring equipment. The steps for performing Leopold maneuvers are as follows:

1. You should perform hand hygiene and provide privacy for the patient.
2. You will position the woman supine with a small rolled towel or pillow under her left side to tilt the uterus to the side, which helps to avoid vena caval syndrome.
3. You will observe the abdomen for fetal movement.
4. For the first maneuver, you will stand at the foot of the woman, facing her, and place both hands flat on her abdomen (Fig. 9.10). Palpation is performed on the uterus fundus to determine the shape, consistency, and mobility. This palpation will determine if the fetal buttocks (will feel soft) or head (will feel firm) is located in the fundus.
5. For the second maneuver, you will face the patient's head and place the left hand on the right side of the uterus and hold it still while palpating the left side of the uterus with the right hand (Fig. 9.11). The process is repeated on the right side. This palpation locates the back of the fetus, which feels firm and smooth. In contrast, the side of the uterus with arms and legs will feel bumpy.
6. For the third maneuver, you will face the patient's head and grasp the lower portion of the abdomen above the

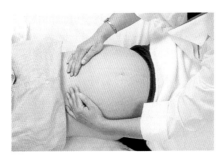

FIGURE 9.10 Leopold first maneuver determines whether the buttocks or fetal head is in the fundus.

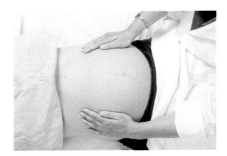

FIGURE 9.11 Leopold second maneuver determines on which side of the uterus the fetal back is located.

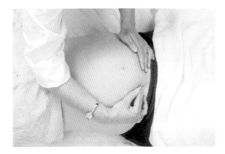

FIGURE 9.12 Leopold third maneuver shows whether the buttocks or fetal head is at the inlet of the pelvis.

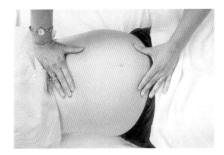

FIGURE 9.13 Leopold fourth maneuver is used only for cephalic presentation to determine fetal attitude and position in the pelvis.

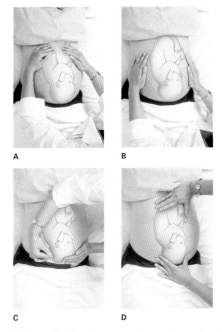

FIGURE 9.14 Assessing fetal presentation and position utilizing Leopold maneuvers. A, Leopold first maneuver. B, Leopold second maneuver. C, Leopold third maneuver. D, Leopold fourth maneuver.

symphysis pubis and gently press the thumb and fingers together (Fig. 9.12). This palpation determines which part of the fetus is at the inlet of the pelvis. A head presentation will be firm, and buttocks will feel soft to the examiner. If the presenting part is upwardly movable, it is not engaged in the pelvis.

7. The fourth maneuver is only completed if the fetus is in a cephalic presentation. You will face the patient's feet and place the fingers on both sides of the uterus about 2 inches above the inguinal ligaments and press downward and inward in the direction of the birth canal (Fig. 9.13). This palpation provides information regarding the fetal attitude and extension into the pelvis (Fig. 9.14).

After performing Leopold maneuvers, you will obtain a baseline FHR assessment using a handheld Doppler device. The patient should be monitored for a minimum of 20 minutes to determine fetal well-being and to establish baseline information (Murray & Huelsmann, 2021). After the baseline is determined, the health-care provider, nurse, and patient can discuss a plan to intermittently or continually monitor fetal well-being.

After completing the admission assessment, the registered nurse should notify the health-care provider of the assessment data and report any of the following signs or symptoms that can indicate a problem:

- Temperature greater than 38°C (100.4°F)
- Blood pressure greater than 140/90 mm Hg or lower than 90/60 mm Hg
- Maternal heart rate greater than 110 bpm
- Respiratory rate greater than 24 breaths per minute
- Vaginal bleeding
- An abnormal FHR pattern
- Uterine contractions lasting 2 minutes or longer or contractions of normal duration but occurring within 1 minute of each other
- Any abnormal finding from physical assessment
- Impending delivery

Medication Facts

To protect the fetus from GBS infection during delivery, penicillin G is usually given to the woman in labor at an initial dose of 5 million units IV, followed by 2.5 million units every 4 hours until delivery. Ampicillin may be used as an alternative choice and is given with an initial dose of 2 g IV followed with 1 g IV every 4 hours until delivery. For women allergic to penicillin, cefazolin, erythromycin, or clindamycin may be prescribed (Vallerand & Sanoski, 2023).

Team Works

Some laboring women have a doula at the hospital to assist with labor support. The word *doula* comes from a Greek word meaning maidservant or female slave. The modern usage of doula refers to a trained and experienced professional who provides physical, emotional, and informational support to the laboring woman. Doulas are not usually nurses but are trained to assist the woman during labor and act as an advocate for carrying out the patient's birth plan. Some doulas are certified by DONA International (formerly Doulas of North America).

CONCEPTUAL CORNERSTONE
Oxygenation

Fetal monitoring is an important assessment tool used in labor and delivery to provide information regarding the oxygenation status of the fetus during labor. Oxygen is transported from the maternal lungs, heart, and blood vessels to the uterus, placenta, and umbilical cord to the fetus. Any disruption of the path of oxygen from the mother to the fetus will cause a deceleration of the FHR and possible hypoxia for the fetus. Any abnormal FHR deceleration is caused by a disruption in oxygenation to the fetus. Abnormal decelerations require prompt nursing interventions to promote oxygenation of the fetus and prevent a brain injury caused by hypoxia.

FETAL MONITORING

Fetal monitoring can detect signs that the fetus is not tolerating the stress of labor. Changes in FHR and contraction patterns alert nurses and health-care providers to intervene to prevent injury or death of the fetus. Nurses who provide bedside care in labor and delivery must receive additional education and become experts on reading fetal monitoring strips and implementing appropriate interventions based on the FHR pattern.

Intermittent Fetal Monitoring

Intermittent fetal monitoring can be done with a handheld Doppler device. A handheld Doppler uses ultrasound waves that bounce off the fetal heart, producing echoes that reflect the FHR. This device is used in hospitals, birthing centers, and clinics to monitor the FHR. Intermittent monitoring can also be accomplished by applying the fetal monitor, obtaining a 20-minute evaluation, and then removing the monitor. Intermittent monitoring allows the woman to move around and change position easily. A disadvantage of intermittent monitoring is that if done with a Doppler, you cannot evaluate **variability** (beat-to-beat intervals of the fetal heart that represent a healthy sympathetic and parasympathetic nervous system in the fetus) and types of **decelerations** (drops in the FHR from the baseline). Another disadvantage of intermittent fetal monitoring is that if the fetal condition changes between scheduled monitoring sessions, early signs of deterioration of the fetal health may not be detected.

Continual Fetal Monitoring

Continual monitoring can be done with a fetal monitor applied externally or internally. Continuous fetal monitoring during labor should be considered for high-risk women. Maternal or fetal conditions that indicate to the health-care provider that continuous fetal monitoring is necessary to provide safe and effective care include the following:

- Hypertensive disorders
- Preterm labor
- Postterm pregnancy
- Maternal cardiac disease
- Oligohydramnios
- Polyhydramnios
- Multiple gestation
- Induction of labor
- Administration of epidural anesthesia
- Vaginal birth after cesarean (VBAC)
- Diabetes

Procedure for Applying the Fetal Monitor

Explain to the woman that fetal monitoring will detect changes in heart rate patterns during labor. If problems are detected, you can initiate interventions to prevent problems for the fetus.

External Monitoring

The procedure for external monitoring is the following:

1. You should start with hand hygiene and perform Leopold maneuvers to determine the position of the fetus.
2. Ultrasound gel is applied to the ultrasound transducer, and the transducer is placed over the area where the fetal back is located. This is the best location to obtain a clear signal of the heart rate. The transducer is then secured with a belt around the woman's abdomen.
3. External monitoring of the FHR provides information about heart rate baseline, variability, **accelerations**

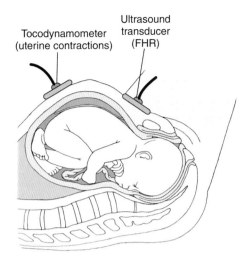

FIGURE 9.15 External FHR monitor and tocodynamometer.

(short increases in the FHR above the baseline), and decelerations.

4. A **tocodynamometer** is used to measure the frequency and duration of uterine contractions. It is placed on the fundus of the uterus and secured with a belt.

5. The fetal heart transducer and the tocodynamometer send a signal to the fetal monitor, and it is recorded on monitor paper. In the United States, the standard paper speed for fetal monitoring is 3 cm per minute. On the fetal monitoring paper, each dark vertical line represents 1 minute, and each lighter color line represents 10 seconds (Fig. 9.15).

Table 9.5 notes the advantages and disadvantages of using external monitoring for the fetus.

Internal Monitoring

Internal monitoring requires the application of a fetal scalp electrode (FSE) to directly monitor the fetal heart. A vaginal examination is performed, and an experienced nurse advances the electrode through the vagina and attaches it to the presenting part. Internal monitoring may be initiated by the nurse if the external method does not provide reliable information regarding the condition of the fetus.

Contractions can be monitored with an **intrauterine pressure catheter (IUPC)**, a small flexible tube inserted into the uterus along the uterine wall that provides exact measurement of contraction length and intensity. Most hospitals require the obstetrician or the nurse midwife to insert the IUPC.

A vaginal examination is performed, and the IUPC is inserted via a guide tube through the cervix and into the uterus. IUPC monitoring may be initiated if more information is required regarding uterine activity, especially the intensity of

• WORD • BUILDING •

tocodynamometer: toco–birth + dynamo–force + meter–measure

Table 9.5
Advantages and Disadvantages of Using External Monitoring for the Fetus

Advantages of External Monitoring	*Disadvantages of External Monitoring*
• The transducers are easy to apply quickly. • External monitoring does not require that the membranes be ruptured and is considered noninvasive.	• The woman may find the belts across her abdomen uncomfortable. • External monitoring cannot measure the pressure or intensity of the contractions. • FHR recordings may have gaps or artifacts caused by movement of the fetus and poor conduction through the maternal tissues. • Uterine contractions may not be monitored correctly if the tocodynamometer slides off the uterus with maternal position changes.

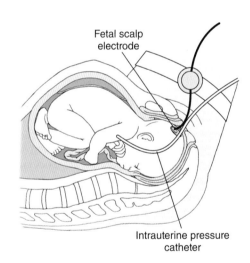

FIGURE 9.16 Internal fetal monitor.

the contractions (Fig. 9.16). Table 9.6 notes the advantages and disadvantages of using internal monitoring for the fetus.

Interpretation of Fetal Monitoring

The nurse in labor and delivery who evaluates the information provided with fetal heart monitoring must have clinical judgment skills and expertise in fetal monitoring. Initiation of fetal monitoring must only be performed and evaluated by licensed experienced health-care professionals (Association of Women's Health, Obstetric and Neonatal Nurses [AWHONN], 2018).

Table 9.6

Advantages and Disadvantages of Using Internal Monitoring for the Fetus

Advantages of Internal Monitoring	*Disadvantages of Internal Monitoring*
• Internal monitoring does not require belts around the abdomen and continual readjustment.	• Internal monitoring is invasive and increases the risk of uterine infection.
• Accurate information is available about FHR, variability, accelerations, and decelerations, regardless of fetal activity.	• Internal monitoring requires extensive training for safe application.
• The IUPC detects the frequency, duration, resting tone, and strength of the uterine contractions.	
• The internal scalp electrode can be combined with external contraction monitoring.	

The purpose of fetal monitoring in labor is to determine the fetal oxygenation. According to Miller (2022), there are principles that can be applied to FHR interpretation:

1. All significant decelerations indicate an interruption in oxygen to the fetus.
2. A disruption in fetal oxygenation can result in hypoxia for the fetus. The first step that occurs is hypoxemia, which is decreased oxygen in the blood. Hypoxemia, if not corrected, leads to hypoxia, which is a state of decreased oxygen levels in the tissues. Tissue hypoxemia can lead to metabolic acidosis in the fetus. An acidotic fetus will show signs of minimal or absent variability and absent accelerations.
3. Fetal neurological injury will not occur if hypoxemia is corrected and significant fetal acidemia does not occur.

The interpretation of the FHR should follow a systematic approach, starting with the baseline FHR; the interpretation of FHR variability; the presence of accelerations; **periodic decelerations** (decelerations associated with contractions); changes or trends in the FHR pattern over time; and the frequency, duration, and intensity of uterine contractions.

Baseline

The normal FHR during labor is 110 to 160 bpm. The baseline is evaluated during a 10-minute segment, not including periods of marked variability and episodic changes (Fig. 9.17).

• An FHR below 110 bpm is considered bradycardia and may be caused by an occiput posterior or transverse position of the fetus or severe deterioration of the health of the fetus (Miller, 2022).
• An FHR greater than 160 bpm is considered tachycardia. However, if the FHR indicates good variability, it is not a sign of fetal distress. Tachycardia may be caused by maternal fever, medications, early fetal hypoxia, or fetal heart failure (Table 9.7).

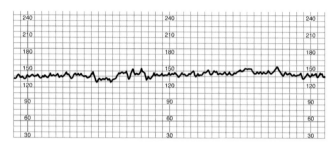
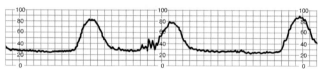

FIGURE 9.17 FHR baseline. The normal baseline FHR is 110 to 160 bpm. Top, FHR. Bottom, Uterine contractions.

Variability

FHR variability is defined as fluctuations in the baseline that are irregular in frequency and amplitude. Variability is an indicator of fetal oxygenation and reserve during labor (Miller, 2022).

Variability is graded as follows:

• Absent variability = fluctuations are undetectable
• Minimal variability = fewer than 5 bpm
• Moderate variability = 6 to 25 bpm
• Marked variability = greater than 25 bpm

Persistently absent or minimal variability is the most significant sign of fetal distress in labor. Causes of absent or minimal variability are as follows:

• Fetal metabolic acidosis
• Fetal sleep cycles
• Prematurity
• Congenital anomalies
• Central nervous system depressant medications
• Betamethasone: a medication used to prepare the preterm fetal lungs for delivery

Table 9.7
Medical Management and Nursing Interventions Related to Treating Tachycardia

Medical Management	Nursing Interventions
• Treat the cause, such as by decreasing or stopping the infusion of oxytocin.	• Decrease or stop oxytocin if applicable. • Change the maternal position. • Administer a tocolytic medication if ordered. • Increase the IV rate to improve hydration. • Support the laboring woman and her family. • Evaluate fetal oxygenation.

Table 9.8
Medical Management and Nursing Interventions Related to Treating Fetal Heart Rate Variability

Medical Management	Nursing Interventions
• The health-care provider may elect to rupture the membranes to allow initiation of internal fetal monitoring. • If known, treat the cause of the minimal or absent variability.	• Change the maternal position to promote fetal oxygenation. • Provide fetal scalp stimulation. • Apply an FSE for more accurate information regarding variability. • Increase IV fluids to promote maternal hydration and increase uterine perfusion. • Notify the health-care provider about minimal or absent variability.

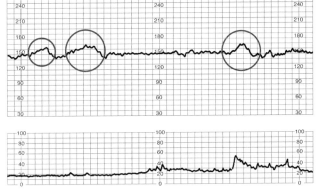

FIGURE 9.18 Top, FHR, with accelerations circled in red. Bottom, Uterine contractions.

Table 9.8 notes the medical management and nursing interventions related to treating FHR variability.

Accelerations
Accelerations are an abrupt increase in FHR above the baseline (Fig. 9.18). Accelerations predict adequate fetal oxygenation. Fetal movement usually results in accelerations.

An absence of accelerations for more than 80 minutes has been associated with increased neonatal morbidity (Weiss, 2022).

Table 9.9 notes the medical management and nursing interventions related to treating FHR accelerations.

Decelerations
A deceleration is a decrease in FHR from the baseline. **Episodic decelerations** are drops in the FHR not associated with uterine contractions. In contrast, periodic decelerations are drops in the FHR that are associated with uterine contractions.

EARLY DECELERATIONS. Early decelerations are caused by the compression of the fetal head in the pelvis and are not considered to be dangerous for the fetus. No nursing interventions are required, excepting observation and documentation (Fig. 9.19).

LATE DECELERATIONS. Late decelerations can be caused by maternal hypotension, uterine hyperactivity, or placental insufficiency, leading to a decrease in oxygen to the fetus and causing a possible hypoxic state (Fig. 9.20; Miller, 2022). Table 9.10 notes the medical management and nursing interventions related to treating late FHR decelerations.

VARIABLE DECELERATIONS. Variable decelerations are an abrupt decrease in FHR of 15 beats or more. On the fetal monitor, the variable deceleration can resemble a U, W, or V in appearance. Variable decelerations can be caused by cord compression, which disrupts the oxygenation of the

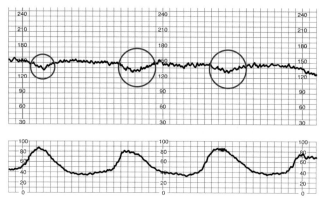

FIGURE 9.19 Top, FHR, with early decelerations circled in red. Bottom, Uterine contractions.

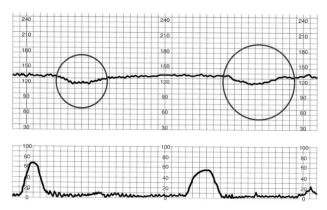

FIGURE 9.20 Top, FHR, with late decelerations circled in red. Bottom, Uterine contractions.

Table 9.9

Medical Management and Nursing Interventions Related to Treating Fetal Heart Rate Accelerations

Medical Management	Nursing Interventions
• If no accelerations are noted, the health-care provider should evaluate fetal oxygenation.	• If accelerations are not noted, the nurse can stimulate the fetal scalp to cause accelerations. • Change the maternal position to awaken a sleeping fetus and observe for accelerations. • Notify the health-care provider of an absence of accelerations.

Table 9.10

Medical Management and Nursing Interventions Related to Treating Late Fetal Heart Rate Decelerations

Medical Management	Interventions
• Determine the cause of the decelerations and treat. • If caused by uterine hyperactivity, **tocolytic medications** that suppress uterine activity may be prescribed. • Cesarean delivery should be considered for recurrent late decelerations with minimal or absent variability.	• Place the patient on her side to promote optimal placenta perfusion. • Discontinue oxytocin to decrease uterine activity, if applicable. • Correct maternal hypotension by changing her position and increasing the rate of IV fluids. • Monitor maternal hydration and increase IV fluids if appropriate. • Notify the health-care provider. • Consider an internal FSE for more accurate data about the fetal condition. • Provide support to the patient and her family to manage anxiety.

fetus (Fig. 9.21). Table 9.11 notes the medical management and nursing interventions related to treating variable FHR decelerations.

PAIN MANAGEMENT IN LABOR AND BIRTH

Laboring women report a wide range of pain levels, and every patient reacts differently to pain. Physical and psychosocial factors may influence the woman's response to pain. The laboring patient's pain level is influenced by the following:

• Women who have supportive care in labor cope with pain more successfully (Diddams, 2022).
• Anxiety related to labor has an important role. Women who are anxious and worried about giving birth have longer, more painful labors (Diddams, 2022).
• Past pain experiences influence current perceptions of pain.
• Cultural concepts of childbirth and pain vary.

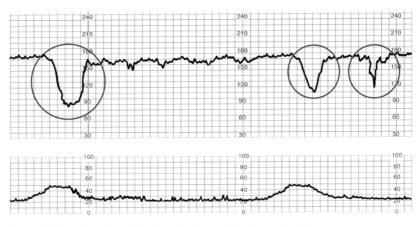

FIGURE 9.21 Top, FHR, with variable decelerations circled in red. Bottom, Uterine contractions.

Table 9.11

Medical Management and Nursing Interventions Related to Treating Variable Fetal Heart Rate Decelerations

Medical Management	*Nursing Interventions*
• Administer tocolytic medications to stop preterm labor by decreasing uterine activity. • Perform **amnioinfusion**, which is a procedure in which room temperature normal saline is infused into the uterus through an IUPC to increase the volume of fluid in the uterus. The increase in fluid may relieve the compression of the fetal body on the umbilical cord (Miller, 2022). • Consider delivery if the fetal condition is deteriorating.	• Change the patient's position to decrease cord compression. • Discontinue oxytocin to decrease uterine activity, if applicable. • Monitor maternal hydration and increase IV fluids if appropriate. • Notify the health-care provider. • Consider an internal FSE for more accurate data about the fetal condition. • Perform amnioinfusion, if ordered, to correct umbilical cord compression. • Provide support to the patient and her family to manage anxiety.

• Past birth experiences, either positive or negative, have an influence.
• A long labor can lead to exhaustion and poor coping.
• A woman who does not understand labor may be fearful of her experience.
• A large fetus and a fetus in the posterior presentation can lead to an increase in pain perception.

Patients need to be educated about the different methods of labor-pain management available. Health professionals can support the woman in labor by providing up-to-date, objective, and evidence-based information on the advantages and disadvantages of the various methods of pain relief.

No pain management method, either nonpharmacological or pharmacological, should be forced upon a patient. You should make it clear from the onset of labor that the patient has a choice in pain management and she should ask for whatever she needs during labor and childbirth.

You will support her choice and provide appropriate nursing care.

The Physiology of Pain

Pain in the first stage of labor, particularly during the active and transition phases, consists of visceral pain from the stretching and dilation of the cervix and uterine pain from a decrease in blood supply during contractions. *Visceral pain* refers to pain in internal organs and is caused by activation of receptors in the chest, abdomen, or pelvic area that send signals to the spinal cord and on to the brain (Yarnell, 2021).

When the fetal head begins to descend and stretching of the perineum occurs, somatic pain is activated through the pudendal nerve, which originates through the second to fourth sacral nerves. **Somatic pain** is caused by activation of pain receptors in the body surface or musculoskeletal tissues. At this point in labor, the patient is experiencing both visceral and somatic pain (Yarnell, 2021).

Nonpharmacological Pain Management

There are a variety of childbirth preparation methods that a woman may use in labor. These methods have the goal of making labor a positive experience with the woman actively participating in managing her pain. They are very effective for the first stage of labor.

- *Dick-Read method:* This method emphasizes relaxation during labor and childbirth using hypnosis. The theme of this method is childbirth without fear. Women using hypnosis report feeling relaxed, calm, and in control during labor. This method is not widely used in the United States.
- *Bradley method:* See Chapter 7 for more information on the Bradley method.
- *Lamaze method:* See Chapter 7 for more information on the Lamaze method.

All methods of childbirth preparation include nonpharmacological techniques that promote relaxation and the release of endorphins; however, not all techniques work with every woman. Some techniques that you can provide or assist the support person to implement for the patient in labor include the following:

- Creating a relaxing environment with low lighting, warmth, and quiet
- Displaying a picture of a relaxing scene or baby's first outfit for the woman to view during labor
- Playing relaxing music or sounds, such as a bubbling stream or birds singing
- Using aromatherapy with lavender, sage, or jasmine
- Stimulating the skin with massage to the lower back or light fingertip massage of the abdomen; stroking of the arm to shoulder or knee to thigh is also relaxing
- Talking the woman through progressive relaxation by having her focus on relaxing her neck and shoulders, and then progressing the relaxation throughout her body

Evidence-Based Practice

A study was conducted to determine if laboring primipara patients reported less pain than a control group after watching a guided imagery video or receiving foot reflexology treatment during labor at 4 cm dilation. The findings indicate that the patients in both groups reported lower pain scores than the control group. Participants who watched the guided imagery video reported lower pain scores than patients who received the foot reflexology treatment. In addition, the guided imagery group experienced a significantly shorter first and second stage of labor and reported higher birth satisfaction scores.

Kaplan, E., & Cevik, S. (2021). The effects of guided imagery and reflexology on pain intensity, duration of labor and birth satisfaction in primiparas: Randomized control trial. *Healthcare for Women International, 42,* 440–454. https://doi.org/10.1080/07399332.2021.1880411

- Positioning pillows under the uterus to relieve some of the strain on the lower back during labor
- Walking, swaying, or rolling on a birthing ball to help her to relax and to ease labor pain
- Using diversion and distraction methods, such as counting or focusing on a task during a contraction
- Applying a cool washcloth to the forehead, which is comforting when she is tired and hot from the work of labor
- Providing ice chips or clear liquids, if permitted by the health-care provider, to soothe her dry mouth and throat
- Assisting her to use breathing techniques, which are a tool that promotes relaxation and diversion in labor

Pharmacological Pain Management

Pharmacological methods of pain management include systemic analgesics, regional analgesics and anesthetics, local anesthesia, and general anesthesia. The patient needs to be involved in choosing the method that will be effective for her.

Systemic Analgesics

Systemic analgesics commonly used in labor include butorphanol, meperidine, morphine, fentanyl, and nalbuphine hydrochloride. Table 9.12 lists the types and dosages of systemic medications used in labor.

These medications may be given IM but are most commonly given IV. Analgesics given in labor do not totally eliminate the pain, but they do make the woman more comfortable and able to use relaxation and breathing techniques to cope with labor. The advantages of IV administration of analgesics are a prompt onset and the ability to use smaller doses of medication to control pain (Yarnell, 2021).

Side effects that may occur are as follows:

- Nausea and vomiting
- Drowsiness
- Sedation
- Respiratory depression with meperidine, morphine, and fentanyl
- Neonatal respiratory depression

NURSING CARE. Nursing responsibilities for managing pain and systemic analgesics include the following:

- Reviewing the patient's medication allergies before administration
- Assessing pain with the 1 to 10 pain scale as well as obtaining information regarding the location, radiation, pattern, and description of pain
- Ensuring that labor is well-established before administering analgesics (or else labor may slow down)
- Not administering narcotic analgesics within 1 hour of delivery because they may cause neonatal respiratory depression
- Providing a higher dose of medication to women with a history of substance use disorder (higher tolerance) to provide pain relief

Table 9.12

Medication Dosages in Labor

Medication	*Dose*
Butorphanol	2–4 mg IM or 0.5–2 mg IV
Meperidine	50–100 mg IM or 25–50 mg IV
Morphine	5–10 mg IM or 2–5 mg IV
Nalbuphine hydrochloride	10 mg IM or IV
Fentanyl	50–100 mcg IV

Source: Vallerand, A. H., & Sanoski, C. A. (2023). *Davis's drug guide for nurses* (18th ed.). F. A. Davis.

Inhaled Nitrous Oxide

Inhaled nitrous oxide is safe for the mother and fetus. It does not diminish uterine contractility and can be used for painful procedures such as perineal repair or manual removal of the placenta (Yarnell, 2021).

Regional Analgesics and Anesthetics

Regional anesthesia has become a very popular method of pain management in labor. In the United States, approximately 60% of laboring women choose regional analgesia for labor pain (Satpathy, 2020). Regional analgesic techniques include **pudendal block** (injection into the pudendal nerve), epidural, spinal, or a combination of epidural and spinal analgesia (Fig. 9.22). These methods of analgesia and anesthesia are provided by a physician or nurse anesthetist. The nurse is responsible for assisting the health-care provider and monitoring the patient's care before, during, and after administration of these types of analgesia and anesthesia.

PUDENDAL BLOCK. With a pudendal block, anesthetic is injected into the pudendal nerve, which anesthetizes the vulva and perineum. It is typically injected in the second stage of labor right before the birth. The advantages of pudendal block are that it

• Controls pain from perineal stretching
• Is quickly administered for a forceps delivery
• Provides continuous anesthesia for episiotomy repair

NURSING CARE. Nursing care for the patient with pudendal anesthesia includes monitoring for urinary retention and for signs of infection.

EPIDURAL ANESTHESIA. The epidural is an effective form of pain relief in labor. An epidural is administered with a small needle and catheter between the fourth and fifth vertebrae into the epidural space. An anesthetic medication, analgesic medication, or a combination of both are injected or infused into the epidural to decrease pain perception. The epidural space surrounds the spinal cord where the nerves branch off. The sensation of pain is blocked in that area.

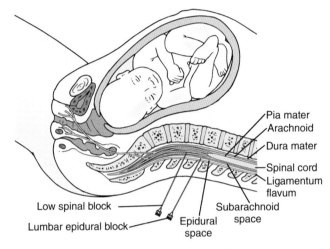

FIGURE 9.22 The spinal canal: Injection sites for regional anesthesia.

The advantages of epidural analgesia and anesthesia are that they

• Provide complete pain relief
• Do not produce respiratory depression for the fetus

Disadvantages of epidural analgesia and anesthesia are that they

• May slow labor for about an hour after administration
• Drop the patient's blood pressure immediately after medication infusion begins
• Require a urinary catheter because of lack of feeling in the bladder area
• May cause the patient's legs and feet to feel numb or tingly
• Will most likely prevent the patient from walking
• Prolong stage 2 of labor (Murray & Huelsmann, 2021)
• May cause fever and itchiness
• Make pushing difficult. Often, the epidural is allowed to wear off before the woman feels the urge to push

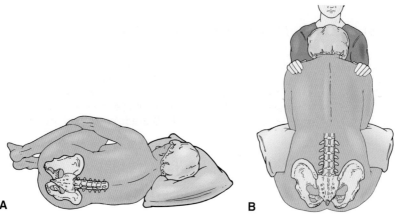

FIGURE 9.23 A, Lateral position for spinal or epidural administration. B, Sitting position for spinal or epidural administration.

- Can inadvertently penetrate the dura and cause a small leak of spinal fluid, leading to a spinal headache
- May lead to vacuum extraction or forceps delivery of the fetus (Yarnell, 2021).

NURSING CARE. Nursing care before administration of epidural analgesia and anesthesia includes the following:

- Assessing the patient's knowledge of epidural anesthesia and obtaining consent
- Obtaining a baseline temperature, heart rate, respiratory rate, blood pressure, and FHR, and confirming the FHR pattern
- Administering a bolus of IV fluids, if ordered, to decrease the risk of hypotension

Nursing care during the administration of the epidural is as follows:

- Providing verbal support and encouragement to the patient
- Assisting the patient to maintain a lateral position with the head and chin flexed onto the chest, or sitting with the head flexed, knees bent, and feet supported on a stool (Satpathy, 2020; Fig. 9.23).

Nursing care after administration of an epidural is as follows:

- Monitoring the blood pressure and FHR every 5 minutes for 15 minutes (Murray & Huelsmann, 2021) to detect hypotension
- If patient-controlled anesthesia (PCA) is used, assessing the patient's understanding about how to use the device
- Positioning the patient in the lateral or upright position with uterus displacement to avoid hypotension
- Inserting a urinary catheter to prevent urinary retention
- Monitoring for pruritus (itching) and notifying the health-care provider for a medication order to treat the itching
- Assessing the effectiveness of the epidural and pain relief

SPINAL ANESTHESIA. Spinal anesthesia is used less often than an epidural because it is fast-acting but short-lasting. **Spinal anesthesia** involves placing a needle into the

> ## Safety *Stat!*
>
> A major complication of epidural anesthesia is the inadvertent infusion of the anesthetic into the intravascular space instead of the epidural space. If this occurs, the patient will exhibit signs of tachycardia or bradycardia, hypertension, tinnitus (ringing in the ears), dizziness, and/or a metallic taste in the mouth. If any of these signs are noted, the health-care provider must be notified immediately (Yarnell, 2021) as this complication can lead to cardiac arrest.

intrathecal space (within the spinal canal), injecting medication, and removing the needle. Spinal anesthesia has the increased risk of spinal headache because of the possible leakage of spinal fluid. Spinal headache can be treated by having the patient lie flat for 8 hours after the injection and providing adequate IV hydration to assist the body in replacing the missing cerebral spinal fluid (Landon et al., 2019; Satpathy, 2020).

COMBINED SPINAL-EPIDURAL ANESTHESIA (CSE). It is possible to combine the fast action of spinal anesthesia with the duration of the epidural. This technique involves first placing the epidural catheter and then advancing a spinal needle through the catheter into the intrathecal space, where a small amount of medication is injected. Afterward, the spinal needle is removed and the epidural catheter remains for continual infusion of medication (Yarnell, 2021). Nursing care appropriate for the epidural patient is also appropriate for the patient receiving spinal anesthesia or CSE.

Local Anesthesia

Local anesthesia is injected into the perineum between the vagina and rectum for fast, temporary relief of the stretching pain during delivery, repair of any tears, or an episiotomy.

· **WORD** · **BUILDING** ·

intrathecal: intra–inside + thecal–sheath or anatomic space

Nursing Care Plan for the Unprepared Adolescent Patient

Angie, a 15-year-old with a term pregnancy, arrives in early labor with mild contractions at the labor and delivery unit. She is accompanied by her father, Bill. The baby's father is not involved in Angie's life. Angie is an only child and lives alone with her father. Because she is obese, she was able to hide her pregnancy from her father until she was in her seventh month. Because of her denial of the pregnancy, Angie's prenatal care began late in the pregnancy, and she did not attend childbirth classes. She has never been in a hospital. Angie and her father are anxious about labor, and Angie asks, "Can you knock me out until it's over?"

Nursing Diagnosis: Anxiety caused by anticipating labor contraction pain
Expected Outcome: The patient will state that her pain is at an acceptable level.

Interventions:	Rationale:
Discuss safe pain management options with Angie.	Angie will understand her choices in pain control.
Provide nonpharmacological pain control and comfort measures.	Angie may need less medication to control her pain.
Teach Bill nonpharmacological comfort measures to use with Angie.	Women with labor support can manage the pain of labor better (ACOG, 2019).
Teach Angie simple breathing techniques.	Breathing techniques assist with relaxation and aid in coping with painful contractions.

Nursing Diagnosis: Powerlessness because of an inability to cope with contractions
Expected Outcome: The patient will demonstrate the ability to make choices for her labor and delivery care.

Interventions:	Rationale:
Provide Angie with options regarding her care whenever possible.	Educating her on the options allows her to make her own choices.
Give positive feedback regarding her choices.	Positive feedback reinforces behaviors.

Nursing Diagnosis: Fear because of the unfamiliar hospital environment
Expected Outcome: The patient will demonstrate decreased fear, evidenced by her ability to ask questions, cooperate with care, and relax.

Interventions:	Rationale:
Explain procedures and expectations to Angie in nonmedical terms.	Simple explanations of procedures will decrease her fear of the unknown.
Encourage questions.	Encouraging questions will assist with building rapport with Angie and information will reduce her fear.

The medication is commonly injected while the woman is pushing. Local anesthesia numbs the area that is infused but provides no relief of pain from the contractions. Local anesthesia does not harm the baby. The medications commonly used by health-care providers are lidocaine, procaine, or tetracaine.

General Anesthesia

General anesthesia is used when an emergency arises and the woman or the fetus needs a cesarean birth quickly, leaving insufficient time to start epidural or spinal anesthesia. Medication is given IV to cause the patient to lose consciousness, and then an endotracheal tube is placed in the trachea to allow the administration of oxygen and gas to keep her unconscious until the birth is over.

Disadvantages to general anesthesia are as follows:

- The anesthesia affects the fetus, and the infant may be less alert when born.
- Rarely, the woman may aspirate foods or liquids from the stomach if she ate or drank within 8 hours of the cesarean. Aspiration can lead to pneumonia.

Labor Stage 2: Pushing and Birth

As soon as the cervix is completely dilated, the woman enters the second stage of labor, which ends with the birth of the baby. The contractions during this phase may be 2 to 3 minutes apart and last about 60 seconds. Generally, the contractions are not as intense as during the transition phase of labor, and the woman may experience the urge to push. Women who have chosen epidural anesthesia may not experience the urge to push and may not be able to actively push. If so, the medication may be decreased to allow the patient to feel and use the muscles required for pushing. The woman, who may have felt tired and discouraged during the active phase, often gets a renewed sense of energy.

Safety *Stat!*

The Urge to Push
Pushing without a nurse or health-care provider present could result in an unattended birth and lead to complications for the woman and her baby.

Medical Interventions

Some health-care providers massage and apply warm compresses to the perineum as the head descends to assist with gentle stretching and to avoid large tears in the perineum. Small tears may still occur, but they can be repaired if needed. As the woman pushes, the health-care provider will determine if an episiotomy is necessary to allow more room for the fetal head and to prevent large tears in the perineal area. An **episiotomy**, which is an incision into the perineum, can be done without the injection of an anesthetic, but anesthesia is necessary for repair. Two types of episiotomies are done: (1) a midline episiotomy is an incision between the vagina and rectum and (2) a mediolateral episiotomy is an incision from the vagina diagonally to the left or right (Fig. 9.24). Because studies have shown that episiotomies are more likely to cause third- and fourth-degree tears, ACOG recommends that episiotomies be avoided if at all possible (ACOG, 2019).

Cleansing of the perineum is ongoing as the woman pushes. Occasionally, some fecal matter emerges as she pushes, and this is wiped away.

As the head emerges from the birth canal, the health-care provider will check for a tight umbilical cord around the neck. If there is a tight cord, it may need to be clamped and cut before the body emerges from the birth canal. Next, the health-care provider may suction the mouth and airway thoroughly before the chest emerges from the birth canal. Some providers prefer not to use suction because of the fear of causing bradycardia and apnea. Current evidence does not support or refute the benefit of suctioning the baby's oropharynx at this time (Funai & Norowitz, 2022).

• WORD • BUILDING •
episiotomy: episio–vulva or perineum + tomy–incision

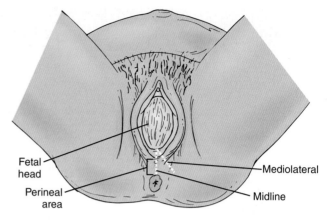

FIGURE 9.24 An episiotomy is a surgical incision of the perineum performed to allow more room for the birth. The most common method is the midline episiotomy: An incision is made from the vaginal opening to the rectum.

After the baby is born, the umbilical cord is clamped and cut. Early clamping may sometimes be necessary to evaluate the baby, but rushing to clamp the cord is not recommended. Delaying clamping of the cord results in higher hemoglobin and hematocrit values and possibly allows greater iron stores for the newborn (ACOG, 2020a). The parents may have a preference regarding the timing of the cord cutting and may wish to participate in it (Fig. 9.25).

A cord blood specimen may be sent to the laboratory. Practices vary, but the specimen is typically sent to the laboratory for a CBC, blood type, Rh, and antibody screen.

After the cord is cut, the infant should be thoroughly dried and placed skin-to-skin with the mother to promote bonding. If the support person wishes to hold the infant, the child should be wrapped in a warm blanket with the head covered with a cap to maintain warmth.

Nursing Care

Nursing care appropriate for this stage of labor may include the following:

• Monitoring the FHR every 5 to 15 minutes
• Providing comfort measures and remaining with the patient
• Giving encouragement and positive reinforcement for pushing efforts
• Providing perineal hygiene; as the woman pushes, she may pass fecal material
• Being an advocate for the patient's desires regarding her birth plan
• Assuming care for the baby after the cord is cut

Labor Stage 3: Birth Through Delivery of the Placenta

The third stage of labor is from the birth of the baby until the completed delivery of the placenta and the attached membranes. The length of this stage of labor is typically 5 to 15 minutes (Smith, 2020). The mother and her support person

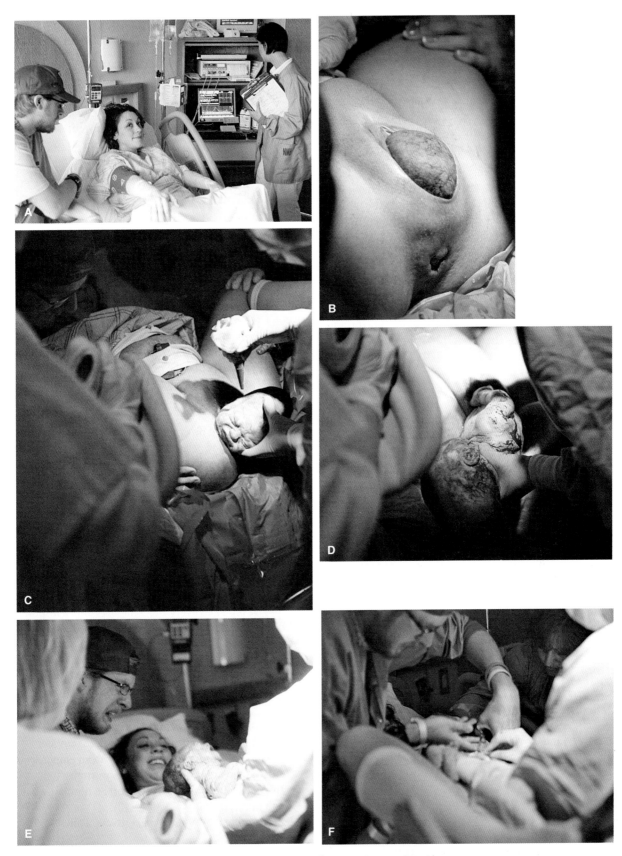

FIGURE 9.25 Vaginal birth sequence. A, Pushing in an upright position allows gravity to assist with fetal descent. B, Crowning. C, Birth of the head. D, Expulsion. E, The infant is shown to the parents. F, The baby's father cuts the umbilical cord.

are usually very excited about the birth, and she may not even notice the delivery of the placenta. Following delivery of the baby, uterine contractions continue, causing the release of the placenta. The patient may describe the contractions as a cramping sensation. As the placenta detaches, it moves into the lower uterine segment, leaving arteries exposed. The anatomy of the uterine muscle and the contractions apply pressure on these vessels, preventing hemorrhage. The health-care provider looks for the following signs that the placenta is detaching:

- The umbilical cord lengthens.
- The uterine shape becomes firmer, rounder, and moves up in the abdomen.
- A gush of blood occurs because of the separation from the uterus (Funai & Norowitz, 2022).

Some health-care providers order a bolus of oxytocin given IV or IM to promote strong uterine contractions and decrease risk of hemorrhage. It is commonly administered after delivery of the baby's anterior shoulder, or after delivery of the baby but before delivery of the placenta, or after delivery of the placenta. There is insufficient data to identify optimal timing for this medication and it is given per the health-care provider's preference (Smith, 2020).

When the placenta delivers, it usually presents with the fetal side facing up. The health-care provider turns the placenta over to inspect the maternal side to determine if any pieces are torn or missing (Fig. 9.26). Missing pieces should be identified because they can lead to hemorrhage or infection if left inside the uterus.

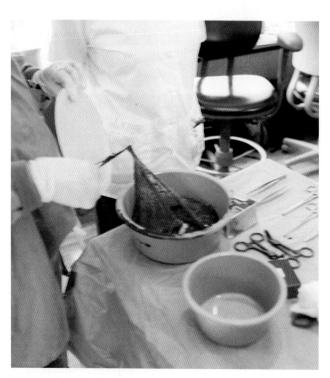

FIGURE 9.26 Examination of the placenta.

Medical Interventions

Medical interventions for this stage of labor may include:

- Clamping the cord with two hemostats and cutting the umbilical cord about 8 to 10 inches from the infant's umbilicus
- Obtaining a cord blood specimen for the laboratory
- Ordering oxytocin infusion or IM injection
- Managing the delivery of the placenta
- Inspecting the cervix, vagina, and perineum for tears
- Suturing of any tears or an episiotomy repair
- Completing a 1-minute Apgar score

Apgar Score

The **Apgar score** was developed by Virginia Apgar, an American obstetrical anesthesiologist, as a quick, systematic method of assessing a newborn's physical condition at birth (Venes, 2021). The Apgar method assesses the newborn's heart rate, respirations, muscle tone, response to stimuli, and color by assigning a score of 0 to 2 to each category. The newborn is evaluated at 1 minute and again at 5 minutes after birth. A 1-minute Apgar assessment that scores between 7 and 10 indicates that the newborn is adjusting to extrauterine life. A score below 7 indicates that medical or nursing interventions may be needed to improve the newborn's cardiorespiratory status. If the 5-minute Apgar score is below 7, the newborn should be evaluated every 5 minutes until the score is 7 or above (Venes, 2021; Table 9.13).

> ### Safety *Stat!*
>
> **Naloxone**
> Naloxone should be available at every delivery. This medication can be administered to a newborn to reverse the effects of opioid pain medication administered too close to delivery. For newborns, 0.01 mg/kg is given IM. The dose may be repeated every 2 to 3 minutes until a response is obtained (Vallerand & Sanoski, 2023).

Nursing Care

Nursing care during stage 3 includes the following:

- Administering oxytocin if ordered
- Providing assistance to the health-care provider
- Assuming care for the newborn with an emphasis on assessing the airway and providing warmth
- Inspecting the umbilical cord for the normal two arteries and one vein
- Performing a 5-minute Apgar assessment

Labor Stage 4: Recovery

The first hour after birth, sometimes called "the Golden Hour," is a critical time of bonding for the mother and infant. But this does not mean that your job is done. The mother's

Table 9.13

Apgar Score

Physiological Parameter	0	1	2
Heart rate	Absent	Slow: below 100	Above 100
Respiratory effort	Absent	Slow: irregular, weak cry	Good; strong cry
Muscle tone	Flaccid	Some flexion of extremities	Well-flexed
Reflex irritability	No response	Grimace	Vigorous cry
Color	Blue, pale	Pink body, blue extremities	Completely pink

Range of Apgar score: from 0–10

A 5-minute Apgar score of 7 to 10 is considered normal. Scores of 4, 5, and 6 are intermediate and not markers of increased risk of neurological dysfunction because such scores may be the result of physiological immaturity, maternal medications, the presence of congenital malformations, and other factors (ACOG, 2021a).

Medication Facts

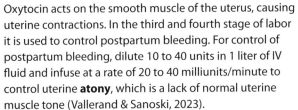

Oxytocin

Oxytocin acts on the smooth muscle of the uterus, causing uterine contractions. In the third and fourth stage of labor it is used to control postpartum bleeding. For control of postpartum bleeding, dilute 10 to 40 units in 1 liter of IV fluid and infuse at a rate of 20 to 40 milliunits/minute to control uterine **atony**, which is a lack of normal uterine muscle tone (Vallerand & Sanoski, 2023).

uterus tends to relax after the delivery of the placenta, and bleeding problems can occur. The infant is also making the transition from intrauterine life to extrauterine life. The first hour after birth requires close observation of the mother and frequent assessments of the newborn to note any early warning signs of trouble.

Nursing Care of the Mother

The goals of nursing care for the first hour are to provide safe care for the mother and to promote bonding with the infant. Expected physical findings during this stage include the following:

- The uterus is firm, and the fundus is located midline, halfway between the symphysis pubis and the umbilicus.
- Lochia (vaginal discharge) is heavy with bright-red blood mixed with clots.
- Mild uterine cramping (afterpains) may be noted as the uterus contracts to return to prepregnancy size, especially if breastfeeding is initiated.

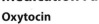

· WORD · BUILDING ·

atony: a–without + tony–stretching

Appropriate nursing care for this period includes the following:

- *Providing a warm blanket:* Immediately after delivery, hormone levels begin dropping, endorphins are released, and the adrenaline level decreases, causing some women to shiver. The shivering is not harmful to the woman and will pass, but most women appreciate a warm blanket during this time.
- *Monitoring blood pressure and pulse every 15 minutes:* Notify the health-care provider if there are significant changes in the vital signs.
- *Palpating the uterus for firmness every 15 minutes or more often if needed:* The uterus should be round, firm, and located between the umbilicus and the symphysis pubis during the first hour.
- *Massaging the uterus:* Perform gentle massage of the uterus with the palm of the hand on the fundus and the other hand supporting the lower uterine segment (Fig. 9.27).
- *Monitoring lochia:* Monitor the patient's lochia every 15 minutes for the amount, color, and odor of the discharge and for the presence of clots. Usual blood loss in the first hour requires no more than two saturated obstetrical peripads and has only a few small clots. Alert the health-care provider if more than two peripads are soaked with blood during the first hour.
- *Promoting bonding:* Promote bonding by allowing the new family time alone to get acquainted with the baby. The baby's mother can also place the newborn skin-to-skin for bonding and warmth.
- *Promoting breastfeeding:* To promote breastfeeding, assist the mother to latch-on the infant.
- *Providing perineal comfort:* Provide perineal comfort with an ice pack.

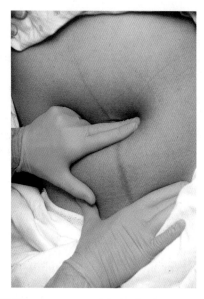

FIGURE 9.27 The nurse massaging the fundus.

Safety *Stat!*

The newborn has been immersed in body fluids, so standard safety precautions must be followed. Until the first bath, you should wear gloves when touching the newborn.

Nursing Care of the Infant

The immediate goals of newborn care are to monitor the infant's transition to extrauterine life and to promote bonding and attachment with the parents. Appropriate nursing care for the newborn in the first hour of life includes:

- *Maintaining the infant's warmth:* Maintain thermoregulation by wrapping the infant in warm blankets, covering the head with a cap, or placing the infant skin-to-skin with the mother. The infant should be placed under a warmer for any procedures.
- *Maintaining the infant's airway:* Maintain a clear airway in the infant by gently suctioning excess secretions with a bulb syringe.
- *Encouraging infant/mother bonding:* Assist the mother to position and latch the newborn on her breast. Provide verbal feedback on positive maternal behaviors, such as touching the newborn and talking to the newborn. Answer the mother and partner's questions.

The following nursing tasks can be completed after the first hour postdelivery, before the family is transferred to the postpartum unit.

- *Properly identifying the infant:* Follow hospital procedures for identifying the infant and attaching hospital security mechanisms to the infant.
- *Providing umbilicus care:* Apply the umbilical clamp closer to the umbilicus and trim off excess cord.
- *Administering vitamin K:* Administer vitamin K IM in the vastus lateralis muscle. Vitamin K is necessary for blood clotting.
- *Administering erythromycin:* Administer erythromycin 0.5% ophthalmic ointment within 2 hours of birth to prevent eye infections known as ***ophthalmia neonatorum*** from untreated sexually transmitted infections (STIs).

Medication Facts

Vitamin K

Vitamin K is a fat-soluble vitamin that promotes blood clotting and is generally synthesized by microorganisms in the intestines. A newborn cannot produce vitamin K until microorganisms are established in the newborn's intestines after feedings. To prevent neonatal hemorrhage, 0.5 to 1 mg IM of vitamin K is administered (Vallerand & Sanoski, 2023).

Patient Teaching Guidelines

Why Does My Newborn Need a Vitamin K Shot?

- Vitamin K is needed to help the blood clot if bleeding occurs.
- Babies are born with very little vitamin K and cannot form clots. In high-risk babies, bleeding can occur in the intestines or brain, locations where bleeding is not easily detected.
- Vitamin K deficiency bleeding can occur in newborns up to 6 months old.
- A single vitamin K shot can protect the baby from vitamin K deficiency bleeding.

• WORD • BUILDING •

ophthalmia neonatorum: opthalm–eye + ia–condition [inflammation] + neo–new + natorum–born

Key Points

- Several theories exist to explain the possible causes of the onset of labor. These theories focus on oxytocin, prostaglandins, progesterone, cortisol, estriol, and the overstretched uterus.
- During labor, the woman experiences changes in the following body systems: cardiovascular, respiratory, renal, gastrointestinal, and hematopoietic.
- Every woman is unique, but common signs of labor are lightening, contractions, cervical changes, SROM, bloody show, and a burst of energy.
- During labor, the cervix must efface and dilate to allow the fetus to leave the uterus.
- There are seven critical factors, the "Seven Ps," that are involved in labor. These factors are *passage, passenger, powers, position, psyche, pain,* and *patience.*
- There are four stages of childbirth:
  - The first stage of labor ends with complete dilation of the cervix.
  - The second stage of labor ends with the birth of the newborn.
  - The third stage ends with the delivery of the placenta.
  - The fourth stage ends 1 to 2 hours after delivery of the placenta.
- Nursing interventions in early labor focus on admission procedures, establishing rapport with the patient and her family, and explaining procedures.
- Medical interventions in active and transition phases of labor may include an amniotomy to rupture membranes and ordering IV pain medication or epidural anesthesia.
- Nursing interventions in active and transition labor focus on pain management. You should assist the patient and her support person by using nonpharmacological comfort measures and educating the patient about her options for pharmacological strategies for relieving pain.
- During the second stage, the fetus moves through positional changes to fit through the pelvis.
- Every woman reacts to pain in labor differently. There are a variety of factors that influence pain response, including support in labor, length of labor, past experiences with pain, and cultural responses to pain.
- Immediate postdelivery care of the patient involves the assessment of uterine tone, monitoring the amount of bleeding, and promoting bonding with the infant.
- Apgar score is a systemic method to determine the physical status of the newborn.
- The placenta should separate from the uterus within 5 to 15 minutes after the birth. Signs of placental separation are a sudden gush of blood, cord lengthening, and the uterine shape becoming firmer and rounder and moving up in the abdomen.
- Care for the newborn immediately after birth includes thermoregulation, maintaining a clear airway, and promoting bonding and breastfeeding.

Review Questions

1. You are describing true and false labor to a patient. Which of the following statements made by the patient indicates that she understands the difference?
   1. "A false labor contraction usually starts in the back and radiates around to the front of my abdomen."
   2. "True labor contractions cause cervical changes."
   3. "True labor contractions will go away with a warm shower."
   4. "False labor contractions get stronger if I take a walk."

2. The longest phase of labor is usually the:
   1. Pushing phase
   2. Early phase
   3. Active phase
   4. Placental phase

3. Which maternal positions are considered appropriate for labor? **(Select all that apply.)**
   1. Side-lying
   2. Supine
   3. Sitting
   4. Standing
   5. Walking

4. Powers, as one of the "Seven Ps," refers to:
   1. The fetal descent in the pelvis
   2. The uterine contractions and pushing efforts
   3. The fetus and placenta
   4. The pelvis and soft tissues

5. Signs that the placenta is separating from the uterus are: **(Select all that apply.)**
   1. A gush of blood comes from the uterus.
   2. The uterus stops contracting.
   3. The maternal pulse slows.
   4. The umbilical cord lengthens.
   5. The uterus rises upward.

6. Immediately after birth, the primary way to promote mother–infant bonding is to ensure _____.

7. What is the stage of labor when it is most appropriate to push?
   1. The first stage
   2. The second stage
   3. The third stage
   4. The fourth stage

8. What does a station of –1 mean?
   1. The fetus is very close to delivery.
   2. The fetal head has passed through the ischial spines by 1 cm.
   3. The fetal head is 1 cm above the ischial spines.
   4. The fetus is unlikely to be born vaginally.

9. A woman is admitted in labor. Her hemoglobin is 12.6 g/dL. What does this indicate to you?
   1. The patient has an infection.
   2. The patient may have problems with excessive blood loss.
   3. The patient has a normal hemoglobin level.
   4. The patient is anemic.

10. A contraction began at 11:00:00 and ended at 11:00:30. The next contraction began at 11:05:00. How far apart were the two contractions?
    1. 30 seconds
    2. 5 minutes and 30 seconds
    3. 4 minutes and 30 seconds
    4. 5 minutes

11. A patient in the active phase of labor begins to experience nausea and has become very irritable. What does this suggest is happening?
    1. She is going to have a long labor.
    2. She is getting closer to full dilation of the cervix.
    3. She is not satisfied with the nonpharmacological comfort measures.
    4. She is going to require more pain medication.

12. A patient's membranes ruptured, and the contractions have become more intense over the last few minutes. Her blood pressure is 122/80 mm Hg, and the respiratory rate is 32 bpm. She is 6 cm dilated. She reports a feeling of numbness and tingling of her fingers. Which nursing action is appropriate for this situation?
    1. Check the FHR.
    2. Turn her to her left side.
    3. Ask her to breathe into a paper bag.
    4. Recheck her blood pressure.

13. A nurse is providing care for a patient in active labor. Which of the following signs should be reported to the charge nurse immediately? **(Select all that apply.)**
    1. FHR of 200 bpm.
    2. Membranes rupture with greenish fluid noted.
    3. The patient states that her low back hurts when she has a contraction.
    4. The patient states that she drank an orange juice before coming into the hospital.
    5. The patient has vaginal bleeding.

14. The laboring patient wants medication for pain management. The health-care provider has ordered butorphanol 1 mg IV. The patient asks you if it is safe for the baby. What is your best response?
    1. "Of course, it is; trust me! I have been working in this department for 20 years. You'll be glad you took it."
    2. "It's such a small dose that I could give it to a 10-year-old. The baby is getting his oxygen through the umbilical cord."
    3. "Don't worry. The baby will be fine. My goal is to help you have a safe labor, and I am watching out for your baby."
    4. "I am giving you a small dose so that the peak effect wears off before the baby is born. That reduces the risk of harm to the baby."

15. You note on the fetal monitor that the fetus is experiencing a late deceleration. Which nursing actions are appropriate in this situation? **(Select all that apply.)**
    1. Continue to observe the fetal monitor for three more contractions.
    2. Turn the patient to her side.
    3. Apply oxygen via face mask.
    4. Increase the oxytocin to speed up labor.
    5. Assist the patient into a pushing position.

CRITICAL THINKING QUESTIONS

1. Prepare a discussion on the pros and cons of hospital and home births for a prenatal class.
2. The *Healthy People 2030* goal is to reduce the number of cesarean births in the United States. Explore ways that nurses can contribute to achieving that goal.

3. A laboring patient's mother comes to the nurse's station and insists on speaking to the charge nurse. The mother states, "I want the doctor called! She has been in labor too long. I can't stand to see her suffer. She needs a C-section." How should you respond to this request?

Resources

For additional resources and information, including Postconference Questions and Activities, Answers, and References, visit www.FADavis.com.

   Student Study Guide

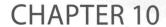

CHAPTER 10
Nursing Care of the Woman With Complications During Labor and Birth

KEY TERMS

amniotic band syndrome (am-nee-OT-ik BAND SIN-drohm)
cephalopelvic disproportion (CPD) (SEF-al-oh-PEL-vik DIS-pro-POR-shun)
chorioamnionitis (KOH-ree-oh-AM-nee-oh-NYE-tiss)
external version (eks-TER-nuhl VER-zhun)
fetal demise (FEE-tuhl de-MYEZ)
fetal fibronectin (fFN) (FEE-tuhl FYE-broh-NEK-tin)
macrosomia (MAK-ruh-SOH-mee-uh)
nuchal cord (NOO-kuhl KORD)
precipitous delivery (prih-SIP-ih-tuss dih-LIV-uh-ree)
premature rupture of membranes (PROM) (pree-mah-CHOOR RUP-chur uv MEM-braynz)
preterm premature rupture of membranes (PPROM) (PREE-term pree-ma-CHOOR RUP-chur uv MEM-braynz)
retained placenta (rih-TAYND pla-SEN-tuh)
shoulder dystocia (SHOHL-duhr dis-TOH-shee-uh)
uterine inversion (YOO-tuh-reen in-VER-zhun)
uterine rupture (YOO-tuh-reen RUP-chur)

CHAPTER CONCEPTS

Clinical Judgment
Perfusion
Professionalism
Reproduction and Sexuality
Stress and Coping

LEARNING OUTCOMES

1. Define the key terms.
2. Identify 10 risk factors associated with preterm labor.
3. Discuss nursing care and the common tocolytic medications used to manage preterm labor.
4. Identify the major complication of PROM.
5. Define *postterm pregnancy* and the possible fetal consequences of postterm pregnancy.
6. Differentiate between oligohydramnios and polyhydramnios and describe potential complications of each.
7. Describe the variations in the passage, passenger, powers, position, psyche, pain management, or patience that can contribute to complications in labor.
8. Discuss the risks of a vaginal breech delivery.
9. Define *macrosomia* and describe nursing care for the patient and fetus.
10. Describe umbilical cord prolapse and the potential risk to the fetus.
11. Define *precipitous labor and delivery* and explain nursing care that promotes safety for the woman and her fetus.
12. Identify risk factors for shoulder dystocia.
13. Formulate an emergency nursing care plan for a patient experiencing uterine rupture.
14. Discuss the causes of a uterine inversion.
15. Identify signs and symptoms of amniotic fluid embolism (AFE) and discuss medical interventions.
16. Using the nursing process, formulate a plan of care with appropriate nursing diagnoses for a patient experiencing a complication of labor and birth.
17. Discuss the grieving process and patient-centered nursing care of the family experiencing perinatal loss.

CRITICAL THINKING & CLINICAL JUDGMENT

Colette is 16 years old and at 30 weeks' gestation with her first pregnancy. She kept the pregnancy a secret from her mother until recently and just began prenatal care 3 weeks ago. Colette's mother calls the clinic and tells you she is concerned because Colette is having mild back pain and has been experiencing mild uterine contractions for a few hours.

Questions

1. Based upon Colette's pregnancy history, what do you need to think about in this situation?
2. What questions should you ask Colette's mother before reporting the phone call to your supervisor?
3. If the health-care provider is not readily available, what instructions should you give Colette's mother?

CONCEPTUAL CORNERSTONE

Stress and Coping

Complications during labor and delivery cause stress for the patient and her family. Fear of the unknown, a feeling of loss of control, and concern of possible risks to the fetus or patient increase stress. The patient may verbalize anxiety and difficulty with coping. She may cry, exhibit clinging behaviors, and be unable to problem-solve or make decisions. As her nurse, you may note physical signs of stress such as increased blood pressure, pulse, and respirations as well as increased perspiration, nausea, and diarrhea.

Stress can be contagious. During stressful situations, you must remain calm. By using therapeutic communication, you can assist the patient to control stress. Communication with the patient should be simple, honest, direct, and concrete with reassurance that the safety of the woman and her fetus is the priority.

The birth of a child is a life event that often proceeds without complications or deviations from the norm. During labor, nurses play a vital role in ensuring the safety of the patient and her fetus by being alert for the signs and symptoms of possible complications. The earlier the complication is identified and the health-care provider notified, the better the chance the complication can be addressed and treated. This chapter discusses preterm labor complications, labor-related complications, emergencies during birth, and care of the family experiencing perinatal loss.

CARE OF THE WOMAN AT RISK OF PRETERM LABOR

Preterm labor is defined as the presence of uterine contractions with enough frequency and intensity to cause effacement and dilation of the cervix before 37 weeks' gestation.

Preterm birth is the leading cause of neonatal mortality in the United States (Ross, 2021).

The exact causes of preterm labor are unknown, but the following risk factors have been identified:

- Late or no prenatal care
- Previous preterm birth
- Maternal age younger than 17 years or older than 35 years
- Domestic violence
- Placenta abruptio
- Overdistention of the uterus because of multiple gestations or polyhydramnios. (See Care of the Woman With Abnormal Amniotic Fluid Volume later in this chapter.)
- An incompetent cervix because of multiple traumas, such as abortions, or cone biopsy for diagnosis and treatment of cervical dysplasia or cancer
- Cervical inflammation because of bacterial vaginosis or trichomonas. (See Chapter 3.)
- Maternal inflammation because of an infection, such as a urinary tract infection
- TORCH infections. (See Chapter 7.)
- Hormonal changes because of maternal or fetal stress
- Inadequate perfusion of the placenta because of hypertension, diabetes, smoking, substance use disorder, or alcohol use
- A short cervix length of fewer than 25 mm during the second trimester (Ross, 2021)

Medical Interventions

Medical interventions start with verification of the gestational age of the fetus by reviewing the date of the last menstrual period (LMP) and obtaining ultrasound verification of fetal size. The goal of medical management is to delay delivery for several days to allow the fetal lungs to mature.

True diagnosis occurs after monitoring labor contractions, evaluating for changes in effacement and dilation of the cervix, and confirming the presence of **fetal fibronectin (fFN)** in vaginal fluid. fFN is a protein that helps the amniotic sac to adhere to the uterine wall. It is detected before 22 weeks' gestation and after 37 weeks' gestation. If the protein is not detected, it is a sign that delivery is not imminent; detection between 22 weeks and 37 weeks indicates preterm labor (Lockwood, 2022). Medical interventions for preterm labor include the following:

- Progesterone supplementation, particularly for women with a short cervix (fewer than 15 mm) and a prior history of preterm birth (Suman & Luther, 2022)
- Treatment of any infections, such as group B streptococcus (GBS) or urinary tract infections, that may be the cause of the onset of premature labor
- IV hydration to increase vascular volume and decrease uterine contractions
- Bedrest to decrease uterine stimulation
- **Tocolytic** medications suppress uterine contractions (Table 10.1). [Tocolytic medications are used only for

---

• **WORD · BUILDING** ·

tocolytic: toco–childbirth + lytic–stopping, slowing

Table 10.1

Tocolytic Medications

Medication	Action	Dose	Maternal Effects	Fetal Effects	Nursing Considerations
Magnesium sulfate	Relaxes smooth muscle; therefore decreases uterine activity	IV infusion of loading dose of 4–6 g IV over 20 minutes followed by a maintenance dose of 1–4 g/hour depending upon uterine response and urine output	Flushing, head-ache, drowsi-ness, blurred vision, respira-tory depression	Duration of longer than 5–7 days may cause hypocalcemia in the neonate and possible skeletal abnor-malities related to osteopenia	Obtain a magnesium level 1 hour after loading dose and then every 6 hours to mon-itor for magnesium overdose. Serum level of 4–8 mg/dL is acceptable. Monitor for signs of toxicity: respira-tory rate lower than 14 breaths per minute; hypotension; absent or minimal DTRs.
Indomethacin	Prostaglandin in-hibitor that stops the production of cytokines that initiate labor	50 mg loading dose followed by 25–50 mg every 6 hours for 48 hours	GI upset	Can cause oli-gohydramnios because of a decrease in fetal renal blood flow Can constrict the patent ductus arteriosus if used after 32 weeks' gestation	Monitor contractions and treat GI upset.
Nifedipine	Calcium chan-nel blocker that inhibits smooth muscle contrac-tions of the uterus	10–20 mg PO ev-ery 4–6 hours	Hypotension and tachycardia	May decrease uteroplacental blood flow	Monitor maternal blood pressure and FHR.

Sources: Ross, M. G. (2021). *Preterm labor.* Medscape. https://emedicine.medscape.com/article/260998-overview; Vallerand, A. H., & Sanoski, C. A. (2023). *Davis's drug guide for nurses* (18th ed.). F. A. Davis.

a short time while waiting for the fetal lungs to mature (Ross, 2021). The American College of Obstetricians and Gynecologists (ACOG, 2022) does not recommend the use of tocolytic medications beyond 34 weeks' gestation or before 24 weeks' gestation.]

- Corticosteroid therapy to accelerate fetal lung maturity. (These medications stimulate the production of mature surfactant in the fetal lungs, which decreases the risk of respiratory distress syndrome in the newborn.)

Nursing Care

Nursing care for the preterm labor patient includes the following:

- Checking the patient for signs of infection and rupture of membranes
- Checking cervical effacement and dilation
- Monitoring fetal heart rate (FHR) and uterine contraction activity and notifying the health-care provider of any non-reassuring patterns
- Obtaining fluid for fFN testing, if ordered by the health-care provider
- Providing oral and/or IV hydration
- Administering antibiotics if ordered

Medication Facts

Progesterone may be given to high-risk women to prevent preterm labor. The dose is 250 mg IM weekly, started between 16 and 21 weeks' gestation and continuing until 37 weeks' gestation (Ross, 2021).

- Administering tocolytics as ordered and monitoring for effectiveness and side effects. (See Box 10.1 for contraindications for the use of tocolytics):
  - Checking vital signs according to hospital protocol, which is usually every 15 minutes
  - Notifying the health-care provider if systolic blood pressure is greater than 140 mm Hg or lower than 90 mm Hg
  - Notifying the health-care provider if diastolic blood pressure is greater than 90 mm Hg or lower than 50 mm Hg
  - Observing for the presence of deep tendon reflexes (DTRs)
  - Monitoring urine output every hour; notifying the health-care provider if fewer than 30 mL/hour (Griggs et al., 2020)
- Administering corticosteroids as ordered
- Providing emotional support to the woman and her family, including allowing them to verbalize fear, anger, and frustrations
- Answering questions directly and honestly
- Explaining all medications and diagnostic tests to the patient
- Determining if the patient and her family understand the plan of care
- Monitoring the patient's responses to treatment
- Providing diversional activities
- Providing hygiene and self-care, depending upon activity restrictions
- If preterm birth is imminent, notifying the neonatologist and intensive care nursery
- If the patient will be sent home, preparing discharge instructions and determining the patient's understanding of discharge instructions

Health Promotion

Prevention of Preterm Labor

The pregnant patient can promote a healthy pregnancy and reduce her risk of preterm labor by following these guidelines:

- Seek early and regular prenatal care.
- Eat a healthy diet.
- Avoid smoking or vaping, drinking alcohol, and using illicit drugs.
- Get the health-care provider's advice before taking any medications, even over-the-counter medications.
- Get immediate medical care for any infections.
- Work closely with the health-care provider to manage any chronic conditions such as diabetes and hypertension.

Safety *Stat!*

Calcium gluconate, 1 g administered by slow IV push, is the antidote for magnesium toxicity that could occur if magnesium sulfate is used to stop preterm labor.

Box 10.1

Contraindications for the Use of Tocolytic Medications

- Severe preeclampsia
- Placental abruption
- Intrauterine infection
- Fatal fetal chromosomal abnormalities
- Advanced cervical dilation
- Evidence of placental insufficiency
- Signs of fetal distress

Source: Ross, M. G. (2021). *Preterm labor.* Medscape. https://emedicine.medscape.com/article/260998-overview

Patient Teaching Guidelines

Strategies to Prevent Preterm Labor
Teach the patient to do the following:

- Follow activity restrictions imposed by the health-care provider.
- Drink eight glasses of fluid each day.
- Eat a healthy, balanced diet.
- Follow the medication schedule.
- Perform a daily kick count and notify the health-care provider if she notices fewer than 10 kicks or fetal movements in 2 hours.
- Place fingers on the fundus of the uterus and note any tightening of the uterine muscle. Notify the health-care provider if more than five contractions are noted in an hour.
- Notify the health-care provider if she experiences any of the following:
  - Membranes rupture
  - Low backache
  - Cramping or pelvic pressure
  - Fever higher than 38°C (100.4°F)

Medication Facts

Betamethasone is a corticosteroid used to stimulate the production of mature surfactant in the fetal lungs. Its use before birth reduces the risk of respiratory distress in the newborn. The usual dose given to the mother is 12 mg IM every 24 hours for two doses (Vallerand & Sanoski, 2023).

Evidence-Based Practice

Health-care providers and nurses endeavor to prolong gestation time and prevent early preterm birth and the subsequent complications. A study was conducted to determine if organized planned relaxation-focused nursing care would help to prolong the gestation and avoid preterm birth. Women were divided into a control group

Continued

Evidence-Based Practice—cont'd

that received standard medical and nursing care and a group that received the same care with the addition of a 2-day formal intensive relaxation training. The group with the relaxation training had lower cortisol levels, decreased contraction severity, reported less anxiety, and experienced prolonged pregnancies.

Ozberk, H., Mete, S., & Bektas, M. (2021). Effects of relaxation-focused nursing care in women in preterm labor. *Biological Research for Nursing, 23*(2), 160–170. https://doi.org/10.1177/1099800420941253

CARE OF THE WOMAN WITH PREMATURE RUPTURE OF MEMBRANES

The term *premature rupture of membranes* (**PROM**) refers to the patient who is at 37 weeks' gestation or later and whose membranes rupture before the onset of labor. **Preterm premature rupture of membranes (PPROM)** is the rupture of membranes before 37 weeks' gestation (Dayal & Hong, 2022).

Patients experiencing PROM will have a leakage of fluid, vaginal discharge, and pelvic pressure but no contractions. A vaginal speculum is used to examine the cervix and to observe for leaking or pooling of fluid in the vagina. To verify the presence of amniotic fluid, nitrazine paper, which turns a dark purple color when it absorbs amniotic fluid, is typically used. Microscopic observation of a fernlike pattern in a sample of the dried fluid can also confirm the diagnosis.

CRITICAL THINKING

Your neighbor **Janelle** is pregnant at 36 weeks' gestation. She mentions to you that she has noticed that her underwear is frequently wet. She first noticed it yesterday. She says to you, "I don't think my water broke. It's too early, and isn't it usually a big splash when that happens?"

Questions

1. What do you need to think about when you respond to your neighbor?
2. What other information do you need to know before you answer your neighbor? How could you know if it is amniotic fluid?
3. What is the best advice for your neighbor based upon your scope of practice?

Medical Interventions

Medical interventions of PROM may include expectant management or the induction of labor. *Expectant management* is waiting for the woman to begin labor without additional interventions. If the mother or fetus demonstrates instability, expectant management is followed by the induction of labor or cesarean birth to deliver the fetus. PPROM is more difficult to manage than PROM at term because the premature fetus faces more potential problems.

Expectant management of PPROM and PROM includes:

- Ultrasound evaluation of the fetal weight, presentation, gestational age, and amniotic fluid index
- Obtaining informed consent from the patient regarding the plan of care and risks of PPROM
- Monitoring the FHR and contractions for 24 to 48 hours
  - If the FHR is reassuring, the patient will be placed on bedrest and monitored at least once a day.
- Monitoring for maternal signs of tachycardia and fever, which indicate possible **chorioamnionitis** (infection of the amniotic and chorionic membranes), requiring antibiotics and a plan for delivery of the fetus
- For the patient with PPROM who is managed expectantly, providing 7 days of antibiotics (Duff, 2022)
- If needed, ordering corticosteroids to accelerate fetal lung maturation

Nursing Care

Nursing care for the patient with PROM includes:

- Providing emotional support and education to the patient and her support person
- Avoiding vaginal cervical examinations, which increase the risk of infection
- Monitoring FHR and uterine activity, and notifying the health-care provider of any nonreassuring FHR patterns
- Monitoring maternal vital signs every 4 hours
- Administering antibiotics and corticosteroids if ordered by the health-care provider
- Notifying the health-care provider of any signs of maternal infection or bleeding

Chorioamnionitis (Intraamniotic Infection)

Infection is the most serious complication associated with PROM. Chorioamnionitis, also known as intraamniotic infection, can involve the amniotic membranes, amniotic fluid, fetus, umbilical cord, and placenta. The risk of infection increases after 24 hours postrupture. With the onset of chorioamnionitis, the mother is also at risk for endometritis, sepsis, and death (Tita, 2022). In addition, the neonate is at increased risk of fetal distress and infection.

The clinical signs and symptoms of chorioamnionitis are as follows:

- Fever greater than 38°C (100.4°F)
- Maternal tachycardia (greater than 120 bpm)
- Fetal tachycardia (greater than 160 bpm)
- Purulent or foul-smelling amniotic fluid or discharge
- Uterine tenderness
- Increased white blood count (greater than 15,000 cells/mm^3; Tita, 2022)

• WORD • BUILDING •
chorioamnionitis: chorio–chorion + amnion–amnion + itis–inflammation

Medical Interventions

Medical interventions include delivery of the fetus as soon as possible, supportive care, and antibiotic administration. Antibiotics most commonly ordered for the patient with chorioamnionitis are penicillin, clindamycin, ampicillin, cefotaxime, or gentamicin.

Nursing Care

Nursing care for the patient with chorioamnionitis includes the following:

- Recognizing and reporting abnormal vital signs and signs of infection
- Administering ordered antibiotics
- Providing an explanation of the infection and plan of care to the patient
- Continuing vigilant monitoring of maternal and fetal vital signs and response to treatment
- Providing emotional support to the patient and her support person
- Notifying the neonatologist of the impending birth of the fetus, who may be infected because of maternal infection

---

Patient Teaching Guidelines

Signs of Premature Rupture of Membrane Infection

Signs of infection from ruptured membranes include the following:

- Elevated temperature greater than 38°C (100.4°F)
- Offensive odor of the amniotic fluid
- Rapid heart rate
- Flu-like symptoms

CARE OF THE WOMAN WITH A POSTTERM PREGNANCY

A *postterm pregnancy* is defined as a pregnancy that extends past 42 weeks' gestation (Caughey, 2021). Risk factors for having a postterm pregnancy are a family history of postterm births and maternal obesity.

The fetal consequences of a postterm pregnancy can be serious:

- Placental insufficiency, which causes fetal distress and a risk for meconium aspiration
- Increased risk of being stillborn
- Increased mortality
- **Macrosomia** (excessive newborn weight), which leads to complications such as **cephalopelvic disproportion (CPD**; the fetal head is too large for the maternal pelvis), prolonged labor, and shoulder **dystocia** (fetal shoulders are wedged or stuck in the maternal pelvis)

• **WORD** • **BUILDING** •

macrosomia: macro–large + som–body + ia–condition
cephalopelvic: cephalo–head + pelv–pelvis + ic–pertaining to
dystocia: dys–abnormal + toc–labor or childbirth + ia–condition

Maternal risks of posterm pregnancy are significant as well:

- Slower and more difficult labor
- Increased perineal injury because of the larger size of the fetus
- Increased rate of cesarean delivery (Caughey, 2021)

Medical Interventions

Medical interventions for the posterm pregnancy begin with the correct identification of the fetal due date. The date of the LMP is compared with the ultrasound dating to estimate the fetal age. Ultrasound dating during the first trimester is the most accurate, unlike ultrasound dating later in pregnancy, which has a margin of error of plus or minus 10 days (Doshi, 2022).

If the health-care provider considers the fetus to be posterm, they have three options for medical management:

1. Elective induction of labor
2. Expectant management of the pregnancy, allowing labor to begin spontaneously
3. Monitoring of fetal well-being with more frequent testing, such as stress tests, nonstress tests (NSTs), and biophysical profiles (BPPs)

The mother should be fully informed of the risks of a posterm pregnancy and should participate in the choice of intervention along with her health-care provider.

Nursing Care

Nursing care for the woman with a posterm pregnancy includes the following:

- Assisting with any ordered testing to determine fetal well-being
- Notifying the health-care provider of any nonreassuring test results
- Providing patient teaching regarding the risks of posterm pregnancy
- Answering patient questions regarding testing
- Providing emotional support to the patient and her support person

CARE OF THE WOMAN WITH ABNORMAL AMNIOTIC FLUID VOLUME

Amniotic fluid serves several functions. It cushions the fetus, allows lung growth and contributes to pulmonary development, allows for fetal movement, and provides a barrier against infection. Before 8 weeks' gestation, amniotic fluid is produced by the passage of fluid across the amnion membrane. At around 8 weeks' gestation, the fetus begins to urinate into the uterine cavity, and fetal urine becomes the source of amniotic fluid production (Keilman & Shanks, 2022). Amniotic fluid volume increases with gestational age, reaching its peak amount of 800 to 1,000 mL around the 37th week of gestation (Fitzsimmons & Bajaj, 2022). The volume of amniotic fluid is an indication of fetal well-being. An abnormally high level of fluid is termed *polyhydramnios,* and an abnormally low level of amniotic fluid is termed *oligohydramnios.*

During a normal pregnancy, the fetus swallows amniotic fluid, which reduces the amount of fluid in the amniotic sac and balances the production of urine by the fetal kidneys. If the fetus does not swallow or has a gastrointestinal (GI) blockage, it can lead to polyhydramnios.

The most common cause of oligohydramnios is rupture of the membranes surrounding the fetus. Because fetal urine makes up the majority of the amniotic fluid, a fetal renal anomaly or urinary tract obstruction can also lead to oligohydramnios.

Abnormal amniotic fluid volume is usually diagnosed by alterations in fundus growth during the pregnancy and by ultrasound evaluation. The patient with oligohydramnios may have slower uterine growth, a small-for-gestational-age (SGA) fetus, and risk for cord compression during labor. On the other hand, the patient with polyhydramnios demonstrates rapid uterine growth. The patient with polyhydramnios is more likely to have preterm labor, a fetal anomaly, a malpresentation of the fetus, and a cesarean delivery (Fitzsimmons & Bajaj, 2022). Ultrasound evaluation of the amount of fluid present, as well as visualization of the internal organs of the fetus, can identify potential causes of the abnormal amniotic fluid volume, such as lung, kidney, and GI anomalies.

Medical Interventions

Medical interventions for abnormal amniotic fluid volume include the following:

- Bedrest to reduce the chance of preterm labor
- Maternal oral hydration of 2 liters of fluid per day, which increases amniotic fluid volume in those with oligohydramnios (Belooseky & Ross, 2022)
- Removal of fluid via amniocentesis, which may provide abdominal comfort
- Serial ultrasonography to monitor fetal growth and the amount of amniotic fluid
- Administration of indomethacin for those with polyhydramnios (See Medication Facts: Indomethacin.)
- Administration of steroids to enhance fetal lung maturity if preterm delivery is expected
- Consultation with a maternal-fetal medicine (MFM) specialist when significant abnormal amniotic fluid volume is diagnosed
- Plan for delivery if the BPP is nonreassuring
- During labor, potentially utilizing amnioinfusion to provide fluid in the uterine cavity to prevent cord compression (See Chapter 11 for more information about amnioinfusion.)
- After the birth, referral to a neonatologist, pediatric surgeon, pediatric cardiologist, or pediatric nephrologist if required

Potential complications of abnormal amniotic fluid volume are as follows:

- Oligohydramnios
  - Preterm labor
  - Fetal distress because of cord compression
- **Amniotic band syndrome**, a rare condition in which adhesions between the amnion and fetus occur, causing deformities such as limb amputation
  - Musculoskeletal deformities such as club foot because of compression (Keilman & Shanks, 2022)
- Polyhydramnios
  - Preterm labor because of increased uterine size
  - Amniotic fluid embolism (AFE). (See the section Emergencies and Complications During Birth later in this chapter.)
  - Maternal hemorrhage because the uterus fails to contract after delivery of the placenta. The lack of muscle contraction is caused by the overdistended uterus.

Medication Facts

Indomethacin

Indomethacin is a prostaglandin inhibitor that reduces fetal urine output and therefore reduces the amount of amniotic fluid. The usual dose is 25 mg orally every 6 hours. It should be administered with food to decrease GI irritation (Vallerand & Sanoski, 2023).

Safe and Effective Nursing Care

Indomethacin is an NSAID. Patients who have an aspirin allergy are at increased risk for developing a hypersensitivity reaction. Monitor for urticaria and respiratory distress (Vallerand & Sanoski, 2023).

Nursing Care

Nursing care for the patient with abnormal amniotic fluid volume includes the following:

- Providing emotional support to the patient and her family
- Answering questions with terms that the patient will understand
- Monitoring maternal vital signs and FHR and notifying the health-care provider of any abnormal results
- Teaching the patient signs of preterm labor
- Teaching the patient signs of ruptured membranes
- Assisting with amniocentesis, if indicated
- Administering indomethacin, if ordered
- Assisting with amnioinfusion if ordered by the health-care provider

LABOR-RELATED COMPLICATIONS

A pregnancy that has gone smoothly can still develop an unexpected complication in labor. These late complications can have a devastating effect on the outcome of the pregnancy. Nurses must be alert to signs of a complication and must intervene to promote a safe outcome for the woman and her fetus.

Care of the Woman With Dysfunctional Labor

Dysfunctional labor is defined as difficult labor or an abnormally slow progress of labor. Other terms that are often used interchangeably in the obstetric literature are *dystocia*, *failure to progress* (lack of cervical dilation), and *cephalopelvic disproportion* (Olsen, 2022).

Dysfunctional labor constitutes any labor pattern that falls outside the normal labor curve. Published in 1955, the Friedman curve described the average amount of time it took women to dilate during labor. Dr. Emanuel Friedman determined that normal nulliparous active labor should progress at 1.2 cm per hour, and multiparous labor should progress at 1.5 cm per hour. For decades, the Friedman curve was used by obstetricians to evaluate labor progress.

New data have shown that Friedman's labor curve is no longer applicable to many women of the 21st century. Zhang and colleagues (2010) and Laughon and colleagues (2012) came to the conclusion that labors are longer than they were 60 years ago because childbearing women are older, have higher body mass indices (BMI), use epidurals, and have labor induced. Based on current research, the ACOG (2021) has published guidelines encouraging health-care providers to allow women to labor longer without interventions. ACOG does not advocate the Friedman curve as the only guideline for evaluating progress in labor.

Dysfunctional labor can usually be attributed to one of the Seven Ps of labor: passage, passenger, powers, position, psyche, pain management, or patience (see Chapter 9).

Passage

The passage contributes to dysfunctional labor when the pelvic bones are too narrow to allow the passage of the fetus through the birth canal. In the case of the obese patient, the fetus has more tissue to pass through for delivery.

MEDICAL INTERVENTIONS. Medical interventions for problems with the passage may include the following:

- Allowing a trial labor to evaluate labor progression
- Taking a pelvic x-ray to determine the size of the passage through which the fetus must pass for vaginal delivery
- Possibly using forceps or vacuum extraction for delivery

NURSING CARE. Nursing care for a laboring patient with problems with the passage includes monitoring labor progress and reporting slow dilation to the health-care provider as well as encouraging the patient to empty her bowel and bladder to reduce soft-tissue obstruction in the pelvic area.

Passenger

The size of the passenger may contribute to dysfunctional labor. A large fetus can cause labor to progress more slowly because it cannot pass through the pelvis for a vaginal delivery.

MEDICAL INTERVENTIONS. Medical interventions for problems related to the passenger may include the following:

- Leopold maneuvers to estimate fetal weight and position
- Ultrasound examination to determine fetal size

- Allowing a trial labor and, if fetal descent and engagement do not occur, scheduling a cesarean birth

NURSING CARE. Nursing care for a laboring patient with problems with the passenger is as follows:

- Monitoring fetal descent through vaginal examination and reporting slow progress to the health-care provider
- Anticipating possible forceps or vacuum-assisted delivery
- Emotionally supporting the patient through a long labor and pushing stage
- Preparing the woman for a cesarean birth if it is determined necessary by the health-care provider

Powers

The term *powers* refers to labor contractions. A woman may experience contractions that are too mild to produce cervical dilation. Additionally, the uterine muscle may not contract in a coordinated manner because of the disruption of communication between uterine segments from scarring or fibroids (Olsen, 2022).

MEDICAL INTERVENTIONS. Medical interventions for problems related to the powers may include the following:

- Artificial rupture of amniotic membranes (AROM) to stimulate labor contractions
- Augmentation of labor with oxytocin to stimulate effective labor contractions
- Planning a cesarean birth if AROM and oxytocin are not successful in producing effective uterine contractions

NURSING CARE. Nursing care for a laboring patient with problems with the powers of labor includes checking for poor or ineffective uterine contractions and reporting them to the health-care provider and administering IV oxytocin per the health-care provider's order to augment labor. (See Chapter 11.)

Position

The term *position* refers to fetal presentation. A posterior, brow, shoulder, or breech presentation will cause slower cervical dilation and labor progression. Most women cannot deliver a posterior, brow, or shoulder presentation vaginally because of the size and shape of the female pelvis.

MEDICAL INTERVENTIONS. Medical interventions for problems related to the position may include the following:

- For a posterior presentation, the mother will be informed that labor will progress slowly until the fetus rotates to an anterior presentation. Failure to rotate may lead to a cesarean birth.
- For a breech or brow presentation, an external version may be attempted. **External version** is a procedure in which the health-care provider applies external pressure to change the fetal position. If the version is not successful, a cesarean birth is scheduled.

NURSING CARE. Nursing care for a laboring patient with a fetus in posterior position includes the following:

- Anticipating severe back pain until the fetus rotates to the anterior position

- Providing comfort measures, such as sacral massage and the application of low back counterpressure during contractions
- Encouraging position changes to promote fetal rotation, such as the side-lying position; sitting, kneeling, or standing while leaning forward, to move the fetus away from the posterior pelvis; and squatting while pushing
- Explaining the fetal position to the patient and her support person
- Providing ongoing positive reinforcement of the patient's coping mechanisms
- Providing nonpharmacological comfort measures
- Administering pain medication as ordered by the health-care provider
- If the patient requests an epidural, notifying the anesthesiologist and assisting with epidural administration

Nursing care for a laboring patient with a fetus in breech or brow position is as follows:

- Assisting with external version if attempted by the health-care provider
- Explaining the fetal position to the patient and her support person
- Preparing the patient for a cesarean birth if the version is not attempted or is unsuccessful

---

Therapeutic Communication

The Impatient Patient

A laboring patient or her family may get discouraged by a slow labor and begin asking for interventions or a cesarean birth. You can communicate therapeutically with the patient and family by:

- Demonstrating a genuine interest in the patient's and family's concerns
- Listening attentively
- Not minimizing their concerns
- Providing labor updates and fetal wellness updates and pointing out progress that has been made
- Praising the patient for her patience
- Encouraging the family to continue to support her in labor
- Reassuring the family that the health-care provider is aware of labor progress

---

Psyche

The woman's psyche contributes to labor progression and can contribute to dysfunction. Some women may have extreme anxiety because of past birthing experiences or a lack of knowledge of the birth process. Women with a history of sexual abuse may have increased anxiety and flashbacks of previous abuse. It is important for caregivers to always ask permission of the patient before touching her, to allow her to make decisions regarding her care, to avoid rushing the patient, to explain every procedure, and to allow her to have any family and friends in the room that she desires (ACOG, 2021).

MEDICAL INTERVENTIONS. Medical interventions for problems related to the psyche may include reassuring the patient that she will be well cared for during labor and emphasizing to the patient that the health-care team will monitor her care and the well-being of her fetus.

NURSING CARE. Nursing care for a laboring patient with problems related to the psyche may include the following:

- Providing nonpharmacological comfort measures
- Encouraging the patient's support person to participate in providing encouragement and comfort measures
- Providing positive encouragement and reassurance to increase the patient's self-esteem and her ability to manage her labor and delivery
- Assisting with relaxation techniques
- Providing appropriate pharmacological pain control
- Monitoring fetal well-being and reporting any nonreassuring FHR patterns to the health-care provider
- Listening to the concerns of the patient regarding her labor and delivery

Pain Management

Pain management, although desirable, can contribute to a dysfunctional labor. IV narcotic medication given too early in latent labor may slow down the contractions and labor progress. In addition, epidural anesthesia during labor contributes to slower dilation and a longer labor (ACOG, 2021). Women with epidural anesthesia experience a longer second stage of labor because of their inability to push effectively.

MEDICAL INTERVENTIONS. Medical interventions for problems related to pain management may include these:

- Providing clear guidelines to the nurses for the use of narcotics in labor and the appropriate timing of epidural administration
- Allowing the effects of epidural anesthesia to decrease before encouraging pushing during the second stage of labor

NURSING CARE. Nursing care for a laboring patient with pain management problems is as follows:

- Implementing nonpharmacological comfort measures to delay the need for narcotics and epidural anesthesia
- Ensuring that the patient is well-established in active labor before administering narcotic medication or initiating epidural anesthesia

Patience

Patience is important if labor is progressing slowly. Health-care providers should allow labor to progress without interventions, such as a cesarean, as long as the mother and fetus are closely monitored and show no signs of distress.

MEDICAL INTERVENTIONS. Medical interventions for problems related to patience may include the following:

- Monitoring the patient and her fetus for well-being and, if no problems are evident, allowing labor to progress without medical interventions

• Reassuring the woman that even though her labor is progressing slowly, the fetus is stable with no signs of distress

NURSING CARE. Nursing care for a laboring patient with problems with patience is as follows:

• Providing the patient with updates on labor progress
• Providing positive encouragement to the patient and her support person as she manages a long labor
• Monitoring the fetus for distress and reporting any nonreassuring FHR patterns to the health-care provider

Care of the Woman and Fetus at Risk Because of Breech Presentation

Breech presentation occurs in 3% to 4% of all pregnancies and is defined as a fetus in a longitudinal lie with the buttocks or feet closest to the cervix (Fischer, 2022). There are three types of breech presentations:

1. *Frank breech:* The hips are flexed and the knees are extended.
2. *Complete breech:* The hips are flexed and the knees are flexed.

3. *Footling or incomplete breech:* One or both hips are extended and the foot presents (Fig. 10.1).

Vaginal breech deliveries were common until 1959, when it was proposed that cesarean delivery would reduce complications (Fischer, 2022). The current practice is that before 36 weeks' gestation, a vaginal delivery may be possible (Fig. 10.2). However, the parents should be

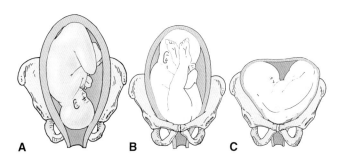

FIGURE 10.1 Breech presentations. A, Normal cephalic. B, Complete breech. C. Transverse.

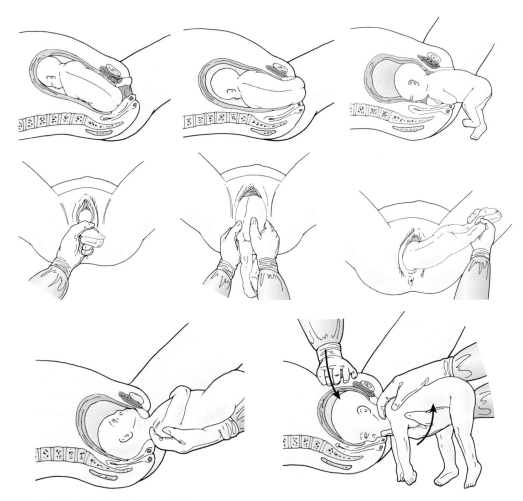

FIGURE 10.2 The mechanisms of labor in a breech presentation.

informed about the risks of breech delivery and decide with the health-care provider whether to proceed. After 37 weeks, the current practice is to try an external version of the fetus and, if that is unsuccessful, to plan a cesarean delivery (ACOG, 2020).

The risks of a vaginal breech delivery are as follows:

- Low Apgar scores because of cord compression
- Cord prolapse
- Fetal head entrapment because the fetal head does not have time to mold in the maternal pelvis
- Neonatal trauma because of malposition of the fetal arms

Medical Interventions

Medical interventions begin with ultrasonography to confirm fetal position, age, and size. Some health-care providers attempt a cephalic version procedure to reposition the fetus. This procedure is discussed in Chapter 11. However, most breech presentations are delivered by cesarean section. Nonetheless, vaginal deliveries do occur when a second twin is breech or when birth is precipitous (rapid).

Nursing Care

Nursing care for the woman with a breech fetus includes the following:

- Notifying the health-care provider as soon as a breech presentation is suspected based on physical assessment of the mother
- Monitoring the mother's vital signs and the FHR
- Assisting with a cephalic version if attempted by the health-care provider
- Preparing the woman for a cesarean birth. (See Chapter 11 for nursing care related to cesarean birth.)
- Reassuring and providing emotional support to the woman and her support person

Care of the Woman and Fetus at Risk for Macrosomia

Macrosomia refers to a newborn that is significantly larger than average for gestational age. The diagnosis of fetal macrosomia can only be made by weighing the newborn. Fetal macrosomia is defined as a birth weight greater than 4,000 g. Macrosomia is associated with an increased risk for neonatal morbidity, neonatal injury, maternal injury, and cesarean birth (Patel, 2020).

Contributing Factors

Factors that are associated with fetal macrosomia include:

- Genetics
- Maternal obesity
- Excessive maternal weight gain
- Postmaturity (gestational age greater than 40 weeks)
- Gestational diabetes, which stimulates insulin and growth factors, leading to fetal growth and the storage of fat and glycogen

- Male fetus
- Hispanic ethnicity of the mother (Patel, 2020)

Medical Interventions

Medical interventions to avoid macrosomia focus on decreasing risk factors by controlling maternal gestational diabetes and excessive weight gain and avoiding postmaturity by inducing labor before the fetus becomes too large.

During labor, the health-care provider will monitor for labor progress and descent of the fetus into the pelvis. Indications that the fetus may not be descending may lead to cesarean delivery.

Nursing Care

Nursing care for the woman and fetus at risk for macrosomia include:

- Monitoring FHR for nonreassuring patterns and reporting them to the health-care provider
- Preparing the woman for a cesarean delivery (See Chapter 11.)
- Providing emotional support, comfort measures, and pain control to the patient as she labors

Care of the Woman With a Prolapsed Umbilical Cord

An *umbilical cord prolapse* is an obstetric emergency that occurs when the umbilical cord passes through the cervix at the same time as or before the presenting part. The prolapse is termed *occult* when the cord passes through the cervix at the same time as the presenting part but cannot be seen or felt by an examiner. In contrast, an *overt* prolapsed cord is visible or palpable in the birth canal or extending beyond the vagina.

The diagnosis of an overt umbilical cord prolapse is made during a vaginal examination when the examiner notices a soft, pulsating mass in the vagina. The diagnosis of a covert cord prolapse is more difficult and may be suspected based on the FHR tracing. Prolapse of the cord is an emergency because it leads to compression of the cord by the fetal presenting part (Fig. 10.3). Compression of the umbilical cord causes a decrease in blood flow and oxygen to the fetus. Severe, sudden FHR decelerations with prolonged bradycardia or variable decelerations are observed on the fetal monitor (Layden et al., 2023; Fig. 10.4).

The primary cause of cord prolapse is the rupture of membranes, either spontaneously or artificially by the health-care provider. The risk factors for a prolapsed cord are the following:

- Fetal malposition, such as breech or brow presentation
- Rupture of membranes when the head is not engaged in the pelvis
- Prematurity
- SGA fetus
- Polyhydramnios
- Multiple gestation
- PROM

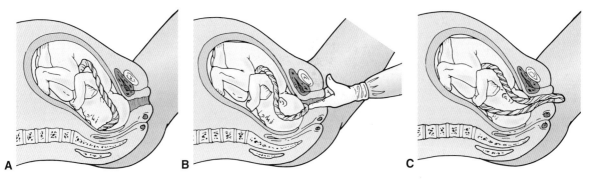

FIGURE 10.3 Umbilical cord prolapse. A, Occult; the cord cannot be seen or felt during a vaginal examination. B, Complete; the cord is felt as a pulsating mass. C, Frank; the cord precedes the fetal head or feet and can be seen protruding from the vagina.

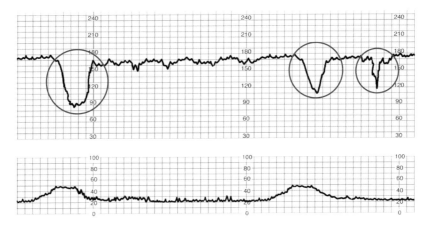

FIGURE 10.4 Variable decelerations from umbilical cord compression (circled in red).

- Grand multiparity (commonly defined as having had at least five births at greater than 20 weeks of gestation)
- Placement of an intrauterine pressure catheter or fetal scalp electrode. (See Chapter 9.)
- Attempted rotation of the fetal head
- Placement of a cervical ripening balloon catheter (See Chapter 11.)
- External cephalic version (Fischer, 2022)

Medical Interventions

Medical interventions for an umbilical cord prolapse include:

- Arrange for an immediate cesarean delivery.
- Place two fingers into the vagina to elevate the presenting part off the umbilical cord.
  - Care is taken to avoid palpating the cord, which could lead to vasospasm. The person manually elevating the presenting part maintains this position until the uterine incision is made.
- Position the mother in the knee–chest or Trendelenburg position to allow gravity to assist with elevation of the fetal presenting part (Bush et al., 2022; Fig. 10.5).
- If there will be a delay of more than 30 minutes before delivery, some health-care providers fill the bladder with 500 to 750 mL of fluid to assist with elevation of the fetal presenting part (Bush et al., 2022; Layden et al., 2023).

- If the cord is outside the mother's body, cover it with wet gauze and replace it gently in the vagina.
- Provide oxygen via face mask to increase the oxygen levels for the fetus.

Nursing Care

Nursing care for the patient with a prolapsed umbilical cord includes the following:

- Elevating the presenting part if diagnosed by the nurse during a vaginal examination
- Repositioning the woman into knee–chest or Trendelenburg position
- Applying high-flow oxygen via face mask
- Notifying the nursing chain of command and the health-care provider of the cord prolapse and the impending cesarean birth
- Preparing the mother for a cesarean birth
- Notifying the pediatrician or neonatologist of the impending cesarean birth
- Monitoring the FHR pattern and reporting nonreassuring heart rate patterns
- Assisting the health-care provider as needed
- Providing emotional support to the woman and her family

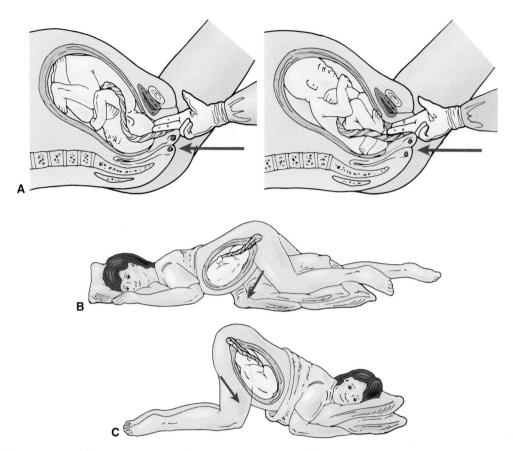

FIGURE 10.5 Interventions to relieve pressure on a prolapsed umbilical cord until birth. A, Two fingers of a gloved hand are placed in the vagina to lift the presenting part off the cord. B, The maternal hips are elevated with two pillows; this intervention is often combined with the Trendelenburg position. C. The knee–chest position uses gravity to shift the fetus out of the maternal pelvis.

There is the potential for a poor outcome for the fetus with an umbilical cord prolapse. However, prompt intervention, especially if delivery is achieved within 30 minutes of diagnosis, leads to good outcomes for the fetus (Dobiesz & Kerrigan, 2021).

Therapeutic Communication

How to Provide Emotional Support
When unexpected complications arise, you can provide emotional support to the patient and her family in the following ways:

- Explain what is happening in nonmedical terminology.
- Explain why procedures are done.
- Reassure the patient that everyone is working as a team to provide the best care for her and her baby.
- Use therapeutic touch by holding her hand or placing a hand on her shoulder.
- Stay with her as much as possible.
- Provide updates to the waiting family members.

Care of the Woman Experiencing Precipitous Labor and Birth

A **precipitous delivery** refers to an unusually rapid labor of fewer than 3 hours and ending with a rapid spontaneous delivery of the infant (Dobiesz & Kerrigan, 2021). A precipitous labor can occur in the labor and delivery suite of the hospital or may occur in the home or car on the way to the hospital. Factors that may predispose a woman to a precipitous delivery include the following:

- A multiparous woman with relaxed perineal floor muscles
- A multiparous woman with unusually strong and forceful contractions
- A woman with a high pain threshold
- A multiparous woman with a history of short labors

A precipitous labor and birth can cause complications for the woman and the infant. Possible complications for the woman include lacerations to the cervix, vagina, and perineum as well as hemorrhage because of uterine atony. The infant is at risk for intracranial hemorrhage because of rapid expulsion of the head and also risks aspiration of amniotic fluid and infection because of unsterile delivery.

Nursing Care

Nursing care for a precipitous labor includes the following:

- Obtaining a thorough history of previous labor lengths and complications to identify a woman at risk for precipitous labor and delivery
- Observing the patient for an impending delivery:
  - Reports of a sudden desire to push
  - Sudden increase in bloody show
  - Sudden bulging of the perineum or crowning of the fetal head
- Remaining calm and notifying the health-care provider
- Not leaving the patient alone
- Obtaining a precipitous delivery pack, which contains towels, scissors, cord clamp, gloves, and a bulb syringe for suction
- Washing hands and applying gloves
- Cleansing the perineum if time permits
- Giving clear directions to the woman and available assistants
- Checking for the amniotic sac; if it is still intact, it must be ruptured before the head emerges and the infant's first breath occurs
- Supporting the perineum and the infant's head as it emerges; instructing the mother to pant-blow to avoid forceful pushing of the head out the birth canal
- After the head emerges, using the bulb syringe to suction the mouth and nose of the infant
- Allowing the infant to spontaneously complete the birth movement of external rotation
- Checking for a **nuchal cord** (umbilical cord around the fetus's neck)
  - If present and tight around the neck, clamping and cutting the cord before the shoulders emerge
  - Assisting the patient to pant-blow while allowing a controlled delivery of the shoulders; the infant will be expelled rapidly after the posterior shoulder emerges
- After delivery, thoroughly suctioning the infant's mouth and nose
- Preventing hypothermia of the infant by drying the infant and placing the infant skin-to-skin with the mother
- Determining the 1- and 5-minute Apgar scores
- Checking the placenta for intactness after delivery (should occur within 30 minutes; never pull or tug on the cord)
- Massaging the uterus immediately after the delivery of the placenta
- Placing the infant to breastfeed to promote the release of oxytocin to enhance uterine involution
- Documenting the following:
  - Fetal presentation and position
  - Presence of nuchal cord and management
  - Color of amniotic fluid
  - Time of delivery
  - Sex of infant
  - Apgar scores
  - Time of placenta delivery and appearance of placenta
  - Maternal condition

Safety *Stat!*

If a delivery is imminent, never leave the patient alone and never attempt to delay delivery by applying pressure to the fetal head.

EMERGENCIES AND COMPLICATIONS DURING BIRTH

Emergencies and complications that occur during the birth can be stressful and dangerous for the patient or the fetus. As a nurse, you must calmly but quickly assist the health-care provider with interventions and provide emotional support for the patient during these situations.

Shoulder Dystocia

A **shoulder dystocia** occurs when one or both fetal shoulders become wedged in the maternal pelvis. After the fetal head is delivered, the shoulders need to rotate within the pelvis in a winding manner to leave the pelvis. If the shoulders are too large or the maternal pelvis is too small, the anterior shoulder can become wedged behind the symphysis pubis, or the posterior shoulder can become wedged at the sacral promontory.

Risk factors for shoulder dystocia are as follows:

- History of shoulder dystocia in a previous delivery
- Fetal macrosomia
- Diabetes
- Excessive maternal weight gain
- Obesity
- Postterm pregnancy
- Precipitous second stage of labor
- Prolonged second stage of labor
- Induction of labor for potential macrosomia

Possible complications of shoulder dystocia include the following:

- Postpartum hemorrhage (PPH) from uterine atony because of fetal macrosomia
- Third- or fourth-degree perineal laceration
- Neonatal clavicle fracture
- Neonatal fractured humerus
- Brachial plexus (nerve supply to the upper extremities) injury

Medical Interventions

Medical interventions for shoulder dystocia involve repositioning the laboring patient and the fetus. In the United States, McRoberts maneuver is the usual first-line maneuver for shoulder dystocia (Layden et al., 2023). To perform this maneuver, the health-care provider requires two assistants to hyperflex the mother's thighs against her abdomen. This movement raises the symphysis pubis about 9 mm, which may provide enough room to release the fetus's shoulder from the pelvis. The flattening of the lumbar spine may help with advancing the posterior shoulder (Fig. 10.6).

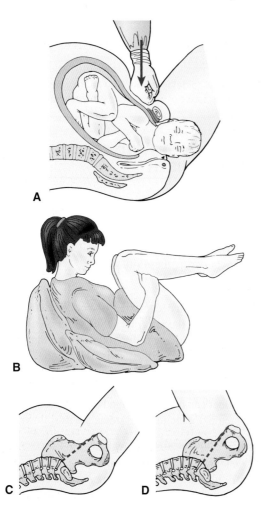

FIGURE 10.6 Methods to relieve shoulder dystocia. A, Pressure is applied immediately above the maternal symphysis pubis to push the fetal anterior shoulder downward. B, McRoberts maneuver; the woman's thighs are sharply flexed on her abdomen to straighten the pelvic curve. C, Angle of the pelvis before the maneuver. D, Angle of the pelvis after the maneuver.

Along with the McRoberts maneuver, the health-care provider may request that you provide firm downward pressure to the maternal abdomen just above the symphysis pubis. The suprapubic pressure compresses the soft tissue that may be making the situation worse and helps to rotate the anterior shoulder away from the symphysis pubis.

Nursing Care

Nursing care for a shoulder dystocia includes the following:

- Assisting the patient into positions requested by the health-care provider
- Providing suprapubic pressure as directed by the health-care provider
- Providing encouragement and support to the patient
- Checking the newborn for complications of shoulder dystocia and notifying the pediatrician or pediatric nurse practitioner

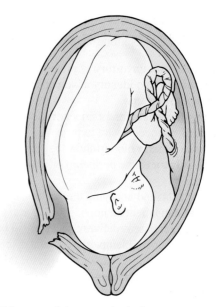

FIGURE 10.7 Rupture of the uterus in the lower uterine segment.

Uterine Rupture

Uterine rupture is the nonsurgical opening of the uterus (Fig. 10.7). A complete rupture includes all layers of the uterine muscle: the endometrium, myometrium, and serosa. A partial or incomplete rupture happens when one or two layers separate. Risk factors for uterine rupture include the following (Landon & Frey, 2022):

- Uterine manipulation for a version
- Abdominal trauma
- Previous cesarean birth
- A birth interval of fewer than 18 months
- Overstimulation of the uterus with oxytocin
- Amnioinfusion

Diagnosis and Symptoms

A uterine rupture can only be definitively diagnosed with a surgical incision to view the uterus. Suspected uterine rupture is based on maternal and fetal symptoms:

- Nonreassuring FHR pattern with variable and late decelerations
- Fetal bradycardia
- Change in uterine shape
- Constant abdominal pain
- Uterine tenderness

If a uterine rupture is suspected, the health-care provider must be notified immediately. In the operating room, the physician will determine the degree of rupture and repair if possible. If the rupture is large, a hysterectomy may be performed.

Nursing Care

After notifying the health-care provider of the suspected uterine rupture, the nursing care for the patient includes the following:

- Notifying the anesthesiologist, neonatologist, and intensive care nursery of the impending birth

- Monitoring fetal and maternal vital signs
- Giving the mother oxygen by mask or nasal cannula
- Preparing the patient for a cesarean birth
- Inserting an indwelling urinary catheter
- Reassuring and providing emotional support to the patient and her support person
- Performing blood type and crossmatch for a possible transfusion
- If no IV line is started, inserting an 18-gauge line for possible blood transfusion

Uterine Inversion

Uterine inversion is a rare complication but can lead to hemorrhage, shock, and death if unrecognized and not treated promptly. During a uterine inversion, the uterus inverts, and the uterine fundus prolapses to or through the dilated cervix. In severe cases, the entire uterus and vagina may invert and prolapse out of the patient's body. In about 60% to 70% of cases, the placenta remains attached at the moment of inversion (Kumari et al., 2022). The patient will experience uterine bleeding that varies depending upon the severity of the inversion.

Acute inversions occur within 24 hours of delivery, and subacute inversions occur more than 24 hours after delivery but before the 30th postpartum day. Possible causes of uterine inversion are a flaccid uterus, excessive pressure on the fundus during delivery of the placenta, a placenta accreta, and the application of too much traction on the umbilical cord in an attempt to deliver the placenta (Kumari et al., 2022).

The signs of a uterine inversion are these:

- PPH
- Sudden appearance of a vaginal mass
- Signs of shock (hypotension and tachycardia)

Medical Interventions

Medical interventions of an inverted uterus are as follows:

- Rapid diagnosis and aggressive management to reduce blood loss and return the uterus to its correct position
- Moving the patient to the operating room
- Infusing IV fluids and possibly blood products to manage the hypotension
- Attempting transvaginal replacement after the woman has been given uterine tocolytics to relax the uterine muscle
- If manual transvaginal replacement is not successful, administering anesthesia and preparing the woman for a surgical procedure to repair and replace the uterus
- After the uterus is replaced, administering medications that cause uterine contractions, such as oxytocin or methylergonovine maleate, to assist the uterus to stay in position
- Some physicians place a Rusch balloon catheter into the uterus for 12 hours after replacement to exert pressure on the placental site and therefore control PPH and maintain uterine position (Dobiesz & Kerrigan, 2021).

Nursing Care

Nursing care for the patient experiencing a uterine inversion includes the following:

- Calling for assistance immediately
- If the health-care provider is not present, notifying them immediately
- Monitoring vital signs and blood loss
- Assisting with notification and coordination of care with the operating room and anesthesiologist
- Administering fluids and blood products as ordered by the health-care provider
- Assisting with transfer to the operating room
- Providing emotional support to the patient and her family

Retained Placenta

After delivery, the placenta should deliver within 30 minutes. Occasionally, after a vaginal delivery, a **retained placenta** occurs. The entire placenta may not detach from the wall of the uterus; or, as the placenta separates from the uterus, small pieces or fragments of the placenta may be left attached to the uterus. Risk factors for retained placenta include mismanagement of the third stage of labor with excessive pulling of the umbilical cord before a complete separation of the placenta, entrapment of the placenta by a constricting ring of uterine muscle, or abnormally adherent placenta tissue (Smith, 2020). A retained placenta prevents the uterus from contracting, causing uterine atony. This can lead to complications of hemorrhage and infection. The health-care provider should carefully inspect the placenta after delivery to notice if any placenta lobules or pieces of tissue are missing and possibly adhered to the uterine wall.

Medical Interventions

Medical interventions for a retained placenta include the following:

- Ordering oxytocin or methylergonovine maleate, which produce uterine contractions to assist the uterus to expel the placenta
- Attempting manual removal of the placenta. A gloved hand and lower forearm are inserted in the uterus, and the health-care provider gently separates the placenta from the wall of the uterus.
- Possibly ordering IV pain medication or spinal or epidural anesthesia for manual removal of the placenta
- If manual removal of the placenta is unsuccessful, performing a dilation and curettage (D&C) with the patient under general or epidural anesthesia
- Ordering a blood transfusion if bleeding is excessive
- Rarely, performing a hysterectomy

Nursing Care

Nursing care for the patient with a retained placenta may include the following:

- Administering oxytocin or methylergonovine maleate as ordered by the health-care provider

- Administering pain medication if ordered by the health-care provider
- Administering medications that relax the uterus if oxytocics are not effective
- Monitoring vital signs and blood loss
- Ordering blood type and crossmatch of packed red blood cells (PRBCs) if ordered by the health-care provider
- Anticipating surgical interventions if manual removal is not successful
- Explaining the situation to the patient and her support person
- Providing emotional support and reassurance to the patient and her support person

Amniotic Fluid Embolism

AFE, sometimes referred to as anaphylactoid syndrome of pregnancy, is a rare obstetric emergency in which maternal mortality is near 80%, with 50% of patients dying within the first hour of the onset of symptoms (Layden et al., 2023). The exact pathophysiology of AFE is poorly understood. The current theory is that during labor or other procedures, amniotic fluid and fetal debris enter the maternal circulation, triggering a massive anaphylactic reaction. The disorder progresses in two phases:

1. In phase one, hypoxia is the major problem. It is caused by pulmonary artery vasospasm with pulmonary hypertension and elevated right ventricular pressure. The patient may progress into left-sided heart failure and respiratory distress.
2. Women who survive phase one enter into phase two. In phase two, the primary problem is massive hemorrhage with uterine atony and disseminated intravascular coagulation (DIC) (Arnolds, 2022).

The signs and symptoms of AFE are the following:

- Dyspnea with labored breathing
- Altered mental status and confusion
- Severe hypotension
- Seizures
- Cyanosis around the mouth and peripherally
- If undelivered, fetal bradycardia because of maternal hypoxia
- Pulmonary edema seen on chest x-ray
- Uterine atony that does not respond to bimanual massage after delivery
- Severe hemorrhage
- Cardiac arrest

Medical Interventions

The following are medical interventions for AFE:

- Administering oxygen to keep oxygen saturation normal
- Initiating cardiopulmonary resuscitation (CPR) if the patient arrests
- Treating hypotension with crystalloids and blood products
- Arranging cesarean birth if the mother is unresponsive to resuscitation, remains severely hypotensive, or FHR analysis indicates a nonreassuring pattern
- Ordering arterial blood gas analysis, complete blood cell count (CBC), and coagulation tests
- Admitting the patient to the intensive care unit (ICU)

Nursing Care

Nursing care for the patient with AFE includes the following:

- Promptly recognizing symptoms and calling for assistance from the health-care provider and the hospital rapid response team if available
- Initiating CPR if the patient arrests
- Arranging for assistance from laboratory personnel and the respiratory therapy department
- Initiating orders from the health-care provider for fluids and blood products
- Arranging transfer to the ICU
- Providing emotional support for the patient and her family

CARE OF THE FAMILY EXPERIENCING PERINATAL LOSS

Perinatal loss, also called *pregnancy loss,* includes ectopic pregnancy, spontaneous abortion or miscarriage, late pregnancy loss, stillbirth, or newborn death up to the 28th day of life (Maslovich & Burke, 2022). (See Chapter 8 for more on ectopic pregnancy and spontaneous abortion.) The death of a fetus at any stage is a **fetal demise.** Fetal demise very early in pregnancy may occur before the woman even knows she is pregnant. However, perinatal loss later in pregnancy can be devastating because it occurs at a time that is usually associated with joy and celebration. The parents' dreams and hopes for their child and the future suddenly disappear.

In most patients, the only symptom of a fetal demise is a decrease or loss of fetal movement. Although you may be unable to obtain fetal heart tones, this alone is not diagnostic of a fetal demise. An ultrasound examination can confirm fetal loss by direct visualization of the fetal heart with the absence of cardiac activity (Layden et al., 2023).

If the diagnosis of fetal demise occurs before labor begins, termination of the pregnancy will be scheduled by the patient and physician. Early fetal loss can be managed by cervical dilation and surgical evacuation (D&E). Late pregnancy loss requires cervical ripening and the induction of labor.

Causes of Perinatal Loss

The cause of fetal demise is unknown in 60% of all cases (Layden et al., 2023). In cases in which a cause is clearly identified, it is usually related to maternal, fetal, or placenta pathology:

- Prolonged pregnancy beyond 42 weeks
- Poorly controlled diabetes
- Hypertension
- Preeclampsia
- Eclampsia
- Uterine rupture

- Maternal trauma or death
- Infection
- Multiple gestations
- Congenital abnormality
- Genetic abnormality
- Intrauterine growth restriction (IUGR)
- Listeria and cytomegalovirus
- Umbilical cord accident, such as a cord that is prolapsed or wrapped around the fetus
- Placenta abruptio
- Fetomaternal hemorrhage
- Maternal substance use disorder
- PROM

After the fetal demise, the health-care provider will want to investigate the cause if it is not readily identifiable. A careful maternal history should be obtained along with antibody screens and a CBC. The placenta and membranes should be inspected, and an autopsy and chromosomal analysis should be completed on the fetus.

The Grieving Process

Grief is the response to loss of someone or something; everyone grieves differently. The grief process is highly personal; there is no specific timeline for mourning and healing. The couple who suffer a perinatal loss will likely grieve in different ways because men and women typically have different patterns of managing grief. Family and friends may not understand the intensity of the grief and the behavior of the parents while they work through their grief.

It is common for parents and families who suffer a pregnancy loss to experience a range of emotions:

- *Denial:* The woman and her family may express disbelief and be unable to grasp the reality of the circumstances. The parents may react with numbness and an inability to acknowledge the death or impending death of their baby. In the event of fetal demise, the mother may request repeated confirmation of an absence of FHR or may question the nurse's or health-care provider's accuracy or skill in assessment. Denial will diminish as the parents slowly acknowledge the loss.
- *Guilt:* The woman may wonder if she did anything to cause the fetal death. She may review her pregnancy in her mind, searching for the possible cause with which to blame herself. The parents may become preoccupied with identifying activities or choices that could have contributed to the death. The mother may feel as if her body failed her. Self-blame may prolong the grieving process, especially if the mother was ambivalent about the pregnancy (Farrales et al., 2020).
- *Anger:* The parents may experience anger toward each other, the health-care provider, the nurses, or a higher power. They may feel resentful about the unfairness of their loss.
- *Depression:* The parents may experience loss of sleep, appetite disturbances, loss of energy, or crying spells and may be unable to concentrate. During a depressive state,

the parents lack joy in any pleasure of life and may feel lonely and empty. These are normal feelings; and, for many people who are grieving, this phase must occur before acceptance and adjustment can begin.
- *Acceptance:* When the parents and family accept the loss as a part of their lives, healing occurs. They are then able to function normally and experience joy in life's events. Even when they have achieved acceptance, individuals will typically return to earlier feelings for a short time throughout their own lifetime. Those feelings will be triggered by holidays such as Mother's Day or Father's Day, the date the fetus was due or died, or observing families with babies.

Nursing Care for the Family Experiencing Perinatal Loss

Support provided by nurses can have a positive effect on the long-term adjustment of couples coping with perinatal loss (Farrales et al., 2020). Interventions vary, depending upon the gestational age at the time of loss. Cultural needs should be considered in planning nursing interventions for the family. Nurses can assist parents who experience a stillbirth or newborn death while in the hospital by doing the following:

- Providing privacy
- Acknowledging the family's grief
- Providing a quiet environment by minimizing interruptions and turning off alarms and monitors if possible
- Assisting the family with contacting funeral homes
- Remaining present with nonverbal behaviors that communicate that you are willing to sit, listen, and support the patient and her family
- Honoring cultural beliefs and rituals
- Facilitating spiritual support if requested by the family
- Allowing the family members to gather significant others such as grandparents and siblings
- Cleaning, dressing, and wrapping the baby in a clean blanket or allowing the parents to care for the baby
- Allowing the family to hold the infant as long as needed
  - Touching and holding the baby assist the parents to create memories, which facilitate the grief process (Fernández-Férez et al., 2021).
- Providing a Cuddle Cot®. This cooling pad slows deterioration of the infant's body and allows the parents to keep the baby with them longer before transferring the baby to the morgue or funeral home.
- Encouraging the family to talk about their experience
- Connecting the family to a social worker, grief counselor, or support group before discharge
- Creating a memory package for the parents:
  - A lock of the baby's hair
  - A photo
  - ID bracelets
  - Footprints and/or handprints
- Providing information regarding grief support, such as community support groups, for after the mother leaves the hospital

Nursing Care Plan for the Woman With a Labor Complication

Deepa is at 30 weeks' gestation and has arrived in the labor and delivery unit after her routine prenatal visit at the clinic. She states that she has been having cramping pains for several hours. At the clinic, the health-care provider determined that Deepa may be starting preterm labor and advised her to go directly to the hospital for evaluation in labor and delivery. She is waiting for her partner to arrive. As you assist her into bed, Deepa expresses fear and anxiety about the situation.

Nursing Diagnosis: Fear because of uncertainty about the pregnancy outcome
Expected Outcome: The patient will verbalize that her fear is under control.

Interventions:	Rationale:
Allow the woman to verbalize fears and anxiety.	*Discussing the patient's fears gives you the opportunity to answer questions honestly without minimizing those fears.*
Provide a quiet environment and give full attention to her concerns.	*A quiet environment is calming to the patient.*
Encourage the participation of the woman's spouse or partner in providing care.	*The spouse or partner can provide ongoing emotional support to the patient.*

Nursing Diagnosis: Anxiety because of unfamiliar medical procedures
Expected Outcome: The patient will verbalize that her anxiety has reduced regarding procedures.

Interventions:	Rationale:
Ask her what is helpful to her in managing anxiety.	*This provides patient-centered care.*
Monitor vital signs and report abnormalities.	*Elevated heart rate, blood pressure, and respirations are physical signs of anxiety.*
Promote relaxation with music, lighting, and massage.	*Music, low lights, and massage can relax patients and reduce anxiety.*
Explain any procedures in simple, nonmedical terminology.	*Understandable explanations of the procedure will reduce the fear of the unknown.*
Provide written and verbal information regarding the procedure.	

Team Works

Teamwork is important when assisting a family to cope with perinatal loss. In addition to the nurses and health-care provider providing direct care to the grieving family, other health-care team members should be included in the plan of care. A pastor or spiritual leader, grief counselor, and social worker should be invited to participate in caring for the grieving family.

Therapeutic Communication

A Grieving Family

- Allow the family to express their feelings without judgment.
- Listen to the patient and family. They need to talk about their loss and the emotions that accompany that loss.
- Be patient.
- Do not use medical terms such as *products of conception, dead fetus,* or *stillbirth.* These terms do not describe the "baby" or the human experience of the parents.
- Ask the parents if they had chosen a name for the baby and use that name when talking about the baby.

Therapeutic Communication:

- "I am so sorry."
- "Your baby is beautiful." (If true and appropriate for the circumstance of the loss)
- "This is not what you expected . . ."
- "Is there someone you would like me to call for you?"

Nontherapeutic Communication:

- "It was for the best."
- "It was God's will."
- "In time you will forget."

Key Points

- Preterm labor that is diagnosed early can be managed with medical and nursing care to prevent preterm birth and possible perinatal loss.
- Nursing care for the preterm labor patient includes monitoring of contractions and the fetus, bedrest, administration of tocolytic medications, hydration, and corticosteroids to accelerate fetal lung maturity.
- The most serious complication of premature rupture of the membranes is chorioamnionitis.
- Postterm pregnancy is linked to increased fetal mortality and an increase in cesarean deliveries.
- Abnormal amniotic fluid volume is usually first noticed by alterations in fundal height during the pregnancy. Polyhydramnios and oligohydramnios are both associated with possible fetal anomalies of the lung, kidney, and GI tract.
- Dysfunctional labor can usually be attributed to one of the Seven Ps of labor: passage, passenger, powers, position, psyche, pain management, or patience.
- Breech presentations increase the risk for umbilical cord prolapse and difficulty delivering the fetal head. Most breech presentations are delivered via cesarean birth.
- A prolapsed umbilical cord is an emergency because of the risk of fetal hypoxia.
- A precipitous labor occurs with fewer than 3 hours of labor and a rapid spontaneous delivery of the infant.

- A precipitous labor can result in vaginal, cervical, and perineal lacerations for the mother and intracranial hemorrhage and amniotic fluid aspiration for the newborn.
- Shoulder dystocia is a complication that occurs when the fetal shoulders are wedged in the pelvis after the delivery of the head. You may assist the health-care provider with maneuvers to produce delivery of the shoulders.
- Women with previous cesarean delivery, abdominal trauma, or closely spaced births are more at risk for uterine rupture. Uterine rupture is the nonsurgical opening of the uterus.
- Uterine inversion is a rare complication in which the uterus inverts and the fundus prolapses through the dilated cervix.
- A placenta that is not delivered within 30 minutes of the birth is a retained placenta. A retained placenta can lead to hemorrhage and infection.
- AFE is a rare emergency with a high mortality rate. The early signs of AFE are dyspnea, hypotension, altered mental status, and cyanosis. AFE can quickly progress to seizures, hemorrhage, and cardiac arrest.
- Fetal demise is a death of the fetus at any stage of pregnancy. Nurses can assist the family in coping with the traumatic and devastating loss. The family will experience a range of emotions as they work through the grieving process.

Review Questions

1. Which of the following are risk factors for preterm labor? **(Select all that apply.)**
   1. Multiple gestation
   2. Urinary tract infection
   3. Rh-negative mother
   4. Bacterial vaginosis
   5. A previous spontaneous abortion (miscarriage)

2. A patient at 37 weeks' gestation is admitted to labor and delivery. Her membranes ruptured 12 hours ago at home. The monitor indicates that the FHR is 150 bpm with moderate variability, no variable or late decelerations, and no uterine contractions. The patient asks you, "Why can't I stay at home until my labor begins?" What is your best reply?
   1. "It looks like the baby may be experiencing some distress."
   2. "We want to monitor you for signs of infection."
   3. "Your doctor wants you here."
   4. "We can keep you comfortable until labor starts."

3. Which of the following statements regarding oligohydramnios is true?
   1. There will be at least 1,500 mL of amniotic fluid.
   2. Throughout the pregnancy, the placenta is the chief source of amniotic fluid.
   3. The patient may experience a postterm pregnancy.
   4. The fetus may be small for gestational age.

4. Nursing care for a patient with PROM includes which of the following? **(Select all that apply.)**
   1. Monitoring FHR and contractions
   2. Frequent vaginal cervical examinations
   3. Administration of antibiotics if ordered
   4. Monitoring the patient's vital signs
   5. Placing the patient in the knee–chest position

5. Which of the following are signs of an imminent precipitous delivery? **(Select all that apply.)**
   1. A bulging perineum
   2. The mother stating a desire to push
   3. Nausea and vomiting
   4. Increase in bloody show and mucus
   5. Contractions that are 3 minutes apart and strong

6. Which pregnant patient is at greatest risk for macrosomia?
   1. The primigravida woman who has diabetes
   2. The multigravida woman who is Rh-negative
   3. The primigravida woman who abuses alcohol
   4. The multigravida woman who works as a hairstylist

7. After a patient's membranes rupture, you perform a vaginal examination and notice that the umbilical cord has fallen through the cervix into the vagina. Which of the following should you do? **(Select all that apply.)**
   1. Manually elevate the fetal head off the cord.
   2. Leave the patient and immediately call the doctor.
   3. Place the patient in the knee–chest position.
   4. Ask the woman to empty her bladder.
   5. Apply oxygen via face mask.

8. Which of the following patients is at highest risk for uterine rupture?
   1. A 15-year-old primigravida woman with a large fetus
   2. A multigravida woman scheduled for her fourth cesarean birth
   3. A primigravida woman pregnant with triplets
   4. A multigravida woman delivering her second child in 2 years

9. You suspect that the patient may be developing an infection called chorioamnionitis. Which of the following could be the cause of this infection?
   1. The patient is a poorly controlled diabetic.
   2. The patient's membranes ruptured 3 days ago.
   3. The patient has been using cocaine during the pregnancy.
   4. The patient is at 42 weeks' gestation.

10. A dysfunctional or abnormally slow progress in labor may be caused by which of the following? **(Select all that apply.)**
    1. A narrow pelvis
    2. A premature fetus
    3. A morbidly obese patient
    4. A brow presentation of the fetus
    5. Narcotic pain medication

ANSWERS 1. 1, 2, 4; 2. 3, 4; 4. 1, 3, 4; 5. 1, 2, 4; 6. 1; 7. 1, 3, 5; 8. 2; 9. 2; 10. 1, 3, 4, 5

CRITICAL THINKING QUESTIONS

1. A woman at 32 weeks' gestation is in preterm labor. Efforts to slow labor have failed, and significant cervical dilation has occurred. The woman states, "What is happening? I don't understand labor. I was supposed to start childbirth classes tonight!" Formulate a nursing plan for preparing this patient for labor.

2. Discuss the fetal and maternal risks associated with a postterm pregnancy.

Resources

For additional resources and information, including Postconference Questions and Activities, Answers, and References, visit www.FADavis.com.

Student Study Guide

CHAPTER 11
Birth-Related Procedures

KEY TERMS

augmentation (AWG-men-TAY-shun)
Bishop score (BISH-op SKOR)
collaboration (ko-LAB-uh-RAY-shun)
external cephalic version (eks-TER-nuhl se-FAL-ik VER-zhun)
forceps (FOR-seps)
labor induction (LAY-ber in-DUK-shun)
Pfannenstiel incision (FAN-en-steel in-SIH-zhun)
trial of labor after cesarean (TOLAC) (TRY-uhl uv LAY-ber AF-ter sih-ZA-ree-uhn)
vacuum extraction (VAK-yoom eks-TRAK-shun)
vaginal birth after cesarean (VBAC) (VAJ-in-uhl BERTH AF-ter sih-ZA-ree-uhn)

CHAPTER CONCEPTS

Collaboration
Professionalism
Stress and Coping

LEARNING OUTCOMES

1. Define the key terms.
2. Describe the amniotomy procedure and discuss nursing responsibilities.
3. Explain the purpose of an amnioinfusion.
4. Prepare patient teaching for the patient undergoing an external cephalic version.
5. Describe how a Bishop score is calculated and explain the significance of the score.
6. Discuss methods used to ripen a cervix and induce contractions.
7. Prepare a patient-centered nursing care plan for the woman undergoing labor induction or augmentation.
8. Differentiate between vacuum extractor–assisted and forceps-assisted vaginal delivery.
9. List common indications for a cesarean delivery.
10. Discuss nursing responsibilities when preparing a patient for a cesarean birth.
11. Plan patient teaching for a cesarean birth.
12. Identify the factors that indicate a patient is a good candidate for a VBAC.
13. Plan nursing care for the patient undergoing a TOLAC.

CRITICAL THINKING & CLINICAL JUDGMENT

Wendy is a gravida 2, para 1 at 41 weeks' gestation. Wendy is obese and has gestational diabetes that is controlled with medication. She is at the clinic today and her health-care provider performs a vaginal cervical examination and calculates a Bishop score. Wendy is dilated 2 cm, and the cervix is soft, in a midposition, and 50% effaced. The fetal head is at 0 station. The health-care provider states that her Bishop score is 7. After discussion with Wendy, she is sent to the hospital for induction of labor with oxytocin. The health-care provider leaves the room and Wendy has questions about having her labor induced.

Continued

CRITICAL THINKING & CLINICAL JUDGMENT—cont'd

Questions

1. Based upon the information provided about Wendy, do you think induction of labor is appropriate for her?
2. Wendy says, "I was so nervous when induction was mentioned, and I can't remember everything. Would you explain to me again how my labor is going to be induced in the hospital?" How can you explain labor induction to Wendy?

CONCEPTUAL CORNERSTONE

Stress and Coping

Stress is a natural reaction that arises to entering a different environment, such as an operating room for a cesarean delivery. The patient's stress response can lead to vasoconstriction of the uterine arteries and fetal distress. Preoperative medications that may be given before other surgeries are not an option for the pregnant patient because of the effects of sedatives on the respiratory effort of the newborn. A nurse can assist the patient to manage stress by clearly explaining the operative process, staying with the patient as much as possible, and allowing the support person to join the patient in the operating room as quickly as possible.

CONCEPTUAL CORNERSTONE

Collaboration

The word **collaboration** means "to work together." True collaboration involves working across professional boundaries. Obstetric nurses work together with obstetricians, nurse midwives, obstetrical technicians, anesthesiologists, neonatologists, pharmacists, social workers, and patients to restore and maintain health. The nurse respectfully values the expertise of each member of the team because their common goal is a safe birthing experience for the mother and baby. Communication is a core aspect of collaboration. Individuals in the health-care team and their patients come from diverse backgrounds; therefore, the professionals all need openness and clear communication skills for collaboration to occur and to assist the patient to make informed decisions regarding her care. The health-care team that empowers its members to listen actively and to share opinions freely will promote safety, patient-centered care, and an improvement in the quality of health care (Giddens, 2021).

The nurse caring for a patient in labor and delivery may be assisting with or performing various procedures to promote a safe labor and delivery. Before, during, and after the procedure, you will need to be alert for possible complications and be prepared to provide safe and effective nursing care for the patient. Therapeutic procedures covered in this chapter include amniotomy, amnioinfusion, external cephalic version, induction/augmentation of labor, cervical ripening, vacuum-assisted delivery, forceps-assisted delivery, cesarean birth, and vaginal birth after cesarean (VBAC).

AMNIOTOMY

Amniotomy is the artificial rupture of the amniotic membranes (AROM). In the term patient, amniotomy usually stimulates labor or starts labor within 12 hours after rupture of the membranes (O'Connell, 2021). AROM may be indicated if labor is progressing slowly. Once the cushion of amniotic fluid is gone, the fetal head will press directly on the cervix, causing faster effacement and dilation and promoting labor progress.

Amniotomy is considered by many health professionals to be safe and harmless. However, it should not be attempted when the fetal head is not engaged in the pelvis or if the fetus is in a breech presentation because of the risk of umbilical cord prolapse when the amniotic fluid flows out of the uterus. In addition, women with prolonged time between rupture of membranes and delivery are at increased risk of infection.

The health-care provider uses a disposable plastic hook (amniohook) to break the amniotic sac (Fig. 11.1) and then performs a vaginal examination to determine cervical dilation, effacement, fetal station, and fetal presentation.

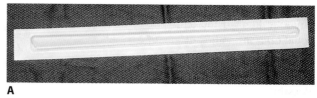

A

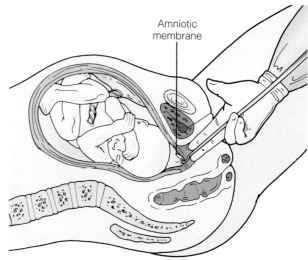

Amniotic membrane

B

FIGURE 11.1 An amniohook (A) is used to rupture the membranes in an amniotomy (B).

Nursing Care

Nursing care for a patient receiving an amniotomy includes the following:

- Explaining the procedure in nonmedical terms to the patient and her support person
- Providing sterile gloves, sterile lubricant, and a sterile amniohook to the health-care provider
- Placing disposable pads underneath the patient to absorb the fluid
- Monitoring the fetal heart rate (FHR) and pattern for 1 full minute after membranes rupture
- Notifying the health-care provider of any abnormal or nonreassuring FHR patterns
- Documenting the time of the amniotomy and the color, quantity, and odor of the amniotic fluid
- Changing the pads regularly as they become saturated
- Monitoring the woman's temperature every 2 hours and reporting elevations greater than 38°C (100.4°F) to the health-care provider

AMNIOINFUSION

Amnioinfusion is the procedure of infusing 0.9% normal saline into the uterus through a catheter placed through the cervix into the amniotic cavity. Amnioinfusion is done to relieve cord compression or to add fluid because of oligohydramnios (see Chapter 10).

Amnioinfusion may also be used to dilute meconium-stained fluid, which occurs when the fetus experiences hypoxia and releases the contents of its intestinal tract into the amniotic fluid. If the fetus inhales the meconium fluid, it could cause aspiration pneumonia (Goldfarb, 2022).

Possible Complications

Possible complications of amnioinfusion include the following:

- Overfilling the uterus, causing high intrauterine pressure
- Prolapsed cord
- Placenta abruptio
- Uterine infection
- Uterine rupture
- Maternal chilling, if cold solution is used
- Fetal bradycardia, if cold solution is used
- Fetal tachycardia, if hot solution is used

Nursing Care

The nursing care for a patient undergoing an amnioinfusion procedure includes the following:

- Explain the procedure in nonmedical terms to the patient and her support person.
- Place disposable pads underneath the patient to absorb fluid.
- Connect the IV solution to IV tubing and flush.

- If the fetus is preterm, warm the solution with an infusion warmer before and during the infusion. For term pregnancies, room temperature solution is acceptable.
- Assist the health-care provider to insert the intrauterine pressure catheter (IUPC).
- After insertion, note uterine resting tone with the patient on her left side, right side, and back. Record the findings.
- Attach the IV tubing to the amnioport on the IUPC. Bolus with 250 to 500 mL as ordered by the health-care provider.
- Place the tubing in the infusion pump and set at the ordered rate. Commonly, the maintenance rate is from 100 to 150 mL/hour (Goldfarb, 2022).
- Document the procedure in the medical record.
- Check and record uterine resting tone every 30 minutes. A resting baseline of fewer than 25 mm Hg should be maintained (Landon, 2020).
- Monitor the FHR pattern and notify the health-care provider of any nonreassuring patterns.
- Observe and record the amount, color, and odor of fluid on the patient's underpad every 30 minutes.
- Discontinue infusion before delivery.

EXTERNAL CEPHALIC VERSION

An **external cephalic version** is the attempt by the health-care provider to move a malpositioned fetus, such as a breech or transverse lie, into a vertex cephalic presentation after 37 weeks' gestation. The health-care provider manipulates through the abdominal wall to reposition the fetus. See Box 11.1 for contraindications for an external cephalic version.

Fetal position will first be confirmed with ultrasound imagery. The health-care provider will locate the umbilical cord, determine the placental location and the amount of amniotic fluid, evaluate the fetal age, and check for any fetal anomalies. External fetal monitoring is conducted to confirm a healthy FHR pattern.

Box 11.1

Contraindications for an External Cephalic Version

- Uterine abnormalities
- Multiple gestation
- Oligohydramnios
- Previous cesarean birth if a classic incision was performed
- Cephalopelvic disproportion
- Nonreassuring FHR
- Hyperextended neck in the fetus
- Placenta previa
- Maternal obesity
- Severe preeclampsia

Sources: Hofmeyr, G. J. (2022). External cephalic version. *UpToDate.* https://www.uptodate.com/contents/external-cephalic-version; Layden, A., Thompson, A., Owen, P., Madhra, M., & Magowan, B. A. (2023). *Clinical obstetrics and gynecology.* Elsevier.

Next, tocolytic medications are administered to relax the uterus. Once the uterus is relaxed, the health-care provider will use two hands on the surface of the abdomen. One hand is placed on the fetal head, and the other is placed on the fetal buttocks (Fig. 11.2). The health-care provider will push and roll the fetus into a head-down position (Layden et al., 2023).

External cephalic version has a success rate of 58%. It is more likely to be successful if the mother has had at least one pregnancy and childbirth, there is normal amniotic fluid volume, and the procedure is done after 36 weeks and before labor begins (Hofmeyr, 2022). If the first attempt is not successful, a second attempt with epidural anesthesia to improve uterine relaxation and reduce pain may be scheduled.

Risks and Complications

Potential risks or complications of an external cephalic version include the following:

- Twisting of the umbilical cord, causing decreased oxygenation to the fetus
- Rupture of amniotic membranes, causing the onset of labor
- Placenta abruptio
- Rupture of the uterus
- Bleeding that could lead to a mixing of maternal and fetal blood

Nursing Care Before and During the Procedure

Nursing care for the patient undergoing an external cephalic version includes the following:

- Obtaining informed consent from the patient
- Providing emotional support and answering patient questions

- Confirming that RhoGAM was given at 28 weeks' gestation to prevent isoimmunization if the patient is Rh-negative
- Performing a nonstress test (NST) to evaluate the fetus
- Administering IV tocolytics to relax the uterus
- Continuously monitoring FHR patterns
- Monitoring maternal vital signs and pain

CRITICAL THINKING

You are assisting the health-care provider during a cephalic version. The patient is placed in a supine position for this procedure, which can take several minutes.

Question

1. What do you need to think about during this procedure?

Nursing Care After the Procedure

After the procedure, the patient should be observed and the fetus monitored for at least 1 hour. Labor may be induced, or the patient may be discharged to wait for spontaneous labor to begin. Nursing care after the external version includes the following:

- Performing an NST on the fetus
- Monitoring for contraction frequency, duration, and intensity
- Monitoring for a decrease in fetal activity
- Monitoring the FHR for abnormalities

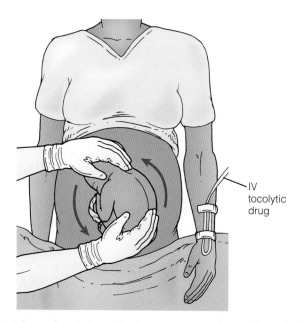
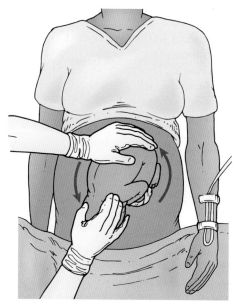

IV tocolytic drug

FIGURE 11.2 External cephalic version is a maneuver performed through the maternal abdominal wall in an attempt to change the fetal position from a breech to a cephalic presentation.

- Monitoring for rupture of amniotic membranes
- Evaluating for pain and discomfort
  - Notify the health-care provider if the patient reports increased abdominal pain; this could be a sign of a placenta abruptio because any abdominal pain should diminish after the procedure.
- For Rh-negative patients, obtaining an order for a Kleihauer-Betke test to detect the presence of fetal blood in the circulation
  - Administer RhoGAM if more than 15 mL of fetal blood is present to suppress the patient's immune response.
- Reviewing signs of labor and ruptured membranes, including guidelines for returning to the hospital, before discharging the patient
- Providing information to the patient to promote safety and health for the patient and her fetus if the patient does not remain in the hospital

Teaching points should include the following:

- An external version is not always successful; sometimes the fetus returns to its original position.
- If vaginal bleeding begins or fetal movement decreases, contact the health-care provider immediately.
- An external version may stimulate labor or rupture membranes.
- If contractions begin, time them from the beginning of one contraction to the beginning of the next (see Chapter 9). If they become regular for an hour, contact the health-care provider.
- Signs of ruptured membranes include either a sudden gush or a slow leak of fluid from the vagina.

Labs & Diagnostics

Kleihauer-Betke Test

The Kleihauer-Betke test is a blood test that measures the amount of fetal hemoglobin in the mother's bloodstream. This test is usually ordered for Rh-negative mothers who have suffered a traumatic injury or procedure that could cause bleeding. Normal values are fewer than 1% of fetal cells present. If more than 15 mL of fetal blood is detected, RhoGAM is usually administered to the patient (Van Leeuwen & Bladh, 2021).

CARE OF THE WOMAN UNDERGOING INDUCTION OR THE AUGMENTATION OF LABOR

Induction and augmentation of labor use artificial methods to stimulate uterine contractions. The process of **labor induction** uses chemical or mechanical methods to start cervical effacement, dilation, and contractions. **Augmentation** of labor is needed if labor has begun but the contractions are ineffective in producing dilation and labor progression.

Indications

Indications for the induction of labor include the following:

- Postterm pregnancy
- Prolonged rupture of membranes
- Pregnancy-induced hypertension (PIH)
- Diabetes
- Chorioamnionitis
- Fetal demise
- Hypotonic contractions that do not produce dilation and labor progression
  (Gill et al., 2022)

Labor cannot be successfully induced if the cervix is not ready or "ripe" enough to respond. The **Bishop score**, a tool used by many health-care providers to evaluate cervical ripening, is predictive of readiness for the induction of labor (American College of Obstetricians and Gynecologists [ACOG], 2022). The score is based upon the findings of a cervical examination. Points are given for cervical dilation, cervical effacement, station of the fetus, consistency (soft to firm), and position of the cervix. A Bishop score of 5 or more is significant for successful induction of labor. Table 11.1 provides details for calculating the Bishop score.

Table 11.1
Calculating the Bishop Score

Criteria	Score
Dilation of the cervix	• 0 cm = 0 points • 1–2 cm = 1 point • 3–4 cm = 2 points • 5–6 cm = 3 points
Effacement of the cervix	• 0%–30% = 0 points • 40%–50% = 1 point • 60%–70% = 2 points • 80%+ = 3 points
Station of the fetal head	• –3 = 0 points • –2 = 1 point • –1 and 0 = 2 points • +1 and +2 = 3 points
Consistency of the cervix tissue	• Firm = 0 points • Medium = 1 point • Soft = 2 points
Position of the cervix	• Posterior position = 0 points • Midposition = 1 point • Anterior position = 2 points

Cervical Ripening

Cervical ripening, the softening of the cervix before the onset of labor, is necessary for dilation and birth. The softening is caused by physiological changes to the collagen fibers caused by enzymes and hormones. Cervical ripening by mechanical or chemical means are methods of inducing labor.

Contraindications

Contraindications to cervical ripening include the following:

- Fetal malpresentation, such as breech or transverse lie
- Active herpes infection
- Regular uterine contractions
- Nonreassuring FHR pattern
- Placenta previa
- Unexplained uterine bleeding
- Previous cesarean delivery
  (Wheeler et al., 2022)

Foley Catheter

The most commonly used mechanical method of cervical ripening and inducing labor is the use of a Foley balloon catheter. This is a safe and cost-effective method of cervical ripening; most women deliver within 24 hours of the insertion of a Foley balloon. Using aseptic technique, the health-care provider inserts a 16F transcervical Foley catheter balloon to or past the internal os of the cervix. The balloon is filled with 30 to 50 mL of sterile water or saline. Gentle traction is applied, and the catheter is taped to the inner thigh. The direct pressure of the balloon on the lower uterine segment tissues causes the release of prostaglandins that result in cervical softening (Layden et al., 2023).

Hygroscopic Dilators

Hygroscopic dilators dilate the cervix by expanding after absorbing fluids from body tissues and causing an outward force to open the cervix. Several dilators are placed in the cervix, and they expand over 12 to 24 hours, producing effects similar to those of the Foley balloon.

COMPLICATIONS. Complications of a transcervical Foley catheter and hygroscopic dilators for cervical ripening and labor induction are rare. Reported complications have included infection, vaginal bleeding, fever, nonreassuring FHR pattern, and pain (Wheeler et al., 2022).

NURSING CARE. Nursing care of the patient undergoing cervical ripening with a transcervical Foley catheter or hygroscopic dilators includes the following:

- Explaining the procedure in nonmedical terms to the patient and her support person
- Assisting the health-care provider with insertion of the Foley catheter or the dilators

- Monitoring the patient's vital signs and the FHR pattern as ordered by the health-care provider or hospital policy; reporting any abnormalities immediately to the health-care provider

Prostaglandin Gel

The chemical method of cervical ripening involves applying prostaglandin gel around the cervix. This method is as effective as mechanical methods of cervical ripening and labor induction. Prostaglandin gel works on the fibers of the cervix to relax, soften, and dilate it. The gel also increases intracellular calcium levels, causing contraction of the uterine muscle.

The room temperature gel is placed in and around the cervix with an applicator. The patient should remain in the lateral recumbent position for 15 to 30 minutes after insertion of the gel to prevent leakage from the vagina.

Medication Facts

Prostaglandin E1 analog (misoprostol) is a synthetic prostaglandin that can be used for cervical ripening. One quarter of a tablet (25 mcg) can be crushed and placed on the cervix. This medication can be repeated every 4 hours (Wheeler et al., 2022).

SIDE EFFECTS AND COMPLICATIONS. Side effects and complications of prostaglandin gel include the following:

- Fever
- Nausea and vomiting
- Headache
- Diarrhea
- **Tachysystole** (uterine hyperstimulation), which is five or more uterine contractions in 10 minutes (Fig. 11.3)
- FHR decelerations in response to the tachysystole

NURSING CARE. Nursing care for the patient receiving prostaglandin gel for cervical ripening and labor induction includes the following:

- Obtaining a baseline FHR pattern and uterine contraction activity before insertion
- Obtaining baseline maternal vital signs before insertion
- Informing the patient that she will need to lie on her side for 15 to 30 minutes after the insertion to prevent leakage of the gel and that she may notice a feeling of warmth in her vagina
- Monitoring the FHR pattern, uterine contractions, and maternal vital signs every 30 minutes
- Obtaining orders for medication to control nausea and vomiting if occurring

---

• WORD • BUILDING •
hygroscopic: hygro–wet + scop–examine + ic–pertaining to

• WORD • BUILDING •
tachysystole: tachy–rapid + systole–contraction

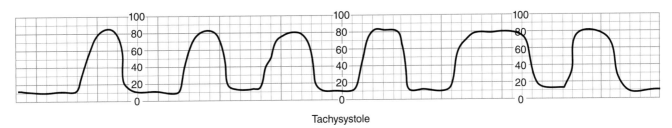

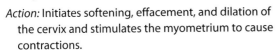

FIGURE 11.3 Uterine tachysystole.

- Providing comfort measures and emotional support to the patient and her support person
- Repeating the dose in 6 hours if no uterine or cervical response occurs

Medication Facts

Dinoprostone

Action: Initiates softening, effacement, and dilation of the cervix and stimulates the myometrium to cause contractions.

Dose: 0.5 mg (contents of preloaded syringe) inserted around and in the cervical os. The dose may be repeated 6 hours later if needed. The maximum dose is 1.5 mg per 24 hours.

Oxytocin Infusion

Oxytocin infusion is a chemical method of inducing labor. Nursing care for the patient with an oxytocin infusion involves close monitoring and a thorough understanding of the procedure of infusing IV oxytocin to ensure a safe labor induction or augmentation of labor. Oxytocin may also be administered to augment labor if contractions are not strong enough to dilate the cervix. Oxytocin improves the strength of the contractions and helps labor to progress. The oxytocin is diluted in 1,000 mL of lactated Ringer's solution or normal saline and infused by IV with a pump to control the rate.

NURSING CARE. Nursing care of the patient receiving oxytocin includes the following:

- Obtaining a Bishop score rating before starting oxytocin infusion
- Connecting the oxytocin intermittent infusion to the main IV line and administering it via an infusion pump
- Monitoring maternal blood pressure, pulse, and respirations every 30 minutes and every time an increase in dosage occurs
- Monitoring the FHR and contraction patterns every 15 minutes and every time the dose is increased
- Increasing oxytocin as prescribed and then maintaining the dose if there is:

- Reassuring FHR between 110 and 160 bpm
- Cervical dilation of 1 cm/hour
- Contraction frequency of every 2 to 3 minutes
- Contraction duration of 60 to 90 seconds
- Contraction intensity of 40 to 90 mm Hg (if an IUPC is inserted)
- Uterine resting tone of 10 to 15 mm Hg (if an IUPC is inserted)

Safe and Effective Nursing Care

When a patient is receiving oxytocin, you need to closely monitor the contractions and fetal well-being. Hyperstimulation of the uterus can be unsafe for both mother and fetus. Oxytocin should be immediately discontinued if hyperstimulation of the uterus occurs, and the health-care provider must be notified. The following are signs of uterine hyperstimulation:

- Contractions that occur more frequently than every 2 minutes
- Contractions that last longer than 90 seconds
- Contraction intensity greater than 90 mm Hg as shown by IUPC
- Uterine resting tone over 20 mm Hg between contractions as shown by IUPC
- No relaxation of the uterus between contractions
- A nonreassuring FHR pattern

Medication Facts

Oxytocin

Oxytocin acts on the uterine fibers to produce contractions. For labor induction, the recommended dose is 1 to 2 milliunits/minute, increased by 1 to 2 milliunits every 15 to 60 minutes until an effective labor pattern is established. Oxytocin has a short half-life of 3 to 12 minutes; therefore, when the medication dosage is reduced or stopped, uterine contractions very quickly reduce in strength, duration, and frequency (Wheeler et al., 2022).

ASSISTED VAGINAL BIRTH

The term *assisted vaginal birth* refers to the use of instruments, such as vacuum extraction or forceps, to expedite a vaginal delivery. There is controversy among health-care providers regarding if and when assisted vaginal deliveries should be performed and which instrument is the best to use (Garrison, 2022). Vacuum extractor delivery and forceps delivery are used in modern obstetric management for approximately 5% of vaginal deliveries (Ross, 2020). However, the vacuum extractor is preferred by most practitioners.

Indications and Prerequisites

Indications for assisted vaginal delivery include the following:

- Maternal exhaustion
- Inadequate maternal pushing efforts, such as those caused by a spinal cord injury or neuromuscular disease
- Fetal distress or a nonreassuring FHR pattern
- A prolonged second stage of labor

Prerequisites for an assisted delivery include the following:

- The fetal head must be engaged and the position known to the practitioner to promote safe placement of the forceps or cup device.
- The cervix must be fully dilated.
- Amniotic membranes must be ruptured.
- The pelvis must be an adequate size for delivery.
- The patient must have adequate analgesia to manage the discomfort of the procedure.
- The patient must be in the lithotomy position.
- The patient's bladder should be empty to allow more room for application of the device.
- Verbal consent, if possible, should be obtained from the patient (Garrison, 2022).

Vacuum Extraction–Assisted Birth

A **vacuum extraction**–assisted delivery involves the use of a cuplike device that attaches to the fetal head with suction. The cup is lubricated with sterile lubricant or surgical soap, the labia are spread, and the cup is attached to the fetal head. Vacuum suction at 450 to 600 mm Hg is applied, and the health-care provider applies traction to assist with delivery of the fetal head. Traction is timed with uterine contractions, and the patient assists by pushing during the contraction (Fig. 11.4; Garrison, 2022).

Safety *Stat!*

When using a vacuum extraction device, you and the health-care provider must follow the manufacturer's instructions and hospital policy on the amount of suction pressure to be used for the extraction to avoid injury to the fetus or patient.

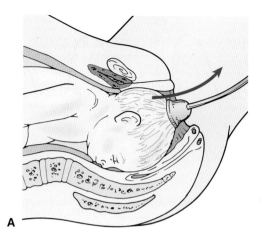

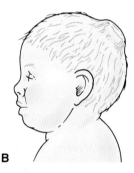

FIGURE 11.4 Vacuum extraction facilitates the delivery of the fetal head and is associated with fewer lacerations of the maternal birth canal. A, The vacuum extractor is applied with a downward and outward traction. B, A caput succedaneum is formed from the suction cup.

Possible Complications

Possible complications that can occur with a vacuum-assisted birth include the following:

- Fetal scalp bruising and lacerations
- Fetal scalp injuries that cause either a cephalohematoma or, rarely, a hematoma. (See Chapter 15 for more about cephalohematoma.)
- Maternal lacerations of the cervix, vagina, or perineum (Layden et al., 2023)

Nursing Care

Nursing care for the patient undergoing vacuum-assisted delivery includes the following:

- Explaining the procedure in nonmedical language to the patient and her support person
- Assisting the health-care provider by setting up the vacuum extraction device correctly and according to manufacturer instructions and hospital policies
- Assisting the patient into the lithotomy position
- Palpating for bladder distention and catheterizing if needed; a full bladder can hold back fetal descent
- Monitoring FHR before and during the procedure
- Observing the newborn for any signs of complications

Forceps-Assisted Birth

A **forceps**-assisted delivery involves the use of a metal instrument that has two curved spoonlike blades with locking handles that fit on either side of the fetal head and assist with delivery of the head. The health-care provider applies the blades to each side of the fetal head and then gently applies traction during contractions (Fig. 11.5).

Possible Complications

Possible complications of a forceps-assisted delivery include the following:

- Lacerations of the vagina and perineum, with an increased risk of incontinence of flatus and feces (Ross, 2020)
- An increase in pelvic floor disorders such as bladder and rectal prolapse (Layden et al., 2023)
- Bruising of the fetal head
- Brachial plexus injury and facial nerve injury to the fetus. (See Chapter 17 for more about brachial plexus injury.)

Nursing Care

Nursing care for the patient undergoing a forceps-assisted birth includes the following:

- Explaining the procedure in nonmedical language to the patient and her support person
- Providing the health-care provider with the requested forceps
- Assisting the patient into the lithotomy position
- Palpating for bladder distention and catheterizing if needed; a full bladder can hold back fetal descent
- Monitoring the FHR before and during the procedure:
  - Observing for decelerating FHR occurring from compression of the cord between the fetal head and forceps
  - Notifying the health-care provider to remove the forceps if variable decelerations or bradycardia occurs
- Observing the newborn for bruising and abrasions at the site of forceps application
- Monitoring the woman postpartum for possible lacerations of the cervix, vagina, and perineum

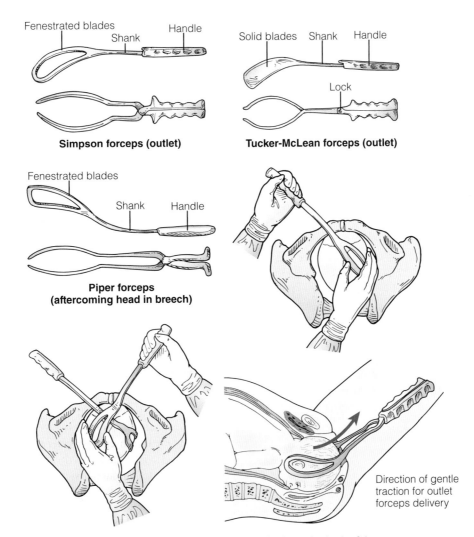

FIGURE 11.5 Forceps are instruments with curved blades that are used to facilitate the birth of the fetal head.

Nursing Care Plan for Induction of Labor

Monica is 20 years old. This is her first pregnancy and she is at 41 weeks' gestation. She is admitted to the labor and delivery department for induction of labor with oxytocin. She is accompanied by her boyfriend. They are anxious and have many questions about induction.

Nursing Diagnosis: Insufficient knowledge regarding induction of labor
Expected Outcome: The patient will verbalize understanding of the process of labor induction.

Interventions:	Rationale:
Explain the expected procedures of vaginal cervical examination, intravenous oxytocin to start labor, and fetal monitoring.	*The patient will understand the process and equipment in the room and know what to expect.*
Encourage questions from the patient and her support person.	*This intervention will allow Monica and her boyfriend to feel free to ask questions and helps to establish rapport with you.*

Nursing Diagnosis: Fear and anxiety because of having her labor induced
Expected Outcome: The patient will demonstrate and verbalize reduced anxiety regarding the induction of labor.

Interventions:	Rationale:
Determine Monica's psychological and emotional status.	*These interventions will decrease her anxiety by providing patient-centered care.*
Encourage verbalization of fears and feelings.	
Answer questions clearly and honestly.	
Provide opportunities for Monica to participate in decisions.	
Use therapeutic communication, verbally and nonverbally.	

Nursing Diagnosis: Risk for injury because of induction process
Expected Outcome: Develop and maintain a good labor pattern with contractions every 2 to 3 minutes, lasting 40 to 60 seconds, with uterine tone relaxing between contractions and the FHR pattern demonstrating a reassuring pattern.

Interventions:	Rationale:
Apply electronic fetal monitoring and obtain a 20-minute record of the FHR.	*This establishes a baseline and determines fetal well-being before beginning the induction of labor.*
Obtain baseline vital signs of the patient including temperature, pulse, respirations, and blood pressure.	*This establishes a baseline for comparison with subsequent vital signs.*
Continue to monitor the FHR and contraction pattern every 15 minutes while infusing oxytocin.	*This detects possible hyperstimulation of the uterus and prevents hypoxia and potential injury to the fetus.*
Monitor maternal vital signs every hour and monitor the maternal temperature every 2 hours.	*This detects early signs of infection.*

CESAREAN BIRTH

In 2020, the cesarean delivery rate in the United States was 31.8% of all births. This is only a small decline from 32.0% in 2017 (Centers for Disease Control and Prevention [CDC], 2022). Approximately 50% of cesarean births are repeat cesareans. Lowering the cesarean rate in the United States is a goal of *Healthy People 2030*.

Indications

A cesarean birth is usually performed when complications arise during labor in which a vaginal birth could compromise the health of the mother or fetus. Common indications for a cesarean birth are as follows:

- Labor dystocia
- Persistent nonreassuring FHR patterns
- Breech or transverse lie presentation
- Fetal macrosomia
- Cephalopelvic disproportion
- Occiput posterior and occiput transverse positions of the fetus
- Maternal obesity
- Multiple gestations
- Active genital herpes at the time of birth
- Prolapsed umbilical cord
- Placenta previa
- Placenta abruptio
  (Berghella, 2022)

Health Promotion

Preparing for a Scheduled Cesarean Birth

Women who have a scheduled cesarean birth can prepare for the birth by doing the following:

- Discussing the desired birth plan with the health-care provider, such as anesthesia, lighting, music, support person, skin-to-skin contact with the baby, and early breastfeeding
- Obtaining preoperative laboratory work
- Completing preregistration with the hospital
- Packing for 3 to 5 days in the hospital
- Arranging for help at home after discharge

The Procedure for a Cesarean Birth

After the decision has been made for a cesarean delivery, the patient will sign an operative consent agreeing to the surgical delivery. Some hospitals have an operating room for cesarean delivery within the labor and delivery department; other hospitals use the general hospital operating rooms. You will usually make the call to the operating room or notify the charge nurse of an impending cesarean delivery. The usual sequence of events for a cesarean delivery includes the following:

- The patient signs consent for a cesarean delivery.
- An indwelling catheter is inserted to keep the bladder empty and urine away from the surgical site. In most cases, this procedure is done in the labor and delivery department before moving the patient to the operating room.
- Preoperative medications may be ordered by the physician.
- An epidural or combined spinal-epidural (CSE) is administered, unless the birth is an emergency; in that case, general anesthesia may be the fastest option.
- After administration of the epidural, the support person is usually allowed to enter the operating room.

- The patient is positioned on her back with a wedge under the hip, tilting the uterus off the vena cava to prevent maternal hypotension and decreased placental perfusion.
- Intermittent monitoring of the fetal status is continued until the cesarean begins.
- The patient's lower abdominal hair near the incision site may be clipped.
- A grounding pad is placed on her thigh to prevent shock from the electrocautery used to manage bleeding during the procedure.
- A sterile abdominal prep to kill organisms that may cause infection will be done before application of the sterile drapes.
- Two incisions are made by the surgeon. In the abdominal wall, the surgeon may make a transverse incision (**Pfannenstiel incision**, also called a *bikini cut*) above the symphysis pubis. In the uterus, a low vertical incision is the most common location, unless the fetus is large or in distress, in which case the surgeon may opt for a midline incision. The uterus incision does not always match the skin incision. For example, a woman may have a transverse abdominal incision and a low vertical incision on the uterus (Fig. 11.6).
- After the incision, the amniotic fluid is suctioned out, and the baby is quickly removed from the uterus. Then, the newborn's airway is suctioned, and the umbilical cord is clamped and cut.
- If the mother is awake and the baby is stable, the baby is placed skin-to-skin with the mother. A nurse will monitor the baby's airway and transition on the mother's chest.
- The placenta will be removed and the incisions sutured.
- The patient will be transported to the recovery room for monitoring (Layden et al., 2023).

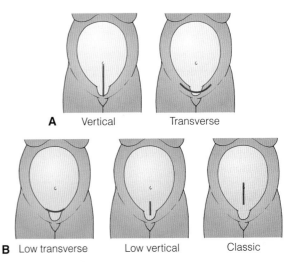

FIGURE 11.6 Abdominal and uterine incisions. A, Skin (abdominal wall) incisions. Vertical and transverse (Pfannenstiel incision). B, Uterine wall incisions: low transverse, low vertical, and classic.

- If the baby is unstable, to promote patient-centered care, you should encourage the mother to see and touch the newborn before the baby is taken from the operating room to the newborn nursery. As soon as the baby is stable, you should reunite the mother and baby in the recovery room for bonding and breastfeeding.

Safety *Stat!*

Most women who deliver by cesarean are given spinal or epidural anesthesia; however, be aware that general anesthesia may be required. Obtain a diet history for the previous 8 hours before delivery and report this information to the anesthesiologist to prevent aspiration during the procedure.

Risks

The risks and complications of a cesarean delivery may include the following:

- Hemorrhage
- Surgical wound infection
- Postoperative endometritis
- Anesthesia complications
- Venous thromboembolism
- Shock
- Cardiac arrest

Serious long-term risks are also associated with cesarean delivery:

- Placenta previa or accreta in future pregnancies
- Uterine rupture
  (Burke & Allen, 2020)

Nursing Care

Nursing care for the patient before a cesarean birth includes the following:

- Alerting the operating room team of an impending cesarean birth
- Obtaining the signed operative consent from the patient
- Monitoring the fetus throughout preparations for the operating room
- Providing emotional support to the patient and her support person
- Administering any ordered preoperative medications
- Inserting an indwelling urinary catheter
- Inserting an IV catheter of sufficient size to allow a blood transfusion, if required
- Preparing the support person for the operating room
  - If it is hospital policy, inform the support person that they are not allowed into the operating room until the epidural or spinal anesthesia is complete.

Evidence-Based Practice

Women with a negative birth experience can develop symptoms of posttraumatic stress disorder. In this study of first-time parents, emotional memories at 4 months postpartum were obtained from the mother and her birth father or partner. Symptoms of anxiety and depression were found in both the mother and the father/partner. When labor and delivery become complicated, possibly ending with an assisted birth or cesarean birth, the mother and the fetus are the focus of the medical and nursing care. The partner is frequently ignored because of the gravity of the situation. This study recommends that the partner be included and provided emotional support throughout labor and delivery in order to prevent anxiety and depression after the birth.

Hughes, C., Foley, S., Devine, R.T., Ribner, A., Kyriakou, L., Boddington, L., & Holmes, E. A. (2020). Worrying in the wings? Negative emotional birth memories in mothers and fathers show similar associations with perinatal mood disturbance and delivery mode. *Archives of Women's Mental Health, 23,* 371–377. https://doi.org/10.1007/s00737-019 -00973-5

Medication Facts

Preoperative Medications

The pregnant patient does not receive a sedative before surgery because of the risk of the medication causing respiratory depression in the newborn. However, it is usual to administer an antacid such as famotidine 20 mg IV or citric acid–sodium citrate solution 30 mL orally. These medications reduce gastric acid and decrease the risk of nausea, vomiting, and possible aspiration when anesthesia is administered. An antibiotic such as cefazolin 1 g IV is frequently ordered to reduce the risk of infection.

Vaginal Birth After Cesarean

A **vaginal birth after cesarean (VBAC)** may be an option for some women. The decision to try for a vaginal birth is based upon a careful physical examination and a thorough obstetric history. The health-care provider gives the patient an estimate of her chance of a successful vaginal birth and advises her of the major complication of a VBAC, which is a ruptured uterus.

Indications and Contraindications

The woman desiring a VBAC has an increased chance of success if she has

- Had a prior vaginal delivery
- Had a prior VBAC
- Spontaneous labor
- Cephalic presentation of the fetus

Contraindications for a VBAC include (Habak & Kole, 2022) the following:

- A large-for-gestational-age fetus
- Malpresentation, such as a breech, brow, or transverse lie
- Cephalopelvic disproportion
- More than two prior cesarean births
- Gestational age greater than 41 weeks
- Gestational diabetes
- Macrosomia
- Maternal obesity
- Short interpregnancy interval

Nursing Care

A woman desiring a VBAC is typically instructed to come to the hospital as soon as spontaneous labor begins. This is termed a *trial of labor after cesarean (TOLAC)*, during which she and the fetus will be closely monitored for signs of a ruptured uterus or fetal distress. During TOLAC, hospitals typically require the health-care provider to be onsite and a team on call for a cesarean delivery in the event of an emergency. If the labor progresses normally and the FHR pattern is reassuring, the patient will continue to a vaginal delivery.

Nursing care for the patient undergoing a TOLAC for a VBAC includes the following:

- Providing routine care of a laboring patient with careful monitoring of the FHR, contraction pattern, and maternal vital signs
- Conducting vaginal cervical examinations and reporting a lack of progress to a health-care provider
- Observing closely for signs of uterine rupture and reporting any of the following findings to the health-care provider:
  - Acute abdominal pain
  - Reports of a "popping" sensation by the patient
  - Palpation of fetal parts outside the uterus
  - Repetitive or prolonged FHR deceleration
  - Vaginal bleeding

Key Points

- Maternal stress during procedures can lead to fetal distress. You need to provide emotional support to reduce stress for the patient.
- Safe and effective patient-centered care requires collaboration between you, other health-care team members, and the patient.
- Nurses must be familiar with obstetric procedures and be ready to assist the health-care provider or, in some cases, perform the procedures. They also must be able to provide emotional support and monitor the patient for complications.
- Amniotomy is using AROM to stimulate labor. After an amniotomy, contractions usually become more intense and labor progresses faster.
- Amnioinfusion is the procedure of infusing fluid into the amniotic cavity to relieve cord compression.
- An external cephalic version is a procedure that uses pressure on the abdomen to manipulate the fetus into a head-down presentation.
- The induction of labor is a process that can involve mechanical or chemical means to soften and dilate the cervix and stimulate uterine contractions.

- The labor and delivery nurse takes an active role in initiating the induction of labor and needs to have an understanding of the safe administration of oxytocin.
- Augmentation of labor is the stimulation of hypotonic uterine contractions if labor has begun but the contractions are ineffective in producing dilation.
- The Bishop score is a tool used by health-care providers to determine if the cervix is ready or "ripe" for labor.
- A vacuum-extraction device attaches to the fetal head with suction to allow the health-care provider to apply traction and assist with the delivery.
- Forceps are metal, spoonlike instruments that fit around the fetal head to allow the health-care provider to assist with the delivery.
- A cesarean birth is usually performed when complications arise during labor.
- A VBAC is possible for many patients. A TOLAC is begun; and, if no complications occur, the patient delivers vaginally.

Review Questions

1. A patient is admitted to labor and delivery. She has had limited prenatal care, is pregnant with her second child, and is Rh-negative. She is prepared for an external cephalic version. You expect the health-care provider to order which of the following medications?
   1. Prostaglandin gel
   2. Oxytocin
   3. Magnesium sulfate
   4. RhoGAM

2. Nursing care following an amniotomy would include which of the following? (**Select all that apply.**)
   1. Observe the color and amount of fluid.
   2. Observe the FHR pattern.
   3. Monitor the patient's temperature every 8 hours.
   4. Change pads underneath the patient.
   5. Administer IV antibiotics.

3. You explain to the patient that the purpose of the Bishop score is to:
   1. Determine the well-being of the fetus.
   2. Determine progress during labor.
   3. Determine the readiness of the cervix for labor.
   4. Determine maternal well-being.

4. A patient asks what a "trial of labor" means. What is your *best* response?
   1. "You need to make progress in the next hours or a cesarean will be scheduled."
   2. "The doctor is giving you time to make progress in labor before considering a cesarean delivery."
   3. "Your pelvis is a little small, but we are going to let you labor and see if you make it."
   4. "A cesarean delivery will be done, but we are going to let you experience labor first."

5. The patient having her labor augmented asks, "What do you mean by 'hypotonic contractions'?" What is your *best* response?
   1. "Your contractions are infrequent and have decreased in intensity."
   2. "Your contractions are not hard enough."
   3. "Your labor is not progressing as it should."
   4. "Don't worry about that. We'll get your contractions going."

6. A patient is receiving oxytocin to induce her labor. You note that the patient has had two contractions 90 seconds apart and each contraction lasted 90 seconds. The FHR has dropped to 100 bpm following the second contraction. What nursing interventions should be implemented? **(Select all that apply.)**
   1. Reduce the dose of oxytocin that is infusing.
   2. Apply oxygen via face mask to the patient.
   3. Place the patient on her left side.
   4. Stop the infusion of oxytocin.
   5. Notify the health-care provider.

7. Which of the following are contraindications for a VBAC? **(Select all that apply.)**
   1. One prior cesarean delivery
   2. Maternal obesity
   3. Macrosomic fetus
   4. A prior vaginal delivery
   5. Gestation of 42 weeks

8. You are preparing to assist the nurse midwife with an amnioinfusion. The patient asks, "Why do I need this?" What is your *best* response?
   1. "You need extra fluid in your uterus to allow the baby to move around."
   2. "The decreased fluid in the uterus is causing the baby to lie on the umbilical cord."
   3. "You need extra amniotic fluid to prevent a dry birth."
   4. "This will replace fluid in your uterus to prevent an infection."

9. Which of the following is a possible side effect of prostaglandin gel?
   1. Frequent urination
   2. Leg cramps
   3. Nausea
   4. Backache

10. Which of the following is a major responsibility of the nurse caring for a patient receiving oxytocin for labor induction?
    1. Monitor the IV site.
    2. Monitor the patient's urinary output.
    3. Monitor the patient's coping mechanisms for labor.
    4. Monitor for tachysystole.

ANSWERS 1. 4; 2. 1, 2, 4; 3. 3; 4. 2; 5. 1; 6. 2, 3, 4, 5; 7. 2, 3, 5; 8. 2; 9. 3; 10. 4

CRITICAL THINKING QUESTIONS

1. A good friend who is pregnant at 38 weeks' gestation tells you that she is planning to have her labor induced "a little early" because her doctor is going on vacation. What is your best response, as a nurse, to your friend?

2. A patient is having her labor induced with oxytocin. She is obese, and you must palpate contractions because the external fetal monitor is not effective in recording the contractions. You note that the patient's cervix is 5 cm dilated, and the contractions are every 3 minutes and last 90 seconds. With palpation, you note that the uterus does not seem to fully relax between contractions.
   a. What additional information do you need in this situation?
   b. What interventions are appropriate?

Resources

For additional resources and information, including Postconference Questions and Activities, Answers, and References, visit www.FADavis.com.

Student Study Guide

CHAPTER 12
Postpartum Nursing Care

KEY TERMS

afterpains (AF-ter-paynz)
attachment (a-TACH-ment)
bonding (BOND-ing)
diaphoresis (DYE-uh-fo-REE-siss)
diastasis recti (dye-ASS-tuh-siss REK-tee)
diuresis (dye-yoo-REE-siss)
engrossment (en-GROHSS-ment)
exfoliation (eks-FOH-lee-AY-shun)
fundus (FUHN-duhss)
involution (IN-vo-LOO-shun)
lochia (LOH-kee-uh)
lochia alba (LOH-kee-uh AL-buh)
lochia rubra (LOH-kee-uh ROO-bruh)
lochia serosa (LOH-kee-uh see-ROH-suh)
puerperium (POO-er-PEE-ree-uhm)
rugae (ROO-gye)

CHAPTER CONCEPTS

Communication
Family
Growth and Development
Health Promotion
Reproduction and Sexuality

LEARNING OUTCOMES

1. Define the key terms.
2. Identify the normal physiological changes following childbirth in the mother's reproductive, integumentary, gastrointestinal, cardiovascular, respiratory, urinary, and musculoskeletal systems.
3. Explain the process of involution of the uterus after delivery.
4. Discuss the effect of a full bladder on uterine involution.
5. Explain afterpains to a multiparous patient.
6. Describe the phases of lochia progression.
7. Demonstrate the correct method of uterine massage for postpartum assessment.
8. Outline postpartum care in the first hour after delivery.
9. Demonstrate a focal postpartum assessment using the BUBBLE LE mnemonic.
10. Plan patient-centered care that addresses the special needs of the adolescent postpartum patient.
11. Describe a therapeutic approach for managing the psychosocial needs of a patient who is relinquishing her infant for adoption.
12. Plan discharge teaching for the postpartum patient.
13. Describe the postpartum psychological adaptations including the taking-in phase, the taking-hold phase, and the letting-go phase.
14. Identify signs that the mother is bonding with her newborn.
15. Distinguish between bonding and attachment.
16. Plan nursing interventions that can facilitate family-centered care and family attachment.

CRITICAL THINKING & CLINICAL JUDGMENT

Scenario #1: **Camila** is 23 years old and gave birth to her first child, Javier, after a long labor and vacuum extraction assistance for the delivery. It has been 4 hours since the birth, and Camila reports perineal pain and fatigue. You observe Camila talking quietly to her infant as she strokes his body with her fingertips. After a short visit in her room, she sends Javier to the nursery.

Questions

1. What do you need to think about while observing Camila's behavior?
2. What would be the best thing to do in this situation?

Nurses today emphasize family-centered care, particularly in the areas of labor and delivery, postpartum, and the nursery. A family can consist of parents and their children, single parents and their children, and grandparents raising grandchildren. The birth of a new family member causes the relationships and the interactions (dynamics) between the existing family members to change. The word *dynamics* in this context means change or growth. When two people add a child to the relationship, family dynamics become more complicated with the couple, the grandparents, and other extended family members. Family dynamics change with each child who is born.

The nurse caring for a patient in the postpartum or mother–baby unit can support the changes in the family dynamics by including family members in caring for the newborn and in teaching about newborn care and breast-feeding. You can provide information for the parents about sibling rivalry and can encourage the siblings to visit the mother and to meet the new baby in the family. You can also observe interactions between family members, identify problems, and make recommendations or appropriate referrals if needed to facilitate the change in family dynamics (Giddens, 2021).

The postpartum period, also known as the **puerperium**, is the period following the delivery of the placenta and lasting until the reproductive organs return to a nonpregnant state, usually about 6 weeks. Nurses need to be aware of normal physiological and psychological changes that take place during this period to provide safe and effective care.

POSTPARTUM PHYSICAL ADAPTATIONS

Immediately after delivery, the woman's body begins to change anatomically and physiologically to return to a nonpregnant state. Postpartum shivering, which occurs in 25% to 50% of women, is noticeable and may frighten the woman. It may occur anytime from 1 to 30 minutes after delivery and lasts for 2 to 60 minutes. The exact cause of the shivering is not known, but several mechanisms have been proposed. The cause could be a reaction to a fetal-maternal transfusion that occurred when the placenta was delivered and maternal and fetal blood mixed. Others hypothesize that the cause is small amounts of amniotic fluid that enter the bloodstream. Still others suggest that the mother experiences a thermal imbalance caused by the delivery of the placenta or a drop in body temperature after birth (Berens, 2022). Providing the patient with a warm blanket and reassurance that the shivering will pass is all that is required to provide for patient comfort.

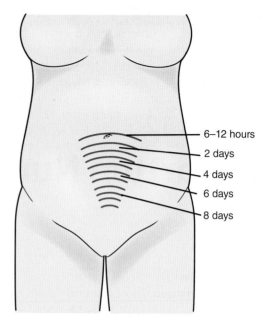

FIGURE 12.1 Location of the fundus at 6 to 12 hours postpartum and at 2, 4, 6, and 8 days postpartum.

The Reproductive System and Associated Structures

The reproductive system experiences the most changes immediately after the delivery and requires the knowledge and attention of the nurse to differentiate normal from abnormal adaptations.

Uterus Involution

Immediately after the placenta is delivered, estrogen and progesterone levels drop quickly. Oxytocin continues to be released, which causes the uterus to contract and begin shrinking down to a nonpregnant size. This process is called *involution*. The uterus weighs 1,000 to 1,200 g immediately after birth. The weight decreases to 500 g by day 7, and to 50 g by 6 weeks because of the decrease in size of the myometrial cells (Layden et al., 2023).

After delivery, the uterus is the size of a grapefruit; the top portion, known as the *fundus*, is located midline and halfway between the umbilicus and symphysis pubis. Within approximately 1 hour, the fundus is firm and even with the umbilicus. The uterus continues to descend approximately 1 cm (a fingerbreadth) per day. Usually, by day 10, the uterus is not palpable above the symphysis pubis (Fig. 12.1; Lopez-Gonzalez & Kopporapu, 2022).

The intermittent uterine contractions that some women describe as cramping are called *afterpains*. Afterpains, which are caused by the release of oxytocin, are more noticeable for multiparous women because the uterus has been stretched before and must work harder to regain tone and return to a nonpregnant size.

· **WORD · BUILDING ·**

involution: in–in + volu–rolling or turning + tion–the act of

Immediately after the delivery of the placenta, the interlacing uterine muscles contract the blood vessels that were attached to the placenta to prevent hemorrhage. In addition, the large blood vessels at the site where the placenta was attached thrombose, which means that blood clots close the vessels, preventing hemorrhage from the placental attachment site. At the placental site, the process of **exfoliation** begins. Exfoliation is the sloughing of dead tissue at the placental site, leaving the site smooth and without scar tissue. This allows the successful implantation of a fertilized ovum in subsequent pregnancies.

Patient Teaching Guidelines

Afterpains
Afterpains can be quite intense and painful for women who have given birth previously because of a decrease in uterine muscle tone. Afterpains can also be noticed while breastfeeding because of nipple stimulation, which causes the release of oxytocin. Oxytocin causes the uterine muscle to contract. The afterpains usually last for a few days and can be alleviated with ibuprofen.

Medication Facts

Ibuprofen
Ibuprofen inhibits prostaglandins, which cause the afterpains. Prostaglandins are produced as part of the inflammatory process. The patient receives the pain relief as well as the anti-inflammatory properties from this medication. The most common side effect is gastrointestinal discomfort; therefore, ibuprofen should be given with food.

Lochia
The inner lining of the uterus begins to slough off, resulting in a vaginal discharge known as *lochia* made up of blood, mucus, and tissue. The total volume of postpartum lochia is approximately 200 to 500 mL, and the process of discharging it may last up to 6 weeks. The lochia gradually gets lighter in color and amount over time.

Cervix
After delivery, the cervix is open and lacks tone. The cervical os (opening) closes slowly and by day 14 is usually barely dilated. A parous cervix will have a slitlike opening instead of the small round opening of a nonparous cervix.

• WORD • BUILDING •
exfoliation: ex–away from + foli–leaf + ation–action

Vagina
After delivery, the vagina lacks tone. Gradually, over the next 4 weeks, the edema decreases, and the vaginal folds, known as *rugae*, appear. The vaginal tissue may not lubricate easily until hormone balance is restored. The vagina will never return to a prepregnant size but does decrease in size and return to near–prepregnancy size as recovery continues.

Perineum
The area between the vagina and anus stretches and thins to allow the birth. Perineal lacerations may occur during delivery, or the health-care provider may perform an episiotomy (surgical incision) to enlarge the birth canal. After delivery, the perineum is usually bruised and edematous, and the muscle tone is weak; however, the tone will gradually be restored over the next 4 to 6 weeks. Kegel exercises can promote the return of tone to the perineal and vaginal areas. These exercises are easy to do, and every patient should receive information about how to perform Kegel exercises to improve perineal tone (see Patient Teaching Guidelines for Kegel exercises in Chapter 5).

Ovaries and Ovulation
The resumption of normal function of the ovaries is variable and influenced by breastfeeding. Menstruation is usually delayed and may not resume for weeks or months for breastfeeding women, and that depends on how much and how often the infant is breastfed. The delay is caused by the suppression of ovulation by the hormone prolactin.

The mother who does not breastfeed may ovulate as early as 27 days after delivery. In general, menstruation, which marks the beginning of ovulation, begins in 6 to 12 weeks for bottle-feeding women (Berens, 2022).

Patient Teaching Guidelines

Postpartum Menstruation
The first menstrual period for a postpartum woman can occur anytime from 6 to 12 weeks after childbirth or even longer if the patient is breastfeeding. Ovulation occurs before menses, so it is important for you to discuss birth control and family planning with patients before discharge from the hospital. For more about contraceptives that are safe to use while breastfeeding, see Chapter 3.

Breasts
Before milk production begins, the breasts secrete colostrum—a thin, yellowish fluid that provides nutrition and antibodies to the breastfeeding infant. The nipple stimulation provided by the infant causes a release of prolactin from the anterior pituitary. The hormone prolactin initiates milk production, and between the second and fourth day the breasts become engorged with milk. The breasts may feel warm and tender. Mothers refer to this as having their milk "come in." Women who choose not to breastfeed will also experience the milk coming in.

Integumentary System

The abdominal skin will resume its prepregnancy state with the exception of abdominal striae (stretch marks), which may take weeks to fade to a silvery color. The linea nigra down the middle of the abdomen will fade but may never completely go away. The effects of melanocyte-stimulating hormones, which cause skin hyperpigmentation called *melasma* on the face, will fade away over a period of days and weeks. Hair loss over the postpartum period is also common but usually resolves without medical intervention (Rajab, 2022).

Gastrointestinal System

After delivery, most women are hungry and thirsty because of the amount of energy exerted during the birthing process. In addition, food and fluids may have been restricted during labor. The combined effects of restricted intake, elevated progesterone levels during pregnancy, and anesthesia often lead to sluggish intestinal peristalsis and constipation. Internal and external hemorrhoids caused by the weight of the uterus and by pushing during childbirth can cause pain with defecation.

Medication Facts

Stool Softeners

A stool softener, such as docusate, may be prescribed to the postpartum patient to prevent straining. The onset for oral stool softeners is usually 12 to 72 hours. This medication is safe to use for breastfeeding women. The most common side effects are diarrhea and abdominal cramps (Vallerand & Sanoski, 2023).

Cardiovascular System

Expected blood loss from a vaginal delivery is 250 to 500 mL; from a cesarean birth, it is 800 to 1,000 mL. Immediately after the birth, fluid changes occur that allow the body to adjust to postpartum blood loss and to prevent hypovolemia. A 60% to 80% increase in cardiac output occurs immediately after delivery and decreases to nearly normal by 1 hour postdelivery. The high output state is caused by the following circumstances:

- After the placenta is delivered, 500 to 700 mL of blood enters the circulation.
- The uterus becomes smaller, which causes more blood to enter the circulation.
- There is improved blood flow to the vena cava because of the reduction in the size and weight of the uterus.
- There is rapid mobilization of extracellular fluid by the body.

After delivery, there is a loss of plasma volume that is greater than the loss of red blood cells, which causes a temporary rise in the hemoglobin and hematocrit. An accurate determination of these two levels may be difficult to obtain (Layden et al., 2023). Along with the increase of circulating blood volume, fibrinogen levels increase and remain increased for several days after delivery.

Safety *Stat!*

Because of increased levels of fibrinogen, the postpartum patient is more susceptible to blood clots. Therefore, ambulation is important for the patient to prevent venous stasis in the legs.

The postpartum patient's body begins to remove excess fluid stored during the pregnancy by the process of **diuresis**, which is the secretion and passage of large amounts of urine. The woman may excrete up to 3,000 mL of fluid per day for the first few days (Berens, 2022). Fluid is also lost through **diaphoresis**, which is excessive perspiration.

Labs & Diagnostics

An increase in neutrophils, which are white blood cells that fight infection, is normal in the postpartum period. This is because of inflammation, pain, and the stress of birth. The white blood cell count may increase to levels as high as 30,000 cells/mm³.

CRITICAL THINKING & CLINICAL JUDGMENT

Scenario #2: Four hours after delivery, a postpartum patient wants to get up out of bed and go to the bathroom to urinate. It will be her first time out of bed since her delivery.

Questions

1. What do you need to think about in this situation?
2. What do you need to do to keep the patient safe?

Respiratory System

The elevated diaphragm in late pregnancy will return to its normal position, reducing shortness of breath and making breathing easier. The postpartum patient's respiratory rate will return to the prepregnancy level. Pregnancy nasal congestion also disappears quickly.

Urinary System

The urinary bladder and urethra are edematous after delivery because of the effects of the fetus passing through the birth canal. The bladder tone decreases, and the woman may not

- **WORD · BUILDING ·**
diuresis: diure–urinate + sis–process

feel the urge to urinate. Therefore, the bladder can become distended and push the uterus upward and to the side. Displacing the uterus can interfere with involution and can lead to hemorrhage for the postpartum patient.

Safety *Stat!*

Poor bladder tone and poor emptying of the bladder can lead to urinary tract infections (UTIs). Monitor the patient for signs of a UTI, including dysuria (painful urination), urinary urgency and frequency, fever, and tenderness over the costovertebral angle. Teach the patient to report any of these symptoms immediately.

Musculoskeletal System

The hormone relaxin, which is responsible for relaxing the pelvic ligaments and joints during pregnancy in anticipation of delivery, begins to subside. The woman may feel hip pain for a few days as the hips recover from overflexion during pushing and as she experiences the effects of the tightening of her pelvis to the prepregnant state.

The abdominal muscles lack tone right after delivery. Some women experience a separation of the abdominal wall muscles called *diastasis recti* (Fig. 12.2). In some cases, this can be corrected with abdominal exercises. For some women, surgical correction may be needed if exercises are not effective to tighten and bring the muscles close together again.

Health Promotion

Abdominal Exercises

Abdominal exercises to regain muscle tone can generally be started at 4 weeks postpartum for vaginal deliveries and 6 weeks postpartum for cesarean deliveries. But it is important to follow the health-care provider's recommendations.

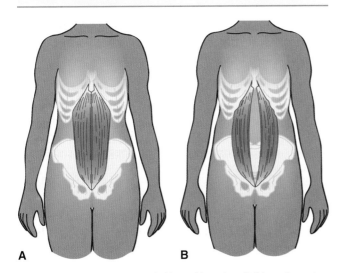

FIGURE 12.2 Diastasis recti. A, Normal location. B, Diastasis recti: a separation of the rectus muscles.

NURSING CARE DURING THE EARLY POSTPARTUM PERIOD

Immediate postpartum care most often occurs in a hospital. Most women remain in the hospital for 1 to 2 days after a vaginal delivery and 3 to 4 days after a cesarean delivery. During this time, women are recovering from childbirth and assuming care for their newborns. Nurses use this time in the hospital to provide physical care and to monitor for complications. Nurses also teach the woman about self-care before discharge.

Uterine Assessment

To palpate the fundus, position one hand at the base of the uterus just above the symphysis pubis and the other hand at the umbilicus. Press downward with the hand at the umbilicus until the fundus is palpated as a firm, hard, globular mass in the abdomen (Fig. 12.3). Note the position of the fundus and document the location.

Safety *Stat!*

Never palpate a uterus without supporting the lower segment because the uterus could invert if not stabilized.

Next, palpate the consistency of the mass. If it is soft or "boggy," support the lower uterine segment and gently massage in a circular pattern with the flattened other hand until the uterus becomes firm. If massage is not effective, there may be a large blood clot in the uterus or extreme uterine atony. *Atony* refers to a lack of muscle tone, which could lead to postpartum hemorrhage (PPH). Many women receive oxytocin after delivery to promote uterine contractions. If the uterus does not remain firm with the administration of oxytocin and massage, the health-care provider should be notified.

Another problem that could lead to uterine atony is a full bladder, which can displace the uterus and make involution

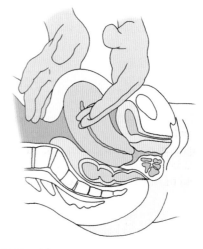

FIGURE 12.3 Fundal massage.

difficult. Palpate the patient's bladder. If bladder distention is noted, assist the patient to urinate and then recheck the uterus to determine if it is firm and has returned to the midline of the abdomen.

Lochia Assessment

Immediately after delivery of the placenta, a large amount of dark red blood flows from the uterus. As the uterus contracts to control bleeding, the volume of vaginal discharge, or lochia, slows. Lochia goes through three stages. This first discharge of dark red blood is termed **lochia rubra**. The lochia progressively changes to a brownish red and then a lighter color called **lochia serosa** around the third to fourth day. Over a period of 1 to 2 weeks, the lochia becomes even lighter and more of a yellowish color, called **lochia alba**. The time that the woman will experience lochia may last from 3 to 6 weeks.

While checking for uterine tone, observe the patient's lochia (Fig. 12.4). View the peripad (similar to a menstrual pad) to inspect the amount and character of the lochia while massaging the uterine fundus. Doing so allows you to visualize any sudden expulsion of clots or blood caused by a boggy uterus. The amount is determined by estimating the diameter of the lochia spot on a peripad after 1 hour (Lopez-Gonzalez & Kopporapu, 2022). Nurses document the amount of lochia by using the following terms:

- *Scant* is less than 1 inch of lochia on the pad.
- *Light* is less than 4 inches of lochia on the pad.
- *Moderate* is less than 6 inches of lochia on the pad.
- *Heavy* is when the pad is saturated within an hour.

The character of the lochia refers to the color (rubra, serosa, or alba) and the presence of clots. It is common for small clots to be present because of blood pooling in the lower

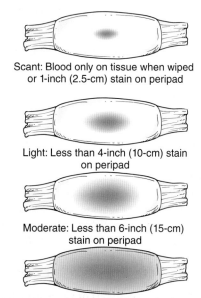

Scant: Blood only on tissue when wiped or 1-inch (2.5-cm) stain on peripad

Light: Less than 4-inch (10-cm) stain on peripad

Moderate: Less than 6-inch (15-cm) stain on peripad

Heavy: Peripad saturated within 1 hour

FIGURE 12.4 Assessment of lochia.

uterine segment. Turn the patient to her side to make sure that blood is not pooling under her thighs instead of being absorbed by the peripad. If small clots occur, it is sufficient just to document them, but because large clots can interfere with involution or indicate signs of hemorrhage they should be reported.

During the first hour after delivery, it is common for two peripads to be saturated. After the first hour, bleeding is considered excessive if the patient saturates more than one pad per hour.

Nursing Care During the First Hour After Delivery

The newly delivered patient will remain in the labor and delivery area for a minimum of 1 hour after delivery. The first hour after delivery is the most dangerous hour in child bearing because of the risk of hemorrhage after delivery. During this first hour, the following nursing interventions should take place:

- Check vital signs, including pulse and blood pressure, every 15 minutes.
- Palpate the fundus of the uterus for firmness and location every 15 minutes.
- While checking the uterine tone, note the amount of vaginal bleeding. Observe the peripads for the amount of lochia, color, odor, and the presence of clots.

When the labor and delivery nurse is confident that the patient is stable and exhibiting no signs of hemorrhage, the patient is transferred to the postpartum or mother–baby unit. Upon arrival, the patient is assessed and close monitoring is continued according to hospital protocol.

Postpartum Assessment and Nursing Interventions

Each time the postpartum registered nurse assumes care for a postpartum patient, an appropriate physical assessment with the focus on the reproductive system should be performed. A mnemonic for remembering the postpartum focal assessment is BUBBLE LE: **b**reasts, **u**terus, **b**ladder, **b**owels, lochia, **e**pisiotomy/laceration, **l**egs, and **e**motions.

Breasts

You should inquire about breast and nipple pain. The breast should be lightly palpated to check for engorgement, and the nipples inspected for redness, irritation, blisters, or bleeding.

Nursing interventions include the following:

- Suggest that the woman wear a bra with good support to promote comfort as the milk comes in.
- If nipple soreness is present, observe the woman breastfeed and correct latch-on problems.
- Provide pain relief such as acetaminophen for sore nipples before breastfeeding.
- Determine her knowledge of breastfeeding and provide appropriate teaching if needed.

- Arrange for the lactation specialist to assist the patient if the woman is experiencing problems that cannot be handled by you.
- Remind her that frequent breastfeeding every 2 to 2½ hours will help prevent engorgement when her milk comes in.

Patient Teaching Guidelines

Managing Engorgement for the Nonbreastfeeding Patient

Women who do not plan to breastfeed will still produce breast milk and will experience engorgement. Patient teaching to promote comfort and reduce milk production includes the following:

- Wear a supportive bra 24 hours a day until engorgement subsides.
- Apply ice packs to the breasts for 20 minutes several times a day.
- Place cold inner cabbage leaves on the breasts; research has shown this will decrease engorgement (Aprilina et al., 2021).
- Avoid any stimulation of the nipple; for example, do not stand in a warm shower and let the water run over the breasts.
- Do not pump or hand express milk; the breast will replace the milk, which will make the engorgement worse.
- Take an analgesic, such as acetaminophen or hydrocodone/acetaminophen, for the pain.
- Note that engorgement usually subsides within 48 hours.

Uterus

Palpate the uterine fundus for location and consistency. It should be firm and in the midline. Document the location of the fundus in relationship to the umbilicus (see Fig. 12.1). For example, if the fundus is 1 cm (1 fingerbreadth) beneath the umbilicus, it is documented as U-1 in the medical record. Inquire about cramping and abdominal pain.
Nursing interventions include the following:

- Some cramping is expected, but abdominal pain or tenderness should be reported to the charge nurse or health-care provider.
- If the uterus is not involuting as expected, note lack of tone or signs of infection and report findings. (For involution delay related to bladder distention, see next.)
- Show the patient how to feel her fundus while explaining the process of involution.

Bladder

You should palpate the bladder when checking the fundus. Bladder distention should not be present. If the bladder is distended, you will note a raised area over the bladder.
Nursing interventions include the following:

- If bladder distention is noted, assist the patient to the bathroom to urinate before completing the assessment.
- If the fundus is not firm, do not let the patient get out of bed.
- If the patient cannot urinate, obtain an order for catheterization from the health-care provider.
- Question the patient about frequency and amount of urination.
- Instruct the patient to drink at least eight glasses of water a day to decrease the risk of a UTI.
- Teach the patient about the normal diuresis process after childbirth.
- Teach the patient about proper perineal care of patting dry from front to back after urination and defecation. Many health-care providers order a peri-bottle for cleansing the perineum. The bottle is filled with warm water and squirted over the perineum after urination and defecation to cleanse the perineum before applying a clean peripad.
- Remind the patient to change her peripad after each urination and defecation.

Bowels

Bowels are assessed by the auscultation of bowel sounds. The patient who experienced a cesarean birth may not have audible bowel sounds for several hours because of the effects of anesthesia on peristalsis.
Nursing interventions include the following:

- Asking the patient when her last bowel movement was; the bowels tend to be sluggish because of the effects of prenatal iron and the decrease in peristalsis from labor
- Encouraging the patient to drink extra fluids and to select fruits and vegetables from her hospital menu
- Administering stool softeners if ordered by the health-care provider
- Encouraging walking to promote an increase in peristalsis

Lochia

Observe and document the amount and type of lochia.
Nursing interventions include the following:

- Ask the patient when her pad was last changed. This provides a better indication of the amount of lochia noted.
- Report any abnormal amount, color, or odor.
- Teach the patient about the progression of lochia.

Episiotomy/Laceration

The episiotomy is best viewed by having the patient turn to her side and bring her upper knee forward. While the patient is on her side, gently lift the upper buttock and inspect the perineum for bruising, erythema, edema, hematoma (a collection of blood in the subcutaneous space), and for intactness of the episiotomy or the repaired laceration. Note if hemorrhoids are present and notify the health-care provider if they are large and painful.
Nursing interventions include the following:

- Ask the patient about her level of perineal or rectal pain and medicate appropriately according to the health-care provider orders.

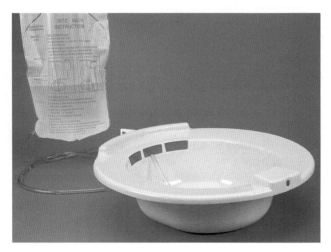

FIGURE 12.5 Sitz bath.

- Report any abnormal findings to the health-care provider.
- Offer an ice pack for the first 24 hours to reduce pain and swelling.
- Teach the patient how to use anesthetic episiotomy spray, if ordered by the health-care provider.
- After 24 hours, warm water soaking (sitz bath) may relieve episiotomy and hemorrhoid pain and aid in healing (Fig. 12.5).

Patient Teaching Guidelines

Preparing a Sitz Bath at Home

Some patients obtain episiotomy pain relief with a warm sitz bath. The word *sitz* comes from the German language and means *to sit*. Some hospitals provide the patient with a round plastic basin that is placed on the toilet seat. It comes with a bag that can be filled with warm water. As the woman sits on the basin, warm water flows from the bag through long tubing into the basin and around her perineum and then into the toilet. The patient can bring the sitz bath home to use. Alternatively, a home sitz bath can be prepared by filling a clean bath tub with 2 to 3 inches of warm water. For added comfort, a clean towel can be placed in the tub for the patient to sit on. No soap, shower gels, or bubble bath should be added. The woman can sit on the soft wet towel in the warm water for 10 to 15 minutes three times a day.

Legs

After questioning the patient about leg pain, determine if there is adequate circulation in the legs by checking the pedal pulses and noting the temperature of the legs. Pedal edema may last for a few days after delivery as body fluids shift (Lopez-Gonzalez & Kopporapu, 2022). Inspect the legs for any red, warm, or tender areas.

Evidence-Based Practice

Researchers conducted a study to determine if a sitz bath or application of infrared lamp therapy was the best method to relieve perineal pain and promote healing of an episiotomy. The study concluded that dry infrared light therapy penetrates deeper into the tissue, promotes faster healing, and decreases pain. Nurses provide most of the postpartum care. Nurses can advocate for change and promote the use of infrared lamp therapy on the postpartum unit.

Choudhari, R. G., Tayade, S. A., Venurkar, S. V., & Deshpande, V. P. (2022). A review of episiotomy and modalities for relief of episiotomy pain. *Cureus, (14)*, 11. https://doi.org/10.7759/cureus.31620

Nursing interventions include the following:

- Report any abnormal findings immediately.
- Encourage the patient to ambulate frequently.
- Teach the patient to avoid crossing the legs.
- Encourage the patient to keep her legs elevated when sitting.
- Encourage high-risk patients to wear compression hose or apply sequential compression devices (SCDs) to the legs.

Emotions

When the placenta is expelled, the woman experiences a sudden drop in progesterone, which can contribute to the "postpartum blues" (Office on Women's Health [OWH], 2021). While providing nursing care, notice the patient's emotions. Emotionally, the patient may range from being excited to apprehensive to tearful and irritable.

Nursing interventions include the following:

- Explain to the patient that the "postpartum blues" are a normal part of postpartum recovery.
- Reassure her and her family that they usually pass within a few days. She or a family member should contact the health-care provider if the "postpartum blues" don't resolve or get worse.
- Encourage the patient to rest frequently, verbalize her needs, and allow her family and friends to assist during the recovery time.

Nursing Care After a Cesarean Birth

The woman who experiences a cesarean birth requires the same monitoring for uterine involution and lochia as the patient who has a vaginal birth with the addition of needing postoperative care. This additional care helps to prevent complications of bedrest, such as atelectasis, thrombosis, and infection. The woman who had a cesarean delivery typically does not have pain in the perineal area but instead from her abdominal incision. Nursing care for a cesarean delivery patient includes the following:

- Evaluating and medicating for pain according to the health-care provider's orders

- Monitoring the incision for signs of infection: **r**edness, **e**dema, **e**cchymosis, **d**rainage, and **a**pproximation of wound edges (REEDA)
- Encouraging ambulation to prevent venous thrombosis when the patient is stable and the urinary catheter has been discontinued
- Discontinuing the urinary catheter as ordered and monitoring the patient for resumption of a normal voiding pattern
- Applying compression stockings or SCDs to prevent sluggish blood flow
- Teaching the patient abdominal splinting with a pillow to decrease pain when coughing or moving in bed
- Encouraging turning, coughing, and deep breathing every 2 hours, along with use of an incentive spirometer, to prevent atelectasis, which could lead to hospital-acquired pneumonia

Nursing Care of the Adolescent

The postpartum adolescent should receive the same physical care as any other postpartum patient; however, she requires more structured teaching about the care of the newborn and herself. She may have limited or no prior contact with babies. Treat the adolescent patient as an adult; do not talk down to her and be careful with the tone of the interactions. A teenager will be especially sensitive to your tone and attitude when receiving teaching about her newborn. Encourage questions and never make the adolescent patient feel embarrassed about any lack of knowledge. Direct the teaching to the teenager, not to her parents or to the support persons who may accompany her. If the father of the baby is present, he should be included in the teaching. Teaching in small segments, using demonstrations, videos, and written material, is appreciated by most teenagers. Providing the patient with periods of rest between teaching sessions and infant care helps to prevent her from becoming overwhelmed.

Whenever possible, role-model infant care and encourage bonding between the new mother and her infant. Be prepared for the patient to be very centered on her own needs. She will require more mothering from you and her family than older patients do. The teen mother responds best to positive reinforcement from the nurses about her attempts at newborn care. Encouragement and praise will increase her self-confidence and self-esteem as she takes on the role of motherhood.

Some adolescents who have had little or no exposure to newborns have unrealistic expectations. For example, a young mother may expect her baby to resemble the perfect baby from infant food commercials on television, or she may be surprised that newborns must be fed around the clock. She may not be prepared for the amount of time that breastfeeding and infant care require. Encourage the patient to verbalize her fears and needs during the postpartum recovery in the hospital and provide education, emotional support, and appropriate referrals.

Teen mothers are at higher-than-average risk for postpartum depression. Teach the patient and her family the signs and symptoms of postpartum depression and instruct them to report these to her health-care provider. The mother (and the father, if he is involved) should be referred to support groups for teen parents for ongoing support (Smithbattle, 2020).

CRITICAL THINKING

You are planning to teach a 16-year-old new mother about self-care and newborn care.

Question

1. What do you need to think about when preparing for the teaching session?

Nursing Care for the Woman Who Relinquishes Her Infant for Adoption

A woman who intends to relinquish or "give up" her baby for adoption usually arrives in the labor and delivery department with a birth plan. The woman may want the adoptive parents present at the birth or want them called afterward. The mother may request to hold her infant only at delivery and then ask that the infant be kept in the nursery. She may not want to hold or see the infant at all. Some women choose to keep the infant in the room until the baby is turned over to the new parents or to the social worker at discharge. It is essential to respect and support the decisions the woman has made about her infant. She will require the same physical care and self-care teaching as any postpartum patient.

How do you communicate empathy to the woman who relinquishes her infant for adoption? Avoid the phrase "giving up the baby" and instead use the phrase "plan for adoption." Encourage the patient to talk by using the following prompts:

- "What can I do to help you?"
- "Share with me your plan for the baby."
- "Tell me how you're feeling today."

Some women have arranged for an open adoption in which the adoptive parents stay in contact with the mother, sending her pictures and updates as the child grows. Other women may choose a closed adoption, in which no identifying information is shared between the mother and the adoptive parents. After a closed adoption is finalized, the records are sealed and may not be available until the child is 18 years old. If a woman decides to relinquish the infant and does not have a plan in place, consult the hospital policy manual for the correct procedure for assisting the woman with her decision.

A woman who relinquishes her newborn will experience grief and loss and will have a higher-than-average risk of postpartum depression (American Adoptions, 2023). She will need to be educated about the signs and symptoms to report to her health-care provider and may require referrals for counseling and support after discharge.

POSTPARTUM PSYCHOLOGICAL ADAPTATIONS

The role of new motherhood may overwhelm some women, whereas others seem to step into their new role without hesitation. Reva Rubin's (1984) classic research on maternal role attainment is helpful for understanding the range of women's postpartum psychological adaptations. Rubin divided postpartum adjustment to motherhood into three phases: (1) the taking-in phase, (2) the taking-hold phase, and (3) the letting-go phase.

Taking-In Phase

In the taking-in phase, the mother is centered on her own needs, such as rest, pain relief, sleeping, and eating. She feels dependent at this time, and she herself needs mothering. During this phase, the new mother often wants to review her labor and delivery experience. This review helps her to integrate it with the reality of her baby being born and the reality of motherhood.

She may not initiate interaction with the newborn, but when handed the newborn to hold, she will stroke the baby with her fingertips and may position the baby facing her so that she can explore the baby's face. This is known as the *en face position*. Fingertip touching and the en face position are signs of positive bonding behaviors. This taking-in of information allows her to identify her infant and begin the **bonding** process. Bonding is the start of a lifelong relationship with the newborn. The mother begins to feel a closeness and a love for the baby. Bonding may occur instantaneously for some women, but for others it is a slower process that grows over a few days or weeks. The taking-in phase may last a day or two.

Taking-Hold Phase

In the taking-hold phase, the mother initiates care of the baby. She wants to be more independent and to make her own decisions, but she is concerned and anxious about her own physical care, breastfeeding, and baby care. The new mother requires praise and positive reinforcement for the things that she does well, such as supporting the baby's head or correctly positioning the baby for breastfeeding. She is open to learning about self-care, newborn care, and bonding, so this is the right time to begin teaching her about these elements. Reassurance of her abilities to be a good mother is important during this time. This phase may last up to 10 days or more.

During the taking-hold phase, many women experience the postpartum blues. This phenomenon is thought to be caused by the decrease in estrogen and progesterone that occurred with the delivery of the placenta as well as exhaustion from lack of uninterrupted sleep and the demands of breastfeeding every 2 to 2½ hours. The woman may feel sad or irritable; she may spontaneously erupt into tears for reasons she cannot explain. Usually this sadness passes after a good cry or in a day or two. Anticipatory guidance for the woman and her support person is important so that they will know that the postpartum blues are common and self-limiting. Occasionally, the blues do not subside, and the woman experiences postpartum depression. Postpartum depression is a serious disorder that requires medical treatment. Postpartum depression is discussed in Chapter 13.

Letting-Go Phase

In this phase, the new mother is adjusting or "letting-go" of her previous childless, more independent role. She must adjust to the responsibility of having her baby dependent on her for everything as well as the lifestyle changes that go along with parenthood. Women who already have children will go through this stage more quickly than first-time mothers as they adjust to resuming infant care and dividing attention between their children. During this phase, attachment with the newborn occurs. **Attachment** is the establishment of an emotionally positive and rewarding relationship between an infant and the parent. The mother learns to understand her infant's cries and body language and receives positive feedback from the infant when the infant's needs are met. The mother learns to trust herself and her instincts when caring for the child and feels confidence in her ability to mother the infant.

Therapeutic Communication

When a new mother expresses anxiety regarding her ability to care for the newborn, be prepared to offer her positive reinforcement, praise, and reassurance. Phrases that may be helpful include the following:

- "You are holding him perfectly."
- "Look! She's looking right into your eyes."
- "Yes, that's the right position for breastfeeding."

Health Promotion

Promoting Bonding With the Newborn
The following nursing interventions can promote bonding after childbirth:

- Promote skin-to-skin contact between the parents and the newborn.
- Encourage breastfeeding.
- Encourage eye contact.
- Allow the baby to stay with the parents as much as possible; avoid unnecessary trips to the nursery.

DEVELOPMENT OF FAMILY ATTACHMENT

Postpartum is a time of change for the family unit. Family attachment, the integration of the newborn into the family unit, takes time.

Typically, the mother's partner begins bonding with the fetus before the birth by attending health-care appointments, ultrasound appointments, and childbirth classes. The partner is often involved in preparing the baby's room and planning for the trip to the hospital. After the birth, the partner should be encouraged to room-in and stay as much as possible with the mother and newborn at the hospital. New parents are often observed staring at their newborns for extended periods. This behavior is known as **engrossment** and is comparable with the en face bonding that is observed with the mother and infant (Fig. 12.6).

The partner should be encouraged to hold the infant and assist with newborn care. They should be included in newborn care teaching before discharge.

Sibling bonding and attachment can be promoted by allowing the sibling to visit in the hospital. Current phone and video technology allow a child to have easy contact with their mother when she is hospitalized, but a visit with her in the hospital will reduce separation anxiety and feelings that the new baby is more important. A visit with mom and the new baby will promote family bonding faster.

The parents need to be cautioned that the older child may exhibit signs of jealously and may regress in their behavior. For example, a 3-year-old who was potty-trained may begin wetting his pants. Even if older siblings are prepared for the birth and the new family member, their behavior may be unpredictable. The child may also express uncomplimentary opinions about the new baby. Often, the sibling vacillates between protective, loving feelings, and dislike for the new family member (Fig. 12.7).

Preparation for Discharge

When preparing the patient for discharge, you should administer a single dose of the MMR vaccine to any woman who tested susceptible to rubella during her pregnancy. If any other immunizations are not current, the patient should contact her health-care provider after discharge to arrange for those vaccines.

All household members, close relatives, and friends who will be in contact with the newborn should be up-to-date with the influenza and tetanus, diphtheria, and pertussis immunizations (Centers for Disease Control and Prevention [CDC], 2021).

At discharge time, the new mother is too excited to focus on teaching. Ideally, teaching should have occurred in small segments throughout the hospital stay rather than being left until the patient is packed and ready to leave her room.

Preparing for discharge requires educating the patient about self-care. Written instructions should be provided along with the verbal teaching.

Self-care instructions should include the following information:

- The sutures used for repairing lacerations and the episiotomy will dissolve over time.
- At first, the perineum may be sore and painful. Use ibuprofen or acetaminophen as prescribed and warm sitz baths to control pain.
- As the perineum heals, it is normal for itching to occur.

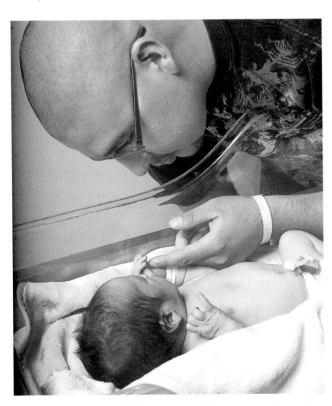

FIGURE 12.6 A father exhibiting a sign of engrossment by gazing at his newborn son.

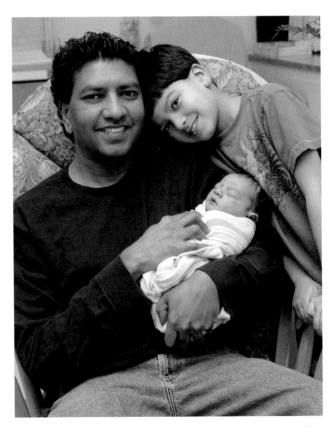

FIGURE 12.7 A new father with the newborn and an older child.

- Purchase menstrual pads and continue to change the pad after each urination or defecation.
- Cleanse the perineum with warm water in the peri-bottle.
- Do not use tampons or douche until after the follow-up appointment with the health-care provider.
- Continue to wear a supportive bra as the breasts adjust to milk production.
- Wash hands before breastfeeding and after every diaper change.
- It is important to keep follow-up appointments with the health-care provider to make sure that postpartum recovery is complete.
- Continue prenatal vitamins and iron as prescribed until the follow-up appointment with the health-care provider.
- Exercise can be started according to the health-care provider's instructions. Walking and stretching are safe starting at 2 weeks postpartum. Vigorous exercise should be started after the postpartum checkup.
- Call the health-care provider if the mother experiences any of the following:
  - A fever of 38°C (100.4°F) or greater
  - Increasing pain, redness, swelling, or discharge from a cesarean incision or episiotomy
  - An increase in vaginal bleeding and a return to lochia rubra after transition to serosa or alba
  - An increase in vaginal bleeding and passing clots larger than a quarter
  - Foul lochia odor
  - Increasing abdominal pain or tenderness

Women usually have questions about sexual activity and contraception but may be too shy to ask. You should introduce the topic in an open, matter-of-fact manner that makes the patient comfortable to ask questions.

Most health-care providers advise that sexual intercourse can resume when bright-red bleeding has ceased, the vagina and vulva are healed, and the woman is physically comfortable and emotionally ready (Layden et al., 2023). The woman needs to be cautioned that ovulation may resume at any time and that she could become pregnant. Suggest that condoms be used until she can discuss birth control options with her health-care provider.

A discussion of family planning and child spacing is appropriate. Research suggests that a pregnancy within 6 months of a prior pregnancy is associated with premature birth, placenta abruption, low birth weight, congenital disorders, and schizophrenia. Also, a pregnancy within 2 years of a previous birth has been associated with an increased risk of autism (Autism Research Institute, 2021).

Health Promotion

Benefits of Exercise After Pregnancy

Exercise after pregnancy has many benefits, including:

- Restoring muscle tone, especially the abdominal muscles
- Aiding in weight loss if combined with reduced calorie intake
- Improving mood and relieving stress
- Improving cardiovascular fitness
- Allowing the new mother to take time for herself

Safety *Stat!*

Rho(D) immune globulin (RhoGAM) is administered intramuscularly (IM) within 72 hours of birth to prevent sensitization to the Rh factor in an Rh-negative woman with an infant who is Rh-positive. This injection will prevent hemolytic disease in subsequent pregnancies.

Key Points

- The maternal reproductive system undergoes the most changes immediately after birth, but all body systems are affected.
- The process of the uterus returning to its prepregnant state is called *involution*.
- The vaginal discharge following childbirth, which is called *lochia*, may last for up to 6 weeks after delivery.
- There are three types of lochia: rubra, serosa, and alba.
- The breasts secrete colostrum first, followed by milk in 2 to 4 days.
- Abdominal striae and the linea nigra will fade but usually do not completely disappear.
- Constipation and hemorrhoids are common after delivery.
- To balance fluids in the body, diuresis and diaphoresis occur for the first few days after delivery.
- Lack of bladder tone can lead to an overdistended bladder, which can prevent uterine involution and cause excessive bleeding.

- Joint and muscle pain is common after delivery as the woman recovers and adjusts to the decrease in relaxin hormone.
- Postpartum assessment can be organized with the mnemonic BUBBLE LE, which stands for **b**reasts, **u**terus, **b**ladder, **b**owels, **l**ochia, **e**pisiotomy/laceration, **l**egs, and **e**motions.
- The woman who experiences a cesarean birth requires the usual postpartum care, along with postoperative care to manage pain and prevent postoperative complications such as atelectasis and thrombophlebitis.
- The postpartum adolescent patient will require positive reinforcement for her attempts at taking on the mother role as well as teaching to prepare her for newborn care.
- Nurses need to provide sensitive and empathetic care to the postpartum patient who plans to relinquish her newborn for adoption.

- Rubin's classic research identified three phases of maternal role attainment: the taking-in, taking-hold, and letting-go phases.
- Nursing interventions can facilitate family attachment and changes in family dynamics.

- All discharged postpartum patients should be provided with guidelines for recognizing complications and knowing when to call the health-care provider.

Review Questions

1. _____ is the process of the uterus returning to its prepregnant state.

2. A multiparous patient asks you, "Why am I cramping? Is something wrong?" What is your best response?
   1. "The cramping is called *afterpains*, and it will go away soon."
   2. "I can get you pain medication, if you'd like it."
   3. "The cramping is called *afterpains*, and they are normal contractions of the uterus as it returns to its prepregnancy size."
   4. "Let's get your mind off that. Would you like to hold your new baby?"

3. How can a woman who does not want to breastfeed suppress milk production? **(Select all that apply.)**
   1. Wearing a tight-fitting bra
   2. Applying ice packs to the breasts
   3. Allowing the baby to nurse for a short time only
   4. Standing in the shower and allowing warm water to soften the breasts
   5. Asking for medication to dry up the milk supply

4. A postpartum woman calls you because she just woke up and her gown and sheets are soaked with perspiration. You know that:
   1. The patient's body is ridding itself of excess fluid through diaphoresis.
   2. The patient has a fever and has probably developed an infection.
   3. The room temperature is too hot for the patient.
   4. The postpartum hormone changes have given her a hot flash.

5. Why would you point out the newborn's positive aspects, such as normal reflexes, to new parents?
   1. To teach the parents the difference between normal and abnormal newborn reflexes
   2. To promote bonding with a newborn whose parents expected it to look "perfect" at birth
   3. To obtain better patient satisfaction ratings from the parents
   4. To encourage the parents to observe, not just hold, their baby

6. At 12 hours after delivery, where do you expect the fundus to be located?
   1. At the level of the umbilicus
   2. Two fingerbreadths below the umbilicus
   3. Three fingerbreadths below the umbilicus
   4. Right above the symphysis pubis

7. A new mother is very interested in caring for her newborn but is concerned about her ability to be a good mother. According to Rubin's phases of role attainment, the new mother is in which of the following phases?
   1. Taking-in phase
   2. Taking-hold phase
   3. Letting-go phase
   4. Attachment phase

8. At 2 weeks after delivery, a patient arrives at the obstetrician's office for a checkup. Which of the following do you expect to see? **(Select all that apply.)**
   1. Lochia alba
   2. Edema of the ankles
   3. Abdominal striae
   4. Diaphoresis
   5. Fundus halfway between the umbilicus and symphysis pubis

9. A postpartum patient, 36 hours after delivery, states that her hemorrhoids are painful. What interventions would be appropriate? **(Select all that apply.)**
   1. Administer pain medication as ordered.
   2. Reassure her that they will go away eventually.
   3. Set up a sitz bath for her.
   4. Suggest that she limit the amount of fiber in her diet for a few days.
   5. Remind her to increase her fluid intake.

10. The patient asks you why she is receiving a stool softener. What is your best response?
   1. "It is ordered by your midwife."
   2. "This medication will make your first bowel movement easier."
   3. "Breastfeeding women often have constipation."
   4. "You haven't been drinking enough fluids."

ANSWERS 1. Involution; 2. 3; 3. 1, 2, 4, 1; 5. 2; 6. 1; 7. 2; 8. 1, 3; 9. 1, 3, 5; 10. 2

CRITICAL THINKING QUESTIONS

1. How can a mother assist her 4-year-old child to bond with the new family member?
2. A new mother is being discharged home. She is accompanied by the baby's father and her mother, who is a new grandmother. The grandmother intends to provide help at home. How can you advise the grandmother about helping the new parents at home?

Resources

For additional resources and information, including Postconference Questions and Activities, Answers, and References, visit www.FADavis.com.

Student Study Guide

CHAPTER 13
Postpartum Complications

KEY TERMS

anhedonia (AN-hee-DOE-nee-uh)
endometritis (EN-doh-met-RYE-tiss)
hematoma (HEE-muh-TOH-muh)
hematuria (HEE-muh-TOO-ree-uh)
mastitis (mass-TYE-tiss)
postpartum psychosis (PPP) post-PAR-tuhm
    (sye-KOH-siss)
subinvolution (SUHB-in-vo-LOO-shun)
thromboembolism (THROM-boh-EM-bo-lizm)
thrombus (THROM-buhss)

CHAPTER CONCEPTS

Infection
Mood and Affect
Perfusion
Professionalism

LEARNING OUTCOMES

1. Define the key terms.
2. Discuss possible causes of uterine atony.
3. Identify the signs and symptoms of postpartum hemorrhage (PPH).
4. Discuss appropriate management of PPH.
5. Discuss the causes, signs and symptoms, and management of a patient with a hematoma.
6. Recognize signs and symptoms of a postpartum infection.
7. Discuss appropriate management of the infection.
8. Identify women at risk for thrombophlebitis as well as nursing interventions to prevent thromboembolism in the postpartum patient.
9. Differentiate between postpartum depression (PPD) and postpartum psychosis (PPP).
10. Identify appropriate nursing interventions for each disorder.

CRITICAL THINKING & CLINICAL JUDGMENT

Scenario #1: **Alice** delivered her fourth child, a baby boy weighing 10 pounds and 2 ounces, 1 hour ago and has been transferred to the postpartum unit. The labor and delivery nurse reports that Alice was 42 weeks' gestation and had her labor induced with oxytocin. She had a long second stage, pushed for 2 hours, and then required an assisted delivery with forceps. Her uterus became soft and boggy between assessments and has required massage and an increase in the rate of the IV oxytocin to maintain a firm fundus. You are assisting the postpartum RN with the physical assessment, and she notes that the uterus is boggy and Alice's peripad is saturated with blood.

Questions

1. What should you think about in this situation?
2. What questions should you ask Alice at this time?
3. Is there anything you should do at this time? Explain your answer.

CONCEPTUAL CORNERSTONE
Infection

An infection occurs when a host is invaded by microorganisms that enter the body, multiply, and cause illness or even death. When an infection occurs, it can be acute or chronic. It can be a localized infection in one area of the body, such as in a wound; or it can become systemic, which means the infection affects the entire body. Postpartum infections are usually localized and can occur in uterine tissue, wound tissue, the urinary tract, and the breast. However, a localized infection that is not identified and treated early can progress into a systemic infection, which could have debilitating effects for the patient.

You need to be alert for patients with risk factors that predispose them to infection in the postpartum period. Regardless of the location of the infection, signs and symptoms include fever, increased pain, redness, swelling, and drainage. Prompt recognition of signs of infection and initiation of antimicrobials, fluids, and nutrition can change the course of the infection and the length of stay for the patient.

Pregnancy and childbirth are considered common events in life. Most women are healthy, and their labor and delivery course is without incident. They spend a short time in the hospital and return home with the new baby, but complications can arise that can have harmful effects on the postpartum patient. It is important that you be alert for signs of complications after childbirth and report them immediately to prevent life-threatening events.

CARE OF THE WOMAN WITH POSTPARTUM HEMORRHAGE

Postpartum hemorrhage (PPH) is the leading cause of maternal mortality in the world (Smith, 2022). PPH is defined as a blood loss of more than 500 mL for a vaginal delivery and more than 1,000 mL for a cesarean delivery. PPH that occurs during the first 24 hours after birth is called *primary hemorrhage*. The most likely time for PPH is the first 4 hours after birth. *Secondary hemorrhage* occurs after 24 hours and before 6 weeks postpartum (Belfort, 2022). Risk factors for PPH include the following:

- Retained placenta
- Failure to progress during the second stage of labor
- Placenta accreta (see Chapter 8)
- Lacerations
- Large-for-gestational-age (LGA) newborn
- Instrumental delivery
- Hypertensive disorders
- Induction of labor
- Augmentation of labor with oxytocin
- Overdistention of the uterus
- Body mass index (BMI) over 40 (Smith, 2022)

Many sources suggest the use of the Four Ts as a mnemonic to remember the causes of PPH: **t**one, **t**issue, **t**rauma, and **t**hrombosis (Layden et al., 2023; Smith, 2022).

Tone

Uterine atony is the most common cause of PPH. The uterus loses tone when the muscles fail to contract after delivery of the placenta. When the muscles do not contract, the blood vessels that connected the placenta to the uterine muscle remain open, causing a rapid blood loss that can lead to hypovolemic shock. The uterine muscles may not contract because of fatigue caused by prolonged or forceful labor, especially one induced or augmented with oxytocin. Sometimes, the uterine muscles may not respond and contract because they have been overstretched (distended) from multiple fetuses or polyhydramnios (Belfort, 2022; Smith, 2022). A common cause of late PPH is **subinvolution**, which is the failure of the uterus to follow the pattern of normal involution; the organ remains large instead of returning to its prepregnancy size.

Tissue

After delivery of the fetus, the uterus contracts to release the placenta. If a portion of the placenta remains attached to the uterine wall, the uterus cannot compress the open vessels and control bleeding. Retained placental fragments are the most common cause of late PPH. Women with abnormal implantation of the placenta, such as placenta accreta and previa, are at high risk for retained tissue.

Trauma

Trauma to the uterus, cervix, or vagina can cause hemorrhage. Forceps delivery is the most common cause of cervical and vaginal lacerations. Lacerations can also occur from manipulation of a shoulder dystocia and by abnormal presentations of the fetus.

Thrombosis

Immediately after the birth, disorders of coagulation and platelets may be missed because uterine contractions are controlling bleeding (Smith, 2022). In the days afterward, fibrin deposits over the placental site and clots within the vessels that supplied the placenta with blood flow are needed to control bleeding. Any preexisting condition such as thrombocytopenia, an underlying clotting disorder, or sepsis could interfere with clotting and cause a late PPH.

Signs and symptoms of PPH include the following:

- Heavy vaginal bleeding with peripad saturation in 15 minutes or less
- Constant trickling or oozing of blood from the vagina
- Uterine atony

· **WORD** · **BUILDING** ·

subinvolution: sub–beneath or less than normal + involu–turning in + tion–action

- Passing of blood clots larger than a quarter in diameter
- Return of lochia rubra after the lochia has progressed to serosa or alba
- Cool, clammy, pale skin
- Tachycardia and decreased blood pressure (These are late signs that may not appear until a significant amount of blood is lost; Smith, 2022)

Care for the woman experiencing a PPH is a collaborative process of the health-care team. The nurse is usually the first person to identify excessive bleeding. Most obstetric units have an emergency protocol for managing PPH, which may include notifying a rapid response team to assist during the crisis. Management for the woman experiencing PPH includes the following:

- When excessive vaginal blood loss is observed, immediately begin fundal massage. Support the lower uterine segment to prevent uterine prolapse. It is important *not* to express clots by over-massage or by applying too much pressure on the uterus if it remains boggy. The clots may be providing pressure at the placental site and reducing blood loss.
- Stay with the patient and continue fundal massage with continual lower segment support, vital signs measurement, observation of the patient's level of consciousness, and monitoring the amount of vaginal bleeding.
- Send another team member to notify the physician or nurse midwife of the suspected hemorrhage and call the rapid response team, if that is hospital policy.
- Weigh peripads and linens on a gram scale to obtain an accurate measurement of the amount of blood lost. Visual estimation of blood has been proven to be inaccurate. One gram equals 1 milliliter of fluid (Layden et al., 2023).
- Observe the patient's bladder and, if distended, insert an indwelling Foley catheter to empty the bladder and to check urinary output and kidney status.
- Maintain or initiate IV fluids. Appropriate fluids are isotonic fluids, albumin, and packed red blood cells

(PRBCs) to maintain blood volume per health-care provider's order.
- Monitor oxygen saturation with a pulse oximeter and apply oxygen at 2 to 3 L via nasal cannula to increase red blood cell saturation. If the PPH continues uncontrolled, increase the oxygen liter flow as needed to increase the oxygen saturation.
- Elevate the patient's legs to a 20- to 30-degree angle to improve venous blood return.
- Provide psychosocial support to the patient and her family.
- Administer oxytocic medications if ordered by the health-care provider. See Table 13.1 for more information about these medications.
- The health-care provider may perform a bimanual compression of the uterus by placing one hand on the abdomen and the other hand as a fist inside the vagina (Fig. 13.1).
- If massage, compression, and medications are not successful in slowing bleeding, the patient may be moved to the operating room. There the patient is sedated, and the vagina and uterus are visualized. Lacerations are repaired, and retained placental fragments are removed via dilation and curettage (D&C). Other procedures that may be performed include occluding the bleeding vessel with a clot, ligating a uterine artery, packing the uterus, or performing a hysterectomy.

Safe and Effective Nursing Care

Rapid recognition of the signs of PPH is essential for successful management. Routine nursing observation and documentation of uterine tone, vaginal blood loss, and vital signs must be performed during the immediate postpartum period.

After the emergency is over, the team should debrief and discuss the management of care for this patient as a way to improve patient care in the future. The patient and her family should be encouraged to ask questions and express their feelings about the emergency. As soon as the woman is stabilized, she should be encouraged to resume bonding with and breastfeeding her newborn.

Labs & Diagnostics

If a patient with PPH requires an emergency blood transfusion, O-negative blood is ordered while the laboratory completes a type and crossmatch of the patient's blood and obtains the correct blood type and Rh. O-negative blood is the universal donor because it will not cause a blood transfusion reaction.

Table 13.1

Medications for Postpartum Hemorrhage

Medication	Action	Dose	Nursing Implications
Oxytocin	Stimulates uterine smooth muscle contractions. Also has a diuretic effect and vasopressor effect (constricts blood vessels and raises blood pressure).	10–40 units in 1,000 mL of IV fluids infused at 20–40 milliunits per minute or 10 units IM	• Infuse with pump for accurate infusion rate. • This medication can cause water intoxication. Monitor for signs and symptoms such as drowsiness, confusion, and headache. • Medicate for uterine cramping if needed.
Methylergonovine	Directly stimulates uterine and vascular smooth muscle.	0.1–0.2 mg IM, then oral 0.2 mg q4–6h for 24 hours	• This medication is not effective if the patient has hypocalcemia. • This medication is usually refrigerated and only stable at room temperature for 60 days. • Use only if clear, colorless, and has no precipitate.
Carboprost	Stimulates the smooth muscle of the uterus and the gastrointestinal tract.	250 mcg deep IM, repeat prn q15–90 minutes, no more than 2,000 mcg or eight doses	• This medication is used after oxytocin and/or methylergonovine have been tried to control PPH. • In addition to cramping, major side effects include nausea and vomiting. Consider an antiemetic if needed. • Keep refrigerated. • This medication is very expensive.
Misoprostol	Acts as a prostaglandin analogue (similar to prostaglandin) to stimulate contractions.	600–1,000 mcg rectally	• This medication is effective to control PPH, but this is an off-label use, which means it is not marketed by the manufacturer for this purpose.

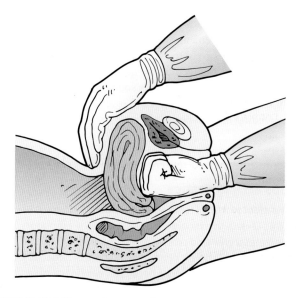

FIGURE 13.1 Bimanual compression.

 ## CARE OF THE WOMAN WITH A HEMATOMA

A **hematoma** is a collection of blood outside a blood vessel. The blood accumulates because the wall of an artery, a vein, or a capillary has been damaged, and blood leaks into tissues surrounding the vessel. The hematoma can be small or large and can cause significant swelling and pain. During childbirth, there is pressure and trauma to the genital tract. Common locations for hematomas are in the vaginal wall or the vulvar area (Figs. 13.2 and 13.3). Risk factors for hematoma formation during or after childbirth are episiotomy, lacerations to the genital tract, instrumental delivery (using forceps or vacuum extraction), nulliparity, and a difficult or prolonged second stage of labor (Oong & Eruo, 2023). The signs and symptoms of a hematoma are as follows:

• Constant pain and pressure in the vagina or rectal area
• Discoloration (bruising) and bulging of the tissue

Nursing Care Plan for the Postpartum Patient Experiencing Hemorrhages

Jasmine delivered her fifth child, a 9 lb 8 oz boy, 3 hours ago. She has saturated four peripads in the past hour despite frequent fundal massage from the postpartum nurse. Jasmine is experiencing a PPH.

Nursing Diagnosis: Decreased fluid volume because of uterine atony and evidenced by vaginal bleeding and increased heart rate and decreased blood pressure
Expected Outcome: Vital signs will return to normal, and bleeding will decrease.

Interventions:	Rationale:
Perform uterine fundal massage with one hand while the other hand supports the lower uterine segment.	*Uterine massage stimulates uterine contractions, and correct hand placement prevents uterine prolapse.*
Change peripads and weigh them on a gram scale to determine the amount of blood loss.	*Observing blood loss on a peripad is subjective. Weighing will give an accurate assessment of blood loss.*
Monitor vital signs.	*Changes in vital signs are late signs of excessive blood loss, so you need to be alert to subtle changes.*
Evaluate the urinary bladder.	*A full urinary bladder prevents uterine involution.*
Infuse isotonic IV fluids per hospital protocol.	*Isotonic fluids will increase fluid volume.*
Infuse oxytocic medications per the health-care provider's orders.	*Oxytocic medications such as oxytocin, methylergonovine, and carboprost are effective in improving uterine muscle tone.*

Nursing Diagnosis: Decreased tissue perfusion because of excessive vaginal bleeding
Expected Outcome: Vital signs and blood gases fall within normal limits.

Interventions:	Rationale:
Monitor vital signs and oxygen saturation levels every 5 to 10 minutes.	*Changes in tissue perfusion will cause changes in vital signs and oxygen saturation levels.*
Note the discoloration of the nailbeds, lip mucosa, gums, and tongue and note the skin temperature.	*With blood being shunted to vital organs, vasoconstriction occurs in peripheral tissues, causing cyanosis and cold skin temperature.*
Monitor blood gas levels and pH per hospital hemorrhage protocol.	*Changes in blood gases and pH levels are a sign of tissue hypoxia.*
Administer oxygen via nasal cannula.	*Supplemental oxygen increases the amount of oxygen in the red blood cells.*

Nursing Diagnosis: Anxiety and fear because of excessive blood loss and the threat of death
Expected Outcome: The patient can verbalize her anxiety; anxiety is under control for the patient.

Interventions:	Rationale:
Evaluate the patient's psychological response to the postchildbirth bleeding.	*The patient's perceptions of the situation influence the intensity of her anxiety.*
Explain the treatments and rationale.	*Anxiety is reduced when the patient understands the treatment plan.*
Remain calm, empathetic, and supportive.	*If you are anxious, the patient will become more anxious.*

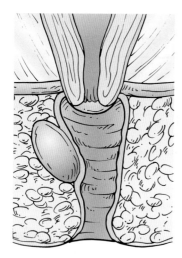

FIGURE 13.2 Vaginal wall hematoma.

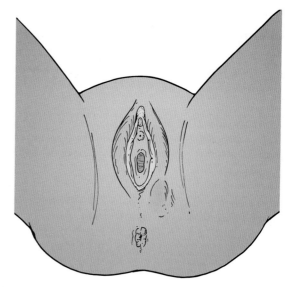

FIGURE 13.3 Vulvar hematoma.

- Tenderness of the tissue
- A feeling of needing to defecate because of pressure on the rectum
- Inability to urinate because of pressure on the urethra
- Possible signs of shock if the hematoma is large

If the signs and symptoms indicate a possible hematoma, carefully observe the perineal area by having the patient turn to her side and gently lift the upper buttock to inspect for swelling and discoloration. Any abnormal findings should be reported immediately to the health-care provider. Medical management of a hematoma includes the following:

- If the hematoma is less than 3 to 5 cm in size, ice is applied for 20 minutes every 2 hours for about 12 hours; then warm sitz baths are prescribed. The sitz bath will provide comfort and assist with reabsorption of the clot.
- Pain medication is ordered.
- If the hematoma is larger than 5 cm, the woman may be taken to the operating room for sedation so that the hematoma can be drained (Barrett, 2020; Layden et al., 2023).
- If significant blood loss has occurred, the patient is managed according to PPH protocol.

Nursing care for the patient with a hematoma includes the following:

- Evaluating pain and administering pain medication
- Applying an ice pack for 20 minutes every 2 hours for 12 hours, followed by a warm sitz bath
- If the hematoma is visible externally, frequently checking it to determine if the hematoma is changing in size
- Monitoring vital signs for signs of shock
- Explaining each treatment and the rationale for it to the patient

CARE OF THE WOMAN WITH A UTERINE INFECTION

Women who experience a prolonged labor or a prolonged rupture of membranes, who undergo internal monitoring, who experience a cesarean delivery, or who have frequent vaginal infections are at risk for a uterine infection, also known as *endometritis*. Bacteria normally present in the vagina and cervix, such as *Escherichia coli* and group B streptococcus (GBS), can enter the uterus and infect the lining of the uterus after the rupture of membranes. The signs and symptoms of endometritis are these:

- Elevated temperature at or above 38°C (100.4°F) for 2 or more consecutive days
- Foul-smelling lochia (Scanty, odorless lochia may be noted when the infection is caused by group A-hemolytic streptococci [Boushra & Rahman, 2022].)
- Lower abdominal tenderness on one or both sides of the abdomen

Medical management for endometritis may include the following:

- Pelvic examination to obtain specimens for culture
- Complete blood cell count (CBC)
- Blood cultures, if severe infection is suspected
- Pelvic ultrasound to detect retained placenta, abscess, or infected hematoma
- Administration of IV fluids and antibiotics (Layden et al., 2023; see Table 13.2 for information about commonly prescribed antibiotics for postpartum infections)

Table 13.2
Antibiotics for Postpartum Infections

Antibiotic and Dosing	Infection Type	Nursing Implications
Cefoxitin 1 g every 6–8 hours IM or IV	Endometritis Wound	• Obtain a history of previous use of cephalosporins and allergic reactions to penicillins. • Observe the patient for signs and symptoms of allergic reaction, such as rash, shortness of breath, or wheezing, and report immediately. • Monitor bowel function. Immediately report diarrhea, abdominal pain, fever, or bloody stools.
Gentamicin 1–2 mg/kg every 8 hours IV	Endometritis	• Obtain a history of allergies and a previous use of aminoglycosides. • Monitor for injury to the eighth cranial nerve, such as tinnitus and hearing loss. Report immediately.
Clindamycin 300–600 mg every 6–8 hours IV	Endometritis Mastitis	• Obtain a history of previous allergies and use of clindamycin. • Monitor bowel function. Immediately report diarrhea, abdominal pain, fever, or bloody stools.
Dicloxacillin 125–250 mg every 6 hours PO	Mastitis UTI	• Obtain a history of allergies and previous use of penicillins. • Monitor for the side effects of diarrhea, nausea, and vomiting.
Cephalexin 500 mg every 6 hours PO	Mastitis UTI Wound	• Obtain a history of previous use of cephalosporins and allergic reactions to penicillins. • Observe the patient for signs and symptoms of allergic reaction, such as rash, shortness of breath, or wheezing, and report immediately.
Cefazolin 500 mg–2 g every 6–8 hours IV	Wound	• Obtain a history of allergies and previous use of cephalosporins and penicillins. • Observe the patient for signs and symptoms of allergic reaction, such as rash, shortness of breath, or wheezing, and report immediately.
Ciprofloxacin 500–750 mg every 12 hours PO	UTI	• Obtain a history of allergies and previous use of fluoroquinolones. • Monitor bowel function. Immediately report diarrhea, abdominal pain, fever, or bloody stools.

Source: Vallerand, A. H., & Sanoski, C. A. (2023). *Davis's drug guide for nurses* (18th ed.). F. A. Davis.

Nursing care for the patient with endometritis includes the following:

• Administering IV fluids and antibiotics
• Administering pain medication and antipyretics for the fever as ordered
• Encouraging fluid intake and foods that boost the immune system such as protein; vitamins A, C, and E; and zinc (Suplee & Janke, 2020)
• Explaining each treatment and rationale to the patient
• Supporting her with bonding and breastfeeding (Chen, 2023)

 CARE OF THE WOMAN WITH A WOUND INFECTION

For the postpartum patient, wound infections can occur in the episiotomy incision, perineal lacerations, and in cesarean incisions. Signs and symptoms of a wound infection for postpartum patients include the following:

• Redness
• Warmth
• Poor wound approximation
• Tenderness

- Pain
- Fever and malaise if wound is untreated (Boushra & Rahman, 2022)

Medical management of a postpartum wound infection usually includes laboratory studies, such as a CBC and wound culture, and the administration of antibiotics.

Nursing care for the patient with a wound infection includes the following:

- Obtaining a wound culture if ordered
- Administering antibiotics as ordered
- Encouraging adequate fluid intake and protein intake to aid in healing
- Evaluating for pain and medicating as ordered
- Teaching the patient proper hand washing to prevent the spread of bacteria

 ## CARE OF THE WOMAN WITH A URINARY TRACT INFECTION

Urinary tract infections (UTIs) are common in the immediate postpartum phase. The urethra and bladder can be traumatized as the fetus moves through the birth canal for delivery. Women who have a Foley catheter during labor and women with prolonged labors are at higher risk for a UTI. The most common organisms causing a UTI are the normal bowel flora, including *E. coli* and *Klebsiella, Proteus,* and *Enterobacter* species (Brusch, 2023). Signs and symptoms of a UTI are as follows:

- Urgency of urination
- Dysuria (painful urination)
- Increased frequency of urination
- Urination of small amounts
- Fever
- Flank pain
- **Hematuria** (blood in the urine)

Medical management for the patient with a UTI is largely based on patient symptoms. It may include a urine specimen sent to the laboratory for a urinalysis, culture and sensitivity test, and oral antibiotics. See Table 13.2 for more information about appropriate antibiotics.

Nursing care for the patient with a UTI includes the following:

- Administering antibiotics as ordered
- Encouraging fluid intake to assist with flushing the bacteria out of the urinary tract
- Teaching the patient to clean the perineum from front to back and to use the peri-bottle provided for cleaning after urination and defecation

· WORD · BUILDING ·
hematuria: hemat–blood + ur–urine + ia–condition

 ### Safety *Stat!*

Sepsis is a life-threatening complication of an infection that can lead to multiple organ failure and death. Be alert for early signs of sepsis and report these symptoms immediately. Early symptoms include fever and chills, a low body temperature, rapid pulse, rapid breathing, nausea and vomiting, diarrhea, and decreased urine output (Cheshire, 2021).

CRITICAL THINKING

You are providing care for a postpartum patient who had a cesarean birth 2 days ago. You are about to remove the urinary catheter and the patient asks, "Can't you just leave it in for another day? It hurts so much to walk to the bathroom."

Question

1. What should you think about when answering this question?

CARE OF THE WOMAN WITH MASTITIS

Mastitis is an infection of the breast tissue. The most common organism to cause mastitis is *Staphylococcus aureus,* which is transmitted from the breastfeeding infant's mouth or throat. *S, aureus* is also present on the woman's hands. The bacteria can enter the mother's breast through cracked nipples caused by improper latch-on of the infant or by the mother touching her own breasts. Mastitis can also develop from blocked milk ducts and milk stasis, also caused by improper latch-on of the infant (Fig. 13.4; Pevzner & Dahan, 2020). Mastitis usually occurs in one breast with a sudden onset of symptoms. Signs and symptoms of mastitis are as follows:

- Red swollen area or mass in the breast
- Fever of 38°C (100.4°F) or higher
- Pain or a burning sensation while breastfeeding
- Skin redness, often in a wedge-shaped pattern
- Malaise
- Inflamed lymph nodes in the axilla

Medical management for mastitis is based upon a breast examination and consideration of symptoms. The health-care provider will determine if a breast abscess has developed, which is a possible serious complication of mastitis. Antibiotics and pain relievers, such as acetaminophen or ibuprofen, are usually ordered.

· WORD · BUILDING ·
mastitis: mast–breast + itis–inflammation

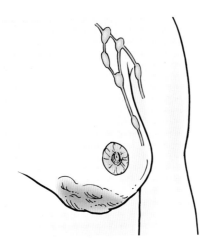

FIGURE 13.4 Mastitis usually occurs several weeks after childbirth. The axillary lymph nodes are enlarged, and there is a warm, tender, hardened area on the affected breast.

Nursing care for the patient with mastitis includes the following:

- Teaching the mother to wash her hands before handling her breasts for breastfeeding
- Observing latch-on of her infant and teaching the correct method of latch-on
- Referring the woman to a lactation specialist if needed
- Teaching the woman to feed the infant regularly to decrease the risk of milk stasis and blocked milk ducts caused by engorgement
- Administering antibiotics as ordered
- Evaluating pain and administering analgesics as ordered
- Reassuring the patient that she can continue to breastfeed while undergoing treatment
- Applying warmth to the breast to cause vasodilation and opening of the milk ducts
- Teaching every breastfeeding patient the signs of mastitis because it can happen anytime while a woman is breastfeeding

CARE OF THE WOMAN WITH POSTPARTUM THROMBOEMBOLIC DISEASE

Pregnancy increases the risk for venous thromboembolism (VTE) four to five times over what is observed in the general population (Springel, 2022). **Thromboembolism** is a condition in which the blood vessel becomes inflamed and a blood clot develops. A postpartum patient's risk for VTE is highest in the first 12 weeks after delivery. This is because of the pregnancy-related hypercoagulability caused by hormones and by sluggish blood flow to the legs during pregnancy and

delivery (Springel, 2022). The major causes of thrombosis are venous stasis, hypercoagulable blood, and injury to the endothelial surface of a blood vessel. A pregnant woman experiences compression of the large vessels in the leg and pelvis because of the weight of the uterus, causing venous stasis. During pregnancy, the fibrin levels are elevated, which can promote clot formation during pregnancy and during the postpartum recovery period. Blood vessels can be damaged by lower extremity trauma and prolonged labor and pushing. All of these factors that occur during pregnancy and delivery greatly increase the risk of thromboembolic disorders. About 1 in 1,000 pregnancies and deliveries is complicated by VTE. This condition includes deep vein thrombosis (DVT) and pulmonary embolism (PE; Mithoowani, 2024).

A **thrombus** is a clot made up of platelets and fibrin that develops on a vessel wall. A thrombus can form whenever the flow of blood is impeded. The vessel wall becomes inflamed because of the presence of the thrombus, and this inflammation is termed *thrombophlebitis*. A DVT is a blood clot that develops in a deep vein of the leg or pelvic region. The clot can become dislodged from the vein and travel to the lungs, causing a PE. A PE leads to extreme respiratory distress and is frequently fatal.

Risk factors for VTE are the following:

- Obesity
- Prolonged bedrest
- Advanced maternal age
- Stillbirth
- Premature birth
- Gestational diabetes
- Cesarean delivery
- Multiparity
- Varicose veins
- Smoking (Mithoowani, 2024)

You can prevent venous thromboembolic disorders by taking the following steps:

- Encouraging all postpartum patients to ambulate frequently
- Carefully observing the legs for signs of thromboembolic problems and promptly reporting any abnormal assessment findings
- Identifying women at high risk for thromboembolic disorders and obtaining orders for compression stockings or sequential compression devices (SCDs) to prevent venous stasis

Although some patients have no signs or symptoms, the typical signs and symptoms of VTE are these:

- Swelling
- Pain or tenderness
- Erythema
- Pain on ambulation
- Stiffness of the leg
- Large, hard, cordlike vein

· **WORD** · **BUILDING** ·

thromboembolism: thrombo–clot + embol–stopper + ism–condition

To definitively diagnose a VTE, the health-care provider will usually order a Doppler ultrasound of the leg or pelvis to identify a clot. If the ultrasound is unclear, magnetic resonance imaging (MRI) is recommended (Springel, 2022). Medical management of VTE includes the following:

- IV heparin therapy (Mithoowani, 2024) is used until the international normalized ratio (INR) has been at therapeutic levels for 2 days, followed by transition to oral warfarin for at least 6 to 12 weeks postpartum.
- Low-molecular weight heparin, such as enoxaparin, may be used instead of heparin.
- Compression stockings are used to improve blood flow in the legs.
- The woman is placed on bedrest with the affected leg elevated.
- Analgesics may be prescribed to control pain.
- Moist heat may be applied to reduce pain and increase circulation.

Labs & Diagnostics

The prothrombin time (PT) and/or the INR should be monitored when the patient is receiving anticoagulant therapy. The desired PT with anticoagulant therapy is 1.5 to 2 times the control PT in seconds. The desired INR is 2 to 3 (Van Leeuwen & Bladh, 2021).

Nursing care for the woman with thromboembolic disorders includes the following:

- Administering heparin or enoxaparin as ordered
- Monitoring the INR and PT and notifying the health-care provider of results
- Applying compression stockings correctly; improper application impedes blood flow, causing venous stasis
- Maintaining bedrest for the patient with the affected leg elevated
- Measuring the calf if the legs are asymmetric to monitor for increased swelling
- Administering analgesics as ordered
- Applying moist heat per hospital policy
- Monitoring for complications such as pulmonary emboli. The symptoms are shortness of breath, chest pain, and cough.

CARE OF THE WOMAN WITH POSTPARTUM DEPRESSION

Postpartum depression (PPD) is more serious and incapacitating than postpartum blues. It can interfere with a woman's ability to care for herself and her newborn. PPD occurs in 10% to 15% of women; although it usually develops during the first 4 months postpartum, it can occur anytime in the first year after childbirth (Mughal et al., 2022).

Women at highest risk of developing PPD are those with a personal history of depression or PPD with a previous birth. Other risk factors that have been identified are recent stressful life events, lack of social support, unintended pregnancy, and financial factors (Mughal et al., 2022).

Recognition of and prompt intervention for PPD are important for maternal and infant well-being. Signs and symptoms of PPD include the following:

- Intense sadness demonstrated by crying more than usual and feeling overwhelmed
- Feeling moody and irritable
- Anxiety or worrying
- Feelings of guilt or inadequacy
- **Ambivalence** toward the baby and family or avoiding the baby and family
- Lack of motivation for self-care or infant care
- **Anhedonia** (lack of pleasure) in everyday things such as the baby's milestones and enjoying time with her partner
- Appetite disturbances; eating too much or too little
- Insomnia, or being unable to sleep when the baby is sleeping
- Fatigue
- Thoughts of hurting the baby
- Suicidal thoughts and preoccupation with death

PPD is usually first noticed by the patient's partner and family. The health-care provider can use screening tools such as the Edinburgh Postnatal Depression Scale, a 10-item questionnaire used to detect postpartum depression. PPD can range from mild to severe. Untreated, it affects the mother, the infant, and the entire family. Early detection and initiation of treatment is associated with improved mother–baby attachment and a decreased risk of suicide.

Medical management of PPD usually includes counseling and antidepressant medications. Selective serotonin reuptake inhibitors (SSRIs) are the first-line treatment. Commonly prescribed SSRIs are fluoxetine, sertraline, paroxetine, and citalopram. Small amounts of these medications do transfer to the baby through breast milk, but medical studies show that the benefits of treating the mother's depression outweigh the small risk to the baby (Lefevre et al., 2022). The patient's symptoms usually start improving in 2 to 4 weeks.

Nursing care for the patient with PPD includes the following:

- Monitoring for signs of suicidal thoughts or thoughts to harm the baby
- Encouraging compliance in taking antidepressant medications

· WORD · BUILDING ·
ambivalence: ambi–in two ways + valence–attraction or feeling
anhedonia: an–without + hedon–pleasure + ia–condition

- Encouraging follow-up visits with her health-care provider
- Encouraging the patient to seek counseling
- Advising the patient to get rest and nap when the baby sleeps
- Making referrals to community agencies such as depression support groups
- Encouraging the patient's partner to locate practical sources of help for the mother such as extended family and friends to support her with socialization, meals, childcare, household help, and errands
- Encouraging the patient to verbalize her feelings and reinforce her personal power and autonomy (Lefevre et al., 2022)

CARE OF THE WOMAN WITH A POSTPARTUM PSYCHIATRIC DISORDER

Postpartum psychosis (PPP) is the most severe form of postpartum psychiatric illness. PPP causes the patient to lose touch with reality and inaccurately perceive the environment. It occurs in 1 to 2 per 1,000 postpartum women. The women at highest risk for PPP have a history of bipolar illness or a previous episode of PPP. This disorder typically has an abrupt onset within 48 to 72 hours of birth; most women who have it will manifest signs and symptoms by 2 weeks postpartum (Payne, 2021). Signs and symptoms of PPP include symptoms of PPD as well as:

- Incoherent conversations
- Rapidly shifting mood from depression to elation

- WORD - BUILDING -
psychosis: psych (mind) + osis (condition)

- Delusional beliefs that may relate to the infant; for example, she may think the baby is better off dead
- Auditory hallucinations that may tell her to harm herself or the infant

CRITICAL THINKING & CLINICAL JUDGMENT

Scenario #2: A patient has arrived for her 2-week postpartum visit at the obstetrics clinic. As you begin to obtain her vital signs and prepare her for her visit with the health-care provider, you ask, "Where's your baby today?" She mumbles incoherently and finally you understand her to say, "They think I'm not a good mother?" "You ask, "Who doesn't think you're a good mother?" She is avoiding eye contact, is restless, and doesn't answer your question.

Questions

1. What do you think is happening?
2. What should you do?

PPP is a medical emergency and requires hospitalization. The woman needs to be admitted to an inpatient psychiatric facility to begin mood stabilizers, antipsychotic medications, and psychotherapy (Raza & Raza, 2022).

Nursing care for the woman experiencing PPP includes the following:

- Immediately reporting any abnormal psychiatric symptoms to the health-care provider
- Reorienting the patient to her surroundings
- Providing for safety for the patient and her baby
- Arranging for admission to a psychiatric facility
- Providing emotional support for the patient and her family

Key Points

- In the first hour after birth, carefully monitor the patient for signs of PPH by palpating uterine involution and observing the amount of lochia.
- PPH is an emergency. Recognize early signs and notify the health-care provider for assistance.
- PPH is usually caused by one of the Four Ts: **t**one, **t**issue, **t**rauma, and **t**hrombosis.
- A hematoma is a collection of blood outside a blood vessel. In the postpartum patient, it is usually caused by the trauma of birthing. It can cause significant pain.
- A postpartum infection can occur in the uterus, lacerations or incisions, bladder, or breasts. Any signs or symptoms of an infection should be reported immediately.

- Preventing thrombophlebitis is important in the postpartum patient. It can be a serious complication that results in death from a PE. Pain, redness, and swelling of the leg must be reported immediately to the health-care provider.
- PPD can be debilitating. Teach the patient and her family the signs and symptoms so that PPD can be identified early and reported to the health-care provider.
- PPP is an emergency situation. Safety for the mother and newborn is the focus of care until the patient can be hospitalized and treated.

Review Questions

1. A patient delivered a 9-pound infant 1 hour ago. She had a forceps delivery and has just been transferred to postpartum care. She puts on her call light and reports severe rectal pain and pressure. The patient is most likely exhibiting signs of a(n) _____.

2. A postpartum patient states that she had PPD with her first baby 3 years ago. What is your best response?
   1. "It will probably not happen again."
   2. "Don't worry about that."
   3. "Have you mentioned this to your nurse midwife?"
   4. "Were you hospitalized last time?"

3. Which patient is at the highest risk to develop a postpartum infection?
   1. The patient who had a 24-hour labor
   2. The patient who delivered a 10-pound infant
   3. The patient who delivered her fifth child
   4. The patient who plans to bottle feed

4. A patient has developed mastitis. Which statement by the patient indicates that further teaching is needed?
   1. "I need to completely finish the antibiotics."
   2. "I need extra rest and fluids while on the antibiotics."
   3. "I must limit the time I feed on the infected breast."
   4. "I need to wash my hands before I breastfeed."

5. A woman calls the postpartum unit 2 weeks after discharge. She reports that her lochia has suddenly become heavier and that she is passing bright red clots. What should you do?
   1. Advise her to rest and call back if the bleeding does not slow down.
   2. Reassure her that it is the normal progression of lochia.
   3. Suggest that she eat a diet high in iron because she is losing more blood.
   4. Advise her to call her health-care provider.

6. During the postpartum focal assessment, you note that the patient has a fever of 38.9°C (102.2°F) and foul-smelling lochia. You report the findings to the health-care provider. Which of the following do you expect the health-care provider to order? **(Select all that apply.)**
   1. Methylergonovine 0.2 mg IM
   2. Gentamicin 1 to 2 mg/kg every 8 hours IV
   3. A culture of the lochia to be sent to the laboratory
   4. Strict isolation of the mother
   5. Pelvic ultrasound
   6. CBC

7. A patient who had a cesarean birth is 3 days postpartum. She reports to you that she gets a sudden urge to urinate and has to hurry to the bathroom and then is only able to urinate a small amount. What should you do?
   1. Report the symptoms.
   2. Reassure the patient that it is normal.
   3. Insert a Foley catheter.
   4. Place a bedside commode near her bed to make it easier for her.

8. A man calls the postpartum unit and says, "My wife had a baby 3 days ago. Today she started crying over nothing! I can't seem to do anything right today. Is this normal? I'm a little worried." How should you respond?
   1. Advise him to call the health-care provider immediately.
   2. Reassure him that it is normal but if she continues to be sad for several days to call the health-care provider.
   3. Tell him to stop worrying.
   4. Advise him to stop any behaviors that may be causing her to be upset.

ANSWERS 1. Hematoma; 2. 3; 3. 1; 4. 3; 5. 4; 6. 2, 3, 5, 6; 7. 1; 8. 2

CRITICAL THINKING QUESTION

1. Why are pregnant women and postpartum women predisposed to develop venous thrombosis?

Resources

For additional resources and information, including Postconference Questions and Activities, Answers, and References, visit www.FADavis.com.

Student Study Guide

CHAPTER 14

Physiological and Behavioral Adaptations of the Newborn

KEY TERMS

bilirubin (bil-ih-ROO-bin)
brown fat (BROWN FAT)
catecholamines (KAT-eh-KOH-luh-MEENZ)
conduction (kon-DUK-shun)
convection (kon-VEK-shun)
direct (conjugated) bilirubin (dih-REKT KON-joo-gayt-uhd bil-ih-ROO-bin)
evaporation (ih-VAP-o-RAY-shun)
glycogen (GLYE-ko-jen)
hypothermia (HYE-poh-THER-mee-uh)
indirect (unconjugated) bilirubin (IN-dih-REKT un-KON-joo-gayt-uhd bil-ih-ROO-bin)
jaundice (JON-diss)
probiotics (PROH-bye-OT-iks)
radiation (RAY-dee-AY-shun)
surfactant (ser-FAK-tent)

CHAPTER CONCEPTS

Comfort
Oxygenation
Reproduction and Sexuality
Thermoregulation

LEARNING OUTCOMES

1. Define the key terms.
2. Identify ways in which heat loss occurs in infants.
3. Describe how infants can produce body heat.
4. List nursing interventions that support thermoregulation in the newborn.
5. Discuss the role of external and internal stimuli in the initiation of breathing in the newborn.
6. Identify the changes that occur as fetal circulation transitions into newborn circulation after birth.
7. Plan appropriate nursing interventions to assist with the transitions of the renal and gastrointestinal systems after birth.
8. Discuss the role of the liver in conjugating bilirubin.
9. Differentiate between indirect (unconjugated) and direct (conjugated) bilirubin.
10. Define normal physiological jaundice.
11. Provide family-centered care by teaching parents about the behavioral changes and wake–sleep cycles of the newborn.

CRITICAL THINKING & CLINICAL JUDGMENT

Scenario #1: **Paloma**, aged 18, delivered her daughter 3 hours ago. You walk into the room and observe Paloma sitting upright on her bed with her legs folded and her newborn baby girl lying on the bed in front of her. The blanket and cap are off the baby, and she is dressed only in a T-shirt and diaper. Paloma is obviously happy about the baby and states to you, "I'm just checking out her fingers and toes again. She is so precious."

Questions

1. What should you think about while observing Paloma and her newborn?
2. What should you do and why?

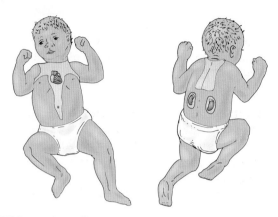

FIGURE 14.1 Sites of brown fat stores in the newborn.

Immediately after birth, the newborn begins critical adaptations to extrauterine life. All organ systems are involved at some level, but the most significant adaptations are in the respiratory and cardiovascular systems. This chapter discusses the physiological adaptations made by the newborn and nursing interventions that support the newborn in this transitional phase. Behavioral adaptations of the newborn are also discussed, along with patient teaching guidelines to assist the parents with understanding newborn behavioral adaptation.

PHYSIOLOGICAL ADAPTATIONS

The transition to extrauterine life actually begins before birth. The fetus is prepared for extrauterine life in the following ways:

- The fetal lungs develop and mature during the last trimester of pregnancy to support gas exchange at birth. **Surfactant**, a mixture of phospholipids and lipoproteins, is produced in the fetal lung cells. The production of surfactant begins around 24 weeks' gestation with distribution throughout the lungs starting at 28 to 32 weeks' gestation. Sufficient concentrations to prevent respiratory complications occur at 34 to 35 weeks' gestation (Khawar & Marwaha, 2022). It is important for the newborn because it prevents the alveoli from sticking together when the newborn takes the first few breaths and makes it easier for gas exchange to occur in the lungs.
- **Brown fat** is a body fat that is used by infants to regulate body temperature. An infant does not shiver to raise body temperature; they burn brown fat instead. The main function of brown fat is to protect the infant from hypothermia. It is deposited during the last few weeks of gestation. Brown fat is located in the scapular area, the thorax, and behind the kidneys (Fig. 14.1).
- Glucose is stored in the liver as **glycogen** to provide an energy source for the newborn at birth.
- During labor, the fetal adrenal glands are stimulated to produce **catecholamines**, which are the hormones dopamine, norepinephrine, and epinephrine. These hormones increase the level of surfactant in the fetal lungs; increase blood flow to the heart, lungs, and brain; increase energy; and stimulate white blood cell production in the immune system (Paravati et al., 2022).

Immediately after birth is a time of significant physiological adaptation for the baby. Physiologically, the infant must adapt or transition from being dependent on the placenta for oxygen and nutrients to independent functioning. Practically every body system undergoes transition at birth with the most significant changes requiring the successful initiation of respiratory function, cardiovascular function, and thermoregulation. Much of the work of transition to extrauterine life is accomplished in the first 4 to 6 hours following delivery (LaMonica, 2022).

Safety *Stat!*

Before the fetus is delivered, it is extremely important to determine if it may need support for the initial transition to extrauterine life. Infants who may need assistance with transition include premature infants, infants with a nonreassuring fetal heart rate pattern in labor, infants with shoulder dystocia, those who went through assistive deliveries, and those with the presence of meconium. Having necessary supplies and personnel on hand will help prevent delay in an infant receiving supportive and resuscitative interventions and will help improve the outcome.

• WORD • BUILDING •
hypothermia: hypo–deficient + therm–heat + ia–condition
surfactant: surf–surface + act–active + ant–agent

• WORD • BUILDING •
glycogen: glyco–sugar + gen–producer

Thermoregulation System

The temperature of a newborn is about 37.2°C (98.9°F) at birth because of the warm environment of the uterus. The infant begins to lose heat immediately after birth through four mechanisms:

- **Evaporation** is the loss of heat as the amniotic fluid on the infant evaporates (Fig. 14.2A).
- **Conduction** is the transfer of heat from the infant's body to cooler surfaces, such as towels or the cold base of a warming unit (Fig. 14.2B).
- **Convection** is the transfer of the infant's body heat to the surrounding cool air (Fig. 14.2C).
- **Radiation** is the transfer of the infant's body heat to a cooler object that the infant is not in contact with, such as a window (Fig. 14.2D).

It can take up to 4 hours for a newborn's temperature to stabilize. Infants do not have subcutaneous fat to provide insulation, and their blood vessels are close to the surface. Therefore, term infants rely on brown fat to provide additional heat if needed. Preterm infants may have no brown fat to assist with temperature regulation. To produce heat, the infant begins to metabolize the brown fat, also known as *non-shivering thermogenesis*. The infant's body constricts blood vessels in the skin, and the deeper vessels pick up heat from the metabolized brown fat to warm the body. The brown fat reserves can be quickly depleted if the newborn experiences prolonged cold stress. When this happens, brown fat breaks down into fatty acids, which can lead to metabolic acidosis in the newborn (Elshazel et al., 2022).

Newborns can also attempt to raise their body temperature by crying and by kicking, but they will quickly become fatigued from this effort (Davidson, 2020).

Careful attention needs to be paid to the thermal environment of the newborn until the infant is able to regulate body temperature. The prevention of cold stress is a priority. As the infant tries to increase body temperature, an increase in the metabolic rate occurs. The consequences of an increased metabolic rate in the cold newborn can be serious:

- An increased need for oxygen
- A decrease in surfactant production
- An increase in the use of stored glycogen, which can lead to hypoglycemia
- Rapid metabolism of brown fat, leading to metabolic acidosis

Nursing interventions for assisting the newborn's thermoregulation transition include the following:

- Drying the infant immediately after birth and removing the wet towels
- Placing the infant skin-to-skin with the mother as soon as possible and covering with a warmed blanket
- Covering the head with a hat as soon as possible
- Monitoring the newborn's temperature every 15 minutes for the first hour
- Avoiding uncovering or exposing the infant's entire body for procedures
- If unable to maintain skin-to-skin contact with a parent, placing the infant under a preheated radiant warmer for procedures
- Not bathing the newborn until the temperature has been stable for at least 2 hours
- Not placing the baby's crib near a draft or a window (Perez & Mendez, 2022)

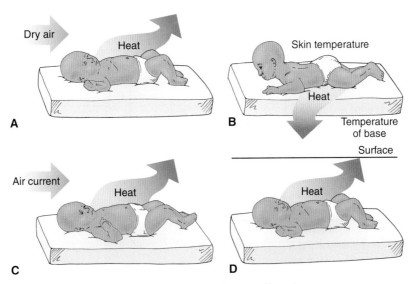

FIGURE 14.2 A, Evaporation mechanism of heat loss. B, Conduction mechanism of heat loss. C, Convection mechanism of heat loss. D, Radiation mechanism of heat loss.

Respiratory System

While in the uterus, the fetal lungs are full of fluid, and the fetus receives its oxygen through the umbilical cord. The fetal circulation picks up oxygen from the placenta, and the umbilical vein transports the oxygenated blood to the fetal heart. Most blood bypasses the lungs because the placenta is supplying oxygen to the fetus. The clamping of the umbilical cord ends the flow of oxygenated blood from the placenta. When the infant is born, a sequence of events must happen in order for the infant to breathe, including internal and external stimuli. The internal stimuli are chemically focused, and the external stimuli are related to mechanical, sensory, and thermal changes in the newborn's body.

First, the external stimuli begin as the fetus moves through the birth canal. Pressure on the chest causes the lung secretions and amniotic fluid inside the lungs to be squeezed out through the airway. Next, when the chest fully emerges from the birth canal, the chest reexpands or recoils, causing an intake of air to fill the lungs. The first few breaths are critical: The lungs are adjusting to pressure changes from the intrauterine environment to outside the mother's body. Blood flow to the lungs increases, and the alveoli are forced open. Surfactant secretion increases to keep the alveoli open after the initial breaths (Ohning, 2021).

After the first few breaths, breathing is easier for the infant. As the infant is dried vigorously, sensors in the skin are stimulated, which further encourage the respiratory center to begin the first sequences of breathing.

Internally, chemical factors influence the newborn to breathe. After the umbilical cord is cut, the newborn experiences a decrease in oxygen concentration, an increase in carbon dioxide, and a drop in the pH in the blood. These chemical changes trigger the medulla to stimulate the respiratory center in the brain to begin functioning (Fig. 14.3; Elshazel et al., 2022).

Nursing interventions for assisting the newborn with the respiratory transition after birth include the following:

• Counting the respirations per minute
• Suctioning the mouth and nose with the bulb syringe to clear mucus
• Monitoring the respiratory effort
• Observing the abdomen because newborn breathing involves the use of the diaphragm and abdominal muscles

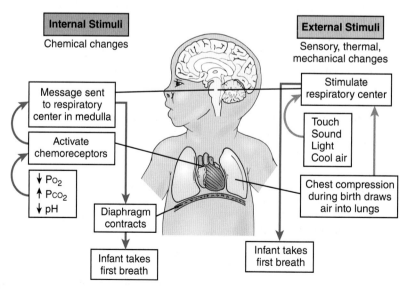

FIGURE 14.3 Chemical, sensory, thermal, and mechanical factors involved in the initiation of respirations. P_{CO_2}, partial pressure of carbon dioxide; P_{O_2}, partial pressure of oxygen.

Nursing Care Plan for Regulating the Newborn's Body Temperature

A 2-hour-old newborn is placed in his crib in his mother's room so that she can rest. Because he is no longer being kept warm by his mother, you will want to prevent heat loss.

Nursing Diagnosis: Risk for decreased body temperature related to a large surface-area-to-body-mass ratio and lack of subcutaneous fat for insulation
Expected Outcome: The newborn's axillary body temperature will remain in the normal range of 36.5°C to 37.2°C. (97.7°F to 98.9°F)

Interventions:	Rationale:
Monitor body temperature frequently.	*Frequent monitoring of the baby's temperature will allow early detection of a body temperature that is dropping.*
Keep the baby wrapped appropriately with a blanket if not skin-to-skin with a parent.	*Wrapping the baby will prevent heat loss through the skin.*
Keep the head covered with a cap.	*An infant can lose body heat quickly through the head.*
Do not place the infant's crib near a draft or a window.	*The infant can lose body heat by convection.*

Safe and Effective Nursing Care

Allowing the newborn short bursts of crying will increase the depth of respirations and aid in opening the alveoli at birth. However, prolonged crying is not safe for the newborn because it will tire the infant and force the infant's body to use up stored glycogen for energy.

Cardiovascular System

After the newborn starts breathing and the umbilical cord is cut, changes occur in blood flow, pressure, and volume within the heart. The fetal circulation is no longer effective, and blood flows in a new route (Fig. 14.4). See Table 14.1 for circulation changes that occur during newborn transition.

A newborn's blood volume is 80 to 110 mL/kg, and a newborn has more red blood cells than the average adult. These red blood cells provide extra oxygenation for the stress of labor. A newborn's hemoglobin averages 14.5 to 22.5/100 mL of blood, and the hematocrit is between 44% and 68% (Van Leeuwen & Bladh, 2021).

After the stress of labor has passed and oxygenation through the lungs is established, the large number of red blood cells is not needed by the newborn. Within days, the extra red blood cells begin to break down. As they are broken down, **bilirubin**, the waste product of the breakdown of the red blood cells, is released, and the serum indirect (unconjugated) bilirubin level rises.

The normal term newborn also has an elevated white blood cell count, ranging from 15,000 to 30,000 cells/mm^3. An elevated white blood cell count in a newborn does not reflect infection but does reflect how stressful the birth was for the infant.

Newborns have a diminished ability to clot blood because of the absence of vitamin K. Vitamin K is essential for the formation of factor II (prothrombin), factor VII (proconvertin), factor IX (plasma thromboplastin component), and factor X (Stuart-Prower factor) in the clotting sequence. In humans, vitamin K is synthesized by bacteria in the intestines. A newborn has a sterile intestine at birth and does not have enough of these bacteria, or intestinal flora, to synthesize vitamin K until about 24 hours after birth. (See Chapter 9 for more information about vitamin K injections.)

Nursing interventions for assisting the newborn with the cardiovascular transition after birth include the following:

- Monitor the heart rate immediately after birth. If lower than 100 bpm, stimulate the baby to breathe. If ineffective in increasing the heart rate, use positive pressure ventilation with room air at a low pressure to increase oxygenation, which will increase the heart rate.
- Begin chest compressions if the heart rate is below 60 bpm. When beginning chest compressions, monitor the color of the trunk and mucous membranes and the capillary refill time of the trunk. Keep in mind that the normal newborn may have decreased peripheral circulation and bluish hands and feet (Ohning, 2021).

· **WORD** · **BUILDING** ·
bilirubin: bili–bile + rubin–red

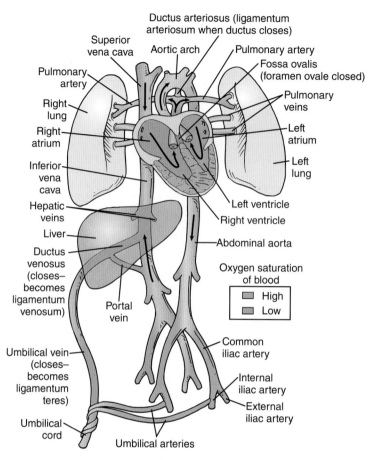

FIGURE 14.4 Neonatal circulation.

Evidence-Based Practice

Newborns frequently undergo painful procedures, such as venipuncture, to check for jaundice. A study was conducted to determine the best method of controlling pain in the newborn during the venipuncture procedure. The newborns were divided into three groups. The first group was swaddled before the procedure. The second group was given sucrose water before and during the procedure. The third group was swaddled and given sucrose water before and during the procedure. A neonatal pain scale was used to monitor the newborn's pain reaction. The third group that was swaddled and given sucrose water demonstrated the lowest pain severity.

Talabi, M., Amiri, S. R. J., Roshan, P. A., Zabihi, A., Zahedpasha, Y., & Chehrazi, M. (2022). The effect of concurrent use of swaddle and sucrose on the intensity of pain during venous blood sampling in neonate: A clinical trial study. *BMC Pediatrics, 22*, 263. https://doi .org/10.1186/s12887-022-03323-0

Renal System

The kidneys of the newborn are immature and do not concentrate urine well until the baby is about 6 weeks old. The urine of a newborn will be odorless and a light color or clear.

The newborn should void within 24 hours of birth with a volume of about 15 mL. For the first 2 days of life, the total daily output should be about 30 to 60 mL. As the newborn ingests more breast milk or formula, the volume should rise to 300 mL per day.

Nursing interventions for assisting the newborn with the renal transition after birth include the following:

- Monitoring the first void
- Weighing diapers if concerned about urinary output
- Encouraging frequent breastfeeding to increase fluid intake and therefore urine output

Patient Teaching Guidelines

Parents do not have a way to measure urine output except by diaper count. They should be instructed to expect the number of wet diapers per day to equal the age of the baby for the first week. For example, a 2-day-old baby should have a minimum of two wet diapers. A 3-day-old baby should have a minimum of three wet diapers. By the end of the week, most breastfeeding mothers have a good milk supply, and the wet diaper count should be six to eight per day, the same as for bottle-fed babies.

Table 14.1
Cardiovascular Changes After Birth

Fetal Circulation	*Postbirth Status*
Pulmonary Circulation	
• Decreased blood flow through the lungs	• Increased blood flow through the lungs
Systemic Circulation	
• Higher pressure in the right ventricle • Lower pressures in the left atrium, left ventricle, and aorta	• Decreased pressure in the right ventricle • Increased pressure in the left atrium, left ventricle, and aorta
Ductus Arteriosus	
• Allows blood to bypass the fluid-filled lungs by shunting blood from the pulmonary artery to the aorta	• Closes almost immediately after birth or may remain open or partially open for up to 15 hours after birth to allow increased blood flow to the lungs to permit oxygenation • May remain open if the lungs fail to expand • Anatomical obliteration within 1–3 months
Ductus Venosus	
• Shunts a portion of the left umbilical vein blood flow to the inferior vena cava, allowing blood to bypass the liver	• When the cord is clamped and blood flow is stopped, it closes completely by day three and forms a ligament
Foramen Ovale	
• An opening that allows blood to flow directly to the right atrium and bypass the lungs	• Functionally closes at birth when increased pressure in the left atrium and decreased pressure in the right atrium occur • Constant circulation leads to permanent closure within a few months
Umbilical Arteries	
• Carry deoxygenated blood from the hypogastric arteries to the placenta	• Blood flow disrupted when the umbilical cord is cut • Closed within hours of birth and permanently gone by 2–3 months
Umbilical Vein	
• Carries blood from the placenta, ductus venosus, and liver to the inferior vena cava	• Closed when the umbilical cord is cut and eventually forms a ligament

Sources: Davidson, M. R. (2020). *Fast facts for the neonatal nurse* (2nd ed.). Springer Publishing Company. https://doi.org/10.1891/9780826184917; Elshazel, M., Anekar, A. A., & Shumway, K. P. (2022). Physiology, newborn. *StatPearls NIH*. https://www.statpearls.com/ArticleLibrary/viewarticle /36205; Layden, A., Thompson, A., Owen, P., Madhra, M., & Magowan, B. A. (2023). *Clinical obstetrics and gynecology*. Elsevier.

Gastrointestinal System

The newborn's gastrointestinal tract is sterile at birth, but bacteria enter the mouth during birth through vaginal secretions and shortly after birth through hospital linens and contact at the breast. These bacteria become **probiotics**, intestinal bacteria that aid in digestion and synthesize vitamin K.

The capacity of the newborn stomach is about 60 to 90 mL. The pancreas is immature in the newborn; the enzymes lipase and amylase, which help to digest fat and starch, are deficient for the first few months of life. In addition, the cardiac sphincter between the esophagus and stomach is weak, which allows the infant to regurgitate easily.

The meconium stool, which is composed of sticky, blackish green material made from mucus, vernix, lanugo, hormones, and carbohydrates that accumulated in the bowel during fetal development, should be expelled within 24 to 48 hours of birth (Davidson, 2020).

· WORD · BUILDING ·

probiotic: pro–for + biot–life + ic–pertaining to

Nursing interventions for assisting the newborn with the gastrointestinal transition after birth include the following:

• Monitoring for the meconium stool and reporting if not expelled within 24 hours
• Teaching parents not to overfeed the newborn
• Teaching parents about the immature cardiac sphincter and regurgitation

Hepatic System

At birth, the liver serves to store glycogen and iron. The immature liver does not detoxify medications or break down bilirubin from red blood cells efficiently. Within days of birth, the extra red blood cells that were necessary to provide oxygenation begin to break down, releasing bilirubin. The liver's job is to remove this **indirect (unconjugated) bilirubin** from circulation and convert, or conjugate, it to a form that can be excreted. Indirect (unconjugated) bilirubin in the circulation causes a yellow discoloration of the skin (**jaundice**).

Therapeutic Communication

You observe a mother bottle feeding her 1-day-old infant. The infant is showing no interest in the feeding and is taking his mouth off the bottle nipple. You notice that the mother is trying to force-feed the infant to finish off the bottle of formula. Using therapeutic communication, you discuss newborn feeding with the mother.

Nurse: "It looks like your little guy is done eating."
Mother: "But he hasn't finished. I want him to get enough to eat."
Nurse: "Actually, it looks like he has taken in about an ounce. That's about all his tiny stomach can hold today."
Mother: "Really? That's not much."
Nurse: "Yes, he can hold about an ounce or a tiny bit more. Every day his stomach gets a little bigger. He will give you cues when he is hungry or done eating. Sometimes overfeeding makes babies spit up even more. If he wakes up and acts hungry, offer him more."

During the conjugation process, the liver changes the yellow pigment from the breakdown of the red blood cell into a water-soluble pigment that can be excreted by the body. **Direct (conjugated) bilirubin** is excreted into the common duct and duodenum. Once the direct (conjugated) bilirubin is in the intestine, the normal intestinal flora reduce it further, and it is excreted mainly as yellowish-brown stool. A small amount of direct bilirubin is excreted in the urine (Fig. 14.5). Because the newborn liver is immature and the number of unneeded red blood cells is large, the job of breaking down and removing the bilirubin is not accomplished efficiently, causing a large number of babies

• WORD · BUILDING ·
conjugated: con–with + jugated–joined

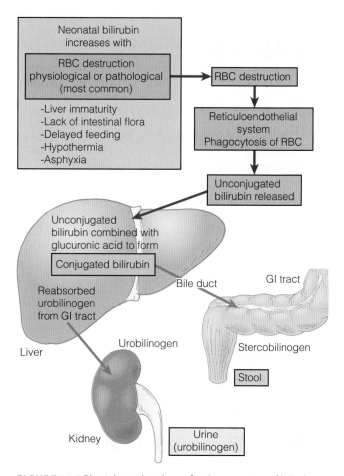

FIGURE 14.5 Physiological pathway for the excretion of bilirubin. GI, gastrointestinal; RBC, red blood cell.

to develop a normal physiological jaundice by days two to four (Rohan, 2020).

Nursing interventions for assisting the newborn with the hepatic transition after birth include the following:

• Monitoring for yellow sclera and skin and reporting findings
• Teaching the parents about normal physiological jaundice

Labs & Diagnostics

The bilirubin and bilirubin fractions laboratory test is also known as the *conjugated/direct bilirubin, unconjugated/indirect bilirubin test*. This test provides the health-care provider with the level of bilirubin in the newborn's body. An expected range for a newborn is lower than 5.8 mg/dL total bilirubin. However, the total bilirubin level will rise and should peak by day five but should be below 11.7 mg/dL to be considered normal physiological jaundice. Elevated levels must be reported (Van Leeuwen & Bladh, 2021).

CRITICAL THINKING & CLINICAL JUDGMENT

Scenario #2: You walk into a postpartum room and see a new mother holding her 8-hour-old newborn. You notice that the newborn has a yellow tint to his eyes and his skin is slightly yellow.

Questions

1. Newborn jaundice is not unusual, but what warning sign do you recognize in this situation?
2. What should you do next and why?

Learn to C.U.S.

You are evaluating a 2-hour-old infant and notice a faint yellow tint to the skin. Knowing that normal physiological jaundice is not visible until days two to four, you are concerned and call the pediatrician, using the C.U.S. method of communication.

C: "Hello, doctor. I am calling because I am *concerned* about baby Ramirez.

U: I noticed that his skin is slightly yellow, and I am *uncomfortable* waiting for you to make rounds later today to see the infant.

S: I feel as if we have a patient *safety* problem. He could be sick. May I order a bilirubin test?"

Immune System

The newborn is born with passive antibodies (immunoglobulin G) passed on from the mother through the placenta. If the mother is fully vaccinated or has had these illnesses, the newborn is protected from polio, measles, diphtheria, pertussis, chicken pox, rubella, and tetanus. This passive immunity from the mother protects the infant for the first 2 to 4 months of life (Davidson, 2020). A newborn does not start producing their own antibodies until about 2 months of age.

Nursing interventions for assisting the newborn with the immune system transition after birth include the following:

- Maintaining strict hand washing for everyone who cares for the newborn

CRITICAL THINKING & CLINICAL JUDGMENT

Scenario #3: You are working at the desk on the postpartum unit. A grandparent of one of the newborn babies has called with a question. "I have a cold sore on my lip. I don't have any other symptoms such as a fever, cough, or runny nose. Is it okay if I visit my new grandson?"

Questions

1. What should you think about in this situation?
2. How should you respond to the grandparent?

- Protecting the newborn from infection
- Screening health-care personnel and visitors for illness
- Teaching the parents about hand hygiene for themselves, family members, and visitors
- **Encouraging the parents to begin immunizations at 2 months of age**

BEHAVIORAL ADJUSTMENT TO EXTRAUTERINE LIFE

Even though babies are nonverbal, they are extraordinary communicators. They initiate interaction by crying, quiet when soothed, and engage in mutual gazing. A newborn will demonstrate that they like something by focusing the eyes and tracking an object or person moving around the room. Newborns also demonstrate behaviors that indicate their dislikes, such as turning away, crying, and yawning. As babies transition into extrauterine life, they also learn to self-soothe by thumb or hand sucking.

Every baby is different, and parents begin to learn the personality and behaviors of their baby from the start. Nurses can assist parents to understand the behaviors of their newborn through education and by providing positive reinforcement to the parents as they care for and interact with their newborn.

Periods of Reactivity

All healthy newborns go through expected periods of alertness and sleepiness. The first period of reactivity occurs in the first 30 to 60 minutes after birth; during this time, the newborn is usually alert, active, and cooperative. A vigorous suck reflex is usually present, which makes this an excellent time to introduce latch-on for breastfeeding.

After this brief period of alertness, the newborn will fall into a deep sleep that can last 2 to 4 hours or longer. This is called *the period of relative inactivity* (Fig. 14.6). During this time, the newborn is unresponsive to external stimuli. The heart rate and respiratory rate both decrease but stay within the normal limits. The parents may have trouble waking the baby for feedings.

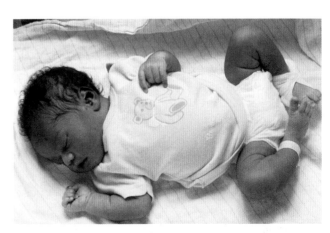

FIGURE 14.6 A newborn in deep sleep.

The second period of reactivity begins when the newborn wakes up from the long sleep and is again alert, active, and hungry. The heart rate will vary depending upon external stimuli, and periods of rapid respirations may be noted in response to stimuli. This is the time to encourage family interaction with the newborn and to educate the parents about hunger cues (Rohan, 2020).

Patient Teaching Guidelines

Sleep and Awake States

Parents can learn about their baby's mood by how they respond to touch, sights, and sounds. Newborn behavior typically falls within the following states:

- *Deep sleep:* The baby lies very still with an occasional twitch. Usually there are no eye movements, and breathing is regular. It is difficult to awaken the baby.
- *Light sleep:* This state is also known as *rapid eye movement sleep.* The eye movements may be visible beneath the eyelids, and the baby may occasionally fuss or make sucking movements. This state typically occurs right before the baby wakes up.
- *Drowsy:* The baby's eyes may open. The baby is not fully asleep and may go back to sleep or wake up more.
- *Alert:* The baby's eyes will be open. Breathing is regular, and the baby is attentive to what is going on. At this time, the baby is most interested in eating.
- *Active alert:* In this state, the baby is more active and may begin to chew on the hands or feet and may try to get in position for feedings. The baby is sensitive to hunger, discomfort, and fatigue. They may require comforting in this state.
- *Crying:* Crying is the way that a baby conveys that something is bothering them. The baby may need to be fed or burped, need to have the diaper changed, be bored or overstimulated, or need close physical contact (Rohan, 2020).

Key Points

- Thermoregulation can be difficult for the newborn because of their inability to conserve heat, which is caused by a large surface area relative to body mass and limited subcutaneous fat for insulation.
- Hypothermia in the newborn is preventable by reducing risks. You need to monitor the environment and the body temperature of the newborn and provide appropriate interventions to maintain a stable body temperature.
- Brown fat aids in body-temperature regulation. It is found in term newborns in the scapular area, the thorax, and behind the kidneys. The infant metabolizes the brown fat to produce heat. This metabolism of brown fat is known as *nonshivering thermogenesis.*
- Glycogen is stored in the liver to provide an energy source for the newborn at birth.
- The infant begins to lose heat immediately after birth through four mechanisms: evaporation, conduction, convection, and radiation.
- The sequence of events that causes the newborn to begin breathing includes internal stimuli and external stimuli.
- After birth, the fetal circulation is not effective, and changes occur that increase blood flow to the lungs and liver. The ductus arteriosus, ductus venosus, and foramen ovale close to redirect the blood flow through the newborn's body.
- The newborn's kidneys are immature and do not concentrate urine well for about 6 weeks. The urine will be odorless and a light color or clear. The newborn should void within 24 hours of birth.
- Bacteria begin entering the gastrointestinal tract during and shortly after birth through vaginal secretions, hospital linens, and contact at the breast. The bacteria aid in digestion and the synthesis of vitamin K.
- The meconium stool, which is composed of sticky, blackish green material made from mucus, vernix, lanugo, hormones, and carbohydrates that accumulated in the bowel during fetal development, should be expelled within 24 to 48 hours of birth.
- The immature liver is unable to change bilirubin released by the breakdown of red blood cells into a form that can be excreted by the body, causing a deposit of bilirubin in the skin (jaundice) to occur.
- The newborn is born with passive antibodies passed on from the mother through the placenta. A newborn cannot produce their own antibodies until about 2 months of age.
- The first period of reactivity occurs in the first 30 to 60 minutes after birth, and this is an excellent time to introduce breastfeeding and encourage bonding.
- The second period of reactivity begins when the newborn wakes up from the long sleep and is again alert, active, and hungry. This is the time to encourage family interaction with the newborn and to educate the parents about hunger cues.
- Newborns have periods of sleep and awake states. Nurses can educate and assist parents to understand the needs and behaviors of their newborn.

Review Questions

1. A newborn is in the active alert state. Which of the following would you expect to see?
   1. The newborn is crying vigorously.
   2. The newborn is attentive to what is going on around him.
   3. The newborn's eye movements are visible under the eyelids.
   4. The newborn is showing signs of hunger.

2. A term newborn has just been born. Which intervention is the highest priority?
   1. Conducting the 5-minute Apgar score
   2. Injecting vitamin K
   3. Removing wet blankets
   4. Applying the identification band

3. A newborn is in the first period of reactivity. Which of the following actions should you take at this time?
   1. Place the infant under the radiant warmer.
   2. Encourage bonding and breastfeeding.
   3. Perform a head-to-toe assessment.
   4. Invite extended family in to meet the baby.

4. A newborn has just been delivered. Which of the following physiological changes is of highest priority?
   1. Passing meconium stool
   2. Closure of the ductus venosus
   3. Spontaneous respirations
   4. Thermoregulation

5. A nurse has been teaching the mother of a 2-day-old infant about the risk for infection in the newborn. Which statement indicates that the mother needs further teaching?
   1. "The baby received some immunity from me through the placenta."
   2. "I plan to drop by my 5-year-old niece's birthday party at the pizza restaurant with my baby tomorrow."
   3. "I will ask any family or friends who want to hold my baby to wash their hands first."
   4. "Anyone who's sick should not visit my baby."

6. A baby can lose heat by evaporation if which of the following situations occurs?
   1. The mother unwraps the baby to show a visitor.
   2. You place the baby crib near the air conditioner vent.
   3. The baby is placed in a cold crib.
   4. The baby is wet from amniotic fluid.

7. How can you determine the successful transition of the respiratory system in the newborn? **(Select all that apply.)**
   1. Count the number of respirations per minute.
   2. Dry the baby thoroughly.
   3. Observe the chest and abdomen.
   4. Observe the capillary refill time of the foot.
   5. Observe the color of the mucous membranes.

8. Which of the following changes occur in the cardio-vascular system when the newborn transitions from the uterus to extrauterine life? **(Select all that apply.)**
   1. The right ventricle has increased pressure.
   2. There is increased blood flow through the lungs.
   3. Blood is shunted from the pulmonary artery to the aorta.
   4. The ductus arteriosus closes.
   5. Blood flow to the liver increases.

ANSWERS 1. 4; 2. 3; 3. 2; 4. 3; 5. 2; 6. 4; 7. 1, 3, 5; 8. 2, 4, 5

CRITICAL THINKING QUESTIONS

1. You are preparing to bathe a newborn. How can you promote the newborn's thermoregulation during this procedure?

2. Describe the adaptations that the heart and blood vessels undergo when converting from fetal to neonatal circulation.

Resources

For additional resources and information, including Postconference Questions and Activities, Answers, and References, visit www.FADavis.com.

Student Study Guide

CHAPTER 15

Nursing Care of the Newborn

KEY TERMS

acne neonatorum (AK-nee NEE-oh-nay-TOR-uhm)

acrocyanosis (AK-roh-sye-uh-NOH-siss)

apnea (AP-nee-ah)

caput succedaneum (KAP-uht SUK-se-DAY-nee-uhm)

cephalohematoma (SEF-al-oh-HEE-muh-TOH-muh)

circumcision (SER-kuhm-SIH-zhun)

dermal melanosis (DER-muhl MEL-uh-NOH-siss)

erythema toxicum neonatorum (air-ih-THEE-muh TOX-ih-kuhm NEE-oh-nay-TOR-uhm)

fontanel (FON-tuh-NEL)

gynecomastia (JIN-uh-koh-MASS-tee-uh)

hemangioma (HEEM-an-jee-OH-muh)

lanugo (la-NOO-goh)

melanocytic nevi (MEL-uh-noh-SIT-ik NEE-vee)

milia (MIL-ee-uh)

nevus flammeus (NEE-vuhss FLAM-ee-uhss)

nevus simplex (NEE-vuhss SIM-pleks)

postterm (POST-term)

preterm (PREE-term)

pseudomenstruation (SOO-doh-MEN-stroo-AY-shun)

retractions (rih-TRAK-shunz)

vernix caseosa (VER-niks KASS-ee-OH-suh)

CHAPTER CONCEPTS

Clinical Judgment
Communication
Growth and Development
Professionalism
Safety

LEARNING OUTCOMES

1. Define the key terms.
2. Define *physical evaluation*.
3. Identify normal newborn vital signs.
4. Demonstrate a head-to-toe evaluation of the newborn.
5. Summarize abnormal findings from the head-to-toe evaluation that must be reported.
6. Identify normal newborn skin variations.
7. Differentiate between cephalohematoma and caput succedaneum.
8. Explain the effects of maternal hormones on the newborn's physical characteristics.
9. Identify the normal newborn reflexes.
10. Discuss nursing care of the newborn.
11. Summarize the usual newborn screenings that are completed for health promotion.
12. Discuss Ballard's tool, which is used to determine gestational age.
13. Demonstrate the correct technique for an infant heel stick.
14. Demonstrate the correct technique for a newborn's bath.
15. Develop a discharge teaching plan on newborn care basics.
16. Plan family-centered care by including the family in discharge teaching.
17. Instruct the parents on newborn safety.

CRITICAL THINKING & CLINICAL JUDGMENT

Scenario #1: You are providing nursing care for a 2-hour-old male newborn at the bedside of a postpartum patient. You notice the following while caring for the newborn: axillary temperature of 36°C (96.8°F), respiratory rate of 42 breaths/min, heart rate of 150 bpm, bilateral crackles in the lower lung bases, the newborn's hands and feet are slightly blue, there are little "white heads" on the nose, and the infant actively moves the left arm but barely moves the right arm. When you removed the diaper, you noticed that the infant had a swollen scrotum and had passed a large, black, sticky stool.

Questions

1. Are you concerned about any of the physical findings? Why?
2. What should you do? Why?

CONCEPTUAL CORNERSTONE

Professionalism

Professionalism in nursing includes assessment/evaluation/data collection. Nursing evaluation is a systematic method of collecting data to identify problems and then plan safe and effective care for the patient. There are three different types of evaluation that you may use while caring for patients in the hospital. The first type is the initial, or baseline, evaluation that is done on admission to establish a baseline for reference and future comparison. This comprehensive evaluation is performed by a registered nurse. The second type of evaluation is problem-focused and is done to determine the status of a particular problem. This type of data collecting can be performed by a licensed vocational nurse who then reports the findings to the registered nurse. The third type is emergency evaluation, which is done to identify any life-threatening problems and may be performed by any nurse. Data-collecting techniques include observation, interviewing, and physical examination.

For this chapter, the concept of evaluation or data collection focuses on the baseline physical examination of the newborn. You will need an understanding of normal newborn physical characteristics and behaviors to be able to identify abnormal findings and potential problems to report to the health-care provider.

The nurse has an important role in the care of a newborn. The nurse is often the first health-care professional to physically examine and provide initial care for the newborn. Nurses also have the responsibility to teach parents basic newborn care so that they are prepared for discharge from the hospital. This chapter provides information about physical evaluation, nursing care of the newborn, and discharge teaching.

PHYSICAL EXAMINATION OF THE NEWBORN

After a baby is born, an Apgar score is given at 1 minute and again at 5 minutes. These scores provide a quick method of evaluating the newborn to determine if any emergency interventions are needed. Within 2 hours of birth, an initial head-to-toe evaluation should be done to determine if there are any problems that require medical or nursing interventions.

Evaluation and observation of the newborn begin at birth and should continue regularly throughout the first 24 hours of life to monitor successful transition to extrauterine life. Nurses need to be familiar with the normal features of the transitional period to detect problems with transition, report the problems, and develop a plan of care.

When providing nursing care, ensure that the infant is in a warm and well-lit environment. Proper lighting is important for observing the skin color. The evaluation consists of observation, auscultation, and palpation. If possible, conduct the observation portion of the evaluation before touching the newborn.

Before stimulating the newborn with touch, you should observe the infant for the following:

- Position
- Sleep or wake cycle
- Skin color
- Respiratory pattern

Vital Signs

Vital signs indicate physiological functioning and include heart rate, respiratory rate, temperature, and blood pressure. Blood pressure is not routinely checked in a newborn unless there are suspicions of a congenital cardiac anomaly. Hospital policies vary on timing for newborn vital signs, but they are usually taken every 30 minutes for the first 2 hours after birth; then every hour for 3 hours; and then every 4 to 8 hours for 24 hours. See Table 15.1 for normal newborn vital signs.

Newborn Measurements

Each newborn should be weighed and measured for length, head circumference, and chest circumference. To prevent inaccuracies, the infant should be weighed on the same scale each day in the hospital. When weighing the infant, be sure to remove the diaper. The standard weight range for term newborns is 2,500 g to 4,000 g (5 lb 8 oz to 8 lb 13 oz; Davidson, 2020; Fig. 15.1).

To obtain an accurate length, fully extend the newborn's leg and record the distance from head to heel. It is easier to obtain an accurate measurement if one nurse holds the infant in place while another nurse measures from head to heel. The standard length for a term newborn is 48 to 53 cm (19 to 21 in.; Davidson, 2020; Fig. 15.2).

Chest circumference is measured by placing the tape measure around the infant's chest at the nipple line and noting the number at midway between inspiration and expiration. The

Table 15.1

Normal Newborn Vital Signs

Vital Sign	Normal Ranges
Temperature	36.5°C–37.4°C (97.7°F–99.3°F) axillary
Heart rate	Asleep: 100 bpm; awake: 120–160 bpm; crying: 180 bpm
Respiratory rate	30–60 breaths per minute
Blood pressure	Not routinely assessed; systolic 50–75 mm Hg diastolic 30–45 mm Hg

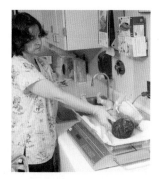

FIGURE 15.1 Weighing the infant.

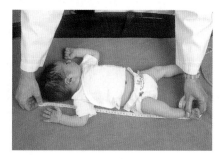

FIGURE 15.2 Measuring the infant's body length.

standard range for a term newborn chest circumference is 30.5 to 33 cm (12 to 13 in.; Fig. 15.3).

Head circumference is measured by placing the tape measure just above the ears and eyebrows. The expected range for the head circumference is 33 to 35.5 cm (13 to 14 in.; Fig. 15.4).

Skin Evaluation

The skin evaluation can give you information about the infant's cardiac function, respiratory function, gestational age, and thermoregulation. Observe the skin color in good natural lighting if possible. There are always variations in skin tone, but an infant with good cardiac and respiratory function

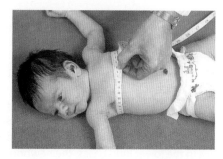

FIGURE 15.3 Measuring the chest circumference.

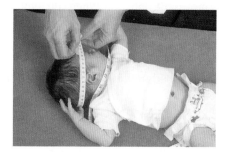

FIGURE 15.4 Measuring the head circumference.

will have pink mucous membranes and nailbeds. In darker-pigmented infants, the mucous membranes may be light pink with a slight yellow or red tinge (Bedford & Lomax, 2021). It is normal for newborns to have acrocyanosis for the first 24 to 48 hours after birth. **Acrocyanosis** is a bluish color of the hands and feet because of immature peripheral circulation. It is also common for newborns to have petechiae on the scalp, forehead, and cheeks. These are tiny pinpoint bruises that occurred from pushing during delivery or from a rapid delivery (Gantan & Wiedrich, 2022).

An axillary temperature range of 36.5°C to 37.4°C (97.7°F–99.3°F) is acceptable for the term newborn. The infant should have good skin turgor to indicate adequate hydration. To evaluate for skin turgor, gently pinch the skin on the thigh or chest. The skin should immediately recoil. If the skin remains "pinched," the newborn has poor turgor and may be dehydrated.

The palms of the hands and the soles of the feet should have creases. The creases in the sole develop from toe to heel. An absence of creases could indicate a motor defect. It is thought that sole creases develop in the uterus because of fetal movement of the lower extremities (McKee-Garrett, 2022). A preterm infant will have minimal creases, and a postterm infant will have increased creasing of the soles.

Lanugo is fine, downy hair that covers the forehead, ears, and body of the newborn (Fig. 15.5). Lanugo develops at 19 weeks' gestation and is very obvious at 27 to 28 weeks' gestation. After 28 weeks, the fetus begins to slowly lose the

• WORD • BUILDING •

acrocyanosis: acro–extremities or tips + cyan–blue + osis–condition

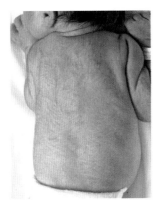

FIGURE 15.5 Lanugo.

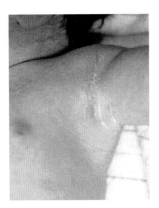

FIGURE 15.6 Vernix caseosa.

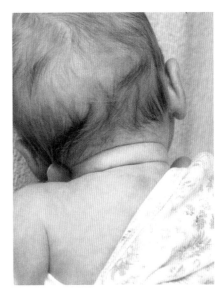

FIGURE 15.7 Nevus simplex, also known as *stork bites.*

hair, and any hair present at birth will fall off within the first weeks of life (Gordon & Lomax, 2021). A postterm newborn will have very little or no lanugo.

Vernix caseosa is a white protective coating on the skin of the newborn. It usually collects in the folds of the legs, arms, and neck (Fig. 15.6). Vernix protects the fetus's skin from the amniotic fluid that surrounds it and disappears as the fetus ages. A term newborn will usually have vernix only in the folds of the armpit or groin area. A premature newborn will have vernix covering the entire body.

Birthmarks, Rashes, and Skin Lesions

Birthmarks are not uncommon and may cause some anxiety for the family. Most birthmarks are benign but some will require further investigation by the health-care provider. Although some birthmarks fade away over time, others persist into adulthood.

A strawberry **hemangioma**, also known as a *nevus vascularis,* consists of newly formed capillaries in the dermal and subdermal layers of the skin. The strawberry hemangioma has sharp demarcation and is raised and dark red. It may be present at birth or may appear in the first few weeks of life. Usually no medical intervention is required unless the hemangioma is larger than 5 cm. The hemangioma gradually fades away over a few years; 50% of hemangiomas are gone by age 5, and 70% are gone by age 7 (Barton, 2021).

Nevus flammeus, also known as *port wine stain,* is usually present at birth and grows with the child. It is made up of dilated skin capillaries. The nevus flammeus is frequently located on the face and is red to purple in color. This birthmark is not raised and does not blanch if pressure is applied. This lesion will not fade on its own, and laser surgery is the treatment of choice if the parents desire to have it removed (Shajil & Das, 2022).

Nevus simplex, also known as a *stork bite, angel kiss,* or *salmon patch,* appears in 40% of all newborns. It may be found on the forehead or nape of the neck. It is pink in color and does blanch when pressure is applied (Fig. 15.7). It may be more prominent when the newborn cries. No treatment is required, and it usually fades by 18 months of age (Rohan, 2020).

Congenital **melanocytic nevi**, also known as *moles,* are uncommon in the newborn but have a potential for malignancy. A nevus may be flat or raised. The congenital melanocytic nevus is usually evenly pigmented and brown or black in color. Hair may be present. A hairy nevus noted along the base of the spine could indicate a spina bifida congenital spine abnormality. (For more information on spina bifida, see Chapter 27.) You should document and report any nevi noted. Melanocytic nevi can be removed surgically for cosmetic considerations or if the parents are concerned about the potential for malignancy later in life (Bodman & Al Aboud, 2022).

Erythema toxicum neonatorum, also known as *newborn rash,* may appear as macules, papules, or vesicles. (For more information on skin conditions, see Chapter 36.) The

• WORD • BUILDING •
hemangioma: hem–blood + angi–lymph or blood vessels + oma–tumor

• WORD • BUILDING •
melanocytic: melano–black + cyt–cell + ic–pertaining to

rash appears on any part of the body except the palms and soles of the feet. It appears suddenly and also disappears quickly, rarely lasting more than 7 days. It does not cause any discomfort for the newborn and does not require any medical treatment (Gibbs, 2020).

Acne neonatorum are clogged hair follicles or pores in the skin. They are found on the forehead, nose, and cheeks and may be white or black. Newborn acne will resolve without treatment and causes no scarring.

Milia are sebaceous glands occluded with keratin. They resemble tiny white papules about 1 mm in size, located on the nose, chin, cheeks, and forehead (Fig. 15.8). Milia usually disappear within 4 weeks and require no special care.

Dermal melanosis, also known as *Mongolian spot*, is a common finding in infants of darker skin, particularly infants of Asian, East Indian, or African descent (Chua & Pico, 2022). The spots are caused by melanocytes trapped deep in the skin. They appear flat and bluish-gray or brown, and are located on the back or buttocks (Fig. 15.9). This lesion can be mistaken for a bruise; however, bruises have yellow, green, and red areas in addition to the dark colors. The presence of dermal melanosis should be documented in the infant's medical record. No medical interventions are required. Most dermal melanosis usually disappears by 1 year of age, rarely persisting to 6 years of age (Chua & Pico, 2022).

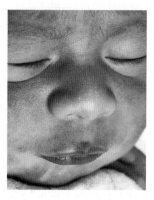

FIGURE 15.8 Milia.

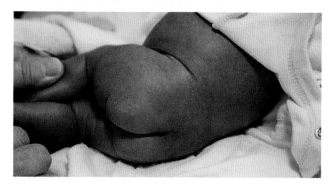

FIGURE 15.9 Dermal melanosis.

• **WORD** • **BUILDING** •
melanosis: melan–black + osis–condition

Report the following abnormal skin evaluation findings:

- Cyanosis, which could be caused by a cardiovascular or respiratory problem
- Thin skin with abundant lanugo, which could indicate prematurity
- Meconium staining, which may be caused by hypoxia in the uterus before birth
- Poor skin turgor, which may be caused by dehydration
- Pallor (paleness), which could be caused by anemia or hypothermia
- Any nevus or mole

Safe and Effective Nursing Care

Pallor refers to pale skin. Possible causes of pallor include anemia, cold exposure, low blood volume, and low thyroid function. When observing for pallor in the newborn, use good lighting. Natural light is best, but artificial light that does not change skin color is acceptable. All skin tones have an underlying red tone. An absence of the red tone may indicate pallor. Skin areas with the least melanin, such as the conjunctivae, the mouth, under the tongue, the palms, and the nailbeds, are best for checking for pallor.

- For light-skinned infants with pallor, the skin and conjunctivae will be pale without any pink tones.
- Infants with naturally yellow skin tones appear more yellow when there is pallor.
- In darker skin-toned infants with pallor, the skin loses its red undertones and may appear ashy gray.

(Lewis et al., 2022)

Head Evaluation

At the beginning of the head evaluation, you should first observe the general appearance, including the shape, circumference, and suture lines. A newborn delivered vaginally will generally have a flattened forehead that rises to a point at the posterior skull over the occiput. This shape reflects the molding that occurred to the skull as the suture lines came together when the head passed through the pelvis during birth. Overriding sutures are normal findings that result from molding and resolve spontaneously. The molding or "cone head" appearance resolves within 3 to 5 days after birth.

Another condition that may be noticed on the head is a **cephalohematoma**, which is a swelling on the head that does not cross the suture line. It develops from birth trauma that causes a rupture of blood vessels between the skull and periosteum. It usually appears by day 2 of life and may worsen over a few days. The cephalohematoma will resolve over days or weeks as the blood is reabsorbed (Rohan, 2020; Fig. 15.10).

• **WORD** • **BUILDING** •
cephalohematoma: cephal–head + hemat–blood + oma–tumor

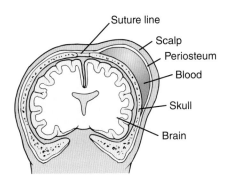

FIGURE 15.10 Cephalohematoma.

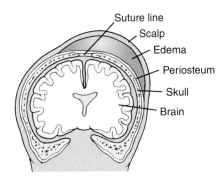

FIGURE 15.11 Caput succedaneum.

Caput succedaneum, a swelling of the scalp of the newborn, is caused by pressure from the uterus or vaginal wall during delivery. The scalp will be soft and spongelike with possible bruising. Caput succedaneum is superficial and does cross the suture lines. No treatment is needed; the swelling will decrease over a few days (Rohan, 2020; Fig. 15.11).

The newborn head circumference, referred to as the *occipital-frontal circumference,* is determined by measuring around the head from the frontal to occipital area by placing the tape measure above the ears. Measure the largest part of the head. As edema and molding from the birth subside, the head circumference may decrease as much as 2 cm over a week. The acceptable head measurement for a term newborn is 33 to 37 cm (13 to 15 in.).

A term newborn will have a diamond-shaped anterior **fontanel** located between the coronal and sagittal suture lines, approximately 4 to 5 cm (1.6–2 in.) in size. A fontanel is sometimes referred to as the "soft spot" on the baby's head. It is a fibrous membrane that lies between the bones of the cranium. The anterior fontanel closes by 18 months of age. In contrast, the posterior fontanel is located midline on the back of the head between the sagittal and lamboid sutures and is approximately 0.5 to 2 cm (0.2 to 0.8 in.) in size. The triangular posterior fontanel should close by 2 months of age. Both fontanels should be flat. Missing or small fontanels could indicate a potential problem of fused cranial bones that could interfere with brain growth. When a newborn cries or vomits, you may observe that the fontanel fluctuates, but it should never be tightly bulging. A tight, bulging fontanel may indicate an increase in intracranial pressure. Sunken

fontanels are associated with dehydration and decreased intracranial pressure (LaMonica, 2022).

Document and report the following abnormal findings:

- Enlarged fontanels
- Abnormally small fontanels
- Bulging or sunken fontanels

Eye Evaluation

Examine the eyes and eyelids for symmetry in size and location on the face. The outer portion of the eye should be at the same height as the top of the ear. The sclera should be white or bluish-white; a yellow appearance indicates jaundice. Birth trauma may cause a subconjunctival hemorrhage. The pupillary reflex can be determined by shining a bright light into the eye and observing an instant constriction of the pupil. The newborn's visual field is approximately 20 to 25 cm (8–12 in.) with a visual acuity of 20/200. Document and report the following findings:

- Yellow or red sclera
- Any exudate noted in the eyes
- Drooping eyelids

Ear Evaluation

Note the ear size, shape, and location. A mature infant will have firmer ear cartilage than a premature infant. You should note any abnormal folds, discharge, or irregularities of the pinna. The placement of the ear should be in a horizontal line from the inner canthus of the eye. If the ears are lower than that line, they are termed "low-set" and may indicate a chromosomal abnormality. Infants with normal hearing should have some response to loud sounds and voices. Document and report the following:

- Any abnormal anatomical findings
- The newborn's lack of response to loud noises

Nose Evaluation

The newborn's nose should be midline with symmetrical nares. A small amount of clear nasal discharge is expected in the newborn. Newborns are obligatory nose breathers, which means that the newborn breathes through the nose much more easily than through the mouth. Check for air movement through the nose by placing a finger under the nose. Newborns who are experiencing respiratory difficulty will often flare the nostrils as an attempt to breathe in more air. Document and report the following:

- Obstructed nasal passages
- Any discharge from the nose that is not clear
- Any anatomical abnormalities
- Any nasal flaring

Mouth Evaluation

Inspect the lips, mouth, tongue, palate, and gums. Note any asymmetrical movement of the mouth or tongue, which could indicate nerve injury from birth trauma. The lips and mucous membranes should be pink, and a small amount of saliva should be present. If the infant has a large amount of mucus that bubbles, suction it with the bulb syringe. If there continues to be a large amount of bubbly saliva, notify the health-care provider to evaluate the patency of the esophagus. A penlight can be used to visualize the palate. Place a gloved finger in the mouth to palpate the palate for intactness and to elicit the sucking reflex from the infant (LaMonica, 2022).

You may notice white papules, known as *Epstein pearls,* on the roof of the mouth or gums. Sometimes they appear as little emerging teeth, but they are really cysts that contain trapped mucous membrane cells. They are commonly found on the midline of the palate and are formed when the palate fused during early fetal development. They are not painful, and they disappear within a few weeks. Document and report the following:

- Asymmetrical movement of the lips or tongue
- Mucous membranes that are not pink
- Excessive bubbly saliva
- Absent suck reflex
- A hole in the palate

Chest Evaluation

Observe the infant's chest for shape and symmetry of movement. The newborn chest should be round and 1 to 2 cm smaller than the head circumference. Note the size, shape, nipple formation, and nipple placement. Frequently, in both sexes, the breasts are enlarged because of the maternal hormones. This condition is called **gynecomastia** and resolves within days as the level of hormones the baby received in utero from the mother declines. Neonatal gynecomastia is sometimes accompanied by galactorrhea, also called "witch's milk." Galactorrhea is a milky appearing discharge from the nipples that resolves spontaneously as the hormone level in the infant drops (LaMonica, 2022). Document and report the following:

- Any variation in chest size from the norm, either too large or too small
- Any abnormalities in the placement or size of the nipples
- Any purulent or bloody discharge from the nipples

Respiratory Evaluation

A respiratory evaluation includes observation of the newborn's breathing effort, chest movement, and auscultation of the lung fields. Newborns experience a breathing pattern known as *periodic breathing.* This periodic breathing pattern is irregular, and the infant can pause breathing for 5 to 15 seconds. When the infant is in a deep sleep, the breathing pattern is generally more even and regular; as the infant becomes more awake, the breathing pattern may change to periodic breathing. The infant's work of breathing should be unlabored, and the infant should appear to be breathing easily. The chest movement should be smooth. Inspect the nailbeds for color; a bluish color indicates decreased oxygenation of the blood.

Infants with respiratory distress may exhibit seesaw movements of the chest and abdomen, nasal flaring, and retractions. **Retractions** are a pulling in of the skin around the ribs and sternum when inhaling becomes hard work for the infant.

When auscultating the newborn's lung fields, use a pediatric or newborn stethoscope. The smaller sized 2.5-cm diameter diaphragm of the pediatric or newborn stethoscope makes it easier to hear the lungs without hearing other body sounds at the same time. Listen to one lung field and cross over to the opposite side to compare the two lung fields. The normal newborn will have wet sounds, such as crackles, for the first 24 hours after birth because of the long immersion in fluid during gestation. Document and report the following:

- A respiratory rate of lower than 30 or more than 60 breaths/minute
- Cessation of breathing (**apnea**) of more than 20 seconds
- Any abnormal sound other than crackles in the first 24 hours
- Any increased work of breathing noted, especially seesaw chest movements and retraction of the skin around the ribs and sternum

Cardiovascular Evaluation

Listening to the heart sounds of a newborn can be difficult because of the normally fast rate. Using a pediatric stethoscope and minimizing extraneous noise and distractions will help. When listening to the heart sounds, first focus on identifying S_1 (closure of the mitral and tricuspid valves) and S_2 (closure of the aortic and pulmonic valves). Next, notice the regularity or irregularity of the rhythm. Finally, systematically listen to the different heart areas using the following sequence:

1. The aortic valve area by placing the stethoscope at the second intercostal space at the right of the sternum
2. The pulmonic valve area by placing the stethoscope at the second intercostal space to the left of the sternum
3. The tricuspid valve area by placing the stethoscope at the fifth intercostal space at the left of the sternum
4. The mitral valve area by placing the stethoscope at the fourth intercostal space at the left of the midclavicular line

One way to remember the positions of heart auscultation is **A**ll **P**hysicians **T**ake **M**oney (APTM). See Figure 15.12 for stethoscope placement for cardiac evaluation on a newborn.

Evaluate the newborn's peripheral pulses for quality and equality by comparing them side to side. The pulse rate and rhythm should match the apical pulse.

• WORD • BUILDING •

gynecomastia: gyneco–female + mast–breast + ia–condition

• WORD • BUILDING •

apnea: a–without + pnea–breath

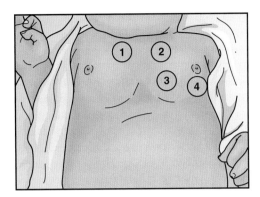

FIGURE 15.12 Stethoscope placement for cardiac evaluation.

The capillary refill time (CRT) can be evaluated by pressing firmly on the foot for approximately 5 seconds, causing the foot to blanch, and then by counting the number of seconds for the skin to return to natural color. Normal CRT should be fewer than 3 seconds. However, the test for CRT in the newborn is controversial because the refill time can be affected by decreased peripheral circulation, the temperature of the foot, and the environmental temperature (Bedford & Lomax, 2021). Document and report the following:

- A heart rate below 110 bpm or above 160 bpm at rest
- Any heart sounds other than the normal S_1 and S_2 heart sounds
- Any abnormal heart sounds, such as blowing, clicking, or mechanical sounds, which could indicate a murmur
- Any discrepancy between the peripheral pulses side to side and with the apical heart rate
- A CRT greater than 3 seconds

Abdomen and Gastrointestinal Evaluation

To evaluate the abdomen, observe its shape, contour, and movement. The abdomen should have a domed appearance owing to immature abdominal muscles. The umbilical stump should be white and gelatinous in appearance and have three vessels, two arteries, and a vein. The umbilical stump begins to dry within hours of birth. Note any bulging around the umbilicus, which could indicate failure of the umbilical ring closure, resulting in an umbilical hernia. The anus should be inspected for patency. Patency can be checked by performing the initial temperature check rectally and thereafter determining temperature by another method.

Auscultate abdominal bowel sounds before touching the abdomen, which could stimulate the bowel, producing peristalsis. There should be bowel sounds within 1 to 2 hours of birth. A stool inspection is an important part of the abdominal and gastrointestinal evaluation. The first newborn stool is the dark and sticky meconium stool, which is made up of bile salts, bile acids, epithelial cells, lanugo, and debris shed from the intestinal mucosa during intrauterine life (Rohan, 2020). The meconium stool should be passed within 24 hours of birth. By the second or third day, the stool is called *transitional* because it will have a green or yellowish

seedy appearance. After a few days, the breastfed infant's stool will have the appearance of mustard, whereas the bottle-fed infant's stool will have a tan, yellow, or greenish appearance. Document and report the following:

- Failure to pass a meconium stool within 24 hours
- A closed anus
- Absence of bowel sounds after 2 hours
- A flat abdomen

Genitourinary Evaluation

During the initial head-to-toe evaluation of the newborn, the health-care provider should include an examination of the genitalia. Inspect the female genitalia for placement of the labia and urinary meatus. In a healthy newborn, the labia will cover the clitoris. Maternal hormones may cause the labia to be swollen and darker than the surrounding tissue. Mucus and blood-tinged vaginal discharge is not uncommon and is called **pseudomenstruation**. The discharge may be present for a few days until the level of maternal hormones in the newborn decreases.

The male infant's penis should be midline and straight with the urethral opening midline at the tip of the penis. The length of the nonerect penis is 2 to 3 cm at birth. Until 3 to 4 years of age, the foreskin is usually tight, but it does not affect the stream of urine. The scrotum will appear large and loose with a dark appearance because of maternal hormones. Lightly palpate for the presence of testes. Testes usually descend by the third trimester and are approximately 1 cm in size at birth (Gantan & Wiedrich, 2022).

Infants with ambiguous genitalia may have underdeveloped external genitals or may have both male and female characteristics. These observations should be reported to the health-care provider immediately. A team of professionals including a pediatrician, urologist, gynecologist, endocrinologist, surgeon, nurse, and psychologist will be involved in the care of the infant.

Urinary output should be evaluated. The newborn should urinate within 24 hours of birth. Normal urine output is 1 to 2 mL/kg/hour. Document and report the following:

- A lack of or decreased urinary output
- Any structural abnormality of the genitalia
- Undescended testicles

Neurological Evaluation

The newborn's neurological system is immature at birth. Periodic jerking or twitching is considered normal. Tremors are not considered a normal finding in a newborn. The newborn's cry can also provide information about the neurological status, as a high-pitched cry can indicate an increase in intracranial pressure. When evaluating the reflexes, consider the gestational age, not the birth weight. Premature infants will have a reduced response to reflex evaluation. Table 15.2

· WORD · BUILDING ·

pseudomenstruation: pseudo–false + menstru–discharge menses + ation–action

Table 15.2

Newborn Reflexes

Reflex	Description	Age the Reflex Disappears
Babinski reflex 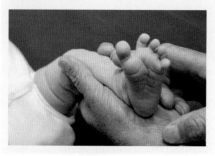	When the sole of the foot is stroked, the newborn's big toe moves upward toward the top surface of the foot and the other toes fan out.	2 years of age
Plantar grasp 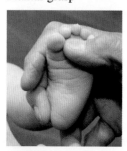	The newborn's toes curl downward in response to pressure applied to the sole of the foot at the base of the toes.	8 months of age
Rooting reflex 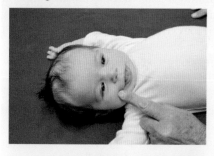 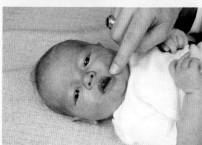	The newborn turns the mouth to the same side of the cheek that is stroked.	Becomes a voluntary reflex around 3 weeks of age
Gag reflex	The newborn coughs in response to stimulation of the posterior oral cavity.	Continues into adulthood

Table 15.2
Newborn Reflexes—cont'd

Reflex	Description	Age the Reflex Disappears
Moro (Startle) reflex 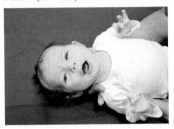	In response to a slight drop, sudden movement of the crib, or a loud noise, the newborn quickly makes a symmetrical abduction of the extremities and places the index fingers and thumbs into a "C" shape.	6 months of age
Palmar grasp 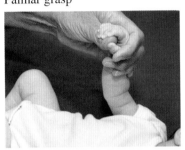	The newborn wraps the fingers around the examiner's finger when it is placed in the newborn's palm.	4–6 months of age
Stepping reflex 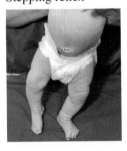	The newborn simulates walking when held in an upright position and the sole of the foot touches a flat surface.	2 months of age
Tonic neck reflex 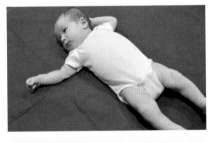	In a supine position, if the newborn's head is turned to one side with the jaw over the shoulder, the arm and leg on the same side extend while the opposite arm and leg flex.	4–6 months of age
Extrusion reflex 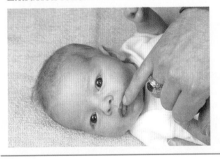	The newborn uses the tongue to push foreign objects out of the mouth.	3–4 months of age

Sources: FamilyDoctor.Org. (2022). *Newborn reflexes and behavior.* https://familydoctor.org/newborn-reflexes-behavior; Rohan, A. (2020). Assessment and care of the newborn. In P. D. Suplee & J. Janke (Eds.), *AWHONN compendium of postpartum care* (3rd ed., pp. 46–81). AWHONN.

provides information about newborn reflexes. Document and report the following warning signs:

- Tremors
- A high-pitched cry
- Abnormal pupil responses
- Hypertonic or hypotonic positions
- Absent newborn reflexes

Musculoskeletal Evaluation

To begin the musculoskeletal evaluation, observe the resting posture. The normal resting posture for a newborn is flexed with good muscle tone. The limbs should be inspected for symmetry, webbing, range of motion, length, and number of digits (Chandran, 2023). Uterine position can sometimes cause the feet to be turned inward. Gently try to straighten the foot. If the foot can be straightened, the issue is usually caused by uterine position and will straighten out over time. If the foot cannot be straightened because of resistance, do not force the foot and report the findings.

Observe the hips for developmental dysplasia of the hip, also known as *congenital hip dislocation.* On observation, one leg may appear shorter than the other, and the thigh and buttock folds do not match. Two tests are recommended to determine hip instability in the newborn. The Ortolani maneuver is performed with the infant in a supine position. Hold the infant's thigh with a thumb and place the index finger of the same hand over the greater trochanter area. Gently lift and abduct the hip while pushing gently down on the knee. If the hip is not stable, you will hear or feel a "clunk." For the Barlow test, place a thumb on the infant's thigh and use the palm of the same hand to press down the knee. While applying gentle pressure, feel for a dislocation with the middle finger of the same hand. If the hip is not stable, you will feel the hip dislocate. Both tests are considered "positive" if a dislocation is observed (Fig. 15.13).

Observe the newborn's spinal cord and back for curvatures and asymmetry. Any nevi, dimples, skin tags, or hairy patches that appear on the midline of the back along the spine could indicate a spinal cord condition and are not considered a normal finding in the newborn. Document and report the following:

- Absence of limbs or digits or presence of extra limbs or digits
- Structural abnormalities of any bones or muscles
- Lack of movement of a limb
- Asymmetrical thigh creases
- Unequal length of limbs
- Positive Ortolani or Barlow tests
- The presence of any nevi, skin tags, or dimples on the spinal cord

Pain Evaluation

Some hospitals require a newborn pain evaluation to be done once a day and before, during, and after a painful procedure. A commonly used pain scale is the Neonatal Infant Pain Scale (NIPS; Lawrence et al., 1993). This pain scale

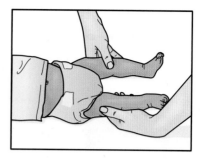

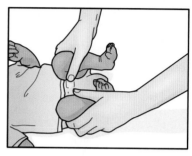

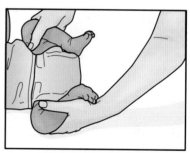

FIGURE 15.13 Barlow and Ortolani maneuvers.

is appropriate for infants younger than 1 year of age. For 1 minute, you observe facial expression, cry, breathing pattern, arms, legs, and state of arousal with a numeric score assigned to each. A score of greater than 3 indicates that the neonate or infant is in pain. See Table 15.3.

Safety *Stat!*

Warning signs observed during the physical examination that must be reported immediately include the following:

- Axillary temperature of lower than 36.1°C (96.9°F) or greater than 37.2°C (99°F)
- Cyanosis of the body, lips, nailbeds (not normal acrocyanosis of the newborn's feet and hands)
- Heart rate lower than 110 bpm or greater than 160 bpm (180 bpm if crying)
- Respiratory rate of lower than 30 or greater than 60 breaths/minute
- Hypotonic or hypertonic muscle tone
- Lack of movement of arms and legs
- Jaundice
- Periods of apnea longer than 20 seconds (Davidson, 2020)

Table 15.3
Neonatal Infant Pain Scale

NPS	0 Point	1 Point	2 Points
Facial expression	Relaxed	Contracted	-
Cry	Absent	Mumbling	Vigorous
Breathing	Relaxed	Different than usual	-
Arms	Relaxed	Flexed/stretched	-
Legs	Relaxed	Flexed/stretched	-
Alertness	Sleeping/calm	Uncomfortable	-

Maximal score of seven points; four or more points indicate pain. Used with permission of Children's Hospital of Eastern Ontario, Ottawa, Ontario, Canada.

Patient Teaching Guidelines

New parents may feel overwhelmed with the number and variety of newborn medications and screenings ordered by the baby's health-care provider. Be prepared to answer questions about and explain the purpose of the following medications and screening procedures:

Vitamin K injection: reduces the risk of bleeding because babies don't get enough vitamin K during the pregnancy or while breastfeeding.

Antibiotic ointment for the eyes: reduces the risk of the baby getting an eye infection from passing through the birth canal.

Hepatitis B injection: starts the immunization process to prevent the baby from acquiring hepatitis B.

Newborn screening blood test: tests for the metabolic disorder phenylketonuria (PKU; see Chapter 32) and up to 40 other disorders. The blood is obtained from a heel stick.

Critical congenital heart defect (CCHD) screening: a noninvasive test with a pulse oximeter measuring the baby's oxygen levels on their limbs. This test is for early detection of a heart problem.

Hearing screening: a noninvasive test for early detection of a hearing problem.

NURSING CARE OF THE NEWBORN

Most hospitals encourage rooming-in of the newborn with the mother. In addition, the mother's partner or other support person is often encouraged to stay with the new mother. Even though the infant spends most of the time in the mother's room, the nurse has the ultimate responsibility for the newborn's care. In addition to the initial evaluation and ongoing evaluations, the nurse provides physical care and completes the basic newborn screenings to promote the health of the newborn. These actions include administering medications, determining the gestational age, completing the first bath, and coordinating newborn screenings before discharge.

Medications

Review the infant's medical record to verify that the vitamin K and erythromycin ointment were given right after delivery. If not, administer those two medications after obtaining parental consent. The Centers for Disease Control and Prevention (CDC, 2018) recommends that all newborns weighing a minimum of 2,000 g receive the first dose of the hepatitis B vaccine within 24 hours of birth. The complete hepatitis B vaccine series is given as three injections over a 6-month period. Starting the hepatitis B vaccine series in the hospital reduces the risk of the newborn getting the disease from family members who may not know that they are infected with the disease (CDC, 2018).

Medication Facts

If the mother has hepatitis B, an additional medication is given within 12 hours of birth to protect the baby against catching hepatitis B. The medication is called *hepatitis B immune globulin (HBIG)*. This medication provides antibodies to help the newborn's immune system fight off the virus (CDC, 2018).

Estimation of Gestational Age

During pregnancy, the gestational age is determined based on the mother's last menstrual period, fundal measurements, and ultrasonography. After birth, not every newborn receives a gestational age evaluation. Most hospitals have a policy regarding which infants should have gestational age evaluations completed. A gestational age evaluation should be completed on babies who are **preterm** (born before 37 weeks' gestation), babies who are **postterm** (born after 42 weeks' gestation), babies of diabetic mothers, babies of mothers who did not obtain prenatal care, and babies weighing fewer than 2,500 g or more than 4,000 g (Rohan, 2020). Classifying the newborn's gestational age provides information that assists the health-care provider and the nurse to plan and provide appropriate care for the newborn.

The most widely used clinical tool for determining gestational age is the Ballard tool. Developed by Dr. Jeanne L. Ballard, it assesses the newborn's gestational age by evaluating six areas of neuromuscular activity and six areas of physical maturity. The scores from the neuromuscular activity evaluation and physical maturity evaluation are combined to classify the newborn as preterm, term, or postterm. The Ballard tool is depicted in Figure 15.14.

Neuromuscular Maturity

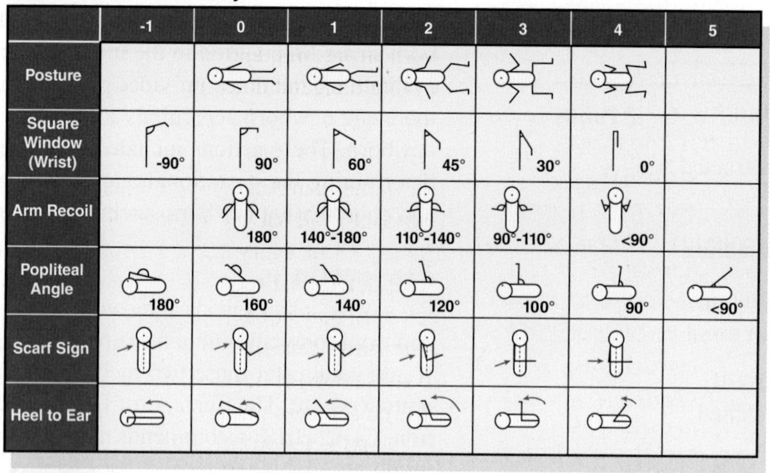

	-1	0	1	2	3	4	5
Posture							
Square Window (Wrist)	-90°	90°	60°	45°	30°	0°	
Arm Recoil		180°	140°-180°	110°-140°	90°-110°	<90°	
Popliteal Angle	180°	160°	140°	120°	100°	90°	<90°
Scarf Sign							
Heel to Ear							

Physical Maturity

Skin	Sticky Friable Transparent	Gelatinous Red Translucent	Smooth pink Visible veins	Superficial peeling or rash, few veins	Cracking Pale areas Rare veins	Parchment Deep cracking No vessels	Leathery Cracked Wrinkled
Lanugo	None	Sparse	Abundant	Thinning	Bald areas	Mostly bald	
Plantar Surface	Heel-toe 40–50 mm: -1 <40 mm: -2	>50 mm No crease	Faint red marks	Anterior transverse crease only	Creases over anterior 2/3	Creases over entire sole	
Breast	Imperceptible	Barely perceptible	Flat areola No bud	Stippled areola 1–2 mm bud	Raised areola 3–4 mm bud	Full areola 5–10 mm bud	
Eye/Ear	Lids fused loosely: -1 tightly: -2	Lids open Pinna flat Stays folded	Barely curved pinna; soft; slow recoil	Well-curved pinna; soft but ready recoil	Formed and firm Instant recoil	Thick cartilage Ear stiff	
Genitals (Male)	Scrotum flat, smooth	Scrotum empty Faint rugae	Testes in upper canal Rare rugae	Testes descending Few rugae	Testes down Good rugae	Testes pendulous Deep rugae	
Genitals (Female)	Clitoris prominent Labia flat	Prominent clitoris Small labia minora	Prominent clitoris Enlarging minora	Majora and minora equally prominent	Majora large Minora small	Majora covers clitoris and minora	

Maturity Rating

Score	Weeks
-10	20
-5	22
0	24
5	26
10	28
15	30
20	32
25	34
30	36
35	38
40	40
45	42
50	44

FIGURE 15.14 Ballard Gestational Age Assessment Tool.

Bath

The purpose of the initial bath is to remove blood and body fluids that could contaminate health-care workers. Amniotic fluid can contain viruses, such as HIV. Practice universal precautions and wear gloves while handling the newborn until the initial bath is given. The risks of bathing the newborn are hypothermia, respiratory distress, and an increased oxygen need. Most babies cry at some point during the bath experience because of stimuli never experienced in the uterus, such as undressing, temperature changes, and the touch of the washcloth and towels (Warren et al., 2020).

The Association of Women's Health, Obstetric and Neonatal Nurses (AWHONN, 2020) recommends that the newborn receive the first bath between 2 and 24 hours after birth if the newborn's temperature is at least 36.8°C (98.2°F). However, the World Health Organization (WHO, 2022) recommends waiting 24 hours after birth. If there are cultural reasons, wait a minimum of 6 hours after birth to avoid interfering with bonding and the initiation of breastfeeding. Delaying bathing is thought to allow nutrients to be absorbed

from the vernix to protect the infant from infection. Moreover, delayed bathing leads to improved breastfeeding rates and reduces hypothermia (Priyadarshi et al., 2022).

Hospitals use a variety of methods to bathe the baby, including sponge bathing, small tub bathing, large tub or immersion bathing, and swaddling immersion bathing. The initial bath can be given at the mother's bedside or in the nursery. When preparing for the bath, ensure that the room is warm and free of drafts. For all methods of bathing, a pH neutral cleanser is used, and the skin is gently washed. Blood and body fluids are removed, but any vernix should not be scrubbed off. Vernix protects the newborn's skin by preventing drying and cracking.

Newborn Screening

Newborn screening is a state-based public health program that tests newborns to determine if a medical condition is present that requires early interventions to maintain health. Newborn screenings are conducted for a variety of genetic, metabolic, and endocrine disorders; infectious diseases; hearing loss; and congenital heart disease. PKU was the first

Evidence-Based Practice

Newborn bathing is a routine procedure in the hospital. Researchers conducted a study to find the most appropriate time for the newborn's first bath. Newborns were divided into groups and received the first bath at either 2 hours, 6 hours, or 24 hours after birth. The newborn's skin temperature, amount of skin-to-skin time, crying time, and the presence or absence of vernix were recorded. Findings indicated that newborns bathed at 2 hours had little or no skin-to-skin contact with the mother and required a longer rewarming time after the bath. Several benefits were found when delaying the bath until 24 hours. This group of newborns received the most skin-to-skin contact after delivery, benefited from the protective and moisturizing properties of the vernix, and required less rewarming after the bath. An additional benefit was that the parents wanted to participate in the bathing, which provided nurses with an opportunity to teach about safe bathing of the newborn.

Mardini, J., Rahme, C., Matar, O., Khalil, S. A., Hallit, S., & Fadous Khalife, M. C. (2020). Newborn's first bath: Any preferred timing? *BMC Research Note, 13*, 430. https://doi.org/10.1186/s13104-020-05282-0

screening test developed for newborns; even though the modern blood test screens for 26 to 40 different disorders, it is still commonly referred to as the PKU test.

The newborn is primarily tested by blood samples obtained from a heel stick at least 24 hours after the first feeding. These samples are placed on special filter paper and sent to the state laboratory. Noninvasive testing is used to test for hearing loss, and an oxygen saturation meter is used to test for congenital heart disease.

Newborn Congenital Heart Defect Screening

The American Academy of Pediatrics (AAP, 2022) recommends that all babies be screened for a CCHD. In the United States, 18 of every 10,000 babies are born with a critical heart defect that requires medical intervention. Because the newborn may not exhibit signs of a heart defect immediately after birth, this simple screening test can help in the early identification of newborns with a heart defect.

The screening is conducted on a 24-hour or older infant. Pulse oximeter probes are placed on the right hand and right foot to obtain a reading of the oxygen saturation of the blood. If there is a difference of more than 3% between the hand and the foot, the test is considered positive. The health-care provider must be notified so that further testing can be ordered.

Newborn Hearing Screening

The National Institutes of Health (NIH, 2021) recommends hearing screens on all newborns. This recommendation has also been implemented by many hospitals. Most states in the United States have implemented mandatory newborn hearing screening programs. Early identification of hearing problems with early treatment can prevent severe psychosocial, educational, and speech problems for a child. Screening is usually completed before discharge.

Nursing Care Plan for Educating Parents About Their Newborn's Appearance

The nurse caring for newborn Ashton notices that Ashton's parents seem unusually quiet and a little sad as they stare at their baby boy. When the nurse asks the parents if they have any questions, they tell her that they are surprised that their newborn does not resemble the babies in television commercials. They are worried that their son has a long head that is slightly misshaped; a hemangioma on the leg; and a red, raised rash on the trunk and legs. "Is he normal?" the father asks.

Nursing Diagnosis: Risk for ineffective parenting as shown by the father's remark of "Is he normal?"

Expected Outcome: Parents will verbalize understanding that their newborn's appearance is normal, the head and rash will improve within days, and the hemangioma will fade over time.

Intervention:	Rationale:
Allow the parents to verbalize their fears without condemnation from you.	*The parents' feelings should not be minimized. Allowing them to verbalize their feelings will help to establish rapport.*

Interventions:	Rationale:
Educate the parents about normal newborn characteristics.	*Explain the process of molding that occurs as the fetus moves through the birth canal.*
Explain that hemangiomas usually fade over a few years.	*Education regarding normal newborn skin will reduce their anxiety.*

Intervention:	Rationale:
Point out the positive physical characteristics of the newborn.	*This will encourage parents to accept their newborn's appearance.*

Labs & Diagnostics

The following is the correct technique for obtaining blood specimens for newborn screening:

1. Warm the newborn's heel to increase circulation.
2. Cleanse the newborn's heel with alcohol and allow to dry.
3. Use a spring-activated lancet to puncture the skin no deeper than 2.4 mm on the outer aspect of the heel.
4. Collect the blood directly on the collection paper or pipette.
5. Apply gentle pressure to the heel with gauze and cover with an adhesive bandage.
6. Provide comfort to the newborn.

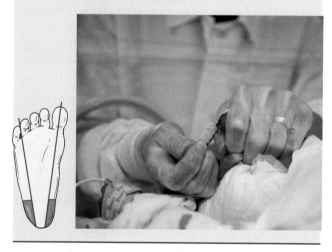

One method of evaluating hearing is the automated otoacoustic emission test (AOAE), which measures a response produced in the inner ear by placing a probe in the ear. Other tests are the automated auditory brainstem response (AABR) or the brainstem auditory evoked response (BAER), which measures the hearing from the ear to the brainstem. Information is obtained by placing headphones on the infant's head or, alternatively, placing electrodes on the infant's head. Both tests are easy to perform in the newborn nursery, and the infant is scored as a pass or a fail. Occasionally, a newborn does not pass the first hearing screen because of fluid in the ears from birth. If the infant did not pass the first time, most hospitals repeat the test one final time before discharge. The health-care provider must be notified if the infant failed the hearing screen on the second attempt. Infants who fail the newborn screen should be retested in 1 month (Delaney, 2022).

DISCHARGE TEACHING FOR NEWBORN CARE

Preparing parents for discharge by teaching and demonstrating basic newborn care is an ongoing process. Establishing rapport with the parents will make them feel more comfortable to ask questions. Encourage parental participation in

Checklist for New Parents Bringing an Infant Home From the Hospital

Before a newborn leaves the hospital, the health-care team should work together to teach the family to care for their infant so that they can be confident and comfortable:

1. Ensure that the family has a federally approved infant car seat and that the harness fits the infant appropriately.
2. Double-check the safety of the infant car seat while it is situated in the center seat, rear-facing position. Ensure that the parents are able to secure and release the car seat.
3. Ensure that the infant will be warm enough on the car ride home; keep the newborn's head covered.

Safety checks to do at home:

- Make sure that the crib/bassinet is not close to a window or an air conditioning vent where a cold draft could reach the baby.
- Keep a bulb syringe near the infant for rapid nasal clearing.
- Keep pets away from the infant.
- Keep parents' and caregivers' fingernails trimmed to prevent scratching the newborn.
- Make sure that smoke detectors and carbon monoxide detectors have fresh batteries and are working properly.

newborn care while they are in the hospital. There is more than one correct way to provide basic newborn care, and the parents should be encouraged to modify the care to meet their needs or cultural preferences. Reassure the parents that a baby does not know or care if the parents are experts at baby care; the infant just needs basic love, food, warmth, and safety needs to be met. Focus on safety and basic care while reassuring parents that they will become more comfortable in their new role of providing newborn care. Box 15.1 gives a safety checklist for bringing a newborn home.

Determine the parents' readiness to learn and their teaching needs. Ideally, teaching should occur in short segments. It is difficult for new parents to absorb all the information if you wait until an hour before discharge to begin the teaching. Experienced nurses know that effective discharge teaching is started well before discharge and that printed material to take home for reference is also important. This section focuses on discharge teaching for the healthy term newborn.

Use of the Bulb Syringe

Parents should be instructed about when and how to gently use a bulb syringe. The bulb syringe can be used to remove excess mucus, breast milk, or formula if the infant chokes. The bulb in the syringe should be compressed to remove the air, with the tip placed along the cheek or gently into the nostril, and then the fingers should release the bulb to provide suction. The mucus or milk can be squeezed out onto a tissue. The tip of the bulb syringe can scratch the throat, so the parents should never stick the syringe straight back into the mouth and throat area (Fig. 15.15).

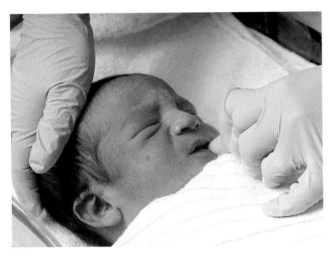

FIGURE 15.15 Bulb syringe used to remove mucus.

Car Seat Safety

A baby should ride in a rear-facing seat that is compliant with current safety standards for car seats until the highest weight or height allowed by the car seat manufacturer is reached (AAP, 2023). The car seat's harness cradles and protects the child's neck and spinal cord in the event of a crash. The car seat should be installed according to the manufacturer's instructions. A car seat that is involved in any accident should be replaced.

Trimming the Baby's Nails

At birth, some babies have long nails. Because of that, they can easily scratch and cut their own skin. Nurses in the hospital do not cut fingernails. Instead, long-sleeved undershirts with cuffs are used to cover the nails and protect the skin. The parents can be instructed to trim the nails with baby nail scissors or baby clippers. The nail edges should be rounded to avoid sharp edges. It is sometimes easier to cut the nails when the baby is sleeping.

> ### Safety *Stat!*
>
> Instruct the parents that if they accidentally draw blood or cut the finger when trimming nails, they should apply pressure with a sterile gauze pad. Never apply an adhesive bandage because babies put their fingers in their mouths and can dislodge the bandage and choke on it.

Diaper Rash

Diaper rash can be caused by persistent wet or soiled diapers or by use of some baby products such as commercial baby wipes or creams. If the baby develops diaper rash, the recommended treatment is as follows:

- Change diapers often.
- Clean the skin with warm water and avoid commercial premoistened cleaning cloths.

> ## Box 15.2
> ### Caring for the Umbilical Stump
>
> The AAP (2020) recommends that parents do the following:
>
> - Keep the stump dry by folding the diaper below the stump so that it is exposed to air.
> - Sponge bathe the baby until the cord falls off.
> - Apply no antimicrobial cream to the stump.
> - Keep the cord clean. If the cord becomes soiled, clean with warm water and pat dry.
> - Allow the dried cord to fall off on its own. Avoid pulling on the cord to dislodge it.
> - Be aware that when the cord falls off, a small amount of bleeding may occur.
> - Report any signs of infection such as pus or redness around the umbilical stump.

- Apply a barrier of zinc oxide cream to the skin.
- Keep the diaper area open to air as long as possible before applying a clean diaper (American Academy of Dermatology, 2023).

Umbilical Cord Care

The baby's umbilical cord will slowly change from whitish blue to black over a period of several days. The umbilical stump will fall off within 10 to 21 days. Care of the stump is presented in Box 15.2.

Circumcision

Circumcision is the surgical removal of the end of the foreskin of the penis. The parents may choose circumcision for the newborn because it is a personal preference or a cultural practice. Circumcision is a controversial topic; however, your role is to provide information, not to offer a personal opinion about whether or not the newborn should be circumcised. Newborn circumcision may be performed in the hospital nursery or at the pediatrician's office.

Before the procedure, a member of the medical staff obtains informed consent from the mother. The health-care provider may apply a numbing cream to the penis 30 to 40 minutes before the procedure. Some physicians also inject an anesthetic before the procedure. In studies, sucrose solution in small amounts has been shown to be effective in reducing the pain response in infants undergoing painful procedures and may be given to the infant (Omole et al., 2020). In one method of circumcision, a ringlike clamp is tightened over the foreskin, and the skin is removed with a scalpel. Another method of circumcision involves the use of a ring called a Plastibell that is left on and falls off on its own, along with the dead foreskin, after 10 to 12 days. After circumcision, the doctor will usually wrap the penis in petroleum gauze to prevent the penis from sticking to the diaper (Fig. 15.16).

· WORD · BUILDING ·

circumcision: circum–around + cis–cutting + ion–action

A small amount of blood-tinged drainage may be noted on the diaper after the procedure, and a yellow crust may form on the circumcision site. Document when the newborn urinates for the first time after a circumcision. Care of the circumcised penis is presented in Box 15.3.

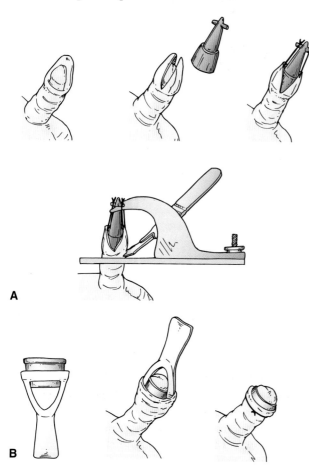

FIGURE 15.16 Removal of the foreskin during circumcision. A, Yellen clamp procedure. B, Plastibell procedure.

Box 15.3

Caring for the Circumcised Penis

Instruct the parents of a circumcised newborn to do the following:

- For a few days, wrap the penis in a small amount of gauze with a dab of petroleum jelly to keep it from sticking to the diaper.
- Do not remove or try to wash off the yellow crust that forms. It is not a sign of infection.
- Give sponge baths until healing is complete and the "ring" falls off, if a Plastibell appliance was used.
- Keep the penis clean and dry.
- Call the doctor if any of the following are noted:
  - Discoloration of the penis
  - Discharge from the penis or surgical site that includes pus
  - A spot of blood in the diaper larger than 2 inches
  - Lack of urination
  - A fever greater than 37.8°C (100°F) axillary occurs
  - The baby cannot be calmed or soothed

Health Promotion

Preventing Flat Spots on the Newborn's Head

A baby sleeps flat on the back several hours a day, which can lead to the formation of flat areas on the back of the head. Parents can prevent flat spots on the newborn's head by arranging for "tummy time" each day. Placing the baby on their tummy on a blanket on a clean floor for several minutes each day will prevent flat spots. Tummy time also makes the neck and shoulder muscles stronger so that the baby can start to sit up and crawl.

Feeding Schedules

Feeding consumes most of the day with a newborn. It is difficult to get a newborn on a schedule; therefore, the AAP recommends feeding the baby "on demand" for the first few weeks. When the baby shows signs of hunger such as crying, rooting, and chewing on hands, the parent or caregiver should feed the baby. The general guideline is that a breast-fed baby should nurse every 2 to $2\frac{1}{2}$ hours and a bottle-fed baby should be fed every 3 to $3\frac{1}{2}$ hours during daytime and evening hours. Unless recommended by the health-care provider, the baby does not need to be awakened at night for a feeding. The baby can wake the parent if hungry.

Elimination

The breastfed newborn should be passing four to five seedy yellow bowel movements per day by day five. A breastfed newborn may have a bowel movement at each feeding or at every other feeding. Once the mother's breast milk supply is established, the infant should void clear or pale yellow urine six to eight times daily. The bottle-fed infant should have at least one large tan or yellow bowel movement per day and six to eight wet diapers (Rohan, 2020).

Positioning and Holding

The caregiver should always support the infant's neck when holding or positioning the infant. The neck is weak, and the infant has no control over the head. In the infant seat or car seat, the neck can be supported with a rolled blanket or towel placed around the outside of the head and neck.

There are two ways to safely hold an infant: the cradle hold and the football hold. In the cradle hold, the infant is supine across the adult's chest with the infant's head in the elbow area, which supports the head and neck, with the other arm supporting the back and lower body. The football hold allows the adult to hold the infant with one arm. The infant is placed along the inner aspect of the adult's forearm with the hand and wrist supporting the head and neck. The rest of the infant's body is supported by the forearm and held snuggly against the adult's body.

Clothing

Any new clothing should be washed before dressing the newborn. To prevent a skin rash, parents should use detergents that are hypoallergenic and free of dyes and perfumes.

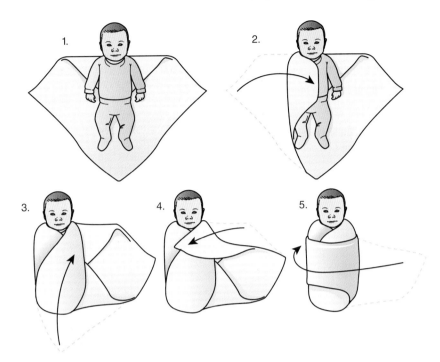

FIGURE 15.17 Swaddling.

Caution parents about overdressing the newborn. Typically, the healthy newborn requires only about one layer more of clothing than the parent. The newborn's head accounts for a significant amount of heat loss; therefore, encourage parents to place a cap on their infant to prevent heat loss when the infant is taken outside or if the room is cool.

Swaddling

Swaddling (Fig. 15.17) is a method of wrapping the baby to provide security and warmth. It is recommended that swaddling for sleep be discontinued when the baby is around 2 months old and becoming more active, to avoid the risk of the blanket twisting around the baby (Moon & Glassey, 2022). Parents can swaddle the newborn using the following steps:

1. Place the blanket on a flat surface with one corner of the blanket pointing away. Fold that corner down a few inches.
2. Place the baby face up on the blanket with the neck at the edge of the folded-over corner.
3. Fold the left corner of the blanket over the baby and tuck it under the back. The newborn's hands can be left close to the face to allow hand-to-mouth behaviors, which are calming for the newborn.
4. Fold the bottom corner over the feet and chest. Allow the baby to be in a comfortable position, such as flexing their legs.
5. Bring the right corner around the baby's body, covering the bottom corner.
6. Make sure the hips can move and the blanket is not too tight.

CRITICAL THINKING & CLINICAL JUDGMENT

Scenario #2: Your next-door neighbor Cora invites you to see her newborn nursery. Her first baby is due in a week. She excitedly shows you the crib which is lined with stuffed animals and has baby blankets ready to use.

Questions

1. What do you notice when looking at the crib?
2. What should you do?

Sponge Bathing

Sponge bathing should be done until the umbilical cord falls off and the circumcision site is healed. A newborn does not require a complete bath every day. However, the genitals and buttocks should be cleaned daily to prevent irritation in the diaper area. Guidelines for giving a sponge bath are presented in Box 15.4.

Skin Care

Babies have delicate skin. Encourage parents to avoid baby bath or skin-care products that have fragrance or unnecessary additives. Some commercial baby wipes can be irritating to the skin. If that is the case, plain water with cotton squares is sufficient for cleansing the diaper area. Talcum powder is not used for babies because of the risk of inhaling the talcum into the lungs.

Box 15.4

Sponge Bathing a Newborn

The procedure for sponge bathing is as follows:

- Gather all supplies before beginning the bath: a mild or hypoallergenic baby soap, washcloths, towel, clean diaper, and clean clothes.
- Place a towel on a firm surface next to the sink or basin of water filled with lukewarm water. Always test the temperature of the water on a forearm.
- Undress the baby and cover with a towel. To avoid chilling the baby, only the parts of the body being washed should be exposed.
- Always keep one hand on the baby.
- Start with the eyes. Using a clean cloth and no soap, wipe gently from the bridge of the nose outward.
- Move next to the ears and the rest of the face. No soap is needed for the face.

- Uncover the chest and, using gentle soap, clean the neck, chest, arms, and hands. Pay attention to creases in the skin. Rinse carefully, keeping the umbilical stump dry. Pat the skin dry.
- Cover the chest and uncover the lower body. Wash, rinse, and pat dry the toes, feet, and legs.
- Turn the baby over and wash and rinse the back.
- Wash the genitals and buttocks last. For a girl, wash from front to back. If the boy is circumcised, do not wash the penis until it is healed.
- After drying the baby, place a clean diaper on them and wrap the baby in a towel before washing the hair.
- To wash the hair, hold the baby in the football hold, supporting the neck and head; use the other hand to wash and rinse the hair. Tilt the head slightly back to keep water and shampoo from running into the eyes.

CRITICAL THINKING & CLINICAL JUDGMENT

Scenario #3: You walk into a postpartum patient's room just as the newborn's aunt is changing the diaper. She says to you, "Where is the baby powder? I don't want him to get a diaper rash."

Questions

1. What should you consider before answering the aunt?
2. What should you do?

Infant Follow-Up Care After Discharge

Most pediatricians and pediatric nurse practitioners schedule a 2-week follow-up appointment for the newborn. However, a newborn who is not feeding well and has lost 10% or more of the birth weight will probably be scheduled for an appointment 2 days after discharge for a weight check.

Patient Teaching Guidelines

Before discharge, parents should be educated that any of the following signs of newborn illness requires a call to the pediatric or family practice office:

- Breathing more than 60 breaths/minute
- Grunting sounds when breathing
- Blue color of the face, tongue, or lips
- Abdominal distention (a hard belly) accompanied by vomiting or no bowel movement for more than 1 day
- Jitters or shakiness of the whole body
- Vomiting that is forceful and shoots out several inches
- Persistent choking during feedings
- Head-to-toe yellow skin color
- An umbilical stump that is red and has pus around the base
- Diarrhea (more than six watery stools per day)
- Poor feeding
- Excessive crying (the baby is not easily consoled by the parents)

Key Points

- An assessment is a systematic way of obtaining data to identify problems. The newborn should have a complete head-to-toe evaluation within 2 hours of birth.
- Initial measurements of the newborn include head, chest, length, and weight.
- A complete head-to-toe evaluation includes vital signs and evaluation of the skin, head, eyes, ears, nose, mouth, chest, and abdomen as well as the respiratory, cardiovascular, genitourinary, neurological, and musculoskeletal systems.

- Throughout the newborn evaluation, you should identify warning signs to report.
- There are a variety of normal newborn skin variations, including rashes, birthmarks, and lesions.
- There are many newborn reflexes that indicate healthy neurological functioning.
- A gestational age evaluation may be indicated if the newborn appears preterm, postterm, small for gestational age, large for gestational age, or if the mother did not obtain prenatal care.

- Nursing care for the newborn includes medications, the initial newborn bath, and coordination of newborn screening for health maintenance.
- You are responsible for discharge teaching regarding newborn care, including umbilicus care, circumcision care, feeding schedules, and elimination.

- To promote safety, the parents need to be instructed about the use of the bulb syringe, sleeping positions, holding and positioning, trimming the nails, bathing, car seat safety, and skin care.

Review Questions

1. _____ is the white protective coating on the skin of the newborn.

2. A mother asks you, "Why does my baby have blue hands?" What is your best response?
   1. "He is just cold."
   2. "He may have been born with a heart problem."
   3. "The circulation in the hands is not fully developed."
   4. "The hands are always blue in the newborn."

3. The grandparents of a 6-hour-old newborn burst loudly into the mother's hospital room and bump the baby's crib. The newborn quickly makes a symmetrical abduction of the extremities and places the index fingers and thumbs into a "C" shape. The mother is alarmed and asks you if this movement is normal for a baby. What is your best answer to give?
   1. "The baby just woke up when the crib was bumped."
   2. "I'm going to take the baby to the nursery to check his blood sugar."
   3. "The baby was just demonstrating the Moro, or startle, reflex and that's normal."
   4. "The baby may have a neurological problem, and I should take him to the nursery."

4. Swelling on the head caused by birth trauma that does not cross the newborn's cranial suture lines is termed:
   1. Molding
   2. Caput succedaneum
   3. Cephalohematoma
   4. Melanosis

5. You note that the newborn's respiratory rate is 42 breaths/minute, the pulse is 140 bpm, and the CRT is fewer than 3 seconds. Which action by you is most appropriate?
   1. Report the findings to the charge nurse.
   2. Document the findings as normal.
   3. Repeat the examination to verify abnormal findings.
   4. Return the newborn to the nursery for observation.

6. You are most concerned about which evaluation finding?
   1. Gynecomastia
   2. Positive Ortolani test
   3. Pseudomenstruation
   4. Dermal melanosis

7. A tub bath should not be given to the newborn until what time? **(Select all that apply.)**
   1. The baby is able to sit up on their own.
   2. The umbilical cord falls off.
   3. Both parents can help with the bath.
   4. The circumcision is healed.
   5. The infant is 1 month old.

8. Which evaluation findings should be reported? **(Select all that apply.)**
   1. Undescended testicles
   2. Periodic mild twitching
   3. Yellowish skin color
   4. "Stork bites" on the forehead
   5. Bulging anterior fontanel
   6. Absent Moro reflex
   7. Irregular breathing pattern

9. What is the purpose of starting the hepatitis B vaccine series before a newborn is discharged home?
   1. To prevent the infant from contracting hepatitis while in the hospital
   2. To comply with state law regarding immunizations
   3. To prevent the infant from contracting hepatitis B from family members
   4. To prevent the infant from acquiring a sexually transmitted infection later in life

10. A new mother asks you if she should get her baby circumcised. Which is your best response?
    1. "Of course, everyone does it."
    2. "What are your questions or concerns about it?"
    3. "I didn't circumcise my son."
    4. "It's up to you; you're the mom."

ANSWERS: 1. Vernix; 2. 3; 3. 3; 4. 3; 5. 2; 6. 2; 7. 2, 4; 8. 1, 3, 5, 6; 9. 3; 10. 2

CRITICAL THINKING QUESTIONS

1. Gracie, a new mother, questions why her baby needs to have the newborn screening tests. She states, "He is perfect. He had 8 and 9 Apgar tests at birth, and he doesn't look sick." How should you answer the patient about the newborn screening tests?

2. Why should an infant of a diabetic mother receive a gestational age evaluation?

Resources

For additional resources and information, including Postconference Questions and Activities, Answers, and References, visit www.FADavis.com.

Student Study Guide

CHAPTER 16
Newborn Nutrition

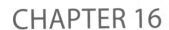

KEY TERMS

areola (ah-REE-o-luh)
engorgement (en-GORJ-ment)
foremilk (FOR-MILK)
galactosemia (ga-LAK-toh-SEE-mee-ah)
hindmilk (HYEND-MILK)
immunoglobulin (IM-yuh-noh-GLOB-yuh-lin)
inverted nipples (in-VER-tuhd NIH-puhlz)
lactoferrin (LAK-toh-FAIR-in)
lactogenesis (LAK-toh-JEN-ih-siss)
prolactin (proh-LAK-tin)

CHAPTER CONCEPTS

Growth and Development
Health Promotion
Nutrition
Professionalism

LEARNING OUTCOMES

1. Define the key terms.
2. Discuss infant nutritional needs.
3. Describe the process of human milk production.
4. Describe the stages of milk production.
5. List the advantages and disadvantages of breastfeeding.
6. Identify contraindications for breastfeeding.
7. Identify cues of infant readiness to nurse.
8. Teach a mother how to correctly latch-on a baby for breastfeeding.
9. Discuss common breastfeeding problems and how to manage those problems.
10. Identify warning signs of inadequate breastfeeding in the newborn.
11. List the advantages and disadvantages of bottle feeding.
12. Teach bottle-feeding parents how to prepare formula.
13. Discuss bottle feeding and safety issues for parents.
14. Identify signs of bottle-feeding problems.
15. Provide patient-centered care when assisting parents to implement their choice of feeding method for their newborn.

CRITICAL THINKING & CLINICAL JUDGMENT

Scenario #1: **Samantha** is 25 years old and pregnant with her first baby. She is planning to return to her job as a kindergarten teacher after a maternity leave of 4 months. At her 20-week prenatal appointment, you introduce the subject of breastfeeding. Samantha is interested in breastfeeding, but no one in her family has ever breastfed before, and she does not really know much about it.

Questions

1. What should you think about in this situation?
2. What should you do and why?

CONCEPTUAL CORNERSTONE

Nutrition

Nutrition is a fundamental concept for nursing practice because it is directly related to health. Good nutrition is important for a healthy lifestyle. The newborn who receives proper nutrition will grow appropriately and is more likely to meet physical, mental, and emotional developmental milestones. Underfed or improperly fed infants run the risk of organ damage and dehydration. They fail to thrive and are less likely to meet developmental milestones. What places infants at risk for altered nutrition? Their immature organs require certain specific nutrients for maturation, and infants must rely completely on others for feeding. Nurses can support the nutritional needs of the newborn by educating parents about infant nutrition, encouraging breastfeeding, supporting correct bottle feeding, and monitoring the growth and development of the infant. Early support of healthy nutrition can set the foundation for a lifetime of healthy food choices.

Whether parents decide to breastfeed or bottle feed, lack of knowledge and skills about how to feed their infant can produce some anxiety for them. Parents look to nurses to provide education, guidance, and support when choosing a feeding method. Infant nutrition is important because it has an effect on the infant's growth and brain development. This chapter focuses on feeding the full-term infant of normal birth weight in the context of both breastfeeding and bottle feeding.

RECOMMENDED INFANT NUTRITION

The American Academy of Pediatrics (2022b) recommends exclusive breastfeeding for the first 6 months of life with the addition of solid foods along with breastfeeding for another 6 months. Breastfeeding with the addition of solid foods should continue into the second year of life. In contrast, the World Health Organization (WHO, 2022) recommends exclusive breastfeeding for 6 months and then the addition of appropriate foods along with breastfeeding for 2 years or more. Breastfeeding is the normal "gold" standard against which all research and recommendations for infant feeding should be measured (Zhang et al., 2021). Women who receive education and family support are more likely to continue breastfeeding to 6 months or longer postpartum. Nurses play a crucial role in facilitating success with lactation. The mother makes her decision about whether or not to breastfeed before delivery in most cases. Therefore, her choice of feeding should be discussed with her starting in the second trimester and throughout the pregnancy and postpartum (Kellams, 2022).

In 2019, the percentage of infants breastfed at birth in the United States was 83.2%. At 6 months of age, only 55.8% were still being breastfed; and at 12 months of age, only 35.9% were being breastfed (Centers for Disease Control and Prevention [CDC], 2022).

Box 16.1

Calorie and Fluid Requirements of the Newborn

Estimated Calorie Requirements
Term infant: 105 to 108 kcal/kg/day
Preterm infant: 110 to 120 kcal/kg/day

Estimated Fluid Requirements
Term infant: 140 to 160 mL/kg/day
Preterm infant: 60 to 80 mL/kg/day

Consolini, D. (2022). Nutrition in infants. *Merck Manual.* https://www.merckmanuals.com/professional/pediatrics/care-of-newborns-and-infants/nutrition-in-infants?query=newborn%20nutrition

Nutritional Needs of the Infant

Calorie needs per kilogram of body weight are higher during the first year of life than at any other time. For the first 4 to 6 months of life, breast or formula feeding can provide sufficient calories. The infant's health-care provider will measure weight and length and plot this information on a standardized growth grid to determine the adequacy of an infant's caloric intake. (See Chapter 18 for examples of growth charts.) The estimated calorie need for infants is based on their age, size, and sex (Box 16.1).

The calories in an infant's diet are provided by protein, fat, and carbohydrates. Of the protein requirement, 50% is used for growth in the first 2 months of life, which declines to 11% by 2 to 3 years of age. Fat provides 40% to 50% of the calories supplied during infancy and is a source of essential fatty acids. Carbohydrates, primarily lactose, are the principal source of dietary energy. Water requirements for the first 6 months are met when adequate amounts of breast milk or infant formula are consumed.

The newborn typically eats only small amounts the first few days; parents should be educated that the infant has a small stomach and cautioned to avoid overfeeding. Overfeeding will lead to more regurgitation after feedings.

Safe and Effective Nursing Care

Nurses who work with low-income women and children should be aware of community resources available to support them. The Special Supplemental Nutrition Program for Women, Infants, and Children (WIC) is a government-funded program that provides supplemental nutritious food such as infant cereal, baby food, eggs, milk, cheese, yogurt, whole grain foods, vegetables, and fruits. The agency also provides screening and referrals to other health and welfare services. This program targets low-income nutritionally at-risk women who are pregnant through 6 weeks' postpartum, breastfeeding women, non-breastfeeding women, infants, and children up to 5 years old (USDA Food and Nutrition Service, 2022).

THE BREASTFEEDING MOTHER AND INFANT

The CDC and WHO encourage exclusive breastfeeding to promote infant health and reduce mortality. The Academy of Breastfeeding Medicine (2021) recommends that all health-care professionals promote breastfeeding early in prenatal care and recognize that breastfeeding is superior to bottle feeding. The promotion of breastfeeding by health-care providers may help to increase support from families and employers, making it easier for the woman to continue breastfeeding. Parents need to be provided with complete and current information on the benefits of breastfeeding and breastfeeding techniques.

After delivery, postpartum and mother–baby unit policies on breastfeeding should support and encourage the mother who chooses to breastfeed. Whenever possible, the newborn should be placed in direct skin-to-skin contact with the mother and the mother assisted with latch-on during the first hour after birth. The mother and infant should not be separated and should be encouraged to sleep in close proximity to facilitate breastfeeding. Supplements such as water or formula should not be given unless medically indicated and ordered by the health-care provider. Women can be successful with breastfeeding when nurses and lactation specialists provide education and support as the new mother learns breastfeeding techniques.

Therapeutic Communication

Not all women choose to breastfeed their infants. It is very important that nurses who are enthusiastic about breastfeeding do not make a patient feel bad about her choice to bottle feed. You should educate and support the patient's decision regarding feeding methods. When discussing breastfeeding choices, use open-ended questions and general leads. Some examples are these:

"What are your thoughts about breastfeeding?"
    (Open-ended question)
"Tell me what you know about breastfeeding."
    (General lead)
"What are your concerns about breastfeeding?"
    (Open-ended question)

Lactogenesis

Milk production, or **lactogenesis**, includes all the processes needed to transform the mammary gland from its nonproducing state to one of milk production.

At puberty, estrogen stimulates breast tissue to enlarge through the growth of mammary ducts into the mammary

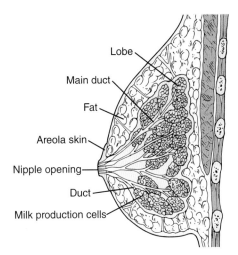

FIGURE 16.1 Cross section of a lactating breast.

fat pad. The effects of estrogen and progesterone enable the formation of the structure of the adult female breast, but full alveolar development and maturation of the epithelium requires the hormones of pregnancy.

The basic unit of the mammary gland is the alveolus that connects to a ductule. Each ductule drains to a duct, which then empties into the lactiferous sinuses. Milk is stored in the lactiferous sinus. At the end of each ductule is a cluster of small, grapelike sacs called *alveoli*. A cluster of alveoli is called a *lobule;* a cluster of lobules is called a *lobe.* Each breast contains between 15 and 20 lobes with one milk duct for every lobe. The 15 to 20 milk ducts merge with eight or nine ending at the tip of the nipple to deliver milk to the baby (Tauber, 2021; Fig. 16.1).

After childbirth and the delivery of the placenta, estrogen and progesterone levels drop quickly. Nipple stimulation from latching-on the infant to the breast signals the pituitary gland to trigger a rise in the hormone **prolactin**. Prolactin causes the alveoli to take proteins, sugars, and fat from the blood supply and make breast milk (Fig. 16.2).

The first substance produced by the breasts is colostrum, which is produced in very small amounts during the second and third trimesters. During that time, the pregnant woman may notice a small amount of a sticky substance on her bra or nightgown occasionally. Colostrum is the perfect first food for the newborn. It is easy to digest and highly concentrated with carbohydrates and fat. It also contains secretory **immunoglobulin** A (IgA), which is a new substance to the newborn. IgA protects the baby from infections in the mucous membranes in the throat, lungs, and intestines. Leukocytes in colostrum also protect the newborn from infections. In addition, colostrum has a laxative effect, which aids in the passage of the first meconium stool after birth (Tauber, 2021).

· WORD · BUILDING ·
lactogenesis: lacto–milk + genesis–beginning

· WORD · BUILDING ·
prolactin: pro–for + lact–milk + in–hormone or chemical
immunoglobulin: immuno–safe + globulin–plasma protein

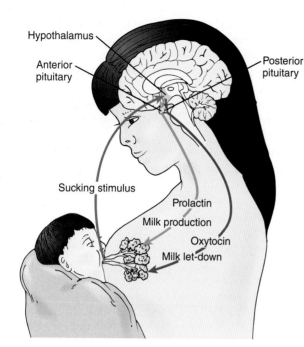

FIGURE 16.2 Mechanism for milk production.

Frequent breastfeeding, at least 8 to 12 times a day, stimulates the pituitary gland to increase levels of prolactin, causing an increase in the volume of breast milk. Mature milk is produced around the third and fourth postpartum day.

For the baby to receive the milk from the breast, the let-down reflex must occur. Suction on the nipple stimulates the pituitary gland to release prolactin to produce milk and oxytocin. Oxytocin causes the cells around the alveoli to squeeze the glands to push the milk into the ductules and into the ducts. The mother may notice the let-down reflex and a tingly or warm sensation in her breasts. She may even notice the milk drip or spray during let-down. The let-down reflex can also be triggered by the mother hearing a baby cry or thinking about her baby. As the baby suckles, the combination of the let-down reflex, compression of the areola, and negative pressure created by suction allows the milk to be delivered to the infant (Pillay, 2022).

Components of Breast Milk

The following list provides an overview of the components and nutrients in breast milk:

Proteins: The balance of the proteins, approximately 60% whey and 40% casein, allows the infant to digest breast milk easily. Other specific proteins in breast milk are:
- **Lactoferrin**, which has bactericidal and iron-binding properties
- Secretory IgA, which protects the infant from viruses and bacteria
- Lysozyme, an enzyme that promotes the growth of healthy intestinal flora and has anti-inflammatory functions

• WORD • BUILDING •
lactoferrin: lacto–milk + ferrin–iron compound

Bifidus factor supports the growth of lactobacillus, which creates an acidic environment in the intestines.
Cholesterol and fats are essential for brain development and the absorption of fat-soluble vitamins and are a primary calorie source.
Vitamin amounts and types in breast milk are directly related to the mother's dietary intake.
Carbohydrates, especially lactose: Lactose is the primary carbohydrate found in human milk, accounting for approximately 40% of the total calories provided by breast milk.
Antibodies from the mother reduce the risk of neonatal infections (Tauber, 2021).

Stages of Human Milk

During the establishment of lactation, there are three stages of milk production: colostrum, transitional milk, and mature milk.

STAGE 1: COLOSTRUM
- This yellowish fluid is present for 2 to 3 days.
- It contains high levels of protein and lower levels of carbohydrates, fats, and calories than mature milk.
- Colostrum is high in immunoglobulins G and A, which protect the infant from infections.
- It has a laxative effect to promote passage of the meconium stool.

STAGE 2: TRANSITIONAL MILK
- This stage is from day 3 to day 10.
- Transitional milk contains increasing levels of carbohydrates and fat with decreasing levels of protein.

STAGE 3: MATURE MILK
- *Foremilk* is the milk produced and stored in the breast between feedings. It has higher water content than hindmilk.
- *Hindmilk* is produced after several minutes of feeding and has a higher fat content and contributes to the feeling of fullness and satisfaction for the infant (Pillay, 2022).

Advantages of Breastfeeding

The advantages of breastfeeding for the mother and infant include the following:

- Breast milk provides the exact nutrients required for an infant's growth and development.
- Breast milk provides immunologic protection. A mother will pass on some of her immunities to the baby.
- Breast milk is convenient and economical for the mother. She does not need to prepare bottles. It is always ready and available for the infant.
- Breastfeeding promotes close physical contact between a mother and child to enhance bonding and attachment.
- Breastfeeding women have lower risks for developing premenopausal breast cancer and ovarian cancer (Perez-Escamilla et al., 2023).

Disadvantages of Breastfeeding

The disadvantages of breastfeeding for the mother and infant include the following:

- The mother must be available for feeding or provide pumped milk if she is absent.
- Feeding in public may cause embarrassment.
- Certain medications can interrupt breastfeeding.
- Early breastfeeding may be uncomfortable.
- Leaking of breast milk may occur and require nursing pads to be worn in the bra.

Medication Facts

Most medications pass from the mother through the breast milk to the baby. If the mother requires medication while breastfeeding, the health-care provider should check for risks to the baby before prescribing the medication and fully inform the mother of the risk.

Contraindications for Breastfeeding

There are some contraindications for breastfeeding. The health-care provider and nurses should be aware of the following contraindications:

An infant diagnosed with **galactosemia**, a rare genetic metabolic disorder that makes it difficult for the infant to metabolize milk sugar; breastfeeding an infant with galactosemia can damage the liver, kidneys, and brain.
The infant whose mother:
- Is HIV+
- Is taking antiretroviral medications
- Has untreated, active tuberculosis (TB)

Learn to C.U.S.

Kari, aged 28, gave birth 1 day ago at the local hospital. She did not have prenatal care and admits to alcohol and drug use. She plans to breastfeed and states, "I can't afford to buy formula; I have to breastfeed." You are concerned about breastfeeding and the probability of continued substance use disorder. You use the C.U.S. method of communication with the health-care provider.
Nurse:

C: "I am very *concerned* about Kari and her baby.
U: I am *uncomfortable* with assisting her with breastfeeding.
S: I feel that we have a *safety* issue because Kari admits to substance use disorder and alcohol use."

- WORD - BUILDING -

galactosemia: galactos–galactose + em–blood + ia–condition

- Is infected with human T-cell lymphotropic virus type I or type II, which is the virus that causes some leukemias and lymphomas
- Is using or is dependent upon an illicit drug
- Has a herpes lesion on her breast
- Is taking prescribed cancer chemotherapy agents, such as antimetabolites that interfere with DNA replication and cell division
- Is undergoing radiation therapies; however, such nuclear medicine therapies require only a temporary interruption in breastfeeding (Perez-Escamilla et al., 2023)

Breastfeeding Techniques

The breastfeeding mother benefits from a relaxed and supportive environment. Be available to assist with positioning, education, and positive feedback during the process. Minimizing interruptions and visitors will facilitate the process. The mother's partner should be included in education and feeding sessions. Women with partners who support and encourage breastfeeding are more likely to choose this method of infant feeding.

Newborn Cues

The new mother needs to be taught signs that the newborn is interested in nursing. However, if the newborn does not demonstrate signs of hunger, she should still offer the breast every 2½ hours until breastfeeding has been established. Infant hunger cues include rooting, making hand-to-mouth movements, and making mouth and tongue movements while in an awake/alert state (Rohan, 2020).

Patient Teaching Guidelines

Mothers who are breastfeeding may experience occasional "leaks" of milk that dampen their clothing. If the mother senses milk let-down happening at an inconvenient time, teach her to cross her arms in front of her breasts and apply gentle pressure to stop the flow.

Positioning

The position of the infant is an important part of successful breastfeeding. First, the mother should wash her hands to avoid transferring bacteria to her breast. Next, she should be in a comfortable sitting position or side-lying in bed. Pillows should be placed around the mother to support the baby and prevent the mother from hunching her back. Pillows can be placed to support her arm. The infant should be placed in the mother's arm with their stomach flat against the mother's abdomen (Fig. 16.3).

Another position is the football hold, in which the infant is cradled in the mother's arm with the infant's head in her palm and the buttocks toward the mother's elbow. This position puts less stress on the abdomen if the mother is recuperating from a cesarean birth.

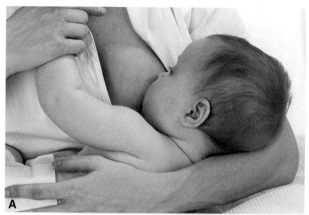

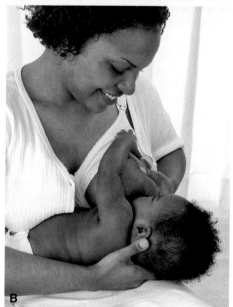

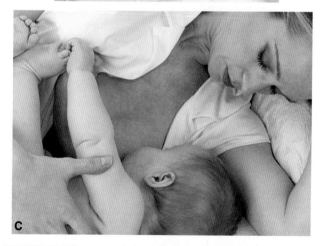

FIGURE 16.3 Common positions for breastfeeding. A, Cradle hold position. B, Football hold position. C, Side-lying position. *(All images are Copyright ©2015 Medela, Inc.)*

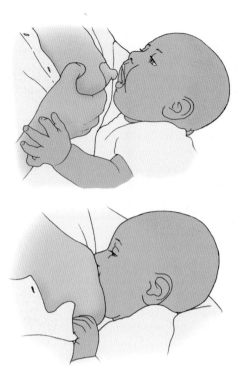

FIGURE 16.4 Correct latch-on position. When properly latched-on, the tip of the infant's nose, cheeks, and chin should all be touching the breast.

Achieving Latch-On

The mother should position her hand around the breast, cupping it with her fingers close to the chest wall. Her hands are usually in a "C" position as she supports her breast: The thumb is on top, and her fingers are underneath the breast. She should avoid covering the **areola**, the dark area around the nipple, which goes into the infant's mouth. After positioning her hand, the mother should lightly brush her nipple across the lips of her infant to elicit the rooting reflex. The infant will instinctively open their mouth and extend the tongue. The mother should bring her baby to her breast and maneuver the nipple and areola into the infant's mouth. These actions will initiate the sucking reflex (Figs. 16.4 and 16.5).

The mother should put the infant on the breast every 2½ hours during the first 4 to 5 days after birth to assist with creation of the milk supply. Generally, it takes about 30 to 40 minutes of sucking for an infant to have a complete feeding. If the infant falls asleep on the breast, the mother should be encouraged to take the infant off the breast, change to the other breast, and resume the feeding session. The baby should be burped between breasts. The mother should alternate the breast at which each feeding begins. This helps to stimulate the production of breast milk. She should avoid offering supplemental formula or water because some babies will suck on a bottle even if full of breast milk (Rohan, 2020).

The new mother should be reassured that even though feeding a newborn can take up much time initially, after breastfeeding is established, the infant becomes stronger and feedings proceed much faster. Instruct the breastfeeding woman that her baby should have several wet diapers and two to three dirty diapers per day. The stools of breastfed infants are looser than those of formula-fed infants.

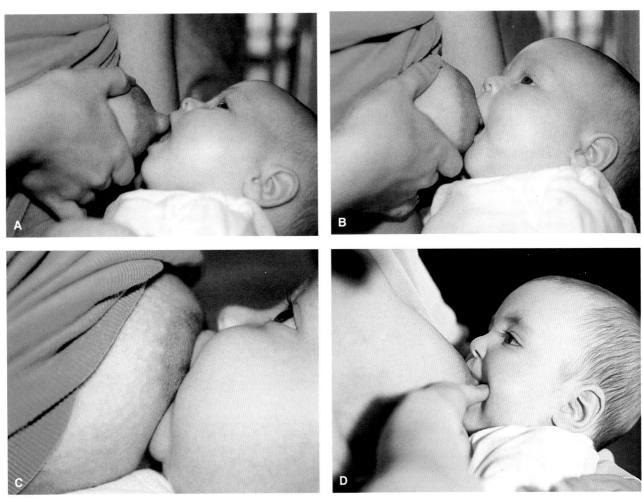

FIGURE 16.5 Infant latch-on. A, Nipple is aligned with the baby's nose. B and C, As the baby latches to the nipple, the baby's mouth is placed 1 to 2 inches beyond the base of the nipple. D, To remove the baby from the breast, the mother inserts her finger into the corner of the baby's mouth to break the seal.

Health Promotion

Checkpoints for Correct Latch-On

- Observe the position of the mother. Is she comfortable with pillows in appropriate locations? Reposition if needed.
- Observe the position of the baby. Is the baby lying "tummy to tummy" with the mother? If not, reposition.
- Observe the position of the baby on the areola. Usually the lips need to be 1 to 2 inches beyond the base of the nipple.
- Observe the infant's lower lip. It should not be folded in.
- Observe the motion of the masseter muscle and listen for sounds of swallowing. A clicking sound indicates improper positioning.
- Observe the comfort level of the mother. If she is experiencing any nipple pain, she should take the infant off the breast and latch-on again.

Signs of Effective Breastfeeding

The infant is getting sufficient intake from breastfeeding if the following are observed:

- The mother's breasts soften during and after a feeding.
- The mother can hear the infant swallowing during the feeding.
- The number of wet diapers increases to at least six to eight by the time the infant is 6 days old.
- The infant has two to three yellow stools per day by the fifth day after birth.

Breastfeeding Challenges

Breastfeeding can be a challenge in the first few days or weeks. You can provide guidance to support the breastfeeding mother with common problems.

Sore Nipples

Sore nipples are a common occurrence but can be prevented or managed with the following interventions:

- Make sure that the infant has correct latch-on every time the baby is placed on the breast.

- Try changing positions from sitting to side-lying or football hold to move the infant's mouth to a different position on the breast.
- Gently insert the little finger between the breast and infant's mouth to break the seal and prevent pulling the infant off the nipple.
- Change nursing pads often to avoid trapping moisture on the nipple areas.
- Expose the nipple to air to promote healing.
- Avoid harsh soaps on the breast.
- Apply modified anhydrous lanolin after nursing to keep the skin soft.
- Gently massage colostrum or breast milk into the nipple to soothe an irritated nipple.

Nipple Confusion

A latex nipple fits into the infant mouth differently than a breast nipple. An infant who is learning to breastfeed can have difficulty with learning how to place their jaws and tongue if a latex nipple is introduced too early. If the mother wants to avoid nipple confusion and be able to later give the baby a bottle, she should establish breastfeeding *for at least 2 to 3 weeks before introducing a bottle.*

Low Milk Supply

Most women make plenty of milk, but during the baby's growth spurts at 3 weeks, 6 weeks, and 3 months, the supply may be a little low to satisfy the baby. To accommodate the baby's increased hunger, the mother should breastfeed more often and allow the baby to decide when to end the feeding, a method that is sometimes called "cluster feeding." In this approach, the baby feeds as often and as long as wanted. This method of feeding increases stimulation to the breast, therefore increasing milk supply for the growing baby. The mother can also try offering both breasts at each feeding. Have the baby stay on the first breast as long as suckling and swallowing continues. Offer the second breast when the baby slows down.

Engorgement

Engorgement can happen when the body is adjusting to the amount of milk to make. It can also occur the first time the baby sleeps through the night. The breasts may feel heavy

Nursing Care Plan for the Patient With Ineffective Breastfeeding

Elaina has arrived at the hospital lactation clinic with concerns about breastfeeding. Even though she is feeding her infant every 4 hours, she reports that he often falls asleep on the breast and only nurses for 10 to 15 minutes. She is concerned that her 5-day-old son is not getting enough milk. She reports that he is having only two wet diapers a day and has not had a bowel movement since yesterday.

Nursing Diagnosis: Inadequate nutrition for body requirements, because of ineffective breastfeeding as shown by infant's inadequate number of wet and soiled diapers
Expected Outcomes: The infant will have at least six wet diapers and two to three stools per day. The infant will breastfeed every 2½ hours with 30 to 40 minutes of sucking time at each feeding.

Interventions:	Rationale:
Provide verbal encouragement.	*Support is needed so that Elaina will not quit breastfeeding.*
Weigh the infant and compare the weight with the birth weight.	*This provides objective evidence of adequate intake.*
Review infant cues of hunger with the mother.	*If the mother is aware of the infant's cue of being awake and hungry, she can encourage feeding when the infant is more likely to be interested.*
Review feeding requirements of offering the breast every 2½ hours and encouraging the infant to nurse for 30 to 40 minutes each feeding.	*Many new mothers do not realize the amount of time that breastfeeding requires for a newborn.*
Encourage her to wake the baby up if he falls asleep while nursing and have him latch-on again.	*Encouraging a longer feeding time will increase intake.*
Observe the mother latch-on the infant and give suggestions if needed.	*Incorrect latch-on can reduce the amount of milk expressed from the breast and cause the mother to have sore nipples.*
Provide written instructions and links to appropriate instructional videos that she can view at home.	*Elaina can have a reference for remembering breastfeeding techniques.*
Ask Elaina to maintain a feeding diary to monitor the infant's intake as well as the number of wet and soiled diapers.	*A feeding diary and record of wet and soiled diapers will provide objective data to determine if feedings are adequate.*

and swollen with a flat nipple. To prevent or minimize engorgement, the mother should breastfeed every 2½ hours when the baby is awake. If her breasts become engorged, she can soften them with a warm cloth or in the shower and then express enough milk by hand to allow correct latch-on by the infant. If the infant latch-on is done correctly, the feeding will take care of the engorgement.

Flat or Inverted Nipples

Flat or **inverted nipples** may make it difficult for the baby to latch-on the breast. Flat nipples do not stand out from the areola; inverted nipples tend to retract or pull inward. Women with these types of nipples may require more assistance with breastfeeding.

- A breast pump may be used to evert or "pull out" the nipple.
- Before delivery, the lactation specialist may recommend that the pregnant woman wear a special device called a *breast shield* or a *supple cup* to encourage the nipple to protrude from the breast.

Warning Signs of Breastfeeding Problems

Warning signs in the healthy term breastfed newborn include:

- Losing more than the normal 5% to 7% of birth weight (Spencer, 2021)
- Not gaining back birth weight by 10 days of age
- Not having at least two to three bowel movements per day after day 2
- Not having four or five wet diapers per day by day 4 with clear or pale-yellow urine, which indicates adequate hydration (Spencer, 2021)

Evidence-Based Practice

The WHO recommends exclusive breastfeeding for 6 months or more. A study was conducted to determine if complete 24-hour rooming-in immediately after birth or partial rooming-in (baby goes to the nursery for periods of time) influenced the rate of breastfeeding at 1 month postpartum. In the study, all first-time mothers who experienced complete rooming-in were still exclusively breastfeeding at 1 month postpartum. At 3 months postpartum, none of the first-time mothers with partial rooming-in were breastfeeding. The study concluded that rooming-in helps mothers learn newborn cues and practice breastfeeding more often in the hospital where they could also receive support from the nurses and is an effective strategy to improve breastfeeding success rates.

Wu, H., Lu, D., & Tsay, P. (2022). Rooming-in and breastfeeding duration in first-time mothers in a modern postpartum care center. *Journal of Environmental Research Public Health, 19,* 11790. https://doi.org/10.3390/ijerph191811790

THE FORMULA-FEEDING PARENTS AND INFANT

The infant formula industry acknowledges the importance of human milk and recognizes breastfeeding as the preferred method for feeding babies. The formula industry is committed to producing infant formulas modeled on breast milk. Commercially prepared formulas meet the nutritional requirements based on the recommendations of the Committee on Nutrition of the AAP to provide the infant with the right combination of protein, fat, carbohydrates, vitamins, and minerals.

The AAP (2022a) states that cow's milk is not suitable for infants under 1 year of age. Cow's milk contains a higher level of protein than the infant requires; the fat is difficult for the infant to digest; it is a poor source of iron; it contains only a small amount of vitamins C, E, and copper; and the sodium level is too high for an infant.

Bottle feeding can be a warm, loving experience for the parents and their infant. If the parents choose this method of feeding, they should be supported and educated without disapproval from the nursing staff.

Advantages of Formula

The advantages of bottle feeding for the parents and infant include the following:

- It may be the appropriate choice for a mother with a chronic illness who requires medications harmful to the infant.
- It provides adequate and acceptable nutrition for the infant.
- Anyone can feed the infant.
- The mother does not need to worry that her food or alcohol intake may affect the baby.
- It may be easier to leave the infant with a sitter or family member to give the parents a break.

Disadvantages of Formula

The disadvantages of bottle feeding include the following:

- The woman's breast milk may come in anyway, causing breast engorgement and pain. (See Chapter 12 for ways to prevent this.)
- Formula costs can be expensive for parents on a budget.
- Bottles, nipples, and formula must be purchased.
- Bottles and formula must be carried along with the infant.
- There is increased risk for serious illness because of improper dilution or home additives.
- There is an increased risk for gastrointestinal illness (Perez-Escamilla et al., 2023).

Types of Formula

If correctly prepared, most infant formulas have 20 calories in each ounce. Prepared formula should be in a covered container in the refrigerator, and unused formula should be thrown out after 24 hours. Hypoallergenic formula should be given if an allergy to milk-based formula is suspected. Soy-based formula should be given to infants who cannot take dairy-based products for health, cultural, religious, or personal reasons, such as a family's vegan lifestyle.

Parents should be taught the following about formula:

- *Ready-to-feed formula* is available in a can or carton and should *not* be diluted.
- *Liquid concentrated formula* is formulated to be diluted with equal amounts of water.
- *Powder formula* should be dissolved in water.

CRITICAL THINKING & CLINICAL JUDGMENT

Scenario #2: A postpartum patient has decided to bottle feed her newborn. She is planning to use the powdered formula that is reconstituted with water because it is less expensive. She and her partner are vegetable and fruit farmers and live in a rural farming area outside of town and get their water from a well.

Questions

1. What should you think about when preparing the discharge teaching for this patient?
2. What should you do regarding their plan of using well water for making formula?

Bottle Feeding the Infant

When educating parents about bottle feeding, include the following information:

- Before purchasing formula, check the expiration date on the container. Do not buy expired formula.
- After purchasing, sterilize the bottles and nipples. After initial sterilization, bottles do not need to be sterilized unless the family water supply is not safe. Washing bottles and nipples with soap and water or in the dishwasher is sufficient to kill bacteria.
- Make sure to follow the package directions exactly to dilute the formula or to mix the bottles correctly.
- If the water supply is not proven to be safe, the water for mixing the formula should be boiled first.
- Wash the outside of the formula container with soap and water before opening it.
- Some babies will drink a bottle straight from the refrigerator. Others prefer a bottle warmed in a bowl of warm water or in a bottle-warmer device. Parents should always check the temperature of warmed formula on their inner wrist to avoid burning the infant.
- Make sure that the nipple is not too large to cause gagging or too small to cause frustration for the infant.
- Parents and caregivers should wash their hands before every feeding.
- Before feeding the infant, find a comfortable place to sit and have a burp cloth nearby.

- Cradle the baby in one arm, with the head slightly elevated, and hold the bottle with the opposite arm.
- Angle the bottle so that the baby is not sucking in air.
- Keep the nipple filled with formula.
- Stop and take burping breaks.
- Try different nipple shapes to see what the baby prefers.
- Discard the contents of any bottle that has been out of the refrigerator for more than 2 hours.
- Continue to feed until the newborn gives indications of being full, such as a decrease in sucking, spitting out the nipple, turning away, or pushing away the bottle.
- Never force a baby to finish a bottle.
- When the baby begins to cut teeth, do not let the baby fall asleep with a bottle in the mouth because this can lead to tooth decay from the milk sugar.

Safety *Stat!*

Warming a Bottle

Never warm a bottle of formula or breast milk in the microwave. Microwaves heat unevenly and a baby could be burned.

Safety *Stat!*

Propping a Bottle

Bottle-fed babies should never have the bottle propped for feedings. There are two major problems with this practice. First, the baby could choke and aspirate without adult observation. Second, the baby who falls asleep with a propped bottle has residual milk left in the mouth that pools around the teeth. The milk sugar can cause breakdown of the teeth and cause nursing-bottle syndrome (CDC, 2021).

Bottle-Feeding Problems

Parents should be warned about the following practices that are not healthy or safe for the infant:

- Infant cereal fed through a bottle increases the risk of choking.
- Water or fruit juice given before 6 months of age does not meet the calorie and nutritional needs of the infant.
- Overdiluting the formula to reduce expense decreases the calorie content and reduces the nutritional value of the formula.
- Formula mixed with private well water that has not been tested for safety can pose a hazard.
- Allowing a baby to sleep with a bottle in the crib can lead to tooth decay.

Key Points

- Parents need to be informed of the nutritional needs of the newborn.
- Newborns should receive breast milk or commercially prepared infant formula for the first year of life. Cow's milk is not appropriate nutrition until the child is 1 year old.
- Breast milk is convenient and economical for the mother. The milk is always ready and available for the infant.
- Teaching the mother correct latch-on technique will promote successful breastfeeding and help the mother to avoid sore nipples.

- Breastfeeding challenges such as engorgement and inverted nipples can be overcome by the mother with assistance from nurses.
- Bottle feeding is an appropriate option for feeding if the mother chooses not to breastfeed, has a chronic illness that requires medications, is HIV positive, or has an addiction problem with alcohol or drugs.
- Parents who bottle feed need education about formula preparation and bottle-feeding techniques to be successful with bottle feeding.

Review Questions

1. A new mother is concerned because her 2-day-old infant is taking only ½ ounce of formula at each feeding. What is your best response?
   1. "The baby is not getting enough to eat."
   2. "You need to feed the baby less often so that he can eat more at each feeding."
   3. "His stomach is small right now; that's about the right amount for a 2-day-old infant."
   4. "There must be a problem with the baby's digestive system."

2. A breastfeeding mother is reporting that she has sore nipples. Which of the following should you do? **(Select all that apply.)**
   1. Observe her latch-on technique with the infant.
   2. Suggest that she only breastfeed for 5 minutes on each side.
   3. Suggest that she change breastfeeding positions.
   4. Suggest that she give the baby a bottle for a couple of feedings.
   5. Suggest that she switch to bottle feeding.

3. A new father states, "As soon as we take the baby home, I am going to be feeding him a little bit of cereal between feedings." What is your best response?
   1. "Babies don't need solid food until about 6 months of age."
   2. "Your baby should sleep through the night if you do that."

   3. "That's the wrong thing to do."
   4. "You'd better ask your pediatrician about that."

4. A new mother is excited and wants to begin breastfeeding her infant son as soon as possible. How should you help the mother to hold her baby to facilitate the first breastfeeding?
   1. With her hand holding the cheeks
   2. With the baby turned in toward her body, in straight head and body alignment
   3. With the baby flat on his back and his head turned toward the breast
   4. With his arms folded over his chest

5. What should be included in teaching for bottle-feeding parents? **(Select all that apply.)**
   1. Warm the bottle in the microwave.
   2. Formula is available in three forms: ready to eat, concentrated liquid, and powder.
   3. Never prop a bottle.
   4. Discard unused formula in a used bottle after 2 hours.
   5. Store prepared bottles in the refrigerator.

ANSWERS 1. 3; 2. 1, 3; 3. 1; 4. 2; 5. 2, 3, 4, 5

CRITICAL THINKING QUESTION

1. What hospital policies could have a detrimental effect on supporting and encouraging breastfeeding?

Resources

For additional resources and information, including Postconference Questions and Activities, Answers, and References, visit www.FADavis.com.

Student Study Guide

CHAPTER 17
Nursing Care of the Newborn at Risk

KEY TERMS

anoxia (an-OKS-ee-uh)
brachial plexus (BRAY-kee-uhl PLEK-suhss)
echocardiography (EK-oh-KAR-dee-AWG-ruh-fee)
hematochezia (HEE-muh-to-KEE-zee-uh)
hypercapnia (HYE-per-KAP-nee-uh)
hyperinsulinism (HYE-per-IN-suh-lin-izm)
hypocalcemia (HYE-poh-kal-SEE-mee-uh)
hypoglycemia (HYE-poh-glye-SEE-mee-uh)
hypomagnesemia (HYE-poh-MAG-nih-SEE-mee-uh)
hypoparathyroidism (HYE-poh-PAR-uh-THYE-roy-dizm)
hypoxic-ischemic encephalopathy (hye-POK-sik-iss-KEE-mik en-SEF-uh-LAW-pa-thee)
intrauterine growth restriction (IUGR) (IN-truh-YOO-tuh-rin GROHTH rih-STRIK-shun)
large-for-gestational age (LGA) (LARJ-for-jess-TAY-shuhn-uhl AYJ)
necrosis (nek-ROH-siss)
necrotizing enterocolitis (NEK-ro-TYE-zing EN-tuh-roh-ko-LYE-tiss)
neonatal sepsis (NEE-oh-NAY-tuhl SEP-siss)
polycythemia (POL-ee-sye-THEE-mee-uh)
respiratory distress syndrome (RDS) of the newborn (RESS-pih-ruh-TOR-ee dis-TRESS SIN-drohm)
small-for-gestational age (SGA) (SMOL-for-jess-TAY-shuhn-uhl AYJ)
spina bifida (SPYE-nuh BIF-ih-duh)

CHAPTER CONCEPTS

Collaboration
Family
Growth and Development
Nutrition
Oxygenation
Professionalism
Thermoregulation

LEARNING OUTCOMES

1. Define the key terms.
2. Identify factors present at birth that can help identify a high-risk newborn.
3. Identify possible causes of birth asphyxia.
4. Recognize signs of respiratory distress in a newborn.
5. Plan nursing care for transient tachypnea of the newborn (TTN).
6. Identify physical signs of a newborn with meconium aspiration syndrome.
7. Discuss the underlying pathophysiology of persistent pulmonary hypertension of the newborn (PPHN).
8. Plan nursing interventions to manage cold stress in the newborn.
9. Recognize signs of hypoglycemia in the newborn.
10. Discuss nursing interventions for the newborn with hypoglycemia.
11. Plan nursing interventions for a newborn with a brachial plexus injury.
12. Discuss the nursing interventions for the jaundiced newborn undergoing phototherapy.
13. Summarize the risk factors, medical management, and nursing interventions for the newborn with sepsis.
14. List risk factors that can lead to a small-for-gestational-age (SGA) newborn.
15. Compare and contrast the SGA newborn and the premature newborn.
16. Discuss possible complications that can occur at birth for the large-for-gestational-age (LGA) newborn.
17. Discuss potential complications of prematurity.
18. Describe the physical characteristics of a postterm newborn.
19. Explain possible complications for the infant of a diabetic mother (IDM).
20. Discuss nursing interventions for a chemically exposed infant.
21. Discuss medical management and nursing interventions for the newborn exposed to HIV.
22. Formulate a plan to provide family-centered care in the neonatal intensive care unit (NICU).

CRITICAL THINKING & CLINICAL JUDGMENT

Scenario #1: Baby **Daniel** was born a few hours ago. He is in a crib at his mother's bedside. You notice that he has dry skin, no lanugo, long fingernails and toenails, and his umbilical cord is stained yellow. Daniel's birth weight was 5 lb 8 oz. (2,495 g). His mother states that she did not have prenatal care, "He is my fifth baby. I know all about pregnancy." She says that he was 2 weeks overdue, and she admits to smoking throughout the pregnancy.

Questions

1. Do you think Daniel's mother is correct about Daniel being a postterm baby? Why?
2. What could be a possible cause of Daniel being small for gestational age (SGA)?
3. What should you do?

CONCEPTUAL CORNERSTONE
Professionalism

An important aspect of professionalism in nursing is ethics. *Ethics,* as applied to nursing, is defined as a system of moral principles governing behaviors and relationships that is based on professional nursing beliefs and values. Simply put, *ethics* refers to standards of right and wrong that influence human behavior. Morals, similar to ethics, are private, personal standards of right and wrong in conduct and character that are based upon one's values and beliefs.

Nurses have a code of ethics that includes respect for human rights and the right to life, choice, dignity, and being treated with respect (Haddad & Geiger, 2022). Nurses are human and, when providing care to high-risk newborns and their families, you may personally disagree with choices a parent has made. For example, you may feel angry at a woman who used illicit drugs during pregnancy and caused harm to her fetus. However, that patient, whose morals and values differ from your own, deserves the same high-quality care as any other patient.

Other situations that may test your professional ethics are when the parents decide to stop care for a critically ill preterm infant, or choose to continue care when there is little likelihood that the newborn will recover. When parents are faced with difficult decisions regarding care of their newborn, you can assist them with thinking through their values and beliefs, but you should not offer an opinion based upon their own beliefs.

This chapter provides an overview of the care of the high-risk newborn. Care of these newborns is a subspecialty of maternity nursing. Nurses who work in this highly specialized area are registered nurses (RNs) with an in-depth knowledge of the care of high-risk newborns.

CONCEPTUAL CORNERSTONE
Oxygenation

To survive, all cells need a regular supply of oxygen and a regular removal of waste. Lack of oxygen or a buildup of waste can cause cell death. Gas exchange is the process in which oxygen is transported to cells and carbon dioxide is transported from cells. The terms *hypoxia* (insufficient oxygen reaching the cells) and **anoxia** (no oxygen reaching the cells) relate to this concept. *Ventilation,* the process of inhaling oxygen into the lungs to the alveoli to exchange oxygen for carbon dioxide that is exhaled, can become a problem for the at-risk newborn.

Many problems can interfere with gas exchange. Newborn hypoxia may be related to delivery problems, such as placental insufficiency or cord compression. After delivery, a lack of surfactant or the presence of fluid in the lungs or of meconium plugging the bronchioles or alveoli can contribute to hypoxia. Regardless of the exact cause, the newborn will exhibit many of the same signs and symptoms of respiratory distress. The basic nursing interventions to treat hypoxia are the same even if you may not know the exact cause of the hypoxia. If you are alert regarding subtle and early signs of hypoxia in the newborn, you can promptly implement care that can prevent a state of anoxia and possible long-term health consequences for the newborn.

IDENTIFICATION OF THE AT-RISK NEWBORN

During pregnancy, women should be screened for factors that could place the newborn at risk for problems. Factors such as premature labor, diabetes, hypertension, placenta abnormalities, HIV infection, and an unhealthy lifestyle can place a fetus at risk. On the woman's admission to labor and delivery, you should review the pregnancy health of the woman and be alert for possible risk factors for newborn problems. Predicting a possible high-risk situation for a newborn allows you to plan appropriate interventions and arrange for enough help at the time of birth. Advanced planning and swift action may prevent long-term complications for the high-risk newborn (Fig. 17.1).

CARE OF THE NEWBORN AT RISK BECAUSE OF BIRTH ASPHYXIA

Birth asphyxia is also known as *perinatal asphyxia, asphyxia neonatorum,* or **hypoxic-ischemic encephalopathy** and is described as acute brain injury caused by asphyxia when the baby did not get enough oxygen during the birth process

· WORD · BUILDING ·
anoxia: an–without + ox–oxygen + ia–condition

(Gillam-Krakauer & Gowen, 2022). Possible causes of asphyxia during the birth process include the following:

- The mother does not get enough oxygen during labor.
- The mother's blood pressure is too high or too low during labor.
- The placenta separates from the uterus too quickly, resulting in loss of oxygen.
- The umbilical cord becomes wrapped too tightly around the neck or body.
- The fetus is anemic and does not have enough red blood cells to tolerate labor contractions.
- The newborn's airway becomes blocked.
- The delivery is too long or too difficult.

Whatever the cause, when the baby becomes asphyxiated and breathing slows or ceases, there is a lack of perfusion of blood to the brain and other organ systems. Hypoxia forces cells to undergo anaerobic respiration, which produces less energy than aerobic respiration. Lactic acid forms as a by-product of cellular respiration, the cells cannot function normally, and tissues become affected and damaged. Initially, the lack of oxygen affects the brain, muscles, and heart. The heart dysfunction causes hypotension, leading to damage in a variety of organs. If adequate blood perfusion returns, the newborn's brain can begin to swell, which causes more neurological problems.

At birth, the infant may exhibit cyanosis, difficulty breathing, gasping respirations, umbilical cord blood pH less than 7, and an Apgar score of less than 3 for more than 5 minutes. Immediate medical care may include performing neonatal resuscitation if needed. The newborn with birth asphyxia may be transferred to the neonatal intensive care unit (NICU) if symptoms are severe or persist (Fig. 17.2). For more about caring for infants with hypoxia, see Table 17.1.

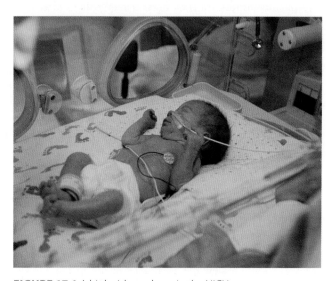

FIGURE 17.1 A high-risk newborn in the NICU.

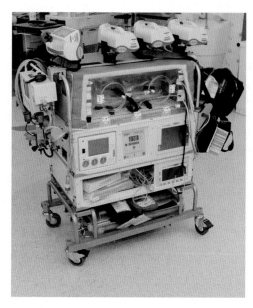

FIGURE 17.2 Neonatal transporter. (Courtesy McLeod Regional Medical Center, Florence, South Carolina.)

Table 17.1
Care and Complications of the Infant With Hypoxia

Medical Management	Nursing Care	Long-Term Complications
• Blood pressure management with medications • Ventilation support and oxygen therapy if needed • Careful fluid management • Avoidance of hypoglycemia or hyperglycemia • Avoidance of hyperthermia • Treatment of seizures • Hypothermia therapy (33°C–33.5°C [91.4°F–92.3°F] for 72 hours), followed by slow rewarming to reduce brain swelling (Rohan, 2020)	• Administering ordered medications and fluids • Monitoring ventilation and oxygenation of the baby • Monitoring fluid balance • Monitoring and reporting signs of hypoglycemia, hyperglycemia, and hyperthermia	• Cerebral palsy • Epilepsy • Blindness • Delayed motor development • Intellectual disability • Learning disabilities

CARE OF THE NEWBORN WITH RESPIRATORY DISTRESS

Respiratory distress is a common problem of the neonate. It can be caused by asphyxia at birth, a lack of surfactant in the lungs with a premature birth, fluid in the lungs, meconium aspiration, pulmonary hypertension, cold stress, and other conditions that affect the ability of the newborn to breathe. Nurses need to be able to identify early signs of respiratory distress and initiate care to provide oxygenation and improve gas exchange to prevent more complications or death for the newborn.

Respiratory Distress Syndrome of the Newborn

Respiratory distress syndrome (RDS) of the newborn is caused by a lack of surfactant in and immaturity of the fetal lungs. RDS is seen almost exclusively in premature infants, but it can occur in infants experiencing birth asphyxia, those born to diabetic mothers, and those born by cesarean section.

RDS was formerly known as *hyaline membrane syndrome* because of the formation of hyaline membranes that line the alveoli and impair ventilation. The function of surfactant in the lungs is to decrease surface tension in the alveoli and assist the alveoli to stay open for ventilation. If surfactant is absent (as in premature infants), the alveoli cannot open for oxygenation; therefore, hypoxemia and **hypercapnia** (elevated carbon dioxide) occur, leading to respiratory acidosis. Acidosis causes vasoconstriction and damages the epithelium of the lungs, causing the formation of a hyaline membrane inside the alveoli that impairs oxygen exchange.

The signs of RDS will be evident either at birth or within 8 hours of life (Pramanik, 2020). The most common signs are the following:

- **Tachypnea**
- **Dyspnea**
- Grunting with expirations
- Nasal flaring
- Intercostal retractions
- Cyanosis

Medical management (Yadav et al., 2022) includes:

- If a premature birth is likely, administration of antenatal corticosteroids will reduce the risk of RDS (Martin, 2023)
- Transfer to NICU
- Surfactant therapy
- Oxygen therapy (Fig. 17.3)
- Continuous positive airway pressure (CPAP) to keep the alveoli open at the end of respiration

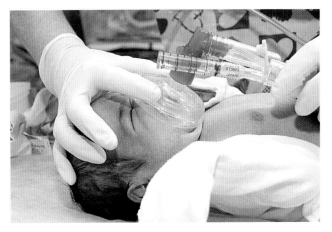

FIGURE 17.3 During respiratory distress, some newborns require oxygen administered through a mask. (Courtesy St. Luke's Hospital, Bethlehem, Pennsylvania.)

- Mechanical ventilation support if needed
- Vapotherm: heated and humidified high-flow oxygen through a nasal cannula

Nursing interventions for a newborn in respiratory distress would include the following:

- Administering neonatal cardiopulmonary resuscitation (CPR) if indicated
- Administering ordered medications and fluids
- Monitoring respiratory and oxygenation status
- Providing emotional support to the family

Transient Tachypnea of the Newborn

Transient tachypnea of the newborn (TTN) is a common self-limiting condition of infants in which tachypnea, increased oxygen needs, and mild respiratory distress occur. TTN occurs more often in infants sedated from maternal pain medications in labor, prolonged labor, macrosomia, and babies born via cesarean section. TTN is thought to be caused by incomplete reabsorption of fluid in the lungs and usually resolves within 3 to 5 days (Alhassen et al., 2021). Table 17.2 provides information on medical management of and nursing interventions for TTN.

Meconium Aspiration Syndrome

During labor and delivery, a fetus may become stressed by placental insufficiency, cord compression, or infection. Any of these stressors may decrease oxygen and cause the fetus to pass meconium into the amniotic fluid. Meconium is rarely found in the amniotic fluid before 34 weeks' gestation; therefore, meconium aspiration mainly affects term and postterm newborns. The meconium can block the infant's bronchioles, causing poor oxygenation, triggering inflammation, and inactivating surfactant, leading to pneumonia and pneumothorax (collapsed lung; Sayad & Silva-Carmona, 2022).

Observe the infant for signs of possible meconium aspiration if the newborn has a greenish-yellow staining of the

- **WORD · BUILDING ·**

hypercapnia: hyper–excessive + capn–CO_2 in the blood + ia–condition

tachypnea: tachy–swift + pnea–breath

dyspnea: dys–abnormal + pnea–breath

Table 17.2

Care of the Infant With Transient Tachypnea of the Newborn

Medical Management	Nursing Interventions
• Supportive care with IV fluids and gavage feedings until the respiratory rate has decreased enough to allow breast or bottle feedings • Oxygen support to maintain oxygen saturation levels above 93% • Chest x-ray • Arterial blood gas (ABG) assessments (Subramanian, 2020)	• Administering and monitoring ordered IV fluids • Monitoring oxygenation by physical assessment, ABGs, and O_2 saturation levels • Administering gavage feedings • Minimizing stimulation • Preventing hypothermia or hyperthermia • Providing emotional support to the family • After TTN has resolved, focusing on bonding and breastfeeding support

Box 17.1

Medical and Nursing Management of the Infant With PPHN

Medical Management

Echocardiography (a test that looks at how blood flows through the heart vessels, valves, and chambers) to diagnose heart defects
Chest x-ray to diagnose lung defects
ABGs to monitor oxygenation
Oxygen therapy
Dopamine to elevate blood pressure
Surfactant, if caused by lung disease
Vasodilators after the infant is stable to reduce lung hypertension
Mechanical ventilation
(Stark & Eichenwald, 2022)

Nursing Care

Administering medications
Continuous monitoring of vital signs and oxygenation
Maintaining a normal body temperature
Nutritional support
Minimal handling of the newborn to reduce oxygen consumption
Teaching and emotional support of the family

skin, nailbeds, or umbilical cord at the time of birth. Additional signs to look for are as follows:

• Tachypnea
• Retractions
• Nasal flaring
• Grunting
• Decreased oxygen saturation levels
• Decreased breath sounds

If meconium is evident at birth, thorough suctioning should occur with the first breath. If the newborn progresses into respiratory distress, endotracheal intubation and mechanical ventilation may be required (Garcia-Pratts, 2021). The infant will be transferred to the NICU, and the medical and nursing care is the same as discussed for the newborn with respiratory distress.

Persistent Pulmonary Hypertension of the Newborn

When the fetus is delivered and takes its first breath, the fetal circulation begins the transition to normal circulation. Blood flows from the right ventricle into the pulmonary arteries to the capillaries in the alveoli for gas exchange. Oxygen is picked up and carbon dioxide is released. In persistent pulmonary hypertension of the newborn (PPHN), the fetal circulation persists, or remains, as it was in the uterus. The ductus arteriosus and/or foramen ovale remain open, blood is shunted away from the lungs, the lungs have high pressure, and there is inadequate blood flow to the lungs for oxygenation of the newborn (Nandula & Shah, 2022). This condition can be life-threatening. The most common causes of PPHN are the following:

• Perinatal asphyxia
• RDS
• Neonatal sepsis
• A congenital defect of the heart or lungs

Signs and symptoms of PPHN are similar to those of RDS except for the additions of cyanosis that does not improve with administration of oxygen, symptoms of shock (low blood pressure and tachycardia), and the possibility of a heart murmur caused by the open ductus arteriosus and/or foramen ovale. Medical and nursing care will begin with transferring the infant to the NICU. Additional medical and nursing management is presented in Box 17.1.

• WORD • BUILDING •

echocardiography: echo–echo + cardio–heart + graphy–writing

The prognosis of PPHN depends upon the initial cause. It may resolve, or the infant may have ongoing health problems. Because of the hypoxemia the infant experienced, survivors of PPHN have a higher risk of neurosensory hearing loss and neurodevelopmental problems later. These babies should be monitored closely for problems and receive early interventions.

Learn to C.U.S.

A newborn was just delivered in his parents' car 20 minutes ago on the way to the hospital. The parents and the newborn arrive in the emergency department (ED) with the baby wrapped in the father's shirt. The ED physician places the infant on a bed and begins a quick assessment of heart rate and respirations. The newborn is breathing, but not crying, and seems lethargic. You note that the newborn has been uncovered for several minutes. Using the C.U.S. method of communication, you address the safety issue.

C: "Doctor, I am *concerned.*
U: I am *uncomfortable* seeing this examination done on a regular bed.
S: We have a *safety* issue. The infant may be cold stressed. We need to move him under a radiant warmer."

CARE OF THE NEWBORN WITH COLD STRESS

Thermoregulation is extremely important for any infant but even more so for the high-risk infant. See Chapter 14 for the four ways that infants can lose body heat. The risk of cold stress is highest during the immediate transitional period after birth. Normal rectal temperature for term and preterm infants is 36.5°C to 37°C (97.7°F–98.6°F). Cold stress is more likely if a newborn is born outside of the hospital environment. Table 17.3 discusses the effects of cold stress on the newborn and interventions to treat it.

NEONATAL HYPOGLYCEMIA

Neonatal hypoglycemia is defined as a plasma glucose level of lower than 30 mg/dL in the first 24 hours of life and lower than 45 mg/dL thereafter. It is the most common metabolic problem in newborns (Cranmer, 2022). Both healthy and ill-appearing infants can be affected by hypoglycemia during the first few days of life. Table 17.4 covers identifying and treating hypoglycemia in the newborn.

Newborns need glucose for energy, and 95% of the available glucose is used for brain function (Cranmer, 2022). Long-term complications from frequent or prolonged hypoglycemia are neurological damage such as intellectual disability, developmental delays, personality disorders, decreased head size, and seizures (Mishra et al., 2022). If the newborn has risk factors for hypoglycemia, check the blood sugar with a heel-stick blood sample. Be aware that the newborn's blood glucose levels can drop if the newborn:

- Has no glycogen stored in the liver; for example, a premature newborn
- Has used up stored glucose for heat production or a birth stress, such as asphyxia
- Is an infant of a diabetic mother (IDM) and has **hyperinsulinism** (increased levels of insulin)
- Cannot feed enough to keep the glucose level in an acceptable range

Most hospital nurseries have standing orders or protocols instituted by the health-care providers on the unit for nurses to follow in the event of hypoglycemia. This saves time and allows you to begin prompt treatment of hypoglycemia.

CRITICAL THINKING & CLINICAL JUDGMENT

Scenario #2: You are working in the newborn nursery. A 10-lb infant born via cesarean birth was just brought into the nursery. The nurse accompanying the newborn reports that his mother is a diabetic and all his vital signs are normal.

Questions

1. What should you think about in this situation?
2. What should you do and why?

CARE OF THE NEWBORN WITH BIRTH INJURIES

Injuries to the newborn can occur because of traction and compression during the birthing process. These injuries are known as *birth trauma.* The overall incidence of birth trauma has declined because of improvements in obstetric care and prenatal diagnosis. The current incidence is 1 in 1,000 births (Dumpa & Kamity, 2022). Risk factors for birth trauma include the following:

- Fetal macrosomia
- Cephalopelvic disproportion
- Prolonged or very rapid delivery
- Use of forceps or vacuum extraction
- Abnormal presentation, such as breech
- Large fetal head
- Extreme prematurity and very low birth weight

· **WORD** · **BUILDING** ·

hyperinsulinism: hyper–excessive + insulin–insulin + ism–condition

Table 17.3

Identifying and Treating Newborn Cold Stress

Who Is at Risk?	What Is the Newborn's Physiological Response to Cold Stress?	What Are the Signs of Cold Stress?	What Interventions Should the Nurse Anticipate?
• Premature infants • SGA infants • Infants who require resuscitation • Infants who have an infection or a congenital anomaly	When the infant's body temperature drops, the body attempts to adapt and raise the temperature by the following means: • Peripheral vasoconstriction conserves heat for the core of the body. • Core blood volume increases, causing an increase in heart rate and blood pressure. • An increase in metabolic rate can lead to increased oxygen needs and hypoglycemia. • Brown fat is metabolized, causing a release of fatty acids and subsequent acidosis.	• Temperature below 36.3°C (97.7°F) • Weak cry • Respirations that become slow and shallow • Jitters from low blood sugar • Refusal to eat • Lethargy • Respiratory distress	• Monitoring the temperature every 15 minutes • Providing skin-to-skin contact with the mother • Placing the infant under a radiant warmer • Double-wrapping the newborn • Placing the infant in an incubator and gradually rewarming • Using special rewarming blankets • Infusing warmed IV fluids • If bottle-fed, warming the formula • Treating hypoglycemia according to the nursery protocol (Kyokan et al., 2022; Rohan, 2020)

Table 17.4

Identifying and Treating the Newborn With Hypoglycemia

Who Is at Risk?	What Are the Signs and Symptoms of Neonatal Hypoglycemia?	What Interventions Should the Nurse Anticipate?
• Premature or postmature infant • IDM • SGA infant • LGA infant • Infant stressed at birth, for example, cold stress or asphyxia (Rozance, 2023)	• Jitteriness or tremors • Lethargy or irritability • Hypotonia • Weak or high-pitched cry • Apnea • Hypothermia • Poor feeding	• Obtaining a blood sample via heel stick as soon as possible after birth for high-risk infants; if results are normal, repeating 30 minutes, 1 hour, 2 hours, 4 hours, 8 hours, and 12 hours after birth (Rozance, 2023) • Obtaining a heel-stick blood sample on any infant who exhibits signs and symptoms of hypoglycemia • If the glucometer reading is between 30 and 40 mg/dL, the infant should be breastfed or bottle-fed • Recheck the blood glucose 20 minutes after a feeding • If the glucometer reading is lower than 30 mg/dL, follow hospital protocol for notification of the health-care provider, a possible blood draw for a STAT blood glucose, administration of glucose gel, or IV administration of D10W (10% dextrose in water; Rohan, 2020; Rozance, 2023)

Common soft-tissue injuries are cephalohematoma, caput succedaneum, and abrasion or lacerations from instrumental deliveries. (See Chapter 15 for more information on these types of injuries.) These injuries resolve within days and cause no long-term problems for the infant. Brachial plexus injuries, cranial nerve injuries, and fractures are less common but have the potential for more complications for the newborn.

Brachial Plexus Injuries

A **brachial plexus** injury to the newborn occurs from an increase in the infant's neck-shoulder angle, resulting in a traction force to the brachial plexus. The brachial plexus is a network of nerves that originate in the neck area and branch off to form the nerves that control movement and sensation in the shoulders, arms, and hands. Brachial plexus injuries occur in 2 infants per 1,000 live births and are associated with large birth weight, long labors, vaginal breech delivery, and shoulder dystocia (Dumpa & Kamity, 2022).

Nurses are usually the first to suspect or detect a brachial plexus injury right after delivery or when completing the first physical evaluation. Symptoms of a brachial plexus injury in the newborn are as follows:

- Limited movement on one side of the body
- No Moro reflex on the affected side
- Clawlike appearance of the newborn's hand on the affected side
- Abnormal muscle contractions on the affected side

Definitive diagnosis of a brachial plexus injury may include x-rays to determine if there is a fracture of the clavicle, shoulder, or arm; imaging studies; and nerve conduction studies. Medical management of a brachial plexus injury will depend on the severity of the injury. Approximately 93% of infants with brachial plexus paralysis demonstrate spontaneous improvement by 4 months of age (Shah & Coroneos, 2021). Medical management may include:

- Physical therapy such as range-of-motion activities, massage, and stretching to help the infant develop muscles on the affected side
- Surgical treatment, such as grafting a nerve from a less used muscle to the affected area (Wells et al., 2022)

Nursing care for the newborn with a brachial plexus injury includes:

- Reporting symptoms of a brachial plexus injury immediately
- Protecting the affected arm from dangling when held or moved
- Not lifting the infant under the axillae
- Teaching the parents how to support the affected arm with rolled blankets when the infant is in the car seat and crib
- Monitoring for signs of pain and reporting to the health-care provider

---

Team Works

When a newborn has a brachial plexus injury, teamwork is an important part of promoting a good outcome and recovery. You will be providing the initial care and educating and supporting the parents. The health-care provider will make the diagnosis along with consultation with neurologists and physical therapists. The parents will be part of the team because they will be learning exercises from the physical therapist that can be done at home with their baby. Later, if complete recovery does not occur, a surgeon will join the team.

- Positioning the infant with good body alignment to prevent complications from muscle contractures
- Providing emotional support to the family

Fractures

The clavicle is the most frequently fractured bone in the newborn during delivery (Mumtaz Hashmi et al., 2021). This injury is associated with macrosomic infants and infants with large shoulders, which can make a vaginal delivery difficult. After the delivery, you will notice that the newborn does not move the affected arm. In addition, a palpable bone irregularity may be noted during physical evaluation. Diagnosis is made with an x-ray of the clavicle and affected arm.

Healing occurs in 7 to 10 days. To decrease pain, the arm is immobilized by using safety pins to attach the undershirt sleeve to the shirt. The newborn should also be observed for a possible brachial plexus injury associated with a fractured clavicle (Mumtaz Hashmi et al., 2021).

HYPERBILIRUBINEMIA

Hyperbilirubinemia is also known as jaundice. Jaundice is the most common condition that requires medical attention in newborns (Rohan, 2020). (See Chapter 14 for information on physiological jaundice.)

In some infants, the serum bilirubin level rises excessively and requires treatment to accelerate the removal of bilirubin from the blood before complications can occur. This type of hyperbilirubinemia is known as pathological or nonphysiological jaundice. When the serum bilirubin is excessively elevated, the skin becomes saturated with bilirubin, causing the yellow coloration. After the skin is saturated, the bilirubin begins to deposit in the brain and can cause a neurotoxicity, known as *kernicterus.*

Risk factors for pathological jaundice include:

- Prematurity
- A blood-type incompatibility with the mother
- Lack of effective breastfeeding
- Excessive bruising from an extended labor or a malpresentation in labor, such as face presentation

Detection and diagnosis of pathological jaundice begins with a physical assessment. Jaundice can usually be detected visually when the level reaches 5 to 6 mg/dL (Rohan, 2020). Jaundice first appears on the face. The sclera may be tinted yellow also. As the bilirubin level rises, the yellow color spreads down the body. A transcutaneous bilirubinometer is a noninvasive instrument that can give an estimate of the total bilirubin before a serum bilirubin test is performed. Definitive diagnosis of hyperbilirubinemia is made through laboratory testing. See Table 17.5 for common laboratory tests that may be ordered to determine the severity of the hyperbilirubinemia and possible causes of the problem.

Medical management is based upon the infant's gestational age, weight, and bilirubin level. Breastfeeding or bottle feeding, phototherapy, and exchange transfusions are the usual

Table 17.5

Laboratory Tests for the Newborn With Jaundice

Test	Purpose
Total or direct bilirubin level	Measures the amount of bilirubin in the blood that is produced when the liver breaks down red blood cells
Direct and indirect Coombs	Detects antibodies against red blood cells seen in Rh and ABO blood incompatibilities
CBC	Detects anemia or infection, which would raise the bilirubin levels
Albumin	Detects the amount of albumin available to bind with bilirubin for excretion
Blood culture	Detects infection that could raise bilirubin levels
Peripheral smear	A follow-up test if the CBC is abnormal; used to closely evaluate the blood cells under a microscope
Reticulocyte count	Useful if the infant is anemic; measures red blood cell production by the bone marrow

Source: Van Leeuwen, A. M., & Bladh, M. L. (2021). *Davis's comprehensive manual of laboratory and diagnostic tests with nursing implications* (9th ed.). F. A. Davis.

medical management. Home phototherapy may be used if the newborn is full term and has overall excellent health except for the jaundice. A home health nurse would monitor the care.

Breastfeeding at least 8 to 12 times or bottle feeding 8 to 10 times a day will help with decreasing bilirubin levels. A baby who is having at least six wet diapers and three stools per day will be able to eliminate the bilirubin through the gastrointestinal tract and kidneys.

Generally, many health-care providers will institute phototherapy when the total serum bilirubin level is at or above 15 mg/dL in infants 25 to 48 hours old, 18 mg/dL in infants 49 to 72 hours old, and 20 mg/dL in infants older than 72 hours (Ansong-Assoku et al., 2023). Phototherapy using a "blue light" converts bilirubin molecules into water-soluble compounds that can be excreted by the body (Ansong-Assoku et al., 2023). The infant can be exposed to the blue light through overhead lights, pads, or blankets (Fig. 17.4). The infant can be removed from the light for feedings, especially because feedings are an important part of the treatment plan.

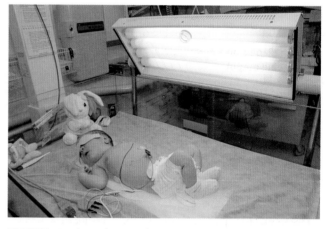

FIGURE 17.4 A newborn undergoing phototherapy. The eyes and genitals are covered for protection. (Courtesy St. Luke's Hospital, Bethlehem, Pennsylvania.)

A blood exchange transfusion in the NICU may be required if the bilirubin levels are rising so quickly that kernicterus may occur. Serious neurological damage may result if the bilirubin levels do not drop with feedings and phototherapy.

Nursing interventions for the infant with jaundice requiring phototherapy may include:

- Encouraging breastfeeding 8 to 12 times a day or bottle feeding 8 to 10 times a day
- Monitoring the number of stools
- Weighing diapers to obtain accurate urine output information
- Placing eye patches on the newborn's eyes to protect the retina from damage from the phototherapy light
- Undressing the newborn except for the genital area to expose the maximum amount of skin to the light

CRITICAL THINKING & CLINICAL JUDGMENT

Scenario #3: Catalina's baby is being treated with phototherapy for jaundice. She is sitting by the crib, touching and talking quietly to him. You notice when you walk by that the eye patches are off the baby's eyes. This is the second time today that you noticed the eye patches were off during the phototherapy.

Questions

1. What should you think about in this situation?
2. What should you do and why?

Nursing Care Plan for the Infant With Jaundice

Caleb is 3 days old and has jaundice. His serum bilirubin is 20 mg/dL, and he is being treated with a bili-light in the nursery.

Nursing Diagnosis: Potential for hypothermia or hyperthermia
Expected Outcome: The infant will maintain an axillary temperature between 36.5°C and 37.4°C (97.7°F–99.3°F).

Interventions:	Rationale:
Check the body temperature and vital signs every 2 hours.	*Prevention or early recognition of hypothermia or hyperthermia will prevent complications.*
Dress the baby appropriately when removing from phototherapy.	

Nursing Diagnosis: Deficient fluid volume related to phototherapy and poor feeding
Expected Outcome: The infant will produce six wet diapers per day.

Interventions:	Rationale:
Encourage breastfeeding 8 to 12 times per day.	*Sufficient fluid volume helps the infant's body to eliminate the bilirubin.*
Document the number of wet diapers.	
Weigh diapers on a gram scale to get an accurate measurement of urine output.	

Nursing Diagnosis: Risk for injury from the effects of phototherapy
Expected Outcome: The jaundice will resolve without injury to the patient.

Interventions:	Rationales:
Place the newborn at the appropriate distance from the light source per hospital protocol.	*Prevents damage from the bili-light (phototherapy).*
Cover the infant's eyes and genitals.	
Ensure that the eye patches do not cover the nose and mouth.	
Turn the infant every 2 hours.	*Exposes more skin to the bili-light to promote success of the phototherapy.*
Note the infant's activity level every 2 hours.	*Lethargy or irritability are early signs of kernicterus.*

- Monitoring the newborn's behavior; irritability or lethargy could be signs that the bilirubin level is irritating the brain
- Monitoring the infant's body temperature for hypothermia from being undressed

CARE OF THE NEWBORN WITH AN INFECTION

Newborns can be exposed to infection from the mother, from organisms that enter the vagina during labor, from contaminated hospital personnel and equipment, and from family and visitors. Nurses need to be constantly on the watch for signs of infection. A newborn has an immature immune system that is unable to mount an attack against a severe infection before it becomes systemic. The newborn may exhibit only subtle signs of infection that an experienced nurse can observe and report immediately to begin appropriate care. This section discusses neonatal sepsis and infection from herpes virus.

Sepsis

Neonatal sepsis is a blood infection that presents within the first 28 days of life (Rohan, 2020). Sepsis is an invasive infection in which chemicals released into the blood to help fight the infection cause inflammation over the entire body. The source of the pathogen may be the hospital environment, maternal flora, or the community. The most common

Table 17.6

Identifying and Treating the Newborn With Neonatal Sepsis

Who Is at Risk?	What Are the Signs and Symptoms of Neonatal Sepsis?	What Might Medical Management Include?	What Interventions Should the Nurse Anticipate?
• Preterm newborns • Maternal infection with GBS • Amniotic membranes ruptured for longer than 24 hours • Chorioamnionitis (infection of the amniotic membranes) • Frequent vaginal examinations during labor in which the examiner inadvertently transports *E. coli* from the rectal area into the vagina and cervix	• Poor temperature control (hypothermia or hyperthermia) • Irregular respirations • Dyspnea • Expiratory grunting and retractions • "See-saw" retractions (the abdomen lifts, and the chest sinks) • Cold clammy skin • Abnormal heartbeat • Lethargy • Poor feeding • Diminished activity or hyperactivity • Bulging fontanel • Diarrhea • Abdominal distention	The septic newborn may require transfer to the NICU. Medical management of sepsis could possibly include: • Cardiopulmonary support • IV fluids • Placement of a central venous line for antibiotic administration • IV antibiotics, such as aminoglycosides, penicillins, and vancomycin • Antiviral medication, such as acyclovir, may be given if the infection may be from herpes • IV parenteral nutrition (PN) during the acute phase to support the immune system as well as growth and development (Kanishiro, 2021)	• Monitoring vital signs and laboratory results, and reporting abnormalities promptly • Promoting thermoregulation • Administering IV fluids, antibiotics, and antiviral medications as ordered • Monitoring fluid balance • Administering PN and observing for complications • Supporting the family emotionally and providing opportunities for bonding

causes of neonatal sepsis are group B streptococcus (GBS), *Escherichia coli,* and herpes (Kanishiro, 2021). For information about identifying and treating newborn sepsis, see Table 17.6.

Herpes

Newborns can become infected with the herpes virus during pregnancy, labor, or delivery. The herpes virus type 2 (genital herpes) is the most common cause of herpes infection in the newborn, but type 1 (oral herpes) can also cause infection. If the mother has an active case of herpes type 2 at the time of delivery, the fetus can be exposed while passing through the birth canal. The newborn may only develop a skin infection that blisters, crusts over, and then heals. However, the herpes infection can become systemic, similar to neonatal sepsis, and be life-threatening to the newborn. The symptoms of a systemic neonatal herpes infection are identical to the signs and symptoms of neonatal sepsis. The medical management and nursing interventions are also the same, except for antibiotics. Antibiotics are not effective against a virus. The newborn would receive antiviral medications instead (Allen et al., 2020).

Safety *Stat!*

If a woman has an active case of genital herpes, she should have a scheduled cesarean birth to reduce the risk of transmission of the herpes infection to her newborn.

CARE OF NEWBORNS WITH PROBLEMS RELATED TO GESTATIONAL AGE AND DEVELOPMENT

The length of a term pregnancy is 40 weeks (280 days), measured from the first day of the last menstrual period to the estimated date of delivery. In the past, the period from 3 weeks before the estimated due date to 2 weeks after the due date was considered "term." However, research has shown that respiratory complications for the newborn vary upon the exact time that a baby is born in that 5-week range. To facilitate delivery of quality health care for the neonate, specific terminology has been created for identifying preterm, term, and postterm births:

• A preterm birth is fewer than 37 weeks, 6 days.
• An early term birth is from 37 weeks, 6 days through 38 weeks, 6 days.

- A full-term birth is from 39 weeks through 40 weeks, 6 days.
- A late-term birth is from 41 weeks through 41 weeks, 6 days.
- A postterm birth is 42 weeks and beyond
  (National Institutes of Health [NIH], 2022)

The following section discusses problems related to gestational age and development.

The Small-for-Gestational-Age/Intrauterine Growth Restriction Newborn

A **small-for-gestational-age (SGA)** newborn is defined as an infant whose weight is less than the 10th percentile for gestational age. The SGA newborn may have been affected by **intrauterine growth restriction (UGR)**, limited fetal growth caused by a decrease in placenta perfusion during gestation. There are many possible causes of SGA:

- Abnormalities of the placenta or vessels that restricted nutrients and oxygen to the developing fetus
- Maternal hypertension
- Uncontrolled, severe maternal diabetes
- Poor maternal nutrition
- Maternal illegal drug use
- Heavy maternal smoking
- Exposure to teratogenic substances
- Maternal alcohol consumption
- Multigestation
- Parents of small stature (Ross, 2020)

IUGR is often diagnosed during pregnancy at routine visits when the health-care provider measures fundal height and through ultrasound examinations. If poor placental perfusion is thought to be the cause, labor may be induced and the fetus delivered early.

Physical findings of an infant diagnosed with IUGR include the following:

- Weight, length, and head circumference all below the 10th percentile for gestational age
- Large head in relationship to the rest of the body
- Thin extremities and trunk
- Loose skin caused by absence of subcutaneous fat
- Thin umbilical cord

Term SGA infants do not have complications related to immature organs such as a premature baby does; however, they are at risk for other complications:

- Perinatal asphyxia during labor if the SGA was caused by placental insufficiency; the fetus may not receive enough oxygen during the stress of labor.
- Meconium aspiration may occur during asphyxia. The infant may pass meconium into the amniotic fluid and then aspirate it into the lungs at birth, causing respiratory distress.
- **Hypoglycemia** (low blood sugar) may occur because of a lack of stored glycogen. *Neonatal hypoglycemia* is

· WORD · BUILDING ·

hypoglycemia: hypo–deficient + glyc–sugar + em–blood + ia–condition

defined as a plasma glucose level of lower than 30 mg/dL in the first 24 hours of life and lower than 45 mg/dL thereafter (Rozance, 2023).

- Hypothermia may occur because of a lack of subcutaneous fat (Osuchukwu & Reed, 2022).

Nursing interventions for the SGA infant are as follows:

- Performing a gestational age evaluation
- Observing for respiratory distress
- Detecting tremors or jitteriness, which are early signs of hypoglycemia
- Instituting early feeding to prevent hypoglycemia
- Monitoring for hypothermia
- Monitoring vital signs and daily weight
- Teaching the parents about the need to keep the infant warm and to provide frequent feedings

Health Promotion

Prognosis for a Small-for-Gestational-Age Newborn
- If asphyxia was avoided at birth, the neurological prognosis for the SGA infant is excellent.
- If the growth restriction was because of placental insufficiency, adequate nutrition after birth will allow the infant to "catch up."
- An SGA situation caused by maternal illegal drug use or smoking may contribute to a smaller child and adult.

The Large-for-Gestational-Age Newborn

The **large-for-gestational-age (LGA)** newborn is an infant whose weight is greater than the 90th percentile for gestational age (Fig. 17.5). The predominant cause of LGA is maternal diabetes (Patel, 2020). Complications can occur during a vaginal delivery because of the large size of the fetus. A cesarean delivery should be considered to prevent injury to the

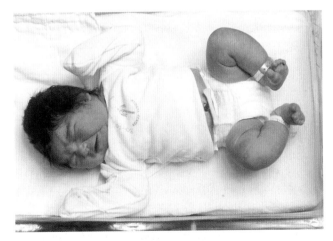

FIGURE 17.5 An LGA newborn.

large infant. The most common complications for an LGA newborn are as follows:

- Shoulder dystocia
- Fracture of the clavicle or limbs
- Perinatal asphyxia
- Meconium aspiration
- Respiratory distress
- Hypoglycemia

Assessment findings would include:

- Large, obese baby
- Listless, apathetic baby

Nursing interventions for the LGA newborn include:

- Performing a gestational age evaluation
- Determining respiratory status
- Checking for signs of birth injuries and reporting them immediately
- Monitoring for tremors, which are an early sign of hypoglycemia
- Providing frequent feedings to decrease the risk of hypoglycemia

The Preterm Newborn

The length of gestation and birth weight are two important predictors of an infant's ability to survive outside the uterus. Preterm infants are born before 37 weeks' gestation and have an increased risk of complications and mortality. In the United States, 10.5% of infants are born prematurely (Centers for Disease Control and Prevention [CDC], 2022).

Risk Factors

There are many risk factors for a premature birth. However, sometimes the cause of a premature birth is never really known. Known risk factors for a premature delivery include the following:

- Low socioeconomic status
- Cigarette smoking
- Prior premature births
- Multiple prior therapeutic or spontaneous abortions
- Little or no prenatal care
- Poor nutrition
- Untreated infections
- Preeclampsia
- Multiple gestation (Robinson & Norowitz, 2023)

Determining Gestational Age

Confirmation of prematurity is based upon a gestational age assessment. The Ballard Gestational Age Assessment Tool (see Chapter 15) is the main tool used to determine gestational age.

During physical evaluation of the premature infant, you will also notice the following:

- The skin is thin, and arteries and veins are visible.
- The skin is fragile and looks smooth and shiny.

- A moderately premature infant will have abundant lanugo.
- Fingernails and toenails may only be partially formed.
- The ears may fold over because the cartilage has not developed.
- Very preterm infants have less muscle tone.
- The premature baby does not lie in a "fetal position" until 35 weeks.

Team Works

When a premature delivery is expected, a team of professionals should be at the delivery to provide prompt stabilization, which is crucial to the long-term outcome for the newborn. In addition to the obstetrician and labor nurse, there should also be a neonatologist, NICU nurses, a laboratory technician, and respiratory care practitioners in attendance.

Potential Complications

Being born too early predisposes the newborn to short- and long-term complications. The age and weight of the premature newborn influence the severity of the complications. In the first few weeks, the premature newborn can experience a variety of short-term complications.

- *Respiratory distress:* The immature respiratory system lacks surfactant to keep the alveoli open.
- *Hypothermia:* Thermoregulation is difficult for the premature infant because of the lack of subcutaneous fat, and the infant may not have developed brown fat to assist with heat production during stress. Cold stress can occur easily in a premature newborn.
- *Heart problems:* The most common problems are a patent ductus arteriosus (PDA) and hypotension. The PDA is supposed to close on its own to allow more blood flow to the lungs; however, in a premature infant, it may stay open, causing heart failure (Fig. 17.6).
- *Intraventricular hemorrhage in the brain:* In the very premature infant, these can occur because of the fragile, underdeveloped blood vessels in the brain. These blood vessels may rupture and bleed into the ventricles of the brain. Although there may be no symptoms, you may observe:
  - Apnea
  - Decreased muscle tone
  - Decreased reflexes
  - Excessive sleep
  - Weak suck
  - Seizure and other abnormal movements

There is no way to stop the bleeding. The health-care team will keep the infant stable and treat any symptoms. The prognosis depends upon the amount of bleeding that occurs and

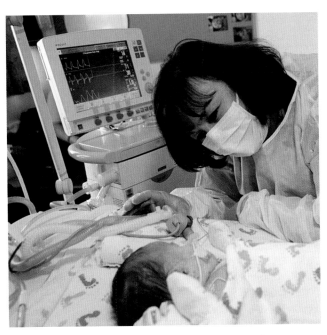

FIGURE 17.6 Most premature newborns are on a cardiore-spiratory monitor. (Courtesy St. Luke's Hospital, Bethlehem, Pennsylvania.)

if there is accompanying swelling of the brain (deVries & Leijser, 2021).

- *Necrotizing enterocolitis:* This complication occurs in the second to third week of life. The exact cause is unknown, but it is associated with formula feeding and characterized by damage to the intestinal tract that may have occurred from abnormal intestinal flora, immaturity of the intestinal mucosa, intestinal ischemia caused by decreased placental blood flow, and possibly a genetic predisposition. The damage may affect only the mucosal lining, or there may be full-thickness **necrosis** (death of the tissues) and perforation of the bowel. The signs and symptoms are as follows:
  - Vomiting
  - Diarrhea
  - Delayed gastric emptying
  - Decreased bowel sounds
  - Lethargy
  - Increased abdominal girth
  - Visible intestinal loops
  - Palpable abdominal mass
  - **Hematochezia** (bright-red blood in the stool)

Medical management includes stopping formula feedings, insertion of a nasogastric tube (NGT), feeding with breast milk, and the administration of antibiotics. Surgical

· WORD · BUILDING ·
enterocolitis: entero–intestines + col–colon + itis–inflammation
necrosis: necr–corpse + osis–condition
hematochezia: hemato–blood + chez–defecate + ia–condition

intervention may be required to remove perforated or necrotic intestinal tissue (Ginglen & Butki, 2022).

- *Anemia:* All infants experience a drop in red blood cells after birth, but it may be more profound for the premature infant if frequent blood draws are required for tests.
- *Infection:* Because of the premature newborn's immature immune system, infection can quickly spread to the bloodstream, causing sepsis.
- *Fluid and electrolyte imbalances:* These can be a problem for the premature infant because of the immature circulatory and renal systems. Close monitoring of IV fluid intake and electrolyte balances is important to prevent fluid overload and heart failure.
- *Apnea of prematurity:* The most common problem of the premature neonate is apnea, the cessation of breathing for more than 20 seconds, or the cessation of breathing for fewer than 20 seconds accompanied by bradycardia or oxygen saturation levels of lower than 85%. Apnea of prematurity is related to immaturity and/or depression of the central respiratory drive to adequately stimulate the muscles of respiration (Nimavat, 2022). Medical management of apnea of prematurity includes tactile stimulation, administration of oxygen, the use of CPAP, and pharmacotherapy. As the infant matures, the apnea will resolve.

Medication Facts

Caffeine is the preferred medication for treating apnea of prematurity. Caffeine stimulates the respiratory center and relaxes smooth bronchial muscles. It can be administered IV or by mouth and has a rapid onset. The usual dose is 5 mg/kg every 24 hours (Vallerand & Sanoski, 2023).

Possible long-term complications of prematurity include:

- *Retinopathy of prematurity (ROP):* A premature birth results in the cessation of normal growth of the blood vessels of the retina. Long-term outcomes include visual impairment and blindness. The American Academy of Pediatrics recommends that all premature infants be tested for retinopathy. Early surgical laser treatment is the treatment of choice (Hong et al., 2022). See Chapter 28 for more information about ROP.
- *Cerebral palsy:* This disorder of muscle tone and movement can be caused by infection or by inadequate blood flow to the developing premature infant's brain. Recent studies indicate that there may be a genetic component that influences whether prenatal or birth stressors will cause cerebral palsy. This may explain why newborns with similar prenatal or birth stressors may have no disabilities or different types of cerebral palsy (Lewis et al., 2020).

- *Delayed development:* In the beginning, premature babies are usually behind on meeting developmental milestones; however, most will catch up by 12 to 18 months. Premature babies typically meet developmental milestones within normal ranges for their corrected ages. To obtain a corrected age, subtract the baby's number of weeks (or months) of prematurity from their actual age in weeks (or months). For example, a baby born 2 months premature who is 6 months old would be expected to meet developmental milestones for a 4-month-old baby. Premature babies are at risk for learning disabilities and are more likely to have neurological problems such as attention deficit-hyperactivity disorder (ADHD; Pravia & Benny, 2020).

The Postterm Newborn

A postterm newborn is born after 42 weeks' gestation. The cause of postmaturity is unknown, but a previous postterm delivery increases the risk. Usually, fetal growth between 39 and 43 weeks' gestation results in a large infant. However, in some cases, the placenta begins to detach and break down, causing placental insufficiency syndrome for the fetus (Caughey, 2021). The fetus receives inadequate nutrition and oxygen from the placenta, resulting in an SGA infant who is undernourished. The fetus may use stored glycogen for energy before birth. In addition, the amniotic fluid volume begins to decrease with postmaturity.

Characteristics of the Postterm Infant

A gestational age assessment should be done to confirm that the newborn is postmature. Physical characteristics of a postmature newborn include the following:

- More alert after birth than a term infant
- Decreased subcutaneous fat
- Loose skin
- Dry and peeling skin
- Lack of vernix and lanugo
- Long fingernails and toenails
- Meconium staining on the umbilical cord (Rohan, 2020)

Potential Complications

Postterm infants have a higher rate of death and disease than term infants. The following are possible complications that can occur:

- The incidence of stillbirth or neonatal death is increased in postterm infants.
- The larger body size can lead to prolonged labor and birth trauma.
- Hypoglycemia can occur owing to lack of stored glycogen.
- During labor, the postterm infant is more likely to have a bowel movement in the uterus because of stress (Cunningham et al., 2022). This increases the risk of meconium aspiration.

CARE OF THE INFANT OF A DIABETIC MOTHER

Neonatal complications for the IDM are directly related to inadequate glucose control in pregnancy (Moore, 2022). Fetal malformations, including cardiomegaly, can occur because of poor glucose control in the first trimester. High levels of glucose in late pregnancy can lead to macrosomia, hypoglycemia, hypoxia, polycythemia, hypocalcemia, and hypomagnesemia.

Congenital Malformations

High blood-sugar concentrations are toxic to cell growth in the first trimester of pregnancy and can cause cardiac and central nervous system (CNS) abnormalities of the fetus. Cardiomegaly with an enlarged left ventricle occurs in approximately 30% of IDMs; the risk of **spina bifida** (see Chapter 27) is 20 times higher for the IDM (Al-Biltagi et al., 2021; Bhandari & Thanda, 2022).

Nursing interventions are the following:

- Promptly identifying the congenital abnormality, if obvious, at birth
- Notifying the health-care provider of any physical abnormalities or abnormal vital signs

Fetal Macrosomia

Macrosomia, or an infant weighing more than 4,000 g at birth, occurs in 15% to 45% of diabetic pregnancies (Akanmode & Mahdy, 2022). High levels of maternal glucose during gestation lead to fetal hyperglycemia and hyperinsulinemia (excess insulin), which causes increased growth in the fetus. If delivered vaginally, the large infant is at risk for birth injuries caused by shoulder dystocia; therefore, the macrosomic IDM is typically delivered via cesarean birth. At delivery, the macrosomic IDM appears ruddy, fat, and puffy and may have decreased muscle tone (Kokhanov, 2022).

Nursing interventions for the macrosomic infant include the following:

- Notifying the pediatrician or pediatric nurse practitioner of birth weight and signs of macrosomia
- Performing a gestational age evaluation
- Observing for signs of birth injuries
- Observing for signs of hypoglycemia

Hypoglycemia

IDMs often have a rapid fall in glucose within an hour of birth. In fact, hypoglycemia can occur faster in an IDM than in normal infants. This is linked to fetal hyperinsulinism that occurs during gestation. In pregnancy, maternal glucose crosses the placenta, but insulin does not. Therefore, the fetus produces high levels of insulin in response to the maternal

· WORD · BUILDING ·

spina bifida: spina–spine + bifida–split into two parts

glucose. When the cord is cut, the glucose influx is over and the fetus is left with high levels of circulating insulin, causing hypoglycemia (Moore, 2022).

Fetal Hypoxia

Poorly controlled maternal diabetes can lead to fetal hypoxia, a decreased supply of oxygen to the fetal tissues. Uncontrolled high levels of glucose can cause vascular disease in the mother, leading to decreased blood flow to the placenta. In addition, the fetus needs more oxygen because of the high levels of glucose coming from the mother. Chronic fetal hypoxia can lead to intrauterine death or to respiratory depression at birth. While in the uterus, the fetus attempts to compensate for the decreased oxygen by producing extra red blood cells, a condition called **polycythemia**.

Polycythemia

Polycythemia is diagnosed when the hematocrit is greater than 65% (Rosenkrantz & Oh, 2021). The extra cells make the blood more viscous (thicker and stickier), which can cause strokes or seizures in the fetus or newborn. Polycythemia contributes to an increased risk of hyperbilirubinemia after birth, when the extra red blood cells break down and the immature liver cannot manage the breakdown of the bilirubin.

Signs of polycythemia in the newborn are the following:

- A "ruddy" (red) appearance of the skin
- Sluggish capillary refill time
- Respiratory distress
- Poor feeding
- Lethargy
- Seizures
- Apnea
- Cyanosis
- Hematuria

Medical management of polycythemia is controversial. The vital signs, hematocrit, and blood glucose will be monitored frequently. The hematocrit levels usually peak 6 to 12 hours after birth and then decline until the infant is 24 hours old. More than 60% of infants with a hematocrit level greater than 64% at 2 hours will have a high value 12 hours later (Rosenkrantz & Oh, 2021).

Some physicians will perform a partial blood exchange transfusion with saline to decrease the hematocrit quickly in symptomatic infants. In asymptomatic infants, the common approach is to observe for the onset of any symptoms and let the newborn's body adjust the hematocrit. Some physicians will hydrate the newborn with IV fluids to decrease the hematocrit.

· **WORD** · **BUILDING** ·

polycythemia: poly–many + cyt–cells + hem–blood + ia–condition

Nursing interventions for the polycythemic infant include the following:

- Notifying the health-care provider immediately of any signs and symptoms of polycythemia
- Infusing IV fluids, if ordered, and observing closely for signs of fluid overload

---

Safety *Stat!*

Newborns are at risk for fluid overload. Calculate appropriate fluid amounts based upon the infant's weight, and always confirm your calculations with at least one other licensed nurse.

Mineral/Electrolyte Metabolism

Hypocalcemia and **hypomagnesemia** can occur in the neonate if the mother had poorly controlled diabetes. In the newborn, *hypocalcemia* is defined as a calcium level lower than 8 mg/dL; *hypomagnesemia* is defined as a magnesium level lower than 1.7 mg/dL (Abrams, 2022). The mother's poor glycemic control leads to maternal glycosuria (glucose in the urine), which is accompanied by magnesium loss. Low maternal levels of magnesium lead to fetal deficiency. Magnesium and calcium metabolism are closely related. If the magnesium level is insufficient, calcium will be lost in the urine and not deposited in the bones and soft tissues. Severe hypomagnesemia causes a secondary hypocalcemia and **hypoparathyroidism** because magnesium is needed for the appropriate secretion of the parathyroid hormone (PTH). Medical management includes screening for hypocalcemia and hypomagnesemia and administering calcium and magnesium to obtain normal levels.

Signs and symptoms of mineral/electrolyte imbalances in the newborn include the following:

- Poor feeding
- Lethargy
- Tremors
- Seizures
- Cardiac arrhythmias
- Respiratory distress

Nursing interventions for the infant with an abnormal electrolyte balance are as follows:

- Recognizing abnormal signs and symptoms and reporting them immediately to the health-care provider

· **WORD** · **BUILDING** ·

hypocalcemia: hypo–deficient + calc–calcium + em–blood + ia–condition

hypomagnesemia: hypo–deficient + magnes–magnesium + em–blood + ia–condition

hypoparathyroidism: hypo–deficient + parathyroid–parathyroid hormone + ism–condition

- Maintaining close observation of the newborn to detect deterioration
- Administering calcium and/or magnesium as ordered by the health-care provider
- Providing education and emotional support to the family

CRITICAL THINKING & CLINICAL JUDGMENT

Scenario #4: You see a 4-hour-old newborn at the mother's bedside in his crib. You observe that his hands have tremors, and he is breathing rapidly. You suspect that he might have hypoglycemia and check his blood sugar. His blood sugar is 42 mg/dL.

Questions

1. Why did you suspect the newborn might have hypoglycemia?
2. What should you do?

CARE OF CHEMICALLY EXPOSED INFANTS

Prenatal substance abuse is a significant problem in the United States. Almost all medications cross the placenta and have an effect on the fetus. In early gestation, medications can have a teratogenic effect, causing structural birth defects. After that initial period of development is complete, medications have a subtler effect, displayed through alterations in neurotransmitters, their receptors, and brain organization (NIH, 2020).

Caring for a newborn who was prenatally exposed to illicit or prescription medications can be challenging for you. The mother may admit her use of medications during the pregnancy or may be fearful of losing custody of her newborn and not report her use. The health-care provider may order a medication toxicology screen on a newborn's urine, cord blood, or meconium to plan appropriate care for the infant in withdrawal.

Neonatal abstinence syndrome (NAS) is a group of similar behavioral and physiological signs and symptoms in the neonate caused by withdrawal from various pharmacological agents. Withdrawal symptoms will vary depending upon the age of the neonate, the medication, the medication's half-life, and the time of the mother's last use (Anbalagan & Mendez, 2023). See Table 17.7 for information on approximate withdrawal onset and symptoms of withdrawal from various medications.

Newborn nurseries and NICUs use neonatal abstinence scales as tools to evaluate newborn reflexes and behaviors that indicate the severity of withdrawal symptoms and help you and health-care providers to plan for medical intervention.

Medical management of the newborn with NAS may include the following:

- Transferring any infant with signs of NAS to the NICU
- Providing supportive therapy with IV fluids to prevent dehydration from nausea and vomiting
- Providing pharmacological therapy to reduce symptoms and gradually wean the newborn from the substance; morphine is the most frequently used medication for opioid-addicted newborns to reduce symptoms and to wean slowly (Shukla et al., 2022)
- Administering phenobarbital, which is effective in controlling seizures

Safety Stat!

Avoid the use of naloxone at the time of delivery if the mother is suspected to be opioid dependent. Naloxone will cause abrupt withdrawal and seizures for the neonate.

Nursing interventions for a newborn with NAS are as follows:

- Observing daily for signs of withdrawal and reporting any signs and symptoms immediately
- Administering and monitoring pharmacological treatment
- Monitoring for skin breakdown and applying barrier ointments for prevention of diaper rash from diarrhea
- Bottle feeding with high-calorie formula to promote weight gain
- Encouraging breastfeeding, if not contraindicated
- Providing parenting education to the caretakers of the infant
- Communicating with and providing a referral to a social worker for postdischarge care and follow-up

Some medication exposures during gestation do not cause severe withdrawal symptoms for the newborn. However, it is likely that brain chemistry and function have been changed because of the exposure. Long-term effects related to prenatal medication exposure may include the following:

- Poor growth through childhood
- Hyperactivity and attention-deficit disorder
- Impaired cognition, leading to learning disabilities
- Poor language development
- Higher rates of criminal behavior and substance use disorder (Shukla et al., 2022).

Table 17.7

Medication Withdrawal for the Neonate

Medication	Onset of Withdrawal Symptoms	Symptoms of Withdrawal
Opioids	24–72 hours	Hyperirritability Tremors High-pitched cry Nasal congestion Hyperthermia Tachycardia Poor feeding Regurgitation Diarrhea
Alcohol	3–12 hours	Jitteriness Irritability Hypertonia Hyperreflexia Seizures Poor suck Poor sleep Tremors Diaphoresis Hyperactivity
Cocaine	2–3 days	Irritability Hyperactivity Tremors High-pitched cry Some neonates have no symptoms of withdrawal
Marijuana	Depends upon mother's last use (symptoms may occur if the mother used marijuana heavily during pregnancy and during labor)	Hypoglycemia Jitteriness Tremors Exaggerated startle reflex Disturbed sleep cycles
Selective serotonin reuptake inhibitors (SSRIs)	Hours to days	Continuous crying Restlessness Sleep disturbances
Barbiturates	1–14 days	Irritability Tremors Excessive crying Restlessness Increased muscle tone Vomiting Diarrhea
Caffeine	At birth	Jitteriness Vomiting Tachypnea Bradycardia

Sources: Anbalagan, S., & Mendez, M. D. (2023). Neonatal abstinence syndrome. *StatPearls NIH*. https://www.ncbi.nlm.nih.gov/books/NBK551498; Rohan, A. (2020). Assessment and care of the newborn. In P. D. Suplee & J. Janke (Eds.), *AWHONN compendium of postpartum care* (3rd ed. pp. 65–69); Shukla, S., Zirkin, L. B., & Gomez Pomar, E. (2022). Perinatal drug abuse and neonatal drug withdrawal. *StatPearls NIH*. https://www.ncbi.nlm.nih.gov/books/NBK519061

Safe and Effective Nursing Care

Care for the Chemically Exposed Newborn

Care for a newborn who has been exposed to medications in the uterus can be challenging. Nursing care should include:

- Provide a calm, quiet environment.
- Practice swaddling, because it is usually very calming for the newborn.
- Avoid unnecessary handling.
- Use a light dimmer to keep lights low.
- Respond quickly to cries.
- Limit stimuli such as stroking, direct speech, and strong fragrances.
- Provide "space" by positioning the baby to face outward, away from the caregiver's body.

CARE OF THE NEWBORN EXPOSED TO HIV

HIV can be transmitted from mother to child during pregnancy, labor and delivery, or breastfeeding; this is known as perinatal transmission. Transmission of HIV from mother to child is the main way by which HIV infection is acquired by children. The risk of perinatal acquisition is 25% to 30% without interventions, such as antiviral therapy (Peterson, 2022).

The CDC (2023) recommends that infants born to mothers with unknown HIV status should receive rapid HIV testing as soon as possible immediately after birth with immediate implementation of prophylactic medication.

The following presents the medical management of the HIV-exposed newborn:

- Zidovudine (ZDV) 4 mg/kg twice a day through 6 weeks of age, if the mother received antiretroviral medications during pregnancy
- If the mother did not receive prenatal antiretroviral medications, the newborn should receive:
  - ZDV 4 mg/kg twice a day through 6 weeks of age plus nevirapine (NVP)—three doses in the first week of life, 12 mg PO per dose if birth weight is greater than 2 kg and 8 mg per dose if birth weight is 1.5 to 2 kg (HIV.gov, 2023)
- Follow-up consultation with a pediatric infectious disease specialist
- Obtaining a complete blood count (CBC) for a baseline

Nursing interventions for the HIV-exposed newborn include the following:

- Strictly maintaining standard precautions to avoid exposure
- Making sure gloves are worn by anyone handling the newborn (including family members) until the first bath
- Notifying the health-care provider of any abnormalities noted during physical evaluation

- Administering medications as ordered
- Educating parents about the importance of following the medication prophylaxis plan after discharge
- Advising the mother not to breastfeed

CARE OF THE FAMILY OF AN AT-RISK NEWBORN

As most parents plan for the birth of their baby, they expect a normal birth and a healthy newborn. Even a woman who experiences complications during her pregnancy holds on to the hope that her newborn will be born without problems and leave the hospital with her. Admission of their baby to the NICU places the parents and other family members in a stressful situation. When the unexpected complication of having a sick newborn happens, the parents will experience a range of emotions:

- Fear of the unknown and the environment of the NICU
- Anger that the birth experience was not what was planned
- Guilt because the mother often blames herself
- Loss of bonding and attachment time because the parents and child are separated
- Loss of control because the staff does not always communicate openly with the parents
- Frustration because the other women on the postpartum unit have their babies in their rooms
- Anxiety about the baby's health
- Helplessness because the baby needs high-level skilled care and the parents cannot provide care to their infant

In addition to caring for a newborn with complex health issues, nurses must provide family-centered care and reduce the stress and anxiety that the parents are experiencing. Some nursing interventions that support family-centered care in the NICU include the following:

- Providing opportunities for the parents to hold and bond with their newborn
- Developing a therapeutic relationship with the parents
- Providing positive reinforcement for the concerns the parents demonstrate
- Encouraging the parents to talk about the NICU experience
- Never behaving as if the parents are in the way or interrupting
- Answering all questions honestly
- Including the parents in an open dialogue with the entire NICU team
- Demonstrating care for the parents and the baby
- Using the baby's first name
- Allowing the parents to provide care such as bathing and feedings
- Starting to teach home health care before discharge so that the parents will not be overwhelmed

Allow skin-to-skin time whenever possible to promote temperature control, glucose stabilization, and bonding.

Evidence-Based Practice

Parents of babies admitted to the NICU experience fear and anxiety much worse than parents of healthy newborns. Psychological distress can continue after the baby is discharged and home with the parents. A study of parents of infants admitted to the NICU concluded that the parents exhibited a high number of symptoms of depression and posttraumatic stress while the newborn was a patient in the NICU. Furthermore, 80% of the participants screened positive for posttraumatic stress a year later. Nurses should recognize the need to support parents of infants in the NICU and to provide appropriate referrals to support groups and social workers.

Salome, S., Mansi, G., Lambiase, C. V., Barone, M., Piro, V., Pesce, M., Sarnelli, G., Raimond, F., & Capasso, L. (2022). Impact of psychological distress and psychophysical wellbeing on posttraumatic symptoms in parents of preterm infants after NICU discharge. *Italian Journal of Pediatrics, 48*, 13. https://doi.org/10.1186/s13052-022-01202-z

Therapeutic Communication

It is very important to establish a therapeutic relationship with the parents of a sick newborn. Communication with the parents needs to be sincere and honest. False reassurance is not therapeutic for the parents. Some examples of therapeutic communication include the following:

"Tell me how you're feeling today."
"What questions do you have?"
"You look worried, what's on your mind?"
"I have time. May I sit with you and talk about your baby and your concerns?"

Key Points

- Early identification of risk factors for a high-risk newborn will facilitate rapid interventions at birth to help prevent complications for the newborn.
- Birth asphyxia occurs when the newborn's brain does not receive enough oxygen during the birth process.
- Respiratory distress can be caused by lack of surfactant, immature lungs, fluid in the airways, meconium blocking the airways, and other conditions that make it difficult for the newborn to initiate or maintain respirations after birth.
- The most common signs of respiratory distress are tachypnea, dyspnea, nasal flaring, grunting, and chest retractions.
- Prompt recognition of the signs of respiratory distress is required so that interventions can be started before resuscitation is required.
- TTN is self-limiting and manifested by mild respiratory distress and tachypnea.
- Meconium aspiration syndrome is caused by the fetus inhaling meconium during the birth process. The meconium can block small bronchioles, thus inhibiting gas exchange.
- Cold stress can compound problems for an ill newborn. Careful management of the newborn's temperature is extremely important.
- Neonatal hypoglycemia is the most common metabolic problem for newborns. Long-term complications from untreated or poorly treated hypoglycemia include developmental delays, seizures, and intellectual disability.
- Birth injuries most often occur with macrosomic infants delivered vaginally. The most common birth injuries are fractured clavicles and brachial plexus injuries.
- Hyperbilirubinemia that is excessive can cause neurological problems for the newborn if not treated. Hyperbilirubinemia is treated with breastfeeding or bottle feeding, phototherapy, and exchange transfusion.
- Newborns can become infected in a variety of ways, but their immature immune systems often cannot produce obvious symptoms. You need to be alert for subtle signs of neonatal sepsis and report promptly to initiate care.
- An *SGA newborn* is defined as an infant whose weight is less than the 10th percentile for their gestational age. The SGA newborn will have mature organs but can have complications related to asphyxia and thermoregulation.
- The LGA baby's weight is greater than the 90th percentile for gestational age. The predominant cause of an LGA infant is maternal diabetes.
- For a preterm infant (born before 37 weeks' gestation), the gestational age and weight are important factors in determining the infant's ability to survive outside the uterus.
- Confirmation of gestational age is based upon a gestational age assessment.
- Premature infants are at risk for problems related to almost every body system.
- The most common problem for the premature infant is apnea of prematurity.
- A postterm newborn is born after 42 weeks' gestation. Postterm infants have a higher rate of death and disease than term infants.
- Complications for the IDM include hypoglycemia, polycythemia, and electrolyte imbalances.
- Fetal exposure to medications in early pregnancy can cause fetal anomalies, and exposure throughout

pregnancy can alter brain chemistry and cause long-term effects on the child.
• Some medications cause severe withdrawal symptoms in the newborn that require medical and nursing interventions.

• Newborns who have been exposed to HIV during pregnancy should receive prophylactic medications to reduce the chance of acquiring HIV from the mother.
• You have an opportunity to provide family-centered care by including the parents in the care of the ill newborn.

Review Questions

1. Which evaluation finding may cause you to suspect a brachial plexus injury?
   1. The newborn has tremors.
   2. The newborn cries continually.
   3. The newborn does not demonstrate a Moro reflex.
   4. The newborn has hypotonia.

2. What are signs of hypoglycemia in a newborn? **(Select all that apply.)**
   1. Tremors
   2. Hunger
   3. Weak cry
   4. Lethargy
   5. Jaundice

3. You check the blood sugar of a 2-hour-old newborn, and the glucometer reading is 32 mg/dL. Which action should you take next?
   1. Recognize that this is a normal reading and document it.
   2. Initiate breastfeeding.
   3. Call the laboratory for a STAT blood glucose level.
   4. Transfer the newborn to the NICU.

4. A nurse has been explaining TTN to the newborn's mother. Which statement indicates that the mother understands the teaching?
   1. "My baby will probably go home on oxygen therapy."
   2. "I cannot breastfeed my baby while he is breathing so fast."
   3. "This breathing problem may have happened because I had a cesarean birth."
   4. "My baby may be in the NICU for about 2 weeks."

5. What are risk factors for neonatal sepsis? **(Select all that apply.)**
   1. Preterm birth
   2. Cesarean birth
   3. Precipitous delivery
   4. Frequent vaginal examinations
   5. A mother with a GBS infection

6. What is a sign that a newborn may be at risk for meconium aspiration syndrome?
   1. Acrocyanosis
   2. Yellow-green tint on umbilical cord
   3. Asymmetrical breathing
   4. Born before 38 weeks' gestation

7. Which physical signs could indicate a risk for hyperbilirubinemia?
   1. Acrocyanosis
   2. Cephalohematoma
   3. Newborn rash
   4. Tremors

8. Which of these is a physical characteristic of a preterm infant?
   1. Dry skin
   2. Lanugo
   3. Long toenails
   4. Hypertonia

9. What are possible complications of prematurity? **(Select all that apply.)**
   1. Retinopathy
   2. Color blindness
   3. Apnea
   4. Cerebral palsy
   5. Learning disabilities

10. When observing a medication-exposed newborn, what symptom suggests that the newborn may be exhibiting withdrawal symptoms?
    1. Sleepiness
    2. Constipation
    3. Irritability
    4. Absent Moro or startle reflex

ANSWERS 1. 3; 2. 1, 3, 4; 3. 2; 4. 3; 5. 1, 4, 5; 6. 2; 7. 2; 8. 2; 9. 1, 3, 4, 5; 10. 3

CRITICAL THINKING QUESTIONS

1. Why is it important to maintain good glucose control throughout pregnancy?

2. Why would it be beneficial to place the IDM at the breast immediately after delivery?

3. Discuss the signs that you would notice if gas exchange is impaired in a newborn.

Resources

For additional resources and information, including Postconference Questions and Activities, Answers, and References, visit www.FADavis.com.

 Student Study Guide

CHAPTER 18
Health Promotion of the Infant: Birth to 1 Year

KEY TERMS

anthropometric measurements (AN-thro-po-MET-rik MEZH-er-ments)
chromosomes (KROH-muh-sohmz)
failure to thrive (FTT) (FAYL-yuhr too THRYEV)
genetics (je-NET-iks)
genomics (je-NOH-miks)
hereditary (huh-RED-ih-tair-ee)
immunizations (IM-yoo-nih-ZAY-shunz)
myelination (MYE-uh-lih-NAY-shun)
separation anxiety (SEP-uh-RAY-shun ang-ZYE-uh-tee)
stranger anxiety (STRAYN-jer ang-ZYE-uh-tee)
thermoregulation (THER-moh-REG-yoo-LAY-shun)

CHAPTER CONCEPTS

Cognition
Comfort
Elimination
Family
Growth and Development
Health Promotion
Nutrition
Safety

LEARNING OUTCOMES

1. Define the key terms.
2. Evaluate the unique needs of the newborn and infant as compared with older children in relation to safety, bonding, communication, and development.
3. Describe the differences between infants, older children, and adults in relation to body systems, rapid growth, anatomy, and physiology.
4. Compare the nutritional needs and eating patterns of the infant, including accurate kilocalorie and fluid maintenance calculations.
5. Discuss the elimination patterns of the newborn, young infant, and older infant.
6. Describe the need infants have for stimulation, play, and sleep to promote normal growth and development.
7. Differentiate the various schedules, infectious diseases, and care required for infants undergoing immunizations.
8. Differentiate various nutritional disorders that can be found during infancy, including organic and nonorganic FTT.
9. Describe respiratory distress in the infant, including assessment and interventions.
10. Describe the phenomenon of sudden infant death syndrome (SIDS) and the needs of the family immediately after the infant's death through the period of grief and loss.
11. Discuss the interventions that can assist a caregiver who is caring for an infant experiencing colic.
12. Describe key assessments and interventions for an infant demonstrating dehydration.
13. Understand the importance of discussing safety issues for infants with parents, including maintaining a clear airway and preventing severe injuries such as shaken baby syndrome.

CRITICAL THINKING

Danielle is a 9-month-old experiencing expected growth and development. Danielle's parents do not "believe" in immunizations; at all of her well-child checkups to date, they have not agreed to any of the childhood immunizations that are recommended by the Centers for Disease Control and Prevention (CDC). Many should have been administered thus far. Her parents say they are concerned with the safety and side effects of childhood vaccines and plan on keeping her exempt from receiving childhood immunizations when she starts school. Danielle and her family live in a county where pertussis is considered an epidemic, and annual influenza has been commonly found across the life span.

Questions

1. What are possible consequences for Danielle of not having childhood vaccines administered according to the recommended schedule?
2. What are overall nursing concerns for older infants whose required immunizations have not been given?
3. After searching for reputable sources that provide information on parental vaccine refusal, how can you incorporate the most common concerns expressed by parents who refuse childhood vaccines into your wellness teaching (also called anticipatory guidance)?

grows and develops in their own timeline and within their own unique growth pattern. No two infants develop in exactly the same way. Each infant also has their own unique temperament and personality. Parents need to understand that each infant is unique; therefore, nurses teach parents about ranges in the expected development of their infant. For instance, a pediatric nurse would explain to new parents that the expected time frame for walking is 10 to 16 months, emphasizing that expectations for each child during the infancy period will be unique and they should not try to compare children's unique development.

One of the most important topics to cover with parents of an infant is keeping well-child checkups (Fig. 18.1). A healthy infant needs a series of **immunizations**; measurements, including head circumference (HC), weight, and length checks; and developmental milestone checks, assessing for dysfunctions or delays in the infant's development. The earlier that a health-care provider identifies problems in growth and development, the sooner they can make referrals for interventions to assist the child. Nurses must encourage parents to maintain all records of infant well-child checkups so that important information is available as needed.

Another important topic is safety. Nurses must teach families ways to prevent injuries in their developing child. Anticipatory guidance, or education focusing on what to expect and planning a safe and healthy environment before an incident or injury happens, is paramount.

CONCEPTUAL CORNERSTONE
Family
The concept of family-centered care provides a foundation on which to base interactions with and support for new families. Family-centered care encourages collaboration, engagement, and respect and promotes the concept of enabling parents to care for their child through demonstration and education, especially if the child has special needs or a chronic illness. Infants are born very dependent, yet rapidly progress and change over the 12 months of this first developmental stage. Family-centered care provides a foundation for interacting with new families with young infants to reduce anxiety, promote safety, and provide guidance about what to expect of their infant.

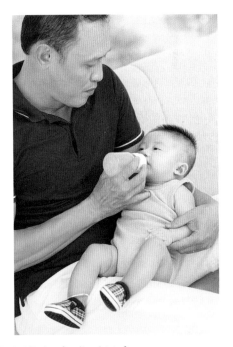

FIGURE 18.1 Father feeding his infant.

The period of infancy is a remarkable experience for the child and caregivers. Infants not only grow exceptionally fast, but they achieve a large number of milestones all within the first year of life, including holding up the head, rolling over, crawling, standing, and beginning to walk.

Milestones are defined as general patterns of growth and development achievements during the stages of life. Infants grow with an expected series of orderly steps, but the growth of an infant does not occur at a steady pace. Each infant

• WORD • BUILDING •
immunization: immuniz–safe + ation–action

GROWTH AND DEVELOPMENT OF THE INFANT

Infancy begins with the newborn period, the first 30 days after birth. Following the newborn period, infancy is categorized as *early infancy,* the first 6 months, and *older infancy,* the second 6 months. After infancy, the child moves to the toddler period. See Box 18.1 for a description of all of the developmental stages.

Heredity and Genetic Influences

Genetics is the study of how our genes, chromosomes, and genotypes, or sequencing and combinations of genes, are expressed and responsible for health or disorders. During fetal development and in the early infancy period, assessment for genetic abnormalities occurs. Although rare, genetic abnormalities (see Chapter 6) should be identified early so that appropriate medical care can be implemented right away. Genes are the elements of **chromosomes** responsible for **hereditary** characteristics (characteristics transmitted from the parent to the offspring). Each parent contributes one gene for each hereditary property. Genes determine the infant's characteristics, such as hair color, skin color, eye color, and height. Some inherited, or genetic, disorders are evident at birth; other genetic disorders will not manifest or become apparent until later in childhood or adulthood. **Genomics** is the study of how genetics influence disease. Genomics is concerned with the study of the structure and function of genes, and how genetics weigh-in on complex diseases and health conditions influenced by one's genetic background and environmental factors.

"Carriers" are children or adults who carry the defective gene but usually do not experience the symptoms of the disease or disorder. A carrier has one defective gene and one healthy gene. Parents need to understand that when one parent is a carrier, there is a 25% chance of having a child with a disease or disorder, a 50% chance of having a child who is a carrier of the genetic trait, and a 25% chance of having a child who does not have the genetic disease or disorder.

In *autosomal dominant diseases and disorders* (ones carried on the first 22 pairs of chromosomes), only one defective gene or set of genes needs to be passed on for the child to have the condition. Examples of autosomal dominant disorders include osteogenesis imperfecta, night blindness, and neurofibromatosis. In *autosomal recessive diseases and disorders*, both parents must pass the defective gene or set of genes to their child. Examples of autosomal recessive diseases are sickle cell disease, phenylketonuria (PKU), and albinism. Genetic counseling is offered to parents who are known to carry a defective gene or who have previously given birth to a child with a genetic disorder.

Some genetic disorders found in infants are sex-linked. These disorders are carried on the X chromosome and are passed only by women to their children. Examples of sex-linked disorders include hemophilia, glucose-6-phosphate dehydrogenase (G6PD), and color blindness.

Genetic abnormalities that are not inherited can also occur. Down syndrome, also known as trisomy 21, is a genetic condition caused by an extra chromosome 21. There is a strong connection between having Down syndrome and having intellectual disabilities, congenital heart disease, obstructive sleep apnea, thyroid disease (hypothyroid), acute lymphocytic leukemia (ALL), visual and hearing defects, intestinal malformations, and increased susceptibility to infections. The care of a child with Down syndrome spans all of childhood and requires a multidisciplinary approach.

A primary physician needs to follow the child carefully; however, many specialists will become involved. The child with Down syndrome may require care from any of the following: ophthalmologist, cardiologist, speech therapist, social worker, dietitian, occupation and physical therapist, teacher, counselor, and gastroenterologist. The goal for care and treatment is to provide an optimal level of functioning, developmental growth, illness management, and chronic care of complications. Children with Down syndrome will process through the developmental stages of childhood, but they do so at their own pace and timetable.

The Newborn Period: Physical Growth and Development

During the newborn period, the physiology of the child is different than at any other developmental stage. Newborns are susceptible to a variety of injuries and health problems, including hypoglycemia and hypothermia. The newborn period has a higher mortality rate (death rate) than any other time period during childhood. Assessing the newborn requires knowledge in each of the body systems because the newborn has unique needs for the first hours, days, and weeks of life. A review of each body system aids the nurse in identifying areas of concern for the vulnerable newborn infant.

Transition to Extrauterine Life

Transition to extrauterine life refers to the first 24 hours of life. The newborn leaves the stable, warm, and nourishing environment of the womb and enters life. The newborn faces profound physiological changes, including the transition from fetal or placental circulation to newborn circulation patterns, closure of the fetal ducts, and development of an

---

Box 18.1

The Nine Stages of Childhood

1. *Premature infants:* Born before 36 weeks' gestation
2. *Newborn infants:* Birth to 28 to 30 days
3. *Early infancy:* 1 to 6 months
4. *Older infancy:* 6 months to 1 year
5. *Toddler:* 1 to 3 years
6. *Preschooler:* 3 to 5 years
7. *Early school-aged:* 6 to 10 years
8. *Late school-aged:* 11 to 13 years
9. *Adolescent:* 13 to 18 years

independent respiratory pattern. Complete metabolic support from the mother stops, and the newborn adjusts to an independent supply of oxygen, nutrients, and thermal regulation. For more about the newborn's adaptations to extrauterine life, see Chapter 14.

Several factors can interrupt the normal transitional period from fetal life to newborn life. Incomplete removal of the amniotic fluid can lead to respiratory distress and tachypnea of the newborn. Fetal asphyxia, hypercapnia, and subsequent acidosis will contribute to a troubled adjustment to postfetal life. The most critical first step in the transitional period from fetal life to newborn life is the onset of breathing and the establishment of a successful breathing pattern. Although some infants require mild tactile stimulation to induce a regular breathing pattern, few require a resuscitative effort to assist the newborn to independent breathing. The simple act of drying off the newborn's skin may be enough stimulation to assist the infant. Gentle and brief back, arm, or trunk rubbing (can use soft, prewarmed towels) and gentle flicking of the soles of the infant's feet are acceptable means to stimulate a newborn to breathe (Kalaniti et al., 2018).

Cardiovascular System

It is important for you to review the newborn's cardiac system as follows:

- Inspect for cyanosis, mottling, edema, discolored or blue nailbeds, and clubbing as signs of cardiac abnormalities and poor perfusion.
- Inspect for heaves and lifts of the chest.
- Auscultate heart sounds starting at the aortic area and moving to the pulmonic, Erb's point, tricuspid, and then mitral areas; check the quality, rate, intensity, and rhythm of the heart; normal innocent heart murmurs may be found in up to 50% of infants.
- Palpate all central and peripheral pulses and compare femoral with brachial, looking for discrepancies in rate and rhythm.
- Percuss the heart; in infancy, the heart is large in relation to body size.

Thermoregulation

The newborn has an important need for the preservation of the core body temperature. **Thermoregulation**, which is the process of maintaining a core body temperature, is a challenge for the newborn and is considered absolutely crucial for survival.

Thermoregulation is important to prevent fluctuations in blood glucose. While trying to regulate their body temperature, newborns can experience hypoglycemia. For more about thermoregulation in the newborn, see Chapter 14.

Newborn temperature assessments should include the following:

- Check rectal or axillary temperatures with a calibrated thermometer.
- Note temperatures above 37.5°C (99.5°F) or below 36°C (96.8°F); these temperatures should be reported and an intervention initiated.
- Wrapping a newborn in extra blankets or removing a layer of blankets may be enough to support thermoregulation. Continue to check the newborn's temperature until stable.

Respiratory System

The newborn has a proportionally large head for the body size with a short neck, small mandible, and large tongue. This makes them more susceptible to airway compromise, and they may require a sniffing position for comfort during periods of respiratory distress.

The newborn also has a compliant rib cage with poorly developed intercostal muscles, which allows the infant to progress from respiratory distress to respiratory failure to respiratory arrest very quickly. If retractions are noted, they must be reported immediately so that an intervention can be initiated.

The newborn has cartilaginous tracheal rings, and the cricoid ring is the narrowest part of the airway. This is in contrast to the adult, in which the larynx is the narrowest part of the airway.

Newborns are obligate nose breathers and have narrow nasal passages that are easily obstructed by mucus. They need to be suctioned in the presence of increasing nasal mucus. Teaching parents how to use a bulb suction device is appropriate. Even a small amount of resistance to airflow from edema or mucus will cause increased work of breathing (WOB).

Newborn respiratory assessments should include the following:

- Inspect the lip color, nail color, and pulse oximetry; blood gases and hemoglobin (Hgb) may be ordered as part of the assessment of the respiratory system if the newborn demonstrates respiratory distress.
- Inspect for retractions, nasal flaring, use of accessory muscles, tachypnea, head bobbing, and shoulder rolling, which all can indicate respiratory distress.
- Auscultate for adventitious or abnormal breath sounds such as rales, rhonchi, wheezing, or stridor.
- Inspect for irregular respiratory rates and patterns.

Gastrointestinal System

Newborns have an absence of normal gut flora and reduced gastric enzymes, which puts them at risk for infection of the

Patient Teaching Guidelines

Teach new parents that swaddling or wrapping the newborn in clean, dry blankets is essential to maintain body temperature. Newborns should consistently wear a soft hat and be dressed in appropriate layers of clothing. One tip is to dress the infant in one layer more than the adults are wearing in the same environment, plus a blanket.

Table 18.1

Stool Patterns of Infants in the First Year of Life

First stool: Meconium	• Usually passes in first few days of life. • Consistency is thick and sticky. • Color is black/green; composed of amniotic fluid, mucosal cells, ingested blood, and secretions from intestinal lining.
Transitional stool	• As the meconium is passed, the stool changes in color and consistency. • Occurs at about the third day of life. • Consistency is less thick and sticky. • Color is green/brown to yellow/brown.
Breast milk stool	• Color is orange-yellow. • Consistency is soft and even. • Appears after the fourth day of life. • Breastfed newborns will have several stools a day.
Formula stool	• Color and odor of formula stools depend on the formula fed. • Consistency is soft.

gastrointestinal (GI) system. Breastfeeding is a natural way of introducing normal gut flora.

Newborns are also at risk for fluid and electrolyte imbalances. At no time should a newborn be given free water unless specifically ordered. If a small amount of water is ordered, it should always be sterile water. Any formula given should be mixed with sterile water during the first few months of infancy to prevent the introduction of unwanted microbes that lead to diarrhea. Overall fluid requirements for the newborn and young infant up to 6 months of age are, on average, 125 to 150 mL/kg/day. Solid foods should not be introduced until 6 months of life. The infant's first solid food should be iron-fortified infant cereal mixed with breast milk to form a slightly thickened liquid to prevent choking. See Table 18.1 for details of the stool patterns of infants.

Newborn GI assessments should include the following:

• Inspect for visible peristalsis.
• Auscultate bowel sounds in all four abdominal quadrants.
• Palpate for masses.
• Note the frequency, quantity, and consistency of stool.

Genitourinary System

The newborn's bladder capacity is about 15 to 20 mL. The newborn's urine is very light yellow because the newborn's kidneys do not concentrate urine effectively. This leaves the newborn at risk for fluid loss and dehydration. Newborns do not cope well with electrolyte fluctuations because their kidneys are immature and unable to concentrate or excrete electrolytes well.

The newborn girl's urethra is very short, which leaves her at risk for the development of urinary tract infections (UTIs). It is important to show parents how to clean the infant girl's genitalia so that they thoroughly cleanse the area, removing all stool.

Newborn assessments of the genitourinary system are as follows:

• Inspect the outer genitalia for hygiene and rashes.
• Inspect the quality and color of urine.
• Sniff for malodorous urine.

Musculoskeletal System

At birth, the newborn's skeletal system has more collagen present than it does ossified bone. Rapidly, the bones mature and become less pliable. The musculoskeletal system is intact and growth occurs via hypertrophy, not hyperplasia or new cellular growth. Because of the risk of injury, careful handling of the newborn is essential. Parents need to be taught how to carefully position, dress and undress, and carry their infant with head support.

Newborn assessments of the musculoskeletal system include the following:

• Inspect for skeletal deformities.
• Inspect bilateral muscle movements.
• Palpate extremities for masses and deformities.

Endocrine System

The newborn's endocrine system is influenced by the mother's hormones. It is not uncommon to see a newborn's nipples secrete a small amount of milky substance called "witch's milk," or a newborn girl's vagina produce a small amount of blood-colored secretion called "pseudomenstruation." The newborn's blood glucose levels fluctuate widely as the pancreas adjusts to secreting insulin. Other hormones are produced, but the endocrine glands are immature. The pituitary gland can secrete only limited amounts of antidiuretic hormone, leaving the newborn at risk for dehydration caused by diuresis. Assessment of the newborn endocrine system includes inspection for symptoms of fluctuating blood sugars, such as hypothermia, poor muscle tone, apnea, shakiness, poor feeding behaviors, and lethargy.

Safety *Stat!*

Stressed or sick newborns require their blood glucose levels to be monitored because they are prone to hypoglycemia. Interventions will be required when a newborn or young infant demonstrates hypoglycemia. Regular feedings (at least every 3 hours or on-demand in shorter intervals of time) will assist a sick or stressed infant to maintain their blood glucose levels. If an infant is too sick to suck, breastfeed, or take a bottle, a small nasogastric or naso-oral tube may be placed to gavage breast milk or formula if breast milk is not available to keep a stable blood glucose level. Hypoglycemia is dangerous for newborns and infants. Prolonged hypoglycemia can lead to harm to the brain and affect the infant's ability to function. Hypoglycemia can lead to serious brain injuries and seizures (Stanford Medicine Children's Health, 2021).

Integumentary System

The newborn's skin is thin, but all structures within the skin are present and functional. Because of the skin's thin nature, any topical medications or ointments will be readily absorbed. Care should be taken to clean the newborn's skin gently but thoroughly to prevent tissue injury, rashes, or tears because the dermis and epidermis are loosely bound. The newborn is at risk for skin breakdown and should be checked regularly.

Assessments of the newborn's integumentary system include these:

- Inspect for rashes, clogged sebaceous glands (milia), and bruises.
- Palpate the skin for lesions and masses.

Neurological System

Maturation of the neurological system takes time because the newborn has immature nerves. **Myelination**, the process of a myelin sheath growing around nerve fibers, continues during *cephalocaudal–proximal-distal development,* and the young infant slowly masters movement. The first movements are primitive reflexes that, over time, become purposeful movements. The most important aspect of the newborn's neurological system is the autonomic nervous system (ANS); this is what stimulates the initiation and maintenance of a respiratory pattern after birth. For more about the ANS, see Chapter 27.

Assessments of the newborn's neurological system include the following:

- Inspect primitive reflexes (see Chapter 15).
- Inspect for equality and symmetry of movements.

Sensory Organs

At birth, the sensory organs are all present. In most newborns, olfactory, tactile, taste, and hearing abilities are all intact; however, vision is not mature for quite some time. The eyes are structurally incomplete with immature ciliary muscles. This means the newborn will have trouble accommodating and fixating on an object. Parents are encouraged to hold their infant close, also known as the *en face* position. (See Chapter 28 for more about the development of vision.) The newborn's sense of smell is well developed. They will react strongly to unpleasant odors. Moreover, newborns are able to distinguish their mother's breast milk from someone else's and will cry for their mother's milk if they smell their mother's unique milk scent (Office on Women's Health, 2022).

Nutrition

Infant nutrition changes rapidly throughout the first year of life.

- The newborn starts with breastfeeding or formula feeding exclusively until the infant is 6 months old. Feedings number about 8 to 12 per day in the newborn period and then slowly become larger and less frequent as the infant grows.
- Foods are then introduced one at a time to allow for the assessment of food sensitivities or allergies. Iron-fortified infant cereals are introduced first, only after the infant both shows an interest in the food and accomplishes the developmental milestone of being able to swallow a small bolus of food placed on the tongue (HealthyChildren.org, 2022).
- Green vegetables are introduced after cereals are well established, followed by the yellow and orange vegetables. Although there is no evidence to say that infants who are introduced to fruits first will turn away from vegetables introduced second, most pediatricians recommend introducing vegetables first (HealthyChildren.org, 2022).
- Pureed fruits are introduced one at a time after eating vegetables is well established.
- Lean meats and egg yolks can be given starting at about 10 months. Vegan options include mashed tofu, pureed beans, and soy or other nondairy yogurt and cheeses (Hayes & Klemm, 2021).
- Egg whites are introduced after 10 months.
- No cow's milk should be given to an infant until after 12 months of age because it can cause inflammation and microbleeds in the intestines. Cow's milk also contributes to milk anemia when young children consume more than 32 ounces a day, replacing iron-rich foods. When cow's milk is introduced, the young child should be given whole milk for the first 2 years to provide the fat needed for brain growth. After 2 years, the child should be offered whichever milk the family drinks, preferably skim milk.
- Soy milk, almond milk, and homemade infant formulas should not be administered to infants as their

Table 18.2
Benefits of Breastfeeding

Benefits for the Infant	Benefits for the Mother
1. Breast milk allows for faster gastric emptying, reducing the likelihood of reflux.	1. Breastfeeding can provide the mother more rapid post-partum weight loss.
2. Breast milk provides host defense immunity factors, immunoglobulin A (IgA), growth factors, cytokines, lactoferrin, lysozymes, and nucleotides. All of these substances provide protection from infections. Breast milk will change in volume and composition to adapt and meet the growing newborn and infant's needs.	2. Breastfeeding allows faster uterine involution after birth, reducing the chance of excessive postpartum bleeding.
3. Breastfeeding reduces the incidence of OM, GI diseases, obesity, respiratory diseases, atopic conditions (asthma, eczema, and dermatitis), and SIDS.	3. Breastfeeding can contribute to the spacing of subsequent pregnancies, although this phenomenon is quite unreliable and should not be promoted as a form of birth control.
4. Breast milk helps protect against necrotizing enterocolitis.	4. Breast milk is sterile and provides economic advantages in comparison with formula. Mothers can breastfeed anytime and anywhere without supplies.
5. Breastfeeding improves long-term cognitive and motor abilities.	5. Breastfeeding can reduce the mother's risk of diseases later in life such as ovarian cancer, breast cancer, hypertension, and type 2 diabetes (CDC, 2021).

compositions do not support the correct carbohydrates, fats, and proteins needed during this critical time of development (Hayes & Klemm, 2021).

BREASTFEEDING. The American Academy of Pediatrics (2022) and the National Institute of Child Health and Human Development (2017) recommend breastfeeding for all infants for at least the first year of life, and the CDC Breastfeeding Report Card (2022) recommends human milk as the exclusive food for full-term infants for no less than the first 6 months. For more about breastfeeding, see Chapter 16. See Table 18.2 for a list of benefits of breastfeeding.

When an infant requires even a short hospitalization, breastfeeding may be disrupted. During an infant's hospitalization, the mother should be supported with a breast pump and given a place to store her milk. Follow institutional policy for breast milk labeling and storage. Typically, extra pumped breast milk can be stored as follows:

- In a freezer compartment with its own door for 3 to 6 months
- In a freezer that is part of the refrigerator compartment for 2 weeks
- In a refrigerator compartment for 4 to 5 days
- In an insulated cooling bag for 24 hours
- At room temperature for 6 to 8 hours (Academy of Breastfeeding Medicine, 2017; La Leche League International, 2019)

USING FORMULA. Although nurses consistently promote breastfeeding and provide education and support for it, an infant's health status may require formula feeding, or the mother may choose to use formula. Examples of conditions in which infants require formula include enteric tube feedings, anatomical abnormalities, GI diseases, or severe **failure to thrive** (**FTT;** see Table 18.8 later in the chapter). On the other hand, the mother may not be able to perform breastfeeding because of birth injuries, breast disease or infection, a medication she takes that may be transmitted through breast milk, or lack of production of breast milk. Formula that is going to be the infant's primary nutrition or a supplement to breast milk should be fortified with iron. Iron stores acquired during fetal development are depleted in the infant by 6 months of age.

Some infant formula is prescribed by the primary care provider to replenish specific vitamins or electrolytes or to provide specific levels of kilocalories or protein. Newborns with congenital anomalies or those with feeding disorders are provided with premade and premeasured formula.

During the newborn and young infant period, all formulas should be mixed with sterile water, and the baby bottle should be warmed in a bottle warmer or a water bath. Even with the use of a warmer or water bath, teach the family to consistently test the temperature of the formula before giving it to the child.

Therapeutic Communication

Nurses and all health-care providers who work with new mothers should show sensitivity while encouraging and educating about breastfeeding. Never shame or blame mothers who choose to formula feed, and never suggest, verbally or nonverbally, that a mother who cannot or does not choose to breastfeed "failed" or is a bad mother. Breastfeeding, although best for the baby, is not everyone's choice. Ultimately, what matters is that the baby is fed.

Safety *Stat!*

Under no circumstances should a microwave be used to warm formula. Microwaves are inconsistent in their power. Therefore, microwaving formula leaves "hot spots" within the liquid and can cause a severe burn. This education should also be provided to the infant's family and other caregivers. What action would you take if you witnessed parents warming breast milk or formula? What would you say to educate the family?

The type of formula used is based on several factors, including the quantity of calories, water, and nutrients the infant needs. Pediatricians or other health-care providers can recommend an appropriate formula. Families should be encouraged to follow the manufacturer's specific instructions for preparing formulas. Deviations from the exact recommended mixture can lead to the infant failing to gain weight if it is too dilute or to dehydration and metabolic acidosis if it is too strong.

To calculate an infant's formula needs, begin with the quantity of calories needed. Table 18.3 lists calorie needs by age. Then multiply the infant's weight in kilograms by the number of calories required per day. Remember to divide the number of daily calories needed by the number of feedings per day to determine calories per feeding.

Table 18.3
Kilocalorie Requirements

Developmental Age	Kcal Requirements
0–30 days	100–110 Kcal/kg/day
1–4 months	90–100 Kcal/kg/day
5 months to 5 years	70–90 Kcal/kg/day
Older than 5 years	1,500 Kcal for first 20 kg of weight, plus 25 Kcal for each additional kg/day

CULTURAL INFLUENCES ON INFANT NUTRITION. Decisions about breastfeeding or bottle feeding, the introduction of foods, and the selection of foods during infancy are highly influenced by the family's cultural background. Your responsibility is to ensure that the newborn and infant are being provided appropriate nutrition for optimal growth and development and are being fed safely.

Sleeping Patterns and Requirements

Young infants require about 22 to 23 hours of sleep a day for the first few weeks of life. Rest is imperative for health, growth, and development. Older infants require about 16 hours of sleep a day, including two naps. Typically, an older infant will nap for 1 to 2 hours in the morning and nap again in the later afternoon.

Patient Teaching Guidelines

To improve an older infant's night sleep behaviors, encourage the parents to schedule the child's naps earlier in the day. Although waking a napping infant is difficult for many caregivers, longer afternoon naps will cause the infant to stay up too late or have difficulty with a bedtime routine.

Infants will begin to sleep through the night at 4 to 6 months, but children vary greatly in this. Parents need to understand that each of their children will be unique in their sleeping patterns and flexibility is warranted. Parents can feel frustrated if they expect siblings to have similar sleeping patterns. Tips for successful infant sleeping include the following:

- Expect **separation anxiety**, a situation in which the child expresses anxiety when parents leave or the child is taken from the parents, to start at 8 to 10 months. Separation anxiety intensifies at about 12 months; therefore, going to bed becomes more difficult. Use routines and be firm and consistent. Provide a safe bed where the infant cannot easily crawl or climb out of the crib.
- Place the infant on the back to sleep; this greatly reduces the incidence of sudden infant death syndrome (SIDS). For up-to-date information on SIDS, see the website of the American Association of SIDS Prevention Physicians.
- Do not place pillows, stuffed animals, blankets, or bumper pads in the crib because they may cause suffocation.
- Rather than covering an infant in a blanket for warmth, dress the infant for sleep in a warm fleece onesie or a light cotton onesie, depending on the weather.
- Do not place infants to sleep on waterbeds; this may cause overheating and provides a suffocation risk.
- Although some families choose to, do not sleep with an infant because injuries can occur. The infant should have a safe and separate sleeping area.
- Do not use electric blankets in an infant's crib because this can cause overheating.

- Do not leave on a TV or radio because this might influence quality of sleep.
- Provide a consistent sleeping situation by establishing a routine before bedtime with a positive interaction.
- Help the infant to feel safe and secure at bedtime by using a night light.

Infant Development

Infants need psychosocial interaction and bonding to support their physical, cognitive, and communication development.

Physical Growth and Development

The physical development of the infant from the newborn period through the first year is astounding. The infant will triple their birth weight and double the birth length in the first 12 months. The infant's weight increases by about 0.68 kg (1.5 lb) per month for the first 6 months of life, then increases by about 0.34 kg (0.75 lb) per month the second 6 months. The infant's length grows at an average of 2.54 cm (1 in.) per month in the first 6 months, reaching an average length of 73.66 cm (29 in.) by 12 months of age. Measurements of children's growth are also called **anthropometric measurements** and can include weight, height, and HC. National standard growth charts are used to follow the natural physical development of the infant and are kept as records for referral if problems are identified. Figures 18.2 and 18.3 provide examples of growth charts.

Several factors influence the infant's physical development. These factors include hereditary influences such as the height and weight of the parents, the infant's nutritional status and overall health, cultural factors, and growth patterns known as *spurts* and *lags*. An infant who is born prematurely will take several months to match the average size of other infants the same age. Growth measurements are followed and plotted from birth to 3 years, and then new charts are used to follow growth from 3 to 18 years. The plotted measurements are interpreted as percentiles; an infant's measurements that fall within the 5th to 95th percentile are considered acceptable.

The infant's HC is measured at each well-child visit and plotted on standardized growth charts as well. The nurse uses a clean, disposable paper measuring tape and places the tape at the level of the largest part of the head, usually right above the brow line. The infant's HC, also known as the *occipital frontal circumference (OFC)*, increases by 1.25 cm (0.5 in.) per month for the first 6 months and increases a total of 33% by the end of the first year. The average value for the HC is 43.18 cm (17 in.) by age 6 months and 45.72 cm (18 in.) by age 12 months. The infant's posterior fontanel closes at

2 to 3 months of age, and the larger anterior fontanel at 12 to 18 months of age. Fontanels come in a variety of shapes and sizes and are therefore unique for each infant. The purpose of the fontanel is to allow the infant's cranium to expand or contract as needed during the birth process.

The nurse will also measure the infant's chest circumference. The chest circumference is typically 2 cm (0.78 in.) less than the infant's HC. To measure the chest circumference, the nurse places the paper measuring tape at the level of the nipples.

The infant will produce six to eight teeth during the first year with central incisors erupting first at about 5 to 7 months. See Figure 18.4 for a description of development of the infant's dentition. Parents should begin daily dental health by cleaning the infant's teeth with a damp cloth as soon as they erupt. Infants are at risk for dental caries (cavities) if they have a bottle or are breastfed while they sleep. This practice should be discouraged, and infants should be weaned from a bottle by 12 months of age to promote dental health.

Normal vital sign ranges in infancy are a heart rate of 120 to 160 bpm in the newborn period, slowing to 100 to 120 bpm by the first year. The respiratory rate is 30 to 60 breaths/minute, fluctuating greatly in the first few weeks of life. The axillary temperature ranges from 36.5°C (97.7°F) to 37.5°C (99.5°F). Blood pressure (BP) in the newborn ranges from 50 to 75 mm Hg systolic over 30 to 45 mm Hg diastolic; pressure rises to an average of 90/60 mm Hg by 12 months.

An infant's metabolic rate is almost twice that of an adult. Infants require more calories, nutrients, and water for their body size in comparison with an adult. The gross and fine motor milestones of an infant are noted in Boxes 18.2 and 18.3.

Play is a wonderful means to promote fine motor development. The pincer grasp, which is mastered by 7½ to 8½ months, can be encouraged by providing a food treat, such as Cheerios, and giving positive reinforcement for success in picking up the food treat and placing it in the mouth. This is now a dangerous time because the infant has mastered locomotion and will get around the floor, picking up any small item and placing it in the mouth. Infants require constant supervision when they move around the home.

Cognitive Development

The infant is experiencing the sensorimotor cognitive developmental period according to Piaget. During this period, the infant is beginning to discriminate between persons, comprehend word meaning, and learn object permanence (an object exists even when it is no longer in view).

According to Freud, the infant is experiencing the oral stage. Here the infant finds enjoyment, pleasure, and satisfaction from sucking and meets the world orally, bringing most

---

- WORD · BUILDING ·

anthropometric: anthropo–human being + metr–measure + ic–pertaining to

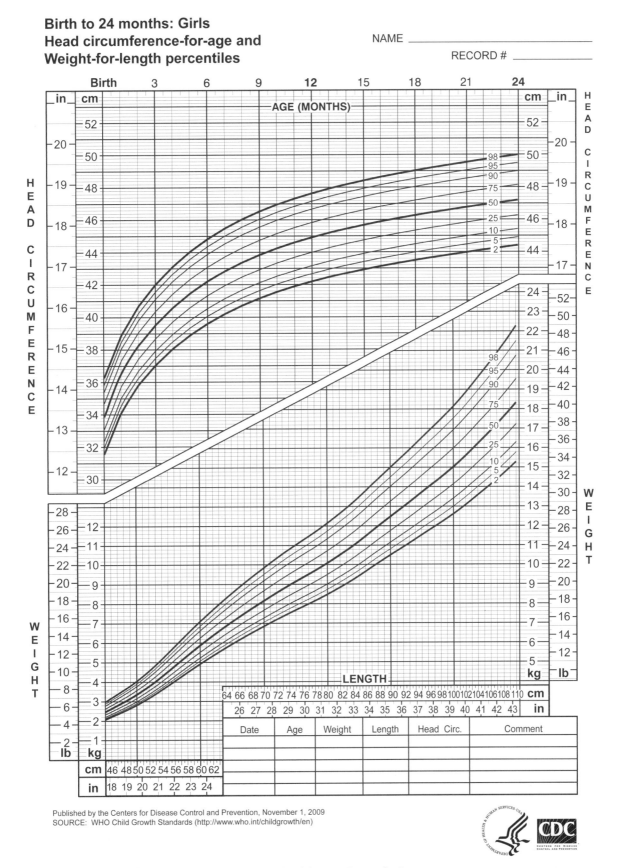

Birth to 24 months: Girls
Head circumference-for-age and
Weight-for-length percentiles

NAME _____

RECORD # _____

FIGURE 18.2 WHO growth chart for girls from birth to 24 months old. (From Centers for Disease Control and Prevention. Published by the Centers for Disease Control and Prevention, November 1, 2009. Source: WHO Child Growth Standards, www.who.int/tools/child-growth-standard/standardRetrieved from www.cdc.gov/growthcharts/who_charts.htm#The%20WHO%20Growth%20Charts.)

Birth to 24 months: Boys
Head circumference-for-age and
Weight-for-length percentiles

NAME _____

RECORD # _____

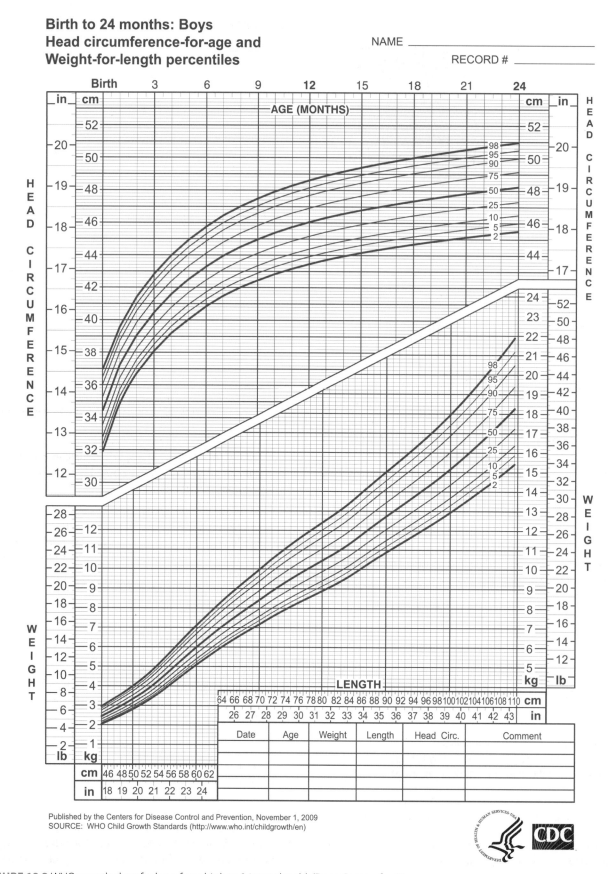

Published by the Centers for Disease Control and Prevention, November 1, 2009
SOURCE: WHO Child Growth Standards (http://www.who.int/childgrowth/en)

FIGURE 18.3 WHO growth chart for boys from birth to 24 months old. (From Centers for Disease Control and Prevention. Published by the Centers for Disease Control and Prevention, November 1, 2009. Source: WHO Child Growth Standards, www.who.int/childgrowth/en. Retrieved from www.cdc.gov/growthcharts/who_charts.htm#The%20WHO%20Growth%20Charts.)

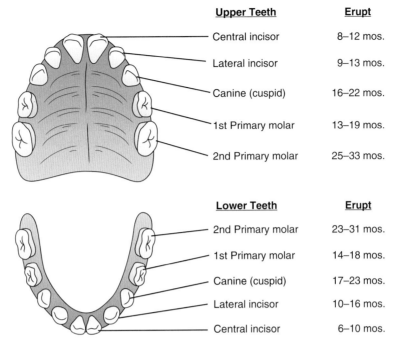

Upper Teeth	Erupt
Central incisor	8–12 mos.
Lateral incisor	9–13 mos.
Canine (cuspid)	16–22 mos.
1st Primary molar	13–19 mos.
2nd Primary molar	25–33 mos.

Lower Teeth	Erupt
2nd Primary molar	23–31 mos.
1st Primary molar	14–18 mos.
Canine (cuspid)	17–23 mos.
Lateral incisor	10–16 mos.
Central incisor	6–10 mos.

FIGURE 18.4 Dentition in children (tooth eruption pattern).

Box 18.2

Gross Motor Milestones of the Infant

1. Holds head up by 3 months while lying prone
2. Rolls over by 5 to 6 months, starting from prone to supine
3. Holds head steady when sitting by 6 months
4. Sits leaning forward by 7 months
5. Sits unsupported by 8 months
6. Gets to a sitting position alone by 9 months
7. Pulls up to a stand by 9 months
8. "Cruises" by standing and holding on to surfaces such as a coffee table by 10 months
9. Stands alone by 12 months
10. Begins to walk independently between 9 and 12 months

Box 18.3

Fine Motor Milestones of the Infant

1. Identifies hands by 3 months
2. Brings hands together by 3 months
3. Grasps rattle voluntarily by 4 months
4. Transfers objects from hand to hand by 6 months
5. Uses finger and thumb to grasp items by 9 months; called prehension
6. Bangs two lightweight items together by 9 months
7. Drinks from a cup at 9 months (needs sippy cup or covered cup to accomplish this task)
8. Begins to nest two items by 12 months
9. Builds two-block tower at 12 months

Safety *Stat!*

New parents need to receive explicit guidelines about maintaining safety for their newborn. Topics to cover include, but are not limited to:

- Head support while handling the newborn
- Maintaining an appropriate body temperature to avoid heat loss, including covering the newborn's head at all times
- Laying the newborn on their back to sleep to reduce the incidence of SIDS
- Never drinking hot liquids near or above an infant, especially when holding the infant
- Using a bulb syringe to clear secretions in the nose and mouth, thereby preventing choking
- Safety while changing the infant's clothes to prevent overextending joints and causing injuries
- Using only an approved newborn-ready car seat and installing the seat safely (rear-facing, in the center of the back seat)
- Preventing falls, burns, suffocation, sunburns, animal bites or scratches, or other home injuries
- Never, ever shaking the baby

items encountered to the mouth for exploration and stimulation. Parents should be taught examples of safe toys for oral play for their infant. See Figure 18.5 for infant toy ideas. Table 18.4 provides information on the key developmental theorists.

Communication Development

The development of communication throughout infancy is a marvelous achievement. As caregivers play with the infant, the infant will express delight by cooing at 1 to 2 months and laughing at 2 to 4 months. The infant will make consonant sounds at 3 to 4 months of age. As the infant continues to interact with caregivers, the infant will make imitative sounds at 6 months, demonstrating the importance of frequent interactions in language development. Communication for families with members who are deaf can also take the form of sign language. Finally, at the end of this first developmental stage, the infant will be able to say one to two words at 12 months. These first words will carry meaning to the infant. The first words may be "Ma-Ma," "Da-Da," "No," "Ba-Ba," or some word that the primary caregiver has emphasized and that the infant associates with something they want.

Interacting with the primary caregivers is an easy and effective way to learn language. When others attempt to interact with the older infant, **stranger anxiety** may prohibit the interactions between the nurse or other stranger and the child. With stranger anxiety, the older infant cries and becomes fussy when a stranger (unknown other) interacts closely with the child.

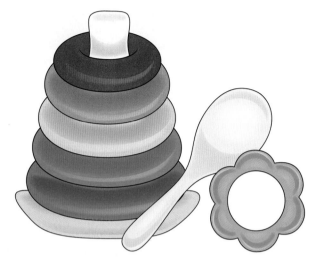

FIGURE 18.5 Appropriate and safe toys for the infant include items such as rattles, teething rings, noisemakers, stuffed animals without buttons, crib mirrors, and crib busy boxes.

Psychosocial Needs and Bonding

Bonding is a process of developing a meaningful relationship between the infant and the caregiver. Bonding provides

Table 18.4

Developmental Theorists

Developmental Theorist	Theory

Psychosocial Development: Erik Erikson	• The crisis of infancy is "trust versus mistrust."
	• The infant must develop a sense of trust as a foundation for future psychosocial tasks across childhood.
	• Having a sense of predictability assists the infant with mastering a sense of trust in the caregiver's behaviors and in the environment. This can be done by providing warmth, nutrition, elimination needs, and play/stimulation upon demand in a predictable manner.
	• Social interactions are very significant for the infant. Progression of socialization occurs monthly:
	  • Socially smiles at 2 months
	  • Recognizes familiar faces at 3 months
	  • Smiles at a mirror at 5 months
	  • Fears strangers at about 6 months

Psychosexual Development: Sigmund Freud	• The child is in the oral stage of development between birth and 18 months of age. • The infant displays the desire to suck, bite, chew, taste, and swallow, and learns about the environment through the mouth.

Cognitive Development: Jean Piaget	• Infancy is the sensorimotor stage, where the infant gains knowledge of the environment through the senses:
	  • Birth to 1 month: The infant demonstrates survival sucking reflexes.
	  • 1–4 months: The infant explores own body as the center of interest.
	  • 4–8 months: The infant now focuses on the environment and gives great attention to objects within reach.
	  • 8–12 months: The infant actively searches for hidden objects and readily explores the environment for stimulating objects and play items. Object permanence is now intact, and the infant sees themselves as separate from others.

a sense of security that is needed for the infant to feel safe. Bonding should be encouraged right after birth by having the parents hold the infant skin-to-skin, talking to the infant in a quiet, nurturing, and calm tone. The infant quickly learns to connect those close feelings with the parents and develops a sense of connection. The infant's sensory organs assist the infant in recognizing the parent and developing their bond. Even ill infants should have the opportunity to bond with their parents, and all steps to promote close physical contact should be provided, as medically indicated.

ANTICIPATORY GUIDANCE FOR NEW PARENTS OF AN INFANT

The rapid development that occurs during infancy is accompanied by many concerns about safety. Anticipatory guidance, or education about what to expect and how to plan a safe and healthy environment before an incident or injury happens, becomes paramount. See Box 18.4 for information about how to guide and educate the parents of an infant.

During infancy, taking purposeful steps to promote a child's health is imperative. Parents and the pediatric

---

Box 18.4

Anticipatory Guidance for Parents of an Infant

- Promotion of overall health and well-being:
  - Well-child checkup appointment schedule
  - Immunization schedule
  - Guidelines for nutrition in the first year of life; introduction of new foods after 6 months and no cow's milk during the first year
  - Safe sleeping areas and patterns; no cosleeping with infant; place infant on the back to sleep to help prevent SIDS
  - Promotion of infant/child CPR classes
  - Preventing sun exposure; use sunscreen with SPF 30 or higher after 6 months of age
  - Avoiding television, smartphones, and tablet computers for children under 2 years old
- Promotion of a safe home environment:
  - Safety sweep of entire home for hazards (see Home Safety Checklist at www.safekids.org)
  - Prevention of exposure to air pollution, mercury, lead, water contaminants, chemicals used for hobbies, bleach-containing cleaning solutions, and mold
  - Assessment for the presence of lead in and around home to prevent poisoning
  - Avoiding the use of pesticides in and around the home or garden
  - Maintaining smoke alarms and carbon monoxide monitors
- Promotion of healthy growth and development:
  - Providing for the need for sucking
  - Encouraging sensorimotor learning and play
  - Encouraging and fostering language development
  - Promoting daily dental hygiene
  - Fostering bonding and a trusting relationship

---

health-care team work collaboratively to form a foundation of health for the rest of the childhood years. Adequate nutrition, an appropriate sleeping pattern, balance between play and napping, proper hygiene, and bonding are all important to promote health in the infant. A benefit of this collaborative approach is that deviations in health can be identified early. Categories of health promotion in the infant stage include well-child checkups and immunizations, dental care, pacifier safety, car seat safety, infant device safety, and toy safety. Toy safety is of particular concern because infants are at such high risk for aspiration, choking, and injury from toys that are developmentally inappropriate.

Dentition

Teaching parents how to care for an infant's emerging teeth is very important. The health of a child's teeth impacts many aspects of overall health. Understanding the growth of teeth and how to care for them provides a foundation for good dental care throughout childhood.

Teething

The infant will have about six to eight teeth erupt during the first year of life. This causes discomfort for the infant as the baby teeth, or deciduous teeth, break through the gum line. Parents should be taught to expect this discomfort and to talk to their caregiver about ideas for comforting the infant. Infant teething rings, including those that can be frozen, should be used under supervision. Infants should not teeth on frozen foods such as bagels because of the aspiration risk.

Safety *Stat!*

Use only commercial teething rings and teething products to promote safety. Allowing the infant to chew on other items may cause choking.

As soon as the first tooth erupts through the gum line, nurses need to teach parents to clean the new tooth and gum line. Cleaning the infant's teeth with a wet washcloth is sufficient. Fluoridated toothpaste should not be used because the fluoride level may be high and cause poisoning, especially if the child swallows toothpaste. Providing this daily routine prepares the infant for appropriate tooth care later in childhood.

Using Bottles

An infant who is formula fed should be weaned from the bottle completely before their first birthday. Juice or other sweet beverages should never be given through a bottle. Infants who are put to bed with a bottle of juice or milk may develop early tooth decay because of the liquid bathing the infant's teeth during sleep. A bottle of water may be given to the older infant at bedtime but should be removed from the infant's bed after they fall asleep.

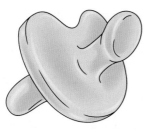

FIGURE 18.6 Example of a safer one-piece pacifier.

Using Pacifiers

Specific guidelines should be followed if a pacifier is introduced to an infant. Only pacifiers that are made of one piece of plastic should be offered to prevent a teething infant from chewing the pacifier into parts and creating a choking risk (Fig. 18.6). Always obtain parental permission before introducing a pacifier to an infant because some parents do not want pacifiers given to their infant.

Safety Measures in the Home

Nurses must promote a safe home environment. Providing anticipatory guidance concerning what to expect as an infant rapidly grows and becomes mobile can save lives. Parents should perform entire-home safety sweeps before an infant is brought home, and they should anticipate the child's motor abilities 1 year in advance. Babysitters and other childcare providers must be able to prevent injuries and to respond to emergencies rapidly. Older siblings need supervision around a new baby, and parents must ensure the infant's safety around strangers.

The Use of Infant Devices in the Home

Parents have a variety of infant feeding, sleeping, resting, mobility, and play devices to choose from. These include high chairs, bouncy seats, walkers, swings, strollers, and play stations. It is imperative that infants not be left alone in these devices; lack of supervision can lead to accidents and injuries. Explain to parents that safe, intact, and approved devices placed in a safe environment with constant supervision are part of a healthy start. Older infants left in high chairs can rock themselves over, pets can have access to unsupervised infants in these devices, and walkers can plunge down stairs if left unsupervised or if safety gates are not installed. If parents have questions about the safety of a certain device, they should contact the manufacturer for specific safety checks and recommendations for use. Parents must be reminded never to leave a child unattended on a changing table or in a swing, highchair, bouncy seat, or wagon. For up-to-date guidelines on the safety of specific types of infant devices, see the American Academy of Pediatrics (AAP) website.

Sun Safety

Sunscreen of any SPF should not be applied to infants under the age of 6 months because their skin absorbs the chemicals. Instead, keep infants out of the sun. Encourage parents to choose a stroller, child backpack carrier, or carriage with a sun-protecting hood and to start placing a wide-brimmed hat on the infant to allow the child to become accustomed to hats.

Toy Safety

Parents should provide safe toys for the teething infant. Infants should not be given toys that have unsafe buttons or any small item that can be gummed or chewed off, creating an aspiration and choking risk. When choosing appropriate toys, parents should keep in mind that the infant experiences the world through their senses and benefits highly from solitary play, visual and auditory stimulation, and touch.

While playing with older siblings and their toys, family members need to supervise younger children to prevent access to hazardous toys. Many toys that are used as building sets pose safety risks for young children. Furthermore, toys with strings or cords longer than 6 inches pose a strangulation risk for young children.

Crib Selection

Parents need to be instructed in safe crib selection. Older cribs may not be safe if there is peeling paint (risk of lead poisoning) or intricate carved designs that may trap limbs. The space between crib rail slats should not be wider than 2 3/8 inches because the young child might place their head between the bars and suffocate. If the crib has wheels, they should be lockable. The crib should not have drop-gate sides because these can cause injury. Top rails should be plastic covered so that when the infant starts teething, there is not a risk of wood splinters. The crib should have a firm mattress and be free from toys, stuffed animals, bumper pads, blankets, or any other suffocation risk.

Car Seat Safety

Health promotion includes providing infants with safe car restraints. Infants should be placed in the center of the back seat, facing backward. In pickup trucks where there is no back seat, the infant should be placed in the middle, facing backward. Infants should always be placed in certified car seats appropriate for their age and size. Children with special needs, or those with orthopedic devices such as spica casts, need specialized car seats.

Children die each summer from heat deaths when parents leave their child in their car unsupervised. Children should never be left, even just for a few minutes, to run into a store or to run an errand—the inside of a car heats up much more than the outside environmental temperature.

 SCREENING AND HEALTH PROMOTION FOR THE INFANT

Infants require several well-child checkups during their first year of life. Attending regularly scheduled appointments allows for measurements, immunizations, nutritional checks, education, and anticipatory guidance to promote healthy growth and development as well as safety. First-time parents need a lot of guidance and support during this year of rapid change.

Well-Child Checkups and Immunizations

One of the most important topics to cover with the parents of an infant is the importance of keeping well-child checkups. A healthy infant needs to have a series of immunizations; measurements, including HC, weight, and length checks; and developmental milestone checks that identify dysfunctions or delays in the infant's development. The earlier problems in growth and development are identified, the earlier referrals can be made for interventions to assist the child. Nurses should encourage parents to maintain all records of infant well-child checkups (Table 18.5) so that important information is available as needed.

CLINICAL JUDGMENT

During the 6-month well-child visit, a family member tells you that their baby loves playing with their cat and is beginning to follow the cat wherever he goes, even to the litterbox. They say that it "might be time to cover it."

1. Based on what the family member has told you, what safety concerns do you have about their home environment?
2. How would you respond to them?

Table 18.5
Schedule for Well-Infant Checkups and Immunizations

Patient Age	Well-Infant Checkup	Immunizations
Neonate	Infant may need weight, HC, and hepatitis B (hep B) vaccine if not administered after birth; may need hearing screening if not conducted within the first few days of life	Hep B
1 Month	Immunizations if not administered at the first visit, and weight, HC check	N/A
2 Months	Immunizations and weight, HC check	Hep B Rotavirus Diphtheria, tetanus, and pertussis (DTaP) *H. influenzae* type b (Hib) Pneumococcal vaccine (PCV) Inactivated poliovirus
4 Months	Immunizations, growth and development	Rotavirus DTaP Hib PCV Inactivated poliovirus
6 Months	Immunizations, growth and development, interactions with caregiver, achievement of expected milestones	Hep B Rotavirus DTaP Hib PCV Inactivated poliovirus Influenza COVID-19
12 Months	Immunizations, growth and development, possible laboratory analysis for anemia if concerns exist, interactions with caregiver, achievement of motor and language milestones	DTaP Hep A Hib PCV Varicella Measles, mumps, rubella (MMR) RSV (CDC guidelines for RSV vaccination are based on the mother's vaccine status or the infant's risk status.)

Immunizations are given to infants to produce antibodies (active immunity) against various diseases that can be acquired in the community. The purpose of immunizations is to prevent the acquisition and spread of infectious diseases and their complications, some of which can be quite profound. Immunization schedules are published regularly by the CDC. See the CDC website for more information including consultation and printed materials on the vaccines required for all healthy infants. Although immunizations are administered at set intervals for healthy infants, schedules may vary because of office visit timing, the wellness state of the infant, missed doses, and a limited vaccine supply.

Immunizations may take weeks to months for a full effect, but then offer lasting protection against specific infectious diseases. Make sure that families receive written information about each disease and immunization, possible side effects, and schedules. Document the discussion of concerns, questions, refusals, or delays. Informed consent from a parent or guardian must be secured before an immunization can be administered.

Some parents or guardians refuse immunizations for their infants. Any refusal must be reported to the physician or primary caregiver for further evaluation. See the latest CDC immunization guidelines for information on the following:

- Schedules and off-schedules when doses are missed
- Guidelines for administration
- Guidelines for premedications such as antipyrectics
- Care for the child after immunizations

SAFETY AND THE HOSPITALIZED INFANT

When infants are hospitalized, a safe environment must be provided (Table 18.6). Many necessary medical equipment devices and situations can place an infant at risk. Nurses provide a clean, safe, and well-protected environment for the infant to recover and rest (Table 18.7). Some common safety precautions are listed next:

- *Identification:* All hospitalized infants must have a hospital-provided identification wrist band or ankle band. The band information should include the infant's full name, date of birth, medical record number, and any other identifying information required by the particular institution. A second band should be added if the infant has demonstrated an allergic reaction to any medication

Table 18.6
Checklist for Maintaining Safety in the Pediatric Treatment Room

Introduction to Treatment Rooms	• Many pediatric units have a treatment room where minor procedures are conducted that do not require a surgical team. Saving the crib as the child's "safety zone" and using the treatment room aids in developing a trusting environment. • Treatment rooms can be stocked with toys and visual distractions to use during procedures. • Whenever possible, members of Child Life should be included in any procedures performed on children in a treatment room.
Equipment Used in Treatment Rooms	• The health-care team should be well prepared for an untoward reaction of a child to a procedure. Having clean resuscitative equipment in close proximity to the child is lifesaving. Even during simple procedures such as an IV insertion, an infant with a respiratory infection can become distressed, cry, and demonstrate respiratory compromise. Being prepared is essential.
Safety Checklist for Treatment Rooms	1. Pediatric crash cart fully loaded and locked 2. Manual resuscitator bags and pediatric masks at hand 3. Source of suction with clean tubing, collection bucket, and new suction tip still in packaging 4. Source of oxygen with tubing and various delivery devices, including pediatric nasal cannula, simple mask, partial rebreather, and nonrebreather masks 5. Cardiac monitoring equipment with adequate supply of three-lead chest leads (small and regular size) 6. Blankets for restraining (mummy wrap) procedures 7. Vital sign equipment with a variety of BP cuff sizes 8. Blood drawing devices, storage bags, and labels 9. Stool/seat for parents 10. Distraction equipment, safe toys, bubbles 11. Proper source of flexible overhead light 12. Functioning call light equipment to rapidly get help/assistance 13. Functioning code button and information to call rapid response team 14. Time-out reminder poster to use before procedure

Table 18.7

Safety Checklist for Hospital Nurses Caring for Infants

Patient Identification	• Infants must always have a secure hospital wrist or ankle band that identifies their full name, medical record number, and birth date. At no time should you remove the identification band and place the band on any surface, around crib rails, or on IV poles or bedside equipment. • The infant's identification must be checked before all medications are administered or any procedures are performed. • Parents are often required to wear a wrist band with the infant's identification information.
Crib Safety	• Older infants will try very hard to climb out of their crib. It is important that the side rails are up to their maximum height at all times. Infants close to 12 months of age should have a high-top crib where they are boxed into the crib for safety. • Every time the crib rails are lowered, you should anticipate the infant trying to immediately climb out of the crib or roll to the edges. • At all times, you should have a firm hand on the infant and all equipment within easy reach. • Every year infants fall out of hospital cribs onto hard floors and suffer injuries. Prevention is key, and you should anticipate a distressed infant trying to climb, roll, or push out of the hospital crib. • Older infants may try to pull themselves to a standing position; climb on top of toys, stuffed animals, or equipment; and attempt to climb out of the crib if these items are left in the bed. The only items that should be in the crib at any time are blankets and one personal item such as a "blankie" or favorite stuffed toy that the child brings from home. Be aware of older infants trying to get out of their crib any way they can, especially during diaper changes.
Airway Safety	• Every hospital crib or isolette should have airway resuscitation equipment within reach. This includes a manual resuscitator bag and three sizes of masks. • Each bed should have a newborn size mask, a pediatric mask, and an adult mask. This equipment should be stored in a clean clear plastic bag out of reach of the infant and should be checked for integrity on a regular basis. • A source of oxygen should always be available for respiratory emergencies, and a complete suction setup should be available at all times for emergency aspirations or other emergencies.
Parental Involvement	• Parents or a significant caregiver, such as a grandparent, should be highly encouraged to stay with the child during the entire hospitalization. • Young children without parents present require high-top cribs because they will climb out of bed to search for family members. • Hospitalized children have better clinical outcomes if they are comforted by the presence of their family.
Monitoring Systems	• If medically indicated, hospitalized children will be monitored for heart rate, respiratory rate, and oxygen saturation. • As the child's vital signs demonstrate stress, the monitor system alarms notify the nursing staff of the clinical change. • Monitoring systems to prevent infant/child abduction can be used to alert the nursing staff if the child is taken off the unit.
Use of Car Seats in Cribs	• Some nurses ask the family to bring in the child's car seat and place the seat safely within the crib with the crib rails up. This sitting up position helps some children who are in respiratory distress. • Check with your institution's guidelines about this practice because not all hospital policies allow for the use of the car seat.
Hot Water Bottles, Hot Pads	• The only heating devices that should be used for children are those that are commercially made and approved by the hospital. These approved devices have a mechanism of temperature control and can be set at a safe temperature for infants and children. • Homemade heating pads should not be prepared on the unit and microwaved. These devices may lead to burns. • Hot water bottles, if approved for use by the institution, should only be used according to the manufacturer's instructions.

Continued

Table 18.7

Safety Checklist for Hospital Nurses Caring for Infants—cont'd

Microwaving Formula and Infant Foods	• Infant formula and breast milk should never be placed in the microwave for heating. Only warm water baths or facility-approved bottle warmers should be used to slowly warm any form of infant nutrition. Microwaving leads to unpredictable "hot spots" that can cause burns. Microwaving breast milk can destroy valuable immunoglobins needed for immune protection. The temperature of any infant nutrition should never be more than 37°C (98.6°F). Many institutions have hospital-approved bottle warmers to warm infant nutrition (Fig. 18.7).
Tubes and Cords; Preventing Strangulation	• Active older infants in cribs are at risk for strangulation by medical tubing and cords. These children must be monitored frequently to prevent strangulation. IV tubing and oxygen tubing, as well as nasogastric tubes (NGTs) and urinary catheters, all provide an opportunity for injury or strangulation.

or food. Many institutions also require that each parent or primary caregiver also wear a band for safe identification. Learn your institution's child-abduction policy and procedure.

• *Prevention of infection:* Hospital environments place the infant at risk for acquiring a nosocomial, or hospital-acquired, infection. Meticulous hand washing before all patient contact and the use of aseptic technique during any medical procedures is imperative. Young infants are considered immuno-immature and are at a higher risk for acquiring infections.

• *Safe handling and neck support:* Nurses are role models for parents to learn proper neck support during handling of the young infant. Care must be taken when dressing the infant to ensure that the limbs and neck are protected from injury. When an infant is ill, you should follow precautions to position the infant into the proper body position to provide alignment and support for the limbs and the neck.

• *Body temperature control:* Young infants are at particular risk for hypothermia. Nurses must take precaution to ensure that the infant's temperature is stabilized during medical procedures and interventions. Infant blanket warmers can be used to warm blankets, but you should always check the temperature of the blanket. Under no circumstances should a nurse prepare a hot pack and place it against an infant's skin for temperature stability because burns can occur.

• *Crib selection:* Several styles of cribs are available for infants during hospitalization, ranging from small isolettes for newborns to high-top cribs for standing infants to prevent climbing and falls.

• *Infants sleeping in a large hospital bed:* Hospital policies exist to ensure that infants do not sleep in a large bed with an adult. Even if the infant shares a "family bed" at home, in the hospital, infants must sleep in an appropriately sized crib with side rails up at all times.

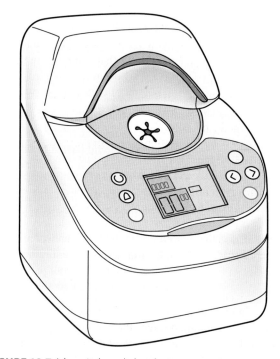

FIGURE 18.7 A hospital-grade bottle warmer.

Safety *Stat!*

Because medication errors in pediatrics can have serious consequences, many hospitals and health-care settings that care for infants require that two nurses double-check medications. This double-check includes the safe dose range for each medication and a double-check of the final concentration before administration. Always follow the "rights" of safe medication administration (right patient, right medication, right dose, right date and time, right indication, right documentation, and right route).

- *Falls:* Infants are at risk for falls in the hospital setting. Nurses must keep crib rails up when not with the child or with their hands on the child for safe holding. Infants who roll over or lunge at the caregiver when the rails are down can suffer head injuries if they fall to the hospital floor. Parents must be reminded to have all infant supplies readily available within easy reach so that they do not turn their back on the infant who can then suffer a fall.

DISEASE AND INJURY PREVENTION FOR THE INFANT

Because infants are anatomically and physiologically different than older children and adults, pediatric health-care team members must evaluate an infant for diseases and injuries common to this vulnerable age.

Otitis Media

Otitis media (OM), a middle ear infection, is a common diagnosis in infancy and early childhood. OM, also known as acute otitis media (AOM), is inflammation of the area behind the eardrum and is caused by pathogens such as *Streptococcus pneumoniae, Haemophilus influenza*, or a variety of viruses. In the neonate, *Staphylococcus aureus* may be the culprit. Occurring most often in children between 3 months and 3 years of age, OM is typically diagnosed in children who are bottle fed, especially while they are in the supine position. Prevention of OM includes instructions to the family about the importance of breastfeeding to provide immunity and only bottle feeding while the infant is held in an upright angle. Because the majority of OM cases are viral in nature, antibiotics likely will not be ordered.

Aspiration

Because infants are focused intently on mouthing anything within their reach and because they are teething, they are at high risk for aspiration. Carpets and wood floors must be kept free from any debris; the crawling infant will pick up and place anything found into the mouth. The infant is also at high risk for suffocation. Plastic bags, shopping bags, dry cleaning bags, and garbage bags all place the infant at risk because the bag can be easily pulled over the head. Crawling infants must be kept safe from cat litter boxes. In addition to the risk of an infant eating cat feces, litter boxes with plastic liners (under the box and/or under the litter) pose a risk for aspiration or suffocation.

Drowning

Infants are at very high risk for drowning in even just an inch or two of water.

- Infants should never be left unsupervised during a bath. The use of bath rings that prop the infant in a sitting position do not provide water safety. Infants can easily tip, fall forward or backward, and drown.
- Crawling infants can fit through pet doors or faulty gates or fences and fall into swimming pools.

Parents must be instructed to constantly hold their young infant while bathing and to stay within easy reach when the infant is sitting up independently in a tub.

Poisoning

According to the American Association of Poison Control Centers (AAPCC.org), the most common poisons children ingest include:

- Cosmetics, such as nail polish, deodorant, perfume, and soaps
- Household cleaning products, such as carpet and floor cleaners and laundry detergent
- Topical products, such as hydrogen peroxide, diaper rash creams and ointments, calamine lotions, and acne treatments
- Pesticides and outdoor chemicals

The most dangerous ingested poisons include antifreeze; windshield wiper fluid; fuels such as gasoline, tiki-torch oil, and kerosene; and oven cleaners, toilet bowl cleaners, and most corrosive cleaners, such as drain blockage products.

Older infants who spend their time exploring their environments are at great risk for poisoning. Medicines, cleaners, and any other potentially harmful substances must be stored in their original childproof containers behind locked cabinets. Several varieties of child-safe cabinet locks are available. Parents should be instructed to post the national Poison Control hotline phone number by the telephone (1-800-222-1222).

Burns

To prevent burns during the infancy period, family and caregivers should follow these four procedures:

1. Never microwave formula, baby food, or breast milk. Only warm water baths or bottle-warmer devices should be used to heat food or drinks. Within hospital or health-care settings, only institutionally approved bottle warmers (water or air) must be used.
2. Never hold an infant with one arm and hold a hot beverage to drink with the other arm. This balancing act can lead to severe hot liquid burns.
3. Never use hot packs on infants because their skin is particularly susceptible to burns. Under no circumstances should hot packs be microwaved and placed on the infant's skin.
4. Home water heaters should not be set above 48.8°C (120°F). Above this, the infant can suffer a severe burn from bath water.

DISORDERS OF THE INFANT

Specific ailments can affect the child during infancy. Become familiar with common ailments as well as the signs and symptoms of unexpected illnesses to find evidence of disease and report these findings to health-care providers. Disorders of young infants cross all body systems and may be present from as early as the newborn period (Table 18.8). Additional resources for SIDS are provided in Box 18.5. Subsequent chapters discuss other body system-specific illnesses that can also occur during infancy.

Table 18.8
Disorders of Infants

	Sudden Unexpected Infant Death Syndrome (SUIDS)	Dehydration	Colic (Paroxysmal Abdominal Pain)	Failure to Thrive (FTT)
Definition	Deaths that occur among infants younger than 1 year old and have no immediately obvious cause. The three commonly reported types of SUID are the following: • SIDS • Unknown cause • Accidental suffocation and strangulation in bed	The clinical consequences of a negative fluid balance	A term that applies to any healthy, well-fed infant who cries more than 3 hours a day, more than 3 days a week, for more than 3 weeks.	A term used when a child is not gaining weight, growing in height, or thriving in a healthy state. Growth retardation may be accompanied by delayed developmental and emotional functioning.
Incidence	In 2017, there were about 1,400 deaths in the United States caused by SIDS, and 3,600 deaths caused by SUID. The incidence of SUID is higher in infants of African American, Native Alaskan, and Native American descent and lower among those of Asian/Pacific Islander and Hispanic descent (CDC, 2019). The peak is between 1 and 4 months (National Institutes of Health [NIH], 2019).	Infant dehydration is not a reportable condition, so there are no accurate incidence rates.	Occurs in as many as 30% of infants.	About 1% of children admitted to hospitals in the United States present with FTT.
Signs and Symptoms	*Detected upon autopsy:* Deceased infant may present with bloody mucus in the mouth or nares, cyanosis of the nailbeds and lips, and inflammation in the upper respiratory tract; petechiae on the lung pleura, thymus and pericardia, and pulmonary edema (CDC, 2018).	*Mild dehydration:* Hard to evaluate because infant's vital signs will remain close to normal. *Moderate dehydration:* Elevated heart rate, deeper respirations, and decreased urinary output (UOP). *Severe dehydration:* Includes the previous signs plus delayed capillary refill time, absent tears, dry mucous membranes, and sunken fontanels. Lower BP is a late sign of dehydration.	Infants present with what appears to be severe abdominal pain or cramping that is accompanied by persistent, loud crying.	FTT exists when a child's measured weight and height consistently fall below the 5th percentile on a national growth chart.

Table 18.8
Disorders of Infants—cont'd

	Sudden Unexpected Infant Death Syndrome (SUIDS)	Dehydration	Colic (Paroxysmal Abdominal Pain)	Failure to Thrive (FTT)
Cause (If Known, or Hypotheses Being Studied)	Cause unknown. Possibly the respiratory center in the brain is immature and cannot sustain a strong respiratory pattern. Hypotheses for SUIDS include intrinsically abnormal control of the cardiorespiratory center, prolonged cardiac QT interval and poor reflex responses to periods of central apnea, hypoxia, and incomplete CNS development (Burnett, 2022)	Infants are particularly at risk for severe dehydration because of their large body surface area, immature kidney function, and susceptibility to gastrointestinal infections, especially viruses.	Rarely is there an organic cause associated with colic symptoms.	*Organic FTT* is when there is an identifiable underlying medical condition such as a problem with the heart, lungs, or central nervous system (CNS); anemia; or GI conditions leading to poor absorption of nutrients. *Nonorganic FTT* has no identifiable underlying medical condition and is associated with psychosocial factors, such as poverty and maternal depression.
Interventions	At-risk infants (siblings of SIDS victims, survivors of apparent life-threatening events [ALTEs], and infants living in households that smoke) should be checked for inspiratory pauses, impaired arousal, and decreased O_2 or increased CO_2.	Replace fluids and electrolytes rapidly while monitoring for ongoing fluid losses. *For moderate dehydration:* Breast milk (not formula) or oral rehydration solution *For severe dehydration:* IV bolus of 20 mL/kg isotonic fluid (Ringer's lactate or normal saline [NS]) OR oral rehydration solution via nasogastric (NG) tube	Some colicky babies respond well when treated for transient lactose intolerance (avoidance of milk-based formula or breastfeeding mothers' avoidance of all milk products in the diet; Turco et al., 2021)	Complete medical workup to rule out organic causes. Evaluate for sleep disturbances, vomiting, recurrent infections, dermatitis, loss of subcutaneous fat, and reduced muscle mass and tone. Developmental milestones should also be assessed. Prevent associated complications such as vitamin deficiencies, dehydration, electrolyte imbalances. Secure assistance from a nutritionist for screening, education, and support.
Prevention	Warn parents that smoking in the home, putting the infant to sleep in a prone position, and having a sibling who died of SIDS, or having had an ALTE, puts an infant at risk for SIDS.	The infant must consume adequate fluids daily.	There is little one can do to prevent colic. Mothers have reported that a change in infant positioning, rocking, abdominal warmth, white noise, and bringing the baby's legs up toward the abdomen led to reduced colic (Mutlu et al., 2020).	Identify the knowledge base of the parents concerning infant nutrition. Educate them about the nutritional needs of their infant. Evaluate for a history of difficulty with feedings. Evaluate the mother for postpartum depression. (See Chapter 13.)

Continued

Table 18.8
Disorders of Infants—cont'd

	Sudden Unexpected Infant Death Syndrome (SUIDS)	Dehydration	Colic (Paroxysmal Abdominal Pain)	Failure to Thrive (FTT)
Patient Teaching	Infants should be placed on their back to sleep with nothing in the crib that could cover or overheat the infant while sleeping. Check that there are no gaps or spaces between the crib mattress and the crib rails and ensure that the crib mattress is firm and nonmoldable.	Teach families to provide adequate breast milk, formula, and, for older infants, PO fluids. Infants who experience illnesses that cause fluid loss (diarrhea, vomiting) will need additional fluids.	Colic can start in infants as young as 2 weeks of age, and almost all infants stop having colicky symptoms by 6 months of age. Infants with colic eat, gain weight, and thrive. Reassure frazzled parents that colic will indeed stop. Encourage parents to take a break from their crying infant and compose themselves during long crying episodes.	Provide a feeding environment free of stress. Offer high-calorie supplements and formulas that provide more than 20 Kcal/ounce.

Nursing Care Plan for the Child With Failure to Thrive (FTT)

A father brings his 7-month-old infant into a public health clinic pediatric well-child clinic. For two consecutive visits, the infant has fallen below the 5th percentile on a national standardized growth chart. The pediatric team is concerned and diagnoses the infant with FTT.

Nursing Diagnoses: Delayed growth and development related to inadequate calorie intake as evidenced by low percentile weight plot on the national standardized growth chart; altered maternal/paternal-infant interaction related to lack of understanding of the infant's needs as evidenced by poor weight gain

Expected Outcome: The infant will demonstrate growth on a national standardized growth chart, achieving a 50th percentile plot point within the next 6 months.

Intervention:	Rationale:
The family will be provided nutritional counseling by a registered dietitian (RD) and will be provided education on how to increase calories.	*Using a team approach that includes education and counseling by an RD, as well as scheduled follow-up visits, will improve the child's clinical outcomes.*

Nursing Diagnoses: Knowledge deficit related to individualized infant nutritional requirements as evidenced by father's questions on daughter's growth requirements and specific daily nutritional needs

Expected Outcome: The father will verbalize the nutritional needs of the infant to the pediatric health-care team staff, including the appropriate daily caloric needs of the infant, safe feeding practices, and appropriate introduction of solid foods.

Intervention:	Rationale:
Specific educational guidelines will be provided to the father (at an appropriate reading level and in his primary language) to increase calories, provide safety while feeding the infant, and safely introduce solid foods.	*Providing written guidelines that are easy to read and written in the father's primary language will improve understanding and implementation of the teaching provided.*

Evidence-Based Practice

Treating Colic With Probiotics

Many studies associate colic crying with a functional disorder of the infant's GI system, with many stating no association with failure to thrive/weight loss. Some research links colic symptoms with intestinal inflammation and an overabundance of gut bacteria. A recent systemic review and meta-analysis was conducted on research as to whether or not *Lactobacillus reuteri* DSM17938 effectively reduces crying and/or fussing time in infants with colic. The findings showed that the common probiotic did reduce the duration of infant crying spells by as much as 1.98 times in groups where infants were given a probiotic intervention.

Skonieczna-Żydecka, K., Janda, K., Kaczmarczyk, M., Marlicz, W., Łoniewski, I., & Łoniewska, B. (2020). The effect of probiotics on symptoms, gut microbiota and inflammatory markers in infantile colic: A systematic review, meta-analysis and meta-regression of randomized controlled trials. *Journal of Clinical Medicine, 9*(4), 999. https://doi .org/10.3390/jcm9040999

Box 18.5

Resources for Information About SIDS

- Sudden Unexpected Death Organization (SUDC.org) at 1-800-620-SUDC

This organization provides family support, education, retreats, and fundraising for research.

- Centers for Disease Control and Prevention provides information for parents and caregivers about how to help prevent SIDS and SUID. See www.cdc.gov/Sids/Parents-Caregivers.htm.

Key Points

- Infancy is from birth through the first year, ending at the child's first birthday.
- The newborn and infant experience rapid physical growth, development, and the achievement of many new motor milestones.
- The first year of life has increased caloric and fluid requirements that far exceed those of the other childhood developmental stages.
- The infant experiences the world through their senses and benefits highly from solitary play, visual and auditory stimulation, and touch.
- Older infants develop object permanence, which allows them to search for a hidden toy or play object.
- Older infants rapidly acquire locomotion, place everything in the mouth, and become very interested in the environment. These behaviors increase safety risks and require constant supervision of the infant and a safe environment throughout the home.
- Parents and caregivers can develop the infant's sense of trust by providing the child with immediate attention to their needs (warmth, play, rest, diaper hygiene, and oral gratification through sucking and nutrition).

Review Questions

1. While taking an infant's anthropometric measurements, you find that the infant's weight has increased from 7.2 pounds at birth to 21.9 pounds. This finding typically represents that the infant is at what approximate age?
   1. At 6 months
   2. At 12 months
   3. At 9 months
   4. At 18 months

2. While checking an infant with moderate dehydration demonstrating a 10% body-weight loss, what would you expect to find?
   1. Decreased pulse
   2. Bulging fontanels
   3. Lethargy
   4. Decreased urine output

3. While reinforcing a teaching session between the nutritionist and a mother of a 5-month-old infant who has stopped breastfeeding, you explain that the maternal iron stores are present in the infant's body until what time frame?
   1. 3 months of age
   2. 1 month of age
   3. 6 months of age
   4. 12 months of age

4. While teaching a course for expecting fathers, you emphasize that, according to Erikson's theory, the infant needs a sense of:
   1. Belonging
   2. Family
   3. Trust
   4. Warmth

5. When administering medications to an infant in the hospital, the best way to ensure medication administration accuracy and safety is to:
   1. Double-check all medications and calculations with a second nurse
   2. Make sure the parents are present to identify their infant
   3. Have a representative from the pharmacy present to double-check medication calculations
   4. Document with a black ink pen immediately after the medication administration

6. All of these represent ways to communicate with infants *except*:
   1. Emphasizing vowels and consonants
   2. Close contact with primary caregiver
   3. Promotion of security through immediate need gratification
   4. Providing simple conversations that encourage autonomy

7. While assisting an RN to evaluate a 4-month-old during a clinical rotation, the nursing student is asked to explain which psychosocial stage the infant is expected to accomplish during the first year of life. Which response by the student is correct?
   1. Sensorimotor
   2. Trust versus mistrust
   3. Autonomy versus shame and doubt
   4. Oral fixation

8. Which food should you teach the parents to introduce to their infant's diet first?
   1. Pureed fruits
   2. Runny oatmeal
   3. Strained green peas
   4. Iron-fortified cereal

9. Which immunization(s) would be given to a 4-month-old infant? **(Select all that apply.)**
   1. MMR vaccine
   2. Varicella vaccine
   3. Rotavirus vaccine
   4. Hib vaccine
   5. Polio vaccine (IVP)
   6. PCV
   7. DTaP

ANSWERS 1. 2; 2. 4; 3. 4; 4. 3; 5. 1; 6. 4; 7. 2; 8. 4; 9. 3, 4, 5, 6, 7

CRITICAL THINKING QUESTIONS

1. The parent of an infant you are caring for has been diagnosed with an inborn error of metabolism. Where can you go to find information for the family? How would you direct them to find information about the condition and reputable sources for treatment on the Web?

2. How would you check a family home for safety concerns? What would be included on a checklist for a safe home environment?

Resources

For additional resources and information, including Postconference Questions and Activities, Answers, and References, visit www.FADavis.com.

Student Study Guide

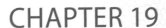

CHAPTER 19
Health Promotion of the Toddler

KEY TERMS

autonomy (aw-TON-uh-mee)
food lags and jags
iron-deficiency anemia (EYE-ern dih-FISH-uhn-see an-NEE-mee-uh)
negativism (NEG-uh-tih-vizm)
parallel play (PAR-uh-LEL PLAY)
stranger anxiety (STRAYN-jer ang-ZYE-uh-tee)
temperament (TEM-per-uh-ment)

CHAPTER CONCEPTS

Cognition
Comfort
Elimination
Growth and Development
Health Promotion
Infection
Mobility
Nutrition
Safety
Self

LEARNING OUTCOMES

1. Define the key terms.
2. Describe the unique needs of the toddler in relation to safety, bonding, communication, and development.
3. Describe the differences between toddlers and older children and adults in relation to body systems, anatomy, and physiology.
4. Compare the nutritional needs and eating patterns of the toddler including accurate kilocalorie needs and socialization at meals.
5. Describe the need toddlers have for stimulation, play, and sleep to promote normal growth and development.
6. Describe cognitive development during the toddler period including causality, spatial relationships, object permanence, and learning through toys.
7. Describe the psychosocial development of the toddler in relation to social engagement, temperament, stranger anxiety, separation anxiety, moral development, and spirituality.
8. Analyze the importance of discipline for the toddler and how anticipatory guidance can be used.
9. Describe child abuse during the toddler developmental period including assessment and interventions.
10. Describe the phenomenon of autism spectrum disorder (ASD), which is often first noticed in the toddler developmental period.
11. Discuss the interventions that can assist a caregiver who is caring for a toddler experiencing iron-deficiency anemia.
12. List the interventions that assist a child experiencing common childhood infectious diseases.
13. State the importance of discussing safety issues with parents including maintaining a safe environment for an active and explorative toddler.

CRITICAL THINKING & CLINICAL JUDGMENT

You are caring for **Callie**, a toddler girl hospitalized for a significant cellulitis of the face requiring IV antibiotics. She has an IV in her left arm with gauze wrapped around the site to prevent her from seeing the site and pulling at it. The parents tell you they are leaving for the day to attend to their other children and check in at work and that Callie can be left in the twin hospital bed for the day because she will be content to watch movies and nap until their return. You explain the hospital's policy that toddlers who are left alone must be placed in a high-top "climber" crib designed to prevent children from crawling over the crib rails, and they become quite upset. They want permission to bypass the policy to make their child happy while they are away.

Questions

1. What safety concerns are associated with this clinical scenario, and what injuries could Callie suffer because of the parents' request that she be left in the twin bed?
2. How should you approach the family to discuss safety concerns?

CONCEPTUAL CORNERSTONE
Safety

Safety is a major concern for toddlers who want to explore their environment and do so independently. Children quickly move from fast crawling to more efficient locomotion, mastering walking and then running. When given the chance, toddlers may run away from parents and adults to explore a new environment or to see a new sight. Toddlers require constant supervision to be kept safe from such things as bodies of water (lakes, pools, and rivers as well as buckets or trash cans with water), playground structures, and traffic. They inherently do not understand and process rules for safety and may rebel against limitations. Toddlers enjoy climbing and quickly learn that by pulling a chair or stool over to a counter, they can climb up and reach items they desire. They are very curious and will open cabinets, storage closets, or any compartment that is not locked. Tantrums, especially after being told "no," are normal toddler behavior but should be handled with care. Parents of toddlers have much to learn about safety and control. Nurses are in the perfect position to offer parents anticipatory guidance about how rapidly toddlers develop, how curious they are, and how inherently unsafe their actions may be.

The period of toddlerhood follows the rapid change and exponential growth period of the infant. Toddlerhood, the time between the first birthday and the third birthday, represents a slower period of physical growth but a faster period of growth in communication and other developmental milestones. The toddler masters mobility and cruises through the environment at a faster and faster pace. With the average age of mastering walking being 9 to 16 months, the toddler may begin this developmental period with walking being the first major accomplishment. Very quickly, the toddler develops a sense of exploration and is determined to get up, walk, steady themselves, and explore every inch of the environment.

Safety *Stat!*

Exploration and curiosity put a toddler at risk for injuries, accidents, and poisoning. You must stress to the parents the importance of providing both a safe home environment and constant supervision for their active and explorative toddler.

Toddlers grow in a steplike pattern rather than a linear pattern. This steplike pattern consists of sudden spurts of growth in height and weight with lags that can be several months long.

The child may approach many interactions with negativity, choosing to use the word "no" as a source of growing independence and **autonomy** (being self-governing). This negativity can cause the parent or caregiver distress, so it is important that they understand this as a normal and healthy process for the child to express themself. Raising a toddler can be exhausting, and the parent or caregiver needs reassurance and support.

Safety *Stat!*

Tantrums are common during the toddler period, and the parents should not give in to the toddler's demands. The best way to handle a tantrum is to ignore the behavior while keeping the toddler safe. Giving in may lead to more tantrums as the child learns that the behavior works to get what they desire. Staying calm, checking on behaviors that the toddler may imitate later, and not raising one's voice may help in these tough situations (Mayo Clinic, 2022).

GROWTH AND DEVELOPMENT OF THE TODDLER

Because the toddler's growth in height and weight slows down, the need for kilocalories is less. Safety becomes the primary concern for the mobile toddler as the growing sense

• WORD • BUILDING •
autonomy: auto–self + nomy–law

of autonomy, the desire to learn and explore, and the lack of safety judgment place the toddler at risk. Parents need to balance safety with encouragement to satisfy curiosity and manipulate objects.

Physical Growth and Development

The toddler grows an average of about 3 inches (7.62 cm) per year. As a general rule, a child's height at 24 months typically represents half the expected height of the child at adulthood. For instance, if the 2-year-old's height is 36 inches, the parents can expect their toddler to be 72 inches (6 feet) tall as an adult. The average 2-year-old is approximately 33 inches tall. Annually, a toddler gains 1.8 to 2.72 kg (4 to 6 lb). Parents should expect their 2½-year-old to have an average weight of 12.24 kg (27 lb) because birth weight quadruples by this age.

Head circumferences (HCs) continue to be measured until at least 24 months of age. From the first birthday to the second, the toddler's HC equals the chest circumference. During the second year of life, the HC will increase on average 1 inch, and then the HC growth slows to 0.5 inch between the second and third birthday.

The toddler presents with a distinct stance. Their abdomens protrude because of their underdeveloped abdominal muscles (lordosis; Fig. 19.1). The bowleggedness (tibial torsion) of the walking older infant continues through early toddlerhood as the weight of their trunk produces a burden on the growing legs. These two distinct toddler characteristics are typically gone by the preschooler period.

The toddler typically walks by no later than 15 months. Some primary health-care providers will want to see the toddler if they are not walking by 16 months. The toddler can walk upstairs, one at a time, holding an adult's hand, by 18 months. By 24 months, the average toddler can walk up and down stairs, one step at a time, placing both feet on each step. Toddlers will jump with both feet at 30 months and ride a tricycle by their third birthday.

Toddlers demonstrate far greater sophistication in their play than infants. The toddler likes to scribble spontaneously at 15 months and will attempt to build a tower with two to three blocks at 18 months. Toddlers are very exploratory (Fig. 19.2). Although quite uncoordinated, the toddler demonstrates increasing mastery of their hands. In early toddlerhood, the child will be clumsy, full of energy, and demonstrate an overwhelming desire to move around constantly. Although the growing toddler may seem to be a supernova of unfocused movement, the development of physical skills follows a predictable sequence from cruising (holding onto furniture) to walking to running to climbing to jumping, all within the course of several months.

Toddlers should be given a spoon to practice feeding themselves. Often, they will hold the spoon in one hand, pick up their food in the other hand, and put the food in their mouths with their fingers. Giving toddlers a chance to eat their food with a spoon gives them a growing sense of autonomy, which is what they need to master. Parents need to allow for self-feeding opportunities and explorations with safe utensils. Finger foods are safe, provided they are not hard and do not otherwise pose a choking risk. A toddler should not be given hot dogs, raw carrots or celery, peanuts, or any hard foods because they carry the risk of aspiration and choking.

Fine motor milestones of the toddler should be encouraged by offering them challenging toys. Placing objects within appropriately shaped slots is a great way to encourage eye–hand coordination while introducing the toddler to shapes, colors, and mental challenges.

The normal vital sign ranges in the toddler period include a heart rate between 70 and 110 bpm, a respiratory rate between 20 and 30 bpm, systolic blood pressure between 90 and 105 mm Hg, diastolic blood pressure between 55 and 70 mm Hg, and an expected temperature of 37.2°C (99°F).

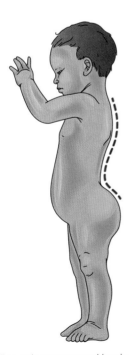

FIGURE 19.1 Toddler with exaggerated lumbar lordosis.

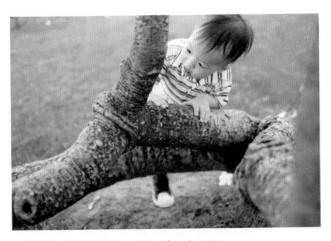

FIGURE 19.2 Toddler in a state of exploration.

Nutrition

During toddlerhood, the child becomes a picky eater and slows their consumption. It is very important that the parents understand that the toddler's milk consumption should be monitored. No more than 24 to 32 ounces of milk should be consumed daily because this will greatly reduce the toddler's consumption of other sources of protein and vitamins. Calorie requirements for the toddler average 70 to 90 Kcal/kg/day, and protein requirements average 1.2 g/kg/day.

During the beginning of the second year of life, the toddler should be eating the foods that the rest of the family is consuming. Parents should be taught to offer smaller portions because of the toddler's decreased appetite and to chop food into small, bite-sized pieces to prevent the toddler from choking. Three complete meals and three snacks per day provide the toddler with needed calories and prevent excessive drops in blood glucose. Toddlers do not have the physiological ability to regulate their blood sugar well, so to prevent fluctuating blood glucose levels, a nutritious no-sugar snack should always be available.

Labs & Diagnostics

Toddlers are at risk for iron-deficiency anemia (fewer circulating red blood cells [RBCs] caused by a deficiency of dietary iron) associated with poor nutritional intake. Too much consumed milk fills the toddler up, leading to reduced interest in eating a variety of nutritious foods. Iron deficiency is confirmed with a hemoglobin, hematocrit, mean corpuscular volume (MCV), reticulocyte count, and mean corpuscular hemoglobin (MCH) laboratory analysis. Dietary changes to increase iron-rich foods as well as oral iron supplementation may be required. Limiting milk will allow more hunger for iron-rich foods. A "milk diet" should be avoided as most toddlers need 7 milligrams of iron daily (Familydoctor.org, 2022).

Some parents worry about getting enough well-balanced nutrition into their toddler's diet. Adding chopped or pureed carrots, spinach, and zucchini to spaghetti sauce; adding chopped fresh fruit to yogurt; making fresh fruit smoothies; or cooking apples with cinnamon and sugar are some ideas to increase intake of fruits and vegetables.

Toddlers may display definite dislikes of certain foods and adamantly refuse to eat them, or they may routinely eat only a limited number of foods. These are known as **food lags and jags**. "Food jags" occur when the child is willing to eat only a few foods for several days (peanut butter and jelly sandwiches, cold milk, and fruits). "Food lags" can be described as a very apparent lack of interest in eating and the missing of meals, much to the parents' distress and concern. These are normal behaviors and should be included in family teaching. Being patient, making meals fun, offering choices, serving new foods with familiar foods, and promoting "dipping" new foods into low calorie salad dressings or hummus may help (Familydoctor.org, 2022).

Toddlers at 1 year of life have an average weight of 10 kg (22.04 lb), and the 2- to 3-year-old's average weight increases to only 12 to 14 kg (26.45–30.86 lb). Over the period from the first to the third birthday, the toddler may only gain 4 kg, or 8.8 pounds. The body weight of a toddler can be estimated using the following formula: Weight in kg = (Age in years + 4) $\times$ 2. The average kilocalorie need for a toddler ranges from 70 to 90 Kcal/kg/day.

A rapid nutritional status assessment of a toddler can be done using the following questions: Is the child's hair evenly dispersed across the head, is the skin not overly dry, and does the child have neither the appearance of being underweight nor overweight (Rudd & Kocisko, 2023)? If the answer to all three questions is "yes," the child is probably receiving adequate nutrition. A "no" answer indicates the need for further assessment.

A thorough assessment of a toddler's nutritional status can be effectively done by conducting an oral intake history over a 3- to 5-day period using a food diary given to the parents or primary caregiver. When the intake history is complete, a registered dietitian should review the diary and make recommendations. The child should be observed for gross changes in body composition including edema, inadequate or excess adipose tissue, dehydration, and increased or decreased muscle mass. The child's height, weight, and body mass index should be assessed and plotted on growth charts (World Health Organization [WHO] charts for children 0 to 2 years of age and the Centers for Disease Control and Prevention [CDC] charts for children 2 years of age and older. See most current WHO and CDC websites for the most updated material). Further evaluation and referrals should be made if the child's growth is below the 5th percentile or above the 95th percentile.

Labs & Diagnostics

If there is an indication of malnutrition in the toddler, laboratory tests should be drawn, including a complete blood cell count (CBC) with differential, comprehensive electrolyte panel, and albumin.

Socialization at the Table

Toddlers should be included at the family dining table. Although their attention span is short, they will benefit from the structure and socialization that occurs at the family meal. A young toddler should be placed in a high chair, and an older toddler may be comfortable in a booster seat. The child should be allowed to participate in the conversation even if their language skills are limited. The child should be praised for participation and then be allowed to leave the table even if the other family members are not done eating. Toddlers have no concept of manners, and they should not be expected to demonstrate them.

Sleeping Patterns and Requirements

The toddler requires, on average, 14 hours of sleep per day. During early toddler months, the child will transition from two naps a day to one nap in the afternoon. Parents should be encouraged to not put their toddler down for a nap too late in the afternoon because this disrupts the bedtime routine. Putting the toddler down to sleep may carry the challenge of separation anxiety. The toddler fears being alone and will fight being put to bed, fearing the separation.

Later in the toddler period, the child may develop a particular desire for a bedtime routine. The child may want the same book read to them a couple of times before bed each night for weeks on end, or the child may want a sequence of events to take place just the same each night. For instance, using the toilet, followed by a story, followed by three kisses, another story, a picture book, and then more kisses, in the same order every night. Parents should be encouraged to follow this routine whenever possible to create a sense of bedtime security.

Security items may become very important to the toddler. Typical security items may be a particular loved stuffed animal, a small soft blanket, or a particular toy. Sometimes the toddler has a surprising security item such as a necktie, a clothing item of the mother's, or some unexpected household item. It is very important that the pediatric nurse respect what is important to the child and protect it from loss or damage.

Patient Teaching Guidelines

During the first year of life, parents should not sleep with their infants because of the risk of suffocation and injury. During the toddler period, in which the child expresses both the fear of the dark as well as separation anxiety, the family may decide to sleep together in the family bed. For young toddlers, the same concerns for injury remain and this should be discussed within the family so risks and benefits can be determined.

Cognitive Development

According to Piaget, the toddler period marks the sensorimotor cognitive development period. This cognitive development occurs in two stages. First, the child must experience trial-and-error experimentation to develop appropriate understanding of the environment. This is also the time of relentless exploration. The independently mobile toddler explores relentlessly and, while awake, needs constant play and stimulation. The second stage of this developmental period is marked by more complex mental combinations. For instance, the toddler's play becomes more complex to include age-appropriate puzzles, stacking items according to size and shape, and language development that includes multiple word combinations.

Mastering the Environment

The toddler moves from crawling to standing to walking to running, all within a short period. This gives the toddler a real sense of autonomy and a deep desire to understand what is around them. It is very common to see a toddler explore the environment, pick up a toy or item, look at it, shake it vigorously to see if it makes noise, listen to it, smell it, lick it to see if there is a taste, and then throw it to see what happens. It is very important that the caregiver allows for this environmental exploration and experimentation because the toddler needs this for new learning and mastery of new skills.

Understanding Causality

Causality becomes important to the cognitive development of the toddler. As children explore their environment, they become aware that there is a causal relationship between two events. Turning on a light switch makes the room bright. Although the toddler learns that x causes y, they cannot then apply this to new situations. Parents will find that toddlers will explore the same cause-and-effect relationship over and over in new situations even if it was experienced in a previous situation. For example, sitting in a high chair at home, the toddler learns that dropping a spoon causes someone to pick it up over and over and become frustrated. When the child is at a grandparent's home or in a restaurant, they will do the same behavior again to see what happens in this new environment.

Exploring Spatial Relationships

Spatial relationships are also being explored by the toddler, who is developing an awareness of shapes and sizes. A very good toy or activity for a toddler to practice these relationships with is a set of nesting cups, where the larger container must be placed below the smaller one to build a tower. A toy that requires the toddler to identify which shape fits into which opening is also an effective way to practice spatial relationships. As the toddler's fine motor skills develop, mastery and speed over these types of activities improve rapidly.

Understanding Object Permanence

Toddlers enjoy the game of hide-and-go-seek, peek-a-boo, and challenges to object permanence. They enjoy searching for a favorite object that has been placed in a drawer, closet, or cupboard. By the end of the toddler period, the child understands that dragging a chair over to a counter or surface will allow access to objects that are otherwise out of reach. The combination of cognitive development with little or no sense of danger poses great risks to the toddler. Therefore, baby gates and locks should be used throughout the toddler period to prevent injuries, burns, and access to toxic or harmful substances. Just telling a toddler "no, do not touch that" does not work to secure a safe environment.

Safety Stat!

It is imperative that parents and other caregivers secure toxic substances, medications, cleaning supplies, and dangerous objects, such as scissors, in locked cabinets or on high enough surfaces that toddlers cannot get them. Adding toilet locks can help prevent explorations around standing water.

Learning Through Toys, Crafts, and Games

Toys, simple crafts, and games should be provided to challenge the toddler in both motor development and cognitive/psychosocial development. An appropriate selection of these activities will help the toddler develop a sense of autonomy by letting the toddler perform developmentally appropriate tasks such as "cleanup," self-feeding, and beginning to self-dress. Undressing skills come long before dressing skills. Toddlers also enjoy imitating adults.

Games and toys for toddlers can be divided into six areas (Table 19.1). All of these promote healthy development and improve motor skills.

Communication Development

Language development occurs rapidly in the toddler period (Table 19.2). The toddler begins the second year with only one to two words, ending the toddler period at the third birthday with between 300 and 500 words. Most toddlers will use two- to three-word sentences, learn to use pronouns, and will state their first and last name by 2½ years of age. Toddlers who are deaf will acquire sign language vocabulary at the same rate that hearing toddlers acquire spoken language if they are raised with parents who use sign language fluently. Deaf children born to hearing parents who do not sign or sign just a few words may experience language delays (Caselli et al., 2021). Even "baby sign language" has been shown to improve communication for young children (Rymanowicz & Cox, 2020).

Multilingual families provide rich cultural experiences for children but may temporarily slow a child's language development. Some research indicates that households where two languages are spoken may cause small delays (only 2–3 months) but is not considered significant in overall child speech development. It just takes children a little longer to

Table 19.1

Toys for Toddlers

Activity	Examples	Rationale
Push/pull toys	Child grocery carts, large trucks/cars, push-pull child's "popcorn popper" with handle	Combines skills of pushing up/pulling
Rocking and rolling	Large plastic balls/soft mats	Provides motor control
Throwing and catching	Soft foam balls	Promotes eye/hand/arm coordination
Climb and balance	Toddler outdoor structures	Encourages confidence and body balance
Running and jumping	Games with music	Promotes large motor coordination
Swimming/splashing	Safety flotation devices/noodles	Promotes large motor coordination and promotes confidence but needs constant parent supervision

Table 19.2

Language Development of the Toddler

Milestones in Expression	Average Age	Notes
First word	11 months	Often "Ma-ma," "Da-da," "No," "Bye-bye"
Second word	12 months	Needs audience, encouragement, and response
Jargon	14 months	Truly enjoys interacting and soliciting a response; will talk in nonsensical language, making up sounds and words
Four- to eight-word vocabulary	16 months	Accumulation of words becomes exponential
Two-word sentences	20 months	Examples include "Daddy bye-bye," "Mo milk"
Three-word sentences	30 months	Toddler puts nouns and verbs together
Use of pronouns	36 months of age	Understands "me," "my," and "you"

learn two words for each object or meaning. Some refer to this phenomenon as simultaneous language learning, not language confusion or language delay. See the Linguistics Society of America for more information (linguisticsociety.org).

A direct link between a young child's language development and positive parenting has been found. Talking, reading, and playing with young children are related to the development of language skills during the toddler period.

Psychosocial Growth and Development

According to Erikson's theory of psychosocial development, the crisis that the toddler is experiencing is "autonomy versus shame and doubt." A parent can be highly influential in the toddler's mastery of autonomy, defined as functional independence, by providing not only opportunities for the toddler to demonstrate independence but also emotional support and encouragement to learn. The toddler may display frustration because this stage is also marked by the need to learn to wait for need gratification and to learn that behaviors have a reliable and predictable effect on others (McLeod, 2018).

The toddler period is marked by distinct psychosocial challenges. The toddler experiences a deep fear of the dark and should be provided a night-light for sleep. The child might protest loudly at bedtime. If they express fear of the dark, the parent should not disagree or challenge the fear, but provide support. If the toddler has mastered the previous developmental stage of trust versus mistrust, then they are ready to start to assert autonomy and control. This may be distressing for the parent because the child will say "no" frequently, have tantrums, and show an ever-increasing sense of individualism. Separation anxiety remains through the early toddler period, even though growing independence is important. The toddler may interpret separation as desertion.

Toddlers do not understand the importance others place on personal items and will test this importance by manipulating others' possessions. This includes jewelry, eyeglasses, car keys, and sentimental home belongings. A typical toddler will identify the importance of an item to an adult, pick the item up, look right at the adult, and throw the item, waiting for the response. The adult must keep calm, verbalize behavioral limits, and be consistent. All valuables must be out of sight and reach from toddlers to keep them safe. Because the toddler period is marked with caregiver challenges and frustrations, a safe environment free of potential catastrophes is essential.

According to Sigmund Freud's theory of psychosexual development, the toddler is now experiencing the "anal" stage. This particular stage can last until the child is in the preschool period, up to 4 years of age. The buttocks and the anus are the sexual centers. The task requiring mastery is the cognitive awareness of the need for expulsion or retention of feces and urine as the toddler learns toilet skills. As the child gains neuromuscular control of the anus, more control is gained over toilet behaviors.

Socialization

Toddlers understand that they are members of a family. The family structure is very important to their development. Observing roles and responsibilities during this time period helps them to understand family dynamics, interactions, and responsibilities. The toddler should be included in all family activities but will need constant supervision. Adapting the family activity to include a toddler may be stressful; the toddler engages in **negativism** (a tendency of having a negative attitude), tantrums, and egocentric behavior. The family should discuss these behaviors and acknowledge the importance of showing patience for the toddler's demands. This is a difficult period for many families because the toddler is unable to share without guidance and is only able to see the world through their own eyes.

Toddlers are slow to warm up to strangers, and this poses specific challenges for health-care providers trying to evaluate an ill child and intervene for them. Physical evaluations are difficult because the young child will not cooperate nor can the child be reasoned with. However, nurses can successfully engage a fearful or uncooperative toddler. Using hand or finger puppets to distract a young child during procedures, reading a simple and familiar book, and providing the child with a "magic wand" full of glitter suspended in oil or water can be helpful if you need cooperation.

Team Works

If a procedure is required, the toddler's safety should be secured first, such as applying a mummy wrap for an IV start. Whenever possible, the child should be provided with a distracting age-appropriate toy. Solicit the assistance of a member of the child life team to come and assist during any procedure. These specialists are masterful in engaging toddlers and distracting them during procedures.

Stranger Anxiety

Stranger anxiety is a very real experience for young children. Starting at about 9 months, the older infant protests when given over to someone else to be held and fears the new person. Stranger anxiety continues throughout the toddler period, typically lessening toward the end of the second year. The parent's response to the new person will greatly influence how the child responds to a caregiver, childcare provider, or person new to the family. For some young children, any unfamiliar situation or person can cause anxiety; for other children, the reaction is milder. Tips to lessen the child's stranger anxiety response are to establish a positive rapport with the parent first, then approach the child in a calm, quiet, and positive manner, encouraging engagement with smiles and soft words. The child should be offered a form of play from you. Whenever possible, the nursing staff should plan care by the same health-care providers to offer consistency and familiarity.

Separation Anxiety

When a toddler must be left alone in a hospital environment, having the parent leave a personal item may reduce the toddler's fear of separation. The toddler is not yet able to understand the function of time, so it is not helpful to explain that the parent will be back "soon" or "at 5:00."

Three stages of separation anxiety can be seen throughout the toddler period: protest, despair, and detachment. These stages of separation anxiety peak at 18 months and are readily apparent during hospitalizations. The duration of separation anxiety varies depending on the child but typically begins in late infancy and lasts until the child is older than 3 years of age.

- *Protest:* In this phase, the toddler protests the separation with loud crying and may demonstrate physical aggression toward others. The toddler fights to cling to the parents before they leave, then becomes agitated and struggles to search for the parents. The toddler in this phase may be inconsolable and may need to be placed safely in a high-top crib to prevent climbing out. No items should be left in the bed other than the toddler's security item(s) because they may stack them to climb out of the crib.
- *Despair:* Here, the young child becomes quiet, may lie on their side facing away from the door or others, and demonstrates behaviors of depression. The child may also be disinterested in eating or refuse to eat. Likewise, the toddler may refuse to participate in play activities or may show great passivity in playing with favorite toys. This phase may last hours to days.
- *Detachment:* The third stage of separation anxiety is detachment, sometimes also referred to as denial. Here, the toddler demonstrates a slow reentry into interactions with others and play. Although the child is still detached, they may demonstrate an artificial adjustment to the separation from the parent. This phase is not always seen in the hospital, because lengths of stay are decreasing.

When nurses are aware of these three phases of separation anxiety, they can provide support and comfort to the child. Encourage the parents never to sneak out of the hospital while the toddler is sleeping or distracted. The toddler should be told in a simple, straightforward manner that the parent must leave and will come back. However, parents and staff should be prepared for the child to protest loudly. Leaving a personal item of the parent with the child can provide comfort. Although the child may be highly resistant to interactions with you in the protest phase, later, as the child recognizes you as the one who will provide for basic needs and play opportunity, improvements in behavior may occur.

Moral Development

Lawrence Kohlberg's theory of moral development describes the toddler period as the preconventional stage (McLeod, 2013). In this stage, avoiding punishment (Mathes, 2021), learning obedience, and obtaining rewards are the central focus of the child's moral development. How and when a parent disciplines the toddler highly affects the young child's moral development. Because of the toddler's egocentrism and inability to see others' points of view, they develop a negative view of morals when privileges are withheld and punishments are applied. It is extremely important that the parent or caregiver provide the young child with a developmentally appropriate explanation as to why they are being punished. Examples include telling the child immediately that running into the street is dangerous because cars might hit them, or that touching the tools in the garage is dangerous because they may get hurt.

Patient Teaching Guidelines

With the increasing need for both parents to work, safe and reliable childcare is very important to secure. Some childcare is provided in private homes with some home care providers licensed by the state and others not. Other alternatives include formal childcare institutions of various sizes as well as childcare facilities offered by city, region, or state offices.

Making the decision about what type of childcare to choose takes considerable planning, and nurses can serve as information resources for parents. To select whether a nanny, a home childcare environment, or a formal childcare institution is most appropriate, parents should review their child's needs, the family's needs, and the child's **temperament** (mental, physical, and emotional traits). Although a nanny provides consistency and one-on-one care, a licensed care facility provides toddler socialization, structure, parent interaction, and a more stable arrangement versus an individual health-care provider.

Suggest that parents enlist the help of organizations such as the National Association for the Education of Young Children (NAEYC) in their search for a local childcare facility. NAEYC and other similar groups offer ideas for selecting childcare sites, choosing curriculum styles, and performing site assessments. Nurses can offer parents a checklist to determine the right fit for their needs and the child's temperament. Using a checklist to evaluate their childcare options can reduce the anxiety parents feel about providing safety for their young child while they work. See Table 19.3 for an example of such a checklist.

Temperament

Parents will often describe to you the "differences" in each of their children. In fact, each child *is* different and unique. Temperament refers to the combination of mental, physical, and emotional traits of a person. The toddler's temperament influences how they view the environment, feel, react, and socialize.

- **WORD · BUILDING** ·

temperament: tempera–mixed properly + ment–state of being

Table 19.3

Checklist for Selecting Safe Childcare

Items to Investigate	*Diversity in Settings*
Types of health-care providers	• Family home health care in private homes • Childcare centers (nursery schools, preschools) • In-home care providers (nanny, babysitter) • Shares, where several families get together to share one health-care provider • Play group exchanges • Babysitting co-ops, where parents rotate caring for their children and others • Childcare facilities that specialize in children with special needs/technology dependence
Licensing and accreditation	• All childcare providers of licensed facilities take a 15-hour course called Early Childhood Education (ECE) that includes cardiopulmonary resuscitation (CPR) and basic first aid
Teacher preparation	• Some facilities have childcare providers with early childhood education degrees
Child-to-staff ratio	• State regulated; often 4:1 for infants, 6:1 for toddlers (check state regulations)
Curriculum	• Structured or free play • Use of standardized toddler curriculum
Napping stations	• Cots versus lying on floor; quiet, clean; flexible for children to rise on their own time
Schedules	• Flexible hours or rigid for all participants
Costs	• Daily, weekly, or monthly fee; early drop-off or late pickup fees • Forms of payment; fees for late payments
Site-visit checklist	• Visit first without child and then second visit with child • Facility philosophy, mission, goals, length of time in business, staff turnover • Written emergency response plan and posted emergency numbers • Published guidelines for child with food allergies • First impressions of safety; first impression of child • Children engaged in play, interacting with health-care providers • Quality, quantity, and safety of toys present • Type of discipline used, consistency and appropriateness, alignment with family values and practices • Well lit, clean, organized, attractive • Toilet-training facilities, hand washing station and practices, support for training, praise/rewards • Kitchen facilities clean, selection of food served, teachers eating with children

Some toddlers are prone to frequent tantrums. Preventing and managing tantrums require skill on the part of the parent. Not giving in to the toddler's demands is very important because the child learns quickly that a tantrum is an effective way to get what they want. Giving in to a tantrum only reinforces the negative behavior. Whenever possible, the parent needs to ignore the behavior while keeping the child safe. Tantrums can be so severe that the child holds their breath or falls to the floor, possibly hitting the head.

An appropriate and successful way to prevent tantrums is to offer two choices. The choices should be visual (this toy or that one) or the choices should be offered in a way the child understands. For instance, if you need to administer an oral antibiotic, the toddler should be offered a choice to have the medication mixed with chocolate syrup or cherry syrup. The toddler *does not* get to choose whether or not to take the medication.

Discipline

Discipline is very important in the toddler stage. The young child becomes frustrated, and then acts out anger or frustration via tantrums. This is normal and universal behavior for a toddler and can be found regardless of culture, ethnicity, or socioeconomic level. These big feelings and the concept of discipline are both new to the toddler. Caregivers should never try to reason with, threaten, make promises to, hit, or give in to a toddler having a tantrum.

Ideas for Discipline During the Toddler Years

- Immediate, positive reinforcement for good or wanted behavior
- Ignoring unwanted behavior and tantrums
- Distracting the young child from participating in unsafe or unwanted behaviors
- Keeping routines simple and consistent, such as at mealtimes and bedtimes
- Setting reasonable limits; giving simple rationales as to why the behavior is unsafe or unwanted
- Trying to provide two-selection choices when possible
- Identifying if the toddler is being intentionally destructive or is exploring the environment with unintentional vigor; decide then if discipline is warranted or if the child needs instructions
- Always following through on discipline, not just stating threats of time-outs or toy removal
- Having a consistent discipline strategy agreed upon by parents and any other caregivers

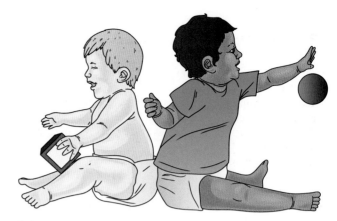

FIGURE 19.3 Parallel play.

When a toddler demonstrates unwanted or unsafe behaviors such as writing with crayons on the wall, jumping on the bed, or running out the front door of the family home, the discipline mechanism of choice is the time-out. A time-out lets a child who is feeling overwhelmed and acting out take a break to regain control of their emotions. Time-outs should be kept brief. As soon as the child is back in control, the child should rejoin the family. Time-outs should begin early in the toddler period with a very short removal of the child from the unacceptable behavior to a quiet place where they can regain composure. As the child gets older, the time-out period can be extended to *no more* than 1 minute per year of age (CDC, 2019). A timer with a bell can be used to alert the child when the time-out is over. It is better for the child if this is used regularly during the time-out.

Consistency is an essential component of positive discipline. All caregivers should be in agreement about providing the toddler with a consistent discipline program. Discipline should be initiated immediately after the misbehavior, planned in advance, oriented to the behavior itself and not to the child, and should be conducted in private and in a non–shame-inducing fashion. The toddler needs to associate the unwanted behavior with the subsequent discipline to learn what is and what is not acceptable. Overcriticizing and restricting may cause increased feelings of shame and doubt. Acknowledging good or desired behavior at every opportunity is essential.

Box 19.1 lists ideas for discipline during the challenging toddler period.

Play

In time, the toddler will move from individual play to **parallel play** (Fig. 19.3). The toddler will desire to play near, or actually alongside, another toddler but will not yet want to share toys or craft supplies. Often the parent or caregiver will see toddlers play back to back, almost touching, but not interacting with their play activities. Sharing is a learned process that requires parental intervention and positive reinforcement. Toys are quickly played with and often discarded for the next new experience. The toddler is happiest with a variety of large, colorful toys all within reach. Toddlers' energy levels allow them to be quite active, progressing from toy to toy, or activity to activity, rapidly.

Appropriate types of toddler play are those that promote learning, challenges, and stimulation of all of their senses. Toys should be large, colorful, and safe by being free of detachable parts. Young toddlers will still explore certain items orally, leaving them at risk for choking and aspiration. Large dolls with clothes that come off and on easily with Velcro and snaps, play phones, busy boards, and cloth books are excellent choices for the toddler. Toddlers are able to build towers of three to four blocks and truly enjoy building, knocking over, and building again. Towers that require the toddler to stack larger blocks on the bottom provide added challenges.

Toilet Training

Toilet training is a universal task of early childhood. The toddler period is the most common time that a child masters this task because the child tends to be both physiologically and psychologically ready (Box 19.2). Readiness for toilet training is demonstrated when the toddler is able to stay dry for 2-hour periods, can sit and squat, and has regular bowel movements. Emotional and cognitive readiness are demonstrated by the child's desire to please the parents and the ability to verbalize the desire to void or produce a bowel movement. Because most young children have full kidney function and anal sphincter control by 2 years of age, toilet training should not be expected to start until after this time. Typically, the child demonstrates fecal control before bladder control.

Wanting to Watch a Family Member

Toddlers often learn about their environment from watching others interact with it and perform duties. Toilet training is no different. It is not uncommon for a toddler to watch how a

Box 19.2

Psychological Readiness for Toilet Training

- Toilet training begins with emotional readiness.
- Toddlers act to please others.
- Toddlers will imitate others they can see using the toilet.
- Feelings of wetness or messiness lead to personal motivation.
- Toddlers will remove clothes, walk to the potty, and sit on it on their own.
- Begin potty sitting at 18 months without expectations.
- Toddlers should achieve day dryness by age 18 months and night dryness by the second to third year.
- If the toddler is not toilet trained by 5 years of age, seek further evaluation.
- Toddlers may fear being sucked into the toilet.
- Toddlers may fear the sound of a loud flush.
- Toddlers will demonstrate great curiosity with excrement.
- Toddler girls should only wipe front to back and must be taught to do so to prevent urinary tract infections (UTIs).
- Toddlers must learn to wash their hands after toileting with the assistance of an adult.
- Stressors such as illnesses and hospitalizations cause regression; toilet training may need to be retaught.

parent or sibling goes to the bathroom. Watching others pull clothing up or down, sit comfortably on the toilet, defecate and urinate, and use bathroom tissue is intriguing to the toddler learning toilet training. This watching may be acceptable to some families and not acceptable to others.

Assistive Devices for Toilet Training

The toddler should have a specific age-appropriate toilet when toilet training. Small plastic or wooden child toilets are available and are an excellent choice to assist the child. The child's toilet should be placed where the toddler has access to it. It may take the child several attempts to learn to sit on the device. At first, the toddler may choose to sit on the potty fully clothed. Later, after a successful attempt, the toddler may want to drag the potty chair around the house and keep it nearby. Praise should be offered at each attempt. The potty should be emptied immediately because the toddler will want to manually explore their "prize" after a successful defecation. Toddlers need supervision with both the child potty chair and the full-size toilet; they may place toys or objects in the toilet or use the water for play.

A wonderful, classic book to recommend to parents of toddlers is *Everyone Poops* by Taro Gomi (2001). This delightful, developmentally appropriate children's book demonstrates the daily regimen of defecation and shows members of the animal world and people participating in toileting. The book can be seen as humorous but is also quite educational for the young child learning to use the toilet.

Positive Reinforcement

The most important aspects of toilet training are providing the young child with enough time to master the act, being patient

with accidents, and providing lots of positive reinforcement. Some families reward the young child with a small treat after each attempt as well as smiling, clapping, and stating, "Good job! We are proud of you!" Using the toilet is a very important step in a child's autonomy and the parent, caregiver, or nurse's response to the child's attempts and successes is very important to the child. Even while hospitalized, toilet training should continue. You need to explain to the family that regressive behaviors are common and toddlers may lose or regress in their toilet training skills while hospitalized.

Patient Teaching Guidelines

Toilet training is challenging, especially if parents have unrealistic expectations for their toddler. Toileting accidents are common during training and can cause parents or caregivers to become frustrated or angry. Support parents by giving them tips to encourage their child's toileting success. Prepare them to handle the child's inevitable accidents calmly and to avoid shaming, blaming, or shouting at the child.

ANTICIPATORY GUIDANCE FOR PARENTS OF THE TODDLER

Preventing injuries in a toddler who wants to exert autonomy can be challenging. Every room of the home, the garage, and the front yard and backyard need to be assessed for potentially dangerous items or situations. Families living in apartment buildings must evaluate for dangers in stairs, elevators, parking lots, laundry areas, trash and recycling areas, and playgrounds as well as the apartment itself.

A trash can with only a few inches of standing water poses a drowning risk because the toddler may fall head first into the receptacle, not be able to push themselves up, and drown. Every year, thousands of toddlers experience severe injuries as their natural tendency to explore without understanding consequences leads them to dangerous situations (drownings, burns, animal bites, falls, etc.). Anticipatory guidance aids you in teaching parents and caregivers of toddlers to identify harmful situations and avoid tragic consequences. Some families use harnesses to allow toddlers to explore within sight and reach of a caregiver (Fig. 19.4).

Dentition

The toddler's tooth-eruption pattern includes the presentation of 10 to 14 deciduous, or baby, teeth for a total of 20 teeth by the third birthday. The first and second molars and canines erupt. Consumption of processed sugar, a **cariogenic** substance, should be limited and the toddler's teeth should

· WORD · BUILDING ·

cariogenic: cario–decay + gen–producing + ic–pertaining to

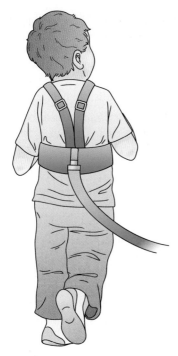

FIGURE 19.4 A single-leash safety harness.

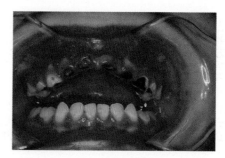

FIGURE 19.5 Tooth decay in a toddler.

be brushed twice a day. To promote success and decrease negativity during toothbrushing, the toddler should be given a large soft-bristled toothbrush to hold and play with while the parent proceeds with actually brushing the child's teeth with another toothbrush. Only a very small amount of nonfluoride toothpaste should be used during this period. Fluoride-containing toothpaste can be toxic if swallowed. Regular toothbrushing at this age prepares the child for tooth hygiene throughout childhood. Flossing a toddler's teeth poses challenges but should be attempted on a regular basis until accepted by the child. The toddler should be seen by a dentist by the third birthday. Parents should be encouraged to investigate if their community water supply is fluoridated. If not, they should discuss with their pediatrician whether to add fluoride supplements into the child's daily nutrition.

Tooth decay can occur during late infancy and toddlerhood (Fig. 19.5). At no time should a young child be put to bed with a bottle of juice or milk. Toddlers do not need refined sugar, and sweets should be eliminated or reduced. Toddlers do not need to experience candy.

Visual and Auditory Acuity

The toddler's sensory organs continue to mature. Visual acuity continues to progress from 20/200 during infancy to 20/40 to 20/60 in the toddler period. A toddler's hearing acuity is completely intact. After completing a hearing screening test in infancy, the child should not need another until they are seen for their prekindergarten well-child check. However, you should question the family about any hearing concerns, especially if there has been a history of inner ear infections. With a pattern of inner ear infections, the toddler may have a conductive hearing loss, which warrants further screening

and possible interventions. Because the period of toddlerhood marks a tremendous growth in vocabulary, it is important that a hearing impairment not delay the toddler's speech development.

Home Safety

The toddler needs constant supervision. Toddlers are at great risk for the ingestion of toxic substances; they continue to mouth many items in their environment, and they will try to explore unsafe areas of the home to make new discoveries. Toddlers are very active and have increasingly accelerated locomotion, so they will often run away when they can. Safety gates are important to prevent toddlers from exploring unsafe rooms such as the kitchen, garage, and bathroom without supervision or attempting to master stairs before they are developmentally ready. Box 19.3 provides a checklist for basic home injury prevention.

Kitchen Safety

The kitchen poses extreme risks for the fast-moving and exploring toddler. It is essential that kitchen cabinets and drawers have childproof locks placed on them. These devices are relatively inexpensive and can be purchased at most drug or hardware stores. Handles from cooking pots must be directed away from the front of the stove and only the back burners should be used. Stove and oven buttons should be removed or have a device placed on them to prevent a toddler from turning the oven or stove on. Drinks that are not hot should be within reach of a toddler so they are not climbing to reach them. Providing one unlocked cabinet with plastic tubs and pots and pans allows toddlers to have their own play center where they can interact with the parent and make loud noises while banging the pots together but still be maintained in a safe environment.

Gates and Barriers

Child safety gates and barriers should be purchased and installed before the infant begins to rapidly crawl and long before the toddler walks. Safety gates should block the child from access to the kitchen area, the bathroom, any pets who are not yet well established with the presence of the child, and the top of any stairs. Several models of safety gate are available that have either swinging doors or levers that allow the parent quick access to the next room. Under no

Box 19.3
Checklist for Home Injury Prevention

1. *Bathroom:* Set water heater to 120°F (49°C) or lower; keep toilet cover closed at all times and use a childproof lock. Never leave bathroom appliances plugged in to the wall socket to prevent electrical shock.
2. *Home:* Place a guard around any heating elements, appliances, or fireplaces; make sure that electrical cords are hidden and out of reach; place safety covers over electrical outlets; test smoke detectors frequently and make sure that they have fresh batteries; maintain a safe and intact fence around the yard and secure double fences around pools; do not use garden fountains if they pose a risk of drowning; mark glass doors with bright-colored decals.
3. *Indoor and outdoor plants:* The following list represents common plants that are dangerous if ingested:
   - *Aloe barbadensis* (aloe vera is often used for mild burns)
   - Amaryllis
   - *Caladium hortulanum* (angel's wings)
   - Chrysanthemum (mums)
   - *Cyclamen persicum* (cyclamen)
   - *Euphorbia pulcherrima* (poinsettia)
   - *Hydrangea macrophylla* (hydrangea)
   - Philodendron (heart leaf philodendron)
   - Rhododendron (azalea)
   - *Solanum pseudocapsicum* (Jerusalem cherry)
     See www.aapcc.org for more information on dangerous plants.
4. *Car:* Do not allow children to play in parked cars; supervise children while in car at all times; do not allow children to unbuckle seatbelts while car is moving. Never leave a toddler in a car by themselves.
5. *Closets:* Children enjoy playing hide-and-go-seek, so make sure that all dangerous items stored in closets are out of reach; do not store items in such a way that a child can experience injuries from falling heavy objects.

circumstances should the toddler have free rein of the house or ever be left without supervision in the kitchen, bathroom, or near the front door.

Pet Safety

Young children cannot be trusted to behave appropriately around animals. And even the most even-tempered animal can lose patience with an aggressive or overly eager child.

Dogs

Children need to be taught not to touch or approach a dog on or off a leash without asking permission to do so. Dog bites are a frequent injury; some require hospitalization with antibiotics administered, whereas others require plastic surgery. Even dogs that are considered "child friendly" may tire of a child's play or attention and snap to stop the child.

Cats

Cat bites are typically deep puncture wounds, making wound hygiene difficult. Common infectious agents include *Pasteurella multocida,* which may very rapidly lead to erythema, pain, and swelling. Cat scratch fever, an infection caused by a scratch from a cat with dirty claws, is a common childhood infection.

Turtles

The feces of turtles have long been known to potentially carry *Salmonella* and other infectious diseases. It is imperative that turtle owners teach their children to wash their hands thoroughly with soap and water after touching, holding, and playing with turtles as well as practicing meticulous hand hygiene after cleaning a turtle's environment.

Swimming Pools

Pools create another level of safety risk. Toddlers are very explorative and fast in their movements. Two locked gates should separate the young child from the household or apartment swimming pool. Toddlers can crawl through a pet door to reach an unsupervised swimming pool (American Academy of Pediatrics [AAP], 2024). If a child falls in, the child may silently drown because they are too young to know to fight to rise to the surface. A complete safety check must be performed on a regular basis. Pool covers are not safety devices because toddlers will walk out on them, fall through, become trapped below the surface, and drown.

Only federally approved swim-safety devices or swimsuits should be used. Before purchasing such a device, the parent should be sure that its label indicates that the device is appropriate for the age or size of their child. At no time should a toddler in a flotation device be left alone in a pool; the parent should have their hand on the child and flotation device at all times.

Preventing Accidental Poisoning

Young children are at risk for ingesting toxic substances, especially during infancy and toddlerhood. Crawling infants, active toddlers, and curious preschoolers are at extreme risk for coming in contact with toxic substances and tasting them as part of their exploration. Common toxic exposures leading to poisoning include the following:

- Acetaminophen
- Salicylate (aspirin)
- Iron or lead
- Carbon monoxide
- Alcohol
- Anticholinergics
- Antihistamines
- Toxic plants
- Muscle relaxants
- Opioids, narcotics, benzodiazepines, and barbiturates
- Cardiac medications such as calcium channel blockers and digoxin
- Tricyclic antidepressants
- Paint thinners
- Certain cosmetics, such as nail-glue removers and nail primers
- Car antifreeze

Patient Teaching Guidelines

Until more clear-cut scientific evidence exists on the effects of infant and toddler aquatic programs, the AAP (2019) recommends the following:

- Children develop at different rates, but, in general, swim lessons may reduce the risk for drowning in children between 1 and 4 years of age. By 4 years of age, most children are ready for swimming lessons.
- Aquatic programs for infants and toddlers should not be promoted as a way to decrease the risk of drowning because even advanced swimmers can drown.
- Parents should not feel secure that their child is safe in water or safe from drowning after participation in such programs. Toddler swim lessons are not considered "drown proof" for young children.
- Whenever infants and toddlers are in or around water, an adult should be within an arm's length, providing "touch supervision." Swimming lessons should be for toddlers and parents together.
- All aquatic programs should include information on strategies for prevention of drowning and the role of adults in supervising and monitoring the safety of children in and around water. Drowning is a leading cause of death in toddlers and research has shown that attentive supervision is critical (arm's reach and high-water safety knowledge; Johnson et al., 2021).
- Hypothermia, water intoxication, and communicable diseases can be prevented by following existing medical guidelines and do not preclude infants and toddlers from participating in otherwise appropriate aquatic experience programs.

Patient Teaching Guidelines

Medication Safety

Teach parents *never* to store medications with the child-proof cap removed or loosened for easy and rapid access. These shortcuts lead to poison exposures. Remind parents to use and secure the childproof cap on medicine bottles, store the bottles up and away from a child's access, and to administer only the correct dose.

CLINICAL JUDGMENT

During your shift at a pediatric clinic, you answer a call from a parent. The parent is very upset and says that they just discovered their 24-month-old son opened the children's vitamins bottle and ate "a lot" of the vitamins. You need to instruct the parent on what to do.

Questions

1. What is the first thing the parent should do in this situation?
2. After the crisis is over, what teaching can you give to the parent to prevent another accidental poisoning?

Managing a suspected overdose or poisoning is a four-step process:

1. *Ensure adequate ABCDs:* Ensure that the young child has adequate airway, breathing, circulation, and disability/mini-neurological examination.
2. *Empty the child's mouth:* Terminate exposure to the suspected substance by emptying the young child's mouth. *Under no circumstances should vomiting be induced until informed to do so by the Poison Control Center.* Poison should be washed from the eyes per instruction, and the child's clothes should be removed and the skin washed as instructed.
3. *Identify the poison:* The child, family, caregiver, and any witnesses should be questioned about the type of substance, amount consumed, and time of consumption. All parties should look for environmental clues such as empty containers, nearby spills, and odor on breath. All evidence, such as containers, vomitus, and urine, should be saved. The child must be taken to the closest emergency department for immediate care; 9-1-1 should be called for transport.
4. *Prevent poison absorption:* The child should be positioned in a side-lying fashion, and the drug antidote or activated charcoal should be administered PO or by nasogastric tube (NGT), as directed by the Poison Control Center. The child may require whole bowel irrigation with polyethylene glycol electrolyte solution, a cathartic such as magnesium citrate or sulfate, or gastric lavage. You should monitor for symptoms of shock and perform a full body systems evaluation. The family will be in great emotional turmoil and will need support and clear communication during the resuscitative process.

Safety *Stat!*

The Poison Control Center should be called immediately for guidance in treatments by calling 1-800-222-1222. The family should attempt to locate the poisonous substance and be able to state the time since ingestion, if possible.

Car Seat Safety

During the toddler period, the young child may transition from a backward-facing infant car seat to a toddler transitional car seat. If the family is going to use a previously owned toddler car seat, they should be instructed to research the product's safety by contacting the manufacturer. The AAP recommends that all infants and toddlers should ride in a rear-facing seat, as long as possible, until they reach the highest weight or height allowed by their car safety seat manufacturer (AAP, 2021). See the National Highway Traffic Safety Administration (NHTSA) most current website for further guidelines.

Medication Facts

Ipecac Syrup

Historically, ipecac syrup was used in the initial management of ingestion of a toxic substance. Ipecac syrup induces vomiting; however, it has not been found to be effective if taken more than 30 to 90 minutes after ingestion of a toxin. Current guidelines for poison exposure management do not promote the use of ipecac syrup, and it should not be used by families unless directly ordered by a Poison Control Center or an emergency department medical team. If a child is further than 1 hour from an emergency department, ipecac may be indicated.

Many contraindications exist in the use of this medication, including the following:

1. Do not use if the child is lethargic or unconscious (aspiration risk).
2. Do not give if the child has ingested corrosives (corrosives cause esophageal tissue damage and erosion when ingested and again when vomited).
3. Do not give if the child is experiencing seizures (risk of aspiration).

A car's airbag can save an adult's life. However, airbags and young children are a dangerous mix. The following guidelines can help keep young children safe (CDC, 2022a; NHTSA, 2018):

- The safest place for all children younger than 13 years to ride is in the back seat of a motor vehicle.
- Never put a toddler in the front seat of a car, truck, sports utility vehicle (SUV), or van with an airbag.
- All children should be properly secured in car safety seats, belt-positioning booster seats, or with the shoulder/lap belts correct for their size.
- Seatbelts must be worn correctly at all times by all passengers who have outgrown booster seats; fit shoulder/lap belts properly to provide the best protection.
- Side airbags improve safety for adults in side-impact crashes, but children who are not properly restrained and are seated near a side airbag may be at risk for serious injury. Vehicle owner's manuals should provide information about side airbags.

SCREENING AND HEALTH PROMOTION FOR THE TODDLER

During the toddler period, the recommendation is for a well child to be seen three times: at 15 months, 18 months, and 24 months. At the first two visits, immunizations are administered. At the 24-month visit, the child will have blood drawn for hemoglobin and lead levels. Wellness promotion is stressed at these well-child visits, and the results of the screening examinations are explained to the parents or caregiver (Table 19.4).

The number of toddlers at risk for protein-energy malnutrition (PEM) can be as high as 39% in some geographical areas of inadequate food supply and can be a significant cause of death (Healthdata.org, 2022). These children are more susceptible to infection and at risk for stunted growth and developmental delay. A single weight is of limited value

Table 19.4

Recommendations for Well-Toddler Checkups

Assessments	15 Months	18 Months	24 Months
History Family routines Sleep habits Nutrition Home safety Toilet training Tantrums/negativity	X	X	X
Physical examination Growth patterns Fine and gross motor skills Skin integrity	X	X	X
Screenings Hearing Lead	X	X	X

Continued

Table 19.4

Recommendations for Well-Toddler Checkups—cont'd

Assessments	15 Months	18 Months	24 Months
Hemoglobin			X
Immunizations	Hepatitis B (Hep B); *Haemophilus influenzae* type b (Hib); diphtheria, tetanus toxoids, and pertussis (DTaP); measles, mumps, and rubella (MMR); vari-cella zoster virus (VZV)	Hep B, DTaP	N/A
Nutrition	X	X	X
Anticipatory guidance education	X	X	X

Patient Teaching Guidelines

Guidelines for Car Travel With Children

- Eliminate the potential risks from airbags by buckling children in the back seat for every ride.
- Plan ahead so that you do not have to drive with more children than can be safely restrained in the back seat.
- For most families, installing airbag on/off switches is not necessary. Airbags that are turned off provide no protection to older children, teens, parents, or other adults riding in the front seat.
- Airbag on/off switches should only be used if your child has special health-care needs for which your pediatrician recommends constant observation during travel, and no other adult is available to ride in the back seat with your child.
- If no other arrangement is possible and an older child must ride in the front seat, move the vehicle seat back as far as it can go, away from the airbag. Be sure that the child is restrained properly for their size. Keep in mind that your child may still be at risk for injuries from the airbag (AAP, 2021; CDC, 2022a).

during nutritional screening procedures for toddlers. Because of growth patterns and eating lags, weight must be documented over time and trends noted. Observations that suggest severely compromised nutritional status include the following:

- Short stature and slowing of lineal growth
- Thin legs and arms
- Poor hair condition, sparse and thinning
- Skin lesions
- Wasted buttocks
- Spinal processes and rib cage visible
- Ascites and edema from reduced albumin, diarrhea
- Lethargy, apathy, irritability, anxiety, decreased social engagement

Safe and Effective Nursing Care

Hospital environments are inherently unsafe for young toddlers who have mastered locomotion. The toddler's incessant desire to move, explore, investigate, and manipulate objects leaves them at great risk for injury while in a hospital setting, whether the setting is an exclusive children's hospital or a traditional hospital serving those across the life span. Toddlers require constant supervision when out of their high-top cribs and frequent monitoring even when in the metal cribs. Nurses need to check on toddlers frequently, and, if medically indicated, the toddler's hospital room door should remain open at all times. For more information, see Chapter 23: Nursing Care of the Hospitalized Child.

 ### INJURY PREVENTION FOR THE TODDLER

Parents must understand the need to provide adequate and constant supervision for toddlers. Table 19.5 provides specific guidelines for parents or caregivers of toddlers in preventing injuries that could be life-threatening or cause serious harm.

 ### DISORDERS OF THE TODDLER

Certain disorders are more commonly found in the toddler period than during the rest of the childhood. Nurses should become familiar with these disorders so that they can be of assistance in early identification and intervention. Four disorders commonly identified in toddlerhood are child abuse, iron-deficiency anemia, autism spectrum disorder (ASD), and infectious diseases. In addition to the information included in the sections that follow, all of these disorders are addressed in more depth in subsequent chapters.

Child Abuse

Child abuse is most commonly seen in the infancy and toddler period. *Child abuse,* also called *child maltreatment,* is

Table 19.5

Injury Prevention Tips During Toddlerhood

Injury	*Injury Prevention Guidelines*
Suffocation	Do not leave any plastic wrapping, dry cleaning bags, plastic grocery bags, or crib mattress plastic covers within reach of the toddler. Explain to the child and older siblings how dangerous it is to place plastic bags over the head. Do not allow young children to play around or in appliances such as the washing machine, dryer, or refrigerator. Do not allow older siblings to place a pillow over the toddler's head during play.
Choking and asphyxiation	Always cut the toddler's food into small bite-size pieces. Toddlers should not be given foods such as hot dogs, carrots, whole grapes, ice cubes, or hard candies that represent a high choking risk. Do not allow older siblings to feed a young toddler until they are old enough to understand the child's need to chew thoroughly before the next bite. Asphyxiation occurs when the child who is choking cannot exchange air and dies. Toddlers should not be allowed to walk around or run while eating or with food in their mouths. It is good practice to insist from an early start that the young child sit throughout all snacks and meals.
Drowning	Toddlers are at high risk for drowning in even a small amount of water. Do not leave toddlers unsupervised in the bathtub. Never leave buckets or trash cans of standing water near the house. Provide the required double-locked gating system around pools. Never allow a toddler to swim alone; always be touching the child or within arm's reach. Only use federally approved swim-safety devices and swim-safety suits.
Electrocution	Place safety covers on all electrical outlets in every room in the house. Do not let toddlers play with electrical equipment or with electrical cords. They are too young to understand the danger of electrical appliances being around water. Do not store curling irons, hair dryers, or electric shavers anywhere near bathroom sinks or tubs. Do not leave electrical appliances plugged in around the kitchen where a toddler can drag a chair over and reach.
Animal bites	Even well-behaved pets can turn aggressive toward a playful toddler. Toddlers do not understand how to be gentle when playing with animals. Do not allow a toddler to approach a restrained dog or pet an unfamiliar dog because many are not comfortable with children and will bite. Cats will readily scratch an aggressive toddler. Cat scratches are especially dangerous because of the potential to transmit bacteria (*Bartonella henselae*) that often requires antibiotic therapy.
Traffic safety and playing outdoors	Toddlers will readily chase a ball out into traffic. It is important to stress to the toddler that they must look before crossing, but *never* trust a toddler around a street. Developmentally, toddlers cannot process the concept of caution and safety around traffic. Toddlers require constant supervision when playing outdoors. Some families choose to use chest harnesses when taking their toddler to busy areas. Harnesses can be basic, where the parent holds a "leash" style handle, or there is also a "belt-to-belt" style. Harnesses allow exploration while avoiding dangers by containing the child. Some parents associate harnesses with animal control practices and are against their use, whereas others say harnesses are less restraining than strollers.
Falls and climbing	Toddlers will readily drag a chair over to reach a taller surface. Prevent injuries in the kitchen, especially around the stove, by using baby gates to keep a toddler away from dangerous home areas.
Motor vehicle accidents	Always use federally approved and size-appropriate car seats when transporting children. Place the child in the center of the back seat. Children younger than 12 years or under 100 pounds should not be in the front seat with an airbag because severe injuries, including decapitation of small children, have occurred. See the most current AAP website for further information on airbag safety.
Burns	Burn injuries can occur during toddlerhood in both the kitchen and the bathroom. Water heaters should be set below 48.9°C (120°F). Toddlers should wear sunscreen with an SPF of at least 30 on all exposed skin while in the sun, even for short periods. And sunscreen should be reapplied after sweating or swimming. Toddlers should be required to wear hats while outdoors.
Bodily damage	Toddlers should never have access to sharp items such as needles or scissors that are not child-safety scissors. Children should not run around the home holding items near their face; impalements occur with such items as pens, pencils, toothbrushes, and kitchen utensils. Never remove an impaled object until the child has been transported to an emergency department because excessive bleeding and further tissue damage can occur.

defined as a nonaccidental injury or trauma that leads to sexual violation, emotional trauma, physical harm, or death. Child maltreatment can take the form of abuse (either physical or emotional abuse) or neglect (such as not providing for the child's medical, nutritional, clothing, and supervision needs). Categories of child abuse include physical, emotional, verbal, and sexual abuse. Infants, toddlers, and preschoolers are the most common victims of physical abuse, whereas school-age children and adolescents encounter emotional abuse and sexual abuse more often.

Contributing Factors

Three general sets of factors contribute to child abuse: child factors, parental/abuser factors, and environmental factors. Although not all of the factors will be present in each case of abuse, these three should be considered as influencing factors.

- *Child factors:* Children who have special needs, are technology dependent, have a difficult or demanding temperament, have learning disabilities, were born premature (with or without a congenital anomaly), or have a chronic illness are at greatest risk of abuse (CDC, 2022b).
- *Parental/abuser factors:* Adults who have substance use disorder or addiction issues, are unemployed, experience frequent moves, are socially isolated, are adolescents, experience multiple stressors, lack parenting skills, have anger control issues and/or a low tolerance for frustration, have low self-esteem or low confidence, and who have experienced abuse in their own lives are at greater risk for becoming abusers (CDC, 2022b).
- *Environmental factors:* Environments that may contribute to child abuse include living in low-income, unsafe neighborhoods; being of low economic status; living in areas of low employment rates; living in crowded conditions; and having a lack of educated adults present. However, keep in mind that child abuse can occur in any socioeconomic level.

Preventing Child Abuse

Prevention strategies include offering parenting classes for young or high-risk parents, encouraging qualified family members to role model parenting strategies, encouraging respite care for stressed caregivers, educating parents to prevent shaken baby syndrome, and offering support groups for parents who are socially isolated.

Assessment and Reporting

Assessment in cases of suspected child abuse includes noting the type, location, and severity of the injury; meticulously documenting all observations; and observing any incompatibility between the history told of the injury and the clinical presentation of the injury. In some cases, failure to thrive (FTT) may be evidence of physical and emotional neglect. Carefully follow state and institutional policies concerning cases of suspected child abuse. Some institutions will want you to initially check the child alone and then include the parents/caregivers. Photographs may be required in the reporting of child abuse. There are several categories of mandatory reports (see state laws). Lack of reporting can lead to heavy fines and imprisonment. See Chapter 26 for an in-depth presentation of child abuse.

Iron-Deficiency Anemia

Anemia is the overall reduction of the number of RBCs or of the hemoglobin that RBCs carry. **Iron-deficiency anemia** is the most common childhood form of anemia. Anemia is not typically classified as a disease process, but rather a manifestation of an underlying condition. When circulating hemoglobin is significantly reduced, clinical symptoms present because of hypoxia. Risk factors include poor nutritional intake of iron. A common cause of reduced iron intake is the overconsumption of milk. Young children whose daily diets include more than 24 to 32 ounces of milk become full and therefore are at risk to consume too little of iron-rich foods, thus leading to iron-deficiency anemia. Mild cases of anemia can be managed via diet; however, moderate cases need iron supplements and severe cases require blood transfusion of packed RBCs.

Autism Spectrum Disorder

ASD generally presents before a child reaches 36 months of age. It can be severely disabling, but its presentation varies widely. The key indicators are impaired nonverbal and verbal communication as well as impaired or absent reciprocal social interactions. Parents report considerable delays in communication patterns and social play compared with other children of the same age and development. The child may display stereotypical body movements and preoccupation with body parts.

Autistic children range from below average to average to above average on the intelligence scale. Autism is somewhat more common in males than in females and may be associated with other neurological disorders. The cause is unknown at this time. Nurses should evaluate the young child for impaired social interactions, impaired communication, repetitive patterns of behavior, and lack of interest in activities expected at the child's age and level of development or an abnormally focused interest in an object or activity. The child with suspected autism may demonstrate abnormal **electroencephalograms** (EEGs) and may display a seizure disorder.

Treatment for younger children with autism focuses on speech and language; the child may require special education. Families should be referred to support groups for caregivers and parents of autistic children. Physical contact should be minimized while the child is in a health-care setting or hospital because it may cause anxiety and distress for the autistic child. For more about ASD, see Chapter 29.

- **WORD · BUILDING ·**
electroencephalogram: electro–electric + encephalo–brain + gram–writing

Nursing Care Plan for the Toddler Who Is Undervaccinated

Two-year-old Jimmy is brought to the clinic for a well-child checkup. As you review Jimmy's health record, you note that Jimmy did not receive his last scheduled immunizations.

According to the file, Jimmy's mother prefers following a delayed immunization schedule. You formulate a plan of care.

Nursing Diagnosis: Knowledge deficit related to mother's request to delay scheduled immunizations

Expected Outcome: The patient's mother will verbalize understanding of the risks associated with delayed immunization.

Intervention:	Rationale:
The pediatric health-care team provides the mother with verbal and written immunization information in the mother's primary language.	*Written material will allow the mother to take the information home for further reading and discussion with other family members.*

Nursing Diagnosis: Risk for infection related to delayed vaccinations

Expected Outcome: The patient's mother will verbalize ways to prevent transmission of infectious illnesses.

Intervention:	Rationale:
The pediatric health-care team teaches the mother the importance of hand washing and safe food preparation and storage.	*Proper hand hygiene and food safety can help prevent several infectious illnesses.*

Common Infectious Diseases

Toddlers are at a particularly high risk for the acquisition and transmission of common communicable infectious diseases. Because toddlers do not demonstrate independent personal hygiene such as effective hand washing, they are at a higher risk for infections than older children. Toddlers who are still in diapers are at risk for becoming infected with or transmitting fecal parasites such as pinworms. Other infectious diseases include the common cold (the most common illness of childhood), influenza, varicella zoster (chicken pox), dermatological infections such as fungus, or infestations such as *Pediculosis capitis* (head lice). Pediatric nurses should always use universal precautions when touching potentially contaminated body secretions and apply standard precautions such as droplet, airborne, and contact precautions for particular illnesses (see Appendix C for infection-control precaution guidelines). Nurses routinely evaluate young children for infectious diseases; apply appropriate infection-control precautions; treat as ordered; and educate family members on the disease process, transmission, incubation period, symptoms, and treatments. For more about communicable and infectious diseases, see Chapter 37.

Key Points

- The toddler period is marked by slower growth, fewer calorie needs, food lags and jags, picky eating, tantrums, and negativity. Families need specific anticipatory guidance during this challenging developmental stage.
- Toddlers need to be introduced to consistent discipline. Time-outs can be used and should last no longer than 1 minute per year of age. Time-outs should be conducted in a private place.
- Because toddlerhood is marked by increasing locomotion and exploration, the toddler requires constant supervision to provide protection against injury, harm, and dangers. The developmental milestone that the toddler is struggling to accomplish is Erikson's psychosocial stage of autonomy versus shame and doubt. Toddlers need opportunities to exert their independence and separation from their primary caregiver.

- A major task for the toddler is toilet training. This task requires instruction, experimentation, support, and patience.
- Toddlers participate in parallel play. They are not able to share naturally and need to be taught how to share. Toddlers are egocentric and cannot process the views or needs of another.
- Toddlers experience both separation anxiety and stranger anxiety. Measures should be taken to reduce the effect of these experiences.
- Toddlers are at risk for aspiration and choking. Foods should be cut into bite-size pieces and only low-risk foods should be served.
- Child abuse is most commonly found in children between the ages of infancy and 3 years. Nurses need to be aware of this risk and evaluate for all types of child abuse (Hockenberry & Wilson, 2013).

Review Questions

1. Which of the following activities within the hospital environment is the child in the toddler developmental stage most likely to be fearful of?
   1. Going into the treatment room for a minor procedure
   2. Having to leave the playroom for a nap
   3. Seeing the parents pack up their belongings to leave for work for the day
   4. Watching a roommate being placed on a gurney to go to surgery

2. According to Erikson, the toddler's psychosocial developmental task can best be supported by which of the following activities?
   1. Activities that support family and sibling interaction and bonding
   2. Creative thinking and play activities that promote exploration
   3. Art activities that promote the sense of completion of a task
   4. Activities that provide the child a sense of individuality and control

3. A frustrating behavior displayed by a toddler that a parent should acknowledge as a normal response to the cognitive development of a toddler is:
   1. The toddler's persistence to eat only what they want
   2. The toddler's lack of sharing with others
   3. The toddler's egotistical thought process
   4. The toddler's need for the consistent presence of a security item

4. The number of words mastered by a toddler by the third birthday is:
   1. 50
   2. 1,000
   3. 300
   4. 750

5. Bedtime fears are a very real experience for the toddler. Which of the following creates the greatest fears?
   1. The unreasonable thought that the toddler's security item will become lost
   2. The fear of monsters under the bed
   3. The loss of time with older siblings who get to stay up later
   4. The fear of separation from parents at bedtime

6. A parent comes into the clinic with a toddler for a well-child appointment. The parent is concerned that the child is not eating enough and is refusing to consume what the rest of the family eats for dinner. Which of the following is the best response by the nurse?
   1. "This is unacceptable and the child should be kept in the high chair until dinner is consumed."
   2. "This is normal because the toddler is experiencing strong food preferences."
   3. "This is worrisome because the toddler experiences exponential growth and requires more calories at this time."
   4. "This is normal and food lags should be expected during this time of slowed growth."

7. Stranger anxiety is a common experience for the toddler. You should practice which of the following to assist in the minimization of stranger anxiety in the hospital? **(Select all that apply.)**
   1. Do not touch the toddler unless absolutely necessary.
   2. Establish a positive rapport with the parents before approaching the child.
   3. Ask the older sibling to hold the child during measurement of vital signs.
   4. Assign as many different nurses as possible to the child's care to get them accustomed to new people.
   5. Call on the assistance of child life specialists to assist with building trust and engagement.

8. Which of the following should be included in teaching parents about car seat safety for their toddler? **(Select all that apply.)**
   1. Maintain the car seat facing backward and in the center back seat until the age of 2.
   2. Maintain the car seat facing forward and in a reclining position.
   3. Use only booster seats because the toddler is tall enough to see out the car windows.
   4. Transition to a convertible seat and place it facing forward when the toddler reaches the highest weight or height allowed by the car seat manufacturer.
   5. Use only toddler car seats that have been inspected and approved for safety.

9. Why is the prevention and identification of child abuse especially important during the toddler years?
   1. The demanding tone of toddlers causes parents to become frustrated and therefore neglect their child.
   2. Tantrums can cause a parent to lose control.
   3. This is the most common age of child abuse in the nation.
   4. Child abuse begins in the infancy period and remains throughout childhood.

10. Iron-deficiency anemia is a common toddler nutritional problem. While teaching a parent how to prevent this disorder, you explain that:
    1. Iron-deficiency anemia is related to the stopping of breast milk at 1 year of life.
    2. Iron-deficiency anemia is correlated with teething.
    3. Food lags and preferences cause the child to stop eating enough iron-rich foods.
    4. Too much milk in the diet prevents the toddler from consuming enough iron-rich foods.

ANSWERS 1. 4; 2. 4; 3. 4; 4. 3; 5. 4; 6. 4; 7. 2; 5; 8. 4; 5; 9. 3; 10. 4

CRITICAL THINKING QUESTIONS

1. During clinicals in a community health center, the student nurse notices that a toddler has a bruise on his right leg. Suspecting child abuse, the student nurse frantically asks her preceptor to call Child Protection Services (CPS). The nurse-preceptor calmly continues their assessment of the child. What should the student nurse do next? Why?

2. How would you evaluate a home for safety concerns for a family with a toddler? How could a checklist be used to guide you in the evaluation of a safe home environment?

3. At a well-child examination, the stay-at-home mother of a toddler reports that she is exhausted. She's so busy supervising her child to keep him safe and thinking of activities for him to do that it's nearly impossible for her to get anything else done around the house. Brainstorm some ways this mother could safely get a break from her active toddler.

Resources

For additional resources and information, including Postconference Questions and Activities, Answers, and References, visit www.FADavis.com.

 Student Study Guide

CHAPTER 20
Health Promotion of the Preschooler

KEY TERMS

anaphylaxis (AN-uh-fih-LAK-siss)
animism (AN-ih-mizm)
artificialism (ar-tih-FISH-uhl-izm)
encopresis (en-koh-PREE-siss)
enuresis (EN-yoo-REE-siss)
imminent justice (IM-ih-nent JUSS-tiss)
intuitive thinking (in-TOO-it-iv THINK-ing)
magical thinking (MAJ-ik-uhl THINK-ing)
nightmares (NITE-mairz)
night terrors (NITE TAIR-ruhs)
preconceptual thinking (PREE-kon-SEP-choo-uhl
   THINK-ing)
selective attention (suh-LEK-tiv uh-TEN-shun)
symbolic functioning (sim-BOL-ik
   FUNG-shun-ing)

CHAPTER CONCEPTS

Comfort
Family
Growth and Development
Health Promotion
Infection
Mobility
Nutrition
Safety
Sensory Perception

LEARNING OUTCOMES

1. Define the key terms.
2. Describe the unique needs of the preschool-age child compared with children in other developmental stages and age groups.
3. Describe the differences between the preschool child and older children and adults in relation to body systems, anatomy, and physiology.
4. Describe the physical growth and development of the preschool period in comparison with other developmental stages.
5. Describe magical thinking in the preschool period and its effect on the child's view of the world.
6. Compare the nutritional needs and eating patterns of the preschooler with those of the infant and toddler.
7. Identify the need to promote hand washing and hygiene practices in the preschool period.
8. Contrast the play needs and socialization practices of the preschooler to other developmental stages.
9. Teach the family of a preschooler anticipatory guidance practices to reduce injury and accidents.
10. Define the phenomenon of enuresis and encopresis in the preschool period and state appropriate resources for the parents of a child with these disorders.
11. Outline a plan of care that focuses on the safety needs of the preschool child, including prevention of illnesses, accidents, and injuries in both home and school settings.

CRITICAL THINKING

Three-year-old **Vanessa** has been hospitalized for cellulitis associated with a spider bite that requires IV antibiotics and wound care. Vanessa is experiencing pain associated with her wound and her peripheral IV site. She demonstrates discomfort by grimacing, moving her legs around in bed frequently, and refusing to get out of bed to sit in a chair or ambulate to the playroom for organized crafts. You use the FLACC objective pain assessment tool (Face, Legs, Activity, Cry, and Consolability) and believe that Vanessa is experiencing a 4 to 6 out of 10. The use of the subjective Wong-Baker FACES pain scale was not successful. When asked, Vanessa says she caused this

Continued

338

CRITICAL THINKING—cont'd

spider to bite her and now caused her hospitalization because she has been "naughty." As a preschool child, her responses to her condition and her hospitalization are very expected because she is demonstrating magical thinking and preconceptual and preoperational thinking.

Questions

1. Taking into account her developmental stage, how would you evaluate the child for her understanding of the reasons for her hospitalization?
2. What actions can you take to encourage Vanessa to get out of bed?
3. What is another subjective pain tool that you can use to gather cues for Vanessa's interpretation of her pain?

CONCEPTUAL CORNERSTONE
Growth and Development

Compared with the toddler period, the preschool developmental period is marked by slower overall growth in height and weight but greater fine motor achievements. Preschool children learn to draw and craft, and they develop skills that require greater eye–hand coordination. Preschoolers are more independent than toddlers, yet they still require frequent reminders about safety issues such as protective gear, street safety, car seat safety, pet safety, and home safety. Growth and development for the preschooler is focused on physical and emotional achievements as they master more complex and creative play. Cognitively, preschoolers rely on magical thinking to explain cause-and-effect relationships that they don't understand.

The preschool developmental period spans the time from the child's third birthday through their fifth year. During this period, many children attend preschool, where they must learn to share toys and attention with others and take direction from adults other than their parents. As a preschool child matures, they display a more even temperament and develop ease and patience, skills not previously shown during the toddler years. This progress is vital for beginning school. By the fifth birthday, most preschoolers are more quiet and contemplative and would rather participate in cooperative play with others than in parallel play.

 ## GROWTH AND DEVELOPMENT OF THE PRESCHOOLER

The preschool period, unlike the infant and toddler periods, is a time when the child is focused on creative play, fine motor achievements, and greater socialization with peers. Physical growth remains slow and steady, but finer movements and motor control become more prominent.

Preschoolers learn to ride a tricycle, jump, skip, draw, paint, write basic letters, imitate roles (dress up), and use their imagination.

Physical Growth and Development

The preschool child is marked by a slowing of physical growth. The preschooler gains only 2.26 kg (5 lb) per year in weight and grows 2.5 to 3 inches (6.35 to 7.62 cm) per year in height. The child's classic stance changes as well. The slightly taller, leaner preschooler stands with an erect posture rather than with a protruding tummy typical of a toddler. Other physical changes include the following:

- By the start of the preschool age, all 20 primary, or deciduous, teeth have erupted. Toward the end of the preschooler period, the child will begin to shed the primary teeth.
- Blood sugar begins to stabilize toward the end of this period, and fewer snacks will be needed.
- Expected vital signs include a heart rate of 65 to 110 bpm, respiratory rate between 20 and 25 bpm, and a blood pressure of 95 to 110 mm Hg over 60 to 75 mm Hg.
- Immunity continues to mature and the administration of immunizations continues. Diseases experienced during this time include lice; influenza; cutaneous staphylococcus infections, such as impetigo; and streptococcus infections, such as strep throat.
- Visual acuity matures; most preschoolers have visual acuity of 20/40 by their third birthday and 20/30 by their fourth birthday.
- Visual disturbances often present during the early preschool period. Both nearsightedness (**myopia**) and double vision (**amblyopia**) can present during this time. (For more about visual disturbances, see Chapter 28.)
- Hearing acuity is 100% intact with no expected deficits. (For more about hearing impairments, see Chapter 28.)

Safety *Stat!*

The continuation of childhood immunizations during the preschool period is essential. During the preschool period, the child is exposed to many more children, increasing the possibility of exposure to infectious diseases (see Chapter 37). The four immunizations that should be administered to the preschool child are varicella zoster (chicken pox), MMR (measles, mumps, and rubella), DTaP (diphtheria, tetanus toxoids, and pertussis), and IPV (inactivated poliovirus).

· WORD · BUILDING ·

myopia: my–shut + op–eye + ia–condition
amblyopia: ambly–dull + op–eye + ia–condition

Gross Motor Development

The preschool child will be able to accomplish new, independent tasks (Table 20.1). The preschool child benefits from mastery of new tasks and will want to showcase accomplishments to parents, caregivers, and nurses (Fig. 20.1).

- Provide praise when a preschooler attempts a new accomplishment, whether or not they actually master it. For example, if a preschooler attempts to tie their shoes, provide praise.
- Do not reprimand a preschooler who fails at a task. When a preschool child hears frequent reprimands, they will be less inclined to attempt a new motor skill.

Nutrition

During the preschool period, the child consumes about half the calories of an adult, approximately 1,200 to 1,600 calories a day, depending on growth and activity level.

- Food preferences may still affect how a preschooler eats; picky eating behaviors may continue well into the preschool period. Food jags and lags can last until the sixth birthday.
- The most important aspect of eating behavior during this period is to teach the parents to ensure that the preschooler is consuming a well-balanced diet, is taking in adequate calories, has limited salt and fat, and is exposed frequently to new foods.
- Preschoolers benefit from two cups of nonfat or low-fat cow's milk or calcium-fortified plant-based milk per day.
- Total dietary intake of fat should not exceed 35% of total daily calories; 25% should be the goal for most children.
- Parents and caregivers should offer fruits and vegetables at every meal; encourage consumption of protein in the

Table 20.1

Gross Motor Skill Development in Preschoolers

3-Year-Old	4-Year-Old	5-Year-Old	Between the Beginning of the Third Year and the End of the Fifth Year
Builds towers of six to nine blocks	Alternates feet going up a flight of stairs	Displays good balance	Buttons and unbuttons
Catches a ball	Gallops	Dresses without help	Draws copies of shapes on paper
Climbs on higher structures	Goes up and down steps easily	Hops and skips well	Draws detailed stick figures
Hops in place	Jumps	Pulls wagons	Learns to write
Jumps horizontally	Pumps on a swing	Rides scooters	Pours from a pitcher
Marches	Runs on tiptoes	Skates	Progresses from holding scissors to being able to cut a line with scissors
Paints in circular motions with whole hands	Skips on one foot	Plays on playground equipment	Progresses from putting on shoes to lacing shoes to tying shoelaces
Rides tricycle	Throws ball over head		Uses eating utensils
Runs	Walks heel to toe		Washes face and hands
Smears or dabs paint			
Stands on one foot briefly			

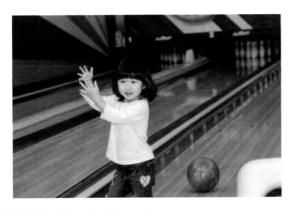

FIGURE 20.1 A preschooler at play.

form of legumes, tofu, lean meats, and fish; and offer only low-sugar cereals.
- Nutritious snacks that are appealing to preschool children include peanut butter on graham crackers (evaluate for food allergies), celery sticks with cream cheese, and carrot sticks dipped in ranch dressing.

Safety *Stat!*

With 6.5% of children having food allergies, trigger foods must be identified and eliminated from an allergic child's diet, potentially in the home, school, and day care environments (Asthma and Allergy Foundation of America, 2021). Preschool children attending childcare or preschool classes and their teachers must be made aware of food allergies to prevent potentially serious reactions. **Anaphylaxis** is a very serious allergic reaction with symptoms including hypotension, severe airway edema, lightheadedness, and bronchospasms. Anaphylaxis can be caused by medications, foods, insect bites, or latex exposure. Specific allergy testing can help determine what allergies a child has. A child with a severe allergy should have access to two epinephrine pens—one at home and one at day care or school. Training in the use of EpiPens must be provided to caregivers at home and school.

Family Meals

The experience of the family meal is very important to the well-being of the preschooler. Parents and caregivers should use meals as an opportunity for the family to become close and demonstrate respect for one another. Children should not be allowed to eat in front of the television but should sit at their own place in their own chair at the family table and engage in conversation during at least one meal per day. The preschooler can add to the family conversation by offering a summary of what they experienced and learned in preschooler class that day.

• WORD • BUILDING •

anaphylaxis: ana–against + phylaxis–protection

Obesity

Childhood obesity rates are increasing as more and more children are being exposed to high-fat diets, including fast food consumption, in combination with decreasing levels of activity. To combat this, the preschool child should be encouraged to eat a variety of nutritious foods and taught the importance of physical activity and vigorous play. Family role modeling is essential.

MyPlate

The older preschool child might enjoy learning about nutrition and physical activity by being introduced to MyPlate for Preschoolers (Fig. 20.2). ChooseMyPlate.gov is a website that provides guidelines for eating well, being active, and being healthy. This family-appropriate site introduces children and their parents to healthy food choices while helping them to understand the calculation of calories and minutes of exercise needed for a healthy lifestyle. In addition, it provides ideas for healthy meals and snacks. The site also assists with teaching young children to follow food safety rules, such as washing their hands before preparing or eating foods, refrigerating foods promptly, not cross-contaminating uncooked foods with cooked foods, and using a food thermometer. Parents can learn about specific food preparation ideas, kitchen safety, and play ideas to enhance the child's experience in food preparation while teaching guidelines for safety (United States Department of Agriculture [USDA], 2021).

Sleeping Patterns and Requirements

The average preschooler needs 12 hours of uninterrupted sleep per night; however, it is common during this stage for the child to wake up and need reassurance from any fears during the night. Providing a bedtime routine and a night-light may assist with the reduction of fears in the middle of the night. Parents need to be educated that their preschooler may demonstrate sleep disturbances, especially if the child is new to preschool, where there is a high level of activity and a new level of intense stimulation. Activities that help a child slow down before bedtime and follow a bedtime routine each night can help the young child understand that bedtime is near and that no delay is acceptable. Young children should not be allowed to watch television before their bedtime because it has been shown to disturb the child's sleep routine.

Nightmares and Night Terrors

Both nightmares and night terrors are common during the preschool period. **Nightmares** are scary dreams that may awaken the child, produce crying, and require reassurance and comfort. **Night terrors** cause the child to demonstrate great fear, which may be displayed through thrashing arms and legs, yelling, and possibly running or walking out of their room or even out of the house. Parents need to be taught that very little needs to be done for the child other than reassurance and safety during the episode.

United States Department of Agriculture

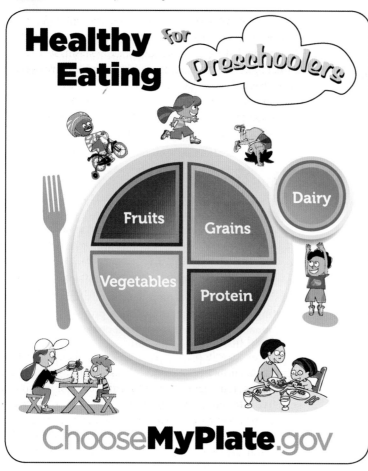

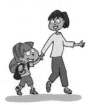

Get your child on the path to healthy eating.

Offer a variety of healthy foods.
Choose foods from each MyPlate food group. Pay attention to dairy foods, whole grains, and vegetables to build healthy habits that will last a lifetime.

Be mindful of sweet drinks and other foods.
Offer water instead of sugary drinks like regular soda and fruit drinks. Other foods like hot dogs, burgers, pizza, cookies, cakes, and candy are only occasional treats.

Focus on the meal and each other.
Your child learns by watching you. Let your child choose how much to eat of foods you provide. Children copy your likes, dislikes, and your interest in trying new foods.

Be patient with your child.
Children enjoy food when eating it is their own choice. Some new foods take time. Give a taste at first and wait a bit. Let children serve themselves by taking small amounts. Offer new foods many times.

Cook together.
Eat together.
Talk together.
Make meal time family time.

Food and Nutrition Service
USDA is an equal opportunity provider and employer.   Based on the Dietary Guidelines for Americans.   FNS-451 Revised December 2016

FIGURE 20.2 MyPlate for Preschoolers. (From choosemyplate.gov. Retrieved from https://www.choosemyplate.gov/resources/myplate-tip-sheets)

Evidence-Based Practice

Night Terrors

Current research on night terrors for young children shows that this is a common sleep disorder, yet there continues to be a lack of explanation or etiology of the experience. Most children do not recall the experience, regardless of the abnormal parasomnias (unusual verbal and physical behaviors that occur). Children experience night terrors during non-REM (rapid eye movement) sleep stages. Non-REM is considered a transitional period between wakefulness and sleep. The only interventions are for the parent or caregiver to soothe the child during the experience without waking them, identify stressors for the child, and promote coping strategies.

Van Horn, N. L., & Street, M. (2022). Night terrors. *StatPearls*. Updated 2022, May 30th. In: *StatPearls* (Internet). StatPearls Publishing. https://www.ncbi.nlm.nih.gov/books/NBK493222

Napping

As the child progresses from toddlerhood to the early preschool developmental stage, they will probably no longer take an afternoon nap. However, this varies greatly among children. Most preschool settings provide the early preschool child with an opportunity to nap or rest during the day. Some schools provide individual cots, and others require the families to bring in a pad. The child gradually needs less rest during the day but needs to obtain sufficient sleep during the night. Instead of a nap, the older preschooler may just need quiet time to lie down and look at a book or play with a stuffed animal.

Cognitive Development

According to Piaget's stages of cognitive development, the preschooler is described as preoperational. However, Piaget identified the preoperational stage as extending from the ages of 2 through 7 years. The preoperational stage is a transitional one during which the young child leaves behind completely egotistical thinking and develops social awareness and the ability to consider other points of view. During this stage, the child thinks symbolically, meaning the child takes one object, word, or thought and attempts to make it stand for something that it may not (preoperational; McLeod, 2018b).

Preschoolers experience three substages of cognitive development:

1. *Preconceptual thinking:* This can be described as the young child's judgment of their environment and objects by sensory experiences and classifying objects by one characteristic only (shape, color, meaning). There are three components: artificialism, animism, and imminent justice (Box 20.1).
2. *Intuitive thinking:* This type of thinking begins around 4 years of age and is defined as the preschooler's ability to classify information while becoming more aware of cause-and-effect relationships. Understanding cause-and-effect relationships allows the child to predict responses to and consequences of actions, which requires a deep understanding of the child's previous experiences.
3. *Symbolic functioning:* This relates to the experience of play and is demonstrated by a child who assigns meaning to an object different than its literal meaning, such as using a pillow for a horsey, a cardboard box for a car, and a blanket for a cape.

Imagination and Magical Thinking

The preschool period is marked by a surge in a child's imaginative life. Preschoolers have rich fantasy lives and deep imaginations; because of this, they have trouble telling fantasy from reality. Through the process of **magical thinking**, preschoolers use their imagination to explain something they do not understand in their complex environments. For example, the preschooler will use magical thinking to explain why a sibling has cancer and is hospitalized and may state that the sibling is being punished for denting their father's car or for poor behavior. Preschoolers may blame their behavior on imaginary friends, or they may believe that their made-up reality replaces and explains their actual reality. Magical thinking also includes the preschooler's ideas that they can influence reality and make things happen.

Box 20.1
Components of Preconceptual Thinking

There are three components of preconceptual thinking:

1. *Artificialism:* The preschooler believes that everything is made by humans.
2. *Animism:* The preschooler believes that inanimate objects are alive or can turn alive.
3. *Imminent justice:* A belief that everything has a determined universal code of law and order.

Patient Teaching Guidelines

Preschoolers will likely struggle with the concept of death. Explain to parents that their child may see death as something temporary. It is important to not use euphemisms such as "went to sleep" or was "put to sleep." As magical thinkers, preschoolers will expect the person or animal to wake up. Give children clear and honest answers and explanations. Parents and other caregivers should be aware that the children's feelings about death may come out in their play activity.

Concept of Time

The preschooler begins to understand the concepts of *today, tomorrow,* and *later,* but struggles to understand the concepts of *past, present,* and *future.* One education goal is to have the preschooler comprehend the days of the week, the months of the year, and the basics of the four seasons before their fifth birthday. By doing this, the child learns to anticipate future events and look forward to particular situations. Birthday celebrations are a classic example of this.

Selective Attention

Parents of preschoolers may question if their child has a hearing impairment when the child does not respond to their voices for certain periods of time. This behavior is known as **selective attention.** The child may not respond to requests or even to their name while playing or concentrating on a craft, puzzle, or fabric book, because the activity has captured the child's full attention. This is normal behavior but can be frustrating to parents (Fig. 20.3).

Language Development

During the preschool period, the child makes great strides in communication:

- *2 years:* The toddler can be expected to say 50 words.
- *3 years:* The child is verbally communicating with up to 900 words.

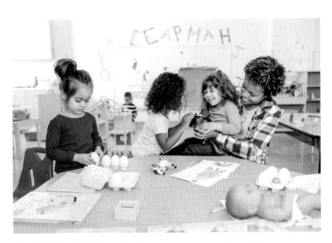

FIGURE 20.3 Child displaying selective attention while engaged in self-play. (kate_sept2004/iStock/Thinkstock)

• *4 years:* The preschooler is answering simple questions with simple answers, and communicates with up to 1,500 words.
• *5 years:* The child rhymes, uses complex and compound sentences, talks in future tense, and states full name and address. At this age, the child may use 2,100 words.

What the preschooler likes to talk about also changes during this period:

• *3 years:* The early preschooler likes to tell simple stories and enjoys describing what they see, hear, and experience. Not all stories told will be completely truthful because the child is in the magical thinking stage.
• *4 years:* The child may talk incessantly while exaggerating and boasting. At this age, the child likes rhymes, silly words, and playing with speech and may also enjoy endlessly questioning parents.
• *5 years:* The child, who is very interested in their environment, tells long tales about daily experiences and may also test parents by using profanity and forbidden words.

See Table 20.2 for more information about the language development of preschool-age children.

Preschool is a period of language growth. With that growth comes the potential for problems. Preschool children need encouragement to speak and explain their thoughts as well as to communicate their questions and their needs. Speech problems, such as stuttering or lisping, should be identified and treated as early as possible.

Numbers, Colors, and Letters

The preschool child is exposed to a new world of symbolic meanings. Numbers are learned after a great deal of practice, sometimes in the incorrect order. Preschoolers delight in learning their numbers and should be able to identify 0 to 10 before their fifth birthday. Identifying colors becomes a game, and learning to mix colors while painting is exciting. Preschoolers learn to copy simple shapes, stick figures, and numbers and should be encouraged to practice this new skill repeatedly. Upon seeing their child begin drawing, some parents and caregivers may push to have the child use one hand rather than the other (right vs. left, left vs. right), which can discourage the child from practicing the skill. Instead, parents and caregivers should encourage their child in this activity, making it a positive experience. By the time the child is 4, the child's dominant hand is well established.

Psychological Growth and Development

Erikson describes the preschool child's psychological and psychosocial developmental crisis as initiative versus feelings of guilt (McLeod, 2018a). The child must master the process of initiating activities that are independent and self-directed. If the child is not given an opportunity to initiate these activities, they may be reluctant to try new processes. As the child takes on new experiences, even if they do not have all the physical abilities to be successful, parents and caregivers need to support the child in the attempts so that the child does not develop guilt over any failures. Frequent experiences of blame or negativity during skill exploration can cause the child to experience guilt and decreased feelings of worth. This period can be a difficult balancing act for parents because they have to guide and support the child while also setting limits and restricting the child from partaking in unsafe situations.

Socialization

The preschool child is now participating in greater social interactions. Unlike the toddler, who is egocentric and participating in parallel play, the preschooler is interacting with

---

Table 20.2

Expected Language Development of the Preschooler

3-Year-Old	4-Year-Old	5-Year-Old
Asks many questions	Asks questions at a peak of frequency	Can state names of coins
Displays a poor use of pronouns	Counts out loud	Enjoys telling long stories
May repeat a sentence of up to six syllables	May use "forbidden" words or mild profanity if in the presence of older children or siblings	Learns time-oriented concepts, such as days of the week, months, seasons
Speaks a total of 300 to 900 words	Names colors	Names most colors
Talks incessantly, even when others are not listening or paying attention	Speaks a total of 1,500 words	Speaks a total of 2,100 words
Uses three- to four-word sentences	States names of animals, people, and places	Uses five-word sentences
	Tells exaggerated stories	
	Uses four- to five-word sentences	
	Uses prepositional phrases, such as "in front of" or "in back of"	

both adults and peers in greater depth during play and school. The development of socialization will depend on the opportunities offered to the child.

Moral and Spiritual Development

According to Kohlberg's theory of moral development (McLeod, 2013), during the preschool period, the child's self-centered understanding of "good" and "bad" is replaced with a basic understanding of what is considered socially acceptable. In addition, the preschooler's conscience is emerging; the child is learning self-control and consequences. The preschooler learns what is right and wrong by listening to, watching, and imitating others. Preschoolers inherently want to please the adults in their lives and will do things to create a positive reaction from parents, teachers, and other adults. Children at this age should be given opportunities to help in small ways and should receive praise for their attempts to please others.

- In general, the preschooler wants to conform to rules, and this desire will increase with age.
- As the preschooler matures through this period, the child becomes easygoing with a positive attitude, is less resistant to change, and is more secure. The child also develops a greater sense of personal identity.
- Children benefit from interacting in a diverse community (Fig. 20.4). The preschool period is an excellent time to provide guidance to a child as their socialization expands and they interact with diverse cultural groups and families (Box 20.2).

The preschooler becomes more self-assured and well-adjusted throughout the fifth year. The child strives to gain inner control while wanting to please those around them. A successful way to teach parents about this age group is to explain that their preschooler needs to know clear and consistent rules and the consequences for breaking those rules.

Spiritual development surfaces during the preschool years as the young child explores the family's faith and religious

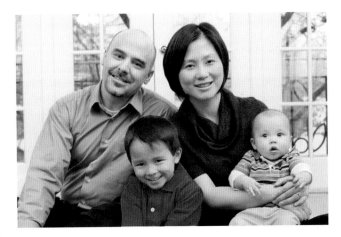

FIGURE 20.4 Cultural diversity in families.

Box 20.2

Diversity and Multiculturalism

The preschool period is considered a prime time to teach children about cultural and ethnic perspectives other than their own because this is when the child begins to develop ideas of the world. At the most basic level, adults should do the following:

- Set a good example by showing respect for all people.
- Encourage children to play with the toys they want to play with, not limiting girls to "feminine" toys or boys to "masculine" toys.
- Point out similarities as well as differences between people.
- Reinforce that people come in all shapes, sizes, looks, colors, and abilities.

Preschool activities that promote cultural awareness and diversity include the following:

- Teaching children how to count in different languages
- Holding parties that celebrate children's different cultures and providing children opportunities to share about holidays, celebrations, art, and music that are special to their culture
- Providing food play sets of ethnically diverse meals
- Providing books that include pictures of children using assistive devices such as wheelchairs, crutches, glasses, or hearing aids
- Reading stories that share the experiences of children from different cultures or regions
- Providing dolls with various shades of skin color

or spiritual practices. Parents should understand that a preschooler's understanding of religious or spiritual matters is limited in the following ways:

- Having a very concrete conception of a god; seeing God as a physical being they can draw, talk to, and think about
- Enjoying simple rituals during worship, such as prayers and spiritual stories
- Potentially finding enjoyment from being able to see and touch religious representations such as statues, crosses, picture books, and crafts

Temperament

As the preschool child's life incorporates more activities outside the home, the child's temperament highly influences their ability to adapt to new social situations, adjust to group situations, adapt to distractions, moderate moods and intensity of reaction, and demonstrate persistence. In order for the child to be successful at school, their temperament must adjust to the new preschool classroom structure and circumstances. Parents can be of assistance by selecting a preschool environment that will support their child's temperament. For example, a classroom that does not restrict movement will better serve a child with an active temperament and extra energy.

Discipline

The preschooler needs to be allowed to develop a sense of initiative while learning self-control and rules. The child should have a consistent discipline experience and be guided by parental desire for appropriate and safe behavior. Teaching self-control takes time and patience, but the rewards include the child being able to behave appropriately while playing with other children or interacting with other adults. Over time, the preschooler learns how to avoid punishment or how to win rewards. Review the family's discipline strategies and maintain consistency while the child is hospitalized.

Family Relationships

Preschool children desire to please the significant people in their lives. They want to conform to the patterns, rules, and expectations of the family structure and fit in as an important part of the family dynamics. The young child is acutely aware of the roles and functions of each member of the family and develops an understanding of sex-role functions. A challenge for a child in the early preschool years is to feel comfortable with separating from parents for increasingly longer periods. This adjustment may start when the child enters a structured preschool educational environment.

Patient Teaching Guidelines

Appropriate Disciplining in the Preschool Period

The preschool child benefits from consistent discipline for unwanted or unacceptable behaviors. Guidelines for disciplining a child within the preschool period include the following:

- Time-outs should last, at maximum, the amount of time it takes for the child to understand and recover from whatever behavior was found to be unacceptable. This time frame varies, but a maximum is 1 minute for each year of age.
- Children in time-out should be placed in a quiet and restricted area where they can regain control of themselves and their behavior.
- Adults who apply discipline should be fair, firm, and consistent.

Tips to avoid situations that require discipline include the following:

- Parents and other authority figures should do their best to prevent children from putting themselves in situations that are unsafe.
- Explanations of the behavior that adults expect should be very clear and concrete.
- Parents and other role models should consistently demonstrate the behaviors that are desirable.
- Parents and other adults interacting with the child should notice when the child engages in desirable behaviors and compliment the child on it.

When the preschool child turns 4 years old, some undesirable behaviors may surface within family dynamics. For example, sibling rivalry may present with either older or younger siblings. The child may become disruptive by invading an older sibling's privacy or touching the sibling's personal possessions. If a 4-year-old perceives that parents or family members are asking too much of them, the child may act rebellious and aggressive, and provoke frustrations. Progressing into the fifth year, the child becomes more in tune with family expectations, desiring to help by doing simple chores or errands around the house. The child may also seek out the company of family members more. It is important that the young preschool child is supervised in their care of younger siblings. For instance, a 3-year-old should not feed an infant sibling without constant supervision because a choking episode can occur.

Enuresis

Enuresis is inappropriate voiding (urinary incontinence) after the child is successfully toilet trained, and it can be quite upsetting for the child and parent. Enuresis can happen during the day (diurnal) or at night (nocturnal). Enuresis may be associated with having diabetes; having a small bladder, a urinary tract infection (UTI), or an overactive bladder; or experiencing decreased antidiuretic hormone (ADH) or other problems. Constipation, if significant, puts pressure on the bladder and can be associated with the development of enuresis.

Preschool children may experience enuresis, or bedwetting, especially if the child is experiencing nightmares, any type of anxiety, or very deep sleep. Enuresis may be related to the child's inability to awaken to the physiological stimulus of a full bladder. It may also be related to excessive nighttime urine production or to the decreased functional capacity of the bladder. There are two main types of enuresis: primary, which is associated with symptoms only at night, and secondary, which involves daytime symptoms. Boys experience enuresis more often than girls. Enuresis can cause extreme frustration and distress and may cause disruptions in the child's social life. The family needs to be committed to management and treatment (Shroff, 2020; Tu & Baskin, 2022).

Enuresis can also be associated with regression, such as when a child is hospitalized or experiencing profound stress; when a child is the victim of abuse, especially sexual abuse; or when a new sibling is born. Parents need to demonstrate patience with their child and attempt to determine what led to the development of the enuresis. Treatment includes changes in evening fluid intake, scheduled night voidings, bladder training, counseling, and/or medications to increase ADH (Liara, 2019). For a complete discussion of enuresis, see Chapter 35.

• WORD • BUILDING •

enuresis: en–in + ur–urine + esis–action or process

Play

The preschool child actively engages in associative play, which does not have a common goal such as cooperative or organized play. In this type of play, preschoolers do the following:

- Interact and engage in a common activity with loose organization and rules.
- Exchange materials, although with hesitation, until each child is finished with materials being played with.
- May attempt to control or limit participation in activities or games.

Parents and caregivers should encourage associative play, but they must also remember that the preschooler needs quiet play that is creative, manipulative, constructive, and educational in nature. Quiet, creative play aids in the development of fine motor movements. Simple sewing projects in which the child uses thick yarn to lace through a design on cardboard, easy construction sets, and coloring projects provide for this type of quiet play.

Ideas for toy selection during the preschool period include toys that allow children to mimic adult activities and pretend-play adult work roles, such as:

- Play kitchens
- Construction kits
- Automobile play kits
- Tool chests
- Medical and nursing kits

Preschoolers should be offered no more than one repetition of a project per year of age. For instance, a 3-year-old will be able to concentrate on and have patience for decorating three holiday cards or coloring three eggs for a spring basket.

Preschoolers learn through play. If facing surgery or another medical procedure, a preschooler can participate in medical play to learn about the upcoming experience and demystify the equipment and procedure. Medical play also helps preschoolers act out their fears and emotions, providing an avenue for release of their feelings.

Team Works

Easing Fears in the Hospitalized Preschooler

Preschool children have great fears associated with body mutilation and require developmentally appropriate explanations in language they can understand. The entire health-care team should refrain from using complex medical terminology in front of a child because this unfamiliar vocabulary will frighten the preschool child.

Here are some ideas for how all the members of the team can ease a preschool child's fears during a hospital stay:

- Give change-of-shift report at the bedside, and direct it toward all members of the family who are present, including the child. Use words that are positive and support the preschool patient's understanding of what is being said. Clinical concerns should be shared without the child listening.
- Incorporate play into all areas of the preschool child's interaction with the health-care team. In a clinic environment, toys and books should be offered that provide appropriate distraction and comfort. In the hospital, play should be designed so that the child can participate regardless of their disease, medical condition, developmental level, or symptoms. Developmentally appropriate books that provide education about the child's condition, disease, and treatments or care should be provided, such as children's books on cancer, sickle cell disease, chicken pox, asthma, or diabetes.
- Respect the child's play time and try to conduct physical examinations and interventions outside of that time. If the nursing unit has a playroom, try not to conduct examinations or hang antibiotics or give medications while the child is in this safe play area.
- Whenever possible, designate the child's hospital bed as a "safe zone" for rest, play, and eating. Use the treatment room to perform painful procedures or examinations that produce discomfort.
- Use a friendly, playful tone when interacting with a preschool child. A playful tone fosters security and demonstrates respect to the child. Baby words or a babyish demeanor should not be used; rather, the health-care team should use a developmentally appropriate and playful conversational tone.
- Consult a child life specialist to provide play ideas and play supplies for preschool children. These developmental specialists are gifted in providing play opportunities to reduce a preschooler's fear surrounding hospitalization, diagnostic examinations, treatments and interventions, and separation from family.

Imaginary Friends

A preschool child may develop imaginary friends as an exercise in creativity or theatrical behavior. These friends or companions may be harmless and somewhat comforting for the child, but parents should be aware of the relationships and monitor their effect on the child's safety. Sometimes an object such as a teddy bear becomes personified; other times it is an imaginary child or pretend pal.

Imaginary friends can be very important if the child experiences periods of actual loneliness. The use of imaginary friends can come and go but may surface with consistency during life-changing circumstances, such as the loss of a grandparent, a geographical move, a divorce, or when a best friend moves away. Children generally have two types of imaginary friends: imaginary companions and objects that become personified. There may be a connection between having imaginary friends and a child's increased social skills, creativity in social interactions, and willingness to socialize with adults and peers (Gleason, 2017).

Parents should be reassured that imaginary friends are fairly common among preschool children (up to 65%; Gleason, 2017). They can ask the child about the imaginary pal, call the friend by name, and include the friend in games.

The child may blame the imaginary friend for certain behaviors, such as a lost item, a broken vase, or some other unwanted or unacceptable behavior. If the child begins to blame the imaginary friend for poor behavior, the parent should intervene. In simple and straightforward terms, the parent should remind the child that they are responsible for the behavior and will experience the consequence of it. For instance, if the child blames the imaginary friend for sneaking restricted food, the parents need to teach the child that, although the imaginary friend was "there," the child will still experience the discipline for the misbehavior.

Games, Arts, and Crafts

One of the joys of the preschool age is that children very much enjoy artistic and creative play. Box 20.3 lists ideas for engaging the preschooler in cooperative activities or solo ideas.

Cheating to Win

During the preschool period, children hate to lose at games or any simple competitive activity. Therefore, children may cheat in order to win. Parents need to understand that this is a normal part of the preschooler's development and not a character defect in their child. Because most of the simple board games or card games for this developmental period are won by chance, not strategy, children should be taught manners and truth-telling while engaging in a game.

Minimizing Technology

According to the American Academy of Pediatrics (AAP, 2020), preschoolers should not have more than 1 hour a day of any type of screen time—television, tablet, smartphone, or computer. Coviewing of high-quality programming with a parent or caregiver is the best way to have screen time, and technology use should never be used as an emotional pacifier. Charging of the device(s) should take place outside of the child's bedroom. Longer screen times have been linked to five negative consequences:

1. Watching a screen more than 2 hours daily has been linked to childhood obesity.
2. When exposed to screen time before bedtime, children have trouble falling asleep.
3. Children in elementary school who have TVs in their bedrooms tend to have poorer academic performance and lower test scores.
4. Children who watch excessive amounts of TV are more likely to participate in bullying behaviors, to have attention problems at preschool, and to show more signs of anxiety and depression as compared with children who have restricted screen time.
5. The more screen time a child participates in, the less creative and imaginative playtime the child has. Unstructured time in play is valuable for developing the brains of young children and improving social skills development and language development (Mayo Clinic, 2022).

Safe Toy Selection

Toy selection should begin with the parent, caregiver, or nurse evaluating the child's motor and cognitive abilities. Because all children are unique and have individual preferences, including the child in toy, game, or craft selection is ideal. When choosing toys, keep these points in mind:

- Preferable toys include those that are large, brightly colored, and challenging but that the child can master.
- Preschoolers enjoy giving the products of their play to important people as gifts. Games, toys, and crafts that require focused attention and produce an item that can be gifted are ideal.

Box 20.3

Preschool-Age Play Activities

All of the following preschool play activities can be easily implemented in a hospital setting:

- Making leaf banners by gluing festive leaves onto pieces of fabric
- Learning simple math by counting small objects of various colors, sizes, and shapes and placing them into organized piles
- Creating "fingerprint trees or animals" that represent the current season, such as a turkey or snow-covered trees
- Making a family photo album by gluing pictures to colorful paper and adding little shapes around them, such as frames with the person's name
- Creating a map of the hospital showing where the kitchen, nursing station, playroom, and elevators are in relation to the child's room
- Building a pinecone bird feeder by placing peanut butter into the cone, rolling it in bird seed, and then attaching a yarn hanger
- Creating jewelry pieces by stringing large beads or flavored cereal loops onto string
- Making tie-dye baby wipes by painting water-soluble colorful paints onto moist wipes and then drying them
- Assembling a sensory table where the child can explore the five senses by squishing, sifting, sorting, digging, and pouring; accept the mess, and let the child explore freely
- Creating a paper plate wind spinner by painting one side of the plate or making glitter-glue patterns, cutting the plate in a spiral, and hanging it with tape; a paper plate face mask can also be created
- Playing dress up with adult-sized clothing to recreate adult occupations (firefighter, police officer, nurse, physician, store keeper, gardener, auto mechanic)

- Because preschoolers have difficulty following rules, it is important to choose games that have simple rules.
- Most preschoolers place items in their mouths, so mouthing behaviors should be evaluated during play to ensure that the child is not placing anything dangerous into their mouth.

Protective Equipment

The preschool child is beginning to attempt greater independence and is graduating from one type of play equipment to the next, such as moving from tricycles to bicycles with training wheels and from scooters to large skateboards. This is the time in the child's life to insist on the use of appropriate protective gear.

- Make sure that the child is using protective gear that is the correct size and type for the sports played, such as shin guards for soccer; helmets for bike riding; and elbow pads, knee pads, and helmets for skateboarding.
- By setting rules for protective equipment early, the child learns their importance and remains safer in play.

Body Image

When speaking with a preschooler who is learning about the body, use correct anatomical language. Teach the child that parts of the body are private, but, in general, the body is normal and everyone is a little bit different. Encourage parents to speak positively about both sexes, teaching about the differences in simple explanations. The preschool child may ask many questions, including where babies come from and why. Using simple, straightforward explanations to answer the child's questions in an age-appropriate way is best.

One activity that can assist the child in developing a positive body image while learning simple anatomy is to have the parent trace the child's body while the child is lying on a large piece of paper. The paper can then be used as an educational tool. The parent names a body part, and the child draws it on the paper outline. Then, the child names the part with the new vocabulary word and colors it.

Sexual Development

According to Freud's theory of psychosocial development (McLeod, 2017), the preschooler experiences the phallic phase. In this phase, the child is finding their sexual identity by exploring the genitalia and masturbating. Although parents and caregivers are often uncomfortable discussing this issue, a preschooler who masturbates is engaged in perfectly normal, healthy behavior. Parents and caregivers must be prepared to encounter this behavior so that they do not pass judgment or show disdain. Parents will benefit from the following anticipatory guidance about the sexual development of the preschooler:

- When the child shows an interest in masturbation, set limits and teach privacy in a nonshaming way.
- The preschooler may cause family conflict as they compete against the same-sex parent, exhibit jealousy and

rivalry with that parent, and try to win the love of the opposite-sex parent.
- This phase typically resolves with a strong identification with the same-sex parent.
- The preschool period is also a time when children want to play doctor to examine the opposite sex. Although they do not understand the function of the genitalia, they want to know the differences between the sexes. Sexual curiosity is normal and can be expected during this period.

Preschool

Preschool is group childcare that occurs before the primary school experience and is not a part of general education mandated for minors. Not all children between 3 and 5 years of age are enrolled in a preschool; some families choose to provide a less structured day-to-day experience. Preschools can be public or private with more expensive preschools exceeding the financial limits of many families.

There are numerous benefits of preschool. It provides the child with social engagement, fine and gross motor development, play opportunities, and skill development in preparation for kindergarten. Children attending preschool have the opportunity to adjust to sociocultural differences and engage in a relationship with a teacher who guides them differently than their parents. Children from a limited peer-group experience, such as an only child, and children from families with limited resources particularly benefit from the preschool experience because it provides extensive stimulation and social interaction.

When is a child ready for preschool? Readiness for preschool is based on the child's emotional maturity, attention span, successful toilet training, and sense of autonomy. All of these factors will influence the child's ability to happily engage in a structured environment in which children are encouraged to participate in a well-planned set of activities, napping periods, shared mealtime, and outdoor play.

Parents who read to their young children, encourage learning, and provide a positive perspective on the preschool assist the child in coping with the newness of the preschool experience. The first day of preschool may pose a particular challenge for both the child and the parent. The parent should behave with confidence, positivity, and support. The preschool child carefully watches the parent's response to the new environment and relies on the parent's support and encouragement to enter and engage. If the parent is confident, excited, and ready, the child will see this and respond to the encouragement.

 ## ANTICIPATORY GUIDANCE FOR PARENTS WITH A PRESCHOOLER

Anticipatory guidance for the family of a preschooler continues to focus on health and safety, as it did for the toddler. Preschoolers, although more cautious than toddlers, can still end up in unsafe situations concerning traffic, swimming, and other hazards. Many preschoolers are at risk for injuries because of their inappropriate belief that they have higher skill levels than they actually do. Box 20.4 contains guidance for promoting the well-being of the preschool child.

Patient Teaching Guidelines

Share the following checklist with parents and caregivers to assist them in evaluating playgrounds for safety:

- Is equipment intact, without broken sections, sharp corners, or unsafe projections?
- Are wooden play structures free from weather damage and splinters?
- Is the general area free from litter, especially glass and motor oil spots?
- Is the area free from animal excrement?
- Do any slides have protective tunnels and an incline of no more than 30 degrees?
- Are slides cool to the touch?

Medical Concerns

The preschool child needs at least one well-child assessment by a pediatric health professional. This is often done as a requirement for entry into formalized childcare or a preschool classroom. Early identification of health problems in this period can assist in the prevention of later poor health consequences. Providing well-balanced nutrition and promoting early care of the child's emerging permanent teeth are important for the growing child's overall health and well-being.

Medication Safety

Preschool children need developmentally appropriate education about medications. For example, the reason they are taking a medication should be explained very simply: "to take your pain away," or "to treat your sore throat." Because preschoolers are magical thinkers, they may believe that they are required to take medication as a punishment for a previous wrongdoing.

Preschool children are unable to swallow pills effectively and may require that the pills be mixed or crushed, or that elixirs be created, which can be incorrectly calculated. In addition, they often refuse medications or fight off taking medications, putting them at risk for not finishing a prescription. Parents must be involved from the very start in the process of administering medications, especially ones that will be continued at home. Tips for parents administering medications to their preschool child include the following:

- Praise the child for adhering to medication scheduling and dosing.
- Never tell the child that medications are candy.

Box 20.4

Promoting Health and Safety of the Preschool Child

At the Clinic
- Evaluate the child's growth and mastery of developmental milestones with the health-care provider.
- Participate in recommended health screenings:
  - Blood pressure
  - Vision
  - Hearing
  - Body mass index (BMI)
  - Hemoglobin/Hematocrit
  - Lead
  - Tuberculosis, if at risk
  - Cholesterol, if at risk caused by obesity or other disease states
  - Evidence of abuse or neglect

In the Home and Community
- Administer scheduled immunizations: DTaP, IPV, MMR, and varicella.
- Evaluate the home for lead-based paint, peeling paint surfaces, or any chewable surfaces painted with lead-based paint.
- Ensure proper storage of household cleaning products, pesticides, and automobile solutions such as antifreeze and windshield wiper solutions.
- Ensure supervision of young preschoolers (3-year-olds) in the bathtub to prevent near or actual drowning accidents; they should not be allowed to play with the water faucet.

- Ensure presence of safety gates at the top and bottom of stairs to prevent falls and serious injuries.
- Maintain safety around pets and teach the child manners and gentle handling of family animals.
- Provide at least 12 hours of uninterrupted sleep per night.
- Promote safe eating habits and prevent choking by always having the child sit down to eat.
- Protect children from excessive sun exposure while outdoors. Protective clothing, application of a sunscreen with an SPF of 30 or higher on exposed skin (applied after swimming), and a hat are essential. Sunglasses protect the eyes from ultraviolet (UV) rays. Limit or avoid exposure to UV rays during the hours of 10 a.m. to 4 p.m.
- Ensure supervision of the child when climbing, swimming, using playground structures, and riding a tricycle or bicycle.
- Reserve both skateboarding and inline skating for children over 5 years of age because younger children do not have the developmental capacity to prevent injuries and protect themselves.
- Insist on the use of protective equipment for sports activities.
- Ensure that any firearms in the house are stored safely by keeping them unloaded, with trigger guards in place, in a locked metal storage container (gun safe) that is inaccessible to children of all ages.

- Do not allow the child to negotiate when to take medications. Minimize stalling behaviors.
- Allow the child to take the medication cup or oral syringe and place the medication into their mouth.

Dentition

Preschoolers shed their primary teeth in preparation for the eruption of their permanent teeth. Dental hygiene practices are important during these years because the enamel on a child's primary teeth is much thinner than that found on permanent teeth. Therefore, the preschooler must brush regularly to prevent caries (cavities), which can occur rapidly because the distance from the tooth's pulp to its surface is so short. Parents and caregivers should encourage the child to brush their own teeth while providing supervision to make sure that the child uses the appropriate amount of toothpaste and is thorough when brushing.

Pediatric nurses need to reinforce to parents that although the primary teeth will be shed, the health of these first teeth is very important to the well-being of the child. If the primary teeth develop caries, the decay and infection can affect the health of the permanent teeth located above or below them. In fact, severe tooth decay in primary teeth can lead to decay in permanent teeth that are budding.

Thumb Sucking

Some children continue to suck their thumbs into the preschool period. This habit provides the young child with a sense of security, but it can be disruptive to the child's tooth alignment. This is especially true if the behavior continues after permanent teeth erupt. It can be difficult to stop when the child is experiencing fears, especially around going to sleep, so some parents choose to apply over-the-counter products to the child's thumb or nails to provide an undesirable taste.

Health-Care Terminology

Because preschoolers are afraid of bodily harm, they may become fearful when around health-care professionals using medical terminology. Follow these tips:

- Make sure that preschool children are not present when parents are discussing specifics about their child's illness or injuries; otherwise, the child will become quite fearful. Have the parent step out of the child's room and discuss clinical status away from the preschooler.
- When the time comes to inform the preschooler of their medical condition or health state, contact a child life specialist. Child life professionals specialize in child development, medical play, typical play, and distractions and strategies for healthy coping. See the Team Works for a summary of child life services.

Medical Play

Preschoolers have a measurable reduction of stress and anxiety while hospitalized if they are offered the opportunity to participate in medical play (Children's Hospital of

Team Works

Child Life Services

Child life specialists are experts in child development. They promote effective coping through developmentally appropriate education, preparation, play, self-expression activities, and family advocacy. In collaboration with members of the health-care team and parents, child life can provide the following:

- Age-appropriate explanations of laboratory tests and other diagnostic tests
- Easing of fears and anxiety because of hospitalization, separation, or the unknown
- Fostering of emotional support, especially with chronic illness
- Advocacy for family-centered care
- Engagement of children and family members in special events, such as holiday celebrations
- Prehospitalization tours of the medical units, operating rooms, and clinics
- Support for siblings of pediatric patients who are affected by the child's illness or trauma
- Provision of health literacy through information and resources as well as engagement of parents whose children have similar health problems
- Collaboration with members of a multidisciplinary care team to provide a comprehensive plan of care and treatment

Philadelphia [CHOP], 2022). Play allows them to work through anxieties and fears associated with the unknowns of the health-care setting.

Beginning 3 or 4 days before the procedure, child life professionals can provide the child with mock situations. Medical kits, plastic syringes, cotton balls, adhesive bandages, tape, gauze, and stuffed animals or anatomically correct dolls can be used to simulate a previous experience or an expected experience (Fig. 20.5). Parents can help by encouraging their child to express themself during medical play. Aggression, anger, and sadness are normal responses that may be expressed during this play. Parents and health-care professionals should listen and watch to see if an explanation or correction is needed, such as when the child is playing out a presurgical experience.

Misconceptions are common in the preschool period, and medical play can be used specifically to help with misunderstanding. After a child is allowed to act out their feelings on the medical play equipment, it is appropriate for a health-care professional to then assist the child with misunderstood words or situations or to correct any magical thinking that has replaced accurate information. For instance, if the child is to have a central venous catheter placed in their chest the next morning, the child can be allowed to play with

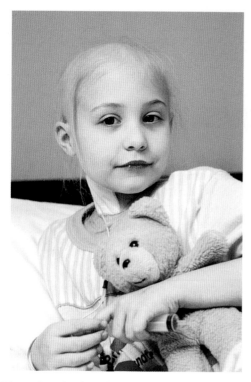

FIGURE 20.5 Preschool child using a syringe and bear during medical play. (From the National Cancer Institute. Photographer, Bill Branson.)

the equipment and medical doll first. Then, a member of child life can guide the child through the expected process to prevent any misunderstandings or provide simple answers to the child's questions about the procedure and after-care.

Special attention should be paid when a preschool child demonstrates fears of the unknown, body mutilation, pain, needles, loss of body function, or bleeding and when a child communicates a belief that the hospitalization or procedure is a punishment for misbehavior. See Box 20.5 for ideas for medical play.

Regression of a preschooler's previously acquired developmental milestones and skills is also a reaction to the stress

Box 20.5

Ideas for a Preschooler's Medical Play

Medical play provides the preschool child with a means of self-expression. When faced with feelings of anxiety about pending medical procedures and the unknown hospital environment, medical play can give the child the opportunity to work through emotions. Medical play includes the following:

- Playing with doctor's and nurse's kits, either made up with real equipment or commercially prepared toy kits for a preschool-age child
- Using medical materials to make collages
- Reading books about health-care experiences
- Painting with watercolors or tempera paints using syringes
- Using an anatomically correct doll to talk through the expected surgical or medical procedure

and anxiety felt during hospitalization. Parents who identify posthospital regression should not reprimand the child but rather assure the child that they acted bravely during a scary experience, and then go back to daily routines (National Child Trauma Stress Network, n.d.). The regression shown by a child after hospitalization may last a while and may be acted out in the preschool environment to teachers. Parents and teachers should remind the child that they are safe.

 ## SCREENING AND HEALTH PROMOTION FOR THE PRESCHOOLER

Health screenings are important to identify health issues in children as early as possible. Most states mandate or promote visual screening for preschool children. Children at this age are particularly vulnerable to myopia (nearsightedness) and amblyopia (double vision). Additional screenings should check for evidence of neglect or abuse, nutrition, obesity, and language development. Head Start programs offer height, weight, and blood pressure screenings for children in their programs. Preschool children also need booster shots for DTaP, IPV, MMR, and varicella.

 ## SAFETY AND THE HOSPITALIZED PRESCHOOLER

Preschool children are curious and explorative. Precautions must be in place to prevent injuries, accidents, and medical and medication errors when children are patients in the complex and often hectic hospital environment. To prevent abduction or wandering off the unit, many institutions require that young children wear a security alarm device on the ankle or wrist for rapid notification of a child leaving the nursing unit. Electrical outlets in the patient's room must have safety covers. And devices to prevent children from playing with IV lines are used to reduce the risk for injuries.

If a preschool child is left alone while hospitalized, measures must be taken to reduce the chance that the child will wander off in search of family members. If there are no hospital personnel who can safely monitor a young preschool child (3-year-old), the child may need to be placed in a high-top crib. Four- and 5-year-olds will need someone at the bedside or to be placed in a bed close to the nursing station for observation.

The best way to maintain an environment that is safe for the preschool-age patient is to have a family member remain with the child. Pediatric nurses should request that an extended family member such as an uncle or aunt, grandmother or grandfather, older sibling, or family friend come and stay with the child if the parents or caregivers cannot remain at the bedside. Under no circumstance should the preschool child be allowed to stay in a nursing unit playroom without constant supervision by an appropriate member of the family, health-care team, or hospital volunteer organization.

INJURY PREVENTION FOR THE PRESCHOOLER

Preschool children are curious and active. Pediatric health-care team members must provide anticipatory guidance to parents and caregivers on how to prevent injuries and accidents in the following six areas: drowning, poisoning, fires/burns, falls, sports injuries, and motor vehicle-related injuries. Preschool children should not play in the garage, kitchen, or yard without adult supervision. Because they do not yet transfer learning from one situation to another, preschool children must be taught safety in both their home environments and at school.

Patient Teaching Guidelines

Parents of preschool children must be taught to secure them in approved, appropriately sized, front-facing car seats in a back seat without airbags. Many preschool children can safely ride in a booster seat with snug-fitting straps over the shoulder and against the top of the legs. Children should not ride in a car with a seatbelt only until they are at least 57 inches tall (4 feet 9 inches, 144.78 cm).

DISORDERS OF THE PRESCHOOLER

During the preschool period, particular health concerns include common infectious diseases and **encopresis**, or soiling after completing potty training.

Infectious Disease

Preschool children are particularly vulnerable to common infectious diseases. These diseases include a variety of viral, bacterial, and parasitic infections (Table 20.3). Parents, preschool teachers, and health-care professionals need to know the basics of prevention and early recognition of the most common childhood infectious diseases to prevent the spread of disease to others and to minimize the risk of complications. Promoting healthy behaviors early in childhood can reduce illnesses.

Health Promotion

Teaching Preschool Children to Avoid Germs

Young preschool children require instruction, supervision, and support in learning how to reduce the chance of acquiring or spreading infections. Following are some healthy habits to encourage in the preschool child:

- Have children wash their hands immediately upon returning home from preschool. Research has shown that

· WORD · BUILDING ·

encopresis: en–in + copr–dung + esis–action or process

the common cold can be reduced by 50% in households with preschool children who are instructed to wash their hands upon coming home from school.
- Have children wash their hands right before sitting down to eat. Preschoolers often use their fingers as well as eating utensils when consuming snacks and meals.
- Instruct children not to share dishes, cups, and eating utensils with others to reduce the chance of spreading germs. Discourage them from feeding younger siblings bites of their food with their own eating utensils.
- Encourage children to wash their hands after they play outside to reduce the amount of soil, dirt, animal dander, and germs from playmates entering the house.
- Teach children to cough into their elbows, not their hands, to reduce the spread of germs.
- Teach children to use tissues when sneezing and blowing the nose. Often, young children wipe their noses on their sleeves or blow their nose into their hands and wipe mucus on their clothing.
- If a child is exposed to a cold or other infectious disease during play, wipe all toy surfaces with a commercial cleaner such as antiseptic household cleaning wipes.
- Clean thermometers after each use, even when used repetitively by the same child.

Patient Teaching Guidelines

Hand Washing for Preschoolers

Parents and caregivers of preschool-age children can use the following guidelines to teach children to wash their hands effectively:

- Provide a stack of paper towels that the child can reach with ease.
- Teach the child to make the water warm, not hot, when turning it on.
- After the child applies a small amount of liquid soap (preferably from a hands-free dispenser), instruct them to sing a song, such as "Happy Birthday," for the duration of lathering the hands up to the wrists.
- Demonstrate the need to pay special attention to the surfaces between the fingers and under the nails.
- Have the child rinse the hands by holding them downward under the flow of water.
- Teach the child to take a small supply of paper towels and dry the hands thoroughly. After turning off the faucet with the used paper towel, the child should then dispose of it directly into a hands-free wastebasket.

Encopresis

Encopresis, also called fecal incontinence or soiling, is a medical diagnosis given to a child 4 years or older who had previously achieved potty training and is now soiling their clothing

Table 20.3

Common Infectious Diseases of the Preschool Years

Disease	Infectious Agent	Spread By	Signs and Symptoms	Nursing Considerations
Chickenpox (Varicella zoster)	Varicella zoster virus	Close contact; airborne exposure via coughing and sneezing	The disease causes fever followed by an intensely itchy rash with lesions. The lesions resemble blisters with characteristic weeping that heal by developing yellow crusts.	The varicella immunization is very effective in protecting the preschool-age group.
Croup (Laryngotracheobronchitis)	Parainfluenza virus	Direct contact; airborne exposure via sneezing and coughing	Croup is marked by a very harsh and repetitive cough that has been compared with the sound of a barking seal. Typically, the coughing begins at night.	Croup is usually not serious and can be treated at home with moist air and oral fluids. Because children younger than age 5 have small airways, the symptoms are worse in these children.
Fifth disease (Erythema infectiosum)	Parvovirus B-19	Respiratory secretions	The virus causes a low-grade fever and a mild rash with a characteristic "slapped cheek" appearance on the child's face and a lacy red rash on the child's limbs and trunk that resolves in approximately 7 to 10 days.	Families must be taught to wash hands frequently and to teach the child to cover the mouth and nose when coughing or sneezing. Once the rash is present, it is unlikely that the child is contagious. Pregnant caregivers should understand potential risks for miscarriage or stillbirth.
Head lice	Pediculus humanus capitis	Close contact, especially when hats, sweaters, play clothes, bed clothes, sports gear such as helmets, and combs and brushes are shared	Lice infestations cause intense itching from the feeding and crawling behaviors of the adult lice.	Over-the-counter pediculicides are effective in the treatment of a lice infestation.

Children should not return to school until they are free of nits (louse eggs). |
| Impetigo | Group A streptococcus or staphylococcus | Direct contact | Small, round bacterial infections are common on the face and have a characteristic yellowish crust. | Young children should not be allowed to touch these lesions because the bacteria can spread or the lesions can get secondary infections.

Impetigo lesions do not produce scars. |
| Pertussis (Whooping cough) | Bordetella pertussis | Airborne exposure via sneezing and coughing | The hallmark symptom is an uncontrollable and violent cough, sometimes followed by vomiting. | The pertussis immunization is very effective in protecting the preschool-age group. |

Condition	Pathogen	Transmission	Clinical presentation	Health information
Ringworm	Dermatophyte (fungus)	A fungal infection spread by direct skin-to-skin contact	The child who presents with ringworm will demonstrate a red scaling ring on the skin, typically appearing 4 to 14 days after exposure. They may also demonstrate hair loss if infestations occur on the scalp.	Early treatment with antifungals can prevent complications of abscesses or cellulitis. Hand washing is the most effective means to prevent transmission.
Respiratory syncytial virus (RSV)	Respiratory syncytial virus	Highly contagious respiratory infection spread by contact with infected respiratory secretions via droplet or contact exposure	Symptoms of RSV infection in preschoolers are typically mild and mimic the common cold, which varies in severity.	Preschoolers do not have as high a risk for complications as infants do but can be very symptomatic. Infection is most common in the late fall and winter months. People are generally contagious for 3 to 8 days, and those with weakened immune systems can remain infectious and shed the virus for several weeks. Hand washing and disinfecting hard surfaces are required to minimize the transmission of the virus.
Rotavirus	Rotavirus	Fecal–oral route, though the virus can survive on surfaces	The child presents with severe diarrhea.	Virus follows a winter seasonal transmission pattern, is self-limiting, and only lasts for a few days for those children with a healthy immune system. The rotavirus vaccine is effective in preventing the associated gastroenteritis.
Strep throat	*Group A streptococcus*	Highly contagious via saliva	The classic infection causes severe sore throat and pain on swallowing.	Parents should seek medical attention for fevers greater than 38°C (100.4°F), pus on the back of the throat, sore throat symptoms lasting for more than a week, or known contact with someone with strep throat. A throat swab confirms the infection. Antibiotics treat this infection and children should not return to preschool until cleared by a health-care provider.

Safe and Effective Nursing Care

Strep throat is associated with pain. Children as young as 3 years can use a Wong-Baker FACES pain scale to rate their pain subjectively. The caregiver provides the child with a tool that depicts a series of face pictures from a smiling face to a crying face; the child picks the picture that most represents their pain level.

The FLACC pain tool can also be used for children from the ages of 7 months through the school age period. Here the caregiver determines the pain level by matching the five areas (expressions on Face, positioning and movement of Legs, Activity level, Cry, and Consolability) to rate the child's level of pain.

during the day. These children experience severe constipation and colon stretching and a decreased sensation that they need to pass stool. A diagnosis of encopresis requires ruling out Hirschsprung disease and megacolon, both of which are much harder to treat (see Chapter 34). This baffling, unexpected, and highly embarrassing fecal soiling is frustrating for both the child and the parents. Encopresis affects up to 3% of children between 4 and 12 years of age (Nemours KidsHealth, 2024).

Stool collection, retention, and impaction in the colon begins the process of encopresis. With the enlargement of the colon, the intestinal walls and the nerves located within them stretch, causing a diminishing of nerve sensation. Eventually, the child will lose the ability to contract and push the stool out. The child with encopresis does not have the sensation or urge to defecate, and the stool is passed without them feeling it until after defecation has occurred. As the intestinal wall continues to stretch, large, hard stools are retained and liquid stool is released by seeping or leaking out around the fecal mass. Typically, soiling occurs in the late afternoon after school.

Risk factors for encopresis include the following (Mayo Clinic, 2019):

- Medications that cause constipation, such as cough syrup
- Anxiety
- Depression
- Attention deficit-hyperactivity disorder (ADHD)
- Autism spectrum disorder

Other symptoms include severe constipation with abdominal pain, lack of appetite, avoidance of bowel movements, and the passage of such large stools that they frequently clog the toilet. Some children are prone to this condition because they are born with colonic inertia, or a tendency toward constipation. Parents often express exasperation that their child neither feels the soiling nor, with daily repeated exposure, notices the odor. However, encopresis is a medical problem that requires intervention and is not an emotional, behavioral, or developmental issue.

Encopresis is a chronic problem, but it is treatable:

- The child must sit on the toilet several times a day in an attempt to pass at least a half-cup–sized stool. Some parents accomplish this by setting a timer in the bathroom and requiring the child to sit for at least 10 minutes.
- The child's diet must include high-fiber foods (fresh fruits and vegetables; dried fruits, such as raisins and prunes; high-fiber cereals, breads, and whole grains) and lots of water.
- The family must work together to diminish the emotional aspect of this condition during the long treatment.
- The overall treatment goals are for the child to have a daily normal bowel movement; to reduce stool retention and heal the stretched large intestine; to have the child gain control of defecation; and to resolve any bad feelings, such as guilt, frustration, and family conflicts, that may have arisen because of the symptoms of encopresis.
- Limiting or eliminating consumption of cow's milk and other dairy products may alleviate symptoms of this disorder.

Nursing Care Plan for the Child With Encopresis

Billy, a 4-year-old boy, is brought to the clinic by his frustrated mother who states, "I thought he was potty trained, but he's started pooping in his pants again!" Billy is experiencing encopresis with expulsion of stool in his clothes on the way home from preschool each day. The mother feels helpless about the situation and has started carrying an "emergency bag" with nitrile gloves, cleansing wipes, zip-top plastic bags, and a change of clothes for Billy.

Nursing Diagnosis: Constipation related to inconsistent patterns of elimination and stool retention

Expected Outcome: Child will produce a daily stool on the toilet.

Interventions:	Rationale:
The family will plan for daily consumption of fiber-rich foods such as fruits, vegetables, and whole grains and will provide the child with adequate oral fluids throughout the day.	*Fiber-rich foods, fluids, and time on the toilet will assist in the passage of normal stools and decrease the chance of stool retention, constipation, and leakage of water stool.*
The child will sit on the toilet no less than three times a day for several minutes to encourage passage of stool.	

Nursing Diagnosis: Bowel incontinence related to watery stool seeping around hardened stool
Expected Outcome: The child will develop, over time, a normal stooling pattern with soft, formed stool passed daily.

Intervention:	Rationale:
The family will assist the child in a process of patiently staying on the toilet for increasing amounts of time until at least a half cup of stool is passed.	*A plan of action to assist the child in passing stools every day will decrease the chance of bowel incontinence and seepage of watery stool in the child's undergarments and clothing.*

Nursing Diagnosis: Anxiety and emotional distress related to the discomfort of incontinence
Expected Outcomes: The parents will verbalize the child's progress in establishing a regular daily stool pattern; the child will no longer experience anxiety, social isolation, or embarrassment.

Interventions:	Rationale:
The parents will describe steps to help their child establish a daily stooling pattern and will provide support to each other and to their child during the process.	*Having education and support during this stressful and embarrassing condition may decrease anxiety about the training process and outcomes.*
The child will be given support and positive reinforcement for consuming high-fiber foods, drinking adequate fluids, and at least three times daily trying to pass a stool on the toilet.	

Key Points

- The preschooler time period begins at age 3 years and ends right before the child's sixth birthday.
- The preschooler experiences rapid language development, often through imitation.
- The young preschooler remains egocentric and slowly learns to identify another person's point of view or feelings. Preschoolers have very active imaginations and enjoy play that allows them to act out adult roles.
- Because of magical thinking, the preschooler makes a minimal distinction between what is reality and what is fantasy, believing they can cause actual events.
- The preschool child fears body mutilation, death, and blood and may show signs of regression in response to these fears.
- Parents and caregivers should allow the preschooler to develop a sense of what Erikson calls initiative by allowing the child to try out new skills and develop new roles.

Review Questions

1. You should explain to the parents of a preschooler that they can expect their 3-year-old child to be able to accomplish which skills? (**Select all that apply.**)
   1. Tie shoelaces
   2. Skateboard
   3. Ride a tricycle
   4. Use a jump rope
   5. Climb a small play structure

2. A 4-year-old child has been admitted to the inpatient pediatric unit for a course of antibiotics to fight cellulitis. Which bed assignment is most appropriate for this preschooler?
   1. In a bed in a single room away from the other children
   2. In a high-top crib
   3. In a multibed room with three other children
   4. In an isolation room to prevent the spread of the infection

3. Which behavior demonstrated by a preschooler would confirm that the child is in an appropriate developmental level?
   1. She takes her oral antibiotic without hesitation.
   2. She cries loudly when her mother leaves the hospital room.
   3. She is distressed about a scar from a previous abdominal surgery.
   4. She is requesting a ballerina bandage after having her blood drawn.

4. Which condition can occur when a preschooler frequently scratches skin lesions?
   1. Secondary bacterial infections
   2. Cellulitis in opposing arm
   3. Scabies infection
   4. Neurological symptoms

5. Which infection experienced by a 5-year-old child in a preschool center must be reported to all parents?
   1. Facial cellulitis
   2. Strep throat
   3. Pediculosis
   4. UTI

6. A preschooler is requesting to have the same lunch for school every day. What would be appropriate teaching for the parent?
   1. "That is unacceptable, and variety is required for sound nutrition."
   2. "That is OK; your young child will change his mind soon enough."
   3. "Try having him take leftovers from last night's dinner."
   4. "Try to have the preschooler pack his own lunch the night before."

7. What would the pediatric nurse most likely think is the reason for a preschooler describing her teddy bear as being in the hospital because she was "naughty"?
   1. Separation anxiety
   2. Magical thinking
   3. Sensorimotor cognitive stage
   4. Egocentrism

8. What heart rate would a pediatric nurse expect to find in a preschooler who is 4 years old?
   1. 65 to 110 bpm
   2. 120 to 125 bpm
   3. 60 to 85 bpm
   4. 50 to 65 bpm

ANSWERS 1. 3; 5. 2; 3. 3; 4. 4; 1. 5; 2. 6; 7. 2; 8. 1

CRITICAL THINKING QUESTIONS

1. What behaviors would you expect from a preschooler demonstrating regression during hospitalization?
2. What health screenings would be worthwhile to conduct in a preschool classroom located in a high-risk neighborhood with families whose incomes are around or below the federal poverty threshold?

Resources

For additional resources and information, including Postconference Questions and Activities, Answers, and References, visit www.FADavis.com.

Student Study Guide

CHAPTER 21
Health Promotion of the School-Aged Child

KEY TERMS

bullying (BUL-ee-ying)
concrete operations (kawn-KREET aw-puh-RAY-shunz)
deciduous teeth (dih-SIJ-oo-uss TEETH)
precocious puberty (pree-KOH-shuss PYOO-ber-tee)
prepubescence (PREE-pyoo-BESS-ents)
puberty (PYOO-ber-tee)
reactivity (ree-ak-TI-vuh-tee)
sexual latency (SEKS-yoo-uhl LAY-ten-see)
temperament (TEM-pr-uh-muhnt)

CHAPTER CONCEPTS

Comfort
Communication
Growth and Development
Health Promotion
Nutrition
Safety

LEARNING OUTCOMES

1. Define the key terms.
2. Describe the unique needs of the school-aged child in relation to safety, socialization, and communication.
3. Evaluate the slower growth period that represents the school-age time period.
4. Compare the nutritional needs and eating patterns of the school-aged child, including accurate kilocalorie and fluid maintenance calculations.
5. Contrast the play and sleep patterns of the school-aged child in relation to the other developmental stages.
6. Discuss the issue of safety for the school-aged child, including the need for education about safety equipment for organized sports, bike riding, skateboarding, and roller skating.
7. Describe the teaching needs of the entire family of a school-aged child in relation to prevention of child abduction, sexual abuse, bullying, and other forms of violence.
8. Define the effects of bullying, including cyberbullying, on a school-aged child's emotional health and well-being.
9. Critically evaluate the health concerns associated with the current epidemic of childhood obesity.

CRITICAL THINKING

Phillip is 10 years old and is at the clinic for a well-child visit. His height is 127 centimeters and his weight is 49.10 kilograms. According to the growth chart, Phillip's height is in the 25th percentile, but his weight is in the 95th percentile. His body mass index (BMI) indicates that he is obese. You document Phillip's measurements, which are reported to the health-care provider. A dietitian is called for a referral for the family and meets with the mother to openly discuss the findings as well as the medical risks and social problems associated with childhood obesity. For 3 weeks, Phillip and his mother record a daily food log of his intake. The log is then analyzed by the dietitian, who notes that the child consumes a lot of fast food and foods high in corn syrup but very few fresh fruits and vegetables. The entire family changes their eating habits and participates in a 6-month-long physical activity program. At the checkup 1 year later, Phillip's height remains in the 25th percentile, but his weight is plotted in the 50th percentile.

Continued

CONCEPTUAL CORNERSTONE
Health Promotion

Because the school-age period is the longest of the five developmental stages of childhood, spanning 7 years, it is important for you to be aware of the child's and family's ongoing health education, nutrition, activity and exercise, well-child checkups, and immunization needs.

Part of educating patients and families about health, wellness, and illness is to understand the developmental and cognitive abilities of children in this stage. Pediatric nurses can provide opportunities for school-aged children to learn about their health and allow them to gain a sense of accomplishment through educational projects and activities. A school-aged child's ethnic and cultural background strongly influences views on life; responses to illness, injuries, and hospitalizations; and participation in health and wellness programs. Making a habit of health and wellness early in the school-age stage will allow the child to enter adolescence in optimal health.

The "school-aged" developmental stage spans from the sixth birthday through the 12th year of life, ending at the child's 13th birthday. This developmental stage, also referred to as "the middle years," is marked by tremendous emotional, linguistic, and cognitive development but slower physical growth than occurs in the younger stages. Growth will speed up again during the adolescent period.

According to Erikson's psychosocial developmental theory (McLeod, 2018a), school-aged children need to master industry, or achievements, and gain confidence. If they fail to navigate this stage successfully, they may experience a sense of inferiority. School-aged children need many opportunities to demonstrate academic, social, and cognitive achievements to learn to perceive of themselves as successfully industrious (Fig. 21.1).

GROWTH AND DEVELOPMENT OF THE SCHOOL-AGED CHILD

Overall growth and development of the school-aged child follows a slower, steadier pattern until the child hits the rapid growth spurt of preadolescence.

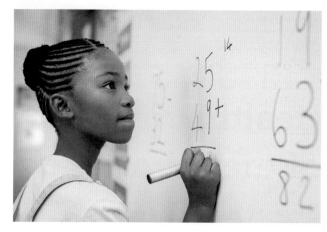

FIGURE 21.1 The school-aged child develops a sense of industry that provides the child with purpose and confidence in being successful.

Physical Growth and Development

Physical development of the school-aged child begins with shedding of the **deciduous teeth** (primary or baby teeth) and ends with the beginning of puberty. During middle childhood, the average weight gain for boys and girls is 1.81 to 2.99 kg (4 to 6.6 lb) per year and the average height increase is 2 inches (5.08 cm) per year. By the end of this developmental stage, children will have doubled their weight and grown 1 to 2 feet (30.48 to 60.96 cm) in height. School-aged children become more graceful in their movements and play and are steadier on their feet. Activities such as bike riding, skateboarding, inline skating, skiing, and climbing become more comfortable and much easier. As the middle years progress, the child becomes taller and thinner in appearance. Muscle tissue replaces fat with the child's body weight gradually representing more muscle tissue and less adipose tissue. In the school-aged child, muscles and bones are still growing and are not as functionally mature as they will be in adolescence. School-aged children experience a decrease in their head circumference growth and an increase in their leg-length growth. The skull itself experiences very little growth over these years, and the growth of the brain also changes relatively slowly.

Body systems become more mature and functional. Blood glucose levels are maintained well, requiring less snacking and less prompt feeding times. The total caloric requirement decreases depending on the level of vigorous activity the child engages in. School-aged children who participate in energetic sporting activities will need higher levels of daily calories. Bladder capacity is variable with girls typically having a larger bladder capacity than boys. The immune system now functions efficiently and can launch both an appropriate antibody response and a localized inflammatory response to the presence of injury or infection.

The greatest variation during the school-age period is at the end, when children are reaching their 13th birthdays. Variations in height, weight, motor ability, coordination, and emotional maturation are noticeable, and many children are quite sensitive

Health Promotion

Musculoskeletal Health and the School-Aged Child
Promoting muscle and bone health in the school-aged child requires some common sense to avoid strains, sprains, and repetitive stress injuries. For everyday wear, children require solid, well-fitting shoes; they require specialty shoes for specific sports. Children should not carry heavy backpacks or book bags to and from school. Ideally, schools should offer children desks that are appropriate for their height and handedness because they spend many hours per day sitting in them.

Children in these middle years need to avoid injuries from overuse or overconfidence. Both soccer and gymnastics are examples of sports where injuries are common in the school-aged developmental period. To prevent injuries, children need to balance practice and games with rest, follow the advice of experienced coaches, and learn their physical limits.

CLINICAL JUDGMENT

Scenario #1: You are providing teaching for parents of a school-aged child on injury prevention related to overconfidence after they tell you they just bought their child a new bike.

Questions

1. What learning needs (cues) would you check for before teaching?
2. What solutions (goals) would you want for the teaching session?
3. How would you know the parents understood the information provided?

to these variations. Be honest about and supportive of these differences. Assure the child that they are just about to enter a time of tremendous growth during adolescence.

Prepubescence, the time period right before puberty, starts toward the end of the school-age period and is marked by the development of secondary sex characteristics. The process takes an average of 2 years, ending with the child's ability to reproduce. Secondary sex characteristics include body hair, breast development, testicular and penile growth, and body odor. This is also a time of rapid growth of bones and muscles. Educate the child and family about the nature and timing of these body changes because prepubescence is a time of great variability, embarrassment, and possibly negative self-image. **Puberty** normally begins in girls between the ages of 8 and 12 and in boys between the ages of 9 and 14. For boys, the first sign of puberty is testicular growth and a

Who Is at Risk for Precocious Puberty?

Factors that place a school-aged child at risk for the development of precocious puberty include the following (Texas Children's, 2024):

1. Female sex; girls are statistically more likely than boys to develop this condition
2. African American descent
3. Being significantly overweight or obese
4. Having medical conditions such as congenital adrenal hyperplasia, hypothyroidism, or McCune-Albright syndrome
5. Being exposed to estrogen or testosterone in creams, ointments, adult medications, or dietary supplements

red-lined scrotum with pubic hair at the base of the penis. For girls, the first signs of puberty are breast buds and pubic hair.

Precocious puberty is puberty that begins before the age of 8 for girls and before the age of 9 for boys. In girls, breast development before the age of 7 in Whites and before the age of 6 in Blacks signals precocious puberty. The cause of this condition often cannot be found; therefore, it is called **idiopathic** precocious puberty (Box 21.1). Rarely, conditions such as hormone disorders, tumors, infections, injuries, or brain abnormalities cause precocious puberty to develop. Symptoms of both puberty and precocious puberty include the following:

- *For girls:* Breast growth and first period (menstruation)
- *For boys:* Enlarged testicles and penis, facial hair starting on the upper lip, and a deepening of the voice
- *For both girls and boys:* Pubic hair, underarm hair, early rapid growth, adult body odor, and acne

If warranted, the treatment for precocious puberty includes the administration of medications to delay further development. The child continues to receive the medication until the normal time of puberty, at which time the medication is stopped and the process of puberty continues. These medications are the same "puberty blockers" that some transgender children take to prevent the development of secondary sex characteristics inconsistent with their identified gender.

Nutrition

Because the school-age period is marked by slower growth in both height and weight, the school-aged child needs to eat responsibly with appropriate portion control. Obesity is a major health problem in the United States, and the school-aged child, if not supported to make healthy decisions, may face this challenge. The school-aged child spends more time away from the family with longer school days and more social events. Food choices become more independent as the child eats more with others, attends parties, and participates in peer-related activities away from the family such as socializing during computer gaming or other types of screen time. Nutrition education should begin in the early school-age period, and the child should be encouraged to share their growing knowledge of healthy eating with the family. Choosing to consume fresh fruits and vegetables as well as whole grains daily is one of the most important lessons the child can learn.

Until the preadolescent growth spurt, school-aged children, on average, need fewer calories per kilogram of body weight than infants, toddlers, and preschoolers (Faizan & Rouster, 2022). School-aged children, on average, need only 1,500 calories for the first 20 kilograms of weight plus 25 calories for each additional kilogram over 20.

Promoting intake of well-balanced meals is a major responsibility of the nurse when working with school-aged children. It is imperative to offer meals that include a variety of healthy, low-fat choices and to discourage consumption of fast foods and candy.

Patient Teaching Guidelines

School-aged children like sweets and are drawn to high-calorie, low-nutrition foods, so the use of sweets as rewards or "bribes" may seem logical. However, food should never be used as a reward for good behavior, whether in the home, hospital, or other health-care settings.

Sleeping Patterns and Requirements

Sleep is very important to the school-aged child's success in school (Fig. 21.2). Children in these middle years may avoid going to sleep, engage in stalling behaviors, have difficulty falling asleep, or experience difficulty staying asleep as they contemplate concerns and worries. School-aged children may seek comfort during the night in the form of a hug or a drink of water. Knowing that they are not alone may help them get back to sleep.

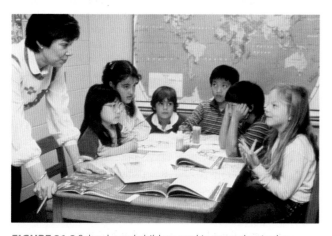

FIGURE 21.2 School-aged children working together in the classroom.

The school-aged child needs 10 to 12 hours of sleep per night. Although they may not sleep in as long as an adolescent, when given the opportunity, they may enjoy staying in bed longer on the weekends. Lack of sleep causes a tremendous decrease in the child's energy at school and may cause poor academic performance. Sleep needs to be prioritized, and the school-aged child needs a predictable routine and a reasonable bedtime each night. Any TV, computer, video game, or music player in the child's room should be turned off while the child is attempting to go to sleep. A child needs time to unwind before sleep, and some children may still enjoy being read to at bedtime.

Patient Teaching Guidelines

One important topic to discuss with families is the need to set limits on the use of technology right before bedtime. Technology use at bedtime may cause the child to have difficulty going to sleep. Parents need to set limits on when the technology, or screen time, should be shut off to allow the child to participate in a relaxing bedtime routine.

Cognitive Development

Cognitive development of the school-aged child is marked by an increase in the ability to think both more abstractly and more concretely and to begin to make rational judgments. Academic work highly influences the child's thinking and cognitive development. Box 21.2 provides examples of tasks

Box 21.2

Tasks Related to Cognitive Development in the School-Aged Child

- Learning to read: The child goes from learning to read to reading to learn, from reading single words to understanding the meaning of what is read, and from stumbling slowly to read aloud to fluency and correct pronunciation.
- Fully developing a sense of time, space, cause and effect, nesting (building blocks, puzzle pieces), reversibility, conservation (permanence of mass and volume), and numbers, including the distance between numbers and their meanings
- Understanding the relationship of parts to the whole (fractions) and being able to focus on projects in which objects are divided into parts, put back together again, and taken apart in a new way, all representing one whole
- Learning to classify objects in more than one way (color and shape and size)
- Becoming interested in collections, board games with rules and rationales, and card games with progressively more difficult challenges (from "Go Fish" to hearts)
- Learning to spell and to use the dictionary
- Moving from very concrete ways of thinking about and interpreting the world to more abstract, logical, and meaningful views
- Moving from a very egocentric, carefree world to one with problems, concerns, worries, and empathy

that influence the cognitive development of the school-aged child. Factors such as nutrition, stimulation, and health can influence the cognitive development of school-aged children (Ranjitkar et al., 2019).

The school-aged child's teacher may be the first important adult in the child's life other than the child's parents. This relationship of teacher and child shapes the child's understanding of who they are, how to interact with others, and how others perceive them. A strong teacher will positively influence the child's cognitive development, social skills, manners, and self-esteem. It is imperative that the child be allowed creativity in the classroom to test out various skills. School is often referred to as the child's "job" during this developmental period. Homework becomes very important, and the middle-school child's sense of identity may be highly influenced by the quality of their work and the grades earned on academic projects.

Psychological Growth and Development

According to Erikson (McLeod, 2018a), the school-aged child must have already mastered the developmental stages of trust, initiative, and autonomy to be ready for the next stage of industry. *Industry* can be defined as the child's sense of worth. A school-aged child's sense of worth can come from within or may be influenced by the social environment or relationships with others, either within the family or outside of it. School-aged children need opportunities to assist with classroom structure and function and to interact positively with adults and those with authority.

Nurses can encourage a child's sense of industry by offering the child a task to perform while hospitalized. Drawing pictures of new ways to design a playroom, coming up with games for younger children, or drawing maps between rooms and the fire alarms/escapes are examples of ideas to promote a sense of accomplishment and success. The child's concepts of successes and failures are very important to the child. If a child is experiencing a chronic illness, encouragement to master a task at the level of the child's ability will be important and should be planned for. For example, children with juvenile idiopathic arthritis (JIA), known previously as juvenile rheumatoid arthritis, or JRA, may experience a sense of accomplishment and industry if they are encouraged to complete their activities of daily living (ADLs) on their own or to take their medications by themselves. These successes should be followed by acknowledgment and praise. Look for situations and opportunities that allow school-aged children to feel that they have contributed to and accomplished important responsibilities and tasks.

Sigmund Freud's theory of psychosexual developmental stages (McLeod, 2017, 2021) identifies the school-age period as one of **sexual latency:** a time when sexual desires are lessened. Sexual drives are dormant or hidden (latent) while the school-aged child focuses attention on schoolwork, hobbies, friends, and expanding socialization and independence. In the early psychosexual stage of infancy, the mouth is the central focus. During toddlerhood, the anus is the central focus. During the latency period, these previous experiences are in the past, and the focus on the genitalia that occurs in adolescence has not yet started.

Piaget's theory of development (McLeod, 2018b) describes the school-age time period as one categorized by **concrete operations,** the beginning of logical thought. This stage begins around age 7 or 8 and continues to about 11 to 12 years of age. Children in this stage of development are gaining a better understanding of their world through logical thinking about concrete events; however, they still struggle with abstract or hypothetical concepts. Piaget believed that school-aged children begin to use inductive reasoning and logic to determine a particular outcome of a certain event. One important development in this stage is the child's understanding of the concept of reversibility, the awareness that actions can be reversed. For example, a child may understand that her pet is a turtle, the turtle is a reptile, and a reptile is an animal. The mental process of reversibility allows the child to understand that the reverse order of the relationship progression in this example is also true.

Socialization

By far the most important social developments of the school-aged child are the relationships they develop with their peers. School-aged children spend less time socializing with their parents and families and branch out to establish new relationships. With these new relationships come certain developmental expectations: (a) The child progresses from free play to play that may be elaborately structured with rules and is able to interrelate with peers according to the rules; (b) the child progresses from informal social structures during play to the demands of formal teamwork, such as baseball, basketball, and soccer; and (c) the child learns to participate in social structures within the classroom, including group projects or group oral or written reports. At this stage, children demonstrate tendencies to be either leaders or followers (Box 21.3).

Box 21.3

Is Your Child a Leader or a Follower?

- *Leaders:* If a child is a leader, the child exhibits confidence in social situations. Leaders are not afraid to take risks in front of their peers and may volunteer to answer questions, take charge in a group project, or be a team captain in a sports activity. A school-aged child leader will be first to volunteer and first to get involved with activities. The child should be praised for this independence but encouraged to learn how to include and involve others who do not demonstrate leadership and would rather "follow the pack."
- *Followers:* If a child is a follower, the child likes to watch how others make decisions and perform. Followers watch and mimic the behaviors of other children and wait to see what others are going to do in an activity. If a child follows the behaviors of someone who is a bully or disrupts class, then the teacher or adult will need to encourage the child to get involved with peers who are a better influence. Followers need to learn assertiveness skills in order to stand up for themselves and not let others control or boss them.

Table 21.1

The Social Domains of the School-Aged Child

Family	*Friends*	*School*
The child wants very much to be accepted in the family structure. As the child spends more time away from the home and family life in other social activities, afterschool activities, and sports, the need to feel part of the activities and togetherness of the family increases.	The school-aged child desires "best friends" as well as membership in social groups. Same-sex friends are the most important. The school environment and friendships made there highly influence a school-aged child's self-perception. Bullying and negative social peer interactions at this time can be devastating with long-term consequences on self-image and self-worth.	School teaches the child what is expected in terms of self-discipline, classroom expectations, and homework performance. Standards of conduct, what is right and wrong, what is acceptable and what is not, and what consequences can happen for undesirable behaviors are all learned during the school-aged child's academic experience.

The school-aged child learns that self-discipline is very important, especially in the area of homework. Completing homework is a requirement for academic success, and the need for self-discipline to do it increases each year as the child progresses in school. If the school-aged child has successfully resolved the crises of the early psychosocial periods and is trusting, autonomous, and full of initiative (Erikson's theoretical stages), then they will easily learn to be industrious and demonstrate the behaviors required to succeed.

The school-aged child learns how to behave and respond to others through interactions with family, friends, and the school environment (Table 21.1). The influence of these three areas affects how children feel about themselves and how they will interact with others later in life.

Moral Development

According to Kohlberg's theory of moral development (Kurt, 2020), the young school-aged child sees rules and behavioral standards as coming from the expectations of those around them. Rules are not established from within but, rather, are created, established, and enforced by others. As children grow and develop, their perception of rules begins to come from within as they interpret actions as either wrong or right. For school-aged children, feelings of guilt may present if they have conducted themselves poorly or made decisions that they consider wrong.

School-aged children need standards in order to learn what is expected of them and whether or not their choices and decisions will be acceptable or perceived as wrongdoings. Experiencing punishment, such as a loss of privileges (recess, playtime, screen time, dessert), will influence the actions of the school-aged child. Rewards provide motivation to behave and can assist in guiding a child's judgment when making decisions between right and wrong. Young school-aged children may still engage in magical thinking (common through the seventh year) when they experience grief (Marie Curie, 2022) and interpret accidents, injuries, and misfortunes as punishment for bad behavior.

Older school-aged children begin to judge a behavior, act, or outcome by the intention of the act, not by just the consequence. Rules are perceived as more authoritarian. Older school-aged children are very keen on learning what exactly the rules are, how they are enforced and by whom, and what the consequences are of breaking the rules. Children can reflect on their intentions to act, contemplate their own reasons for action, and begin to predict the consequences of the act on others' feelings and perceptions.

Children in the school-age period are, according to Kohlberg, in Stage Two of moral development, the emergence of moral reciprocity. They have learned the difference between right and wrong, what makes adults happy, and the basic consequences of actions. In Stage Two, children begin to focus on the instrumental, pragmatic value of an action. The rightness of an action may depend on the child's understanding of reciprocity, the idea that a certain stimulus "deserves" a certain response. For example, the school-aged child can apply the Golden Rule, "Do unto others as you would want done to you," as easily as the statement "If someone hits me, I am going to hit back." According to Kohlberg's theory, the school-aged child is processing situations with the rules but choosing to apply rules only when it is in the child's immediate interest. Deals, agreements, and equal exchanges are prevalent in the child's social interactions. The school-aged child's concrete thinking and individualistic sense of self benefit from guidance to learn that, beyond self-interest, it is important to pursue what is just and right for others.

Spirituality

During this longest period of childhood development, school-aged children explore their thoughts and beliefs around spiritual topics. Religious children's perception of God evolves as they progress toward adolescence. The young school-aged child typically perceives God according to teaching by family members or religious teachers. The older school-aged child begins to develop independent thoughts about their system of beliefs. The young school-aged child prefers spiritual information that is concrete, systematic, and logical, whereas the older school-aged child is able to think about spirituality in a more abstract way. Many children in this developmental period enjoy learning about their family's religion and are comforted by prayer and their beliefs. Participating in spiritual activity may be a coping mechanism for school-aged children who experience stress (Nauli & Mulyono, 2019).

Temperament

Temperament, also called **reactivity**, is a set of traits that influences behaviors. For the school-aged child, temperament is very much related to previous behavioral patterns or reactions to past situations. As children grow, they interact with their environment, having experiences that shape their reactions. Some school-aged children have what is considered a very "easy" temperament. These children fit in smoothly to new social situations, are flexible to schedule changes, do not react with passion when they encounter difficult situations, and generally are easy for peers and adults to relate to. Other children are slow to warm up to new people and situations, which they may perceive as a threat, and they exhibit a certain level of social discomfort. This discomfort may present as shyness or mild aggression. These children need advance notice of change, time to adjust to new circumstances, and encouragement to engage with others at their own speed.

The temperaments of parents and children influence how a family interacts. If a highly organized parent has children whose temperaments express spontaneity, disorganization, impulsivity, and easy distractibility, the parent may find family time a challenge. How siblings relate to each other also is influenced by temperament.

Family Dynamics

School-aged children typically enjoy participating in family activities, regardless of the family's structure or size and regardless of the age difference between or among siblings. School-aged children enjoy planning activities, special events, and even vacations and often request that all family members participate in an activity. This valuable family time brings members together and solidifies the family structure.

Patient Teaching Guidelines

Unlike children with an "easy" or even a cautious temperament, a child with a difficult temperament has strong, negative emotional reactions to new situations and experiences. Teach parents to offer these children rehearsals or practice situations in which they can try out the new situation and become accustomed to the new perceived demands. Raising, teaching, or providing nursing care to a child with a difficult temperament requires special skills, including patience, authoritarianism, consistency, support, firmness, prediction, and great understanding.

Each pair of family members has a unique relationship. A child will relate differently to each parent as well as to each sibling. Because the school-aged child can be quite sensitive to these different relations, family time is paramount. As much as possible, a family should try to spend time together in recreation every week. Participating in family meetings helps with both the planning of recreation and the feelings of togetherness (Box 21.4).

The school-aged child becomes fully aware of the social roles and responsibilities of each family member. The young school-aged child discovers what parents do for a living and takes pride in discussing these roles and responsibilities at school with peers. For older school-aged children, there is a realization of the meaning behind these roles. They learn to understand the experiences behind their parents' working roles and learn to adapt to variable schedules, demands, work time needed at home, and financial limits on family decisions.

Some ideas for family time with school-aged children include the following:

- Family movie night
- Cooking a special meal together
- Playing board games or video games
- Collaborating on larger family chores or projects
- Decorating the home for seasonal holidays
- Making homemade birthday gifts from recycled materials, craft supplies, and found objects
- Looking through old family photos or home movies
- Participating in church camps or special events
- Having a picnic in the park, backyard, or even the living room

Box 21.4

How to Create and Implement a Family Meeting

- The meeting should occur at a regular and convenient time for all family members.
- The parent(s) should serve as the leader(s) of the discussion and make sure that all ground rules are followed, such as allowing all members to have a chance to speak and share ideas and thoughts.
- The meetings should have the goal of emphasizing what members view as family needs, plans, and accomplishments, discussing positive efforts by each member.
- At no time should any family member experience criticism, interruption, or be held back by ridicule when sharing ideas and thoughts.
- All children should understand that the parents have the final say when difficult decisions are being made and that children are considered valuable "consultants" to the family decisions.
- Records should be kept that document goals, ideas, rewards, positive behaviors, and any new agreements.
- The family meeting should end with everyone sharing their perspectives about how the meeting went and what could be done to strengthen or improve future meetings.

Play

Play continues to be an important part of a school-aged child's daily life. Young school-aged children enjoy competitive games in which same-sex teams compete. Through this early team play, children learn to cooperate and negotiate, and they learn how important rules are. Through team play, the school-aged child develops a sense of belonging, cooperation, and compromise. Although a young school-aged child may cheat to win, they quickly learn that cooperation yields greater social rewards than winning alone. School-aged children often join in afterschool sports such as soccer, basketball, swimming, or baseball. Through these activities, the school-aged child learns to participate in group activities and to answer to an authoritative figure other than a parent or teacher. Groups offer a testing ground for the child to experiment with interpersonal interactions, assertiveness and self-concept, and sex-role behaviors.

During the school-age period, the child often develops their first true friendship. The concept of "best friend" becomes important. The child and their best friend share secrets, pass notes, and use private code words. It is important for a parent to determine the impact of this intense relationship to make sure that the child continues to be social and engaged with others.

Play during the school-age period also enhances the development of morality as the child conforms to social norms, customs, and expected behaviors. Despite this newfound moral sense, cheating may continue throughout the school-age period, even when the child knows perfectly well what the rules are. Over time, play may shift from a group focus to the more intimate recreation of video games and handheld devices.

ANTICIPATORY GUIDANCE FOR PARENTS OF A SCHOOL-AGED CHILD

Parents of school-aged children should be taught about safety, nutrition, obesity prevention, good dental practices, and the need for vigorous daily physical activity. Other anticipatory guidance should include the following:

1. Promoting school attendance and the value of consistently being on time and well-prepared for each school day
2. Promoting successful homework behaviors through designated study time, proper lighting, and a good desk/table and comfortable chair
3. Preventing back injuries caused by heavy book bags and backpacks
4. Establishing rules for afterschool activities and about checking in with parents
5. Discussing developmentally appropriate information on keeping safe after school to avoid physical harm, bullying, abduction or sexual assault, and other forms of societal violence
6. Establishing limits on "screen time" whether via video games, TV, or handheld electronic devices

7. Requiring the use of helmets and pads to prevent sport injuries; having the child properly fitted for shoes
8. Teaching the child ways to reject offers to use tobacco, illicit drugs, alcohol, and other illegal and harmful substances
9. Teaching the child ways to set personal boundaries, reject sexual advances, and report unwanted touching or sexual comments
10. Preventing dental caries and gum disease through consistent brushing and flossing at least twice daily
11. Allowing for sufficient high-quality sleep for 9 to 11 hours a night (not less than 7 hours and not more than 12 hours per night; National Sleep Foundation, 2022)

CONCERNS OF THE SCHOOL-AGED CHILD

During the school-age years, children are exposed to several common infectious diseases, viral illnesses, and bacterial infections because they are spending more time away from their family and homes. School-aged children's better hand washing and more robust immune systems prevent them from having many of the respiratory and skin infections that are common to preschoolers. However, school-aged children are still vulnerable to head lice. (For more about head lice, see Chapter 20.) Obesity is a growing health concern in this age group, and overweight and obese children are often the targets of bullying, the other concern discussed in the following section. Asthma, also common to this age group, is covered in detail in Chapter 30.

Obesity

Childhood obesity is defined as a BMI that is at or above the 95th percentile on a national growth chart (Centers for Disease Control and Prevention [CDC], 2022a). Childhood obesity is now considered an epidemic in the United States.

Although it varies geographically, the overall rate of childhood obesity prevalence has reached a range of 19.7% with a range of 12.7% to 22.2% (CDC, 2022b). The causes and consequences of obesity are summarized in Table 21.2.

The severity of childhood obesity is identified by calculating the child's BMI. This calculation is performed by dividing the child's weight in kilograms by height in meters squared. Parents should be shown the result of the child's BMI and growth chart measurements. If the child's measurements are at or above the 95th percentile for weight for two consecutive plots on the growth chart, initiate a referral to a registered dietitian for the child and the family. The dietitian can provide the family with immediate interventions concerning diet, food selections, and ideas to promote activity.

Encourage children to learn good eating and exercising habits by visiting the interactive website at www.MyPlate.gov. The site includes learning activities on nutrition appropriate across the school-age developmental period.

Table 21.2
Causes and Consequences of Childhood Obesity

Causes of Childhood Obesity	*Consequences of Childhood Obesity*
Lack of physical activity related to too much "screen time"	Social difficulties, such as isolation, bullying, teasing
More calories consumed than expended, especially in the form of high-calorie/low-fiber fast foods	Financial costs, such as increased family food and health-care costs, increased national health-care costs
Genetic factors, such as the genetic mutation of leptin-melanocortin pathway, which controls energy regulation and hunger (Children's Hospital of Philadelphia [CHOP], 2021)	Poorer health outcomes, such as development of diabetes, hypertension, heart disease
Family/cultural dietary habits including access, preferences, and preparation	Child obesity may be influenced by family decisions and cultural practices

Team Works

Team Management of Childhood Obesity

- A team approach is required to assist families in committing to a plan of decreased total caloric intake along with increased physical activity. The entire family should be a part of the healthy eating and exercising plan.
- Nurses and health-care providers need to make referrals to health-care specialists in the area of childhood obesity. Making a referral to a registered dietitian is imperative for long-term weight management in children. Nurses can also make referrals to food banks in the community that provide free or low-cost nutritious foods.
- A social worker and/or a child or family psychologist can help the child and family work on the emotional issues that may be related to being overweight or obese and offering support during weight loss.
- An exercise physiologist can work with the child to set goals for exercise that are safe, effective, and individualized and that reduce the chance of injuries.
- At no time should the team working with a family with an obese child use the word *diet* or discuss *dieting*. *Healthy food selection, healthy food preparation, healthy eating,* and *increased physical activity* are phrases that should be used by all team members.
- When an overweight or obese child comes into the clinic or hospital, accurate measurements should be made each time the child is seen, and the results should be shared with the interdisciplinary team.
- The health-care team members must feel confident in talking openly to parents about the risks and long-term consequences of obesity (bullying, hypertension, musculoskeletal disorders, heart disease). Conversations should be open, frank, supportive, and goal-oriented to the child's health.

The emotional factors associated with childhood obesity cannot be ignored. Bullying, discrimination, and social isolation can all occur for a child with obesity. Nurses working with children and their families should evaluate children for these serious emotional factors and with approval from the health-care provider can assist the family by making a referral for additional counseling and support.

Bullying

Bullying is defined as aggressive behavior among children that is unwanted and demonstrates a feeling of perceived or real power imbalance (Stopbullying.gov, 2019). School-aged children, especially children who are overweight or obese, are at risk for experiencing bullying at some time during this developmental period. Many more are at risk for witnessing bullying behavior, which can be traumatic. Bullying is a very real and devastating experience that can have long-term consequences on a child's social life, self-esteem, mental health, and overall life. Nurses must screen for bullying and report findings to parents who may not have been told about the experience (Table 21.3). According to StopBullying.gov (2021b), 28% of 6- to 12-year-olds experienced bullying and 30% of youth admitted to bullying others. In addition, 70% of children have witnessed bullying (StopBullying.gov, 2021b). The child who is severely bullied must be referred for immediate help from parents, teachers, and school administrators. Disclose severe bullying to other members of the health-care team because the child might benefit from a referral to a child psychologist.

Another form of bullying is called cyberbullying. Here, bullies use technology such as e-mails, texts, social media, apps, short message service (SMS), forums, gaming, and photographs as a form of bullying against another child. Cyberbullies use all types of digital devices to humiliate, threaten, or embarrass another child. As many as 15.7% to 16% reported being cyberbullied (StopBullying.gov, 2021b). It is important for nurses caring for children to understand local laws because some forms of cyberbulling

Nursing Care Plan for the Obese School-Aged Child

Tasha, who is 9 years old, presents to the urgent care facility and reports severe back pain and knee pain. Her weight plotted on a growth chart is over the 99th percentile for her age and height. Tasha states that she started an exercise program during the day preceding the visit and experienced the onset of pain late last night. She has made several negative comments about her body since she entered the examination room.

Nursing Diagnosis: Body image; disturbed as evidenced by critical statements of self-image
Expected Outcome: The patient will converse with the staff about a healthy body image.

Intervention:	Rationale:
Health-care staff will openly ask about Tasha's lifestyle and her self-image and allow her to discuss her feelings and experiences.	*School-aged children need to have honest discussions with health-care professionals about how they are feeling and what their needs are. This child needs guidance and support to implement safe and healthy changes to her diet and activity patterns.*

Nursing Diagnosis: Altered nutrition: intake exceeds body needs as evidenced by weight in the 99th percentile on growth chart
Expected Outcome: The patient will verbalize specific, measurable goals for healthier eating and exercise patterns.

Intervention:	Rationale:
You will teach the patient about making healthy nutritional choices and choosing safe, low-impact exercises.	*Tasha needs information about how to eat more healthfully and to exercise safely to avoid injury. This child needs guidance and support to implement safe and healthy changes to her diet and activity patterns.*

Table 21.3

Identifying and Preventing Bullying and Cyberbullying of the School-Aged Child

Examples of Bullying and Cyberbullying Behavior	*Signs of a Bullied Child*	*Ways to Prevent or Stop Bullying or Cyberbullying*
• Punching, shoving, and other acts that hurt people physically • Spreading negative rumors about people • Keeping certain people out of a group • Teasing people in a mean way • Getting certain people to "gang up" on others • Sending mean texts, e-mails, or instant messages • Posting nasty pictures or messages about others in social media • Using someone's username to spread rumors or lies about someone else	• Appearing sad, lonely, anxious; suffering from low self-esteem • Feeling "sick" without other symptoms • Having suicidal thoughts • Coming home with torn, damaged, or missing pieces of clothing, books, or other belongings • Coming home with unexplained bruises, cuts, or scratches • Expressing fear of going to school, walking to and from school, riding the school bus, or taking part in organized activities with peers	• Determine the extent of the problem. • Establish a code of conduct in the home and classroom and on the playground. • Establish and consistently enforce consequences. • Provide supervision before and after school as much as possible. • Build students' sense of community. • Distinguish between "ratting" or "tattling" and "reporting." • Train all school personnel how to evaluate bullying and about antibullying interventions. • Conduct school-wide antibullying activities using role-modeling and play-acting with positive resolutions. • Teach children to maintain a "poker face" (emotionless and expressionless) if they are teased and/or bullied. Showing embarrassment and anger gives bullies what they want—the knowledge that they have upset the child. • Teach children that it is every student's right to inform staff of what is going on and it is every student's right to attend school without being bullied or teased. • Encourage a child who is experiencing cyberbullying to turn off the technology that is providing a means to be cyberbullied, to not respond, and to immediately report the bullying behaviors to a responsible adult.

are unlawful and are seen as a form of criminal behavior (Stopbullying.gov, 2021a).

It is important that when a nurse caring for children identifies evidence of bullying, the child's experiences need to be acknowledged and support provided. A child who is being bullied is at risk for emotional distress and depression and may participate in self-harm. A referral must be made to assist the bullied child, promote their safety, and identify risk factors for further self-harm, self-injury, or lasting emotional distress (Stopbullying.gov, 2019).

CLINICAL JUDGMENT

Scenario #2: You are assisting with a well-child visit for **Kim**, an 8-year-old, when you note that they start to cry when you ask how things are at school.

Questions

1. What questions could you ask Kim to probe for possible bullying?
2. What specific actions should you take when Kim confirms the bullying?

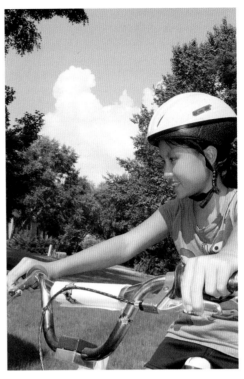

FIGURE 21.3 School-aged child with a protective helmet.

Safety *Stat!*

It is essential for parents of a bullied child to take the problem seriously. Extreme bullying has been associated with depression, anxiety, and suicide. Serious and lasting consequences can occur if a child who is bullied does not receive interventions and support. These consequences include mental health issues, school dropout, substance use disorder, self-harm, and suicide. School shooters, in the majority of cases, had been victims of bullying (Stopbullying.gov, 2021a).

 ## INJURY PREVENTION FOR THE SCHOOL-AGED CHILD

School-aged children are at risk for a variety of injuries. Because of their interest in trying new sports and activities, it is imperative to provide children and their parents with information about injury prevention (Fig. 21.3). Safety information should address topics such as sports and other physical activities, the proper use of protective gear, automobile safety, water safety, caution around strangers, safe and unsafe touching, and firearm and fireworks safety. For information on preventing dog bite injuries, see Box 21.5.

- *Sports safety:* Parents should not allow a child to participate in a sports activity until the child is physically and developmentally ready to do so. School-aged children should try out for sports and have experienced coaches determine if the child is ready to participate. Any child

Box 21.5

Preventing Dog Bite Injuries

1. Never approach a dog that is not known to you.
2. If a dog is tied up, restrained, in a car with the window open, or behind a fence, do not approach the dog.
3. If the dog is accompanied by its owner, ask if you may approach or touch the dog.
4. Do not approach a dog that is eating, chewing on a toy or bone, or that is caring for puppies.
5. Do not yell, squeal, or make loud noises near a dog because it will become startled and will take a defensive stance.
6. Read the dog's moods; if the dog is angry or frightened, do not approach the dog. Look for signs of anger such as bared teeth and fur standing up on the dog's back. Look for signs of a frightened dog such as tail down, ears back, and curled up in a ball. Do not approach any dog that does not show signs of happiness such as relaxed ears and a wagging tail.
7. Allow the dog to smell your hand before you touch the dog anywhere else on the dog's body.
8. If you feel threatened by the dog, do not scream and run. Stay still, keep your arms to your side, face forward to the dog, and look down. If you run, the dog will consider it a chase.
9. If you are attacked by a dog, try to put something between your face and head and the dog's mouth. If you have a backpack, textbook, purse, or jacket, use it as a shield.
10. If you continue to be attacked and are knocked over, curl up in a ball, hold your arms over your head, and put your hands over your ears. Again, do not scream or roll around; you want the dog to get bored and lose interest in you.

who experiences a head injury and loses consciousness must be seen by a health-care provider. Emergency transport may be required.

- *The use of protective gear:* School-aged children must consistently wear protective equipment and padding for contact sports or activities such as scootering, snowboarding, or bicycling. For more about bicycle safety, see Box 21.6.
- *Skateboarding safety:* Children should be taught the importance of not riding in the street and should be brought to skateboard parks and taught the rules. At a skate or skateboard park, supervision is required to prevent injuries to young children who are riding near older children who are faster and have higher levels of skill. Never allow a child to "catch a ride" from a car by hanging on to the back of a moving vehicle.
- *Inline skating and roller-skating safety:* Skaters are prone to injuries. Children should be taught how to slow down and stop and how to protect themselves from falling injuries. They should never go down sloping paths.
- *Avoiding trampolines:* Trampolines are notorious for causing injuries and should be avoided. If necessary, only trampolines with secure-fitting safety nets should be allowed and only with adult supervision.
- *Automobile safety:* School-aged children should always wear seatbelts. Young school-aged children may benefit from using a booster seat if they are petite. Check state laws concerning each age group and required car-safety devices. Some states continue to require booster seats for children between 4 and 8 years of age and up to 80 pounds. Children who weigh less than 120 pounds and who are under 5 feet tall should not be in a seat with an emergency airbag. All children aged 12 years and under should be required to sit in the back seat.
- *Water safety:* School-aged children may act much more independently in water than younger children. They must be reminded about water safety and should not swim alone or unsupervised. Goofing off, rough play, dunking, and unsafe diving must be controlled to prevent water injuries or drownings.
- *Stranger safety:* Many school-aged children are "latch-key children," meaning they are home alone after school. Parents should insist that the child not tell others (in person, on the telephone, or in a text) that they are alone. School-aged children must also be taught to be cautious of strangers. People who prey on children may try to lure them close by asking for directions or seeking help to find a lost puppy. Even though they may want to be helpful, children need to learn how to refuse such requests and to quickly get away from potentially dangerous situations.
- *Touching:* Health-care professionals caring for children must teach them that no adult or older child has the right to touch them in a way that makes them feel unsafe or uncomfortable. Nurses and other health-care providers should offer simple explanations for why they need to touch the child and, whenever possible, ask the child's permission to touch them. It is imperative that children discuss their concerns about unsafe or uncomfortable touching with a trusted adult.
- *Firearm safety:* Guns must be stored unloaded with ammunition in a separate, locked area of the house. Ideally, both firearms and ammunition should be secured in a steel gun safe. School-aged children are particularly vulnerable to firearm injuries and death; therefore, in homes where firearms are present, precautions should include frequent family discussions on gun safety and no-touch rules.
- *Fireworks safety:* Every year, children lose fingers, hands, and sight because of the misuse of fireworks. School-aged children need constant supervision around fireworks and should never be allowed to light them themselves. Parents should model safety precautions used when lighting fireworks and teach children to stand a safe distance from lit fireworks.

Box 21.6

Bicycle Safety

Children must follow the law and wear snug-fitting bicycle helmets that meet national standards. Helmets that are damaged or too small must be replaced. If the child's forehead is showing, then the helmet is too small. Teach your patients the following guidelines for safe bike riding:

- Ride close to the curb or on designated bike paths.
- Use hand signals when turning and allow plenty of time for cars to see the hand signal.
- Ride in single file.
- Yield to pedestrians.
- Only allow one person on a bike at a time.
- Keep both hands on the handlebars.
- Place reflectors and lights on the bike if riding will be done at dusk or at night (however, young children should never ride at night).
- Wear shoes that protect the feet while biking; do not wear loose sandals or flip-flops.
- Be aware of the cars around you; be especially careful in parking lots where cars may be backing up; and look left and right twice before turning.

Safety *Stat!*

Sexual predators pose a very real danger to an unsuspecting child. They find children through social networks and chat rooms and then present themselves as peers with similar interests, sports, and hobbies. Predators gradually gain trust and make the child feel as if they have an emotional investment. Once trust is established, the predator will then seek to set up times to meet the child in person. Children must be taught to be cautious of any virtual friends they "know" only online.

Patient Teaching Guidelines

Tips for Parents for Safe Internet Use

Suggestions for parents to ensure safe internet use include the following:

- Use content blockers and filters for younger children to prevent access to explicit material that may be frightening and shocking.
- Investigate the use of tracking software for older children, which enables parents to see which sites children have visited.
- Periodically verify sites to encourage safe and selective usage. Not all adult sites post industry ratings that can be identified by filter, blocker, or tracker software, so reinforcing family internet usage guidelines is important.

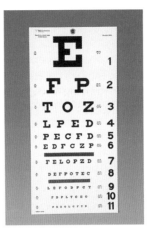

FIGURE 21.4 Visual screening chart used for school-aged children; Snellen standard chart.

 ## SCREENING AND HEALTH PROMOTION FOR THE SCHOOL-AGED CHILD

School-aged children require routine health screenings to ensure positive growth and development in all areas of their life. Simply put, healthy children learn better. Children who don't hear well cannot understand classroom presentations and discussions. A child who cannot see the blackboard or screen will miss out on vital parts of a classroom lesson. School nurses may conduct hearing and vision screenings, or they may help coordinate screening services. School nurses should tell teachers about the types of screenings being conducted so that teachers can help to identify children who display hearing or vision problems in the classroom. The Labs & Diagnostics feature provides information about essential health screenings for school-aged children.

Labs & Diagnostics

Essential Health Screenings for the School-Aged Child

Specific protocols should be followed and may vary per school, district, or state.

- *Immunizations:* Immunization boosters that school-aged children require include tetanus, diphtheria, and pertussis (TDaP); measles, mumps, and rubella (MMR); and inactivated poliovirus (fourth dose). In addition, Gardasil 9 (human papillomavirus [HPV] vaccine) for both boys and girls, meningococcal Group B vaccine, and an annual influenza shot are recommended.
- *Hearing screening:* School-aged children should have their hearing screened annually, or at least four times between kindergarten and eighth grade. The American Speech and Hearing Association recommends that an audiologist train screeners. Children with odorous discharge or drainage from their ears should have their hearing checked as soon as possible. Furthermore, if a child is easily

distracted, frustrated in group learning, has difficulty finding the source of a sound, or needs repeated verbal instructions, hearing screening should be immediately recommended. (See Chapter 28 for more information.)
- *Visual screening:* School-aged children should have their vision screened annually, or at least four times between kindergarten and eighth grade. Most children are visual learners, so it is imperative that vision problems are diagnosed and corrected to promote academic success. According to Prevent Blindness America (2015), one out of four school-aged children is affected by vision problems. If a child's vision is found to be 20/40 or less, a second screening should take place. The Snellen chart is still considered to be the most reliable and is the most widely used instrument for visual screening (Fig. 21.4). (See Chapter 28 for more information.)
- *Scoliosis:* School-aged children should be screened for scoliosis at least once before sixth grade. (See Chapter 33.) This screening checks for any abnormal curvature of the spine and determines its severity. If a curvature is found, the child should be referred for an x-ray. Because the screening often includes forward bending to check for a rib hump; obvious curves; and uneven shoulders, waist, or hips; a similar-gender screener should be used. Privacy is essential because clothing may need to be partially removed or lifted during screening.
- *Child abuse screening:* School-aged children should be evaluated for physical, emotional, and sexual abuse or exploitation as well as neglect. School-aged children should also be evaluated for the presence of safe afterschool supervision and for problems with delinquency.
- *Lice screening:* School-aged children should be screened monthly for head lice. (See Chapter 20.) Some school districts allow and encourage parent volunteers to be trained for lice screening.

Continued

• WORD • BUILDING •

scoliosis: scoli–crooked, bent + osis–condition

Labs & Diagnostics—cont'd

- *Dental screening:* Schools are encouraged to coordinate a volunteer team of dental specialists to screen children's teeth at least once in the early school-age period. Poor dental health may affect a child's academic performance, especially if the child is in chronic pain from dental disease or severe caries.
- *Blood pressure screening:* School-aged children should have their blood pressure screened at least every 2 years. Elevated blood pressure in children is not commonly found. However, early identification and treatment are correlated with the prevention of heart disease, stroke, and kidney disease in later life. It is imperative that a correct-size cuff is used because children in the school-age developmental period can vary greatly in body size and shape. The width of the rubber bladder should cover 75% of the child's upper arm. Only trained health professionals should take blood pressure.
- *BMI screening:* Annual BMI screening is needed in light of the national epidemic of childhood obesity. Volunteer screeners should be trained by professionals, and a national standardized chart should be used to interpret the results. Screening children with potential or actual weight problems can contribute to positive health outcomes. Sensitivity and positivity should be used when discussing results with the child and family.
- *Well-child visits:* Well-child visits need to be encouraged by school staff on an annual basis. The completion of all vaccines and assessments for high-risk areas are covered.

Schools notify parents of upcoming health screenings, and parents have the right to refuse to have their child screened. Confidentiality agreements must be signed for any organization or individual outside of the school system who performs health screenings on children. In addition, states vary in their mandates concerning contacting parents about the findings of the health screening. Many states encourage the nurse to participate in the "rule of threes," attempting to contact a parent or guardian three times concerning the need for a referral if the health screening produces results that require follow-up. It is imperative that the school nurse document the findings as well as the details of contact with, or attempts to contact, the family. Sending written communication home with the child is not recommended and may not be allowed by certain states.

SAFETY AND THE HOSPITALIZED SCHOOL-AGED CHILD

One of the most important areas of nursing care of the hospitalized school-aged child is to observe for maladaptive responses such as anger, resentment, and hostility. Hospitalizations are stressful. Although children in this developmental period do not suffer the same intensity of separation anxiety as younger children do, being apart from family is stressful and frightening and can lead to regression, aggression, and feelings of isolation. Even if a school-aged child acts stoic when parents have to leave the hospital, you should provide the child with company, social interaction, play therapy, and distraction. Observe for behaviors of isolation because of school absenteeism, lack of peer contact, and increased dependence on caregivers.

Providing comfort and pain control is an important role for you when caring for a school-aged child who is hospitalized. Children at this developmental level can use subjective pain tools and should be encouraged to describe their pain, state its location, and respond to a numeric pain scale tool.

Key Points

- The school-age stage of growth, also considered the period of middle childhood, spans the longest developmental period and lasts from the child's sixth birthday to the 13th birthday.
- During this period, physical growth is slower, but social, developmental, communicative, and cognitive growth expand dramatically.
- According to Erikson's theory, the school-aged child must accomplish the task of industry or else feelings of inferiority develop. The feeling of industry is associated with achievements at school. The experience of school is highly influential on the child's self-esteem.
- Younger school-aged children experience the shedding of deciduous, or primary (baby), teeth and the eruption of the permanent or secondary teeth.
- Older school-aged children experience the changes associated with entering puberty, such as the growth of pubic hair, the development of body odor, breast development, menarche, and changes in testicle and penis size.
- School-aged children are prone to musculoskeletal injuries and must be guided to wear protective equipment and padding while participating in sports.
- Parents need anticipatory guidance concerning keeping the school-aged child safe and healthy. Prevention of tooth decay, injuries, and obesity are all important.
- Immunizations needed during the school-age period include TDaP, MMR, inactivated poliovirus (fourth dose), HPV vaccine, meningococcal Group B vaccine, and an annual influenza shot.

Review Questions

1. Evan, an 11-year-old, has been hospitalized for a fractured femur caused by an all-terrain vehicle (ATV) accident while his family was on vacation. The injury requires 2 weeks of traction, and you note that Evan appears bored and restless. Applying developmental theory, which of the following do you select to distract Evan? **(Select all that apply.)**
   1. A multichapter adventure book on pirates in the seven seas
   2. A board game requiring multiple players
   3. A deck of cards to play solitaire whenever he chooses
   4. A video game for two on the large screen in the playroom
   5. An electronic device that plays simple mathematical games

2. The parents of 7-year-old Heather bring her into the clinic for advice on her third pediculosis infestation in the last 6 months. Her mother describes Heather's intense interest in the performing arts and shares that she has been in two musicals in the last year. What advice from you is most appropriate?
   1. Take a break from the theatre performances because it may be taking away from her homework.
   2. Encourage more dress up at home and less participation in children's theatre.
   3. Describe the importance of not sharing costumes with others and keeping personal items in a plastic bin away from other performing children.
   4. Be alert to other childhood parasite infestations because lice are one of many the child might be exposed to in these developmental years.

3. Which of the following factors are associated with the development of childhood obesity? **(Select all that apply.)**
   1. Genetics
   2. A sedentary lifestyle
   3. A high-fat diet
   4. Depression
   5. Social isolation

4. According to Erikson, the greatest influence on a school-aged child's readiness to master this stage of development is:
   1. Mastery of the first three stages of psychosocial development
   2. Acknowledgment of the child's strengths and weaknesses
   3. Participation in school activities so that the child can demonstrate "industry" or accomplishment
   4. Support from parents on taking on new sports challenges

5. While providing care at a summer camp for children, you are approached by a counselor who asks what prepubescence is. What explanation is correct?
   1. The time period of initial sexual organ development
   2. The time period of intense emotional fluctuation
   3. The time period just before sexual maturity
   4. The time period when menses first occurs

6. _____ _____ begins before the age of 8 for girls and before the age of 9 for boys.

7. Six-year-old Josie refuses to play outside with the other children because "Mommy says that I shouldn't get my dress dirty." What developmental theory explains Josie's behavior?
   1. Piaget's theory of cognitive development
   2. Erikson's theory of psychosocial development
   3. Freud's theory of psychosexual development
   4. Kohlberg's theory of moral development

6. Precocious puberty; 7. 4

ANSWERS 1. 2, 4; 2. 3; 3. 1, 2, 3, 4; 5. 3;

CRITICAL THINKING QUESTIONS

1. What factors might lead school-aged children to be at risk for violence, isolation or supervision problems, and delinquency?

2. When does a school nurse need to become involved if a child is experiencing severe bullying?

3. How might a nurse effectively discuss the subject of obesity with a family of an obese child?

Resources

For additional resources and information, including Postconference Questions and Activities, Answers, and References, visit www.FADavis.com.

Student Study Guide

CHAPTER 22
Health Promotion of the Adolescent

KEY TERMS

acne vulgaris (AK-nee vul-GAR-iss)
alcohol abuse (AL-kuh-hol ab-YOOSS)
anorexia nervosa (AN-uh-REK-see-uh
ner-VOH-suh)
bulimia (boo-LEE-mee-uh)
cyberbullying (SYE-ber-BUL-ee-ying)
gender dysphoria (JEN-der diss-FOR-ee-uh)
human papillomavirus (HPV) (HYOO-muhn
pap-ih-LOH-muh-VYE-russ)
LGBTQIA+
obesity (oh-BEE-sih-tee)
overweight (OH-ver-WAYT)

CHAPTER CONCEPTS

Communication
Growth and Development
Health Promotion
Nutrition
Reproduction and Sexuality

LEARNING OUTCOMES

1. Define the key terms.
2. Describe the unique needs of the adolescent in relation to children in other developmental stages and age groups.
3. Describe the differences between the adolescent and adult in relation to body systems, anatomy, and physiology.
4. Differentiate the physical growth and development of the adolescent period in comparison with the earlier developmental stages.
5. Describe abstract thinking in the adolescent period and its effect on the teen's worldview.
6. Compare the nutritional needs and eating patterns of the adolescent with the behaviors of the earlier developmental stages.
7. Identify the need to promote hygiene, self-care, disease prevention, and health-promotion behaviors in the adolescent developmental period.
8. Contrast the recreation, play needs, and socialization practices of the adolescent to the earlier developmental stages.
9. Teach the adolescent and the family of an adolescent anticipatory guidance practices to reduce injury and accidents.
10. Define the phenomenon of sexuality, sexual practices, and sexually transmitted infection (STI) prevention in the adolescent period.
11. Describe the pathology of acne and discuss prevention and intervention practices to assist an adolescent with acne.
12. Analyze the relationship between suicide and depression as it relates to the developmental stage of adolescence. Integrate aspects of safety in relation to rapid evaluations and interventions for adolescent depression to prevent suicide ideation, gestures, and attempts.

CRITICAL THINKING & CLINICAL JUDGMENT

Katie, a 15-year-old girl, has been admitted to your unit for a 2-week inpatient stay. She has a history of cystic fibrosis that has required many prolonged hospitalizations. Her height is in the 55th percentile, and her weight is in the 5th percentile. For this hospitalization,

Continued

CRITICAL THINKING & CLINICAL JUDGMENT—cont'd

Katie requires respiratory treatment every 2 hours, chest vibrating physiotherapy every 4 hours, and triple antibiotics for both pneumonia and a questionable central line infection. Katie expresses a great deal of anger and despair to you about her hospitalization and often tries to refuse her respiratory treatments.

Questions

1. What might be contributing to Katie's frustration, anger, and refusal of care?
2. How can you provide Katie developmentally appropriate care while she is hospitalized for 2 weeks?

CONCEPTUAL CORNERSTONE

Health Promotion

The concept of health promotion is the most important concept to discuss when providing care to the adolescent population. Teenagers experience tremendous physical, emotional, and cognitive growth between the years of 13 and 18. Their personal decisions about their health are highly influential to their overall wellness. Teenagers face many social pressures concerning experimentation with drugs, alcohol, and sexuality and their decisions about these pressures influence their health. Nurses provide straightforward information to teens about health promotion and injury, disease, and infection prevention as well as specific information about pregnancy and sexually transmitted infection (STI) prevention. Anticipatory guidance is given to teens and their family concerning adolescent milestones and expectations of behaviors with an emphasis on the promotion of good nutrition, effective sleep patterns, dental health, and safety.

Adolescence is typically considered to be the time period between a child's 13th and 18th years. However, some child developmental specialists consider adolescence to extend beyond the 18th birthday, referring to this developmental period as "puberty to the 22nd birthday."

Adolescence is a time of rapid physical growth and growing emotional maturity. Yet, popular culture tends to focus on the problems associated with the adolescent time period rather than its positive aspects. For instance, news stories highlight high school drop-out rates, gang involvement, sexual activity, experimentation with drugs and alcohol, and depression rates. In reality, most adolescents succeed in school, have strong attachments to their families, involve themselves in their communities, and emerge without serious problems such as pregnancy, substance use disorder, depression, or involvement with violence.

When interacting with teens, families, and the community, you can help to shift negative perspectives and illuminate the positive aspects of working together to teach, nurture, support, protect, and guide teens through their journeys. Nurses may forge unique relationships with teens in which trust creates a closeness that allows healthy advice, role modeling, and profound emotional support to take place. Helping a family direct an adolescent to healthy pursuits can be a rewarding experience.

Creating open communication is one of the most important aspects of working with adolescents. Teens do not simply "open up" to adults, and a bond needs to form between you and the adolescent for effective communication to take place. Because adolescents display a wide range of maturity, emotions, communication styles, and lifestyles, you need to be open, kind, flexible, and nonjudgmental; you also need to be willing to work on the relationship. The rewards of gaining trust and closeness with a teen are worth the work because you can be highly influential in health promotion and disease prevention behaviors in the teen's life.

Similar to adults, adolescents are increasingly diverse, not just in terms of culture, ethnicity, language, education level, and spirituality, but also in terms of sexuality and gender identity. It is important to evaluate adolescents and their families for all the influences that can affect health-care decision making.

GROWTH AND DEVELOPMENT OF THE ADOLESCENT

As the child progresses from the school-age period through adolescence, the physical changes in height, weight, body hair, and sexual development are dramatic. Girls grow breasts and begin menstruating; boys grow body hair and experience nocturnal emissions, and their voices deepen. Perhaps even more striking are the profound changes that happen in adolescents' brains and in their social structure. Teens develop new cognitive skills, the ability to think abstractly, and an enhanced ability to reason. The frontal lobe neurons become fully myelinated and allow for more critical thinking and reasoning. Myelination of the parietal lobe gray matter has a strong age dependence, is developing during adolescence, and is linked to learning, behavior, and cognitive processing (Corrigan et al., 2021).

Socially, the teen transitions to new relationships with peers and adults with tremendous emphasis on "fitting in." The rapid emotional and physical growth experienced by the adolescent influences the care provided by the health-care team.

Hormones prompt an adolescent's physical changes, such as body mass increase; sebaceous gland activation; and hair growth in the axillary, breast areola, genital, and anal areas. Moreover, hormones affect a teen's emotional state. Stress

Table 22.1

Physical Growth in Adolescence

	Girls	*Boys*
Average Weight Gain	6.8–24.9 kg (15–55 lb)	6.8–29.5 kg (15–65 lb)
Average Gain in Height	2.54–7.62 cm (1–3 inches)/year	5.08–10.16 cm (2–4 inches)/year
Growth Spurt Begins	10 years of age	13 years of age
Growth Spurt Ends	16 years of age	Late teens
Vital Signs (VS)	By 18 years of age, VS are comparable with those of adults	By 18 years of age, VS are comparable with those of adults

hormones, sex hormones, and growth hormones all influence brain development. Teens experience intense sexual feelings and rapid physical changes, and they also demonstrate increasing analytical capacity and emotional maturity. Dramatic changes are occurring in every aspect of the teen's life.

Physical Growth and Development

Adolescence marks a period of rapid physical growth for both boys and girls. The rapid skeletal growth (Table 22.1), usually beginning at about 10 to 12 years for girls and 12 to 14 years for boys, finishes at about the teen's 17th year (Box 22.1).

Nutrition

Teens experiencing a growth spurt seem to be constantly hungry and are frequently eating. In fact, the calorie requirements for 11- to 14-year-olds are 60 to 85 Kcal/kg/day (1,500 to 3,000 Kcal/day). For 15- to 18-year-olds, the calorie requirement jumps to 2,100 to 3,900 Kcal/day! Even more calories are needed if the teen participates in vigorous sports activities.

Be aware that a growing number of teens follow a variety of diets. These include vegetarian or vegan diets, diets that support an athletic lifestyle, or diets specific to a chronic illness such as a gluten-free diet for a teen with celiac disease. Evaluate the child's and the family's knowledge of these diets and provide guidance as needed to ensure that the teen is receiving adequate amounts of both macro- and micronutrients.

Adolescents need more calcium to support their rapid skeletal growth. Between 12 and 18 years of age, they need 1,300 mg/day, which equates to 4 servings of calcium-rich foods per day. To make the best use of calcium, teens need other nutrients as well. Magnesium (410 mg/day) helps the body absorb and retain calcium. Vitamin D (600 units/day) helps to regulate the use and storage of calcium, and vitamin K (75 to 120 mcg/day) helps regulate calcium and form strong long bones.

With increasing independence and individual food/nutritional decision making, teens may gravitate toward

Box 22.1

Normal Vital Signs for Adolescents

Temperature: 36.6°C to 37.2°C (97.7°F–99°F)
Heart rate: 55 to 100 bpm (85 bpm average)
Blood pressure: Systolic <120 mm Hg
Respiratory rate: 15 to 20 breaths per minute

Most adolescents will follow these growth patterns, but some won't. Teens who have any of the following conditions are likely to deviate in their development:

- Down syndrome (trisomy 21)
- Turner syndrome
- Exposure as a fetus to teratogens such as phenytoin or alcohol
- History of extreme prematurity (fewer than 28 weeks' gestation)
- Exposure as a fetus to TORCH (toxoplasma, others, rubella, cytomegalovirus, and herpes) infections (see Chapter 7)

Patient Teaching Guidelines

Calcium

To build strong bones, teens need to consume adequate dietary calcium. Explain to the patient and family the daily requirement of calcium and give examples of foods that are high in this mineral. Ask teens to identify foods on the list that they already consume and help them calculate their daily intake of calcium. If they are not meeting their daily requirement, encourage them to consume additional servings of low-fat options from a variety of food groups.

Foods rich in calcium include the following. The recommended single serving is included.

- Fortified cereals: 250 to 1,000 mg per ½- to 1-cup serving
- Calcium-fortified orange juice: 200 to 400 mg per 1 cup serving
- Sardines: 370 mg per 3-ounce serving
- Dairy products (milk, yogurt, cheese): average 312 mg per serving

Patient Teaching Guidelines—cont'd

- Spinach: 240 mg per 1-cup serving
- Calcium-fortified plant-based milks (soy, almond, cashew, oat) 200 to 400 mg per 1-cup serving
- Salmon: 170 to 210 mg per 3-ounce serving
- Enriched breads: 150 to 200 mg per slice
- Broccoli: 180 mg per 1-cup serving
- Beans and legumes: 50 to 100 mg per ½- to 1-cup serving
- Turnips: 80 grams per 1-cup serving
- Almonds: 50 to 80 mg per 1-ounce serving
- Kale: 55 mg per 1-cup serving

easy meals on the go with friends. These high-fat, high-sodium, and low-nutrition "fast foods" are detrimental to health and may contribute to obesity, high blood pressure, elevated serum cholesterol, and anemia. During the adolescent growth spurt, teens need education about proper diet to match their nutritional needs and their hunger. The teenage years are marked with an increased need for protein, calcium, zinc, and iron. Overall caloric intake should be based on activity level. Teens need to eat a nutritional breakfast, and snacks should be based on nutrition, not accessibility. Teenage girls with heavy menses may be at higher risk for iron deficiency, and teens who are pregnant need even more calories and nutrients to support a healthy pregnancy (see Chapter 7).

Obesity and Overweight

Overweight and **obesity** remain serious concerns throughout childhood in the United States. Today's teenagers are more prone to overweight and obesity than previous generations. Nationwide, 30% of adolescents are overweight or obese, which places them at high risk for developing type 2 diabetes, **osteoarthritis**, chronic kidney disease, and many forms of cancer. These teens also risk social discrimination, low self-esteem, and depression. The greatest prevalence of obesity during childhood is between 10 and 14 years of age when 37% of girls and 38% of boys are obese. What factors contribute to teen overweight and obesity? During adolescence, physical activity levels begin to decline, teens consume fewer fruits and vegetables, and they engage in more hours of "screen time." The data on childhood obesity in America reveal a national health crisis, which may contribute to shorter life expectancies and lower quality of life for today's children. Adolescent obesity is associated with several conditions in adulthood, including obstructive sleep apnea, hypertension, type 2 diabetes, and cardiovascular disease (Chao et al., 2019).

Sleeping Patterns and Requirements

The average teen needs at least 8 to 10 hours of uninterrupted sleep per night; however, research has shown that fewer than 14% of American teens get more than 8.5 hours of sleep each night (Sleep Foundation, 2022). Many teens report that they do not get this amount. Both the quality and length of sleep affect adolescents' ability to perform well in their academic lives. Sleep deprivation has a profound negative effect on the teen's ability to concentrate and perform well in school.

Nursing Care Plan for the Adolescent Patient's Nutritional Needs

Christina, a 16-year-old, decides to stop eating all animal products in her diet. Her mother brings Christina to the clinic, reporting that since her change in diet, her daughter reports fatigue and is demonstrating overall poorer academic performance than usual.

Nursing Diagnosis: Nutrition; less than what the body requires
Expected Outcome: The adolescent patient will consume adequate protein, calories, vitamins, and minerals sufficient for bone growth, disease prevention, and tissue health.

Intervention:	Rationales:
Teach the patient and her family about healthy dietary habits and adequate nutritious food intake, including plant-based protein sources.	*Teens need adequate protein to support appropriate growth and development. Vegan patients get their protein from plant sources only.*
Teach the teen where to find resources on how to prepare healthy vegan food choices.	*To follow any healthy eating plan, including a vegan one, patients require evidence-based nutritional information as well as good recipes to make tasty dishes that they will want to consume.*
Teach the patient to take a vitamin supplement containing vitamin B_{12}.	*Humans need vitamin B_{12} to produce red blood cells and aid in nerve-cell function. Teenage girls need about 2.4 mcg of B_{12} every day. This vitamin occurs naturally only in animal-based foods, so vegetarians and vegans typically need to take a supplement to maintain adequate levels of B_{12} in the body.*

- WORD · BUILDING ·
osteoarthritis: osteo–bone + arthr–joint + itis–inflammation

Lack of sleep has also been associated with emotional troubles, car accidents, poor grades, and illness. Without enough sleep, the body cannot produce adequate amounts of cytokines, which fight infection and control inflammation. For example, when the body experiences chronic inadequate sleep, the flu shot produces ineffective quantities of antibodies to the flu virus (Sleep Foundation, 2019). As many as 89% of adolescents report having electronic devices in their sleeping quarters (Sleep Foundation, 2022).

Adolescents have a different sleep pattern than adults do, based on a different circadian rhythm, or internal biological clock. Teens produce the brain hormone melatonin later at night than adults and therefore may report difficulty falling asleep (Harvard Health Publishing, 2018; Sleep Foundation, 2022).

Tips to help a teen improve the amount and quality of sleep include the following:

- Set a regular bedtime schedule and plan ahead for chores and homework to be done.
- Avoid any stimulants such as coffee, tea, chocolate, and caffeinated beverages or soda, especially after 4 p.m.
- Avoid using tobacco (smoking or chewing) or e-cigarettes ("vaping"); nicotine is a stimulant.
- Keep the lights out or low in the bedroom; computer screens and other sources of blue light should be minimized 2 to 3 hours before sleep (Harvard Health Publishing, 2018).
- Wake up with a bright light as a signal to rise and get going.
- Refrain from napping on a regular basis, or nap no longer than 30 minutes.
- Do not stay up late or all night studying.
- Exercise regularly but not right before bedtime; exercise should be finished at least 3 hours before sleep.
- Unwind the mind before bed; do not play violent video games or watch scary movies or TV shows.

Cognitive Development of the Adolescent

Physical changes in the adolescent, although significant, are less dramatic than the cognitive changes taking place in the teen's brain. How adolescents think, understand, and reason changes radically during the years from age 13 to 18. Teens may now analyze situations logically in terms of cause and effect, yet they do not always display mature decision-making. Cognitively, teens are able to entertain hypothetical situations, use and understand metaphors, and participate in future-oriented and higher-level thinking.

However, adolescents are equally capable of making poor decisions and engaging in risky behaviors. There is a relationship between immature adolescents and the increased likelihood of participating in risky behaviors, such as violence and the use of alcohol. But a teen's age and sex are less predictive of participation in risky behaviors than are cognitive maturity and judgment. Adolescents are also more likely to fear social consequences to risky behavior, such as being shunned by peers, than they are to fear the potential consequences of discipline. As teens become more cognitively mature, their decisions about risky behavior and consequences become more mature.

Several theories exist to explain why adolescents engage in high-risk behaviors. Perhaps it is the excitement of doing something novel. Or maybe they are seeking approval or acceptance from their peers or higher status within their peer group. They may be modeling adult behaviors they have seen in the media, or they may fear teasing or bullying by their peers if they avoid high-risk behaviors.

A trusted nurse can assist an adolescent patient who is at risk of engaging in high-risk behaviors in several ways:

- Being a role model of health and decision-making
- Opening a trustworthy channel of communication and listening
- Providing honest information about the consequences of high-risk behavior
- Not passing judgment when a high-risk behavior has occurred
- Praising and complimenting the teen for well-thought-out decisions
- Helping the teen weigh the risks of the danger with the perceived benefits
- Giving ideas for and promoting healthy alternative behaviors, actions, and interests
- Understanding that any conversation brought up with an adult on these topics is a very positive sign
- Knowing the difference between "normal adolescent experimentation" and troubled high-risk youth
- Identifying when a teen is participating in multiple high-risk behaviors

Safety Stat!

Texting while driving can be dangerous and deadly. According to the National Highway Traffic Safety Administration (2022) in 2020, 3,142 lives were lost to texting and driving (distracted driving), with many of the fatalities being teens.

Because adolescence spans several years, theorists consider there to be three phases of adolescent cognitive development: early, middle, and late adolescence. Each of these phases has specific developmental markers (Association of Maternal and Child Health Programs, 2018).

Early Adolescence, 12 to 13 Years
- Beginning use of formal logical operations in academic work
- Early formation of verbalizing one's own thoughts, opinions, and views
- Early questioning of authority figures and social standards

Middle Adolescence, 14 to 15 Years
- Posing intense questions concerning societal standards and expectations
- Using analysis with more depth and sophistication
- Beginning to develop one's own code of ethics and what one considers right and wrong
- Beginning to think about the long-term aspects of life
- Thinking about making one's own life plans

Late Adolescence, 16 to 18 Years
- Thinking about greater global issues
- Focusing less on one's self but continuing to argue against views that oppose one's own
- Putting a greater focus on future plans for education and career decisions

As teens develop higher levels of cognitive processing, it is very common for them to become argumentative. According to the American Psychological Association ([APA], 2021), it is perfectly normal for adolescents to engage in the following behaviors:

- *Argue purely for the sake of arguing with adults:* Teens need opportunities to experiment with their new skills of reasoning, even when creating frustration in the adults around them.
- *Be self-centered in life and conversations:* Teens are naturally "me-centered."
- *Rapidly jump to conclusions:* Even with the new skill of logical thinking, teens can jump to conclusions and defend their perspectives verbally. They need to be listened to, not corrected during debates.
- *Constantly find fault in positions that adults take (parents, teachers, and others of authority):* Teens experiment with their new critical thinking, focusing on the exceptions, contradictions, and discrepancies they find in what adults say. Teens are known to be most critical to those adults they find particularly safe.
- *Consider everything a "big deal" and display overly exaggerated responses (being "overly dramatic"):* Teens use social drama as a means to communicate, not necessarily as an indicator of worrisome actions.

Even though adolescents display a range of higher-level thinking skills, they still need adult supervision and guidance to help them make positive, healthy, and safe choices.

Adolescents may seek adult input into decisions about finances, college choices, and career considerations. When these conversations come up, adults should give teens their full attention, support, and honest guidance so that trust continues and the lines of communication stay open.

Sexual Development

Puberty and sexual maturity are a slower developmental process than physical growth. *Sexual maturity,* defined as achieving fertility, begins at around the age of 10 for girls and 11 for boys. Girls' development starts with breast budding and progresses to an increase in pelvic girth and the start of menstruation. For boys, the onset of puberty involves enlargement of their testes and progresses to the first ejaculation, which occurs, on average, between 12 and 14 years of age. During mid-adolescence, the teen develops secondary sexual characteristics such as increasing body hair and changes in voice. A male teen's voice changes at the same time his penis grows in length and girth. Nocturnal emissions of seminal fluid (wet dreams) often occur at the same time as the peak growth spurt of the boy's height.

The Tanner Scale

Many health-care providers use the Tanner scale to evaluate and describe the external changes that take place during sexual development. This five-point scale divides into stages the genitalia and pubic hair changes that take place during childhood (Figs. 22.1 and 22.2). The Tanner scale for girls also reviews breast development (Fig. 22.3). When a teen demonstrates late or very early physical and sexual maturity, the health-care team must be alert to the need for an investigation of metabolic health. Research has shown a relationship among depression, substance use disorder, eating disorders, and disruptive behaviors for girls who mature physically and sexually early and for boys who mature physically and sexually late. There is also a higher incidence of bullying for boys who mature late. Research has also shown that boys who mature early are more likely to participate in early high-risk behaviors such as smoking, delinquency, and sexual activity (APA, 2016). Although early maturity for both sexes has been associated with risky behaviors, later maturity has been found to be protective (Hoyt et al., 2020).

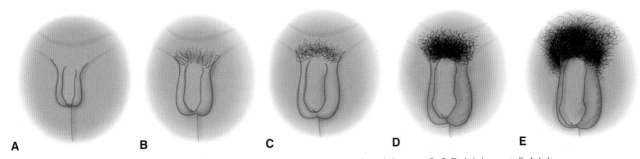

A   **B**   **C**   **D**   **E**

FIGURE 22.1 Tanner stages for male genital and pubic hair development: A, Preadolescent; B, C, D, Adolescent; E, Adult.

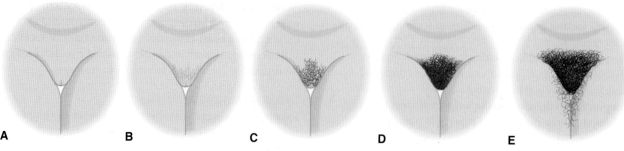

FIGURE 22.2 Tanner stages for female genital and pubic hair development: A, Preadolescent; B, C, D, Adolescent; E, Adult.

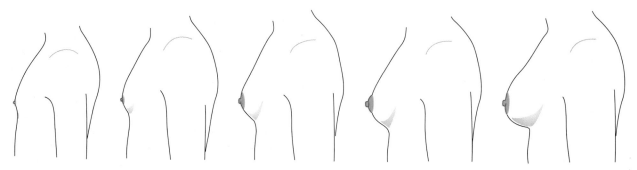

FIGURE 22.3 Breast development.

Adolescence is the time when some teens experiment with sex. Therefore, teens need to have factual information about protecting themselves against pregnancy and STIs. Nurses might find that the teen is more comfortable talking with a nurse than talking to a family member about sex. Offering straightforward information on sexuality, sexual activity, risks, and protection is an important nursing role.

Team Works

Health Care for the Transgender Adolescent

Gender dysphoria (discomfort or lack of identification with one's sex assigned at birth) intensifies during puberty (Kaltiala-Heino et al., 2017) and may be first experienced by many at 7 years of age (Zaliznyak et al., 2020). For young adolescents with gender **dysphoria**, treatment currently consists of suppressing the release of gonadotropin-releasing hormone during early puberty. In that way, adolescents do not develop the secondary sex characteristics of the gender they do not identify with. If the child later changes their mind, the "puberty-blocker" medication can be discontinued, and secondary sex characteristics develop according to the child's sex assigned at birth.

Older transgender adolescents may choose to begin hormone replacement therapy (estrogen or testosterone) to develop the secondary sex characteristics of their identified gender. They may also choose to have gender-affirming surgical procedures.

Children with gender dysphoria and those who identify as transgender require carers who are knowledgeable about transgender health and sensitive to the needs of transgender patients. Ideally, the health-care team should consist of a psychologist or social worker, an endocrinologist or transgender-health specialist, and the child's primary health-care provider. Nurses are essential to teach the child and their family about the medications given and to support the whole family through a life-changing transition, demonstrating the respect and compassion nurses are known for.

Nurses and other health-care personnel should be familiar with current terminology that describes the diversity of sexuality and gender identity that exists among the patients they care for. The abbreviation **LGBTQIA+** is widely used and stands for (LGBTQIA Resource Center, 2023; GLAAD, 2023):

Lesbian
Gay
Bisexual
Transgender
Queer/Questioning
Intersex
Asexual
+ (all other gender identities and sexual orientations not yet defined)

It is important to keep in mind that terminology is constantly evolving, however.

• **WORD** • **BUILDING** •

dysphoria: dys–difficult, bad + phor–state or tendency + ia–condition

Psychological Growth and Development

Psychological maturity for teens involves their developing sense of identity. According to Erik Erikson's theory of psychosocial development, the teens are in the phase of development called *identity versus role confusion.* Here, the teens are examining and redefining self, family, peer group, and community while experimenting with different roles. If they are successful in this stage of development, they will develop confidence in their self-identity and optimism about their future. If they are not successful in this developmental stage, Erikson's theory suggests that they will be unable to have a meaningful definition of self and will therefore develop role confusion. The teens must refine their self-concept and establish healthy self-esteem. Self-concept refers to a person's beliefs about who they are in relation to attributes such as intelligence, physical appearance, and personality. Self-esteem also refers to how people view themselves, but it can be influenced by the comments of others. Low self-esteem has been found to have a direct relationship with eating disorders, depression, substance use disorder, and delinquency behaviors (APA, 2021; Mirror-Mirror.org, 2016).

According to Freud, adolescence is the "genital stage" of development. The teen focuses on genitals as an erogenous zone and will engage in masturbation and possibly sexual relationships. Freud's theory of psychosexual development discusses the conflict that the teen may have between society's expectations of restraint and the need for sexual satisfaction. This is a time for education concerning self-care and protection from pregnancy and STIs.

Piaget's theory of cognitive development describes adolescence as a time of cognitive complexity, formal logical operations, and abstract thinking, all referred to as "formal operations." According to Piaget, the adolescent is able to logically manipulate abstract observable and nonobservable concepts with greater depth. This transition from earlier concrete thinking to formal logical operations occurs over time with each teen developing at their own rate.

Emotional Development

Emotional growth and development during the adolescent period is highly variable. Regardless of where individual adolescents are in their development, their emotional status is influential to their well-being. You must have an awareness of what to expect in relation to emotional variability when interacting with teens. Eight common emotional experiences that can occur anytime during adolescent emotional development are the following:

1. A period of high influence of the peer group on self-esteem, self-image, and self-worth
2. Feelings of invincibility
3. Vacillation between the emotions experienced by children and young adults
4. Craving independence yet needing family time, parental influence, and support
5. Balancing conformity with the peer group and feelings of embarrassment when seen as unique or different than others
6. Feeling "grown-up" when participating in adult-type activities such as driving and voting
7. Feeling restless and reporting being "bored" if not socializing, playing sports, or using technology
8. Feeling tremendous concern about appearance and trying to balance "fitting in" with finding uniqueness and self-expression in relation to their looks

It is important to listen carefully when a teen is expressing concerns about their physical appearance. If the teen is reporting about eyeglasses, acne, weight, or overall features, it is imperative that you listen and offer support, never dismissing the conversation by saying, "You look fine" or "Don't worry; that is normal." To keep communication open, you should be an attentive listener and offer support, allowing the teen to discuss serious concerns.

According to the Centers for Disease Control and Prevention (CDC, 2023) report on youth risk behavior, adolescents are experiencing both emotional distress and emotional trauma at high levels requiring action. In the Youth Risk Behavior Survey (YRBS), teens continue to experience high levels of both physical and sexual violence and continue to demonstrate concerning mental health issues including suicidal thoughts. High levels of bullying continue to impact teens' mental health; according to the 2021 YRBS report, rates of mental health issues are at the point of needing urgent interventions. One finding, that teens have decreased their use of protective sexual behaviors (condom use, STI and HIV testing), is creating alarm across healthcare settings. Nurses can use the findings of this report to make significant impacts on the well-being of adolescents (CDC, 2023). (To find a frequently updated report, see the current CDC website.)

Spiritual Development

U.S. adolescents report a declining prioritization of religion in their lives as compared with their parents' lives, with only 44% of adolescents saying religion is important (Pew Research Center, 2020a). Yet, the majority of teens do "say they believe in God or a universal spirit" (Pew Research Center, 2020a, para. 2). Many teens are now less likely to say there is one true religion and more likely to say that "many religions may be true" (Pew Research Center, 2020a, para. 3). Morality can be thought of as a component of religion or spiritual development. According to 61% of teens, one does not need to believe in God to have values and be a moral person (Pew Research Center, 2020b).

Kohlberg's theory of moral development describes adolescence as a time period when teens seriously question existing moral values and how these values have relevance to themselves, other individuals, and society. According to

Kohlberg, this stage is called the *postconventional level of morality* and is marked by the development of a child's individual conscience and set of moral values. As adolescents attain higher levels of maturity and autonomy, they begin to replace the morals and values instilled by parents and family with their own. Concepts of duty, obligation, right versus wrong, and making amends for mistakes or misdeeds begin to emerge and become influential to decision-making and actions. Some adolescents use the values and beliefs of their families as a foundation upon which to base their own beliefs and values.

Recreation

Adolescents engage with a "social community" as their main form of recreation (Fig. 22.4), and social media has become the main source of their "social communities." Many researchers have determined that the average time spent by a teen in some form of media is 6 to 8 hours a day. Sports, church groups, and, if the teen is old enough, work can also serve as a social community. When interacting with teens, you need to promote positive media experiences while minimizing negative ones. Explain to the patient that rules exist in the pediatric health-care setting concerning what teens are allowed to view or use for recreation and distraction. A child life specialist should be consulted for healthy choices in recreation while a teen is hospitalized.

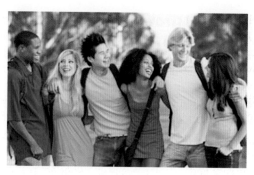

FIGURE 22.4 Teenagers socializing.

LEGAL ISSUES IN ADOLESCENT HEALTH CARE

State laws govern whether or not an adolescent can consent to treatment without parental knowledge. The three widespread requirements for a minor to be exempt from parental consent are emergencies, being an emancipated minor, and being a "mature minor":

1. *Emergencies:* A minor child can be treated without parental consent if the child experiences an emergency need. This is based on the primary health-care provider's (the nurse practitioner's or physician's) good judgment and when a delay to seek parental consent would jeopardize the health or life of the minor.
2. *Emancipated minor:* Minor children who live away from their parents or legal guardians, are fiscally independent, are no longer subject to parental control, are in the military, or are married may seek and secure a legal status of emancipated minor. States vary in their definitions and requirements for emancipation. Many states provide both medical emancipation, which allows for independent medical treatment decision-making, and fiscal emancipation, by which the teen is granted fiscal independence.
3. *Mature minor rule:* Some states have laws that recognize that a minor child may be of sufficient maturity to comprehend their illness, disease, or injury and the need for health care and therefore is allowed to provide consent for treatment.

ANTICIPATORY GUIDANCE FOR PARENTS OF THE ADOLESCENT

Adolescents and their parents require knowledge about what to expect during the teenage years, how to identify early signs of common problems, and how to prevent disease and illness. However, the major cause of morbidity and mortality during adolescence is not illness but rather injuries and self-harming, high-risk behaviors. Consequently, you need to be prepared to discuss a wide range of topics concerning disease prevention and health promotion with parents and their teens. Health education can take place at well-child clinic

---

CONCEPTUAL CORNERSTONE

Growth and Development

Age-appropriate recreational activities for teens include the following:

- Organized and spontaneous sports activities with use of safety gear
- Caring for a pet
- Volunteering
- Reading for pleasure
- Age-appropriate social media
- Movies at home with friends
- Board games at an adolescent's developmental level (Monopoly, Clue, Beat the Parents, backgammon, Ticket to Ride, The Settlers of Catan)
- Video games
- Social events (movies, school dances, parent-supervised parties)
- Development of a secret code or secret languages
- Physical recreation such as surfing, hiking, running, kite flying, or dancing
- Scrapbooking
- Journaling
- Making a "feeling" or "self-history" collage
- Beading and jewelry making

visits; in hospital environments; or at schools, churches, and health fairs.

Because teens need privacy and confidentiality, health interviews and education may be appropriate during an individual session with the teen. Topics for discussion when providing anticipatory guidance for teens and their families include the following:

- *Dental health:* Oral hygiene and regular dental checkups are a part of overall health and well-being. Preventing gum disease and dental caries is an important part of health promotion. Teens should brush their teeth at least twice a day and floss once a day. Visiting a dentist should continue at least annually. The final molars ("wisdom teeth") erupt during the end of the adolescent period and may need to be extracted. It is recommended that needed extractions be done in the mid- to late-teens because extractions done earlier or later than this increase the risk for complications.
- *Hearing:* Many teens enjoy music as part of their daily routine. Teaching families to be aware of the danger of developing cochlear damage from sustained loud music is an important aspect of anticipatory guidance.
- *Posture:* Because of the inverse relationship between rapid skeletal growth and slower muscular growth, many adolescents demonstrate poor posture, or slumping, while seated. Differentiating scoliosis (see Chapter 33) from typical poor posture is important.
- *Preventing motor vehicle accidents:* Teens often have feelings of invincibility and the belief that harmful things, such as motor vehicle accidents, "won't happen to me." Wearing a seatbelt while driving or riding in a motor vehicle is required in every state and should be mandated by parents. Riding with underage drivers or allowing more riders in a car than there are seatbelts is a concern that should be discussed.
- *Tanning and sun exposure:* Some adolescents feel the need to participate in tanning, whether outdoors or in tanning salons. But any exposure to ultraviolet (UV) radiation is associated with skin damage and the early development of skin cancer. Tanning also causes premature aging of the skin. To protect themselves from harmful radiation outdoors, teens should use a broad-spectrum sunscreen with a sun protection factor (SPF) of at least 30 and sunglasses that offer UVA/UVB protection. If the teen has an existing respiratory illness, aerosol sunscreen should be avoided.
- *Social isolation:* Family members need to be able to identify when a teen is demonstrating social isolation. Because adolescence is characterized by social interactions, peer group association, and intimate friendships, the early identification of the lack of these relationships is important. Providing opportunities for teens to interact in groups such as clubs, sports, and youth groups is imperative for healthy social and emotional development.

CLINICAL JUDGMENT

When you enter the room to take vital signs for **Juan**, a 16-year-old, in the office for his annual examination, you hear music and realize it is coming from his earbuds. You have to wave your hands to get Juan's attention and start the appointment.

Questions

1. What do you notice about Juan when you walk in the room and what concerns you?
2. How can you teach Juan about safe use of personal electronics in a developmentally appropriate way?

Patient Teaching Guidelines

Tips for Talking With Teens

Families may need education about how to best talk to their teen.

The following tips provide suggestions for improving communication with teens:

- Listen nonjudgmentally and show a greater interest in their topic than in stating or discussing your own.
- Pose open-ended questions that inquire into the teen's interests and lifestyle.
- Do not ask "why" questions; they can make teens defensive and stop talking.
- Do not "attack" and put the teen on the defensive or make the teen feel accused of something.
- Try to match the teen's emotional state while talking, such as enthusiasm or sadness.
- Be emotionally authentic; do not communicate anger, hurt, or disappointment when you are not experiencing these emotions. Similarly, do not communicate happiness and approval when you do not feel that way. Teens can read parents' emotions well, so express your true emotions.
- Talk about the news; discuss social or ethical dilemmas and interesting global issues of importance.
- Role-model decision making during conversations, such as explaining how you got to your position or how you arrived at a decision.
- Keep it short and simple by keeping the conversation to a reasonable length.
- Be yourself; do not try to act or talk the same as the teen or one of their friends.
- Seize the moment; be ready to identify a relaxing, good moment for conversation or a discussion; be around enough to grab a good moment to connect.
- Show genuine deep respect for what your teen has to say and wants to discuss with you.

SCREENING AND HEALTH PROMOTION FOR THE ADOLESCENT

Health screenings for teens help to identify health problems early and prevent experimentation and risk-taking problems associated with the time period. Screening adolescents should take place during health checks and at school. With budget cuts, many teens are not offered comprehensive health screening sessions. Between the ages of 12 and 18, teens should be screened for the following:

1. Child abuse and neglect
2. Substance use disorder
3. Relationship health and dating violence
4. STIs, if sexually active; follow-up for physical examination or treatment
5. Pregnancy, if sexually active; follow-up for physical examinations and referral
6. Signs and symptoms of depression, suicide risk, and other mental health issues
7. Alcohol, drug, and tobacco use
8. Learning problems, delinquency, and the need for special counseling
9. Blood pressure
10. Cholesterol, if the teen's parents have a serum cholesterol level greater than 240 mg/dL
11. Multiple risk factors associated with cardiovascular disease or diabetes
12. Nutritional risks, such as anemia and eating disorders including **anorexia nervosa** (an eating disorder marked by weight loss and disturbance of body image) and **bulimia** (an eating disorder marked by episodes of binge eating followed by emotional distress and self-induced vomiting and diarrhea), as well as behaviors suspicious of eating disorders, such as fixation on weight

---

Health Promotion

Immunizations and Other Health-Promotion Activities
You should obtain a copy of the teen's immunization record. The teen should receive a single dose of the tetanus toxoid, reduced diphtheria toxoid, and acellular pertussis vaccine (TDap), provided they received the complete set of childhood immunizations. The current CDC guidelines include the first dose of meningococcal serogroup B vaccine and the meningococcal serogroups A, C, W, Y during the school-age period, but after the minimum age of 10. This is now a mandate to begin many colleges. If a second dose of measles, mumps, and rubella vaccine (MMR)

• WORD • BUILDING •
anorexia: an—without + orex—appetite + ia—condition
bulimia: bu—ox + lim—hunger [meaning ravenous hunger] + ia—condition

was not administered earlier, the second dose should be given by the end of the 12th year. Vaccination for the **human papillomavirus (HPV)**, a common STI that is associated with the development of several types of cancer, is also recommended for both boys and girls. The initial dose will need to be followed with two more doses at 2 months and 6 months. Hepatitis B vaccine should be administered if not previously received, and hepatitis A vaccine should be administered in a two-dose series. The annual influenza vaccine should also be administered.

Health-promotion activities may also include breast self-examinations and Pap smears (if indicated) for teen girls and testicular self-examinations for boys. More information about these health-promotion activities for teens is available on the most current American Cancer Society website.

INJURY PREVENTION FOR ADOLESCENTS

Because accidents remain the leading cause of teenage death via motor vehicle accidents (above firearms; Goldstick et al., 2022), families need to have continued teaching about injury prevention for their teens. Teen drug and alcohol use increase the risk of accidental injuries as well as the risk of STI transmission and pregnancy. You must feel confident to bring up these subjects during hospitalization or routine visits to the pediatric clinic and provide teens with accurate information about substance use and abuse.

Safety *Stat!*

Teenagers need role models of safety when they are learning to drive. Parents should be reminded that everyone in the car must wear seatbelts at all times. Parents, especially, can be influential role models for safety by consistently wearing a seatbelt.

Teens must understand the importance of wearing safety equipment. When playing sports, it is imperative that appropriate helmets, protective padding, mouth guards, and safe shoes be worn. Seatbelts must be worn whenever driving or being a passenger in a car or truck, and helmets must be worn when riding a bicycle or motorcycle. The risk of injury increases when a teen's judgment is impaired; therefore, teens should be counseled to avoid drugs and alcohol.

Many teens desire tattoos or body piercings. Because it is illegal for professional tattoo artists to tattoo a minor teen

---

• WORD • BUILDING •
papillomavirus: papill—small protuberance + oma—tumor + virus—virus

without adult consent, some teens seek self-tattooing or tattooing by peers. In schools and wellness visits, nurses should reinforce the permanence of tattoos and the risks of injury from a nonprofessional using unclean practices and instruments.

Safe and Effective Nursing Care

If teenagers are hospitalized, they may be viewed as mature and independent. However, this perception poses risks for injuries, accidents, and high-risk behaviors. Teens need clear guidelines about peer visits, wandering through the halls or off the unit, going outside, and not leaving the grounds of the hospital. Rules concerning use of teen lounges, the unit kitchen, and other common areas may need to be reinforced if the teen is hospitalized for an infectious disease. For more information, see Chapter 23.

CHALLENGES IN ADOLESCENCE

Challenges in adolescence range from acne to violence, depression, suicide, and self-harm. In addition, experimentation with drugs, **alcohol abuse**, and sex are common and should be addressed with teens. Take the opportunity to teach teens about resisting peer pressure, reducing risk and harm, making healthy decisions about sexuality and relationships, preventing alcohol abuse, and preventing STIs and pregnancy. (For more about preventing STIs and about birth control, see Chapter 3.) Issues of gender identity and/or sexual orientation may also become especially challenging during this developmental period. Teens may turn to a trusted nurse to ask questions, to seek assistance in finding community resources and support groups, and to share their emotional reactions to their emerging sexuality.

Patient Teaching Guidelines

State laws differ concerning providing health care and counseling to minors around topics of birth control, treating STIs, and so on. Know and understand the breadth of and restrictions on the laws in your state that govern providing sexual health care to minors. In some states, minors as young as 13 can seek care without notifying their parents or legal guardians, whereas other states require parental consent for all services provided.

Acne

Teens typically have some acne. It is so prevalent during this developmental period that it is often considered a common experience and a normal part of puberty. Although not life-threatening, acne can cause distress in teenagers who are conscious of their appearance and who are worried about how they look to others (Fig. 22.5).

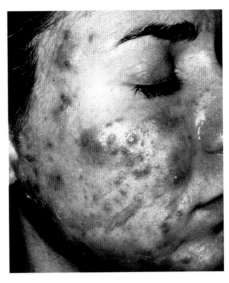

FIGURE 22.5 Acne generally begins in the teen years.

There are four types of skin presentations of acne: (1) blackheads, called *open comedones;* (2) whiteheads that are pustules, also called *closed comedones;* (3) pimples; and (4) cysts. The hormonal changes that occur during adolescence contribute to the development of acne. The form of acne most common in teens is called **acne vulgaris** (*vulgaris* means "common type") and can present on the face, hairline, neck, chest, shoulders, and upper back.

Hair follicles contain *sebaceous glands,* also known as *oil glands,* that produce a substance called *sebum,* whose function is to lubricate the hair and skin. Hormones secreted during adolescence stimulate the sebaceous glands to become overactive. This overproduction of sebum traps dead skin cells and clogs pores. Bacteria get trapped in the pores as well and begin to multiply, causing redness and swelling, which appears as acne. The most common bacteria associated with acne is *Propionibacterium acnes.* Closed, clogged pores become whiteheads; open, clogged pores become dark in color and are called *blackheads.* If the wall of the pore opens up, the sebum, dead cells, and bacteria make their way under the skin and cause a pimple. Very large, infected clogged pores become painful nodules, which are called cysts or boils.

Although some people find that eating certain foods such as chocolate causes more acne, in general, foods consumed do not contribute to the production of acne. The most helpful action one can take to help prevent and treat acne is to wash the face twice a day in lukewarm water with a mild soap. Scrubbing the face with a washcloth or using hot water does not help. Rather, gently cleansing the face is best. Washing one's face after having contact with oil, such as at a job at a fast food restaurant, and not using face products that contain oil may help. Many over-the-counter (OTC) topical products contain benzoyl peroxide or salicylic acid, which help to prevent acne and reduce its presence. Topical and oral prescription medications are also available. A teen should never try to pop or pick at acne because this can cause secondary infections and scarring. Seeing a dermatologist is appropriate if there is cystic acne present, if anti-acne OTC medications and face wash products are not effective, or if the skin condition produces disfigurement.

Violence

For some teens, the threat of violence or actual violence is a daily occurrence. Violence in a teen's life can come from child abuse, intimate partner violence, bullying, sexual assault, gang violence, or street violence in the neighborhood. Being a victim of violence is associated with feelings of insecurity and anxiety. Even though teens are often the size of adults, they are still children who need to be protected from violence to thrive and develop. Teens facing violence need to be referred to counseling and offered support. Teens experiencing violence in their lives need interventions similar to younger children. When interacting with teens, it is appropriate to ask if they feel threatened by violence in their lives. If a teen discloses that someone is threatening them or is causing emotional or physical harm, further investigation and referral are imperative to provide the child with safety and security. Teens must be encouraged to seek help from a trusted health-care professional, administrator, teacher, or adult when they are experiencing bullying or violence. (For more about child abuse, see Chapter 26.)

Health Promotion

Cyberbullying
Cyberbullying is defined as emotional bullying using social media to intimidate, harass, threaten, target, or embarrass another person. Current data show that 43% to 50% of children between the ages of 10 and 15 have been cyberbullied in some form (Bullyingstatistics.org, 2019), with girls being more likely to be involved as victims. Only 10% of children who are cyberbullied tell their parents about it, and only one in five cases is reported to law enforcement agencies (Bullyingstatistics.org, 2019). Nurses must encourage children who are being cyberbullied to take the following actions:

- Talk about their cyberbullying experiences to trusted adults who can reassure them that they are victims and will not be punished.
- Keep cyberbullying texts and e-mails as proof that a crime is occurring.
- Never share pictures they would not want to be made public, and never share their passwords.
- Turn off their technology to enjoy family time and socialization and block those that have hurt them.

Identifying if a child is being cyberbullied may be difficult. Children and teens often hide this form of bullying from parents, guardians, or teachers. Looking for signs such as withdrawing from family and friends; feeling uneasy or resistant to go to school; appearing jumpy or nervous when on the computer; or being angry, frustrated, or hurt after using the computer may help to provide clues if cyberbullying is taking place.

Posing as a child on social media sites, or setting up a website, social media post, or e-mail address to taunt and torment a child are forms of cyberbullying. Several cases of suicide have occurred from children having been teased or ridiculed by others.

Prevention is the best solution for cyberbullying. Parents should know all of the child's login and password information. Limiting screen time and having computer access in open family areas help to prevent overuse of social media and to identify early if cyberbullying is developing. Monitoring interactions on a regular basis also provides information on social media use. Parents must balance being overbearing with providing education and safety.

Depression and Suicide

Adolescence is a period of adjustment and mood changes. Teachers, parents, and health-care providers must distinguish between normal teen emotional states and the development of clinical depression. Sadness is not considered clinical depression. See Chapter 29 for a discussion of adolescent depression.

Patient Teaching Guidelines

Talking to Teens About Dating Violence
Teenagers are at risk for experiencing dating violence, a situation in which an intimate partner attempts to obtain and maintain power and control over them. Mental domineering and manipulation are common and may or may not be accompanied by physical abuse. Abusers will make demands such as having partners account for their whereabouts every minute of the day or every social interaction with others, or setting limits on time away from each other. Teenagers may not know that this is abusive behavior because they have had no or limited dating experience. Social networking has contributed to the ability of an abuser to monitor the activities of the dating victim. Teenagers need parents and adults to talk to them about what constitutes a healthy normal relationship and discuss the warning signs of dating violence.

Self-Harm

The period of adolescence may be associated with emotional pain, suffering, and depression. A teen may feel overwhelmed with a relationship breakup, a tumultuous relationship with a parent, losing someone very close to the teen, or trying to deal with day-to-day interactions. For some, these experiences cause a teen to participate in self-harm. Self-injury is one form of self-harm and can take the form of cutting skin and tissue with utensils such as knives, razors, or sharp objects (Fig. 22.6). The cuts can be repetitive superficial cuts, or they can be deep gashes that cause significant blood loss and require surgical intervention. Whereas most people will ask how someone can cut themselves, some adolescents feel that self-harm allows them to focus on pain other than their emotional pain. Adolescents have reported that the sensation of cutting releases painful emotions, such as anger, sorrow, or rage (Lyness, 2015), and may provide a feeling of relief after experiencing painful emotions (Orchinik, 2022).

Self-harm is serious. Adolescents who feel the need to cut must talk to a mental health professional about their problems. If they are not comfortable with in-person counseling for cutting, they should be encouraged to call a self-injury hotline. Pediatric health-care providers should evaluate for evidence of self-harm, which is often hidden, including burns, cuts and scars, and fresh cuts and wounds on any skin surface.

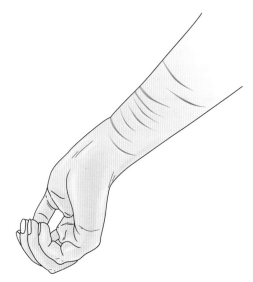

FIGURE 22.6 A teen who participated in self-harm by cutting.

Key Points

- Adolescence, the time period between the 12th birthday and the 18th year of life, is a time of tremendous physical and mental/emotional growth. The adolescent completes puberty and experiences gains in height and weight. Adolescents grow cognitively and begin to process more and more complex and abstract thoughts.
- Teens need information on appropriate self-care including good nutrition, healthy sleeping patterns, dental health, posture, and healthy social interactions. Nurses are in a good position to offer the family anticipatory guidance on what to expect during the teen years.
- Teens face challenges concerning peer pressures, societal expectations, sexual maturity, and their future.
- Erikson's theory of psychosocial development describes the challenge of this time period as "identity versus role confusion"; this childhood stage focuses on the peer group, self-concept, self-esteem, and new roles. If teens do not develop a sense of who they are in their families, peer groups, and society, they may experience the inability to solve conflicts.
- Common fears associated with adolescence include relationships with an intimate partner and whether or not the teen can assume roles associated with being an adult.

- Teens still need their family and can appreciate limit setting and support without interference with their lives.
- Freud's theory of psychosexual development presents adolescence as the genital stage. Here teens focus on their sexual maturity, sexual feelings, need for masturbation, and interest in sexual relationships.
- Piaget describes this developmental stage as the formal operations time period, where the adolescent is developing abstract thinking and reasoning.
- Kohlberg's theory of moral development discusses the postconventional level of morality; teens are influenced by society and family, yet define their own set of moral values.
- Because of their tremendous physical, emotional, and cognitive growth and the demands that accompany this growth, teens face challenges with mental health issues, peer pressures, potential for injuries, and substance use disorder.
- Nurses must develop skills that make them comfortable with talking to teens and offering them nonjudgmental support.
- Challenges in adolescence include acne, dating violence, bullying, depression, suicide, and self-harm. Experimentation with drugs, alcohol abuse, and sex are also challenges that need to be addressed with teens.

Review Questions

1. Which of the following growth and development expectations should a girl and her parents have after she experiences the first menses?
   1. Accelerated linear growth
   2. Accelerated weight gain
   3. Decreased hunger
   4. Delayed breast growth

2. When educating a teenage girl on her expected weight gain during adolescence, you would be correct in stating that the average weight gain between 12 and 18 years of age is:
   1. 6.8 to 24.9 kg (15 to 55 lb)
   2. 9.07 to 18.14 kg (20 to 40 lb)
   3. 6.8 to 29.5 kg (15 to 65 lb)
   4. With the diversity among ethnic groups, there is no national average.

3. A girl will demonstrate sexual maturity by (1) increasing pubic hair, (2) growing breast buds, (3) having her menses, and (4) increasing in height. Place these clinical presentations in the order of occurrence.
   1. 4, 1, 3, 2
   2. 2, 1, 3, 4
   3. 1, 2, 4, 3
   4. 2, 4, 1, 3

4. Cyberbullying prevention includes the evaluation of which of the following signs and symptoms? (**Select all that apply.**)
   1. Appearing nervous when checking social media, texts, e-mail, or instant messages
   2. Closing the computer browser or e-mail windows in the presence of an adult
   3. Needing more time alone or privacy in one's room
   4. Appearing sad or depressed
   5. Demonstrating withdrawal from social interactions with friends and family
   6. Sudden and unexplained stopping of computer use

5. In many states, the adolescent is allowed to give consent for physical examinations and treatments of which of the following?
   1. Emergency treatment of a fractured arm
   2. Required prefootball physical clearance
   3. Treatment for staph infection on skin
   4. Medical treatment for a confirmed STI

6. Hospitalized adolescents' concerns focus on all of the following *except:*
   1. Restricted independence and loss of choices
   2. Separation from peers
   3. Need for parental approval
   4. Missed school assignments and deadlines

7. A young licensed vocational nurse (LVN) is caring for a hospitalized teen. The supervising registered nurse (RN) overhears you tell the patient, "C'mon, bro! Take your pills; then, I'll beat you in a hand of poker!" What feedback is most appropriate for the RN to give the young nurse?
   1. "You did well in establishing a rapport with your patient."
   2. "We have other games that are more appropriate to play than poker."
   3. "Please include all of the other teens in the card game."
   4. "I would rather you not socialize with teen patients close to your age."

8. A minor may seek to become emancipated from their parents. States vary in their definitions and requirements for emancipation. Which of the following are components of emancipation? (**Select all that apply.**)
   1. Teen cares for or lives with grandparents.
   2. Teen lives away from their parents or legal guardians.
   3. Teen is fiscally independent.
   4. Teen is no longer subject to parental control.
   5. Teen is in the military.
   6. Teen is married.

9. Which of the following contribute to the development of acne? (**Select all that apply.**)
   1. Consuming greasy foods
   2. Poor hygiene
   3. Hormones
   4. Picking at pimples
   5. Overuse of antibiotics

ANSWERS 1. 2; 2. 1; 3. 2; 4. 1, 2, 4, 5, 6; 5. 4; 6. 3; 7. 2; 8. 2, 3, 4, 5, 6; 9. 2, 3

CRITICAL THINKING QUESTIONS

1. What programs exist in your community to help teens deal with the social problems of gang violence, school shootings, alcohol-related accidents, drug use, suicides, and date rape? Are these programs being evaluated for their effectiveness? How? What are the outcomes of these prevention programs?

2. In the health-care professional literature, adolescence tends to be portrayed as a negative stage in life, a period of emotional storm, stress, and social survival. What evidence can be used to refute these negative perspectives? How can adolescence be considered a positive growth period that profoundly affects the rest of the person's adult life?

3. Setting boundaries may be difficult for many parents and adults working with teens. How can boundaries be negotiated? How can a nurse implement boundaries and rules within a health-care setting? Do adolescent behavioral contracts work in a hospital setting? Who creates them, implements them, and evaluates these contracts?

Resources

For additional resources and information, including Postconference Questions and Activities, Answers, and References, visit www.FADavis.com.

Student Study Guide

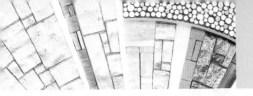

CHAPTER 23
Nursing Care of the Hospitalized Child

KEY TERMS

family-centered care (FAM-lee SEN-terd KAIR)
medical play (MED-ih-kuhl PLAY)
regression (rih-GRESH-uhn)
restraints (rih-STRAYNTS)
therapeutic hugging (ther-uh-PYOO-tik HUG-ing)

CHAPTER CONCEPTS

Comfort
Mobility
Safety

LEARNING OUTCOMES

1. Define the key terms.
2. Describe the unique needs of a pediatric patient across childhood while hospitalized for a variety of acute and chronic conditions.
3. Discuss the safety concerns for young children while hospitalized in fast-paced, chaotic health-care environments.
4. Differentiate between adult hospital units and policies and pediatric units and policies in relation to schedules, play environments, meals, equipment, sleep needs, and specialized staff training for caring for children.
5. Describe how bed selections, room selections, and staffing patterns differ between adult care environments and pediatric care environments.
6. State the three phases of separation anxiety in young children and describe the expected behaviors in each phase.
7. Describe the basic guidelines for working with hospitalized children.
8. Analyze pain evaluations and interventions for pediatric patients and describe both pharmaceutical and nonpharmaceutical nursing interventions to help relieve pain in children.
9. Describe the variations in frequently encountered nursing care procedures for pediatric patients across childhood.
10. State measures to administer medications safely to children who are hospitalized.
11. Describe the various methods for collecting specimens from children who are hospitalized.

CRITICAL THINKING

Katrina, 27 months old, was admitted to a large city hospital pediatric unit for failure to thrive (FTT). Her mother, a 17-year-old, was with her on admission 2 days ago but has not visited the child since a few hours after admission. You have been caring for Katrina on the unit and noted she still is in the state of separation anxiety and "protest" with persistent crying and has not had any visitors since the mother left 2 days ago. The hospitalization is expected to be at least a week because the toddler

Continued

CRITICAL THINKING—cont'd

is being evaluated for the etiology of her FTT, poor eating habits, delayed speech, and listless behaviors. You discussed this with your charge nurse, who made a referral to social services to review the family dynamics and identify how the mother can be helped to be with her child more.

Questions

1. What are your priorities for Katrina's care while she is in the hospital?
2. How can the health-care team prepare for Katrina's discharge to promote healthy growth and development?
3. With which members of the health-care team could you collaborate while caring for Katrina?

CONCEPTUAL CORNERSTONE
Comfort

Being hospitalized is an unfamiliar, stressful, and uncomfortable experience for children with acute illnesses and injuries. Hospitalized children are exposed to frightening surroundings, different schedules, and unfamiliar people. Among young children, regression, protest, and despair are common reactions to being separated from parents. Emotional discomfort is a very real experience for children across the developmental stages. Pain, or physical discomfort, may be caused by many sources of stimuli within a child's hospital experience. Nurses are leaders in pain evaluation, management, and treatment; they must anticipate a child's pain and then manage pain appropriately while a child is hospitalized.

Hospitalization, for a child of any age, can be a very traumatic event. Not only does the illness, disease process, or surgical procedure cause anxiety and fear, but the unfamiliar environment with different rules and lots of strangers can be frightening. In addition, separation from the child's primary caregiver, home environment, and familiar toys can cause stress.

According to Erikson (McLeod, 2018), the primary goal of infancy is the development of trust. Hospitalization reduces the building of trust because the child experiences inconsistent caregivers, fluctuating schedules, and a varying routine. Toddlers, who strive for a sense of autonomy, are confronted by the hospital's limitations and restrictions. Preschool children, in their magical thinking, may believe that they caused their illness or hospitalization by behaving badly and thus experience exaggerated fright. School-aged children, while striving for industry

and independence, feel as if they have less power in the hospital and become frustrated. Adolescents who are hospitalized are still working on their self-identity and should be supported to discuss their school, home, and social lives as well as their dreams for the future and how they see themselves fitting into the world. It is up to you to address the developmental needs of hospitalized pediatric patients and to explain to children and their families why the hospitalization is taking place and what they can expect throughout the experience.

Providing family-centered care helps reduce the negative consequences of hospitalization for the child and family. **Family-centered care** means acting in ways that offer the patient and family consistency, collaboration, and empowerment. A key element of family-centered care is recognizing that the child's family is the constant in the child's life; no matter what is experienced in the hospital, the child will usually go back home to family, unless there is evidence of severe child abuse. Therefore, families need support to learn all aspects of the child's care and should be empowered to care for their child. You need to establish a partnership with the family based on respect, support, education, and encouragement. To do this effectively, you must consider the family's level of function, connectedness, spirituality, cultural practices, economic level, and education. Parents should be included in care conferences during which the child's condition will be discussed and treatment plans will be outlined. See Chapter 1 for an in-depth discussion of family-centered care. Families should also be given access to read the hospital's version of the Bill of Rights for Hospitalized Children (Box 23.1).

Box 23.1
Bill of Rights for Hospitalized Children

1. Right to evidence-based, quality health care based on national standards
2. Right to dignity, respect, and emotional support
3. Right to confidentiality and privacy
4. Right to the application of family-centered care
5. Right to religious and spiritual expression
6. Right to clear communication and use of interpreter services
7. Right to developmentally appropriate play and creative expression
8. Right to participate in informed decisions
9. Right to prompt pain assessment and symptom treatment and management
10. Right to access to the health-care institution's mission statement
11. Right to know the health-care institution's fees and charges
12. Right to access to interdisciplinary teams and social workers
13. Right to a second opinion on treatment plans or options

HOSPITAL SETTINGS FOR CHILDREN VERSUS ADULTS

Not all hospitals offer the specialty of pediatric medical and nursing care. Some hospitals do not have a separate pediatric unit but rather have designated beds within an adult environment. Other hospitals have pediatric units constructed and devoted to helping children feel comfortable while away from their homes. Some hospitals care for children only; these often are health-care institutions with specialty care teams such as pediatric oncology, gastroenterology, burn care, neurology/rehabilitation, and pediatric trauma. No matter what environment the child is hospitalized in, special family-friendly, child-friendly, and child-focused care is required to achieve the best clinical outcomes. Nurses caring for children need specific child-centered competencies.

Hospital Unit Overview and Orientation

When possible, the child and family should be oriented to the pediatric unit before hospitalization. A child life specialist, if available, can provide tours and **medical play**, structured play that allows a child to learn about their diagnosis, procedures, surgery, and diagnostic or medical equipment. A child life specialist can also explain policies concerning visiting hours and sleeping arrangements to make the child more comfortable. During an acute hospitalization or an unexpected surgery, this preorientation tour may not be achievable. If a young child can at least see the hospital unit, playroom, treatment room, vital sign measurement equipment, and even an empty room in the pediatric unit, stress and anxiety are usually reduced.

Designated pediatric units typically have a playroom for both the hospitalized child and the siblings. This is an area where no physical examinations, medication administration, or any medical evaluations or discussions should take place. The child should be allowed, whenever feasible, to have time to enjoy the playroom while hospitalized. Bringing the child to the playroom in a wheelchair, on a gurney, or even in the child's own hospital bed will help the child feel there is an opportunity for recreation and enjoyment. Engaging child life specialists in providing specific play opportunities for children with disabilities is important. For instance, a child with cancer who is immunosuppressed should be allowed to have "neutropenic" playtime in the playroom where surfaces and toys are cleaned and the chance of acquiring an infectious disease from another child is minimized. Children enjoy getting out of their hospital beds and rooms and participating in developmentally appropriate play.

Admission Procedures

Hospitalized children require specialized admission assessments that differ from those of adults. Before conducting a physical evaluation of the child, the admitting registered nurse (RN) follows the institution's admission procedure, usually asking the parents questions about the following topics:

- Demographics, including the local home phone number and cell phone numbers to contact the family
- Chief complaint, associated symptoms, recent illnesses in the home, and past medical history
- Known allergies, including to food, medication, and environmental substances
- Medication reconciliation: List all medications and supplements the child has recently taken or is currently taking
- Developmental milestones
- Toilet training and patterns
- Immunization history and any need for updates
- Pain response, previous pain experiences, how the child expresses pain, and what soothes the child
- Eating patterns and typical diet
- Spiritual needs, religious practices, and cultural influences on the child's care
- Special comfort item such as a blanket or stuffed animal
- Any other concerns the family has

The Three Stages of Emotional Response to Hospitalization

When a child is hospitalized, their relationship with parents and family becomes disrupted. The child experiences an unpredictable routine and is forced to interact with many strangers under frightening circumstances. The hospital experience promotes a feeling of distrust. Children can feel as though they have a lack of control over their situation and the environment around them and therefore perceive the hospital experience as a threat. Infants and toddlers between the ages of 6 and 36 months experience separation anxiety. As shown in Robertson's classic study, separation anxiety can lead to three typical reactions to hospitalization: protest, despair, and detachment/denial (Robertson, found in Yawkey & Pellegrini, 1984). Young hospitalized children were also shown to be frightened, stressed, and have poor sleep habits (Cahayag, 2020; MedlinePlus, 2022).

Patient Teaching Guidelines

Nurses may need to give parents or other caregivers difficult news about their child during the course of a hospitalization. Using the principles of family-centered care, parents should be given news about their child's condition at the bedside, where they can understand what is happening to their child. If the child's developmental level will make them vulnerable to fear, anxiety, or confusion, such as preschool children who engage in magical thinking, the team and parents may decide to step out of the room to discuss the news in a private setting.

Protest

During the first stage, the young child protests loudly. This is displayed by crying, screaming, agitation, or demonstrations of anger. The child is often inconsolable and watches intently for the caregiver(s) to return. This period is difficult for you and the other health-care providers because the child does not readily respond to gestures of play or cuddling or to offerings of comfort. This first stage of protest can last hours up to 1 or 2 days.

Despair

In the second stage of separation, the young child withdraws and becomes inactive and uncommunicative. The child appears very sad and hopeless. Often, the child is lying quietly in despair on their side, turned away from the door or from others, sometimes in a fetal position. When the parents return during this second phase, the child may act ambivalent or sad. This is challenging for the parents and health-care team because they desire to comfort the child.

Detachment/Denial

In the third phase, it appears that the child is adapting to the absence of their parents. The child starts to engage in interactions with others, may play in the bed, or may participate in activities offered in the playroom. The child appears to be adjusting but is actually still experiencing sadness and anxiety. When the parents return during this stage, the child may ignore them as a form of punishment for leaving. Parents may feel surprised, hurt, or guilty from this response to the reunion. Educating parents about how normal the child's reactions are may reduce their alarm and dismay.

Separation anxiety is further complicated by the child potentially having sleep deprivation. The strange environment, noises of the monitoring equipment, nighttime procedures, and the absence of the parents offering bedtime routines are all disruptive. Children with disrupted sleep may have more acute reactions because of their deep fatigue.

The goal for the nursing staff is to build trust with the young child who is experiencing this negative response to separation and hospitalization. Continuing to offer the child support, positive and playful interactions, and consistency through routines helps to build this trust. Even at a young age, the child needs to hear from you that the parents are coming back. Parents who must leave their child in the hospital should be encouraged to ask extended family members to stay with the child when the parents cannot. Leaving a personal item of the parents with the child also may make the child feel safe. This can be an article of clothing, a picture of the family, or a familiar item from the home. Parents need to know that the negative responses to hospitalization are transient.

Stranger anxiety is also common when a young child is hospitalized. Stranger anxiety starts at approximately 8 months and continues through late toddlerhood and sometimes through the early preschool period. The most acute period of stranger anxiety occurs between 8 and 18 months of age. Children display anxiety with the close presence of a stranger, which is exacerbated by their lack of ability to verbalize their protests. Young children do not readily take to a stranger's touch or holding. Consistency in caregivers is one way to reduce stranger anxiety. Children also respond better to the caregiver who establishes rapport with the parents first, then slowly approaches the child, speaking in a soft, quiet voice. Whenever possible, the health-care team should perform evaluations while the infant or toddler is in the parent's arms or lap.

Regression is also a common reaction from a young child being hospitalized and feeling loss of control. *Regression* is defined as a child displaying behaviors associated with a younger developmental stage. Children use regressive behaviors to help cope with stressful events. Behaviors can include bed-wetting and wanting to wear a diaper, desire for sucking on a bottle or pacifier, thumb sucking, frequent temper tantrums, food refusal, and the use of "baby talk." Children should be encouraged to behave according to their age and developmental level but should never be punished for the regression. Parents need to be taught that this is a normal response and that the child will behave again at their developmental level once the stress of hospitalization is over and feelings of loss of control subside.

Childhood Considerations for Hospitalization

Children are not little adults. They have physical, emotional, and play needs that are different than those of adults. Children need more undisturbed sleep, they need to have parents and familiar objects with them, and they need to have a bed selection that works with their medical diagnosis as well as their age and developmental level. Consider the following topics when caring for a hospitalized child.

Time Demands and Potential Sleep Deprivation

Hospitalization can be detrimental to the rest and sleep patterns of children. The hospital's 24-hour work schedule must be balanced as much as possible with the child's rest and sleep needs. For example, posting a sign stating that the child is napping is appropriate to allow uninterrupted sleep time during the day. Children should be encouraged to go to sleep as close to their normal bedtimes as possible because sleep is often disrupted for nighttime vital sign measurement, weight, and phlebotomy.

Health Promotion

Tips for Sleep Success

- Consistent lights out and bedtime while hospitalized
- Minimal nighttime disruptions for vital signs or evaluations, when possible
- Bedtime rituals maintained while hospitalized (bath, bedtime reading)

Health Promotion—cont'd

- Personal comfort items kept at bedside and offered to child at bedtime
- Lighting minimized but adequate for safety (bathroom light on only)
- Noise reduced to allow child to fall asleep and stay asleep
- Assignment of a bed to allow a roommate of a similar age and bedtime
- Fears determined and addressed, such as strangers, monsters, and the dark
- Presence of a parent or an extended family member so that someone familiar to the child is with the child overnight to provide support
- Medications administered before bedtime and as infrequently as possible at night as well as grouped together for minimal sleep disruptions
- Aromatherapy such as a small lavender pillow
- Essential oils such as lavender drops to the spine area; or chamomile, marjoram, or valerian drops to smell (Always dilute topical essential oils with a base carrier oil such as apricot kernel oil to avoid stinging or burning the child's skin.)
- Music therapy such as soothing jazz, light Disney tunes, or classical music before bedtime
- Massage therapy before bed, such as a soft foot rub or back rub with lotion
- Water intake minimized at bedtime, as hydration orders allow, to prevent the need to use the bathroom during the night
- Warmth provided before bedtime, such as a soft blanket from the blanket warmer

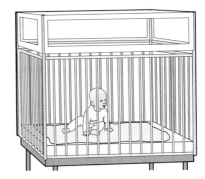

FIGURE 23.1 High-top toddler crib.

Safety *Stat!*

Caregivers of young children who are hospitalized should be given their own safe sleeping bed or convertible sleeping chair. Remind parents never to nap or sleep with their hospitalized infants. Cosleeping with an infant increases the risk of suffocation or injury. Also, infants must never be left unattended on the parent's bed, even for a brief bathroom visit, because of the chance of a fall. Tell parents to notify you when they are going to shower or leave their infant or young child alone.

Bed Selection

Careful consideration is required when making pediatric bed assignments. Medical diagnoses influence how children are placed within the unit. Children with similar diagnoses should be placed together for support if private rooms are not available. Children of similar ages may enjoy similar activities and each other's company. Protect privacy at all times, regardless of the child's age.

Young infants require either an open crib or an incubator. Older infants, in constrast, should be placed in cribs. Toddlers and older infants who can stand and climb must be in cribs with high tops so that injuries can be avoided (Fig. 23.1). Follow your institution's policy about the age that an older toddler or young preschool child can be given a full-size hospital bed.

Visiting Hours

In pediatrics, visiting hours are often adapted to meet the needs of the family. Some hospitals have multiple pediatric patients in one large room; other facilities provide double or single rooms. Visiting hours may be influenced by the type of room provided. For instance, facilities with private rooms may not restrict visiting hours at all, whereas hospitals with shared rooms may limit visitation from 10 a.m. to 8 p.m. Pediatric intensive care units (PICUs) typically limit the number of visitors to two at a time.

Parents at the Bedside

The positive impact of the presence of a child's parents at the bedside during hospitalization cannot be overestimated. Parents are encouraged, and sometimes requested, to stay with their young child around the clock. Parents should be provided with essentials, such as access to unit kitchen areas, internet service if available, meal guidelines or local restaurant menus for takeout or delivery, and privacy as required. Hospitals commonly provide parents with sleeping arrangements next to their child or a boarding room for longer stays. Encourage the family's involvement and support the family's cultural, spiritual, and religious practices whenever possible during the stressful event of a hospitalization.

Children fare better and have more positive clinical outcomes if their parents are present, engaged in the child's care, and offer the child comfort. Every effort should be made to assist the parents in maintaining a presence as much as possible each day. However, nurses need to realize that parents may need to be away from the bedside to maintain employment or care for other siblings at home.

Research has shown many positive effects of parental presence in the hospital. These include increased opportunities for education, increased coping strategies for the parents, and greater adjustment to the hospitalization by the child (Romito et al., 2021), as well as increased collaboration in medical decisions and provision of emotional support to the child (Suparto et al., 2020).

Factors That Affect a Family's Response to a Child's Hospitalization

The factors that influence a family's reaction, adaptation, processing, and ability to stay present during a hospitalization include the child's age, whether the disease process is acute or chronic, family function and structure, the parents' employment status, the availability of extended family members, the family's trust in the hospital system to provide safety, the presence of a child life specialist, and cultural and ethnic norms and practices.

THE CHILD'S AGE. Many first-time parents of newborns or young infants may be very reluctant to leave their child in the hospital without constant supervision. Mothers who are breastfeeding should be encouraged to stay to provide fresh breast milk or to pump at home and bring in breast milk, either fresh or frozen. Parents of young infants often feel emotional distress if they have to leave their infant to attend to other siblings or work responsibilities.

Parents of children of all ages often feel torn when work or family responsibilities pull them from the hospitalized child's bedside. The parents must hear from you that the child will be kept safe, supervised, and cared for in their absence.

NATURE OF THE DISEASE PROCESS. When faced with an unexpected hospitalization of an unknown duration, families of a child with an acute injury or disease process feel thrown off balance. Because there is no time to plan a work absence, distress and frustration may occur when the unexpected event creates havoc in the family's life. You must clearly explain what to expect, such as an estimated length of stay or an estimated length of recovery until the child can return to their normal routine. Parents must be supported when they need to be absent from the hospital to take care of responsibilities that they may not have the power to change.

An exacerbation of a chronic disorder such as sickle cell disease or cystic fibrosis may influence how much family members visit the hospitalized child. Some families may not visit as much when the child has more frequent admissions.

PARENTAL EMPLOYMENT. Working parents may not be able to miss work if the family's financial resources are limited. There are times when parents must juggle other children's needs, transportation, and employment. Explain to the hospitalized child, at their appropriate developmental level, what the circumstances are and exactly when the parents will visit. Encourage the child to keep a picture of the family and to draw pictures of the family, home, and pets to feel connected in their absence.

AVAILABILITY OF EXTENDED FAMILY MEMBERS. Some fortunate families have grandparents, uncles or aunts, church members, neighbors, or good friends who can relieve the parents and stay with the hospitalized child to provide distraction and comfort. But families who have recently relocated or who have a limited social network may not have family or community contacts who can visit the hospitalized child. Engage hospital volunteers to play with the child, read the child books, or help the child with homework to provide some distraction and comfort; but keep in mind that not all children's temperaments accept the presence of strangers.

TRUST IN THE HOSPITAL'S SAFETY SYSTEM. Parents with a perception that their child will be kept safe while hospitalized may feel more secure in leaving to take care of other family matters or work-related issues. However, families who perceive that their child will be unsupervised or feel that their child's safety will be compromised will be less comfortable about leaving. It is acceptable to describe to the family how much supervision can be provided, but it is imperative to communicate that emergencies do happen on the floor and that there may be times when the health-care staff is attending to an emergently ill child and cannot keep an eye on their child. Infants and toddlers must be secured in a high-top crib, or, if able to stand and jump, they must be in a crib with a cover to prevent accidental falls from climbing out.

PRESENCE OF A CHILD LIFE SPECIALIST. Members of the child life department can work with the family to set up a system of communication, play, distraction, and comfort while a child is alone in the hospital. Child life specialists provide visits and not around-the-clock supervision, but they can work with the child to help them feel more comfortable, secure, and engaged in play and activities that lessen feelings of homesickness or of missing the parents.

CULTURAL AND ETHNIC NORMS AND PRACTICES. Cultural norms may prevent a family from leaving a child alone in a hospital. Cultural or ethnic groups who emphasize the family as a collective will ensure the presence of a family member, extended family member, or family friend at all times.

Social customs related to the care of a sick, hospitalized child may involve special foods, prayer sessions, and cultural religious practices, among other things. Call the dietary department to provide culturally acceptable foods and to ensure that any homemade foods follow the hospitalized child's nutritional and other medical orders.

Whether family is present or not, the child's well-being is the focus of the hospitalization, and you must support the entire family unit as they all adapt to the stress of a hospitalization and a disruption of family life and work schedules.

Sibling Reactions to Hospitalization

Siblings may experience negative reactions to a brother or sister being hospitalized. Fear, worry, anxiety, and loneliness may all surface at any time throughout the hospitalization. When parents are absent and preoccupied with an ill child, the sibling may become angry and act out with jealousy and resentment. When possible, older siblings should be included in bedside rounds so that they have a chance to comprehend what is happening to their hospitalized sibling and have a better understanding of the need for the hospitalization.

Meals for Pediatric Units

Hospitals provide pediatric patients with specific diets that are medically indicated and developmentally appropriate. They also provide infant formulas and baby food. The health-care team should consider choking hazards and food allergies when making food selections for toddlers and ensure toddler snacks are safe and follow dietary recommendations for the age group. Food from home is usually allowed but should be discussed with the health-care team. Homemade foods must match the recommended consistency and tolerance ordered by the health-care provider.

Safety With Alarm Systems

Hospitals are required to provide procedures to notify security and all health-care personnel in the unlikely event of an infant abduction. Typically, the hospital provides an electronic-banding system (wrist or ankle) that will notify the nursing station and the security office if the child is taken off the unit or moved far enough away to be considered in danger. Nurses should respond immediately to the sound of the alarm and follow procedures precisely to prevent abduction, harm, or injury. A hospital policy will exist to inform the nursing staff how to handle such an event.

Safety *Stat!*

Under no circumstances should parents or children be allowed to remove their security alarm devices. If a device needs to be removed briefly for a procedure, such as an IV placement or a transport to radiology, you are responsible for replacing the device immediately afterward to maintain safety. When the child is off the unit, the care team should place a temporary name band without the alarm.

Caring for a Child With a Sensory Impairment

Hospitalized children who have a sensory impairment require special care and consideration. Hearing, visual, and tactile impairments place a hospitalized child at greater risk for stress, anxiety, and injuries. Policies must be in place to guide care of a child with a sensory impairment so that communication is maximized and frustrations are minimized. Offer children with significant hearing impairments all available technology to improve their understanding of the environment and care. Staff should encourage the child's use of hearing aids at all times, use sign language interpreters, and access other assistive technology to reduce confusion and anxiety. If a child has learned lip-reading, be sure to engage the child's attention before speaking, face the child directly, and use a clear, slow, even rate of speech without exaggeration. For children with visual impairments, maintain safety with clear verbal communication to reduce anxiety.

PLAY THERAPY AND CHILD LIFE SPECIALISTS

The importance of play while hospitalized cannot be emphasized enough. Children of all ages need opportunities for play and expressive activities. You should work with a child life specialist to ensure a match between the child's medical condition and the form of play suggested. Fatigue, infectious processes, chronic illnesses, disabilities, sensory impairments, and levels of cognitive and motor ability are just a few things that affect the hospitalized child's ability to participate in play. No matter what the medical diagnosis, age of the child, or developmental level, offer some form of play on a daily basis. Play is known to provide six benefits:

1. *Creativity:* Play promotes fantasy, imagination, exploration of talents, and the development of interests.
2. *Sensorimotor development:* Play improves fine and gross motor skills by encouraging the child to explore the environment through visual, tactile, auditory, and kinetic stimulation.
3. *Intellectual development:* Play provides learning through experimentation, exploration, manipulation, and comprehension.
4. *Socialization and moral development:* Play teaches the child about social rules and order, how to share, how to negotiate and interrelate with others, and about socially approved behaviors and moral standards.
5. *Self-awareness:* Play provides an exploration of one's self-identity and tests/expands the child's abilities.
6. *Distraction from stress, anxiety, and tension:* Play while hospitalized provides a source of positive distraction from the frightening environment of the hospital. Play allows the child to express feelings, emotions, and anxiety while facilitating communication. Offering a child the opportunity for mastery over an unfamiliar environment, play allows for decision-making and a sense of control; it also lessens the child's stress.

Types of Play

Play is an essential component of healing for children from infancy through adolescence. The information that follows describes the types of play for each developmental stage.

- *Infants:* Infants participate in solitary play in which the focus is on sensorimotor experiences and pleasure. Mirrors, mobiles, musical toys, and toys with a variety of textures, sounds, and motor challenges are used in the hospital. Because of mouthing in the older infant, toys must be washed thoroughly between infants.
- *Toddlers:* Toddlers participate in parallel play in which children play next to each other but are participating in their own play experience. Play for the toddler is generally a whole body, multisensory experience during which they often imitate adult roles (firefighter, police officer, ballerina, nurse, rock star, mother, or teacher). Fantasy toys such as train sets, block towers, and dress-up clothes allow toddlers to imitate their world experiences.

- *Preschoolers:* Preschoolers participate in associative play in which children play together with loosely regulated or poorly defined rules. Informal games allow preschoolers to learn social norms, sharing, and cooperation. Puzzles, games, and simple arts and crafts provide interactions and stimulate imagination.
- *School-aged children:* School-aged children participate in cooperative play via formal games, contests, competitions, and social groupings. Provide opportunities for a school-aged child to play games with family members, hospital staff, and visitors.
- *Adolescents:* Adolescents continue with cooperative play, focusing on strong social interactions and abstract problem-solving. Teens need a means to keep in contact with their peers and should be provided opportunities to use technology to help them feel connected.

Safety *Stat!*

In the hospital, toys brought from home need to be reviewed for safety hazards. Toys should be inspected for parts that pose aspiration and choking risks. If a child is receiving oxygen therapy, then toys with friction or electrical parts should be evaluated for sparks that might cause the oxygen to ignite. Latex balloons are not allowed in hospitals because a young child may choke and asphyxiate on a small piece of the balloon's latex if the balloon breaks. Signs should be posted to alert visitors that only Mylar balloons are allowed on a pediatric ward.

Functions of Medical Play

Medical play, also known as therapeutic play, is a form of play with a purpose of accomplishing therapeutic goals. The use of toy medical kits that a young child can manipulate and experiment with safely allows for expressions of emotions and mastery of the unknown. Giving a doll a shot with a toy syringe allows a child to express fear and anger. Using anatomically correct dolls permits the child to increase understanding of a medical procedure or surgical outcome. Child life specialists can assist you to teach a child what is going to happen during hospitalization, surgery, or diagnostics. As with all toys, the use of medical toys requires supervision, proper cleaning, and safe storage.

 ### PROVIDING A SAFE ENVIRONMENT

Children who are hospitalized require measures to ensure their safety. Follow hospital policy to instigate safety measures such as identification/name bands, security devices, and bed selection that keeps unattended children close to the nursing station. Teach parents how to provide safety by instructing them about how to use the call bell, what symptoms or clinical signs they should watch out for, how and when to call for help, and how to use side rails on cribs. Patients and family members need to be reminded to have all electrical equipment that is brought in checked for safety by facility employees. With the parents, discuss supervised ambulation policies and the importance of never walking barefoot. Parents should not sleep with their infants or young toddlers in big beds. Any supplies kept in a pediatric hospital room should be out of reach or locked up. Children should not be allowed to touch monitoring or infusion equipment.

 ### PAIN MANAGEMENT

Families are very fearful of their child experiencing symptoms, with pain being the most feared symptom. Unfortunately, even in health care, several myths exist about children's experience of pain. For example, some health-care providers mistakenly believe that infants, because of their immature neurological systems, do not experience pain. To properly treat a child's pain, it is essential for you to rely on facts, not myths. See Box 23.2 to test your knowledge of the evaluation, management, and treatment of pain in children.

CRITICAL THINKING & CLINICAL JUDGMENT

You are checking on **Maya**, a 6-year-old on the pediatric unit, and note the following since your last check: She left half of her dinner on the plate, her heart rate has increased significantly, her breathing seems more labored, and her temperature is the same.

Question

1. What is the most important data to report?

Consequences of Untreated Pain in Pediatric Patients

If left untreated, pain in children of all ages affects their ability to trust members of the health-care team. Untreated pain has detrimental effects in many body systems including the endocrine system, metabolic processes, and inflammatory responses. The physiological demands of adapting to painful injuries place a child in a vulnerable position. Nurses must prioritize identifying and treating pain.

The immediate responses of untreated pain include the following:

- Decreased oxygen saturations
- Increased heart rate
- Increased blood pressure
- Heart rate variability
- Decreased peripheral blood flow and poor wound healing
- Increased caloric consumption; potential for periods of hypoglycemia
- Stress response leading to prolonged hyperglycemia
- Mistrust in the environment and with the health-care team
- Impaired sleep and impaired physical function

Box 23.2

Myths About Pain in Infants and Children

How much do you know about the way infants and children experience pain? Read each of the following statements and decide if it is true or false. The answers are printed upside down after the list.

1. Infants do not feel pain.
2. Young children cannot describe their pain.
3. Young children cannot localize their pain.
4. Infants and children do not need pain medication.
5. Children become easily addicted to pain medication.
6. Assessment of a child's pain is difficult.
7. Children always tell the truth about their pain.
8. Children's vital signs do not demonstrate pain.
9. Children should never be given narcotics.
10. Newborns do not experience pain.
11. Children experience more severe side effects from narcotics than adults.
12. If children are playing, they are not in pain.

1. False! Infants have a definitive presentation of pain, similar to older children and adults.
2. False! Children with language skills can talk about their pain.
3. False! Children can accurately place their hand over the place where it hurts.
4. False! Children need pain medications, similar to adults.
5. False! Children who take narcotics when in pain and not excessively do not become addicted.
6. False! Use age-appropriate objective and subjective pain tools to accurately measure pain.
7. False! Children may lie about their level of pain to avoid injections or oral medication.
8. False! Pulse rate, respiratory rate, and blood pressure may increase, and oxygen saturation may decrease.
9. False! Narcotics such as morphine are important treatments for severe pain during childhood. Always administer narcotics according to safe dose range (mg or mL/kg)
10. False! Even fetuses in the womb react to painful stimuli.
11. False! Children experience side effects similar to those of adults.
12. False! Children play even when in severe pain.

The long-term consequences of untreated pain in children include the following:

• Poor motor performance
• Poor adaptive behavior, learning disorders, and cognitive defects
• Temperament changes and psychosocial problems; reduced quality of life

Box 23.3 provides ideas for pain control by planning ahead for a painful procedure or experience.

• Use topical cream anesthetics if ordered, such as lidocaine and prilocaine, before starting IVs or giving injections (but not on very young infants).

Box 23.3

Pain Control Methods for the Hospitalized Child

Plan ahead and intervene before pain starts:
• Offer a sucrose-dipped nipple or prescribed quantity of sucrose to infants before procedures.
• Use nonpharmacological pain-management techniques as well as pharmacological pain control measures before a painful procedure, including the following:
• Distraction
• Relaxation
• Deep breathing
• Guided imagery
• Heat or cold to site
• Positions of comfort
• Favorite blanket, stuffed animal, toy, or personal possession (ask child or parent for ideas)
• Warm blankets wrapped around child
• Being held or rocked in a rocking chair
• Lowered noise environment
• Reduced lighting

• Use a variety of words to describe pain (ouch, ouchie, booboo, owie, hurtie). Take into account the child's developmental level and the words the family uses. Ask the parents what words they use for pain. Write them on a card kept at the bedside; document for the interdisciplinary team.
• Use a team approach for pain control; involve child life specialists.
• Understand the side effects of narcotics administration including gastrointestinal (GI) distress, constipation, and sedation. Educate parents about what to expect.

Pain Assessment

Thorough pain assessment is the first step in managing both acute and chronic pain. Children who are hospitalized can be expected to have various experiences that cause them pain and discomfort. Providing assessments that are frequent (no less than with every set of vital signs); thorough; developmentally appropriate; and that use standard, well-accepted, and respected pain tools is key. Assessments should be performed immediately when there are indications of pain, and pain should be reevaluated no more than 1 hour after a pain intervention is initiated. Pain assessments, interventions, and reevaluations must be carefully documented.

The assessment of pain considers three areas: (1) physiological indicators of pain, such as changes in vital signs; (2) behavioral aspects of pain, such as withdrawal and physical signs of depression; and (3) the results of pain-tool assessments. Table 23.1 provides possible assessment findings for each developmental stage and the appropriate tools to be used.

Table 23.1

Assessment of Pediatric Responses to Pain

Developmental Age	Patient Response to Pain	Pain Scale Assessment Tool
Neonates	Rigidity, thrashing, generalized body response	CRIES pain scale
Infants	Local reflex withdrawal, high-pitched loud crying with eyes closed, pushes stimulus away after it is applied, localized body response	CRIES pain scale or FLACC scale
Toddlers	Loud crying, screaming, verbal expressions of one word, uncooperative, pushes stimulus away before it is applied, thrashing	CRIES pain scale or FLACC scale
Preschoolers	Loud crying, screaming, may put hand on site or misrepresent actual location of pain, may describe pain but not intensity	CRIES pain scale, FLACC scale, OUCHER pain scale, or the Wong-Baker FACES pain rating scale
School-aged children	Often see stalling behaviors, clenched teeth, body stiffens, closed eyes	• FLACC scale or the Wong-Baker FACES pain rating scale for younger school-aged children (ages 6–10) • Wong-Baker FACES pain rating scale, the numerical version, for older school-aged children (ages 11–13)
Adolescents	May talk about pain openly, less protesting, uses expressive words to describe pain experience	Wong-Baker FACES pain rating scale, the numerical version, or adolescent-specific tools such as the Adolescent Pediatric Pain Tool

Nursing Care Plan for the Hospitalized Child in Acute Pain

A 4-year-old girl is admitted to the hospital for acute abdominal pain of unknown origin (possibly appendicitis). The child demonstrates **tachycardia**, diaphoresis, elevated white blood count (WBC), elevated C-reactive protein (CRP), and a FLACC scale of 7 to 8. You want to include the child in the evaluation of pain and show her the FACES pain rating scale, asking her to point to the face that shows the kind of pain she is having. The child points to the face that represents a pain scale of 6.

Nursing Diagnosis: Pain related to an acute abdominal infection as evidenced by subjective and objective pain scale scores of 6 to 8

Expected Outcome: The patient's FACES pain rating scale report will reduce from a 6 to a 3 or lower within the next 60 minutes.

Interventions:	Rationale:
Place the child in a position of comfort.	*Using a multidimensional approach to treat the child's pain is more effective than using a single modality. By providing positioning comfort, pain medication, the distraction of play, and emotional support, you would expect to resolve as much of the child's pain as possible.*
Administer ordered IV pain medication.	
Provide emotional support and play therapy.	
Encourage the child's parents to comfort child both physically and emotionally.	

• WORD • BUILDING •

tachycardia: tachy–rapid + card–heart + ia–condition

Safe and Effective Nursing Care

Key points to keep in mind when caring for a child who is experiencing pain and discomfort include the following:

- Evaluate pain and discomfort regularly and frequently, at least with every set of vital signs.
- Try to prevent pain, not treat it after it occurs.
- Believe the child's reports of pain.
- Use pain scales that are developmentally appropriate; use behavioral indexes.
- Use the QUESTT protocol (Baker & Wong, 1987):
  - **Q**uestion the child about their pain.
  - **U**se appropriate pain tools.
  - **E**valuate the pain experience: Identify physiological and behavioral changes.
  - **S**ecure the parents' or caregivers' involvement.
  - **T**ake all influencing factors into account, such as the child's previous pain experiences, developmental stage, communication techniques, and abilities.
  - **T**ake action; report; reevaluate after each pain-reducing intervention.

Pediatric pain-assessment tools have been developed and widely tested for validity and reliability. Effective pain management requires you to use a pain tool that is appropriate for the child's developmental stage and then to take action to relieve the pain. For infants and toddlers, use observations of the child's behavior to determine pain level. Preschoolers, school-aged children, and adolescents can actively participate in pain assessment. Therefore, these children can use subjective pain tools to rate their pain and communicate the result to you. Behavioral cues and vital signs also indicate the level of pain a patient is experiencing. It is imperative that you believe the child's pain rating. Common pain tools for children are found in Table 23.2.

Pharmaceutical Interventions for Pain

Therapeutic nursing management of pain may require both nonpharmaceutical measures (see Box 23.3) and pharmaceutical agents. For the sake of the child's safety, the pediatric nurse must understand the indication, action, dosage, administration, side effects, and interactions of pain medications. Extra precautions are needed with the administration of IV narcotic medications. Mild pain can be treated with nonopioids and NSAIDs. Moderate to severe pain requires opioids

Table 23.2
Pain Assessment Tools

Pain-Assessment Tool	Developmental Age of the Patient	Scale Description	How to Use It
Adolescent Pediatric Pain Tool (APPT)	Adolescents	A multifaceted pain assessment tool available online for download that covers numerical values and a variety of categories of descriptive words (burning, stinging, aching, throbbing) and temporal (timing) measurements (constant, infrequent); there is also a drawing outline of the body where the child can note exactly where the pain is located.	Teens have options to use color markers or shades of pencil markings to denote the severity of their pain experience on the body outline; for the descriptive words and temporal words or phrases, they circle the items that match their pain experience.
CRIES Pain Scale	Best used with infants who are 32–40 weeks' gestational age but can be used in young toddlers	• 0 = no pain, 10 = worst pain • Based on assessment of five presentations with a scoring of 0 to 2: • Crying • Requires oxygenation • Increased vital signs, such as heart rate (HR) and blood pressure (BP) • Expressions, especially grimacing • Sleeplessness: Waking at frequent intervals or being constantly awake	• Used for infants who are preverbal. • Used for neonatal postoperative pain. • Evaluate for crying, requirement of oxygen, increased HR and BP, facial expressions, and sleepless state. • A score of 4 or higher indicates need for pain management.

Continued

Table 23.2

Pain Assessment Tools—cont'd

Pain-Assessment Tool	Developmental Age of the Patient	Scale Description	How to Use It
FLACC Scale (Face, Legs, Activity, Cry, Consolability; Fig. 23.2)	Can be used for children between 2 months and 7 years	Based on the assessment of child's: • Facial expressions, such as grimacing, frowning • Legs: Relaxed to tense, restless, or kicking • Activity: Quiet to arched, rigid, or jerking • Crying: None to crying steadily, sobbing • Consolability: Content to difficult to console	Scale is scored between 0 and 2 in each of the five categories for a total score between 0 and 10. Observe child for 2–5 minutes. Observe legs uncovered. Reposition patient if needed to observe. If patient is asleep, observe for 5 full minutes. The revised FLACC scale can be used for children with disabilities.
Numerical Pain Scale, 0–5 or 1–10 (Fig. 23.3)	Children as young as 5 years may be able to conceptualize these numbers and their values.	Use only when a child is old enough and developmentally ready enough to conceptualize numerical values and distance between digits.	Explain to child and family that one side of the scale (0) represents the absence of pain and the other side of the scale (10) represents the child's perception of the worst pain they could imagine.
OUCHER Pain Scale (Fig. 23.4)	Can be used for children as young as 3 years old	Series of photographs used to evaluate pain, scored on 0–10 scale. • Pictures include Caucasian, African American, Hispanic, and Asian children. • Children's faces range from laughing to crying. • Each photograph is translated into a numerical value.	Ask the child to choose the photograph of the child on the tool that best matches their pain experience.
Visual Analog Scale (VAS)	Older schoolchildren (ages 10–13) and adolescents	A straight line or a numbered line is used to describe no pain to the worst pain the child can imagine.	Ask the child to draw a perpendicular line across a horizontal line, with the left side representing zero and the right side of the line representing 100, or worst pain the child can imagine.
Wong-Baker FACES Pain Rating Scale (Fig. 23.5)	Can be used for children as young as 3 years old; revised Faces Pain Scale (FPS-R) is recommended for children 3–7 years of age	• Six cartoon faces ranging from smiling (0) to a tearful face (10). • 0–5 numbers can replace the 0–10 numbers if desired. • The face selected by the child represents a numerical value. • This scale provides three ways to measure pain: expressions, words, and numerical values.	• Tell the child that the faces represent, from left to right, a person with no pain all the way to a person with the worst pain imaginable. Point to each face and describe the words that describe each face. Ask child to select the face that represents their pain.

FLACC Pain Scale

Categories	Scoring		
	0	1	2
Face	No particular expression or smile; disinterested	Occasional grimace or frown; withdrawn	Frequent to constant frown, clenched jaw, quivering chin
Legs	Normal position or relaxed	Uneasy, restless, tense	Kicking, or legs drawn up
Activity	Lying quietly, normal position, moves easily	Squirming, shifting back and forth, tense	Arched, rigid, or jerking
Cry	No cry (awake or asleep)	Moans or whimpers, occasional complaint	Crying steadily, screams or sobs, frequent complaints
Consolability	Content, relaxed	Reassured by occasional touching, hugging, or talking to; distractable	Difficult to console or comfort

Each of the 5 categories—(F) Face; (L) Legs; (A) Activity; (C) Cry; (C) Consolability—is scored from 0 to 2, which results in a total score between 0 and 10.

From: (C) 1997 The Regents of the University of Michigan

FIGURE 23.2 FLACC Pain Scale. From: (C) 1997 The Regents of the University of Michigan.

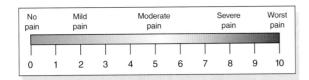

FIGURE 23.3 Numerical Pain Scale

(narcotics) for complete pain control. General procedures for using pharmaceutical interventions for pain include the following:

- Consulting a current medication guide for correct safe dose ranges for both opioid and nonopioid medications; follow institutional policy
- Using the child's most current weight to accurately determine the dose for pain medications; most medications are dosed as milligrams per kilogram of weight
- Following safety procedures for narcotics; children who are narcotic naive (those who have not had narcotics previously) require frequent monitoring for sedation and respiratory suppression; hospital protocols often dictate the documentation of hourly respiratory rates when a child is on narcotic pain control for the first time
- Double-checking infant and young children's pain-medication doses with a second nurse to reduce medical errors

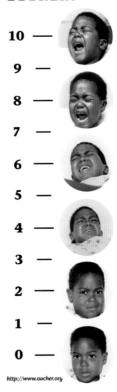

OUCHER!

http://www.oucher.org

FIGURE 23.4 OUCHER Pain Scale

Wong-Baker FACES® Pain Rating Scale

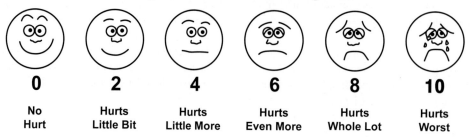

0	2	4	6	8	10
No Hurt	Hurts Little Bit	Hurts Little More	Hurts Even More	Hurts Whole Lot	Hurts Worst

©1983 Wong-Baker FACES Foundation. www.WongBakerFACES.org
Used with permission. Originally published in *Whaley & Wong's Nursing Care of Infants and Children.* ©Elsevier Inc.

FIGURE 23.5 Wong-Baker FACES pain rating scale ©1983 Wong-Baker FACES Foundation. www .WongBakerFACES.org Used with permission. Originally published in *Whaley & Wong's Nursing Care of Infants and Children.* © Elsevier Inc.

Table 23.3

Medications Used in Pediatric Pain Control (Always Follow Institutional Policies and Accepted Formularies.)

Medication	Common Routes
Acetaminophen	PO, IV, rectal
Ibuprofen	PO
Morphine	IV, IM
Codeine	PO
Oxycodone	PO
Hydrocodone	PO
Acetaminophen with codeine	PO
Meperidine	IM
Methadone	PO, IM, IV

- Involving the parents in the assessment and management of pain; teaching parents how to safely administer pain medications to their child
- Understanding that pain is a unique experience and expressions of pain will vary; using many evaluation techniques when deciding pain severity and choosing dosages of pain medications
- Documenting carefully both nonpharmaceutical and pharmaceutical interventions given for pain, and documenting all evaluations of pain, including reevaluation of pain after interventions are administered

Table 23.3 provides the medications and dosages of medications used in pediatric pain control.

Medication Facts

Topical Local Anesthetics

Topical local anesthetics, such as EMLA cream, should be used proactively on pediatric patients to ease pain and lessen fear associated with common nursing procedures such as intramuscular (IM) injections and IV starts. Secure a health-care provider's order for the cream and apply it according to manufacturer's directions, allowing ample time for it to work. Place the cream on several areas where the needlestick may take place in case it takes more than one stick to be successful. These anesthetics may be used on infants but should only be applied on a single site on young infants and neonates. Cover the cream with a clear dressing and remove it completely with a clean dressing before any needlestick.

Culture influences the pain experience, including the expression of pain, verbalization of the pain experience, and the meaning given to the pain experience. Members of some cultures may express concerns about the administration of narcotics to their children. They may not support the use of any narcotics that may change the child's mental status or clarity of thinking. Parents need to be offered education on the importance of managing pain; especially acute pain from surgical procedures. Parents also need to be reassured that addiction to narcotics during childhood is very rare. Ask the family what pain-relief practices are used in their culture

Safety *Stat!*

An accurate weight is the key to safety in calculating and administering pain medications to children. Hospitalized children on pain medications should be weighed daily, not just on admission, because weight fluctuations will change the dose required; this is true regardless of the route of administration (PO, IM, or IV).

and, if appropriate, encourage them to use practices such as prayer, chanting, or laying-on of hands in addition to medications to ease their child's pain.

Procedural Sedation and Analgesia

Children undergoing painful procedures, such as lumbar puncture, bone marrow aspiration, and peripherally inserted central venous catheter (PICC) line placement, may be sedated. These and other procedures require sedation at a level that requires close monitoring both during and after the procedure. Constant airway monitoring and management is imperative, so the child may need to recover in a PICU.

HOSPITAL PROCEDURES WITH CHILDREN IN MIND

Children should be prepared for procedures that will occur while they are hospitalized. First, determine what the child and family understand about the upcoming procedure and then provide a teaching session that is supportive, factual, and at a developmentally appropriate level. Allow time for the child and family to process the information and ask any questions that arise. Explain medical terms in simpler language and use visual aids to assist understanding. Simple, straightforward, and concrete explanations are best. When possible, provide the child and family literature with drawings or pictures or videos that explain upcoming procedures.

Informed Consent

A parent or guardian of a minor child must give consent in order for the child to receive medical care. Hospital admission, medical procedures or surgeries, blood-product transfusions, and diagnostic procedures such as magnetic resonance imaging (MRI) or computed tomography (CT) scans all require the parent's or guardian's signed informed consent. The health-care provider performing the procedure or the anesthesiologist administering the child's sedation is required to explain the procedure, possible risks, expected benefits, and alternatives to the family. Explanations should be done with the use of an interpreter (live or remote) if the family's primary language is not English. Your responsibility is to make sure that parents or guardians have no further questions about the procedure and to act as a witness to their signatures. Explanations should be given at the level of parents' or guardians' understanding, and parents or guardians should then state that they have no further questions.

Special consent is needed for taking photographs of the child. Other reasons a parent's signature is required are when the parent chooses to remove the child from the hospital against medical advice (AMA), when consent for a postmortem examination on a child is requested, or when the child's medical history or records are released to another health-care provider or institution. Also, when a child is asked to participate in a clinical trial or research study, informed consent must be obtained from the child's parents or guardian.

Assent is the term used when a child participates in the consenting procedure. Typically, a child is old enough to give assent on their seventh birthday. The perspective offered in the American Academy of Pediatrics journal, *Pediatrics* (Wasserman et al., 2019), is that a child should participate in the decision-making process to the extent that is appropriate to the child's development, and the child should be honored with respect with the child's best interest kept in mind.

Preparing for Surgery

When not in an emergency situation, you prepare the child emotionally and cognitively as well as physically for surgery. Both you and a member of the child life team should explain the procedure in developmentally appropriate language. The child's emotional well-being should be taken into account with every effort made to comfort the child. Reduce the child's anxiety by talking in a quiet, soft voice and using direct eye contact to establish trust and calm. The child should be with the parent up to the last minute before sedation. Physically, the child should have all jewelry removed, their hair tied back, skin surfaces washed, fingernail polish removed, and any loose teeth reported to **anesthesia**. Make sure the child is wearing readable identification before transport to the procedure. The child should be transported on a gurney or in a wheelchair or should be carried by the parent and accompanied by a health-care team member (Box 23.4).

Postoperative Care

The assessment of a postoperative child begins as soon as the patient arrives on the unit. Have the family stay near the child, touching them if appropriate, so that the child feels supported. Carefully transfer the child from the surgery gurney onto the hospital bed or crib, trying not to jar or move the child too roughly, which could cause discomfort or fear. Lock the gurney and the bed to prevent injury and use a transfer sheet to provide the child with support when transferring.

Implement postoperative care:

- Check the child's airway, breathing, and circulation.
- Evaluate the neurological status, including the mental status and level of alertness.
- Check vital signs, oxygen saturation, and need for oxygen delivery. Postoperative vital signs are more frequent than routine vital signs. Always follow your facility's policy.
- Evaluate for pain using the most appropriate pain assessment tool for the child's developmental level.
- Check patency and functioning of IV lines, pumps, surgical drains, and catheters.
- Observe wound or surgical incision areas, and document the presence of drainage. Many hospitals require that the original surgical dressing be changed by the surgeon; before that time, if wound drainage occurs, the edges of the drainage are marked and dated and the dressing is reinforced.

· WORD · BUILDING ·

anesthesia: an–without + esthes–sensation + ia–condition

Box 23.4

Transporting a Child to Surgery.... *What Should You Keep in Mind?*

For the safety of a child going from the pediatric unit to the surgical suite, always follow your institution's preoperative checklist. Using a checklist improves communication between teams and reduces the chance of medical errors.

- Check and document vital signs (temperature, blood pressure, pulse, respiration rate, oxygen saturation, and pain scale).
- Document the exact time and content of the last oral intake (food and drink consumed or the last breastfeeding session).
- Document the time and quantity of the last stool and urination.
- Using symptom-evaluation tools, check for nausea, general discomfort, fatigue, emotional distress, dyspnea, and sleep deprivation.
- Ensure the presence of a signed and dated consent form for the procedure and, if a transfusion might be needed, a consent form for a blood-product transfusion.

- Check the child's mouth for the presence of loose teeth and report to the surgical team if found; loose teeth can become dislodged during intubation for surgery.
- Check for the presence of any metal in or on the child's body, including implants, implanted central line ports, hardware, screws, and braces.
- Administer ordered preoperative medications, such as presurgical antibiotics.
- Report to the surgical team any concerns that arise before surgery.
- Determine the child's and family member's understanding of the surgical procedure.

- Check safety, ensuring crib rails or upper side rails are up, and rails are padded as needed.
- Position the child for comfort.
- Determine the child's need for elimination.
- Provide emotional support for parents/caregivers.

Safety *Stat!*

The surgical team will need an accurate height and weight to determine safe doses of anesthesia for a child having surgery. They will rely on you to communicate a recent measurement of both on the day of surgery. The best way to obtain a height is to have the child stand and to use the measurement arm. If the child is on bedrest and cannot stand, use a measuring board for accuracy.

Activities for Recovery After Medical Procedures

To help a child cope with recovery following medical procedures, there are many playful ways to engage the child, including the following:

- *Early ambulation:* Prepare a game or age-appropriate craft activity in the playroom and have the child ambulate to the room to participate.
- *Increasing fluid intake:* Offer popsicles, decorate a cup, provide a silly straw, have the child keep track of intake and output (I&O) on a colorful chart, provide stickers as an incentive, or have a tea party for family.
- *Deep breathing and/or the use of an incentive **spirometer** (ICS):* Blow cotton balls across the table, have the child make and use a colorful construction paper pinwheel, blow bubbles, pretend to be a fire-blowing dragon, or use a pediatric ICS decorated as an animal.

- *Dressing changes:* If indicated, use premedicated dressings. Then allow the child to wash their hands, remove the dressing, and decorate the new dressing with colorful stickers. Provide a special prize or activity afterward.
- *Removal of monitoring devices:* Allow the child to participate in postprocedural activities, such as the removal of cardiac leads or oxygen saturation monitoring devices.

Positioning for Procedures

Some medical procedures require the patient to be in a particular position. For instance, with a lumbar puncture, the child is side-lying in the fetal position to maximize the spinal column for needle insertion. For pulmonary toileting, such as chest physiotherapy percussion, the child will be placed in a variety of positions during the procedure to maximize sputum drainage. Before you assist with one of these procedures, check the institutional policy and procedure manuals to identify the position required for the procedure. Positioning can vary according to the preference of the health-care provider performing the procedure.

Restraints

The purposes of safety **restraints** are twofold: (1) The child is prevented from moving during a procedure that could lead to harm; and/or (2) the procedural site, wound, or medical device is kept from being touched, manipulated, or removed by the child. The use of restraints for any situation other than gently holding a child safely and restricting movement during a short procedure requires a physician's order. The family should be informed about the use of a medical restraint, and an explanation of the need for the restraint should be offered.

- Always provide the least restrictive form of a restraint and encourage the family to provide company to the child during the use of the restraint. During the use of a restraint, follow the institutional policy for monitoring the child's skin perfusion and circulation frequently.

- **WORD · BUILDING ·**

spirometer: spiro–breath + meter–measure

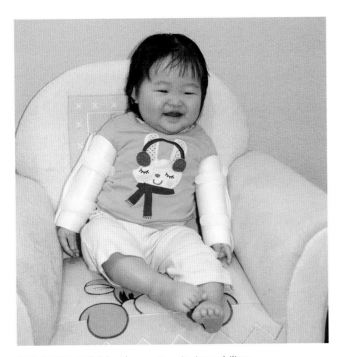

FIGURE 23.6 Child with an extremity immobilizer.

- Follow institutional policy meticulously about the use of restraints and the essential evaluations of a child in a restraint. The Joint Commission (TJC) mandates the use of standards for acute care hospitals. These standards provide the health-care team with guidelines about the use of, orders for, alternatives to, application of, frequency of, assessment of, and documentation of restraints. A medical order must be received within 1 hour of applying a restraint to a child. The medical order must include the indication for use, both the initiation and release times, the date, the type of restraint, and a signature. If needed, an RN can receive a verbal order or telephone order for the initial use of a restraint. Know your institution's policy on restraints and adhere to the mandates of safe care.
- Whenever possible, use **therapeutic hugging** (also called comfort holding) instead of physical restraint during a procedure. Therapeutic hugging includes a chest-to-chest straddle hold in a sitting position by a parent, or a back-to-chest sitting position in which the child's legs are held down securely during the procedure.
- Types of restraints include the following:
  - Pediatric immobilizers, or extremity restraints (elbow restraints), to protect an IV line or to prevent a child from bending an elbow to get access to a nasogastric tube (NGT) or a medical device that could be removed by the child (Fig. 23.6)
  - Mummy (swaddle) restraint, which is used for short-term positioning and extremity control during a minor procedure
  - Leg and arm restraints, which immobilize extremities for healing or during procedures

· WORD · BUILDING ·
therapeutic: therapeu–healing, treatment + tic–pertaining to

Phlebotomy

When a child requires a blood test via venipuncture during hospitalization, special considerations are needed. When possible, the use of a topical numbing cream such as EMLA (lidocaine/prilocaine) helps to reduce the child's pain. Double-checking two patient identifiers helps to prevent an error in handling and processing the specimens. If possible, any painful procedures such as phlebotomy should not be performed in the child's bed, which should be treated as a "safety zone." Use a treatment room for any shots, laboratory draws, or painful dressing changes.

Safety *Stat!*
Newborns and very small infants who require multiple blood draws may need to have their blood loss calculated as output. Keeping accurate records on blood lost per shift may be required. Use only microcontainers for blood collection in infants to minimize loss. Most microcontainers need less than 1 mL of blood. Always check with the laboratory for specimen-submission requirements across the ages of childhood.

IV Therapy and Central Lines

A hospitalized child may require IV hydration or IV medications through either a short-term peripheral line or a central line (Fig. 23.7). It is imperative that safety considerations are implemented to prevent an accident leading to significant injury. When a hospitalized child has an IV, make sure to take the safety steps through frequent assessments of integrity of IV site.

 ## FEEDING CONSIDERATIONS FOR HOSPITALIZED CHILDREN

Children who have had anesthesia, certain procedures with side effects, or many infectious processes, as well as children undergoing chemotherapy, do not have much appetite. Providing food that is visually appealing and tasty may prove challenging. Have the family bring foods from home that are familiar to assist with the child's intake. Allow the child and family to select foods from the hospital's food service, encouraging them to choose foods that are colorful and mild in flavor. Giving the child ample time to complete a meal may increase oral intake. Hot, spicy, strongly aromatic, and greasy foods may deter the child from eating. Smaller portions, with appetizing snacks or fruit smoothies between meals, may help.

Nutrition
Before and immediately after a surgical procedure, children are NPO, meaning that they are to have nothing by mouth to eat or drink. They then progress to the introduction of clear fluids (broth, apple juice, frozen pops). If those are tolerated, children can consume full liquids (milkshakes, yogurt smoothies), and then progress to soft foods (apple sauce,

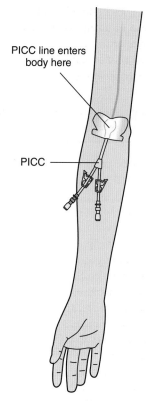
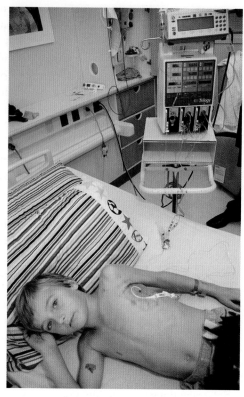

PICC line enters body here

PICC

FIGURE 23.7 Child with a central line. Photo by the National Cancer Institute.

mashed potatoes). If the progression is successful, children will move to regular foods that are appropriate and safe for their age and developmental stage. Before providing food or fluids after surgery, check the child carefully for active bowel sounds in all four quadrants to make sure the child tolerates the food and does not vomit. Passing flatus further demonstrates the child's bowels are active and moving, which makes introducing clear fluids safer.

Safety *Stat!*

Nurses must ensure that patients follow the diets that are ordered. The following list provides examples of food items on each type of diet.

Clear liquid: broth, flavored gelatin, ice pops, clear juices, ice chips

Full liquid: cream soups, milk products, ice cream, liquid yogurt drinks without pulp

Soft: mashed potatoes and other vegetables, soft meats, pureed fruits, yogurt

Regular: any foods considered safe for the child's developmental stage (Infants should have baby foods after they are introduced at home; toddlers should have foods that are considered to have low choking risk.)

Always call the dietary office and speak to a registered dietitian if there are questions about appropriate foods for a child's diet. Some children will have an order of NPO.

Calorie Counts

Because children often stop eating when they are sick, it is important to be aware of the kilocalorie needs of a child based on weight and age. The following guidelines are helpful in determining the number of calories needed on a daily basis. If a child has a gastrointestinal (GI) disorder or a diagnosis of FTT, alternative calorie requirements may be warranted (Table 23.4).

Fluid Maintenance Calculations

Determine the minimum amount of fluid a child needs each day using the following formula:

- If the child weighs between 0 and 10 kg (0 to 22 lb), the fluid requirement is 100 mL/kg/day.
- If the child weighs between 11 and 20 kg (24.3 to 44.1 lb), the daily fluid requirement is 1,000 mL plus 50 mL for each kg between 11 and 20 kg.
- If the child weighs between 21 and 70 kg (46.3 to 154.3 lb), the daily fluid requirement is 1,500 mL plus 20 mL for every kg between 21 and 70 kg (46.3 to 154.3 lb).

Example:

What is the daily minimum fluid requirement of a child weighing 42 pounds?

Divide the pounds by 2.2 to get the weight in kilograms: 42/2.2 = 19.09 kg (round to 19 kg)

Table 23.4
Daily Kilocalorie Requirements for Infants and Children

Age of Infant or Child	Daily Kilocalorie Requirements
0–30 days	100–110 Kcal/kg/day
1–4 months	90 to 100 Kcal/kg/day
5 months–5 years	70–90 Kcal/kg/day
Greater than 5 years	1,500 Kcal for first 20 kg plus 25 Kcal for each additional kg/day

There are 9 kg between 11 kg and 19 kg (including kg 11):
= 9 kg

1,000 mL + (9 × 50 = 450 mL)

Minimal fluid maintenance for a child weighing 42 pounds
= 1,450 mL per 24 hours

Gastrointestinal Feeds

Children whose medical condition requires feedings and medication administration through an NGT or a gastrointestinal tube (G tube or GT) directly into their stomach need specialized care to prevent aspiration and skin breakdown. After the placement of a feeding tube, teach the family how to check the patency of the tube, flush it, and administer medications and feedings through it. Be sure the family also knows how to properly clean the tube. If a child has had an NGT or a GT at home, then the hospitalization period provides an opportunity to determine how the family is doing, to reevaluate their skills, and to provide more teaching as needed. Liquid medications or tablets that have been crushed and mixed with water or formula are administered through the tube. Always check for patency before administering medications or starting a continuous or bolus feeding in either an NGT or a GT.

Calculation of Intake and Output

Children who are medically frail, at risk for fluid or electrolyte imbalance, or receiving medical treatments that affect their fluid status (such as long periods of NPO) are placed on strict I&O measurements. If it is unclear how many mL are in a certain size cup, an ice pop, or a food container, call the dietary office for assistance. The health-care team typically evaluates the child's 24-hour total I&O balance and then makes decisions. The term *positive fluid balance* denotes that the child has had more intake than output and may be at risk for fluid overload. The term *negative fluid balance* describes a child who has lost more fluids than taken in. This occurs with severe **diarrhea**, vomiting, or diuresis. Report

· WORD · BUILDING ·
diarrhea: dia–through + rrhea–flow

discrepancies in fluid balance to the health-care team so that action can be taken to correct a hospitalized child's fluid and electrolyte needs. Calculating a child's average urine output per kilogram per hour may be helpful to determine minimal and desired quantities.

ADMINISTERING MEDICATIONS TO HOSPITALIZED CHILDREN

Hospitalized children often require a variety of medications administered by a variety of routes, including oral; topical; IV; injection; suppositories; and those administered through the ear, eyes, or nose. Safety is paramount because children require very specific doses that are typically based on their most current weight (milligrams or milliliters per kilogram) or by their body surface area (BSA). Follow institution policy about double-checking the "10 rights" of accurate medication administration (Box 23.5).

Medicating children requires a focus on safety. Safe storage, which includes locking medications in cabinets or drawers, is a very important measure to take when caring for children. Check a current pharmacology book for the safe-dose range, safety considerations, and preparation guidelines for all pediatric medications. If a dose is outside the safe-dose range, hold the medication and promptly check with the health-care provider who prescribed the medication and also with the pharmacy for guidance.

Safety *Stat!*

All medications must be stored away from a child's reach and should never be left at the bedside or in a child's hospital room for later administration. If a delay in administration is required, return the medication to the safety of your medication room for storage and make sure that the medication is labeled with the child's name, medical record number, date, time, and dose. *Never call medicine candy.*

Box 23.5
The 10 Rights of Medication Administration

1. Right patient
2. Right medication
3. Right dose
4. Right route
5. Right time
6. Right method of administration for the child's developmental stage and medical need
7. Right preadministration evaluation (heart rate, blood pressure, pain-scale score)
8. Right family education
9. Right postadministration evaluation
10. Right documentation

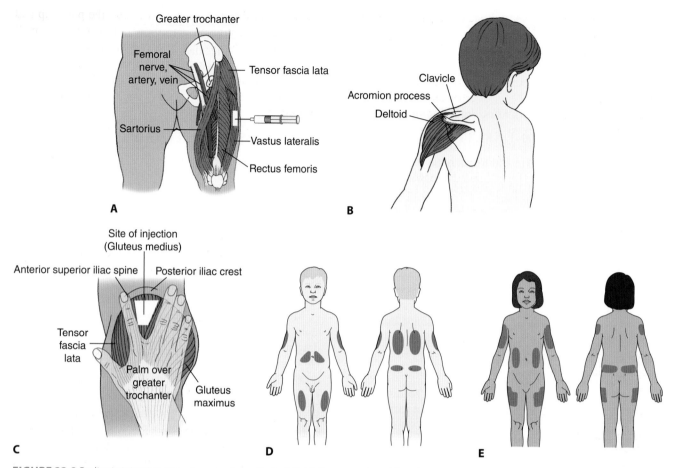

FIGURE 23.8 Pediatric injection sites: A, vastus lateralis; B, deltoid; C, ventrogluteal; D, subcutaneous; and E, intradermal.

Oral Medications

Most pediatric oral medications come in a flavored liquid or a chewable tablet. If the medication is not palatable, mix it in a small amount of flavored syrup. Accurately draw up the medication in an oral syringe and hold the syringe at eye level to check for accuracy in dosing. Older infants and toddlers may prove challenging to medicate. Solicit the assistance of a parent and give choices to the child when able, but do not allow stalling behaviors. *Never force a crying infant or young child to take a medication because this may lead to aspiration.*

Sublingual Medications

Some medications are given sublingually (SL). Here the child places the medication under the tongue or against the buccal mucosa, where it rapidly dissolves and is absorbed.

Subcutaneous and Intradermal Medications

Subcutaneous and intradermal (ID) routes are used frequently in pediatrics for some vaccines, insulin, hormone replacement, allergy desensitization, tuberculosis skin testing, and biotherapies, such as granulocyte colony-stimulating

factor (GCSF). Using the smallest gauge needles (26 to 30), you inject the child with the smallest volume of medication (typically 0.5 mL or less). Using either a 45-degree angle for young children with little subcutaneous tissue or a 90-degree angle for children with adequate tissue, insert the needle carefully with the bevel up. Common sites for both subcutaneous and ID injections in pediatrics are the same as in adults: the upper outer arm, central thigh, or abdomen (Fig. 23.8). Rotate sites to prevent inflammation or soreness.

Intramuscular Medications

IM medications are most commonly antibiotics or pain medication. Three considerations are important when preparing to give a medication IM:

1. The amount of medication to be administered will determine the size of the syringe.
2. The **viscosity** of the medication to be administered will determine the gauge of the needle.
3. The depth of the tissue to be penetrated will determine the needle length.

· **WORD · BUILDING ·**

viscosity: viscos–thick, sticky + ity–state or quality

Most institutional guidelines will state that the maximum amount to be administered into one IM site is 1 mL for infants and young children up to 5 years of age, 1.5 mL for children 6 to 10 years of age, and 2 mL for children 11 to 18 years of age. The volume will ultimately depend on the amount of muscle present. Some medication volumes require two injections. When possible, solicit the assistance of another nurse and give the shots simultaneously to reduce fear.

Common sites for IM injections include the vastus lateralis, ventrogluteal, and, less commonly, the deltoid muscles. The needle is inserted at a 90-degree angle with a quick, dartlike motion. Aspirating for blood with IM injections is no longer common practice because selecting appropriate large muscles will avoid larger veins. Massaging the site is not necessary. Medications should be injected slowly to reduce discomfort. In some situations, nurses may choose to use either the air-bubble technique or the Z-track technique in pediatric patients to prevent leakage of the injected solution through the subcutaneous tissues. These techniques are used in the vastus lateralis and ventral gluteal IM sites. Two caregivers may be required to hold the child during the procedure. EMLA cream may be ordered to provide topical analgesia. Place a colorful bandage over the site and praise the child for cooperating.

IV Medications

Children often receive IV medications while in the hospital. Special care is needed to ensure IV patency, because on many children it is difficult to start an IV. This is especially true for infants. Figure 23.9 illustrates venous access sites for infants.

Ear Medications

Otic (ear) medications are used to treat infections or inflammations of the outer ear and ear canal. Medications are instilled using a dropper to administer the prescribed number of drops. Eardrops should be instilled while the child is side-lying. For children under 3 years, pull the pinna down and back; for those children over 3, pull the pinna up and back for drop administration. After administration, a small cotton ball can be placed in the ear to prevent the medication from running out. If possible, medication administrators should allow refrigerated otic medicine solutions to reach room temperature to prevent causing the child discomfort.

Eye Medications

Eye medications are administered to children in the same fashion as they are administered to adults. If the medication is in a drop form, the child should be placed in a supine position, and the drops should be administered directly into the eye. If the medication is an ointment, the child should be either sitting with their head back or in a supine position. The ointment is placed in a thin line from the inner canthus to the outer canthus on the bottom inner lid. Never touch the tip of the medication bottle onto the eye tissues because this contaminates the tip and may cause reinfection.

Topical Medications

Children younger than 6 months of age readily absorb topical medications directly through their skin. Therefore, it is imperative never to apply topical medications to young infants without an order. Topical medications should be administered in a thin layer, and infants and toddlers should be held or gently restrained so that they do not immediately lick or rub the medication off their skin. Only administer the medications for the duration ordered and carefully instruct parents to follow orders carefully. Apply topical medications only to the affected skin and take care not to stain the child's clothes.

Rectal Medications

Medications administered in the rectum cause most children to be quite fearful. This route is used most commonly when a child is unable to tolerate oral medications, is NPO, or is having a seizure. Suppositories should never be inserted in

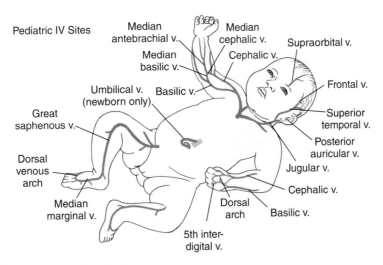

FIGURE 23.9 Preferred sites for venous access in infants.

a child with a bleeding disorder or with a low platelet count. The suppository should be lubricated with a water-soluble lubricant and inserted slowly and gently with a gloved finger. The suppository should be inserted at least 0.5 to 1 inch to pass through the sphincter muscle and stay in place.

SPECIMEN COLLECTION

Specimens are collected on a variety of body fluids to assist the health-care team with an appropriate medical diagnosis or to evaluate the progress of healing. Always wear gloves when handling laboratory specimens. All specimens should be placed in the appropriate container (if there is a question, call the laboratory for guidance) and labeled with the patient's name and medical record number, the collector's initials, and the date and time of collection.

The assessment of a child's urine is a very common diagnostic procedure performed in hospitals and clinics. You will be responsible to collect either a clean sample of urine or a sterile sample of urine.

Clean-catch method: An undiapered child. For a clean-catch urine specimen, the child's genitalia should be gently cleansed with commercial saline wipes or with soap and water, using a clean washcloth. Ideally, the specimen should be collected midstream and in a sterile collection cup that is labeled. The specimen should be immediately sent to the laboratory for processing.

Clean-catch method: A diapered child. When the patient is diapered, cotton balls can be placed in the diaper to collect urine. While wearing gloves, you retrieve the saturated cotton balls and wring them out in a sterile specimen cup. Processing the specimen is the same as for an undiapered child. The use of a urinary collection bag is also common (Fig. 23.10). If a sterile urine specimen is ordered, do not use the cotton ball technique. Instead, use a pediatric urine collection bag (U-bag) for sterile collection.

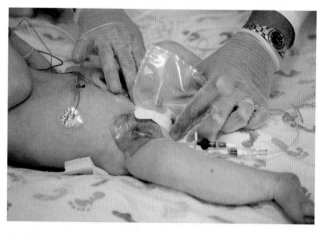

FIGURE 23.10 Pediatric urine collection bag.

Sterile catheterization. When contamination is probable or if the health-care provider orders a specimen for culture and sensitivity, use an in-and-out sterile catheter to retrieve a urine specimen. Some institutions provide catheterization kits, whereas others require you to collect individual equipment. The size of the catheter must be correct for the child's physical size. Cleanse the child's genitalia with a povidone-iodine solution, then insert the sterile catheter to collect urine. Young children may be very frightened of this procedure and may physically protest. Two or three nurses may be required to perform the procedure. A young girl's urinary meatus is very small, and a flashlight may be required to locate the meatus opening.

Twenty-four-hour urine collections. A 24-hour urine collection is done to evaluate the secretion of a material, such as creatinine, over time. The storage container for the 24-hour collection must be received from the laboratory, and the specimen should be timed exactly from when the first urination was collected and stored. The container is kept in a specimen refrigerator, where no breast milk or foods are stored. Check with the hospital environmental services department for storage guidelines.

Stool specimens. Stool specimens are collected in the hospital environment to evaluate the presence of blood, parasites, or ova (parasite eggs). Small amounts of stool are required and should be sent to the laboratory immediately after collection. Either placing a urine-collection hat ("top hat") in the toilet or scraping stool off a diaper is an acceptable collection method.

Sputum specimens. During cold and flu season, many children are hospitalized with respiratory infections. Collecting sputum specimens from young children is difficult because they typically cannot follow instructions to produce sputum and spit in a cup. Instead, children often cough and swallow their sputum. Respiratory therapists are skilled in sputum collection and should be utilized for assistance, especially with young children.

Viral respiratory specimens. Viral illnesses are common in fall and winter seasons, and bronchiolitis caused by respiratory syncytial virus (RSV) is one of the most common. For infants and children with chronic health conditions, an RSV infection can be very serious and require hospitalization. (See Chapter 30 for more about RSV.) When RSV or another viral infection is suspected, you should perform a nasal wash. RSV is very communicable, so you should wear a mask, goggles, gloves, and gown for viral specimen collection. A small amount of sterile saline is injected via a sterile 3-mL syringe without a needle, aspirated right back with the nasal fluid, and capped. Because of the uncomfortable sensation of this collection procedure, a second nurse or nurse aide should assist to restrain the child's arms in a firm but comfortable hold. After collection, the specimen is sent to the laboratory for a rapid enzyme-linked immunosorbent assay (ELISA) evaluation to detect the presence of viral antibodies.

Methicillin-resistant Staphylococcus aureus *(MRSA) specimens.* Because of the rampant spread of MRSA, testing is common in hospital environments. To identify risk and stop the spread, institutions are requesting that patients be tested by a nasal swab upon admission to critical care environments and sometimes to pediatric units. Ask the laboratory for the correct swab because there are differences between swabs for viral and bacterial specimens. The procedure can be frightening to young children, so use a comforting swaddle or a therapeutic hold. Explain to the older child that there is a small level of discomfort that resolves immediately.

Influenza specimen collection. When a child presents with flu-like symptoms, you obtain a nasal specimen for a rapid antibody test. Swab the child's nares with a sterile collection device and send the specimen immediately to the laboratory for evaluation. Wash your hands carefully before and after the procedure. Be sure to follow the institutional policy meticulously to determine if a child's symptoms resemble influenza symptoms; flu spreads easily, and the child must be placed in respiratory and contact isolation.

COVID specimen collection. Because of the ongoing COVID-19 pandemic, hospitalized patients are swabbed on admission to the hospital. Follow institutional policy carefully.

GUIDELINES FOR PARENTS ADMINISTERING MEDICATIONS AT HOME

Before a child is discharged from the hospital, the parents need to understand how to safely administer medications at home. Does the child have a PRN medication based on the presentation of a symptom? Or is the child supposed to have an around-the-clock (ATC) medication regimen? It is your responsibility to determine the parents' ability to comply with dosing instructions, to administer the medication accurately, and to understand any warnings about or side effects of the medication before discharge.

Storage
All medications should be kept out of reach of the children who reside in the home. Medications should always remain in their original containers. Pediatric medications come in child-safe containers and should be kept completely closed at all times to prevent accidental ingestion and potential injury through poisoning.

Calculating Doses
Before discharge, or under the direct instruction and supervision of the pharmacist, the family needs to be taught how to read the medication label and calculate the correct amount of medication to be administered. The medication should be dispensed with simple directions about how to draw up the correct amount of the solution or identify the correct number of pills. The prescription should provide exactly the correct amount of medication for the full prescription, unless it is commercially made, such as eye drops, eardrops, or topical medications. Spoons with measurement markers, syringes with larger fonts, and small medication cups with clear markings can all help the family's accuracy.

Preparation
If the medication prescribed requires any form of preparation, you should demonstrate how to do the preparation before discharge. Medications such as powders, granules, or those that come in packets will require preparation immediately before administration.

Administration
Before discharge, it is essential that the family understands how to administer the medication. Topical medications should be applied sparingly, and eye drops and eardrops must be applied correctly to be effective. NGT and GT medications require teaching and demonstrations, and injections such as insulin require specialized teaching to ensure that the child receives the correct amount through the right administration procedure. Teaching checklists should be used to document the teaching being conducted. Teaching should be done over time, not just on the last day of hospitalization, with ample demonstration, return demonstration, and time for comprehension.

Assessment of Symptoms
Sometimes a home prescription requires that a parent or adult caregiver evaluate the child's symptoms to determine whether a medication should be administered and how much should be given. If possible, provide parents with a symptom scale appropriate for the child's stage of development. For example, request an approved copy of a developmentally appropriate pain-scale tool from the hospital for the family to use at home.

Disposal
After the completion of the home medication regimen, the family should dispose of any remaining medication according to the pharmacist's instructions. Caregivers should not flush medications down the toilet or pour them down the sink. Neither should a prescription medication be saved for future use unless specifically directed to do so by the dispensing pharmacist.

Compliance
Adherence to the posthospital medication regimen is essential. If you suspect that the family will be unwilling or unable to obtain the prescribed medication because of financial, transportation, or social reasons, or if you suspect that the

family will be unwilling or unable to administer the medication correctly, you should notify the nursing supervisor, charge nurse, and the health-care provider. In extreme cases, the child may be kept in the hospital to make sure that a prescribed medication is administered and the prescription completed. In persistent cases of noncompliance with medical treatments, Child Protective Services may need to be notified.

Safety *Stat!*

Completing the Prescription

Antibiotic-resistant microbes are a growing international problem. It is imperative that you emphasize to the family that the entire dose of an antibiotic must be completed, even if the child appears well or healed.

DISCHARGE PROCEDURES

With shorter hospital stays and increased reliance on home health care, discharge procedures have evolved. It is more important than ever for you to provide teaching and discharge instructions about all care required after the hospitalization. Parents may need to learn specific skills, such as dressing changes and medication administration, and will need to arrange to take the child to follow-up visits. When a child is being discharged from the hospital,

the following are imperative for the health-care team to provide to the parents:

- A follow-up appointment to evaluate the child's health after hospitalization; often, this is done with the child's community-based health-care provider who has been following the child's growth and development
- Any needed referrals to specialists or specialized services, such as occupational therapy, physical therapy, developmental screening, or psychosocial care
- Any prescriptions that need to be filled for medications that are being initiated or that are being continued from the hospital stay
- A thorough evaluation of the child's hospital room so that no personal items are lost or left behind

Safety *Stat!*

Discharge procedures are crucial times for the pediatric health-care team to stress important follow-up plans, including further appointments, diagnostic examinations, and laboratory draws. It is vital that parents understand everything that the care team is telling them. For patients or families who do not speak English, use interpreter services as needed to confirm understanding of discharge plans and follow-up appointments.

Key Points

- During hospitalization, pediatric patients across childhood have unique needs for a variety of acute and chronic conditions. These include their reactions to being separated from home, siblings, toys, pets, parents, and familiar environments.
- Young children experience both separation anxiety and stranger anxiety. The three phases of separation during hospitalization are protest, despair, and detachment/denial.
- Safety concerns for hospitalized young children include falls from beds and cribs, aspiration, choking, strangulation, and medical/medication errors. Being at the bedside, nurses are in a unique position to monitor for safety concerns.
- Pediatric and adult hospital units differ in their policies for visiting hours, play environments, meals, equipment, bed assignments, and sleep needs. Children are not considered to be "small adults" and therefore should not be treated as such. Hospitalized children should be supported based on the child's developmental stage and should be provided opportunities for growth, development, play, and social interactions.

- Careful consideration is required when selecting pediatric bed assignments. Medical diagnoses and childhood infections influence how children are placed within the unit. Children with similar diagnoses can be placed together for support.
- Activities for recovery after medical procedures include early ambulation to a fun activity, increased oral fluid intake through play such as a tea party, deep breathing using toys and pinwheels, and having the child assist with postprocedure skills such as bandage application or removal of cardiac monitoring leads.
- Pain is a unique experience for each child. Pediatric-specific assessments and interventions for pain are required. Pain tools developed for each stage of pediatric development have been validated by research and are considered very effective. Hospitalized pediatric patients should be offered both pharmaceutical and nonpharmaceutical nursing interventions to help relieve pain.
- Pediatric-specific calculations must be applied to children in the hospital. This includes calculating accurate medication doses, calorie requirements, fluid maintenance, and I&O, especially with diapered infants.

- Specific measures should be taken to administer medications safely, accurately, and effectively to children who are hospitalized. Double-checking weight-based pediatric medications and preventing choking should all be considered while caring for hospitalized children.
- There are a variety of specimen-specific guidelines for collecting blood, urine, sputum, and other body fluids

from children. Unique collection requirements of children include the inability to produce sputum on demand, emotional responses to having specimens collected, and collecting urine and stool samples from infants and toddlers who are diapered.

Review Questions

1. What is the best way to measure the height of a hospitalized 16-month-old?
   1. Plastic tape measure
   2. Horizontal measuring board
   3. Asking the parents about the results of the last height measurement
   4. Having the child stand on the unit scale and using the measuring arm

2. How do you determine how many calories a child needs on a daily basis?
   1. By asking the dietitian to calculate the child's caloric needs
   2. By asking the parents their average daily meal preparations
   3. By calculating the child's BSA and multiplying the result by 2
   4. By using a child's age to estimate daily calorie need per kilogram of weight

3. Two forms of pediatric pain-assessment tools are used to collect information about a child's pain experience. What are these two forms?
   1. Numerical and visual
   2. Subjective and objective
   3. Physical and emotional
   4. Objective and parent's descriptions

4. Which one of the following pain-assessment tools is used for a newborn?
   1. Wong-Baker FACES pain rating scale
   2. FLACC scale
   3. CRIES pain scale
   4. VAS

5. By what age can most children answer specific questions about the location and severity of their presenting symptoms?
   1. Preschool-aged child, starting at 5 years
   2. School-aged child, starting at 7 years
   3. Older school-aged child, starting at 9 years
   4. Older toddler, starting at age 22 months

6. Oral morphine sulfate has just been administered to a 6-year-old in severe pain after a surgical appendectomy. According to the child's age and developmental level, which pain tool would you use to determine this child's level of pain relief?
   1. 1 to 10 descriptive numerical pain scale
   2. Poker Chip Pain Assessment Tool
   3. Wong-Baker FACES pain rating scale
   4. VAS

7. _____, or returning to behaviors of an earlier developmental stage, is a common response of a young child to the stressors of hospitalization.

8. Children experience negative reactions to hospitalization, including fear, anxiety, and pain/discomfort. Parents also experience reactions. Which of the following are possible responses that parents may have toward the experience of a hospitalized child? (**Select all that apply.**)
   1. Fear
   2. Guilt
   3. Family cohesiveness
   4. Frustration
   5. Loss of control
   6. Normality
   7. Financial concerns

9. Lack of control is one of the most stressful effects of hospitalization on a young child. When a child perceives a decrease in or lack of control of their environment, what does the child experience?
   1. A perception of a threat
   2. An overload of stimulation
   3. A reaction of anger and despair
   4. An acceleration of developmental growth

10. You are preparing a young school-aged child to go to surgery. As you are completing the preoperative checklist, special attention should be given to which of the following?
    1. The presence of braces
    2. An allergy band
    3. Loose teeth
    4. Assent to the procedure

ANSWERS 1. 4; 2. 4; 3. 2; 4. 3; 5. 2; 6. 3; 7. Regression; 8. 1, 2, 4, 5, 7; 9. 1; 10. 3

CRITICAL THINKING QUESTIONS

1. How do children in each of the six developmental stages of childhood (newborn, infant, toddler, preschool-aged, school-aged, and adolescent) differ in their response to being hospitalized for an acute or a chronic disorder? How do children in each of the developmental stages differ in relation to feelings of separation from family; the need for distraction and play; and the need for continued cognitive, social, and emotional development?

2. What nonpharmaceutical interventions can be implemented as adjunct pain-control measures for children in each of the developmental stages?

3. What forms of communication between pediatric nurses and other members of the health-care team work best for reducing errors in the hospitalized setting? For instance, what are ways in which communication can be improved while moving or transferring pediatric patients between departments? What elements of a hand-off (more formally known as a hand-off report) between health-care professionals promote safety and continuity of care?

Resources

For additional resources and information, including Postconference Questions and Activities, Answers, and References, visit www.FADavis.com.

 Student Study Guide

CHAPTER 24
Acutely Ill Children and Their Needs

KEY TERMS

apparent life-threatening event (ALTE) (uh-PAIR-uhnt LIFE-THRET-ning ih-VENT)
Broselow tape (BROHZ-loh TAYP)
central cyanosis (SEN-truhl SYE-uh-NOH-siss)
clinical status (KLIH-nih-kuhl STAY-tuhss)
code blue (KOHD BLOO)
epiglottitis (EP-ih-glot-EYE-tiss)
higher level of care (HYE-uhr LEV-uhl uv KAIR)
peripheral cyanosis (pe-RIF-uh-ruhl SYE-uh-NOH-siss)
rapid response team (RRT) (RAP-ihd ris-PONSS TEEM)
safety precautions (SAYF-tee prih-KAW-shunz)
SBAR (ESS-BAR)
shock (SHOK)

CHAPTER CONCEPTS

Comfort
Communication
Family
Growth and Development
Safety

LEARNING OUTCOMES

1. Define the key terms.
2. Discuss safety concerns when an acutely ill child is hospitalized, including every-shift safety checks for emergency equipment and safety precautions all nurses should perform.
3. Apply the principles of professional interdisciplinary communication through the use of the SBAR system.
4. State typical color-coding systems used within a hospital to call for rapid assistance from a variety of teams (code red, code blue, code pink, code grey, code yellow).
5. Review the most current American Heart Association guidelines for cardiopulmonary resuscitation (CPR).
6. Discuss a comprehensive assessment of an acutely ill child who is hospitalized.
7. Define the system of emergency response with the color-coded, length-based resuscitation tape.
8. Analyze the use of and outcomes of a rapid response team (RRT).
9. Create a care plan that encompasses the needs of the family when a child is acutely ill and has a sudden change in clinical status that requires a higher level of care.
10. Describe the emergency response measures needed to assist a child in shock.
11. Discuss use of a pediatric early warning tool and communication techniques to respond to an acute change in clinical status or an acute emergency.

CRITICAL THINKING

You and a registered nurse (RN) are taking care of 2-year-old **Miguel**, who is being seen in a public health department for difficulty breathing, rapid respiratory rate, and congestion. The parents expressed concern that he caught a viral infection from his sibling. Miguel presents with a respiratory rate of 48 to 56 breaths per minute, a heart rate of 146 to 161 bpm, blood pressure of 92/48 mm Hg, and an oxygen saturation of 88% on room air. He has very dry

Continued

CRITICAL THINKING—cont'd

mucous membranes, no void thus far today (dry diaper), and presents with sleepiness, curling up in the father's lap. His lungs sound congested, and you and the RN identify subcostal retractions. After you take his vital signs (VSs) and report his condition to the RN, the RN comes immediately to evaluate him. Concerned, the RN calls for the physician, who decides to place Miguel on oxygen in the clinic and to continuously monitor him using an oxygen saturation probe. His saturation does not rise with 2 liters of oxygen administered via blow-by, and he is moaning and pushing away the oxygen delivery system. The team calls ahead to the local emergency department (ED), gives a report, and requests that his parents take him to the ED immediately for further evaluation.

Questions

1. What is most concerning for the pediatric health-care team in the clinic?
2. Which primary finding led the team to insist on an immediate transfer to the local ED?
3. Why did Miguel not respond to the oxygen?
4. Is Miguel dehydrated? How do you know?

Nurses working in the acute care environment must confidently respond to emergencies and quickly and smoothly perform skills to ensure a rapid response to a sudden change in **clinical status** (the overall clinical well-being) of the acutely ill child. This chapter presents several strategies and skills to assist you as a part of a health-care team caring for a child whose level of acuity (sickness or injury) requires a team effort to provide safety and avoid harm.

Children, in general, are healthy and strong. When children become very ill from an infectious disease, a severe injury, or an exacerbation of a chronic illness, their internal resources to maintain homeostasis may falter. Acutely ill children may be able to compensate for quite a long time before they suddenly become very much worse. For example, a child with severe dehydration may not demonstrate hypotension until the blood pressure can no longer adjust to the loss of intravascular fluids and therefore suddenly plummets. A child in severe respiratory distress may abruptly go into respiratory failure and then respiratory arrest. Children whose clinical status is "guarded" need to be monitored carefully because they may suddenly need to be moved to a **higher level of care**, where they can receive an increased level of interventions and one-on-one nursing care. Although most pediatric patients presenting to the ED are considered "treat-and-release," meaning care is provided without a subsequent admission and hospitalization (Weiss & Jiang, 2021), some children do not respond to emergency treatment and need the higher level of care of an inpatient hospital stay. Recent data shows that 388 children out of 1,000 visit the ED annually, with 3.2% of those visits leading to hospitalization (Weiss & Jiang, 2021). Pediatric trauma is the leading cause of death in children in the United States, with approximately 12,000 children between 1 and 19 years dying from their injuries (Stanford Medicine, 2022). During the COVID-19 pandemic, pediatric ED visits sharply declined (22% during 2021 and 23% by January 2022), mostly because of parents' perception of risk (Centers for Disease Control and Prevention [CDC], 2022).

CONCEPTUAL CORNERSTONE
Safety

There are always safety concerns when a child is experiencing an acute illness or injury requiring hospitalization. Safety checks must be consistent and frequent. **Safety precautions** is the term used to describe multiple safety measures implemented by the pediatric health-care team to keep a child safe. Checking that emergency equipment functions, is present, and is the right size for the child is a responsibility of each nurse at the beginning of the shift. Being able to identify a change in clinical status for the worse and being able and confident to call for help rapidly will save lives. Safe practice means calling a rapid response team (RRT) or a code blue team, and then clearly communicating the child's status and recent assessments with them. Using a communication tool such as SBAR allows a nurse experiencing a stressful event to think clearly and communicate safely. Hospitals are inherently unsafe, and the provision of safe care across all developmental stages is a major responsibility for all members of the health-care team.

PROVIDING SAFETY AT THE BEDSIDE

It is imperative that a nurse caring for a hospitalized child conduct a safety assessment of the child's room. Is the emergency equipment the correct size for the child? Does the emergency equipment function properly? The following checklist should be used to determine room safety for an acutely ill child who may need an emergency response:

- The bed is in low position with the side rails up and the call light within the child's reach.
- The manual resuscitator bag and a set of masks are in a clean plastic bag away from the child's reach.
- The mask is the correct size for the child for whom you are caring.
- A suction setup with tubing and a clean canister is present; turn on the suction to make sure that the equipment works effectively.
- At least one suction device is present: tonsil tip, olive tip, bulb syringe, or deep sterile suctioning kit (Fig. 24.1).
- A source of oxygen is available, including a green color-coded "Christmas tree" connector that will allow

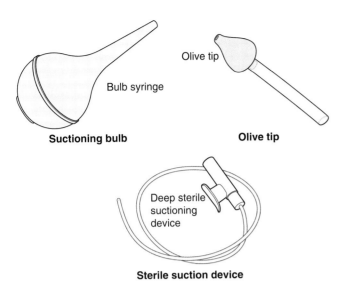

FIGURE 24.1 Suction devices for emergency use.

the rapid placement of oxygen tubing onto the oxygen wall device.

- An oxygen-delivery system, such as a nasal cannula, a simple face mask, or a nonrebreather mask, depending on the severity of the child's illness, is present and correctly sized.
- The **code blue** (cardiopulmonary arrest) call system, such as a code button or a code string/pull, is present and working.
- The numbers for emergency response—code blue (respiratory/cardiac arrest), code red (fire), and the **rapid response team (RRT)**, which responds to an emergency at the bedside—are by the bedside phone.
- Within the child's bathroom, there is a working emergency call button or string/pull.

A variety of color-coded response systems are used in large clinic and hospital settings. It is imperative that a nurse checks with their institution to learn the specific color codes for a particular health-care institution. Table 24.1 provides an example of color codes commonly used by direct caregivers to alert specific individuals, groups, security, or administration of an emergency and to communicate that help is required.

Safety *Stat!*

Four pieces of emergency equipment must be at all hospital bedsides:

- Suction machine setup with tubing and a variety of nasal and oral suction devices
- Source of oxygen and access to a variety of delivery systems and flow meters
- A variety of manual resuscitator bags and different sizes of masks to fit newborns to teens
- A means to call a RRT and a code button to call for a full code blue

Table 24.1
Color-Coded Response System

Code	Response
Code red	Fire or smoke is present on the unit. Identify the exact location and begin patient removal from harm as well as containment procedures.
Code pink	A newborn, infant, or young child is missing or has been abducted. This process initiates a lockdown procedure or security watch of all elevators, stairs, and hospital exit doors.
Code blue	CPR is needed, and a full team is required, including a pharmacist, laboratory personnel, a nursing supervisor, and a pediatric advanced life support (PALS)–certified response team.
Code yellow	A disaster has occurred; prepare for a large number of incoming patients.
Code gray	An adult is missing from their room or unit.
Code Dr. Strong	There is a need for security to come immediately to the unit or location.
Code rapid response	There is a need for an emergency response team, but the child has not fully coded.

SBAR Communication Techniques

Because ineffective communication is the source of many errors in health-care environments, the SBAR tool was developed to allow prompt, organized communication of critical information between health-care team members. **SBAR** is especially effective in communications between the nursing staff and the medical staff. The technique provides a consistent framework to communicate about a patient's condition. It is easy to remember, can be used in person or over the phone, and is useful for communicating information that requires immediate attention. *SBAR* stands for *S*ituation, *B*ackground, *A*ssessment, and *R*ecommendation. Some pediatric health-care institutions add a second R (SBARR) for *R*eading back or *R*estating the recommendations or order given by the primary health-care provider to the nurse. (As soon as possible, all verbal orders must be placed in the electronic health record. Verbal orders that are not entered correctly are a cause of significant errors.)

Team Works

SBAR Communication Tool

Here's how to use SBAR when communicating with a member of a patient's medical team.

Situation

- Identify yourself, giving your name, your title (licensed vocational nurse [LVN], RN), and the location where you are calling from.
- Identify the patient by name, date of birth, age, sex, and reason for hospitalization.
- Describe briefly the reason for the phone call; if urgent, say so.

Background

- Give the patient's presenting report, such as being short of breath, in pain, or bleeding.
- Briefly describe the patient's pertinent past medical history relating to the immediate situation, such as the patient had surgery this morning or is hospitalized for a cardiac procedure.
- Give a brief summary of the background of your concern, such as rapid development of chest pain or evidence of surgical wound infection.

Assessment

- Provide important assessment information such as recent VSs, pain scale (see Chapter 23), a change in status, or a change in level of consciousness (LOC).
- State again if any VSs are outside of parameters, such as in tachypnea, **bradycardia**, or high temperature.
- Describe your impression of the severity of the patient's situation.

Recommendation

- Provide a brief suggestion of what action you think should be taken.
- Provide an explicit list of what you think you need.
- Wait to hear a response and write it down; read back any orders that are given.
- Ask if a health-care provider will be coming to evaluate the child or what next steps are needed to provide safety and follow-through.

Safety *Stat!*

Verbal orders may be necessary in an emergency situation for an acutely ill child, but they are very prone to errors. All orders need to be placed in the child's chart (electronic medical record) as soon as possible. *Always read back or restate a verbal order to confirm it.*

· WORD · BUILDING ·

bradycardia: brady–slow + card–heart + ia–condition

RESPONDING TO EMERGENCIES

Nurses must be prepared to quickly respond to an emergency when an acutely ill child's condition worsens. Children are emotionally, anatomically, and physiologically different than adults. Their ability to compensate for a change in blood pressure, vascular volume, and respiratory status is limited; and their condition can deteriorate quickly. For this reason, it is imperative that a nurse regularly practice emergency response procedures within the clinical setting and be prepared to respond when a child's condition becomes worse. The Pediatric Early Warning System (PEWS) scoring tool allows nurses to objectively evaluate a child's behavior and clinical status. A critical PEWS score can warn the interdisciplinary care team to initiate life-saving interventions, possibly averting the need to call an RRT or a code blue team. Nurse-administered bedside PEWS scoring with an alert to physicians reduced PICU transfers (Mills et al., 2021).

Most acute care institutions offer regular practice code blue scenarios. Practicing how to call for an RRT, call a code blue, initiate a crash cart, and perform cardiopulmonary resuscitation (CPR) across the life span (newborn, infant, child, and adult) are essential nursing skills. Many conditions warrant a skilled emergency response for acutely ill children (Table 24.2). Even for experienced nurses, participating in mock codes is very helpful and allows a review of emergency equipment and procedures that may be infrequently used.

Cardiopulmonary Resuscitation

Because of developmental differences, each age group requires its own set of rapid CPR response skills. It is imperative that the pediatric health-care team apply the correct CPR skills to the age/weight of the child. Figures 24.2 and 24.3 outline the two algorithms required for one person or a two-person team to correctly perform CPR, respectively. It is imperative that a nurse remains certified in CPR (also called Basic Life Saving [BLS]). Changes in the sequence and content of CPR courses and guidelines are made based on the most recent research on clinical outcomes and best practices. Check the American Heart Association's website on a regular basis to review any changes made to CPR guidelines. Implement only the most current guidelines for the best possible outcome and a coordinated team effort. It is your responsibility to stay competent, confident, and ready to respond within a team to an acute pediatric emergency.

The majority of pediatric cardiopulmonary arrests originate from a problem in the respiratory system after a clinically significant respiratory event. Both infants' and small children's airway diameters are significantly smaller relative to their stature than adults' airways. Therefore, even a small amount of thick mucus, inflammation, or a foreign body obstruction can produce symptoms of respiratory distress. Nurses must be prepared to support a young child's airway by rapid suction, airway support, oxygenation, and possible resuscitation.

Table 24.2
Emergencies in Acutely Ill Children

Type of Condition	Examples
Cardiovascular	• Cyanotic newborn • Infant in shock • Complicated postoperative care with bleeding • Cardiac arrhythmias • Septic shock
Metabolic	• Diabetic ketoacidosis • Severe hypoglycemia • Malignant hyperthermia
Neurological	• Change in consciousness • Child abuse/shaken baby syndrome • Increased intracranial pressure
Gastrointestinal	• Peritonitis • Appendix rupture • Gastrointestinal bleeding
Immunologic	• Anaphylaxis • Acute blood-product transfusion reaction
Toxicological	• Poisoning • Ingestion of an unknown substance
Respiratory	• Severe respiratory distress, significant increased work of breathing • Foreign body aspiration • Acute epiglottitis • Status asthmaticus • Dislodged tracheostomy tube
Burns	• Smoke inhalation • Chemical, thermal, or electrical burns

Choking Emergency

In children younger than 1 year old, aspiration, obstruction, and choking are the leading causes of death. A young child's narrow airway contributes to significant choking episodes. The airway remains small for size until the child is about 5 years old. Anticipatory guidance for new parents should include explaining that an older sibling should not be allowed to feed an infant without constant supervision and that the mobile infant's environment should be frequently surveyed for choking and aspiration risks. A tracheostomy may need to be inserted if the child has upper airway obstruction to provide rapid ventilations. See Figure 24.4 for a depiction of tracheostomy equipment. Knowing how to clear a child's airway is a very important skill for a nurse (Table 24.3). Access to a bulb syringe, Yankauer device, olive tip device, or a sterile deep suction device for rapid suction of secretions from a child's airway is essential.

For children of all ages, expect continued airway symptoms after removal of the obstruction because of residual edema, inflammation, and irritation.

Child in Shock

Shock is a serious consequence of an acute or critical illness. It is the clinical outcome of poor perfusion, severe **hypovolemia**, low systemic vascular resistance (severe hypotension), or systemic venous congestion. Shock requires immediate identification and a combination of aggressive treatments or the condition is fatal. There are four types of shock: hypovolemic, cardiogenic, distributive, and obstructive. Children who are hospitalized for trauma, severe infections, severe dehydration, or with cardiac complications are at risk for shock. The highest priority in the early treatment of shock is to restore oxygenation to the tissues and the brain. In general, this is done by providing an oxygen source, improving blood volume and distributing the volume, reducing the increased oxygen demand, and correcting metabolic instability. Any change in perfusion, blood pressure, or LOC must be reported and acted upon rapidly. See Box 24.1 for a list of types of shock found in children.

Safety Stat!

Three common symptoms of early shock are hypovolemia, hypotension, and a change in mental status. If shock is suspected, immediately call for help (RRT, code blue, or 911 emergency services) and begin life-saving interventions. Stay with the child at all times.

General Management of Shock

Associated with poor clinical outcome and death, shock can only be reversed when it is identified early and there is a team effort to stabilize the child's cardiopulmonary system. The following guidelines can help stabilize the child in shock:

- Position the child to increase cardiac output, such as in supine position.
- Provide rapid, high-flow oxygen and prepare for intubation and mechanical ventilation.
- Protect the child's vascular access to allow administration of **vasoactive** medications; child may require a central line placement (Figs. 24.5 and 24.6).

· WORD · BUILDING ·

hypovolemia: hypo–deficient + vol–volume + em–blood + ia–condition

vasoactive: vaso–vessel + active–acting on

BLS Healthcare Provider
Pediatric Cardiac Arrest Algorithm for the Single Rescuer

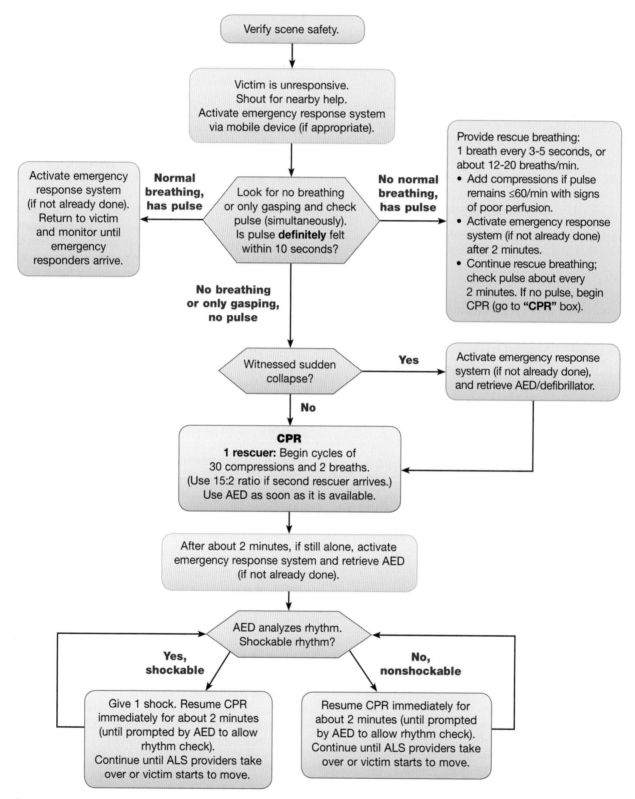

© 2015 American Heart Association

FIGURE 24.2 BLS healthcare provider pediatric cardiac arrest algorithm for the single rescuer. Reprinted with permission. Web-Based Integrated American Heart Association Guidelines for CPR & ECC-Part 11: Pediatric Basic Life Support and Cardiopulmonary Resuscitation Quality © 2015 American Heart Association, Inc.

BLS Healthcare Provider
Pediatric Cardiac Arrest Algorithm for 2 or More Rescuers

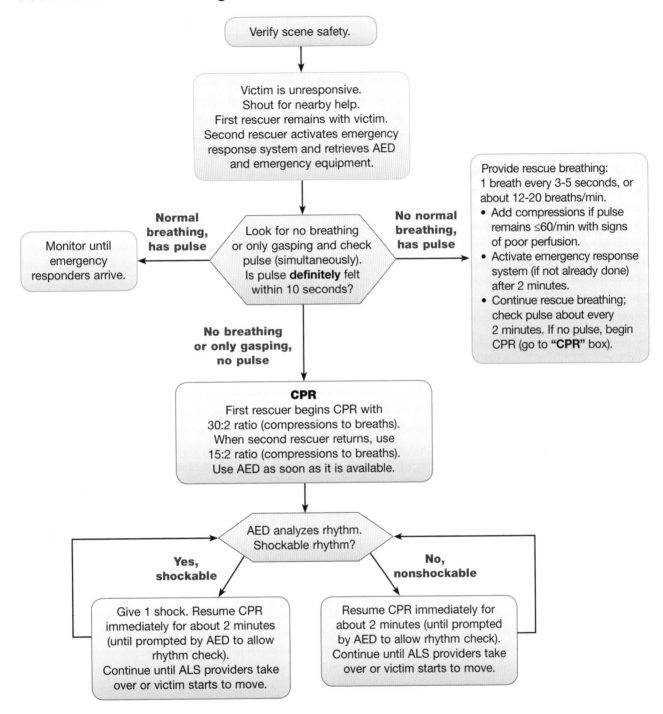

Verify scene safety.

Victim is unresponsive.
Shout for nearby help.
First rescuer remains with victim.
Second rescuer activates emergency
response system and retrieves AED
and emergency equipment.

Normal breathing, has pulse → Monitor until emergency responders arrive.

Look for no breathing or only gasping and check pulse (simultaneously). Is pulse **definitely** felt within 10 seconds?

No normal breathing, has pulse →

Provide rescue breathing:
1 breath every 3-5 seconds, or
about 12-20 breaths/min.
• Add compressions if pulse
  remains ≤60/min with signs
  of poor perfusion.
• Activate emergency response
  system (if not already done)
  after 2 minutes.
• Continue rescue breathing;
  check pulse about every
  2 minutes. If no pulse, begin
  CPR (go to **"CPR"** box).

**No breathing
or only gasping,
no pulse**

CPR
First rescuer begins CPR with
30:2 ratio (compressions to breaths).
When second rescuer returns, use
15:2 ratio (compressions to breaths).
Use AED as soon as it is available.

AED analyzes rhythm.
Shockable rhythm?

**Yes,
shockable**

**No,
nonshockable**

Give 1 shock. Resume CPR
immediately for about 2 minutes
(until prompted by AED to allow
rhythm check).
Continue until ALS providers take
over or victim starts to move.

Resume CPR immediately for
about 2 minutes (until prompted
by AED to allow rhythm check).
Continue until ALS providers take
over or victim starts to move.

© 2015 American Heart Association

FIGURE 24.3 BLS healthcare provider pediatric cardiac arrest algorithm for two rescuers. Reprinted with permission. Web-Based Integrated American Heart Association Guidelines for CPR & ECC-Part 11: Pediatric Basic Life Support and Cardiopulmonary Resuscitation Quality © 2015 American Heart Association, Inc.

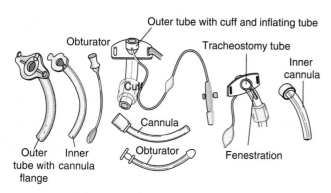

FIGURE 24.4 Tracheostomy equipment.

- Make sure that the team has an accurate height and weight of the child, or secure the use of a color-coded resuscitative tape, such as the Broselow system.
- Collect specimens for STAT laboratory analysis.
- Provide vascular volume expansion through isotonic crystalloid IV fluids (normal saline [NS]) via boluses that may be repeated several times.
- Administer required medications such as vasoactive medications and antibiotics.
- Closely monitor the child for responses to the preceding interventions.
- Secure either a rapid transfer to an intensive care environment or place the crash cart near the child.

Table 24.3
Guidelines for Airway Clearance

Patient Population	Airway Clearance Guidelines
Newborn airway clearance (birth–1 month)	• Do not perform blind finger sweep; rapidly suction secretions or mucus. • Place newborn on flat surface. • Perform five chest thrusts with two fingers. • Monitor respiratory status continuously after removal of object. • Provide low-flow oxygen as required after event. • Position newborn supine in sniffing position for maximal ventilation.
Infant airway clearance (1 month–1 year)	• Do not perform blind finger sweep: remove foreign object via finger sweep only if visible. • Place infant over leg, head down, and start in prone position; support the head and neck with one hand. • Perform five back blows followed by five chest thrusts with the other hand. • Monitor respiratory status continuously after removal of object. • Provide low-flow oxygen as required after event. • Position child side-lying and in sniffing position for maximal ventilation. • Make sure that child is seen by emergency personnel and transfer to appropriate level of care.
Child airway clearance (1–8 years)	• Do not perform blind finger sweep; remove foreign object via finger sweep only if object is visible. • If over 1 year of age, perform Heimlich maneuver (abdominal thrusts). • Continue until successful or child loses consciousness; then begin CPR. • Monitor respiratory status continuously after removal of the object. • Call for emergency backup and assessment (RRT or 911); may require transport. • Position child for adequate ventilation. • Provide low-dose oxygen as required after the event.
Older child/adolescent airway clearance (8 years–adult)	• Do not perform blind finger sweep; remove foreign object via finger sweep only if object is visible. • Perform Heimlich maneuver (abdominal thrusts). • Continue until successful or if patient loses consciousness, then begin CPR. • Monitor respiratory status continuously after removal of object. • Position child for adequate ventilation. • Provide low-dose oxygen as required after event. • Call for medical personnel (RRT or 911) to evaluate older child or adolescent after episode for possible transfer.

Box 24.1

Types of Shock Found in Children

Hypovolemic Shock

Hypovolemic shock occurs when a child presents in severe dehydration and then experiences severe vascular volume depletion. The child will require rapid administration of IV fluids with a reassessment of their fluid status via VSs after each fluid bolus to determine if more is required. Urine output is severely compromised during hypovolemic shock, and IV potassium should not be administered until the child's urine output has been reestablished.

Cardiogenic Shock

When the child demonstrates signs of pulmonary or systemic venous congestion such as increased work of breathing, distended neck veins, grunting, and signs of decreased perfusion, cardiogenic shock must be suspected. The focus of treatment is on the restoration of cardiac output. The child must be transferred to a critical care environment because mechanical ventilation is often required to support the child and vasoactive medications may be needed to maintain adequate blood pressure and circulation.

Distributive Shock

Children who demonstrate a severe low blood pressure may be experiencing distributive shock. This condition is caused by a very low systemic vascular resistance, vasodilation, and the buildup of lactic acid. Monitor the child for change in LOC. The most common causes of distributive shock are an overwhelming infection, leading to sepsis, or a complete loss of vascular tone from conditions such as spinal cord injury or anaphylaxis.

Obstructive Shock

Obstructive shock is identified when a diagnostic examination finds increased central venous pressure. The cardiac output is reduced, and a decrease of blood flow from the heart is suspected. The goal of therapy is to initiate vasoactive medications in an intensive care environment.

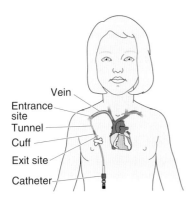

Vein
Entrance site
Tunnel
Cuff
Exit site
Catheter

FIGURE 24.5 Tunneled catheter.

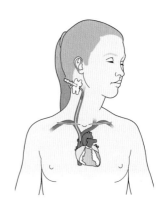

FIGURE 24.6 Jugular line.

Labs & Diagnostics

The pediatric health-care team may request laboratory analysis of a child's blood if the child is demonstrating signs and symptoms of shock. These analyses include venous blood gases, arterial blood gases (ABG), blood cultures, lactate, calcium, complete blood cell count (CBC), chemistry panels, and glucose.

Medication Facts

For a child in shock, these are the most important medications to anticipate for administration:

- Antibiotics
- Vasopressors (vasoactive medications that support blood pressure) such as dopamine, norepinephrine, or epinephrine
- Glucose, for severe hypoglycemia
- Corticosteroids, for adrenal insufficiency and to support hemodynamic stability
- Antihistamines

Cardiovascular Conditions

It is rare that a previously healthy child experiences a significant cardiac event that requires emergency response. Young infants, on the other hand, can experience circumstances where the airway, ventilation, and gas exchange are affected, in which case they demonstrate serious symptoms requiring emergency care. An episode of acute hypercyanosis, tet spells (associated with a serious congenital heart condition called tetralogy of Fallot [TOF]), or acute life-threatening events are three examples of clinical situations where children may need rapid emergency cardiac care provided by interdisciplinary teams.

Cyanotic Infant

Cyanosis is defined as an episode in which a patient suddenly becomes purplish or blue in the skin and mucous membranes. The discoloration is related to a sudden decrease in oxygenation. The child may present with a central cyanosis or peripheral cyanosis. If the child has accompanying respiratory

· WORD · BUILDING ·
cyanosis: cyan–blue + osis–condition

distress, then the health-care team should consider a respiratory cause of the cyanosis. If the patient is tachycardic but otherwise quiet and without respiratory involvement, the team should consider a cardiovascular cause.

- **Central cyanosis:** Discoloration of the trunk caused by reduced hemoglobin; associated with reduced oxygen saturation measurements.
- **Peripheral cyanosis:** Decreased cardiac output with an accompanying decrease in the peripheral blood flow; peripheral cyanosis (in the extremities) may not demonstrate a reduced oxygen saturation measurement.

Safety Stat!

If a nurse encounters an infant with cyanosis, interventions required include the following:

- Checking for breathing and circulation
- Opening the airway and determining the need for CPR
- Stimulating the child
- Giving 100% oxygen via mask
- Suctioning the airway as needed to remove an obstruction
- Monitoring the child: placing on oxygen saturation and cardiac monitor
- Obtaining an ABG, electrolyte panel (also called chemistry panel), and a CBC

Tet Spells

A congenital (existing since birth) heart condition called TOF is an emergency cardiac anomaly. TOF requires open heart surgery for a repair of four conditions: overriding aorta, hypertrophy of the right ventricle, ventricular septal defect, and pulmonary stenosis. This severe condition causes acute and sudden central cyanotic spells referred to as *tet spells*. A tet spell requires the immediate application of oxygen. An RRT should be called to assist with this life-threatening emergency. (See Chapter 31 for more about TOF.)

CRITICAL THINKING & CLINICAL JUDGMENT

While walking in the halls of a busy pediatric unit, you see a toddler walking with his mother suddenly start crying loudly over her refusal to give him a treat. The child becomes quiet, falls to the floor, turns cyanotic, and loses consciousness. You know the child is hospitalized for continued care for TOF.

Questions

1. What is the severity of this event?
2. What should you do immediately after witnessing this event?

Apparent Life-Threatening Event

An **apparent life-threatening event (ALTE)**, also called an *acute life-threatening event* or a *brief resolved unexplained event (BRUE)*, is not a formal medical diagnosis. Rather, it is a sudden, acute, and unexpected change in a young infant's breathing pattern, which leads to a color change (blueness, paleness, flushing or redness), apnea, limpness, and often choking or gagging. An ALTE is frightening to a caregiver who witnesses it. The child appears in acute distress, and it may even appear as if the infant has died. The episode requires immediate interventions from advanced pediatric health-care providers, and the child should be hospitalized and monitored carefully during the diagnostic period. The child may require only stimulation to bring them out of the episode or may require resuscitation efforts. Monitor the child closely for a subsequent event. Risk factors associated with ALTE include a history of cyanosis, difficulties with feeding, and episodes of repeated apnea.

Safety Stat!

Rapid assessments and interventions for a witnessed ALTE include positioning the airway open, stimulating the child, checking for obstruction, checking for bradycardia or other abnormal heart rhythms, checking for an airway obstruction, administering 100% oxygen, suctioning the airway if mucus is obstructing it, and beginning CPR as needed.

Typically, the child's health-care provider will send the infant to the ED, describing the incident of ALTE as the "chief complaint." A thorough investigation into the cause of the ALTE needs to be conducted to rule out sepsis, gastroesophageal reflux, central nervous system (CNS) disorders, airway obstruction, metabolic disorders, or poisoning. ALTE is often associated with obstructive apnea.

The following should be obtained for all infants who present with ALTE:

- Thorough medical history and detailed description of the event
- History of pregnancy, birth, and perinatal period
- Information about any recent fall, injury, or ingestion of a substance
- Physical examination of height, weight, VSs, signs of trauma, developmental assessment, and airway
- If the ALTE is determined to be a laryngospasm after gastroesophageal reflux, then further diagnostics should be performed, including:
  - Blood counts, cultures, and chemistries
  - Urinalysis
  - Metabolic screening
  - Reflux screening
  - Brain neuroimaging
  - Skeletal survey
  - Echocardiogram
  - Chest x-ray

Management of an infant who presents with ALTE should include hospitalization with monitoring. Any serious underlying medical conditions must be ruled out, especially those concerning the child's airway. The family should be taught CPR before hospital discharge. Home-monitoring equipment may be ordered but often is used on a case-by-case basis.

Child in Acute Respiratory Distress

Children in acute respiratory distress need immediate attention and intervention. Young children are dependent on abdominal and diaphragmatic breathing and require rapid interventions to maintain an effective airway, air exchange, and breathing pattern. Early signs of respiratory distress include the following:

- Nasal flaring (Fig. 24.7)
- Head bobbing
- Anxiety
- Lethargy
- Decreased rate of responsiveness
- Retractions (subcostal, intercostal, suprasternal, and sternal)
- Wheezing and stridor
- Increased use of energy and effort needed to breathe
- Feeding problems and refusal to eat (fatigue and decreased ability to suck/swallow)
- Tachypnea and/or **hyperpnea**
- Hypoxia and hypercarbia

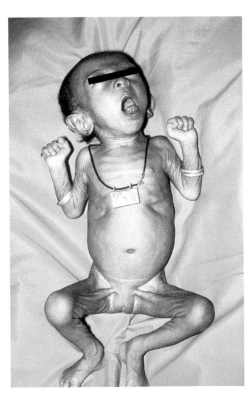

FIGURE 24.7 Infant demonstrating flaring of nares during respiratory distress.

hyperpnea: hyper–excessive + pnea–breathing

Late signs of respiratory distress include the following:

- Poor perfusion
- Bradycardia
- Decreased air movement and diminished breath sounds
- Expiratory grunting
- Apnea (cessation in spontaneous breathing for greater than 20 seconds)
- Sweating

Airway issues are the number one cause of emergency responses in children. Airway obstruction, inflammation, or occlusion will cause the child to have respiratory distress that may lead to the need for ventilation support. Think about airway issues first when a child demonstrates a change in clinical status. Common causes of decreased ventilation and respiratory distress can be found in Table 24.4.

Table 24.4
Common Causes of Decreased Ventilation and Respiratory Distress

Lower Airway	*Upper Airway*
• Respiratory syncytial virus (RSV) • Bronchiolitis • Asthma • Pneumonia • Foreign body in airway • Bronchospasm • Copious mucus	• Tracheal stenosis • Foreign body in airway • Croup • Epiglottitis • Tongue swelling (allergic response)

Safety *Stat!*

Epiglottitis is a life-threatening infectious process that has the potential to cause complete obstruction in a child's airway. Patients who present with epiglottitis may need to have a tracheostomy if antibiotics and corticosteroids are not effective in reducing the infection and inflammation.

Safety *Stat!*

When a child is diagnosed with a severe respiratory illness and is experiencing respiratory distress, the team should place the child's condition on "guarded" or "critical" status. This designation will provide extra monitoring by health-care team members so that a change in clinical status can be identified and rapid airway support provided.

epiglottitis: epi–above + glott–glottis + itis–inflammation

A smooth response to an acutely ill child in crisis is the responsibility of a team. Because an effective response requires more than one person, designated health-care personnel must be available 24 hours a day to respond to emergencies. The following steps outline the actions needed to provide critical care support:

- Initiate compressions, airway, and breathing (CAB) through high-quality and effective CPR.
- Call for backup help immediately; do not hesitate to get help, and do not take a "wait and see" attitude!
- Do not leave the child alone or unsupervised under any circumstances, especially if there is a decline in the child's condition.
- Bring the crash cart to the child's room and position it close to the child; it is much better to have it and not need it than to delay a resuscitative effort to retrieve it.
- Monitor pulse oximetry continuously if you suspect a change in condition.
- Provide supplemental oxygen therapy.
- Position the child for maximal air exchange, such as the sniffing position.
- Monitor the child's blood pressure; hypotension is often a late sign of an imminent emergency.
- Apply a cardiorespiratory monitor; set on lead II for ease of interpretation. See Figure 24.8 for placement of leads.
- Establish patent IV access.
- Be prepared to rapidly draw pertinent laboratory tests (chemistry, CBC, ABG).
- Communicate child's history, present clinical status, and medical diagnosis to responding interdisciplinary RRT or code blue team.
- Provide support to the family.
- Call the nursing supervisor for leadership and coordination of all unit activities during the emergency.
- Call the social worker to come and assist with the needs of the family in crisis.

Children who have severe allergies may need to have an epinephrine injector (EpiPen) prescribed. In an emergency, severe respiratory distress can be treated with epinephrine in an outpatient setting with the child being transferred to an acute setting for further evaluation and treatment. Parents must know how to identify when the EpiPen is needed, how to check for the pen's expiration date, how to administer the medication, and how to call for help after administration. Further guidelines include the following:

- The pen should remain in the original manufacturer's packaging so that the administration instructions can be referred to quickly.
- At least two pens should be maintained so that there is one at home and one stored per protocol at the child's school or daycare.
- The pen's expiration date should be checked on a regular basis and the pen replaced before it expires.
- The parents and any other caregivers for the child should periodically practice administering the medication to maintain competence and confidence.

HIGHER LEVEL OF EQUIPMENT PROVIDED IN THE HOSPITAL ENVIRONMENT

Children who experience a significant change in clinical status that warrants a move to a higher level of care will also need specialized emergency equipment. Becoming familiar with emergency equipment can save lives. Even if you are not directly responsible for using the equipment, a basic level of understanding should be secured. Knowing where the equipment is stored, what it is used for, how to determine what equipment will be used when, and how to determine the right size of equipment for a child's particular height and weight can be extremely helpful for the response team.

Various clinical settings have different emergency equipment available. At the very least, a crash cart and a defibrillator should be made available. The following section describes several pieces of emergency equipment.

Crash Carts

Emergency response carts (crash carts) are available throughout the acute care hospital environment. It is imperative that you know where to locate these carts and be familiar with how the equipment is organized. Some crash carts are organized by the child's weight in kilograms; others are organized in systems such as airway support/intubation drawer, medication drawer, or IV access and fluids drawer. In general, the following list represents what a nurse can expect to find on or in the cart:

- Emergency response medications for various emergency conditions and situations
- Oxygen equipment, including a variety of masks and various sizes of manual resuscitator bags and masks
- Airway supplies, including a variety of sizes of equipment for intubation

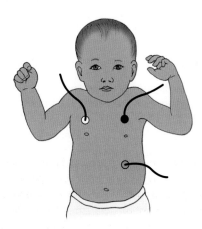

FIGURE 24.8 Child with a cardiac monitor on.

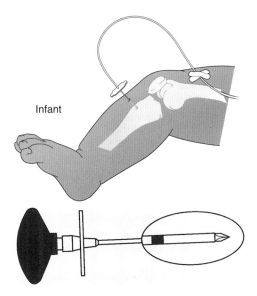

Infant

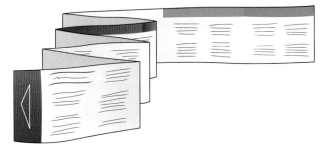

FIGURE 24.10 Color-coded, length-based resuscitation tape.

FIGURE 24.9 Intraosseous needle inserted in bone. (Bottom) Permission for use granted by Cook Medical, Bloomington, Indiana.

- IV therapy/fluids such as NS, lactated Ringer's (LR) solution, and IV start supplies; both peripheral IV catheters and interosseous needles must be present in the cart (Fig. 24.9)
- Laboratory specimen collection equipment and containers for obtaining ABG, CBC, electrolytes, and chemistry
- Back board to rapidly provide a hard surface for efficient chest compressions
- **Broselow tape** in case the child's weight is unknown
- Suction equipment for rapid airway clearance
- Cardiac monitoring equipment and cardioversion equipment
- Oxygen tanks
- Algorithmic charts or cards to guide the team through various emergency situations (bradycardia, tachycardias, asystole, etc.)

Medication Facts

An interosseous needle is used if traditional peripheral or central IV access is not possible or is unsuccessful during the care of a critically ill child. The needle is placed into the marrow of one of the child's long bones, such as the anterior superior area of the tibia. This use of the interosseous needle and the site of the flat area of a long bone has been found to be as effective a system of medication administration and distribution as IV injections.

Crash carts must be checked every 24 hours. One person, such as the charge nurse, will be responsible to check on the function and status of crash cart contents. Checking for expiration dates of the emergency medications is a very important aspect of maintaining emergency response equipment. All crash cart checks must be documented for state or regional inspectors.

Color-Coded, Length-Based Resuscitation Tape

Color-coded, length-based resuscitation tape—for example, Broselow pediatric emergency tape (Broselow-Luten system)—is a tool used to determine the correct equipment and dosage of medication needed for children of various sizes during an emergency response (Fig. 24.10). The tape is recommended for use on any child under the age of 12 years. Because pediatric medications are most often calculated by milligrams per kilogram, rapid decisions can be made more easily and correctly if the child's exact weight is known. In emergency situations in which the child cannot be or has not been weighed, the color-coded resuscitation tape is used to determine the best estimate of the child's weight based on the child's length. The tape is retrieved rapidly from the crash cart and placed next to the critically ill pediatric patient. Where the child's heel falls on the tape determines the color-coded "zone" where medication doses and equipment sizes are presented. The team reads the information given on the zone and then selects the prepared medications, IV fluid boluses, and emergency equipment (endotracheal tubes, suction catheters, and urinary catheters) based on that colored zone. The response team does not need to rely on memory to determine the appropriate size of equipment or medication dosing during an emergency. With increasing rates of childhood obesity, Broselow tape may be less accurate because of underestimation of a child's weight (Waseem et al., 2019). The tape may lead to underdosing medications in children who are obese as the tape estimates weight based on length (Walls, 2018).

Safety Stat!

The child should never be measured for the color-coded length-based emergency resuscitation tape while sitting up or having the head of the bed up. Pull the foot up in a 90-degree flexed position before measuring "Red to Head" (red marking on top denotes where to place tape).

For the color-coded length-based pediatric emergency tape to be effective, it must be used correctly. The child is placed supine on a flat surface with the color-coded side of the tape visible. The team places the red end of the tape even with the top surface of the child's head (Think "Red to Head.") and smooths the tape out along the child's side. The zone appropriate for the child is determined by where the child's heels, not the child's toes, fall on the tape.

Other than a color-coded, length-based, pediatric emergency resuscitation tape, the acute care facility may also have crash carts that are organized according to the color-coded system. Here, instead of being organized by body system, the crash cart will have all of the equipment needed for the child in a particular color zone. For instance, the orange zone cart is for children whose measured height will average a weight that falls between 24 and 28 kg (52.9 and 61.7 lb).

Rapid Fluid Resuscitation

Children whose condition rapidly deteriorates often require the rapid instillation of IV fluids (IVF). A common order is to provide NS (0.9%) IVF boluses at 20 mL per kg. The rate at which the boluses are delivered is up to the emergency response medical team. A common order for a child with a *deteriorating condition* would be to administer between 1 and 3 boluses with VSs rechecked after each bolus. Follow orders carefully for safe clinical practice when caring for a child whose clinical condition is rapidly deteriorating.

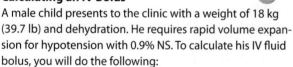

Medication Facts

Calculating an IV Bolus

A male child presents to the clinic with a weight of 18 kg (39.7 lb) and dehydration. He requires rapid volume expansion for hypotension with 0.9% NS. To calculate his IV fluid bolus, you will do the following:

- Multiply his weight of 18 kg (39.7 lb) by 20 mL (IV boluses are typically 20 mL per kg per bolus but may vary between 5 to 30 mL per kg).
- The total is 360 mL of fluid.
- The fluid IV bolus is 0.9% NS.

The rate of infusion is standard; infuse each bolus ordered over 30 minutes to 1 hour unless otherwise directed. You will then take a set of VSs to see if the child's clinical status has improved.

CARING FOR FAMILIES PRESENT DURING EMERGENCIES

The family of an acutely ill child may be in the room when the child experiences cardiac or respiratory failure ("codes"). How do you provide care for the family while activating an emergency response for the patient? Should the family be allowed to remain in the room, out of the way of medical personnel, or should they be asked to leave? Although research is not conclusive, some studies have shown that some family members who witness at least part of an emergency resuscitative response have a shorter period of grief if the child dies (Compton et al., 2011; Dahlin et al., 2016). Witnessing the resuscitative response may help to reduce the experience of pain if death occurs (De Stefano et al., 2016) and has not been found to have a negative impact on the family (Vardanjani et al., 2021). Determining if the family should be present during a code is based on hospital practice or policy.

Follow these principles in providing care to families of critically ill children:

- Know the institutional policy for guidelines on family presence during resuscitation efforts.
- Understand that research has shown that most families want to be present for at least part of the attempted resuscitative process and to see and/or touch the body if the code response was not successful (De Stefano et al., 2016).
- Families may be very reluctant to ask to remain present, so offer the opportunity.
- Discuss the option of being present for resuscitation efforts *before* the child experiences a code blue.
- Notify the nursing supervisor of the family's wishes and provide physical room for them to be present.
- Evaluate the family's reaction and be sensitive to their need to leave during the resuscitation process.
- Provide emotional support after the resuscitation event and answer any questions the family may have.
- Make sure that a referral is made to the social worker for the immediate assistance of professional support and clergy follow-up.

Evidence-Based Practice

Research has shown that family presence during a code blue resuscitative effort on children does not have a negative impact. In a review of literature by Vardanjani and colleagues (2021), families who stay during a resuscitative effort did not hinder the code team, but rather focused on the patient. Most studies found that the presence of the family was helpful to both the family members and to the staff performing the efforts. Being present was found to reduce anxiety and fear and gave them the sense of peace of mind that all was being done that could be done for the child. Vardanjani and colleagues (2021) provided the conclusion that, "Given the strong emotional bond among family members, the opportunity to be present during resuscitation or invasive procedures was comforting for all parties" (p. 757).

Vardanjani, A. E., Golitaleb, M., Abdi, K., Kia, M. K., Moayedi, S., Torres, M., & Dehghan-Nayeri, N. (2021). The effect of family presence during resuscitation and invasive procedures on patients and families: An umbrella review. *Journal of Emergency Nursing, 47*(5), 752–760. https://doi.org/10.1016/j.jen.2021.04.007

Identifying the Decision-Maker Within the Family

When an acutely ill child experiences a change in clinical status, a transfer to a higher level of care, such as an intensive care unit (ICU), may be warranted. During this stressful time, it is very likely that decisions will have to be made. The health-care team needs to identify who the legal decision-maker is for the child and who the primary decision-maker is in the family. These may be two different family members, or they may be the same person.

The primary decision-maker for health-care treatment plans may not be the child's legal guardian. Although the legal parents or guardians will sign the treatment forms and consents, it is possible that a family elder ultimately makes decisions for the family. Including the decision-maker in the family conference is an important gesture of respect for the cultural or ethnic background of the family. Empowering the family to be included in treatment discussions ultimately creates more trusting and respectful collaborative interactions.

According to Citko and Bourne (2002) and Chaet (2017), the following questions should be answered about the family's decision-maker or a surrogate decision-maker:

1. Does the health-care decision-maker have a close, caring relationship with the patient?
2. Is this person aware of the family's and the patient's (child's) values and beliefs?
3. Is this person willing and able to make the needed medical treatment decisions?
4. Is there a consensus among the individuals as to the proper decision or decision-maker?
5. If the decision-maker is not a family member but rather a surrogate, is the person known to the patient?

The health-care team should document how medical decisions were made if someone other than the primary legal guardian or parent is involved with the child's health-care treatment decisions. Because children under 18 years of age are unable to make their health-care wishes known with legally binding documents such as advance directives, it is imperative that the health-care team support the family during difficult decision making and document the entire process that has occurred.

RAPID RESPONSE TEAMS

In acute care settings, a patient's condition can worsen rapidly, and the health-care team needs to have assistance immediately. RRTs were developed to offer family and staff an option to request and receive support from health-care professionals above and beyond those present on the floor. RRTs give nurses support in responding to emergencies in which a patient's condition suddenly becomes much worse but the patient has not fully "coded" or gone into cardiopulmonary arrest. The activation of an RRT can be done by anyone who sees a patient's condition change so dramatically that assistance is required right away to prevent full cardiopulmonary arrest. Most institutions post the number to call for an RRT at each patient's bedside.

Team Works

The Emergency Response Team

Essential members of a code blue team or RRT include the following:

- Pediatric hospitalist in-house; will lead the code
- RN assigned to the patient's care; will have the most current information about the child, including the admitting diagnosis, current medications, most current weight, and clinical picture of the child
- Pediatric Advanced Life Support (PALS)–certified nurse to assist during the resuscitative efforts
- Critical care nurse with expert knowledge of calculating, drawing up, and administering antiarrhythmic medications
- Respiratory therapist to manage the child's airway
- Pharmacist who can assist with the management and replenishing of the emergency medications
- Member of central supply who can provide backup supplies for the crash cart
- Runner (laboratory personnel member) for the specimens to be taken to the laboratory or to run the bedside laboratory evaluation equipment
- Nursing supervisor who can provide staffing support and support for the family

---

RRTs significantly lower mortality (death) and length of stay in pediatric intensive care units (PICUs; Kolovos et al., 2018); research has shown a 21.4% reduction of deaths and a 37% reduction of arrests (Cheng & Mikrogianakis, 2018). In addition, the Institute for Health Improvement (2019) continues to support the development of timely identification of need for RRTs to prevent unnecessary deaths.

Clinical situations in which an RRT should be called include the following:

- Airway compromise
- Grand mal seizures
- Change in neurological status/LOC
- **Dehiscence** of a wound
- Significant fall, resulting in an actual or potential injury
- Any unexpected or rapid change in clinical status in which you or the family becomes concerned for the child's welfare
- Head injuries
- Hemorrhage

· WORD · BUILDING ·

dehiscence: de–apart + hiscence–gaping or splitting

How to Call a Rapid Response Team

Every hospital or health-care institution may have a slightly different procedure to call an RRT. The phone number to call should be posted in each child's room with an explanation of the purpose of the team. The number should also be posted at the nursing station and in the treatment room, the elevators, and the playroom. Typically, the call is transferred to an operator who then sends the emergency notification out to the various team members. Many institutions promote the calling of an RRT by family members who are present during a change in the clinical status of their child. Research has shown that this system is not abused by families and that the RRT is used appropriately.

Patient Teaching Guidelines

Calling for the Rapid Response Team

Many pediatric units and hospitals are now providing the family with a means to call the RRT without waiting to notify you of the child's changing condition. Guidelines for the family should include the following:

- Providing the family with education about what the RRT is and does
- Reminding the family that they may call the RRT for rapid assistance for their child in an emergency
- Teaching the family symptoms and/or clinical signs to be aware of that would warrant calling the RRT
- Providing the number to call the RRT in large, dark print located near the child's hospital room phone
- Letting the family know that if they are uncomfortable calling the RRT, they may call for help from the nursing station and help will be rapidly summoned

HELPFUL EMERGENCY RESPONSE MNEMONICS

Mnemonics (memory devices) are tools to help rapidly remember and organize thinking about the steps to an assessment, response, or skill. The most commonly used medical mnemonic is CAB (compressions–airway–breathing), the steps of basic CPR. It is important to identify mnemonics that have been validated and are supported by professional nursing and medical associations, such as the American Heart Association. Table 24.5 provides a list of mnemonics that are useful to nurses who need to perform rapid assessments or interventions for children whose conditions are clinically unstable.

Safety *Stat!*

The three medications the pediatric health-care team may require when a child is demonstrating acute respiratory distress, such as allergic responses to immunizations or antibiotics, are the following:

- Epinephrine 1:1,000 OR 1:10,000 (depending on the route given)
- Antihistamine, such as diphenhydramine
- Anti-inflammatory, such as methylprednisolone, a corticosteroid

ASSESSING AN ACUTELY ILL CHILD

One method of assessing the stability of an acutely ill child is by using a systems approach. Table 24.6 provides comprehensive assessment information to determine the need to call for assistance from the pediatric hospitalist, RRT, or code blue team for the child. Any abnormal finding must be reported, acted on, and documented carefully.

CHAIN OF COMMAND AND REQUEST FOR A HIGHER LEVEL OF CARE

Nurses must always provide care within their scope of practice. A licensed practical or vocational nurse (LPN/LVN) uses the chain of command to immediately report any significant change in a patient's clinical status to the next appropriate person. If an RN is present and is a part of the health-care team, such as in a hospital or an acute/critical care environment, then the LPN/LVN would immediately solicit the involvement of the RN. If the setting does not include an RN, such as in some long-term care environments, then the LPN/LVN must follow the institutional policy on rapidly reporting a clinical concern. In some environments, such as a blood bank, the LPN/LVN may be required to call 911 for immediate assistance. It is imperative that you know the scope of practice and the reporting chain of command in the facility (Box 24.2).

When a hospitalized child experiences a change in clinical status that warrants a higher level of care, quick and efficient processes must take place to move the child and their belongings. You are responsible for assisting the health-care team to move a child from the acute care pediatric unit to the PICU. Communicating with the family is imperative so that their stress and fears about the move are reduced.

Transferring to a Higher Level of Care

The child should never be left alone during the preparation for the transfer. Ideally, one staff member should be assigned to the child until the transfer is complete, especially if CPR

Table 24.5
Medical and Nursing Mnemonics for Care of the Acutely Ill Child

Mnemonic	Definition
CAB	**The Beginning Steps of CPR** C = **C**ompressions A = **A**irway B = Resuscitative **B**reathing (bag-valve-mask of appropriate size)
ABC COPIME	A = **A**irway assessment, open B = **B**reathing C = **C**ompressions after an assessment of presence of heart rate C = Grab the **C**rash **C**art, open drawers, and attach the equipment to the child. Place on three-lead electrocardiogram (ECG) for monitoring or attach cardioversion pad (age appropriate), attach blood pressure cuff, and prepare suction device and tubing. O = Place the child on an appropriate **O**xygen delivery device and flow rate for condition; if artificial breathing is required, attach high-flow source of oxygen to the manual resuscitator rescue bag. P = **P**lace the child on a backboard, typically located on the back of the crash cart, to provide support for compressions. I = Start **IV** access, rapidly draw laboratory tests, and have a runner take to the laboratory; begin fluid resuscitation with NS boluses (20 mL/kg rapid infusion). M = **M**ove all equipment, other patients, and any physical obstructions to make room for the resuscitative team. E = **E**xplain to the members of the response team the medical history of the child, what happened, how long the child was requiring resuscitation, and what has been done.

Source for CAB: Merchant, R. M., Topjian, A. A., Panchal, A. R., Cheng, A., Aziz, K., Berg, K. M., Lavonas, E. J., & Magid, D. J. (2020). Part 1: Executive summary: 2020 American Heart Association guidelines for cardiopulmonary resuscitation and emergency cardiovascular care. *Circulation, 142*(Suppl. 16), S337–S357. https://doi.org/10.1161/CIR.0000000000000918. Original source for ABC COPIME: Linnard-Palmer, L., Phillips, W., Fink, M., Catolico, O., & Sweeny, N. (2013). Testing a mnemonic on response skills during simulated codes. *Clinical Simulation in Nursing, 9*(6), e191–e197. https://doi.org/10.1016/j.ecns.2011.12.004

Table 24.6
Rapid Assessment of Body Systems

Body System	Signs
General appearance	• Work of breathing • Overall skin color • LOC • Poor feeding behaviors • Inconsolable crying in nonverbal children
Skin	• Presence of a rash • Mottling of skin • Cyanosis: central, peripheral, and/or **circumoral** • Presence of petechiae • Purpura spots on skin • Poor perfusion; delayed capillary refill time (greater than 3 sec)
Head, ears, eyes, nose, and throat (HEENT)	• Sunken eyes • Signs of traumatic head injury • Retinal hemorrhages • Epistaxis (nosebleed) • Inability to swallow, drooling, dyspnea (epiglottitis?)

Continued

· WORD · BUILDING ·

circumoral: circum–around + or–mouth + al–relating to

Table 24.6

Rapid Assessment of Body Systems—cont'd

Body System	Signs
Cardiovascular (CV) system	• Presence of abnormal heart sounds; murmurs • Tachycardia • Apnea (periods of no breathing lasting 20 sec or longer) • Hypotension (often a late sign)
Respiratory system	• Hypoventilation • Wheezing • Rales • Retractions: subclavicular, substernal, intracostal, and/or subcostal • Paradoxical breathing/see-saw breathing • Adventitious breath sounds
Gastrointestinal system	• Abdominal pain • Vomiting • Projectile vomiting • Diarrhea • Abdominal masses • Signs of obstruction or peritonitis
CNS	• Irritability • Lethargy • Altered LOC, especially a reduction in alertness • Seizures • Paralysis • Weakness • Coma

Box 24.2

Case Study: Reporting Chain of Command

A 4-year-old male child is admitted to the pediatric unit of a small community hospital after being stabilized for a fracture of his left femur within the ED. In the ED, a cast was placed on the child's left lower extremity, extending from the child's hips to the ankle (spica cast). VSs are within an expected range, and the child's pain score using the FLACC pain assessment tool and the Wong-Baker pain assessment tool both demonstrated a value of 1/10. The LVN performs VSs and an examination of the child's foot and toes below the site of the fracture. Using a CCSMT (color, circulation, sensation, movement, and touch) tool, you find that the neurovascular status of the child's affected foot is within normal limits (WNL). The child is comforted and given colorful, developmentally appropriate books for distraction.

Two hours after being admitted to the unit, the child's father presses the call button at the child's bedside and requests an urgent response. The LPN/LVN finds the child writhing in bed, diaphoretic, and demonstrating a pain assessment finding of 6 to 7/10. The child's left foot is pale, cool to the touch, and slightly swollen to the point that checking the peripheral pulse is difficult. The pulse is weak. The LPN/LVN immediately notifies the RN who is in charge of the pediatric unit. He comes in and evaluates the child's CCSMT, confirming that there is a critical change in neurovascular status from expected findings. The RN calls the ED physician who placed the cast on the child's left femur and, after using the SBAR communication tool, is told to quickly call the orthopedic technician on call to come to the floor STAT to window the cast and provide relief from pressure. The ED doctor also tells the RN to call the pediatric hospitalist in-house and have her come and evaluate the child's condition immediately. The health-care team is activated within 5 minutes, and the cast is removed to restore adequate circulation and have full visual assessment of the site. The child is taken back to the ED and a new cast is placed. All members of the team debrief quickly and find the chain of command effective. The RN expresses appreciation to the LPN/LVN for the rapid notification of the child's condition and makes it clear that the processes and teamwork were effective.

Therapeutic Communication

When a child needs to be moved to a higher level of care, the family needs to receive an explanation of the situation. The explanation can be brief and should help them understand that the move is for their child's safety. Moving to a higher level of care will allow for closer monitoring and for interventions that are necessary to support the child's airway. The family needs to be talked to in a calm, matter-of-fact manner with direct eye contact. One person should be assigned to support the family and calmly describe the steps of the move.

or other emergency support will be required. The move consists of the following steps:

1. The nurse prepares all of the child's medical records, nursing chart, medication administration records, and identification card. (If all materials are electronic, make sure that the process of transferring access to the PICU is complete.)

2. The nurse calls the receiving unit and gives an oral report directly to the nurse who will be taking charge of the child. The following information should be included in the call for an effective handoff:
   • Child's full name, date of birth, weight and height, date of admission, and admitting medical diagnosis
   • Short history of the hospital stay up to this time, including the severity of the child's condition and/or symptoms from admission to the present
   • Reason for the transfer, including any medical interventions that were attempted to stabilize the child's condition
   • Any pertinent results of laboratory, diagnostic, or radiological studies (ABG, chemistry panels, or hematological panels such as a CBC)
   • Emotional condition of the family, which family members are present, and the depth of their knowledge about the need for immediate transfer

Nursing Care Plan for the Family of a Hospitalized, Acutely Ill Child

An 18-month-old boy was admitted to the pediatric unit yesterday for respiratory distress from rhinovirus and adenovirus lung infections. Today, the child's condition has deteriorated; and he is rapidly transferred to the PICU for further support, high-flow oxygen, anti-inflammatory medications, IV placement, and fluids. The mother, who speaks only Cantonese, expresses great worry about her young son through the interpreter.

Nursing Diagnoses: Anxiety related to child's acute health state; fear related to unknown medical diagnoses; knowledge deficit related to medical treatments; family coping compromised because of acute events; caregiver role strain related to hospitalization and need to care for other family members; communication impaired because of language differences

Expected Outcome: Family members will demonstrate less fear and anxiety by asking clarifying questions concerning the child's acute condition and receiving clear answers concerning the child's medical diagnosis throughout the child's hospitalization.

Intervention:	Rationale:
Pediatric health-care team will ensure the presence of an interpreter, or will use the interpreter phone or streaming video services, for all communication with the family, including frequent updates on the child's condition in the PICU.	*Clear communication that is offered frequently may reduce fear and anxiety. The use of interpreters will allow the family the ability to ask specific questions to the team.*

Nursing Diagnosis: Knowledge Deficit related to child's primary medical diagnosis
Expected Outcome: Parents will demonstrate an understanding of the child's medical condition by being able to ask pertinent questions and describe basic information concerning the medical diagnosis, including diagnostics and treatment plan during the hospitalization.

Intervention:	Rationale:
Using the interpreter, the family will be able to ask questions about the medical condition of the lung pathology and treatments to assist the child in effective ventilation as well as any diagnostics being ordered and performed such as laboratory studies and chest x-ray.	*Families want to know that everything is being done to help their child during an acute phase of an illness, and they want to know what exactly is being done and why.*

Key Points

- The nurse caring for an acutely ill child in the hospital needs to be able to determine a change in clinical status and quickly call for appropriate help.
- Having size-appropriate emergency equipment available in each child's room will provide safe care if a child's condition changes. Suction, oxygen, resuscitation masks of various sizes, and a working code blue button should be in every hospital room. The nurse should check for the presence, function, and size of equipment at the beginning of each shift.
- Using a body-systems approach, the nurse identifies conditions that may warrant reporting up the chain of command and possible transfer of the child to an intensive care environment.
- Using tools such as SBAR for effective communication and mnemonics for rapid recall of emergency response steps allows a nurse to make significant contributions to the acutely ill child's clinical outcomes.
- Supporting the efforts of an RRT contributes to a child's clinical stabilization. Parents need to learn how to call for the RRT and should be encouraged to use this system if their child's condition changes and they become concerned.
- The nurse must make sure to be familiar with the location and use of the pediatric color-coded, length-based resuscitation tape that provides information based on the estimated weight regarding equipment, fluids, and medications to be used during emergencies.
- Basic bedside emergency equipment should include suction, oxygen, a manual resuscitator bag, mask and valve, code button, telephone to call the RRT, and instructions for calling various codes for help (code pink, code gray, code yellow).
- The nurse must be aware that certain conditions, such as severe reactive airway disease and epiglottitis, pose dangerous risks for a child's ability to ventilate. Therefore, the child's condition must be considered "guarded," prompting extra attention, monitoring, clinical care, and concern.
- Shock is a serious condition for children that requires immediate identification, interventions, and transfer to an intensive care environment. Vasopressors, antibiotics, fluid boluses, and constant monitoring are required.

Review Questions

1. SBAR is a system that a nurse can follow to prepare for and implement an effective phone call to a primary health-care provider. The components of SBAR include all of the following *except:*
   1. Situation of the child and the background of the concern
   2. Assessment of the child's current status
   3. Awareness of the parents' educational needs
   4. Recommendation of the pediatric nurse

2. Which of the following items are essential equipment that should be present at every hospitalized child's bedside area? **(Select all that apply.)**
   1. Suction device and tubing
   2. Blood sugar glucose monitoring device
   3. Manual resuscitator bag and correct size mask
   4. Access to code blue button and/or phone
   5. Source of oxygen with connector and tubing

3. For which of the following events should an RRT be called? **(Select all that apply.)**
   1. A 7-year-old girl experiences a grand mal seizure.
   2. A morbidly obese teenager experiences dehiscence of an abdominal surgical wound.
   3. A 4-year-old boy trips, falls, and gets back up again while ambulating in the hall.
   4. A newborn's O_2 saturation varies during the first hour he is being monitored.
   5. A 10-year-old girl who is 2 hours postoperative becomes anxious; her heart rate increases, her blood pressure drops, and she is sweating profusely.

4. When working on a pediatric hospital unit, you teach the family about the RRT. When describing who is allowed to activate the RRT, you would be correct in stating:
   1. Only the medical team who is asking for further team assistance
   2. The immediate family
   3. The nursing team who finds the child in distress
   4. Anyone who identifies the need to request help for the child

5. An LVN must use the chain of command to immediately report any significant change in a patient's clinical status to the next appropriate person. In the hospital setting, who should the LVN report a patient's clinical status changes to?
   1. The hospitalist on duty
   2. The nursing supervisor
   3. The ED attending doctor
   4. The RN working on the unit

6. The LVN and RN nursing team of a busy medical clinic is asked to participate in a "mock code blue." What are the components of this practice session? **(Select all that apply.)**
   1. Practicing how to call for an RRT
   2. Calling a code blue response by call button and phone
   3. Initiating the use of a crash cart
   4. Performing CPR
   5. Documenting admitting assessments from the ED

7. Nurses can assume various roles during an emergency response in an acute care environment. What do these roles include? **(Select all that apply.)**
   1. Airway management
   2. Compressions
   3. Taking serial VS measurements
   4. Running laboratory specimens
   5. Passing equipment from the crash cart to the response team
   6. Providing emotional support to the family

8. Which of the following are interventions you should perform immediately when a child becomes cyanotic? **(Select all that apply.)**
   1. Provide a source of oxygen.
   2. Suction the child's airway.
   3. Stimulate the child.
   4. Phone the parents to come to the hospital.
   5. Call for pharmacy backup.
   6. Plan for impending death.

9. A(n) _____ is not a formal medical diagnosis but a sudden, acute, and unexpected change in a young infant's breathing pattern that leads to a color change, apnea, limpness, and, often, choking or gagging.

ANSWERS 1. 3; 2. 1, 3, 4, 5; 3. 1, 2, 5; 4. 4; 5. 4; 6. 1, 2, 3, 4; 7. 1, 2, 3, 4, 5, 6; 8. 1, 2, 3; 9. apparent life-threatening event (ALTE)

CRITICAL THINKING QUESTIONS

1. Use an online literature database to discover how long, on average, a nurse retains CPR skills after the completion of a mandatory class. What can be done to help nurses retain resuscitation skills? Which skills need frequent practice? Do mock codes help in increasing nurses' reported comfort and confidence in responding to emergencies?

2. Should parents be allowed to stay in a room when a child requires emergency resuscitation? Why or why not?

Resources

For additional resources and information, including Postconference Questions and Activities, Answers, and References, visit www.FADavis.com.

Student Study Guide

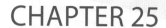

CHAPTER 25
Adapting to Chronic Illness and Supporting the Family Unit

KEY TERMS

brachycephalic (BRAK-ih-sef-AL-ik)
chronic illness (KRON-ik IL-niss)
normalcy (NOR-muhl-see)
technology dependent (tek-NAWL-uh-jee dee-PEN-dent)

CHAPTER CONCEPTS

Family
Safety
Stress and Coping

LEARNING OUTCOMES

1. Define the key terms.
2. Discuss examples of chronic illnesses found throughout childhood.
3. Discuss the health-care concerns that develop when a child has a chronic illness.
4. Analyze the effects of a childhood chronic illness, both positive and negative, on the family unit, structure, and daily life.
5. Demonstrate how to evaluate side effects associated with a chronic illness that causes severe symptoms such as pain, dyspnea, sleep disorders, emotional distress, fatigue, and nausea.
6. Discuss the importance of open and effective communication between the health-care team and the family unit when caring for a child with a chronic illness.
7. Describe the late consequences of a pediatric chronic illness and the impact on growth and development.
8. Acknowledge the effect of death on the family members of a child with a chronic illness.
9. Analyze how membership in local, regional, and national organizations can help a family of a child with a chronic illness cope with the exacerbations, hospitalizations, social isolation, and financial effects.
10. Describe the general safety precautions families need to learn and initiate when taking home a child who is technology dependent. Discuss various scenarios that include home respirators, oxygen delivery systems, cardiac monitoring systems, central venous catheters, and suctioning equipment and the safety issues associated.

CRITICAL THINKING

You are caring for 16-year-old **Carmella** after she was admitted to the outpatient surgical center for placement of a percutaneous feeding device to supplement her decreasing oral intake. She has lost a significant amount of weight and is now diagnosed with failure to thrive. A feeding tube is needed to supplement her poor oral intake because she has had three bouts of aspiration pneumonia in the last 24 months and continues to show clinical signs of aspiration risk.

Continued

CRITICAL THINKING—cont'd

Carmella's 26-year-old sister is her primary caregiver because both of their parents work and commute. Carmella presented with significant joint contracture in a reclining wheelchair because she does not have independent motor abilities.

Questions

1. As you take Carmella's vital signs, what data could help her health-care provider determine that she was experiencing significant failure to thrive?
2. How have her chronic conditions impacted her nutritional intake?

CONCEPTUAL CORNERSTONE
Safety

Safety is the most important concept associated with a diagnosis of a chronic illness during childhood. Children with chronic illnesses experience a variety of consequences for their medical diagnosis that affect their level of safety. A child may experience repeated exacerbations (aggravation or relapse of symptoms) of the illness and subsequently require frequent care encounters or hospitalizations. Families need to be taught how to care for the child's emotional and physical needs, especially if the child is technology dependent (requires medical devices at home). Safety must be in the forefront of all encounters, and anticipating and planning for these safety concerns are paramount.

DEFINING CHRONIC ILLNESS AND ITS SCOPE

A **chronic illness** is an illness that has the potential to last throughout the person's life (Figs. 25.1 and 25.2). The frequency of exacerbations and the severity of the symptoms associated with the chronic illness may change over time. A chronic illness is one that lasts for more than 3 months in a year, causes hospitalizations and increased medical attention (Centers for Disease Control and Prevention [CDC], 2021), and is characterized as an illness that has "quiet" and "active" periods. During the "active" periods, the child may become quite symptomatic and ill and may require prolonged hospitalization for management. Examples of chronic illnesses include cystic fibrosis and asthma (see Chapter 30); type 1 (insulin-dependent) diabetes (see Chapter 32); atopic dermatitis (see Chapter 36); and sickle cell disease, congenital neutropenia, and various forms of childhood cancer (see Chapter 38). It is estimated that approximately 10% to 30% of children in the United States (about 20 million children) have a chronic illness (Healthychildren.org, 2022; Russo, 2022). These children are now experiencing increased survival rates, but with longer lives they are experiencing more comorbidities and new morbidities. Table 25.1 provides definitions of concepts related to childhood chronic illnesses.

A chronically ill child needs to know that the goal of care is to provide a childhood that is as close to normal as possible with play, socialization, academics, sports, and control

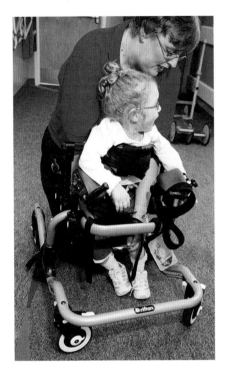

FIGURE 25.1 Chronic illness can last a lifetime.

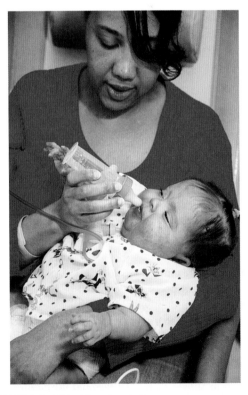

FIGURE 25.2 A child with a chronic illness.

Table 25.1
Definitions of Concepts Related to Chronic Illness in Children

Concept	Definition
Chronic illness	• A condition that interferes with daily function for more than 3 months in any given year, causes hospitalization for more than 1 month of a year, or is likely to do either or both
Congenital disability	• A condition causing a chronic state that has existed since the birth of the child
Developmental delay	• A documented slower rate of development, considered a maturational lag, that causes the child to function at a lower level than expected for their chronological age
Developmental disability	• A physical or mental disability that manifests before the child's 22nd birthday and is very likely to continue throughout the child's adulthood
Disability	• A functional state that causes a limitation with a child's ability to walk, lift, play, or learn
Handicap	• A term used to describe a condition, limitation, or barrier in the child's environment; not used as a synonym for the term *disability*
Impairment	• Refers to any loss or abnormality of a biological structure or function (mobility, sensory organs, or cognitive function)
Technology-dependent child	• A child whose disability or chronic illness requires the use of medical equipment or a medical device on a routine basis, requiring support, education, and access when not hospitalized
Developmental focus of care for a child with a chronic illness or disability	• Both the family and the health-care team working together to concentrate on the child's developmental growth and maturity rather than on the child's chronological age
Normalization	• Intentions and behaviors of a child with a chronic illness or disability to integrate into society by living life as fully as a child who does not have an illness or disability; this includes entering school and enjoying recreation, sports activities, hobbies, and social situations such as birthday parties and camping trips
Anticipated parental stress points	• Points of time during the child's life where considerable stress is experienced by the parents; these points of time include developmental milestones that are not met, times when the child should enter or progress in education, missed proms, missed graduation, and stresses associated with future placement; issues concerning sexuality and reproduction; and issues concerning threat of death caused by chronic illness exacerbations
Denial	• The unwillingness of a parent to accept the child's disorder and the belief that the disorder, chronic illness, or disability does not exist, or the belief that the child will overcome the illness or disability and gain a life similar to peers who do not have the chronic condition or disability
Chronic sorrow	• A set of feelings experienced by parent(s) of a child with a chronic illness or disability that recurs in waves over time

of symptoms. The child needs to be encouraged to do those activities that their peers are doing but perhaps in a slightly modified way. Children with chronic illnesses need consistent care, but they also need independence and support to live their lives as normally as possible. Children with a chronic illness must be supported to achieve milestones in each of the developmental stages. The goal is to minimize disruptions such as illness exacerbations and hospitalizations by managing health issues to maximize autonomy (self-care)

and **normalcy** (attaining normal standards) in their lives. Because chronic illness can interfere with happiness and emotional well-being, nurses must learn how to apply principles of long-term care to support a child to have emotional health and physical well-being (Fig. 25.3). Research has shown that when children with a chronic illness are distressed, anxious, and unhappy, their medical condition is harder to control and manage. In hospital settings, families of children with a chronic illness who have an exacerbation report that they

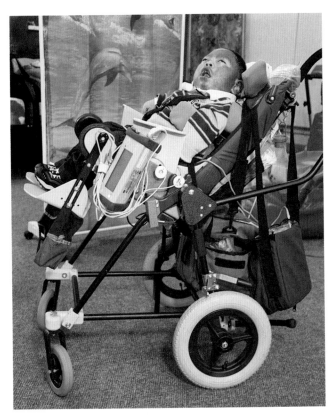

FIGURE 25.3 Support is needed for physical and emotional well-being.

are fearful for their children, feel left alone, fear medical and medication errors (Pordes et al., 2018), and experience fear, loneliness, and anxiety (Sybertz, 2022).

During chronic illness exacerbation, you should evaluate the child for the following concerns:

1. Poor sleeping habits and loss of sleep
2. Fatigue that leads to the inability for self-care, play, academics, and socialization
3. Poor eating habits that lead to poor nutritional intake
4. Emotional distress, mood swings, fear, and anger
5. Talking about their death or death in general
6. Not cooperating with the medical treatment plan, nursing care plan, and illness self-management

Some children may experience frustrations that lead to rebellion against important medical care. Not testing blood sugar regularly, not taking appropriate insulin, and eating poorly for a diabetic can have devastating consequences that lead to hospitalization for diabetic ketoacidosis. Children with severe rheumatoid arthritis who do not take their medications can be hospitalized for severe inflammation, crippling joint disease, and profound pain. Children with severe asthma who do not test their peak flows daily, do not follow their daily prevention medications, or do not take their rescue medications when needed, including identifying the severity of their symptoms, can experience life-threatening asthma attacks requiring a pediatric intensive care unit (PICU) stay

and possible intubation. If family members express concern about managing their young child's care or feel that their teenager is not managing health-care needs, it is imperative that the child be seen for a psychological, emotional, and medical evaluation to prevent complications that can be life-threatening.

 CHRONIC ILLNESSES BY BODY SYSTEM

Children can experience a chronic illness in any of the many body systems. Table 25.2 provides a list of chronic illnesses from various body systems that a nurse may encounter in a variety of different care settings.

 ESTABLISHMENT OF A THERAPEUTIC RELATIONSHIP

Parents of children with complicated medical needs and chronic illnesses may experience a range of emotional responses. Feelings of blame, guilt, anger, despair, and anguish are not uncommon. It is imperative that each member of the pediatric health-care team who interacts with the family attempt to develop a therapeutic relationship. This relationship is based on openness, mutual respect, and honesty, all while being goal-oriented and professional. You and the health-care provider working with the family need to understand that the family needs an effective listener, someone who is engaged and attentive to the parents' concerns and needs.

Establishing a therapeutic relationship can be challenging if the parents blame the health-care system for their child's condition. The pediatric health-care team must continue to attempt to establish an open, honest, and goal-oriented relationship, even when it is difficult, keeping the ill child in mind. Various cultural groups may have different responses when a child develops a chronic illness.

Some families will immediately call others from their cultural group to assist with transportation, childcare for well siblings, meals, prayer, and respite. Members of other cultural groups may not be as inclined to ask for help and may actually be resistant to share their situation with others and ask for assistance. Nurses can be instrumental in determining the family's needs and suggesting that they participate in social resources that can diminish the burden of caring for a child with multiple health needs, hospitalizations, and complex home-care needs. It is important that the health-care team respect the family's cultural background, offer to help contact social networks, and encourage families to work together to provide care for the entire family.

Some families want to hear estimates of the length of life, a description of the course of the chronic illness, and possible responses to treatment. Other families would rather not have these discussions. It is important to ask what information the family wants to know. Providing reputable information about support groups; organizations; and educational books, websites, and videotapes can prove very helpful to most families. It is important

Table 25.2
Chronic Pediatric Illnesses by Body System

Body System	Chronic Illnesses
Cardiovascular	Pulmonary hypertension Congestive heart failure Complications associated with congenital heart disease
Neurological	Long-term effects of a brain tumor Seizure disorder Cerebral palsy Shaken baby syndrome Central nervous system diseases Head trauma Severe sensory impairments Congenital malformations **Brachycephalic**
Respiratory	Asthma Chronic inflammatory lung disease Cystic fibrosis
Renal	Nephrotic syndrome with relapses Chronic kidney disease
Hematological	Sickle cell disease Hemophilia Bone marrow transplant complications
Immune	Juvenile idiopathic arthritis Systemic lupus erythematosus (SLE) Severe allergies Muscular dystrophy
Oncological	Leukemia Lymphoma Long-term consequences of cancer treatment
Gastrointestinal	Crohn disease Short gut syndrome Inflammatory bowel syndromes
Dermatological	Severe atopic dermatitis
Endocrine	Diabetes Severe hormonal insufficiency

for you to discuss the child's estimated length of life (prognosis) with the family only after the health-care provider has discussed it with the parents. Parents may want you to talk to the child about the prognosis, or they may prefer to do it themselves.

• WORD • BUILDING •
brachycephalic: brachy–short + cephal–head + ic–pertaining to

SYMPTOMS ASSOCIATED WITH CHILDHOOD CHRONIC ILLNESS

Chronic illnesses can cause a child to experience a variety of symptoms. These symptoms can come and go and can vary in severity. In a classic body of research on symptom management theory (Dodd et al., 2001; Humphreys et al., 2008; Linder, 2010), it was surmised that the most common reason that patients seek access to health care is for the management of symptoms. Without symptom control, daily activities and quality of life are potentially influenced. Your role when caring for children with chronic illnesses includes the evaluation, diagnosis, and management of symptoms. Nurses must be aware of the three components of symptom management: the symptoms experience itself, the strategies used to manage the symptoms, and the outcomes influenced by the symptoms (emotional and functional status; Dodd et al., 2001; Humphreys et al., 2008; Linder, 2010). Symptoms that should be checked for on a regular basis include the following (Mayo Clinic, 2023; Russo, 2022):

- Discomfort or pain
- Fatigue or extreme tiredness
- Nausea or vomiting
- Emotional distress, anxiety, or depression
- Sleep disorders
- **Dyspnea** or difficulty breathing
- Changes in bowel and bladder function

Discomfort or Pain
Discomfort is a unique experience for each child and assessment includes the character, location, quality, and intensity of the pain. Behavioral distress scales (CRIES, FLACC, and NIPS) are used for infants and young children, and visual tools (Wong-Baker FACES pain scale, numerical scales, and adolescent pain perception tools) are used to determine the older child's perception of pain. Children with chronic pain become more sensitized to the experience and require greater pain-relieving measures (Fig. 25.4).

Fatigue or Extreme Tiredness
Fatigue is a sensation of tiredness and can be determined using physiological indicators, psychological indicators, and self-reports. Fatigue is associated with anemia, pain, exhaustion, sleep deprivation, and prolonged hospitalization. Nurses can assist children experiencing fatigue by allowing breaks between procedures, promoting quality of sleep, administering blood products if the child is anemic, and encouraging rest periods as needed.

Nausea or Vomiting
Unlike vomiting, which is a clinical sign, nausea is a sensory experience associated with many precipitating factors

• WORD • BUILDING •
dyspnea: dys–abnormal + pnea–breathing

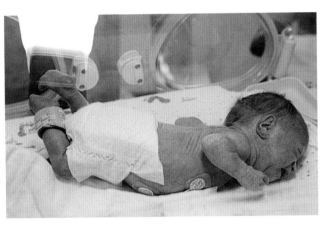

FIGURE 25.4 Children with chronic pain become more sensitized.

for children with chronic illness. Nausea can be associated with the administration of medications such as antineoplastic medications (used to kill cancer cells) as well as procedures and many other stimuli. The older child will report nausea, whereas the younger child may appear pale or refuse to suck, breastfeed, or eat. When known nausea-producing stimuli are present, you should request antinausea medications around the clock, not just as needed (prn).

Emotional Distress, Anxiety, or Depression

Many aspects of chronic illness cause emotional distress for a child. Separation from home, family, siblings, friends, pets, and familiar, comforting surroundings can cause great distress for a child. A young child may not know how to verbalize their feelings and therefore act out or become aggressive or passive. An older child should be encouraged to talk about their feelings. If available, a child life specialist should be called in to support the child. A referral to a clinical psychologist may be beneficial.

Sleep Disorders

Interrupted sleep, poor-quality sleep, and shortened sleep are unfortunately associated within a busy, loud, 24-hour-a-day pediatric unit. Children are awakened by nighttime vital signs, surgical preparations, weighing, intake and output measurements, phlebotomy, noisy roommates, and other disruptive activities. Beds and cribs are often uncomfortable and unfamiliar, and children may have a difficult time getting to sleep or getting back to sleep once awakened in the night.

Dyspnea or Difficulty Breathing

Difficulty breathing, or the feeling of not being able to effectively breathe, catch one's breath, or acquire enough air, is called *dyspnea*. Dyspnea is associated with physiological conditions such as fibrotic lung disease and inflammatory airway/reactive airway disease, but it also has emotional components. Many chronic disorders lead to difficult airway

management; for example, poor swallowing may result in excessive secretions and salivation. Children can become very frightened with the sensation of dyspnea, and health-care providers should offer multifaceted interventions, including suctioning, giving oxygen, positioning, massage, visualization, relaxation training, and guided imagery. Medications such as narcotics, anxiolytics (antianxiety medications), and sedatives may be necessary to reduce the sensation of dyspnea.

Changes in Bowel and Bladder Function

Many aspects of chronic illness or disability can lead to the development of constipation or altered bladder function. Poor diet, changes in diet, reduced fluid intake, or poor bowel habits can influence a change in elimination. Encouraging family to report early changes in bowel or bladder habits can assist a child in rapid resolution.

EXAMPLES OF CARE ENVIRONMENTS FOR CHRONICALLY ILL CHILDREN

Chronic illnesses are lasting experiences for a child. The care and management of a pediatric chronic illness often require that a child be cared for in a variety of clinical settings. Children may be seen first in emergency departments (EDs) or acute care settings, then followed in a clinic environment while the family learns and masters the skills required to care for their child at home. The following section discusses the various clinical settings where chronically ill children may receive care.

Safety *Stat!*

A child with multiple impairments or a complicated chronic illness will benefit from the prevention of secondary problems. Secondary problems include nutritional complications (weight loss), pressure injuries, aspiration pneumonia, urinary tract infections, contractures, and muscle wasting syndromes.

Home Health Care for Chronically Ill Children

Home environments provide the family with a sense of control and familiarity. To be successful in providing care to a chronically ill child at home, the family must have the skills to provide all aspects of care. The adults in the home need to know how to evaluate for complications and have a plan for rapid access to health care if the child's condition becomes acute and a higher level of care is needed.

A child who is **technology dependent** is one who requires a medical device to maintain health and wellness or to support life. Many conditions, from extreme premature birth to congenital abnormalities of the heart or lungs to complications from surgery to illness or injuries or neuro-muscular diseases, may cause a child to depend on medical technology. Common devices that are needed include oxygen and oxygen delivery systems, mobility devices, suctioning machines, **tracheostomy** equipment, apnea or cardiac mon-itors, and central venous catheter devices. It is essential that the family of the child learns how to safely care for and im-plement the devices. Your role is to teach the family how to care for the child, how to use the technological device, and how to maintain the device's integrity. Although some chil-dren with a severe chronic illness will have nursing care at home, the priority safety element for a technology-dependent child is that the family feels comfortable with the child's care and knows how and when to respond to an emergency at home. Research encourages health-care providers to see technology dependence as a way of adapting and function-ing with medical assistance, rather than as problem-focused (Brenner et al., 2021).

Hospitalizations

Many chronic conditions of childhood require hospitaliza-tions because the child's condition moves from stable to an acute episode of complications. Hospital health-care teams are skilled at managing acute exacerbations of childhood chronic illnesses. However, the family should carry with them a list of all medications and treatments currently being used at home and should be able to describe the child's medical his-tory and previous hospitalizations. Not all health-care team members will be familiar with a chronically ill child's past and will need information from which to create a treatment plan while the child is hospitalized. Some conditions, such as cystic fibrosis, chronic asthma, and childhood leukemia, may require several hospitalizations within a year (Fig. 25.5).

Day Respite Centers

Within some communities, families have access to organi-zations or health-care centers where a chronically ill child or a technology-dependent child can spend time safely with knowledgeable and skilled health-care providers. One form of this is summer camps that specialize in children with spe-cific chronic conditions such as cancer, cystic fibrosis, AIDS, asthma, and diabetes.

Long-Term Care Facilities

When a child requires a longer healing time before going home, long-term care facilities and rehabilitative centers can provide long-term care and rehabilitation services for the chronically ill child. Most of these facilities are adult-oriented, but some have pediatric specialty beds to provide children with developmentally appropriate care with cor-rectly sized equipment.

• WORD • BUILDING •

tracheostomy: trache–trachea + ostomy–surgical opening

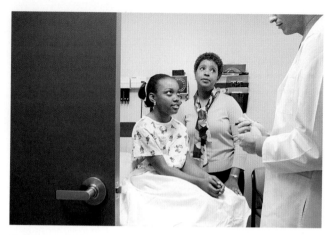

FIGURE 25.5 Many hospitalizations may be required for chron-ically ill children.

Pediatric Hospice Care

Pediatric hospice care is a specialty area of practice imple-mented by nurses and doctors who specialize in the care needed to comfort a child and provide care at the end of life. Unfortunately, pediatric hospice care is not prevalent across the nation. In some urban areas, pediatric hospice care can be secured to provide symptom management and support to families who wish to have their child die at home. Other communities have pediatric hospice facilities where the child and family can live until the child dies.

 ## ASSISTING CHILDREN IN COPING WITH CHRONIC ILLNESS

Children receive cues from their environment that they have a chronic illness, even when they do not receive a formal medical explanation of the illness. Children process the looks of their concerned parents, the hushed responses of family and friends, and their contact with other chronically ill chil-dren. It is important that children understand that they are not valued or their worth measured by others' responses to the illness but are valued as individuals separate from the chronic illness state.

Sometimes a chronically ill child will display a photo-graph taken before becoming ill and say, "This is a picture of me, who I really am." Chronically ill children may perceive the past as a very idealized place, before the confines of med-ical procedures, treatments, office visits, surgeries, and hos-pitalizations (Martini, 2023), and they may be self-conscious or feel left out (Garey, 2022).

It is imperative that the multidisciplinary health-care team provide the child with the highest potential to develop a strong self-image and positive emotional health. Adults in the child's life, as well as peers, can assist in developing and maintaining the child's positive emotional health.

Patient Teaching Guidelines

Families should be encouraged to provide for the emotional support of a child whose life is highly affected by a chronic illness. Emotional support can include the following:

- *Providing routine:* Set expectations of self-care and routine times for medications and treatments, but remain flexible during times of scheduling changes.
- *Acknowledging that emotional turmoil is normal, expected, and acceptable:* Provide support, but also guidelines about what are considered safe and acceptable displays of anger, fear, distress, anxiety, and unhappiness. Determine the severity of emotional reactions and seek help if the child is inconsolable or at risk for self-harm.
- *Showing an understanding of the child's distress:* Say statements such as, "I know that taking so many medications a day is frustrating," "I know you do not like to be hospitalized," or "Having your illness is really rough on you and your friendships with others."
- *Providing a reward system:* Implement rewards when the child is cooperative with medications, treatments, and self-care.
- *Making sure that all adults in the child's life understand the severity of the illness:* This includes teachers, childcare providers, close helpful neighbors, leaders in the family's church, and any health-care providers who are new to the child's medical history and illness management.

Protecting a Child's Emotional Health

Children experiencing chronic illnesses should be treated no differently than their siblings; yet, they are more vulnerable to emotional reactions, including distress. The experience of chronic illness and the frustrations and disappointments that can occur when a child is adjusting to or having exacerbations of the illness can cause vulnerability to a mood disorder such as depression. Furthermore, children with a chronic illness may find themselves frequently encountering and communicating with families of children with similar life experiences. Seeing other children in the hospital or clinics with relapses, complications, or symptoms associated with the illness can be distressing.

Depression and Chronic Illness

Depression in response to having a chronic illness should be viewed as a complication that requires formal evaluation and treatment. A child's depression is not a normal and expected outcome; each case needs individualized care.

Childhood depression is not linked to the number of hospitalizations or to the severity of the illness. It is important to determine if the child had a preexisting affective disorder, or if the development of depression is linked to the experience. Adolescent girls have a greater risk of developing depression than adolescent boys with a chronic illness. The most severe rates of depression for children with chronic illness are for those with orthopedic disorders (23%), severe asthma (15%), cardiac disorders (13%), and burns (13%). Children with cancer have the lowest rates of depression. Warning signs include disrupted sleep, self-blame, withdrawal, and hopelessness (Garey, 2022).

When Another Child Dies

Children with a chronic illness that places them frequently around other children with similar diagnoses become acutely aware when another child gets gravely ill or dies. Feelings of vulnerability develop, and the child will need to process feelings and reactions to the loss. If the child was aware of the dying child's condition, symptoms, and experience, they may become afraid of separation from parents and family. It is important to maintain the principles of the Health Insurance Portability and Accountability Act (HIPAA), which details regulations to protect patient health information and patient privacy: Do not discuss any aspect of the dying child's medical status. However, it is important to acknowledge the feelings of fear that will surface.

THE EFFECT OF CHRONIC ILLNESS ON THE FAMILY

Having a child with a chronic illness affects the family in many ways. Parents carry increased levels of stress, worry, and care for the child. Other children in the family may feel that they are not getting enough support or attention from their parents. The whole family may suffer sleeping problems, separation problems while the child is hospitalized, financial problems, and lack of recreation and play. Adhering to treatment plans can be frustrating for the entire family and may take quality time away from the family unit. During hospitalizations, plans for family time, vacations, meals together, and alone time for parents all become disrupted.

For the health of the family, respite care and assistance may be needed. Trusted childcare providers, medical childcare providers, and babysitters can be helpful in carving time out for family members. Joining support groups, attending sibling summer camps, and soliciting education and support from national organizations can provide much help for all family members. It is important to acknowledge that caring for a child with a severe chronic illness causes disruption in family life. It is imperative that nurses provide guidance to families about how to seek support and assistance from a variety of sources.

Families Experiencing Prolonged Hospitalization

Pediatric hospital environments provide stimulation, play, arts and crafts, technology, and opportunities for socialization. Yet for a family with a child who has a chronic illness,

Patient Teaching Guidelines

Families should have the opportunity for respite from the demands of caring for the medical needs of a child with a chronic illness. However, asking for help from others can be difficult. Nurses can initiate the conversation by asking if the family has thought of the following ideas:

- Asking a trusted neighbor to provide supervision for short periods
- Requesting that grandparents or other close relatives assist in the child's care
- Tapping into support systems at church, work, or other organizations with which the family is involved
- Offering to trade respite care with a family who has a child with a similar disorder

Safety *Stat!*

Nurses must explain to the family that no one knows their child better than they do. With this in mind, it is important to maintain safety when others are providing respite care. The provider of respite care should know how to care for the child, including problem-solving any issues with a technological device, and when and how to call for help. Emergency numbers should be readily available. The family should also secure a back-up respite provider.

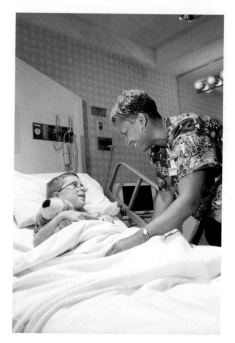

FIGURE 25.6 Care should include caring for a child's emotional needs.

Patient Teaching Guidelines

Although difficult when the child is symptomatic, expectations of behavior must be made clear, limits must be set, and a clear understanding of what is expected of the child needs to be communicated. When the child is quite sick, parents may need to change their expectations.

hospitalization can be stressful. Concerns about numerous diagnostic examinations, surgeries, and medical treatments are distressing. At times, the hospital environment can be traumatic for the child as well. The medical condition and the treatments for it can produce anxiety and pain that make the child more sensitive to subsequent experiences. The longer the hospital stay and the greater the exposure to diagnostics and treatments, the more discomfort the family and child feel (Fig. 25.6).

THE EFFECT OF A CHRONIC DISEASE ON PARENTING

Parenting continues even during periods of exacerbation and hospitalization. Parents need to understand that the child still needs discipline and boundaries when ill. Structure, consistency in parenting, and discipline for inappropriate acting out is very important for the well-being of the child, parent, and family.

Honesty is also very important. Children should learn about their chronic illness and the treatments and management of the illness according to their developmental level. Teach children about the pathology, severity, triggers, medications, treatments, and home health care so that they can be motivated about and included in their care.

Parents of chronically ill children may create unfair expectations for their healthy children. With long absences required to care for a hospitalized child, parents may expect their other children to take over chores, provide for one another, and look after younger siblings in their absence. Parents need to acknowledge this possibility and determine both their expectations of their children and the children's developmental capability to take on more responsibility.

The parents also need to acknowledge that they will need help. Managing both the physical and the emotional challenges of a chronic disease may become overwhelming for a parent. Encourage them to seek means of self-care as well as professional help for their child.

Parents need to carve out time to be together. Trying to provide care, special meals, and trips to doctors' offices, as well as to meet the demands of the illness itself, can be fatiguing. Often, time for parents to be alone together or to pursue individual interests is the first item that is sacrificed. A multidisciplinary health-care team can help overwhelmed parents cope with the needs of a chronically ill child.

CRITICAL THINKING & CLINICAL JUDGMENT

A child with a severe chronic disorder, who has been frequently hospitalized, and the child's parents and siblings are in the waiting area of a pediatric clinic setting. The restless younger siblings are playing with the patient's wheelchair and medical equipment in an unsafe manner. You are working in the clinic and notice the possible safety issues.

Questions

1. What are the potential risks you notice in this unsafe play?
2. How should you address the safety concerns with the family?

Caring for Teenagers With Chronic Illnesses

The impact of a chronic illness on teenagers should not be underestimated. Teens want to become more independent from their parents and siblings and feel good about their body image, but the impact of a chronic illness can dampen their developing independence and their self-image. Encourage teenage patients to be a part of decision-making, to learn about their condition, and to visit privately with friends and peers. Because chronic illness impacts all areas of a teen's life, it is important for you to discuss concerns that the teen and the family may have and to assist them with problem-solving. Concerns such as emotional instability, anger, medication noncompliance, poor body image, or the presence of overly dependent behaviors (regression) warrant a referral to a mental health professional (Children's Hospital of Wisconsin, 2022).

THE EFFECT OF A CHRONIC DISEASE ON SIBLINGS

The siblings of children with chronic disease or disability have their own special needs. Often overshadowed by the child with a chronic illness, siblings are required to adjust to life changes, including feeling left out, left behind, and without opportunities to be the center of attention. Feeling neglected is a common reaction of a sibling to the increased needs of the ill child. Preschool-aged siblings experiencing magical thinking may feel they themselves have caused the illness and complicate their emotions with added guilt. Some younger siblings will express that they wish they were sick as well.

Emotions that siblings may experience include being scared that their family will be separated or that they may lose their ill sibling and have deeply sad parents. Siblings may feel resentful and angry that they are not receiving the same level of attention and feel that they have lost important

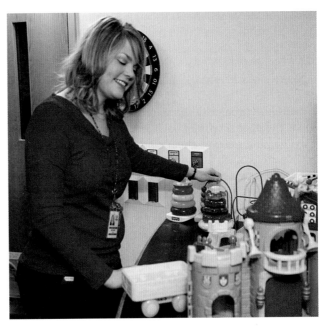

FIGURE 25.7 Child life therapist.

and meaningful moments with their parents. They may feel embarrassed about the level of disability, dependency, or illness of the child. No matter what the reaction is, the response may require special assistance from members of child life, social services, and educators from the sibling's academic setting (Fig. 25.7).

Patient Teaching Guidelines

Gently remind parents of the possible unmet needs of the sibling and encourage them to spend quality time and attention with the sibling. Help guide the parents to identify the unique needs of each of their children and to provide time and attention to each one.

Although sibling rivalry is expected in all families, it is imperative that the pediatric health-care team teach families about the "red flags" associated with severe reactions. The potential for sibling abuse must be identified. Signs of abuse include avoiding or ignoring the ill child, acting out physical or emotional abuse during play, demonstrating increasing roughness/violence toward the ill child or between siblings, and seeking attention in high-risk ways such as sexual promiscuity.

Safety *Stat!*

Other warning signs of a sibling not doing well with adapting to the care demands of a child with a chronic illness include the sibling demonstrating poor sleeping habits, a lack of concentration in school or increased absenteeism, dropping grades, poor self-esteem, withdrawal, and talking about hurting themselves.

Not all of the experiences of being a sibling of a chronically ill child or child with a disability are negative. The experience can cause the sibling to grow in good qualities such as empathy for others, dependability, patience, supportiveness to others, and loyalty while standing up for their brother or sister.

Offering chronically ill children and their families support is an important part of holistic and family-centered care. Providing information about siblings' camps and national organizations, such as the Sibling Support Project, can be life-changing for siblings.

Patient Teaching Guidelines

National Organizations for Assisting Chronically Ill Children and Their Families

Local, regional, and national organizations can help the family of a child with a chronic illness cope with the exacerbations, hospitalizations, social isolation, and financial worries. Many organizations offer support groups, either online or in person, with opportunities to connect with other families for emotional support, education, and ideas for adaptation and acceptance. The nurse caring for families whose child has a chronic illness can be instrumental in providing information about support networks and professional organizations.

The professional organizations noted next provide information about various topics associated with chronic illness during childhood. Other than being informative, some have support networks that connect families with each other either online or via local chapter meetings.

1. *American Academy of Pediatrics:* Information on support for siblings of children with chronic illnesses
2. *American Academy of Pediatrics:* Information on coping with chronic childhood illness
3. *American Lung Association:* Asthma and children fact sheet
4. *American Psychological Association:* Information on how to help a friend or loved one suffering from a chronic illness
5. *Children's Heart Foundation:* Parental resource book and support for children with a congenital heart defect
6. *Crohn's and Colitis Foundation of America:* Comprehensive information on the diagnosis, treatment, management, and prevention of complications of Crohn disease and colitis
7. *Department of Health & Human Services, Office of Women's Health: Illness and Disability for Girls:* Information on chronic illness and disabilities for girls
8. *Nemours Foundation:* Information on care for a seriously ill child, information and ideas on how to best balance academics and serious illness, and information on dealing with a health condition for teenagers
9. *American Chronic Pain Association:* Information for family members to assist a loved one with living with chronic pain
10. *Centers for Disease Control and Prevention:* Information on a variety of chronic diseases and conditions

---

The Realities of Readmission

Readmission refers to the admission of a child back into the hospital, often for complications associated with a previous condition. Because of the complexities of a child with chronic illness, readmission is not uncommon. The challenge for the health-care team is to ensure that the family feels comfortable, empowered, and ready to take the child home and care for the child independently. If the family becomes frightened of a change of clinical status, if the child's symptoms suddenly become worse, or if the family perceives that they are not ready or able to care for the child at home, they may bring the child right back to the ED or pediatric inpatient unit. It is imperative that the health-care team thoroughly evaluate the child's needs and status before discharge. The parents and any other caregivers for the child at home should be questioned about their concerns and home-care needs. Families benefit from having home-health agencies and services/supplies set up and on-boarded before discharge. These services can be coordinated with the institution's discharge planner. Preventing early readmission reduces health-care costs and leads to greater satisfaction for the family and child.

Death of a Child With a Chronic Illness

The terminal phase of a chronic illness requires meticulous nursing care and support of all family members. The terminal phase includes frequent checks of symptoms such as discomfort, dyspnea, fatigue, nausea, emotional distress, and sleep disorders. Most children will understand their situation and will have their own unique way to process and express their feelings. The child may wish to never be alone, yet not wish to be touched a great deal or may even wish for silence. Spirituality can be a great comfort to a child and family. Every effort should be made to offer the assistance of a spiritual leader of the family's choice. Many hospitals have clergy on staff who can be a conduit to providing for the spiritual needs of the family. Nurses must be prepared to help the dying child and be prepared to answer questions about death, dying, heaven, and other topics related to spirituality that may come up. See Table 25.3 for further information about understanding death across childhood.

Nursing Care Plan for the Child With a Chronic Illness

Antony, age 5, is having his first sickle cell crisis and has been admitted to the pediatric unit for treatment. After Mark, an RN, settles Antony and his parents in their room and conducts the admission assessment, he begins to develop a plan of care for his new patient.

Nursing Diagnosis: Pain related to chronic illness, as evidenced by facial expressions and inability to sleep

Expected Outcome: The patient will demonstrate a pain scale score that is zero or that is acceptable to the child and parents.

Intervention:	Rationale:
Administer ordered pain medications and reevaluate pain level after 30 minutes.	*A sickle cell crisis is extremely painful and strong opioid medications are necessary to relieve the pain.*

Nursing Diagnosis: Risk for constipation related to opioid medication use

Expected Outcome: The patient will pass a formed stool within the next 24 to 36 hours.

Interventions:	Rationales:
Provide a diet rich in fiber and encourage adequate fluid consumption.	*A high-fiber diet combined with plenty of fluids will stimulate elimination.*
Encourage movement and exercise as tolerated.	*Moving and exercising promote peristalsis to stimulate elimination.*

Nursing Diagnosis: Anxiety related to first hospitalization and the need for blood draws, as evidenced by the child's expressions, crying, and fighting against the staff during transportation

Expected Outcome: The patient will demonstrate a reduced level of anxiety, as evidenced by calm facial expressions and cooperation.

Interventions:	Rationales:
Provide play therapy, music therapy, and opportunities to express emotions and anxieties.	*Allowing the child creative outlets and opportunities to express emotions will help to alleviate anxiety.*
Explain the need for blood draws in relation to treatment and the healing process.	*Teaching the child about medical procedures may enable him to understand that the hospital staff are working to make him feel better.*

Patient Teaching Guidelines

The death of a child with a complicated chronic illness is very hard for all those involved with the child's care. Many adults or siblings have been long-term caregivers and support systems for the child. Common signs of impending death should be explained to the family to help them prepare. A child who is progressing through the stages of dying can be expected to demonstrate the following physiological responses to imminent death:

• Increasing terminal airway secretions
• Slowing of peristalsis and delay in elimination
• Not wanting to be touched
• Myoclonus (brief, involuntary twitching)
• Irritability
• Mottling of the skin

Safety *Stat!*

Pediatric health-care team members must know institutional policies on postmortem (after death) care. Attending to the family's needs to be with the child is of primary importance, but knowing how to respectfully care for a child's body is essential.

Table 25.3

Understanding of Death Across Childhood

Age Group	Perception of Dying and Death
Infant	Infants have no concept of death or dying. They need close physical contact, and older infants will become distressed with separation. Pain is a very real experience for children across infancy, and you should use age/developmentally appropriate pain evaluation tools to determine if the dying infant is experiencing discomfort.
Toddler	Toddlers have no concept of death or dying. Between the ages of 8 and 36 months, separation anxiety and stranger anxiety are very real experiences. Toddlers need routines and will respond to changes in care providers, daily routines, and their parents' emotional reactions.
Preschooler	Preschool children will see death as temporary and therefore reversible. They may express their feelings about death in terms of degrees, stating, "The dog is just a little bit dead right now." Because preschoolers are in the "magical thinking" phase, they may believe that they are the cause of death or believe that death of an animal, family member, or even their own death is a punishment for something they or someone else did. Toward the end of the preschool period, the young child may be afraid of death and have nightmares and acting-out behaviors in response to death.
Young school-aged child	Young school-aged children will understand that death is irreversible. Not until school-aged children are close to 10 will they realize that death is universal and will eventually happen to them and those close to them. In relation to their own death, they may try to act adultlike and deny their feelings. Experiencing psychosomatic reports and having trouble concentrating are common at this age.
Older school-aged child	For the child between 10 and 12, there is a strong understanding that death is permanent, inevitable, and universal. Older school-aged children often ask their caregivers what they believe in and question their feelings about God and spirituality. Older school-aged children are interested in the details of death and may ask many questions about the death experience, pain, funerals, burials, and what their family will do after their death.
Adolescent	Adolescents may respond to death with grief and strong emotional reactions. They may become very sad while they search for meaning and a deeper understanding of the loss and ramifications of death to those remaining. Some may view death with conflict because they may feel invincible. Teenagers who have experienced death of a close family member or someone important to them may experience acting-out behaviors, risk-taking behaviors, promiscuity, delinquency, and suicide attempts.

Key Points

- A chronic illness is an illness that has the potential to last throughout the person's life.
- Many health-care concerns are associated with a diagnosis of a chronic illness. The frequency of exacerbations (relapses of the primary disease or illness) and the severity of the symptoms associated with the chronic illness may change over time. Children with chronic illness are now experiencing increased survival rates, but with this they are experiencing more comorbidities and new morbidities.
- The family of a child with a chronic illness may experience a variety of struggles and challenges. Because children with a chronic illness have greater emotional, behavioral, and psychiatric symptoms as compared with their healthy peers, the family needs support from health-care professionals and support groups.
- For children with chronic illnesses, symptom evaluation, treatment, and management are primary pediatric nursing responsibilities.
- Establishing and maintaining effective communication is an important aspect of caring for a child with a chronic illness and their family. The focus for care by the interdisciplinary team and multiple medical specialists is to always empower, educate, and include the family in

decision-making as well as to focus on adjustment, coping, and optimal developmental growth.

- Children with a chronic illness need to be supported to reach their maximal potential; progress through the developmental stages to achieve milestones; and be provided positive social, emotional, academic, and recreational experiences.
- Two frequent concerns for family members are the late consequences that can occur when a child has a chronic illness: social isolation and depression.
- The terminal phase of a chronic illness requires meticulous nursing care and support. The terminal phase includes frequent checks of symptoms. Children, if developmentally able, will understand their impending death and will have their own unique ways to process and express their feelings.
- Membership in local, regional, and national organizations can help the family of a child with a chronic illness cope with the exacerbations, hospitalizations, social isolation, and financial worries. Many organizations offer support groups either online or in person with opportunities to connect with other families for emotional support, education, and ideas for adaptation and acceptance.
- Maintaining safety at home is crucial. The nurse assists with educating the family about any medical devices that are used for the child's health and wellness. The family must understand how to implement, care for, and problem-solve all medical devices.

Review Questions

1. A child with a chronic illness is dying. Which of the following are expected physiological responses to death that should be explained to the family? **(Select all that apply.)**
   1. Increasing terminal airway secretions
   2. Slowing of peristalsis and delay in elimination
   3. Increasing sensations of thirst
   4. Not wanting to be touched
   5. Myoclonus
   6. Irritability
   7. Mottling of the skin

2. Which of the following statements about siblings of a child with a chronic illness is *true?*
   1. They often mimic the symptoms of the ill child.
   2. They can demonstrate regression to an earlier developmental period.
   3. They rarely demonstrate empathy because of their anger.
   4. They typically feel engaged and optimistic.

3. While talking to you, the family of a child with a seizure disorder who also has an unusual skull size (brachycephalic) asks what aspect of the child is contributing to the seizures. What is your correct response?
   1. Having a cephalic index of greater than 80%
   2. Having a cephalic index of 50%
   3. Having a cephalic index of less than 75%
   4. Having a cephalic index of less than 50%

4. While the pediatric team is speaking to the parents of a child with a chronic illness, they bring up the topic of respite care. The definition of *respite care* is which of the following?
   1. Developing relationships with long-term care facilities in case the child's condition warrants more care
   2. Involving siblings in the care of a child with a chronic illness at home
   3. Providing supervision to a child with a chronic illness to provide a break to family members
   4. Providing meals and financial support to a family with a child with a chronic illness

5. The term *exacerbation* is used when a child experiences which of the following? **(Select all that apply.)**
   1. The aggravation of symptoms
   2. Relapse of an acute phase
   3. The development of a new chronic illness
   4. The removal of a tumor or cyst
   5. The emotional reaction of an adult

6. Which statement about a chronic illness is *false?*
   1. A child with a chronic illness may have symptoms up to 3 months of a year.
   2. Chronic illnesses in children are resolved by adulthood.
   3. A chronic illness is noted to have quiet and active periods.
   4. As many as 27% of children in the United States have a diagnosis of a chronic illness.

7. Which of the following are considered chronic illnesses?
   (Select all that apply.)
   1. Crohn disease
   2. Appendicitis
   3. Hemophilia
   4. Severe allergies
   5. Pyelonephritis

8. A child who is _____ _____ is one who requires a medical device or skill to maintain health and wellness.

ANSWERS 1. 1, 2, 4, 5, 6, 7; 2. 2, 3, 1; 4. 3; 5. 1, 2, 6, 2; 7. 1, 3, 4; 8. technology dependent

CRITICAL THINKING QUESTIONS

1. Chronic illness in children has severe financial consequences for families. Multiple hospitalizations, clinic visits, consultations with specialists, medications, transportation, loss of days at work, and childcare costs add up to a considerable burden on families. To what services can a nurse refer a family with medical financial burdens? What organizations may be helpful to provide support services to a family with a chronically ill child?

2. Children with a chronic illness are at higher-than-average risk of morbidity and mortality. Discuss the association of chronic illness and childhood death. How do children of various ages comprehend death?

Resources

For additional resources and information, including Postconference Questions and Activities, Answers, and References, visit www.FADavis.com.

Student Study Guide

CHAPTER 26
The Abused Child

KEY TERMS

abuse (ab-YOOSS)
acts of commission (AKTS uv kuh-MI-shun)
acts of omission (AKTS uv oh-MI-shun)
battered (BAT-uhrd)
chain of custody (CHAYN uv KUSS-tuh-dee)
Child Protective Services (CPS) (CHILD pruh-
   TEK-tiv SER-viss-uhz)
factitious disorder imposed on
   another (fak-TIH-shus dihs-OR-der im-POHSD
   on uh-NUH-ther)
human trafficking (HYOO-muhn TRAF-ih-king)
intentional injury (in-TEN-shun-uhl IN-juh-ree)
mandatory reporters of child abuse and
   neglect (MAN-duh-TOR-ee rih-POR-terz uv
   CHILD ab-YOOSS and neg-LEKT)
neglect (neg-LEKT)
sexual abuse (SEKS-yoo-uhl ab-YOOSS)
unintentional abuse or injury (UN-in-
   TEN-shun-uhl ab-YOOSS or IN-juh-ree)

CHAPTER CONCEPTS

Family
Growth and Development
Safety
Stress and Coping
Violence and Neglect

LEARNING OUTCOMES

1. Define the key terms.
2. Describe global perspectives, historical perspectives, and legal aspects of child abuse, including the development of laws aimed at protecting abused children and preventing abuse in society.
3. Discuss the various types of abuse and their incidences and prevalence rates, and give examples of abuse scenarios in each of the developmental stages of childhood.
4. Analyze high-risk children and social/environmental influences on the development of child abuse.
5. Describe the child, parent, and environmental influences on child abuse situations.
6. Create a child abuse nursing care plan for a school-aged child, including physical, emotional, and social implications.
7. State the essential nursing care of the abused child and family, including identifying signs and symptoms, supporting medical assessments, and documenting appropriately.
8. Describe how to maintain safety for a child who has been abused, including essential communication, team membership, and legal steps needed for protection.

CRITICAL THINKING

Scenario #1: Accompanied by her 19-year-old boyfriend, **Katrina**, an 18-year-old single parent, brings her child into the emergency department (ED) because her 10-month-old infant is "sleeping too much, eating poorly, and is too thin." The ED nurse evaluates the infant and notes that the infant has poor hygiene; a dirty diaper with dried stool; a significant diaper rash; lower than expected weight (10th percentile on a national growth chart); lethargy; and large, wide eyes. The infant does not demonstrate stranger anxiety, and she does not smile when you attempt to play with her and present her with a brightly colored toy. Katrina states that she is very stressed, has no support from her parents in the care of the child, has dropped out of high school, and has no childcare for the infant during the day. The mother states that she cares for the infant in her parents' home and "never has time away from her." The boyfriend is not engaged in the child's care and remains focused on his cell phone, texting during the entire time you are interacting with the mother and child.

Continued

CRITICAL THINKING—cont'd

Upon further evaluation, the child demonstrates a yellowish bruise on her low flank and a new bluish bruise on her upper right arm. The ED medical team orders a chest x-ray that shows the child has three rib fractures with evidence of healing. The team suspects child abuse, and **Child Protective Services (CPS)** is notified. Within 60 minutes, a hospital social worker, a sheriff, and a member of the county CPS arrive to the ED and place the child on a 72-hour police hold. The child is transferred to the pediatric inpatient unit and is now awaiting a computed tomography (CT) scan of the body and a magnetic resonance imaging (MRI) of the head. Katrina is not allowed to visit her child without supervision.

The entire health-care team focuses on the well-being and healing of the child. The social worker identifies local support services for the mother, including a parenting class and a local mothers' support group. The team holds a family conference in the conference room on the floor of the pediatric unit, and the following are present during the meeting: the mother, her parents, the social worker, two CPS professionals, the attending physician, the charge nurse, a nutritionist, a child life specialist, and the ED physician. After the case conference, during which a plan of action is made for the mother, CPS allows the mother to reunite with the infant at discharge but will follow the family closely by agency visits and home visits. Mandatory parenting classes are required, and the mother receives both group counseling and individual counseling. The child is discharged after she demonstrates progressive weight gain.

Questions

1. What cues did you identify that warrant a workup for abuse?
2. Which conditions are most indicative of potential child abuse?
3. How did the health-care team provide immediate safety for the infant?
4. Why would the health-care team request the child have an MRI of the head?

CONCEPTUAL CORNERSTONE
Family
Families who are experiencing violence and abuse need help. Providing the abused child with a safe environment is the most important and immediate aspect of care. However, child abuse is a problem for the entire family. When a child presents with evidence or suspicion of abuse of any form, you can expect that the family will need help with parenting, anticipatory guidance, role modeling, counseling, and support services.

Child **abuse**, also called *child maltreatment or **intentional injury***, is a complex social problem. Defined by the World Health Organization (WHO) as "the abuse and neglect that occurs to children under 18 years of age. It includes all types of physical and/or emotional ill-treatment, sexual abuse, neglect, negligence and commercial or other exploitation, which results in actual or potential harm to the child's health, survival, development or dignity in the context of a relationship of responsibility, trust or power" (WHO, 2023, para. 1).

Child abuse may be hidden within the family structure, or it can be exposed by child injury or death. One quarter of all adults report being abused as a child. Nearly three in four young children under 4, or 300 million, endure physical punishment and/or psychological violence (WHO, 2023). Annually, worldwide over 40,150 homicide child deaths are attributed to abuse; however, this figure is only an estimate because of inadequate reporting (WHO, 2023). The U.S. Department of State estimates there are over 24.9 million sex trafficking victims around the world (2022). Nurses can be frontline health-care providers who identify the subtle or apparent evidence of child abuse of any form. Understanding the factors that contribute to child abuse, learning the various types and clinical presentations of each, and understanding the steps required to report child abuse are all essential components in protecting the child from further harm. Nurses are **mandatory reporters of child abuse and neglect**. Mandatory reporters, because of their positions, are legally responsible to report actual or suspected child abuse to the legal authorities. All health-care providers are considered mandatory reporters. Other mandatory reporters include commercial film developers, childcare custodians, and law enforcement agents from all branches of the law such as police officers and correctional personnel. Check your state law for mandatory reporter definitions and requirements.

- *Health-care providers:* All persons involved with the care of the child will be held responsible for evaluating and reporting any actual or suspected symptoms or signs of child abuse. These include nurses, nurse practitioners, physician assistants, physicians, social workers, or anyone involved with the health of the child.
- *Commercial film developers:* Those who develop film are also held responsible to report pictures taken of children in sexually or physically abused circumstances. However, with the widespread use of digital photography and recording, distribution of sexually explicit images of children occurs mostly online nowadays.
- *Childcare custodians:* Although the definition of who is considered a childcare custodian may differ from state to state, those who provide care and supervision for children, whether it is public or private, are considered mandatory child abuse reporters. Childcare providers, clergy, coaches, and teachers are all included under this category of mandatory reporters.

- *Law officers (all branches) and correctional personnel:* Anyone who holds a legal position of authority in any branch of law is considered a mandatory reporter. This includes sheriffs, police, highway patrol, and other staff employed by those divisions. Persons who work for CPS are also mandated to follow up on all actual or suspected child abuse.

Child maltreatment encompasses both abuse (physical, emotional, and sexual) and **neglect** (failure to provide for basic needs even when the means are present). Child maltreatment refers to abuse of children younger than 18 years old by a parent, a person in a custodial role (clergy, coach, or teacher), or a caregiver. The perpetrator of abuse may or may not have been known to the child.

Safety *Stat!*

Nurses are required to report both suspected and actual abuse or neglect. It is not your responsibility to determine who caused the abuse; that is the job of the local Child Protective Services (CPS). This agency provides assessment, interventions, and treatment referrals for families who have a child who has been identified as experiencing maltreatment. After an abuse report is called in to CPS, the person making the report has 24 to 48 hours to submit a written report, depending on state law. Failure to report, or delayed reporting, can result in severe legal consequences for a mandatory reporter. The written report should include all pertinent evidence collected, including verbatim quotes, pictures, radiographs, or any diagnostics that are associated with the child's clinical presentation or injury.

Safety *Stat!*

Sometimes local law officers should be called to the setting to provide immediate assistance. If you suspect that the child, or other family members, are currently at risk for further abuse, hospital security and law enforcement officers should be notified STAT.

 ## CHILD ABUSE GLOBAL PERSPECTIVES

Internationally, child abuse has been recorded throughout history in science, art, and literature in most parts of the world. Reports of neglect, mutilation, infanticide, abandonment, casting out the weak child to fend for themselves, sexual abuse, and many other forms of violence toward children have been documented dating back to ancient civilizations (Bensel et al., 1997). Unfortunately, child abuse did not gain attention in modern times until 1962, when Kempe's seminal work, *The Battered Child Syndrome,* was published. Child abuse remains a global problem with neglect being the most common form of child maltreatment.

Child abuse is a highly complex social phenomenon. Child abuse crosses all cultures, ages, economic levels, races, and religions, but is most prevalent in families with specific parental, child, and environmental characteristics. These include families living in poverty, families who have previously been reported to CPS, and those families composed of adolescent parents with young children (Christian, 2015). However, each case is unique. Therefore, nurses should never make assumptions based solely on a family's characteristics. Rather, nurses must be aware that social, economic, and personal stressors can contribute to child abuse in any type of family.

Culture plays a prominent role in principles of child rearing and childcare. Forms of child discipline accepted in one culture may be acts that are reportable and prosecutable in another. In culturally diverse societies, health-care professionals may be challenged to determine what practices are abusive or neglectful and which might be considered culturally acceptable. You, or any mandated reporter, must follow state laws concerning reporting suspected abuse, even if the evidence is not perfectly clear.

Safety *Stat!*

Protecting the child from further or continued abuse is of immediate importance. No matter the clinical setting in which abuse is suspected, the health-care team must protect the child from further abuse and report the suspicions or signs of abuse to the authorities.

 ## CHILD ABUSE AND PREVENTION

Federal legislation was created in 1974 to provide definitions and guidance for identifying and preventing child abuse. The Child Abuse Prevention and Treatment Act (CAPTA), amended in 2010, offers evaluation, technical assistance, data collection, and supporting research as well as minimal definitions of child neglect and child abuse.

Acts of commission in child abuse are situations in which the responsible person, often the parent, intentionally harms the child via physical, emotional, or sexual abuse. *Acts of omission* in child abuse are situations in which a parent or caregiver, to the best of abilities and often inadvertently, cannot provide adequate nutrition, shelter, warmth, appropriate seasonal clothing (winter coats), safety, and/or education for their child. Both are considered child abuse, and situations that fall in either category must be reported to authorities. The rationale for responding to both acts of commission and acts of omission is to provide safety for the child, or provide what is necessary for the child to thrive and grow in a safe environment.

A parent who expects a very young child to behave outside the child's age or developmental ability, or a parent who expects a young child to perform chores beyond the child's physical, emotional, and cognitive development, may contribute to abusive situations. That parent is at risk for becoming abusive (Smith et al., 2019; WHO, 2023). A challenge for the health-care team is to determine if the abuse was intentional or unintentional. **Unintentional abuse or injury** occurs when a parent or caregiver lacks education on child rearing or basic needs or neglects a child's basic needs because of lack of resources. See Table 26.1 regarding the etiology of abuse.

TYPES OF ABUSE

Child abuse includes physical abuse, emotional abuse or neglect, physical neglect, and sexual abuse. Teamwork is needed to identify the variety of clinical manifestations of abuse (Box 26.1).

Physical Abuse

Physical abuse is defined as acts of commission caused by either a parent or caregiver that result in actual physical

Table 26.1
Etiology of Abuse

Type of Factor	Factors
Parent/ Caregiver	• The parent(s) experienced severe punishment when they were children, or were neglected. • The parent(s) have poor impulse control. • The parent(s) accept free expression of violence within the home. • The family is experiencing social isolation, lack of parenting mentors, and little or no respite care. • The parent(s) have poor social-emotional support systems. • The parent(s) are participating in substance use disorder. • The parent(s) have low self-esteem. • The parent(s) have mental health issues. • The parent(s) have a history of cruelty to animals. • The parent(s) delay seeking medical treatment for the child and lack follow-through. • The parent(s) use multiple health-care providers, yet have a decreasing number of visits or increased no-shows. • The parent(s) have unrealistic expectations for the child's developmental stage or age. • The parent(s) have a low education level and are considered low income. • The caregivers are not the biological parents of the child.
Child	• The child is under 4 years of age. • The child has a difficult and/or demanding temperament. • The child is perceived as a misfit within the family structure. • The child has had numerous illnesses or has a chronic illness/disorder requiring extra demands. • The child has a documented disability or has mental health issues. • The child has developmental delays. • Typically, only one child is being abused; other siblings within the family are not usually abused. • The child was a product of an unplanned or unexpected pregnancy. • There was a difficult or problematic pregnancy and/or delivery. • The child has a hyperkinetic disorder. • There was an early failure to bond between the child and parent. • The child was born prematurely and/or is low birth weight. • The child has a resemblance to someone the parent does not like. • The child is male (greater risk than females).

Table 26.1
Etiology of Abuse—cont'd

Type of Factor	Factors
Environmental	• The environment the family functions in has chronic stress. • Member(s) of the family are going through or have recently been through a divorce. • The family has a nonbiologically related adult male living in the household. • The family has experienced frequent relocation to different geographical locations. • The family is living in poverty and oftentimes is living in a low-income urban or rural area. • The family has experienced the consequences of unemployment. • The family is living in inadequate, poor housing or unstable housing. • The family is living in an unsafe neighborhood. • The family is living in a community in which ongoing violence is experienced; thus, child abuse may be accepted.

Adapted from Centers for Disease Control and Prevention. (2022c). *Violence prevention: Risk and protective factors.* https://www.cdc.gov/violenceprevention/childabuseandneglect/riskprotectivefactors.html; Flaherty, E. G., Stirling, J., Jr., American Academy of Pediatrics. Committee on Child Abuse and Neglect. (2010). Clinical report—the pediatrician's role in child maltreatment prevention. *Pediatrics, 126*(4), 833–841. https://doi.org/10.1542/peds.2010-2087

Box 26.1
Clinical Manifestations or Symptoms of Abuse

Nurses and other health-care team members must be able to identify possible signs of abuse, including incompatibility of injuries noted and the given history of the injury. Other clinical manifestations may include the following:

• Lack of or delayed normal growth and development
• Language delay
• Irritability, resists affection and cuddling, may be unresponsive to nurturing
• Vacant eyes and/or gaze aversion
• Expressionless face, infrequent smile, may demonstrate anxiousness
• Weight is below the fifth percentile or a diagnosis of failure to thrive (FTT; see Chapter 18)
• Shaken baby syndrome (classic symptoms include subdural hematoma, cerebral edema, and retinal detachment or hemorrhage)
• Falls and associated injuries in young children
• Bruises in various stages of healing and of various shapes (the shape of the object used for infliction)

• Slapping or grab marks, bruises demonstrating being tied up (linear bruises on ankles and wrists)
• Gag marks
• Bilateral black eyes, including upper eyelids
• External head, facial, and oral injuries
• Boggy scalp injuries from subgaleal hematomas (caused by lifting the scalp off the skull)
• Thermal injuries such as dry contact burns that are second degree
• Forced immersion burns such as sock, glove, dunking, or donut burns (clear line of demarcation without accompanied splash burn marks)
• Traumatic hair loss (alopecia)
• Unexplained fractures that may be in different stages of healing
• Spiral fractures
• Unexplained dislocations
• Sexual abuse: bruising, discharge, pain, or sexually transmitted infections (STIs)
• Physical neglect, such as very poor hygiene

harm or are considered to have the potential to cause physical harm. Examples of physical abuse include shaken baby syndrome; a **battered** child showing evidence of repeated injury to the skin, nervous system, or skeletal system; and visceral trauma from blunt force, especially with clinical evidence of repeated injury. Children who present with evidence of slapping, hitting, burning, or any other form of physical harm have most likely been experiencing the abuse for an extended period (American Academy of Pediatrics [AAP], 2019). Figure 26.1 provides examples of instruments that have been used for physical punishment and the marks they leave behind. Figure 26.2 illustrates the areas of a child's body where accidental injuries would be unusual.

CRITICAL THINKING

Scenario #2: A 3-month-old infant is brought to the ED by her grandfather. He was visiting the family and found the infant lethargic, unresponsive to his touch or voice, and with two small bruises on both upper arms. The grandfather became concerned when both parents said she woke up in this state in the morning.

Questions

1. What are the critical signs of shaken baby syndrome?
2. What was most concerning about the grandfather's findings?

Burn Marks

| Lightbulb | Curling iron | Car cigarette lighter | Steam iron |
| Knife | Cigarette | Forks | Immersion |

Marks from Instruments

Belt buckle	Belt	Looped cord	Stick/whip
Fly swatter	Coat hanger	Board or spatula	Hand/knuckles
Bite	Paddles	Hair brush	Spoon

FIGURE 26.1 Instruments used for physical punishment and the marks they leave.

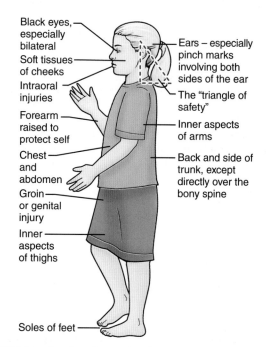

- Black eyes, especially bilateral
- Soft tissues of cheeks
- Intraoral injuries
- Forearm raised to protect self
- Chest and abdomen
- Groin or genital injury
- Inner aspects of thighs
- Soles of feet
- Ears – especially pinch marks involving both sides of the ear
- The "triangle of safety"
- Inner aspects of arms
- Back and side of trunk, except directly over the bony spine

FIGURE 26.2 Accidental injuries in these areas are unusual.

New parents must be taught to never shake their infant. A single episode of shaking can have lifelong devastating effects on a child's neurological system. Shaken baby syndrome may also be referred to as abusive head trauma (AAP, 2020).

Emotional Abuse or Neglect

Emotional abuse or *neglect* is defined as the failure of the parent or caregiver to provide an appropriate supportive environment. The child's emotional health and development suffer. Examples of emotional abuse include denigration, ridicule, intimidation, threats, hostility, discrimination, rejection, and restricting a child's movement (WHO, 2024). A child who is regularly threatened, humiliated, ignored, blamed, called names, made fun of, or found to be at fault is also considered emotionally or psychologically abused. Child Welfare Information Gateway (2019b) further describes emotional abuse as impaired self-worth, rejection, or mental injury.

Physical Neglect

Physical neglect is when a parent or caregiver fails to provide nutrition, shelter, medical care, and/or safe living conditions for the child. However, physical neglect is different from poverty. Parents or caregivers who are neglectful have reasonable resources available, but they do not provide them to the child. Hunger from deprivation of food, a lack of physical development, medical noncompliance, and very poor hygiene are universal symptoms of physical neglect.

Sexual Abuse

Sexual abuse is when a parent, sibling, caregiver, stranger, family friend, relative, or neighbor uses a child for their own sexual gratification. A child who is used in a sexual way by an adult or an older child, whether or not touching or penetration occurs, is considered sexually abused. Sexual abuse occurs when a child is forced to look at an adult masturbating, adult genitalia, or pornography or is forced to be a part of the production of pornographic materials. Some sexually abused children are not forcibly assaulted but are persuaded, tricked, coerced, or bribed to engage in sex acts. See Box 26.2 for factors associated with the sexual abuse of children.

Box 26.2

Factors Associated With Sexual Abuse of Children

- Anyone can be an abuser: father, mother, sibling, member of the extended family, teacher, or coach.
- The person who is sexually abusing a child is typically male and known to the family. "Stranger danger" is much less common.
- Sexual abuse offenders come from all socioeconomic levels, cultures, and races.
- Abusers often choose to work in environments in which children are present.
- Father-daughter or stepfather-daughter abuse situations tend to be prolonged. The eldest daughter is typically the victim.
- Male victims are less likely to admit and report sexual abuse because of social stigmas.

Children who are victims of sexual abuse display classic symptoms of infection, abdominal pain, genital injury, constipation, urinary tract infections, sexually explicit behaviors incompatible with their age, an increased interest in sexuality, and emotional disturbances. Health-care providers who work with children need a high index of suspicion of and familiarity with the behavioral, physical, and verbal indicators of this type of abuse. If sexual abuse is suspected, forensic evaluation should be instigated, urine specimens collected, and tissues evaluated for trauma and swabbed by a specially trained nurse. All documentation must be written in clinical, objective terms. You must maintain the chain of evidence, labeling each photograph taken and each specimen collected and keeping all evidence within sight until it is given to law enforcement.

Team Works

Specialty training is required to lawfully collect evidence of child sexual abuse. Evidence collected by a certified registered nurse (RN) in the field, who can testify in court about what was seen and collected, provides a greater opportunity for the case against the abuser to move forward. The nurse caring for the child victim should immediately provide a safe environment, call the social worker, and call for a SANE (Sexual Assault Nurse Examiner) nurse, who is certified in the required forensic specialty. The child, the nonabuser caregiver(s), and even the health-care team caring for the child will need support from the social worker (International Association of Forensic Nurses, 2019).

FACTITIOUS DISORDER IMPOSED ON ANOTHER

Why would a parent or caregiver intentionally create an illness; fabricate the symptoms of an illness; or describe nonexistent clinical symptoms such as seizures, vomiting, or bloody diarrhea in their child? Having the child admitted into a hospital or health-care setting and receiving praise for the parent's attentive parenting are the rewards for a parent with **factitious disorder imposed on another** (FDIA; formally known as Munchausen syndrome by proxy). This disorder is a mental illness in which one has an inner need for another person (their child) to be seen as injured or ill, and produces this by false claims (Mayo Clinic, 2024). This rare (approximately 1,000 out of 2.5 million child abuse reports) but real mental health disorder is demonstrated typically by a mother who has some health-care knowledge and who displays behaviors of overinvolvement with her child. The perpetrator wants the child to experience multiple invasive tests and treatments, which allows the parent to receive a great deal of attention from the members of

the health-care team. The symptoms described by the parent are not witnessed by members of the health-care team, and the symptoms are not present when the parent is not around the child. Box 26.3 provides indicators of FDIA. The parent is typically viewed as very attentive and caring, until a pattern of bizarre attention-seeking behaviors is identified. You must identify this type of child abuse as soon as possible, preferably before the child is subjected to multiple, sometimes painful, unnecessary diagnostic procedures. Box 26.4 presents a case study on a child identified as a victim of FDIA.

Box 26.3

Indicators of Factitious Disorder Imposed on Another

1. The child is under 6 years of age with a history of many illnesses, frequent hospitalizations, and vague and "strange" symptoms; may present with scars from previous surgical or medical procedures.
2. Perpetrator is usually the mother, who has some health-care knowledge; may have great knowledge of diseases and medical terms.
3. Father is not present in the health-care interaction, is uninvolved, or is absent from the home/family.
4. Possible positive family history exists of parent with factitious disorder or another sibling who has experienced this type of abuse.
5. Claimed medical history of the child by the mother is not supported by evidence found by health-care professionals.
6. Child has both a history of multiple hospitalizations and experiences with multiple blood tests, x-rays, and other invasive procedures.
7. The child does not display the symptoms during hospitalization, symptoms are not witnessed by another, and the child's condition improves when the mother is not present.
8. The child's clinical signs and symptoms cannot be explained or substantiated by a known disease etiology. Conditions do not respond to standard medical treatments as expected by the team.
9. A history of one or more unusual illnesses or death of another child in the family is present.
10. The child's condition improves while in the health-care environment.
11. Specimens of blood do not match a specimen of blood from the child.
12. Chemicals are found in the child's body secretions (urine, blood, or stool).

Sources: American Psychiatric Association. (2022). *Diagnostic and statistical manual of mental disorders* (5th ed., text revision). Author; Cleveland Clinic. (2021). *Factitious disorder imposed on another (FDIA).* https://my.clevelandclinic.org/health/diseases/9834-factitious-disorder-imposed-on-another-fdia; Mayo Clinic. (2019). *Factitious disorder.* https://www.mayoclinic.org/diseases-conditions/factitious-disorder/symptoms-causes/syc-20356028; National Institutes of Health. (2021). *Munchausen syndrome by proxy.* http://www.nlm.nih.gov/medlineplus/ency/article/001555.htm.

Box 26.4

Case Study: Factitious Disorder Imposed on Another

A 35-year-old mother rushes her child to the ED of a large hospital claiming that her infant daughter just had a "blue spell" followed by a long grand mal seizure and then a period of not breathing. A full diagnostic workup is started. The mother claims a history of reflux, bloody stools found in the diaper, and fevers. The mother is praised for identifying the child's condition, and the child is eventually admitted to the pediatric intensive care unit (PICU) for further observation and diagnostic procedures. After a long hospitalization, visits from multiple pediatric specialists, and many complex diagnostic procedures such as upper and lower gastrointestinal (GI) series, blood tests, and electroencephalogram (EEG), no evidence is found to support the mother's claims. While in the PICU, the child experiences none of the symptoms described by the mother. What indicators of FDIA are present?

Safety *Stat!*

If a member of the health-care team suspects FDIA on the part of a parent, an immediate consultation should be requested from a social worker, and pertinent members of the child's health-care team should be notified of the concerns. If the parent believes that they may be a suspect, the parent may leave the health-care facility against medical advice. Family members identified as flight risks should be reported to hospital security and their assistance secured.

ABUSE STATISTICS

According to the Centers for Disease Control and Prevention (CDC), identified cases of child abuse represent only a small fraction of a widespread problem (2022a). According to the CDC's 2022 statistics, one in seven children has experienced child abuse and/or neglect in the last year. CPS found that 686,000 children under the age of 18 were victims of child abuse; and the overall national rates of child abuse are estimated to be as high as 9.2 per 1,000 children. The breakdown of the types of child abuse is reported to be as follows:

- 74.9% neglect
- 18.3% physical abuse
- 8.6% sexual abuse
- Others include abandonment, congenital medication addiction, and threats to harm.

The percentage total is greater than 100% because some children suffer multiple types of abuse (CDC, 2022a).

The effects of child abuse can last long into adulthood. Long-term consequences of child abuse in adults include the following (Child Welfare Information Gateway, 2019a; WHO, 2023):

- Obesity, stroke, and heart attack
- Smoking, lung disease, and chronic bronchitis
- Medication misuse and alcohol misuse
- Malnutrition
- Depression
- High-risk sexual behavior
- Unplanned pregnancy
- Cognitive delays
- Cancer

It is imperative that health-care providers do not miss child abuse in clinical practice, as a significant number of cases are frequently missed (Gonzalez et al., 2022). A useful mnemonic to think about is TEN 4; bruises or injuries on the Torso, Ears, or Neck on children 4 years of age or younger (Gonzalez et al., 2022).

FATAL ABUSE

How often does child abuse lead to the child's death (filicide)? Based on an investigation of death registries and mortality data, between 1,750 and 1,830 children died in the span of 2019 to 2020 because of abuse (ACF, 2022), but this is only an estimate because many cases are not reported to government officials. An accurate number is difficult to determine because routine postmortem examinations are not always conducted. Infants and very young children are at greatest risk for death associated with abuse, with rates that are double those of children 5 to 15 years old. The most common causes of childhood deaths associated with abuse were head trauma, shaking deaths, burns, drowning, smothering, suffocation, choking, and strangulation, and most fatalities were children younger than 6 months of age (National Center on Shaken Baby Syndrome, 2022). Perpetrators of fatal child abuse tend to be the child's biological parent (most often the mother) and to have incomes below the federal poverty threshold; however, demographics of perpetrators vary in different geographical areas (Child Welfare Information Gateway, 2020).

PREVENTION OF CHILD ABUSE

Preventing child abuse before it occurs is the ultimate goal of everyone working to reduce the incidence of child maltreatment. Community education is one important aspect of prevention. After all, 20% of child maltreatment is reported by family, friends, and community members (Spilsbury et al., 2018). Another essential component of child abuse prevention is readily available and affordable parenting classes in which childcare and anger management skills are taught and reinforced. Good communication and parenting skills, knowing when and how to respond to a child's physical and emotional needs, and age-appropriate discipline techniques are helpful aspects of positive parenting. Protective factors such as strengthening financial security, engaging the family in the child's preschool, and providing quality childcare opportunities and parenting classes are all effective prevention strategies (CDC, 2022b). Programs that help to improve the parent–child relationship and those that provide social support, role modeling, tools for prevention, and specific encouragement for success have been successful in reducing the incidence of child abuse (Preventchildabuse.org, 2019).

Patient Teaching Guidelines

Three ideas to communicate to parents struggling with positive parenting are the following:

- Count to 10 before disciplining a child.
- Match discipline techniques with the child's developmental stage. Know what to expect from each stage and do not expect more than the child is cognitively, emotionally, or physically able to do.
- Practice good self-care. To be a good parent means to take care of oneself so that stress, anger, and short-tempered responses can be minimized.

Prevention starts with early reporting of suspected abuse or neglect. If health-care professionals suspect that a child is being maltreated or threatened with maltreatment, they should call the National Child Abuse Hotline at 1-800-4-A-Child (1-800-422-4453).

For a list of child abuse prevention strategies, see the CDC website.

MEDICAL AND NURSING MANAGEMENT OF CHILD ABUSE

In managing child abuse, it is imperative that a comprehensive treatment plan be developed that includes a variety of team members using a family-focused care model. First and foremost, the child should be protected from further abuse. The authorities must be notified to begin the process of identifying the abuser, and careful documentation by the health-care team of all that is heard, seen, and done is imperative. The entire health-care team's role is to provide the child with safety and support and to begin to conduct evaluations and diagnostics to confirm abuse. CPS's role is to identify the perpetrator and to ensure the child's continued safety.

Therapeutic Communication

The pediatric health-care team, as they are establishing a trusting relationship and rapport with the child, must emphasize that the child did not cause the abuse and is not responsible for the abuse that has occurred.

The care team should use the following steps in the care and protection of a child who has been a victim of child abuse:

1. *Stabilization:* The child's physical, physiological, and emotional health need to be stabilized. The early identification and treatment of physical harm (head trauma, shaken baby syndrome, spiral fractures, and bleeding) need to be the priority in the care of a child who has been abused.
2. *Protection from further harm:* The care team needs to set up circumstances to prevent further harm to the child. The child may need a police hold, hospital security may need to be involved, social services will need to talk to the family, and CPS may need to provide temporary medical foster care.
3. *History taking:* The care team must identify if there are inconsistencies between the presentation of the injury and the parent–child history or description of the cause of the injury. The history must be carefully and objectively documented because records can be required in court.
4. *Collection of laboratory specimens:* The collection of specimens needs to take place as soon as possible using protocols that protect the evidence, such as the collection of semen and human hairs from the child's body.
5. *Securing of photographs:* Many health-care environments will have a policy that guides the health-care team in how to document the visual evidence of abuse via photographs. Any evidence and/or photographs must be carefully labeled and kept with you in a secured location until turned over to law enforcement. This is called the **chain of custody** for specimen collection (conscientious handling to prevent tampering), processing, holding, and handing over to officials (Badiye et al., 2022).
6. *Differentiation of child abuse from other medical conditions:* One challenge for the health-care team, social services, and CPS workers is to differentiate suspected child abuse from other medical conditions or from injuries received during normal activities or vigorous play.
7. *Determination of spiral fractures:* Spiral fractures are often associated with violent abuse of young children, so meticulous radiography needs to be taken to determine if the child's fracture is a spiral fracture. This type of fracture occurs very rarely in conditions or circumstances other than abuse.
8. *Ruling out congenital brittle bone disease:* A very rare condition, brittle bone disease must be ruled out in the presence of multiple fractures found in a variety of healing stages.
9. *Distinguishing between abuse and cultural care practices:* Some cultural care practices exist that can leave physical marks that resemble child abuse.

Labs & Diagnostics

Laboratory analysis and diagnostics that can aid the team in confirming or ruling out abuse include the following:

- Skeletal bone surveys
- CT scan
- Ophthalmological examination
- Color photographs
- Examination of cerebrospinal fluid
- Pregnancy tests
- STI screening tests
- Evidentiary examinations of specimens by the local coroner, CPS, or medical examiner

Safety *Stat!*

Do not wash or bathe a child who is a suspected victim of sexual abuse. Many specimens will need to be collected from the child's clothing, orifices, and skin. It is important to obtain these specimens according to strict legal protocols for the evidence collected to be usable in court. If possible, collect the first urination.

Safety *Stat!*

Never use a personal cell phone to collect evidence of child abuse! Instead, contact your administration and follow the institutional protocol carefully.

Nursing Care Plan for the Victim of Abuse

Kyle, age 18 months, is brought to the outpatient clinic by his teenage single mother because "his arm hurts." Upon observation, you note that the child keeps his right arm immobile and cries when you reach for his hand to check range of motion. While checking Kyle's lung sounds, you note bruises in various stages of healing on the child's torso. When asked about the bruises, the mother states that Kyle is "clumsy" and "falls down a lot." X-ray reveals a spiral fracture of Kyle's right tibia. You begin to plan his care.

Nursing Diagnosis: Pain related to fractured right tibia
Expected Outcome: The patient's pain is reduced to a tolerable level.

Intervention:	Rationale:
Administer pain medication as ordered.	*It is essential to meet the child's physical needs first. Relieving the child's pain will make it easier for the health-care provider to set his fracture.*

Nursing Diagnosis: Impaired physical mobility related to fractured right tibia
Expected Outcome: The patient's bone will heal with complications.

Intervention:	Rationale:
Assist the health-care provider to cast the arm to immobilize the fracture.	*It is essential to meet the child's physical needs first. The bone must be set and immobilized in order for the fracture to heal properly.*

Nursing Diagnoses: Altered parenting related to a poor understanding of a child's cognitive and developmental abilities and needs; altered parenting related to use of violence
Expected Outcomes: The child experiences a nonviolent home, the parent understands and uses developmentally appropriate discipline when the child misbehaves, the parent learns and uses anger management techniques to avoid becoming violent, and the parent receives support to give her time for self-care activities.

Interventions:	Rationales:
Report suspected physical abuse to a hospital social worker and to CPS.	*Reporting suspected abuse is the only way to get help for the family.*
Refer mother to parenting and anger management classes; encourage her to join a support group for single parents of young children.	*To address the mother's knowledge deficit, classes in parenting and anger management are needed.*
	A support group may help the mother feel less alone and give her practical suggestions for managing her life.
Brainstorm a list of reliable friends or family members who could babysit the child for a few hours each week.	*Having time for self-care and time away from her toddler will help the mother relax and regain her composure.*
CPS will follow up with home visits to check on the child's welfare and the mother's development of new coping skills.	*It is essential for CPS to follow up with the family to ensure the child's safety.*

NURSING CONSIDERATIONS AND CARE

Identifying and reporting child abuse are difficult aspects of being a nurse. Being able to identify when abuse has occurred when signs and symptoms are vague is difficult for even experienced nurses. Care must be given to protect the child from ongoing abuse, but it's also imperative not to jump to conclusions. If a child has infected wounds, injuries, or disease processes because of a delay in seeking treatment, or if no treatment was sought for such concerns, it is your responsibility to follow up, to discuss the findings with the health-care provider and social worker, and to report to the authorities as indicated. Reporting abuse to the appropriate authorities is essential in the prevention of escalating violence and continued harm.

Safety *Stat!*

Look for behavioral signs as well as physical signs of abuse. A child who has experienced neglect, emotional abuse, or physical abuse may display fear, irritability, aggression, withdrawal, or apathy. Be caring and vigilant. Ask team members to assist you in observing the child's behavior.

Using a team approach can assist all staff members through the difficult and emotionally charged experience of managing care of an abused child. Discussing the case with the charge nurse, nursing supervisor, or nurse manager is appropriate to have support in the reporting process. Nurses must be familiar with institutional policies on reporting child abuse. Team members, childcare custodians, and other mandatory reporters who do not report child abuse are at risk for legal consequences such as heavy fines and/or jail sentences. The consequences to the child of not reporting suspected abuse include the continuation, and sometimes the escalation, of abuse. Families of an abused child will not secure help, such as childcare and appropriate child discipline classes, if the abuse is not reported.

HUMAN TRAFFICKING

Human trafficking is defined as the recruitment, transportation, transfer, harboring, and exploitation of persons by the means of threat, force, or abduction for the use of prostitution, forced labor, slavery, servitude, or the removal of organs for sale (Migrationdataportal.org, 2019; Article 3, para. (b)). Human trafficking is a worldwide humanitarian crisis. The United Nations Office on Drugs and Crime (UNODC, 2018) states that there are approximately 600,000 to 800,000 "modern-day slaves" (laborers, sex workers, and domestic workers) in the United States. According to the International Labour Organization, children make up 25%

of the 40.3 million victims of human trafficking worldwide, and 75% of those children are girls. A significant number of children are sold by their parents or other family members to human traffickers. According to recent data, the proportion of children taken for sexual exploitation has decreased slightly, but the proportion of children taken for forced labor has increased (Migrationdataportal.org, 2019). Those at greatest risk for being trafficked include the following (UNODC, 2016):

• Children who are experiencing homelessness
• Children who have run away from home
• Children living in poverty
• Children living in foster care
• Youths who use illegal drugs or other substances
• Youths who are members of sexual and gender minorities

The most important action a nurse can take is to be aware of the widespread nature of human trafficking. Nurses caring for children should understand the magnitude of the global problem and be astute about identifying child victims.

Identifying Victims of Sex Trafficking

The prevalence of child sex trafficking in the United States is unknown but estimated to be between 15,000 and 50,000, including women and children (DeliverFund, 2022). Victims of sex trafficking experience physical and sexual violence, STIs, pregnancy and unsafe abortions, and chronic medical conditions. For these reasons, they do seek medical care, making health-care professionals ideally situated to connect victims with authorities who can secure their safety. The major challenge so far has been the extreme difficulty in identifying victims. Fear of the trafficker, distrust of authorities, shame, and hopelessness make victim self-identification rare. It is common for the victim to be coerced, forced, or manipulated to secure nonconsensual sex labor. Traffickers use debt bondage, migration issues, or threats to secure participation (State.gov, 2023).

In order to develop a screening tool, Greenbaum and colleagues (2018) set out to describe characteristics of child sex trafficking victims that set them apart from their peers in a high-risk adolescent population. They compared child victims of sex trafficking with similar-aged patients with allegations of sexual assault or sexual abuse. The differences between the two groups allowed researchers to identify variables to turn into screening questions. The quick, six-item screening tool they developed effectively identifies victims of commercial sexual exploitation or child sex trafficking in a high-risk adolescent population. Tips for screening are also provided by the National Child Traumatic Stress Network (NCTSN.org, n.d.) found at https://www.nctsn.org/what-child-trauma-trauma-types-sex-trafficking/screening-identification-and-assessment.

Key Points

- Child abuse happens worldwide and crosses all socio-economic levels, cultures, and religious backgrounds. It is important for nurses to possess strong evaluation skills and follow-through to protect children of all ages.
- Abuse includes physical abuse, physical neglect, emotional abuse, emotional neglect, and sexual abuse.
- Child-related factors that influence child abuse include children who are the result of unplanned pregnancies, have difficult temperaments, have developmental delays, have chronic diseases, or are seen as "different" from their siblings. Parental factors that influence child abuse include experience with severe punishment when they were children, poor impulse control, acceptance of violence within the home, social isolation, a lack of parenting mentors, little or no respite care, low self-esteem, and substance use disorder.

- Classic symptoms and clinical presentations of the various types of abuse include low birth weight; poor weight gain; a lack of normal growth and development, including language delay; vacant eyes and/or gaze aversion; an expressionless face; infrequent smiling; anxiousness; subdural hematomas; fractures; bruises; retinal hemorrhages; bruises in various stages of healing; thermal injuries; traumatic hair loss (alopecia); spiral fractures; STIs; and evidence of physical neglect, such as very poor hygiene.
- Maintaining safety for a child who has been abused includes essential communication, teamwork, and taking the legal steps needed for protection. Health-care team members who do not report child abuse are at risk for heavy fines and/or jail sentences.

Review Questions

1. Which situation would be considered child abuse, or maltreatment of a child, in most states in the United States?
   1. Lack of economic resources within a home
   2. Domestic violence between family members
   3. Intentional harm directed at a child
   4. Negligence in providing safe living conditions

2. A nursing instructor asks a student to define *child abuse.* Which response by the student indicates a need for clarification?
   1. Lack of physical care to the child, such as inadequate food and feedings
   2. Absence of emotional care and stimulation that allows a child to develop normally
   3. Denial of education to a child, such as not enrolling a young child into an appropriate school
   4. Preventing a child from participating in extracurricular activities within a school setting

3. Which acts are types of child abuse or maltreatment? **(Select all that apply.)**
   1. Physical violence
   2. Sexual abuse
   3. Emotional abuse
   4. Emotional neglect
   5. Physical restraint
   6. Physical neglect

4. While checking a young school-aged child suspected of having been sexually abused, which observation would be most significant to you?
   1. Seductive behaviors demonstrated by the child
   2. The child's inappropriate knowledge or interest in sexual activities or acts
   3. The child's fear of a particular family member, neighbor, or friend
   4. The child's obsession with masturbating in private

5. Which is one of the first clues that a child may have experienced abuse?
   1. You hear the stories of abuse from a younger sibling.
   2. You identify that there is a discrepancy between the injury present and the reported history of the injury.
   3. You identify a history of substance use disorder in one of the parents.
   4. You evaluate a history of a difficult and prolonged labor for the mother of the child.

6. Which evaluation is of the highest priority in caring for a young child suspected of being a victim of child abuse?
   1. Testing the child for STIs in cases of suspected sexual abuse
   2. Conducting developmental evaluations to determine the level of cognitive processing
   3. Obtaining skeletal radiographs of a child with a suspected glove burn
   4. Evaluating relationships with siblings and the order of birth

7. A nurse is caring for a 4-year-old boy admitted for observation from the ED. The child's mother reports a history of belly pain, bloody emesis, and seizures dating back 6 months with the latest seizure occurring this morning. The child is slender, pale, and slightly anemic. All other laboratory values are within normal limits. What condition should you suspect?
   1. Intentional child abuse
   2. Shaken baby syndrome
   3. Medical neglect of a child
   4. FDIA

8. The nurse working in a pediatric clinic sees a child with a fading ecchymotic ring around his left eye. What is the most appropriate question to ask the child?
   1. "Did you get that black eye during sports?"
   2. "Who did this to you?"
   3. "Have you been bullied at school?"
   4. "How did you get the black eye?"

9. Which burn marks on a child raise the suspicion of child abuse?
   1. Burns around both feet with edges marked in a line above the ankle
   2. Splash marks on the child's anterior chest and abdomen
   3. A small round burn on the side of one thumb
   4. Large fluid-filled vesicles with erythema on both shoulders

10. When it comes to suspected child abuse, nurses, police officers, teachers, and commercial film developers are all _____ _____.

ANSWERS 1. 3; 2. 4; 3. 1; 4. 6; 4. 5. 2; 6. 2; 7. 4; 8. 1; 9. 1; 10. mandatory reporters

CRITICAL THINKING QUESTIONS

1. What steps are most appropriate for a new nurse to take when they suspect that a child has been physically or emotionally abused?
2. Three factors typically found in cases of factitious disorder are the following:
   • The child is under 6 years of age.
   • The perpetrator is usually the mother, who has some health-care knowledge.
   • The father is not present in the health-care interaction, is uninvolved, or is absent from the home/family.
   What explanations can you think of for why these would be common factors in FDIA?

Resources

For additional resources and information, including Postconference Questions and Activities, Answers, and References, visit www.FADavis.com.

Student Study Guide

CHAPTER 27
Child With a Neurological Condition

KEY TERMS

cranial nerves (CN) (KRAY-nee-uhl NERVZ)
encephalopathy (en-SEF-uh-LOP-uh-thee)
grand mal seizure (GRAND MAL SEE-zhur)
increased intracranial pressure (ICP) (IN-kreest
    IN-truh-KRAY-nee-uhl PRESH-uhr)
ketogenic diet (KEE-toh-JEN-ik DYE-uht)
meningitis (MEN-en-JYE-tiss)
myoclonic (MYE-oh-KLON-ik)
Reye syndrome (RYE SIN-drohm)
status epilepticus (SE) (STAY-tuhss
    EP-ih-LEP-tih-kuss)
tonic-clonic seizure (TON-ik-KLON-ik SEE-zhur)

CHAPTER CONCEPTS

Intracranial Regulation
Neurological Regulation
Oxygenation
Perfusion

LEARNING OUTCOMES

1. Define the key terms.
2. Describe the anatomy and physiology of the peripheral nervous system (PNS) and central nervous system (CNS).
3. Discuss each of the senses and describe the developmental process of sensory organs after birth.
4. State the components of a holistic nervous system evaluation, including the 12 cranial nerves and rapid neurological checks.
5. Analyze the clinical presentation and functioning levels of children with varying degrees of cognitive impairment (CI).
6. Discuss the phenomenon of, and the clinical outcomes of, a child who experiences "near drowning."
7. State the serum value of lead that denotes lead poisoning in children.
8. Define the various types of seizure disorders and describe the evaluations, nursing care, and treatments for each.
9. Analyze the consequences of various nervous system pathologies, including hydrocephalus, neural tube defects, meningitis, Reye syndrome, and intraventricular hemorrhage (IVH).
10. Describe factors associated with a diagnosis of a traumatic brain injury (TBI).
11. Discuss the clinical phenomenon of childhood migraine headaches and describe the various treatment options for this condition.
12. Describe issues of safety relative to a child with a neurological disorder or condition, including safe environments, safety precautions, rapid evaluations for changes in clinical status, and safety around medications for neurological conditions.

CRITICAL THINKING

Scenario #1: **Randal** is a 16-year-old patient admitted to the pediatric intensive care unit (PICU) with an initial diagnosis of bacterial meningitis. He is prepared for a lumbar puncture. His cerebrospinal fluid (CSF) is cloudy, and his temperature increases to 39.3°C (102.7°F). Broad spectrum antibiotics are started STAT. Randal demonstrates focal seizure activity within 1 hour of being admitted to the PICU and is immediately placed on seizure precautions.

Continued

CRITICAL THINKING—cont'd

An appropriate dose of lorazepam is administered through his IV to stop his seizure activity. Randal is placed on droplet precautions with constant supervision in the PICU. You are assisting the RN caring for Randal.

Questions

1. What are the priorities for Randal's care?
2. How do you provide seizure precautions?

CONCEPTUAL CORNERSTONE

Sensory Perception

A child's perception of sensory stimulation is produced by the nerve tissue of the peripheral nervous system (PNS) and the central nervous system (CNS). Sensory perception relates to all neurological structures that take in and process sensory information. The neuron, being the central component of the sensory experience, is protected by a myelin sheath. When a child experiences a sensory stimulation—pleasure, pain, or other sensory information—the stimulus is transformed into an electrical current that runs from afferent (sensory) nerve fibers to the area of the brain that corresponds to interpretation. The brain then processes the sensory stimuli. Efferent (motor) nerve fibers then transmit the brain's interpretation and command to the extremities, which respond with a motor movement. Sensory perception is key to safety. If a child experiences a painful or unpleasant sensation, the brain will process the information and cause the child to move away from, let go of, or recoil from the uncomfortable sensation. Young infants, whose nerve fibers have yet to be myelinated, respond with primitive reflexes that are replaced with purposeful movement as the nerves mature **cephalocaudally**.

Before providing care to a child with a neurological disorder, it is important to review the anatomy of the neurological system. The two main divisions of the nervous system consist of the CNS and the PNS. Each of these two systems has unique functions to regulate all of the systems of the human body. Another system, the autonomic nervous system (ANS), regulates bodily functions without conscious effort and includes the motor and sensory nuclei in the brain and spinal cord.

THE DEVELOPMENT OF THE NERVOUS SYSTEM

During early embryonic development, the nervous system begins to form. During later intrauterine development, the fetus responds to sensory stimuli. After birth, the neonate's nervous system continues to develop; within the first year of life, the infant moves from primitive reflexes to purposeful movement and on to the beginning of fine motor movement. The pincer grasp (using the index finger and the thumb to pick up small objects) presents, on average, at age 7 to 8 months. This grasp is an example of the steady neurological development of the infant from uncontrolled, reactive movements, or reflexes, to fine motor movements, such as being able to pick up a small object with the fingers.

Central Nervous System

The CNS is composed of the brain and the spinal cord. The brain consists of the cerebrum, which is the center of consciousness, and the two cerebral hemispheres (Fig. 27.1). The frontal lobe controls speech; voluntary muscle movements; personality; and areas for behavioral, autonomic, and intellectual functions. The brain also contains the temporal lobe for hearing and smell; the parietal lobe for sensory coordination, interpretation, and taste (some overlap with the temporal lobe); and the occipital lobe for visual stimuli interpretation. Other anatomical components of the brain are the diencephalon, which houses the thalamus (sensory relay for pain, pressure, and temperature), the hypothalamus (controls the ANS; regulates emotion, behavior, hunger, and thirst; and secretes antidiuretic hormone and oxytocin), the cerebellum, and the brainstem. Extending from the brain, the spinal cord is a cylindrical-shaped bundle of nerve tissues and fibers that connects the brain to the nerves in the body.

Peripheral Nervous System

The PNS is composed of all the nerves outside the CNS, including the 12 pairs of cranial nerves and the 31 pairs of spinal nerves. **Cranial nerves (CN)** are numbered by the order in which they contact the brain; they originate in the cranial cavity and innervate the head (Fig. 27.2). The PNS connects the brain to the remote areas of the child's body. The PNS has both afferent neurons that transmit information from the organs, skin, and tissue to the brain, and efferent neurons that transmit regulatory and control information from the brain to the body. Figure 27.3 depicts the nerves of the spinal cord and vertebral structures.

Team Works

Team Assessment of a Child's Cranial Nerves

The pediatric health-care team will work together to assess a child's CNs.

CN I Olfactory: Provides the ability to transmit odorous signals from the nasal cavity to the brain (tested with a cotton ball soaked with stimulus such as vanilla oil)

CN II Optic: Provides the ability to transmit visual signals from the retina of the eye to the brain (tested with various visual cues)

Continued

• WORD • BUILDING •

cephalocaudal: cephalo–head + caud–tail + al–relating to

Team Works—cont'd

CN III Oculomotor: Provides the ability to perform most eye movements (tested by requesting the patient to follow finger commands)

CN IV Trochlear: Provides the ability to laterally rotate the eyeball (tested by asking the patient to rotate the eyeball inward, down, up, and outward)

CN V Trigeminal: Provides the ability to feel sensations in the face and perform mastication (chewing; tested by requesting the patient to perform chewing movements on command and testing the patient's response to cotton ball sensations to the full face)

CN VI Abducens: Provides the ability to perform abducted movements of the eye (tested by requesting that the patient follow commands to move eyes left and right)

CN VII Facial: Provides the ability to demonstrate motor movements of facial expressions and taste of anterior two-thirds of the tongue (tested by requesting the patient to move the face in various expressions and by testing taste on the front of the tongue)

CN VIII Acoustic: Provides the ability to detect sound, body rotation, and gravity (tested by assessing the patient's ability to hear bilaterally, close the eyes, and know where their body is in relation to gravitational pull)

CN IX Glossopharyngeal: Provides the ability to taste in the posterior one-third of the tongue (tested by providing the patient with various tastes by providing stimuli such as salt, sugar, and bitters)

CN X Vagus: Provides the ability to vocalize and swallow effectively (tested by assessing the ability of the patient to vocalize and the effectiveness of the patient's ability to swallow)

CN XI Spinal accessory: Provides the ability to use the sternocleidomastoid and trapezius muscles (tested by asking the patient to shrug and move the head effectively side to side and up and down)

CN XII Hypoglossal: Provides the ability to move all muscles of the tongue (tested by requesting the patient to perform bolus swallowing and speech articulation)

The following is a common mnemonic that helps to remember the CNs:

On Old Olympus's Towering Tops, A Finn And German Viewed Some Hops.

Autonomic Nervous System

The ANS is responsible for involuntary body functions. The ANS regulates salivation, digestion, respiration, perspiration, urination, cardiovascular function, and sexual arousal by way of the hypothalamus, which supervises the sympathetic nervous system (SNS) and the parasympathetic nervous system.

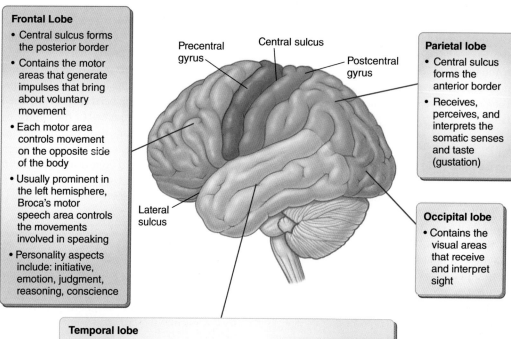

Frontal Lobe
- Central sulcus forms the posterior border
- Contains the motor areas that generate impulses that bring about voluntary movement
- Each motor area controls movement on the opposite side of the body
- Usually prominent in the left hemisphere, Broca's motor speech area controls the movements involved in speaking
- Personality aspects include: initiative, emotion, judgment, reasoning, conscience

Precentral gyrus

Central sulcus

Postcentral gyrus

Parietal lobe
- Central sulcus forms the anterior border
- Receives, perceives, and interprets the somatic senses and taste (gustation)

Lateral sulcus

Occipital lobe
- Contains the visual areas that receive and interpret sight

Temporal lobe
- Separated from the parietal lobe by the lateral sulcus
- Contains sensory areas for hearing and olfaction (smell)
- Visual recognition
- Also in the temporal and parietal lobes, usually only on the left side, is Wernicke's area where comprehension of speech occurs.

FIGURE 27.1 Areas of function in brain.

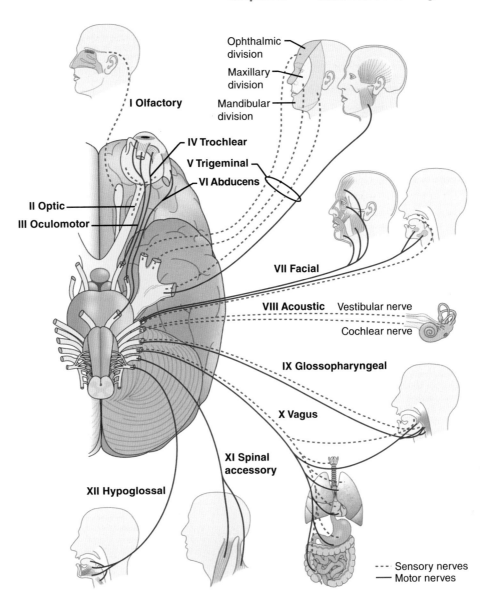

FIGURE 27.2 Cranial nerve origins.

Sympathetic Nervous System

The SNS provides the emergency responses the body needs to respond to stimuli. This includes the "fight or flight" response, which entails decreased peristalsis, increased heart contractions, peripheral blood vessel constriction, increased perspiration, bronchiole dilation for effective breathing, and dilation of the heart and peripheral blood vessels. All of these contribute to a response to physical or emotional stress.

Parasympathetic Nervous System

The parasympathetic nervous system influences muscle tone; decreases heart rate; provides the contractility of smooth muscles; and produces secretions, including intestinal glandular activity. The parasympathetic nervous system is also responsible for the relaxation of the sphincter muscles.

Anatomy of the Brain

The brain, contained within the three protective membranes—dura mater, arachnoid membrane, and pia mater—provides the coordination of the entire nervous system (Fig. 27.4). CSF forms in the brain's lateral ventricles and flows through the third and fourth ventricle to circulate to the subarachnoid space of the spinal cord (Fig. 27.5). Excess CSF is absorbed by the arachnoid membrane to maintain a fluid and pressure balance.

Increased intracranial pressure (ICP) is pressure within the brain's ventricles caused by either an overproduction or a lack of absorption of CSF. After a child's skull bones fuse, the sutures and fontanels (soft spots) can no longer provide a

· WORD · BUILDING ·

intracranial: intra–within + crani–cranium + al–relating to

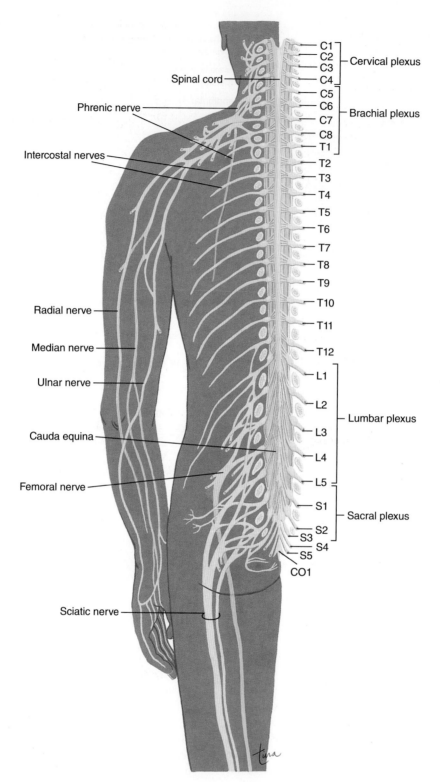

FIGURE 27.3 The spinal cord and vertebral body.

means of adapting to ICP. Instead, the ICP balance is maintained by three homeostatic mechanisms:

- Production or absorption of CSF within the brain
- Blood vessel dilation or constriction within the brain
- Production and circulation of hormones that cause increased or decreased production of urine (aldosterone)

Neurological Development

A child's age and developmental level provide guidance about how to evaluate functioning of the CNS. Although the CNS is one of the first systems to form in fetal development, it is actually one of the last to fully mature during childhood. Myelination, the formation of a protective coating around nerve fibers,

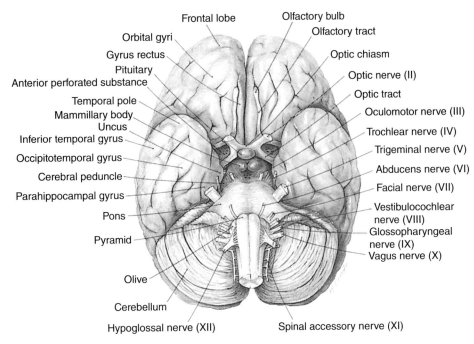

FIGURE 27.4 Brain structures as viewed from the ventral surface.

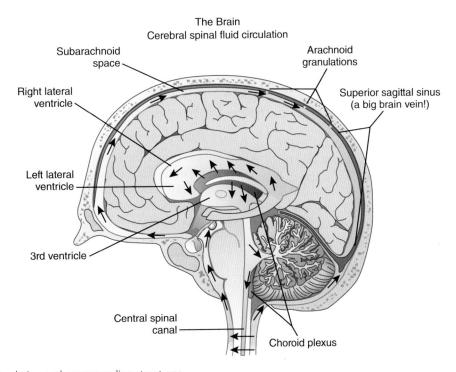

FIGURE 27.5 CSF circulation and corresponding structures.

needs to take place throughout the brain for motor control and coordination as well as for cognitive maturity. The presence of primitive reflexes in a newborn demonstrates an intact spinal cord and brainstem (see Chapter 15). These reflexes disappear at generally predictable intervals during infancy. Environmental factors such as nutrition, maternal infections, hormones, medication use, alcohol, maternal disease, and chemical exposure (lead) influence a child's neurological development.

COMMON NEUROLOGICAL DISORDERS DURING CHILDHOOD

CNS disorders affect one or more of the intricate components of the system: the brain, spinal cord, CNS, PNS, or ANS. Trauma, injuries, accidents, infections, tumors, and congenital anomalies can all contribute to the development of CNS disorders. Figure 27.6 illustrates the common locations of brain infections.

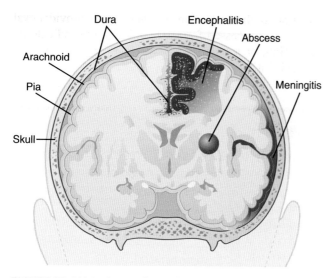

FIGURE 27.6 Major brain infection locations.

Nursing care of children with CNS diseases or disorders requires rapid assessments, followed by comprehensive workups, diagnostic examinations, and careful monitoring for changes in clinical status or the development of complications. Complications associated with CNS diseases or disorders can have devastating effects, leading to permanent brain damage or lasting motor or sensory dysfunction. Nurses must know how to conduct evaluations and then know what observations to report to whom so that the child can be stabilized. Medications are an important part of caring for a child with a neurological disorder.

You must master developmentally focused neurological evaluations to report deviations or changes rapidly to the health-care team. It is imperative to practice these observations and evaluations so that when faced with an emergency, CNS injury, brain infection, or suspected child abuse case, you can identify changes in normal or expected neurological health and report them to the appropriate team member for further diagnostics or interventions. Mastery of neurological observations and evaluations will save lives by decreasing morbidity and mortality.

Team Works

Interdisciplinary Neurological Assessments
Nurses assist the health-care team by providing complete health histories and rapid physical examinations. When a child presents with a neurological concern, the team works together to determine factors that influence the condition and to identify all clinical presentations of the disorder.

Health History
- Risk factors for neurological system injury (accidents, intentional injuries such as child abuse)
- Risk factors associated with perinatal period such as injury, infections, maternal toxic exposures, illicit drug use, alcohol use, and prematurity
- Familial history of seizures, cranial deformities, mental illness, neural tube defects, and chromosomal anomalies

Physical Examination
- Rapid visual observation: Rapid assessment of the level of consciousness (LOC), skin color for cyanosis, and ability to breathe effectively
- Further inspection of the child including LOC (full, confused, disoriented, lethargic, obtunded, coma [Box 27.1]) and posturing (decorticate and decerebrate [see Fig. 27.14, later in this chapter]) as well as abnormal movements such as tremors, seizure activity, or tics
- Vital signs (VSs) evaluating for hypertension or hypotension, widening pulse pressure, bradycardia, and dyspnea/apnea; temperature should be taken to evaluate for abnormal core body temperatures (Do not attempt oral temperatures in a neurologically impaired or seizing child.)

Safety Stat!

A fixed and dilated pupil is a neurosurgical emergency! Brainstem herniation presents with opisthotonos, nuchal rigidity, poor PERRLA (**P**upils **E**qual, **R**ound, and **R**eactive to **L**ight and **A**ccommodation), bradycardia, abnormal respiratory patterns, and increased blood pressure reading for age with widening pulse pressure (widening systolic and diastolic readings).

Box 27.1

Levels of Consciousness

Full (consciousness): Normal consciousness; alert, oriented, communicating

Confused: Reduced awareness of being; bewildered and unable to think clearly

Disoriented: Not oriented to person, place, or time with a deepened state of confusion

Lethargic: Being sluggish, perhaps apathetic, and unable to stay aroused

Obtunded: Loss of sensitivity to one's surroundings

Coma: Deep unconsciousness

When a child first presents with health concerns, rapid examinations are conducted to quickly determine the status of the child's neurological system. A rapid neurological examination includes a quick evaluation of the child from head to toe:

- Overall LOC and ability to respond to verbal and tactile/pain stimuli
- Short- and long-term memory in a verbal child
- Ability to speak without slurring, delay, or regression in a verbal child
- Ability to swallow effectively
- Use of accessory muscles
- Strength of hand grip and strength of movement of legs
- Incontinence in a potty-trained child
- Cerebellar status of balance, coordination, and gait in an ambulatory child

Other evaluations are also used for a child who presents with suspected or confirmed neurological concerns. For the newborn and young infant, primitive reflexes are evaluated to investigate neurological health. Primitive reflexes occur in the infant's brainstem or areas of the spinal cord. However, the absence of reflexes in the newborn or young infant does not confirm the presence of neurological disease, injury, or concern. The evaluation of reflexes is part of a holistic neurological assessment and gives basic information about the communication pattern between the CNS and the PNS as well as the overall health of the system. Exaggerated primitive reflexes may demonstrate a condition of the CNS, whereas diminished primitive reflex responses may indicate a condition of the PNS. Most newborn and infant primitive reflexes are gone by the first few months of life.

The following neonate and young infant reflexes are evaluated:

- *Moro:* Movement with a change in equilibrium, such as a sudden movement down that causes the child to reach the arms up and grasp with the fingers
- *Sucking:* Ability to demonstrate effective sucking movements when an area around the infant's mouth is touched
- *Startle:* Movement when exposed to a loud sound with pulling of the arms and legs in toward the trunk
- *Fencing/Tonic neck:* Movement of the arms with a rapid, small movement of the head; child will pose in fencing position with the arm and leg extended and the fist opened on the side the head is turned toward, bringing in the arm and leg on the opposite side while clenching that fist
- *Dancing/Step:* Small stepping motions when the child is held carefully up by the trunk (not under the arms); child demonstrates small steps when the sole of the foot touches a surface

Evaluation of the infant's fontanels is also part of a neurological assessment. The infant should be in an upright position for the evaluation. The health-care provider evaluates for a recessed fontanel, which could indicate dehydration, or a bulging fontanel, which could indicate increased ICP.

Labs & Diagnostics

Laboratory studies that may be ordered to evaluate a child's neurological health include the following:

- Electrolytes to rule out disturbances such as hypernatremia or hyponatremia
- Complete blood cell count (CBC) to rule out infection
- Serum lead level to evaluate for lead exposure or toxicity
- Blood culture to rule out severe infections

The following diagnostic tests may be ordered to evaluate a child's neurological status:

- Lumbar puncture to collect CSF and cultures for infections
- Electroencephalogram (EEG)
- Urinalysis to rule out toxic exposures

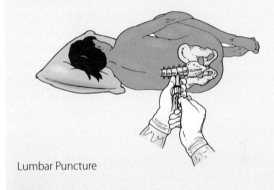

Lumbar Puncture

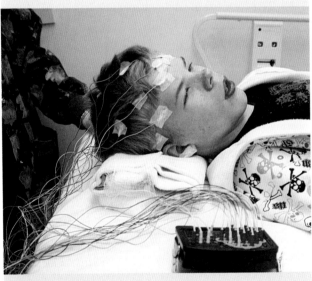

EEG

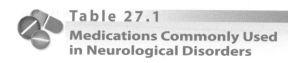

Table 27.1
Medications Commonly Used in Neurological Disorders

Purpose	*Medication Used*
Anticonvulsants are used to prevent or manage seizure activity.	• Gabapentin • Clonazepam
Diuretics are used to decrease increased ICP.	• Mannitol • Furosemide
Neuromuscular blocker to prevent resistance to mechanical ventilation and agitation are used when a child with a neurological impairment requires airway management (TBI or C-spine injury). This medication works by the following three mechanisms: muscular relaxation for a surgery, muscular relaxation for mechanical ventilation, and airway management (Adeyinka & Layer, 2022). This is a high alert medication.	• Rocuronium

Neurological disorders in childhood often require long medical treatment plans and care. The degree of disability and restoration of function depends on the location of the disorder, the amount of damage that has occurred, and the quality and timeliness of medical interventions. Frequently, children are required to be on medications that promote stability of the neurological disease. See Table 27.1 for a list of common medications nurses should be aware of.

THE SENSES

Infants are born with some intact sensory organs and others that must mature with time and exposure. For instance, hearing is considered fully intact at birth after the amniotic fluid is removed from the external ear canal and is considered fully mature at 1 month of age. The sense of smell (olfaction) is also considered fully intact at birth. Visual acuity is dependent on nerve maturation. An infant's visual acuity is thought to range between 20/200 and 20/300 and is not fully intact until close to the child's fifth birthday. The sense of touch is thought to be fully intact at birth, but the sense of taste must develop. Although taste buds are present at birth, taste aversions and preferences develop with experience of breast milk, formula, and early foods. Babies prefer the taste of breast milk over formula (Stanford Medicine Children's Health, 2021a).

The sense of space, also called proprioception, can be considered an additional sense to the five discussed previously.

The brain relays information to the body about where the body is in space. Without proprioception, a child may experience clumsiness and discoordination.

CONGENITAL NEUROLOGICAL DISORDERS

A congenital disorder is one that exists from birth. These disorders can take place during fetal development or during the birthing process. Several conditions that affect a child's neurological health are congenital disorders. The following section outlines the most prevalent congenital conditions within the neurological system.

Cerebral Palsy

Cerebral palsy (CP) represents a group of disorders involving the functioning of the nervous system and brain. CP is considered a birth accident from anoxia before, during, or after the birth process up to the second year of life. Premature infants have a higher risk of developing CP because of their higher incidence of bleeding in the brain, brain infections, severe jaundice, and head injuries. CP is a nonprogressive injury of the brain and nervous system directly related to a low level of oxygen to the CNS structures, which is termed *hypoxia*. Symptoms of CP can be mild to very severe. The degree of disability relates to the severity of the hypoxia episode.

There are five types of CP:

1. *Ataxic:* Poor muscle coordination, poor equilibrium, and unsteady, possibly wide-based gait
2. *Spastic:* **Hypertonicity** with poor posture control, legs scissoring, altered quality of speech, persistent primitive reflexes, and persistent muscle contractions with potential development of contractures
3. *Hypotonic:* Generalized poor muscle control with muscle dystrophy
4. *Dyskinetic:* Also called *dyskinetic-athetoid,* involves constant involuntary wormlike movements that diminish during sleep and that affect facial musculature
5. *Mixed:* Child presents with a variety of CP clinical presentations

Evaluating Cerebral Palsy

The child may have CP involving one or both sides of the body. CP may affect both arms, both legs, or only one arm or leg. Symptoms, if severe, may be detectable at 3 months of life. The child with CP will demonstrate delayed motor growth and delayed mastery of first year skills such as rolling over, sitting up, crawling, standing, and walking.

Assessments for CP include identifying the presence of one or more of the following signs:

• Tight muscles that do not stretch, possibly worsening over time
• "Scissors" movements of arms and legs

· WORD · BUILDING ·

hypertonicity: hyper–excessive + tonicity–muscle tension

- Joint contractures in which the joints do not open and do not have full range of motion (ROM)
- Paralysis or muscle weakness
- The presence of tremors
- Floppy extremities or overextension of joint areas
- The presence of pain

You should also note the following:

- If the motor symptoms are present bilaterally or unilaterally
- If the child is able to suck, swallow, and manage secretions
- If the child demonstrates effective ventilation, airway clearance, and containment of saliva

Interventions for Cerebral Palsy

There is no treatment or cure for CP. The pediatric health-care team provides support, symptom management, and interventions to promote mobility and socialization and to reduce injuries. Medications can assist with spasticity, drooling, and tremors. Surgical procedures may be needed to reduce joint contractures and severe gastroesophageal reflux.

Medication Facts

Treatment for motor spasticity and excessive drooling includes the administration of the botulinum toxin. Baclofen is a pharmaceutical agent that has been effective in reducing spasticity and tremors.

Nursing Considerations for Cerebral Palsy

Nursing considerations focus on assisting the pediatric health-care team to reduce complications for the child with CP. Teaching the family how to maintain a clear airway is imperative. Demonstrating how to perform passive ROM exercises helps to slow the process of contractures. Nurses need to monitor for the development of poor nutrition, failure to thrive (FTT), constipation, bowel obstruction, and osteoporosis.

Safety is a key component to the care of a child with CP and includes all aspects of the child's life, including the prevention of aspiration, falls, and contractures. Maintaining safe equipment for mobility and preventing pressure injuries is paramount.

Neural Tube Defects

Neural tube defects are a group of disorders within the CNS related directly to birth defects. The inappropriate closure of the neural tube during embryonic development can lead to one of several defects. Each defect has varied levels of clinical symptoms and disability associated with the severity of the deficit. Although the origin of a neural tube defect is considered multifactorial, there is a strong association with the lack of sufficient maternal folic acid consumption at the time of conception. The following list represents several types of neural tube defects found in childhood.

- *Anencephaly:* The child is born with a severe brain anomaly that is associated with the absence of both hemispheres and the presence of a brainstem and cerebellum only. If the newborn survives, the child's condition is incompatible with life, and death will occur in time.
- *Microcephaly:* The child is born with an abnormally small head and brain. Fetal exposure to the Zika virus is associated with congenital Zika syndrome, which is characterized by decreased brain tissue, eye damage with macular scarring, congenital contractions such as club foot, hypertonia, and microcephaly. Microcephaly associated with Zika syndrome can lead to such a small brain that the skull partially collapses (Centers for Disease Control and Prevention [CDC], 2024).
- *Encephalocele:* The child is born with an abnormal sac of fluid that causes the brain tissue (brain and meninges) to herniate, or protrude, through an abnormal defect in the skull. The brain tissue may be found within this sac.
- *Spina bifida:* The child is born with a defect within the spinal column. Spina bifida occulta has no signs other than the possibility of skin dimpling at the site of the defect. When the defect is apparent, it is one of two general types of spina bifida:
  - *Type 1: Myelomeningocele:* The child is born with a portion of the vertebral column not closed, leading to the protrusion of a sac containing not only CSF but also the meninges and a portion of the child's spinal cord. Eighty percent are located in the lumbosacral or lumbar areas, which are the last areas of the neural tube to close in fetal development.
  - *Type 2: Meningocele:* The child is born with a defect in the bony spinal column resulting in an abnormal protrusion of a CSF-filled sac located externally to the child's spinal column.

Many myelomeningoceles are associated with Arnold-Chiari malformations, which are brain malformations of the cerebellum and brainstem, associated with hydrocephalus and cysts.

CRITICAL THINKING

Scenario #2: You assisted with a birth and as you observed the newborn, you noticed abnormal hair growth along the spine. Remembering that this can be a concern, you immediately notified the attending birth team.

Questions

1. Why is it important to evaluate every newborn for an abnormal presentation of hair growth on the spine?
2. What pathology or disease process could this observation be associated with?

Evaluating Neural Tube Defects

Assessments of neural tube defects, including spina bifida, start with appropriate and early fetal assessments. Ultrasounds should determine the presence of the abnormality, and a cesarean section for safe delivery is essential.

Evaluate for neurological disabilities below the level of the deficit. Frequent head circumferences will be ordered to evaluate for hydrocephalus. Because nerves for bowel and bladder innervate below the site of the defect, you should also evaluate bowel and bladder function.

Interventions for Neural Tube Defects

After birth, handle the abnormal sac with care and inspect for leaks, rupture, and infection around the sac area or infection in the CNS in general. Keep the sac moist by carefully applying NS-soaked gauze. The family will need support and interdisciplinary team teaching to better understand the consequences of the necessary surgery and the possible long-term deficits the child may have.

After surgery, the child will have routine postoperative care that focuses on providing fluid balance and preventing infection as well as special care to the skin at the operative site. Provide early ROM and support for the lower extremities that may have neurological deficits. The urinary bladder may need intermittent catheterization.

Medication Facts

Although more attention is given to folic acid deficiency as a cause of neurological defects, iron deficiency also has direct impact on neurological development. Without adequate iron, a child's cognitive function, attention span, memory, and attentiveness may all be affected.

Nursing Considerations for Neural Tube Defects

Nursing considerations for neural tube defects include paying special consideration to the development of latex allergy because this population has a much higher incidence than the general population.

Families need to understand that the child with a neural tube defect can have a healthy and productive life but that they will need to be aware of associated motor limitations and the possibility of bladder catheterization. Teach the public about the importance of taking folic acid starting before conception and continuing during pregnancy as part of healthy eating and adhering to prenatal vitamins as indicated by a health-care provider.

NEUROLOGICAL INJURIES

Across the developmental period, children can experience severe injuries that affect the health and function of the neurological system. Injuries can be to the child's PNS or CNS.

Many of these devastating injuries can be prevented by offering appropriate supervision, teaching the child safety rules, and by providing anticipatory guidance to caregivers and parents. The following section outlines several neurological injuries.

Drowning and Near Drowning

Drowning ranks high overall as a cause of unintentional injuries (average 4,000 fatalities a year) throughout childhood (CDC, 2022). The peak period for drowning or near drowning is in the toddler period (CDC, 2022).

Drowning is defined as a submersion in a liquid medium followed by suffocation and asphyxia. With submersion, rapid and irreversible multisystemic injuries occur, which can lead to death. When a child dies within the 24-hour time period after submersion, it is called *drowning*. If the child lives beyond 24 hours, even if the child later recovers or dies, it is called *near drowning*.

Toddlers and preschoolers are at risk when they are unsupervised, which typically occurs in residential pools and bathtubs and around buckets or trash cans of water. Adolescents, especially boys between 15 and 19 years of age, are at risk for drowning or near drowning at natural bodies of water such as lakes, ponds, rivers, and oceans because swimming in them is more difficult than swimming in pools, and people tire more rapidly and get into trouble more readily (Department of Health [DOH], 2021; Seattle Children's Hospital, 2023). In the United States, most drownings and near drownings for children younger than age 5 occur at home pools (CDC, 2022). Sex distribution for drowning fatalities has a ratio of boys to girls of 8:1 (CDC, 2022).

Degrees of disability associated with near drownings are related to the victim's clinical course. The outcome of the event relates to duration of submersion, circumstances surrounding the event, rapid response of the rescue, and how effective the postsubmersion resuscitative efforts are. The pathology of near drowning can be summarized as a multiorgan effect of hypoxemia. Cardiopulmonary resuscitation (CPR) should start at the scene to rapidly restore oxygenation, ventilation, and circulation. Close to 80% of all childhood near drowning victims survive, and close to 92% of those make a complete recovery. According to the CDC (2022), for every child who suffers a drowning fatality, another seven need emergency care for nonfatal drowning incidents.

Evaluating Drowning and Near Drowning

Assessments for a child brought into the health-care arena for postsubmersion injury involve assessing the airway, ventilation ability, quality of respirations, presence of effective heart rate and blood pressure, arterial blood gases (ABGs), and level of hypothermia. Level of neurological intactness and LOC should also be assessed.

Interventions for Drowning and Near Drowning

Interventions for drowning and near drowning victims are rapid and effective advanced resuscitation, including ventilator support using oxygen, restoration of cardiac rhythm, correction of hypercapnia and hypoxia, correction of shock (signs of which are altered mental status, cool extremities, and slow capillary refill), and IV fluid administration with boluses of a nondextrose-containing solution such as lactated Ringer's (LR) solution or NS. It is common for the child to suffer extensive volume depletion because of severe pulmonary edema and intracompartmental fluid shifts. Remove the child's wet clothes, keep the environmental temperature very warm, and wrap the child in warmed blankets.

Nursing Considerations for Drowning and Near Drowning

Nursing considerations include supporting the team during the resuscitative efforts. They also include supporting the family, who will be in great distress and emotional shock. Consider initiating a rapid referral for a social worker, clergy, or other spiritual support system and offering to call extended family.

Intraventricular Hemorrhage

Intraventricular hemorrhage (IVH) is a very severe diagnosis. In IVH, the child experiences a rupture of the vascular network within the germinal matrix, and a bleed develops within the brain. Depending on the severity of the bleed, the child may have full recovery or may experience severe brain damage or death from the anoxia associated with the bleed and ICP. The group most at risk for IVH is premature infants of less than 32 weeks' gestation. Children with IVH can develop secondary to severe neonatal respiratory distress, birth asphyxia, metabolic disorders, or congenital vascular structural anomaly.

Evaluating Intraventricular Hemorrhage

The child with suspected IVH will have a magnetic resonance imaging (MRI) or a computed tomography (CT) scan to confirm the bleed. Serial hemoglobin and hematocrit levels will be drawn to assess the severity and continuation of the bleed. ICP will be measured and assessed on a regular basis. The child with IVH will demonstrate somnolence, very poor muscle tone, and the absence of a Moro reflex. In very severe cases, the child may demonstrate bulging and tense fontanels.

Interventions for Intraventricular Hemorrhage

Interventions for IVH include providing a reduced-stimuli environment and minimal handling of the child. Keep the child's head midline and relaxed to decrease hydrostatic pressure changes, which cause further ICP. The child may require transfusion therapy while being treated for ICP and acidosis. To reduce ICP, a catheter is placed (ventriculostomy) to remove the collected subdural fluid. Maternal steroid administration reduces the chance of IVH in premature infants by 33% (Stanford Medicine Children's Health, 2021b).

Nursing Considerations for Intraventricular Hemorrhage

One of the most important nursing considerations for a child receiving care for IVH is to keep the child's head midline, comfortable, and supported. Any movement of the child's head should be done with great caution and should have the assistance of two staff members. Any stimulation that would produce discomfort or crying should be minimized.

Lead Poisoning

Lead is highly toxic because of its affinity for a group of proteins called sulfhydryl (SH). After binding to this protein group, lead irreversibly impairs brain function. A child with lead poisoning may initially exhibit behavioral changes such as attention disorders, intellectual disabilities, hyperactivity, colic, constipation, and severe abdominal pain. The ensuing **encephalopathy** leads to ataxia, papilledema, seizures, impaired consciousness, and coma. **Encephalopathy** is a generalized brain dysfunction of varying degrees that causes an impairment of arousal, orientation, speech, and cognitive processing. A child with significant lead poisoning must be rapidly removed from the source of exposure and then hospitalized for treatment of the lead poisoning.

Children are exposed to lead in their environments through contaminated soil in play areas; contaminated clothing worn by parents who work in lead-dust environments; lead-based paints in older homes and apartments; and imported candy, jewelry, and pottery that were processed with lead. Although lead paint was banned from consumer use in 1977 in the United States, lead can be released into a child's home environment via peeling or chipped paint, chalking (when a powdery layer forms on the surface of dry paint, caused by ultraviolet [UV] radiation), or renovation activities of older homes. Lead-contaminated household dust from paint remains the major cause of lead exposure for Americans (Halmo & Nappe, 2022). See Box 27.2 for examples of cultural practices that have the potential to increase lead exposures in children.

Different degrees of disability are related to toxic lead exposure. Guidelines for recognizing when a serum lead level shows potential toxicity in children are presented in Table 27.2. See the table for the CDC's serum blood lead levels and recommended subsequent actions.

Evaluating Lead Poisoning

Current recommendations by the American Academy of Pediatrics (AAP, 2016) are to check with local health departments for areas and communities considered to be of increased risk. People living in low-income housing, populations with low socioeconomic status, and people who are eligible for Medicaid tend to have higher risk. Children

· WORD · BUILDING ·
encephalopathy: encephalo–brain + pathy–disease

Box 27.2

Cultural Practices That May Increase Lead Exposure

Families need education about the potential exposure to lead from their culturally based health-care practices. Nurses have the responsibility to identify when complementary or alternative health-care practices or substances are being used to treat a child's health-care condition and rapidly report such use to the health-care team. All alternative, naturopathic, and complementary medical practices should be reported to the pediatric health-care team so that the team can evaluate their indications, dosing, and side effects for safety. Families should be approached with respect so that full disclosure can be secured.

Lead can also be consumed by children through the following sources:

- Root vegetables that uptake lead from contaminated soil
- Imported canned food processed in other countries
- Pottery or ceramics when the layer of protective glaze wears off
- Brass fixtures, lead pipes, solder, and older plumbing in homes built before 1986

Table 27.2

Centers for Disease Control and Prevention Lead Levels Recommendations

Blood Level (Micrograms/Deciliter)	Actions Recommended
0–3	No immediate concerns for the child; follow-up needed.
3.5	Child is considered to have had a lead exposure and requires further evaluation and repeat laboratory analysis via a venous blood draw rather than a finger stick.
3.5–19	Considered lead exposed and lead poisoned. Report finding to local health department. Identify source such as a home evaluation. Educate family on nutrition and provide repeat lead levels within a month.
20–44	Conduct a survey of the home environment and provide education to families about lead exposure and increased health risks with exposure. Perform diagnostic imaging (x-ray) of the abdomen to check for paint chips and foreign bodies. Contact poison control center (1-800-222-1222) for medical guidance.
≥45	Remove the child from the source of the lead (home may be unsafe to return to) and bring the child to the medical facility for a workup and treatment. Perform the previously noted evaluations and diagnostics and initiate chelation therapy.

Information based on most current guidelines from the Centers for Disease Control and Prevention. (2022). *Childhood lead poisoning prevention: Recommended actions based on blood lead levels.* https://www.cdc.gov/nceh/lead/advisory/acclpp/actions-blls.htm

should be tested for lead exposure according to local health department guidelines or at least at 1 year and again at 2 years of age. Initial assessments of a child with suspected lead poisoning include a thorough and accurate assessment of the child's environment, including the year the home was built and the type of paint used. Lead-containing paint in the home places a child at high risk for exposure. Note the child's age and participation in teething on window sills or doorways or the child's participation in pica behaviors. A nickel-size lead-based paint chip will cause blood lead levels to rise. Although there is no safe blood level of lead, 5 mcg/dL indicates possible exposure.

Interventions for Lead Poisoning

Interventions for lead poisoning begin with confirmation of the child's blood lead level and then the immediate identification of the lead source and removal of it. All symptomatic children, regardless of their measured blood lead level, are medically treated in a hospital environment. Emergency treatment for symptoms may include a PICU stay. Current recommendations are to start chelation therapy at blood lead levels of 45 mcg/dL and greater (Halmo & Nappe, 2022).

Nursing Considerations for Lead Poisoning

Nursing considerations while caring for a child with suspected or known lead poisoning begin with evaluating for changes in normal behavior for the child's developmental stage and age, and then promptly reporting any new signs or symptoms. Children with mild lead exposure require the provision of a safe home, school, and play environment with education for the whole family about the hazards of lead exposure. Children with higher levels of lead poisoning require

medical treatments and hospitalization. Monitor children for side effects of medical therapy, including following clinical nursing protocols about monitoring the child's blood pressure during infusions.

Health-care institutions may have a policy to not discharge or release a child to the family home if the home is the suspected source of the lead poisoning. The child and family may need temporary housing until the house is inspected and considered lead-free and environmentally "clean."

Patient Teaching Guidelines

Nationwide, family education programs promote awareness of lead poisoning in communities. These programs can help communities identify high-risk homes and buildings as well as contaminated community spaces. Accurate and reliable home test kits for lead are also available. Because lead poisoning has potential long-term consequences for children, reinforcing the information shared in these widespread education programs is essential. Contact your local public health department to ask how you can become involved with educational programs. Health fairs, presentations to parent meetings at schools, and other community-awareness programs rely on nurses to educate the public about the dangers of lead. Parents need to know that common home renovation activities (demolition, sanding, cutting) can create toxic chips and dust (CDC, 2019).

Meningitis

Meningitis is inflammation of the membranes of the brain or spinal cord and possible cerebral edema often caused by an infectious process. This inflammation can be caused by bacteria, viruses, or chemical agents that enter the bloodstream and spread through the CSF. Causative organisms include *Escherichia coli* and group B streptococcus (GBS) for newborns and infants and *Haemophilus influenzae* type B, *Streptococcus pneumoniae,* and *Neisseria meningitidis* for older children. If bacterial or viral in nature, meningitis can be spread by droplets of mucus during sneezing, coughing, or nasal congestion. The organisms that cause meningitis can enter the child's body via the nasal cavity, the middle ear (if the tympanic membrane is injured), neurosurgery, or trauma. The incidence of meningitis has been greatly reduced in the public since the introduction of the childhood vaccine for *H. influenzae*. Meningitis can be found in all ages across childhood but is much more common in infants and toddlers.

Prognosis with meningitis is dependent on the age of the child during infection, the causative organism, and the response to treatment. The younger the child, the greater chance of acquiring bacterial meningitis, which can be fatal if not identified and treated promptly. If the child has acquired viral meningitis, no treatment is warranted other than supportive care with an expected duration of illness of 6 to 10 days. Without treatment, complications include thrombi, brain abscesses, blindness, deafness, seizures, and paralysis.

The most dangerous form of meningitis is meningococcal meningitis. This type of bacterial meningitis is caused by *N. meningitidis* and leads to a sudden infection, resulting in disseminated intravascular coagulation (DIC), massive adrenal hemorrhages, and purpura. It carries a high mortality rate of 90% or more. If a child of any age presents with abrupt eruption of a purplish rash or petechial rash, the health-care team must suspect meningococcemia and initiate immediate medical attention. Meningococcal meningitis must be identified rapidly with immediate antibiotic administration to save the child's life.

Evaluating Meningitis

Assessments for meningitis include early identification of the following symptoms:

- Poor feeding habits
- Fever
- A child who is irritable, is inconsolable when held, or has a high-pitched cry
- Lethargy
- Bulging fontanels
- **Opisthotonos** positioning: Hyperextension of the child's neck and back, or nuchal rigidity in which the child holds the neck very still
- Kernig sign: Resistance and sudden pain with knee extension when the child is in a supine position with knees flexed up (Fig. 27.7)
- Brudzinski sign: When the child's neck is flexed during supine position, the child will suddenly flex the knees and hips (Fig. 27.8)

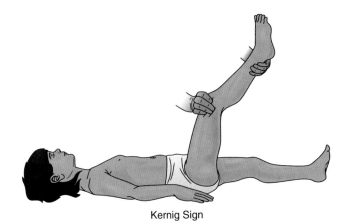

Kernig Sign

FIGURE 27.7 Kernig sign.

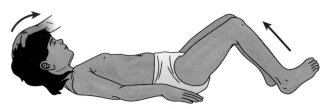

Brudzinski Sign

FIGURE 27.8 Brudzinski sign.

- WORD - BUILDING -
meningitis: mening–meninges + itis–inflammation

- WORD - BUILDING -
opisthotonos: opistho–backward + tonos–stretching

Interventions for Meningitis

Rapidly collect laboratory specimens, including CBC, CSF culture, and blood culture, and start ordered antibiotics immediately. The antibiotic administered must match the causative organism for the best prognosis and rapid recovery. Corticosteroids may also be administered to prevent cerebral edema, and anticonvulsants may be required if the child is seizing from the infection or toxin.

Nursing Considerations for Meningitis

Nursing considerations for meningitis include meticulous maintenance of a patent IV catheter for antibiotic therapy, symptoms management, and fluid as needed. Care should be taken to keep antibiotics administration on time and therapeutic serum values of antibiotics on target. Keep the child's condition guarded, and until the causative agent is identified, maintain the child on strict droplet and contact isolation and leave in place for 24 to 48 hours after the administration of antibiotics begins. Some institutions require that three doses of antibiotics be administered before isolation is discontinued.

Monitor the child for increasing ICP and head circumferences. If there is a change in head circumference, the child may be experiencing the complication of meningitis called *obstructive hydrocephalus*.

Reye Syndrome

Reye syndrome is a nonspecific, noninflammatory encephalopathy with organ involvement, including the liver, spleen, kidney, pancreas, and lymph. Death, although rare, can occur because of brain tissue herniation in association with severe cerebral edema, sepsis, and shock. Reye syndrome is strongly associated with the use of salicylates (aspirin) to treat symptoms of varicella infections or influenza. Warnings to parents and health-care professionals to avoid using salicylates in children with possible infections of varicella or influenza types A or B continue (National Institute of Neurological Disorders and Stroke [NINDS], 2023). However, Reye syndrome can sometimes occur without the use of salicylates.

Evaluating Reye Syndrome

Early symptoms of Reye syndrome may be irritability, diarrhea, and rapid breathing. As the condition progresses, Reye syndrome is associated with six major clinical presentations. Not all of the clinical presentations listed next may be present, but the pediatric team will evaluate for the following in a child with suspected Reye syndrome:

- Frequent vomiting and diarrhea (early stage)
- Rapid breathing (early stage in infancy)
- Encephalopathy (later stage)
- Increased ICP (later stage)
- Metabolic dysfunction (later stage)
- Hepatic dysfunction (later stage)
- Renal damage (later stage)

- Fatty infiltration of the viscera (later stage)
- Confusion, irrational behavior, and loss of consciousness (later stage)

Interventions for Reye Syndrome

A team approach is needed to provide interventions and treatment for Reye syndrome. Interventions include the following:

- Monitoring the child carefully for progression through the stages of Reye syndrome (Table 27.3)
- Monitoring the child for changes in neurological status and immediately reporting any slight change in status, including the LOC, confusion, and neurological deficits
- Evaluating the child for symptoms of GI bleeding, pancreatitis, or liver failure
- Providing hydration with a source of glucose (mainly IV fluids)
- Implementing seizure precautions to keep the child safe if seizures occur
- Monitoring the child's respiratory status and immediately reporting any signs of dyspnea
- Checking the child's Glasgow Coma Scale (GCS) score (Fig. 27.9)
- Evaluating for the presence of increasing ICP
- Elevating the child's head of bed (HOB) by 30 to 45 degrees
- Keeping the child free of discomfort and pain and helping the child to avoid crying
- Providing a quiet environment to rest
- Care of the wound after a liver biopsy is performed
- Reinforcing the patient/family teaching session about the importance of follow-up, including auditory, speech, and potential motor and/or intellectual deficits

Table 27.3

Stages and Symptoms of Reye Syndrome

Stage	Symptoms
I	Lethargy, vomiting, sleepiness, normal posture, brisk pupil reaction, and purposeful response to pain stimuli
II Follows 5–7 days after stage I	Combative, stuporous (not fully conscious), and disoriented, with a normal posture, a sluggish pupil reaction, and purposeful or nonpurposeful response to pain stimuli
III	Coma, decorticate posture, and sluggish pupil reaction
IV	Coma, seizures, decerebrate posture, and sluggish pupil reaction
V	Coma, apnea, limpness, and no pupil reaction

Source: National Institutes of Health, www.nih.gov

Pediatric Modification of the Glasgow Coma Scale

Eye Opening

0–1 year	1 year
4 Spontaneously	4 Spontaneously
3 To shout	3 To verbal command
2 To pain	2 To pain
1 No response	1 No response

Best Motor Response

0–1 year	>1 year
6 Normal spontaneous movements	6 Obeys
5 Localizes pain	5 Localizes pain
4 Flexion withdrawal	4 Flexion withdrawal
3 Flexion abnormal (decorticate)	3 Flexion abnormal (decorticate)
2 Extension (decerebrate)	2 Extension (decerebrate)
1 No response	1 No response

Best Verbal Behavior

0–2 years	2–5 years	5 years
5 Coos, babbles	5 Appropriate words	5 Oriented, converses
4 Irritable	4 Inappropriate words	4 Disoriented
3 Cries to pain	3 Cries/screams	3 Inappropriate words
2 Moans to pain	2 Nonspecific sounds	2 Incomprehensible sounds
1 None	1 None	1 No response

Scoring:
- 13–15: Mild head injury
- 9–12: Moderate head injury
- <8: Severe head injury; intubation may be required

FIGURE 27.9 Glasgow Coma Scale. (Modified from Andreoni, C., & Klinkhammer, B. (2000). *Quick reference guide for pediatric emergency nursing.* Saunders; James, H. E. (1986). Neurologic evaluation and support in the child with an acute brain insult. *Pediatric Annals, 15,* 16; Jennet, B., & Teasdale, G. (1977). Aspects of coma after severe head injury. *Lancet, 1,* 878; Siberry, G., & Iannone, R. (2000). *The Harriet Lane handbook* [15th ed., p. 14]. Mosby.)

Further medical treatments are dependent on the child's clinical status and the severity of the syndrome. The administration of diuretics for improved fluid balance; plasma and vitamin K to prevent bleeding; and airway support, including ventilation, may be required treatments.

Nursing Considerations for Reye Syndrome
Nursing observations for Reye syndrome include the following:

- Symptoms of hypoxia
- Presence of seizures
- Hypoglycemia
- Coagulopathies
- Electrolyte imbalances
- Hyperthermia

The staging of Reye syndrome is a process performed by the pediatric medical team. See Table 27.3 for a listing of the five stages associated with Reye syndrome and the corresponding symptoms.

Spinal Cord Injury
Before the age of 15, spinal cord injuries (SCIs) are rare. Between 17 and 23 years of age, the incidence rises; 53% of all SCIs occur in people between 16 and 30 years of age. The causes of SCI include trauma, tumors, infections, and congenital disorders. Motor vehicle accidents (MVAs) account for more SCIs in younger children than in adolescents, who are more commonly injured in sports. Conditions such as trisomy 21 (Down syndrome), spina bifida, rheumatoid arthritis, and degenerative disc disease put a child at greater risk for SCI. The cervical area of the child's anatomy is the most frequent site of an SCI. The most common etiology of childhood SCI are falls and MVAs. Infants, who have larger heads (25% of body mass) as compared with adults (10%), are more at risk because of their immature and nonossified cervical spine (Hagan et al., 2022).

There are three types of SCI:

1. Complete SCI, which causes a complete loss of sensorimotor and reflex activity below the site of injury
2. Incomplete SCI, which causes the preservation of some motor and/or sensory function below the site of injury
3. Sacral sparing SCI, in which motor/sensory activity at the anal mucocutaneous border exists

The degree of disability depends on the location of the injury and immediate spinal cord stabilization after injury.

Evaluating Spinal Cord Injuries
Assessments of SCIs will depend on the severity of the accident. Typically, the initial emergency team will perform a complete neurological examination followed quickly by

either a CT or an MRI. Because the initial injury may have caused swelling of tissues at the site, it is important to continue to evaluate a child's neurological status to monitor for changes in symptoms. Orders will be written to conduct a variety of neurological examinations at specific intervals. It is imperative that any change in the assessments be reported immediately to the neurologist.

Interventions for Spinal Cord Injuries

Place the child on a straight backboard with neutral head and neck alignment and apply a cervical collar. Stabilize the airway because respiratory insufficiency may not occur right away and instead be delayed after the injury. Monitor the child for neurogenic shock, which presents as bradycardia and hypotension. The treatment often includes high-dose methylprednisolone, which is administered within 8 hours of the injury.

Nursing Considerations for Spinal Cord Injuries

Nursing considerations when caring for children with SCIs include caring for their elimination needs. The child with an SCI may need to be catheterized, and the child and/or family may need to be taught how to catheterize using clean technique for long-term care. Teens should be encouraged to have a frank discussion with their nurse and/or health-care provider about sexuality and sexual function after an SCI.

Traumatic Brain Injury

The term *traumatic brain injury (TBI)* encompasses many types of head injury, including concussions, traumatic injuries from external forces, and fatal TBI. The complications of head injury that lead to severe outcomes relate to both increased ICP and cerebral edema. Minor closed head injuries typically cause no change in mental status, no evidence of skull fracture, and no abnormal findings on a neurological examination. Even with a minor head injury, the child may demonstrate a brief loss of consciousness, headache, lethargy, and vomiting. A major head injury is more complicated because the brain tissue is injured, and the symptoms and outcomes are more severe and may last for weeks. All concussions in childhood are serious because they are brain injuries (Nationwide Children's Hospital, 2023). Common symptoms are headache, sensitivity to light and noise, nausea and vomiting, dizziness, and balance difficulties (Nationwide Children's Hospital, 2023).

Primary brain injuries develop at the time of trauma when the brain tissue suffers initial damage. For instance, a coup-contrecoup injury (Fig. 27.10), which results from accelerated or decelerated motor vehicle movements, is a bruising of the brain within the bony cranium that can lead to increased ICP, apnea, and a loss of consciousness.

Secondary brain trauma develops as the child's body is responding to the injury. Here, brain damage occurs secondary to developing cerebral edema, hypoxia, hypotension, increased ICP, and hemorrhage. Secondary brain trauma can develop hours or days after the injury with irreversible consequences if not treated.

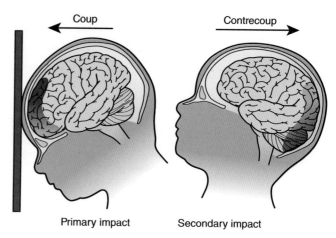

FIGURE 27.10 Coup-contrecoup injury.

CRITICAL THINKING & CLINICAL JUDGMENT

A grandfather is attending an appointment with his infant grandchild at a pediatric clinic. His grandchild is lying on the clinic's changing table after being weighed on an infant scale, and he steps away for a minute. You step in immediately to provide protection from a fall and note the safety issue.

Questions

1. What type of injury could this young child have experienced if the child fell from the table to the hard clinic floor?
2. What should you do to prevent an injury from a fall?

Health Promotion

Protecting the Head From Injury Across Childhood
Parents, especially first-time parents, need instructions about how to handle their infant safely. Early safe practices support a neonate and young infant's head and neck and prevent injuries.
Neonate
- Carefully handle the head; the neonate's head should be supported by one's hand or should lay on one's arm while the infant is being carried.
- Carefully handle the head during dressing, especially with clothes with sleeves.
- Maintain head and neck alignment while sleeping or being held.
- *Never shake the newborn.*
Infant
- Use car seats correctly; an infant car seat should face the rear to prevent coup-contrecoup head injuries.

Health Promotion—cont'd

- Use head-support cushions with an infant car seat to prevent a young infant's head from sagging or drooping.
- Prevent falls after an infant masters rolling from front to back or back to front.
- Do not use baby walkers, especially in the presence of stairs (walkers are not recommended by the AAP [2018]).

Toddler

- Use an appropriate forward-facing car seat with a secure chest harness.
- Prevent falls; a toddler is still head-heavy.
- Prevent falls into buckets of water or water-filled trash cans, which pose a drowning risk because the child is too young and too weak to keep their head pushed up and out of the water.
- Prevent injuries on tricycles; the toddler must be supervised and must wear a helmet.

Preschooler

- Ensure the use of safety devices and protective equipment when participating in any sports or cycling.
- Teach preschoolers to never go into the street; preschoolers must be supervised at all times during play.
- Prevent falls from play structures; provide supervision and the use of foam padding.

School-Aged Child

- Teach bike safety skills and the need for consistent helmet use with the chin strap buckled.
- Use snug-fitting sports safety devices and protective equipment.
- Prevent head injuries from playing with piñatas at parties; keep children back and do not use devices such as golf clubs or baseball bats from which children can experience a severe facial, skull, and brain injury. Use only plastic bats or plastic tubes.

Adolescent

- Insist on proper seatbelt use in cars and note the importance of not texting while driving.
- Teach teens about head injuries when diving into natural water sources.
- Teach about using protective equipment at all times when skating, skateboarding, skiing, and participating in contact sports.

Types of Traumatic Brain Injuries

Children are vulnerable to TBIs. Neonates and young infants are at particular risk because of their large head size and weight-to-body ratio. Beyond infancy, children who participate in contact sports or those who take physical risks during unsafe play or unsafe activities are prone to head injuries. The following sections present common brain injuries that occur anytime during the developmental period.

CONCUSSION. Also called a *mild TBI*, this condition is associated with a transient loss of consciousness from shearing and/or compression of the brain's nerve tissue. Children with concussions tend to have what is called *postconcussion syndrome*, in which they have headaches, difficulty with memory, problems at school, photophobia (extreme sensitivity to light), and possible personality changes. If a child experiences a concussion with a contact sport such as football, protocols must be followed to seek health care immediately.

Therapeutic Communication

Families whose child suffers a concussion need support. Concussions can be mild, with few symptoms, or a concussion can be a temporary but serious injury that affects the child's thinking process and academic performance. Families need education about what to expect for symptoms, rest, and treatments. Family members might feel traumatized and experience fear, grief, remorse, and sadness. Suggesting a visit from a social worker or a clergy member who can provide support is recommended. Staying with the family and providing professional presence, silence, or listening is very therapeutic.

CONTUSION. A contusion is a bruising of the brain tissue. It is typically associated with blunt trauma, which causes tears to the vasculature and tissue. Both head concussions and head contusions are serious. A concussion represents more widespread injury and can be in more than one location, whereas a contusion is considered a localized bruising occurring in one area of the brain tissue.

Evaluating Traumatic Brain Injuries

You must assist the health-care team with preparing to implement rapid neurological assessments for a child who has experienced a TBI. These assessments include the following:

- Assessing airway for patency and effective breathing patterns.
- Monitoring VSs and conducting neurological checks frequently to look for signs of shock, poor perfusion, and increased ICP; the Cushing triad is considered a late sign of ICP and presents as a widening pulse pressure, an irregular breathing pattern, and bradycardia.
- Monitoring LOC with the GCS; children who demonstrate a GCS of 8 or less have significantly poorer outcomes, including significant disabilities.
- Assessing CNs as ordered.

Nursing Care Plan for a Child With a Concussion

While playing in his first varsity football game, 16-year-old Cody was tackled hard and briefly lost consciousness. After conducting a brief on-field evaluation, the team trainer assists Cody to the sidelines where his parents are waiting. The trainer requests that

Cody's parents take him to the ED for a concussion workup. Cody is awake but has difficulty following simple commands. He has no memory of being tackled. His speech is slow and hesitant.

Nursing Diagnosis: High risk of injury related to brain tissue/cerebral trauma
Expected Outcome: The patient will remain free of injury.

Interventions:	Rationales:
Obtain CT scan or MRI and skull x-ray. Initiate ICP monitoring as ordered.	*CT or MRI will reveal presence of hemorrhage, cerebral edema, or shift of midline structure; x-ray will reveal presence of skull fracture; ICP monitoring will provide early information about increasing ICP.*
Make patient NPO (nothing by mouth) as ordered.	*Increased ICP causes nausea and vomiting, placing patient at increased risk for aspiration.*
Start an IV and give fluids as ordered.	*Patient will be NPO and needs adequate hydration.*
Administer medications as prescribed to decrease ICP and pain.	*Increased ICP can cause permanent brain damage, so it is important to take all necessary measures to lower it. Pain may cause anxiety or agitation and increase ICP.*

Learn to C.U.S.

A school nurse is watching a football game in which a freshman student experiences a contact injury to the head and loses consciousness briefly. The child asks the coach if he can continue playing. The school nurse intervenes in the situation and uses the Learn to C.U.S. method of communication to express their concerns:

C: "I have a *concern* that your player wants to return to the game after this head injury.

U: I am *uncomfortable* that a "second hit" to the head can cause serious brain injury.

S: We have a *safety* issue here. The child cannot continue to play and, because of the loss of consciousness, needs to be seen by a health-care provider now."

Interventions for Traumatic Brain Injuries

Medical treatments for a TBI depend on the seriousness of the injury and the presenting complications. Complications include brain hypoxemia with swelling, increased ICP, enlarging hematomas, seizures, and hyperthermia. Airway management is the priority intervention. Typically, after diagnostics are undertaken to determine the location, severity, and associated complications of the injury, the child will be monitored in a PICU for severe injuries or on the pediatric unit for milder injuries. The child will rest, may be sedated, and will be provided a low-stimulation environment. Steroids might be ordered. Intubation and airway support on

a ventilator may be required. TBI can cause posttraumatic hyperthermia, so the child's core body temperature must be managed. The child will need the HOB raised to help decrease ICP. In severe cases, the child will have ICP monitoring through cranial bolts and a transducer. This equipment allows the neurologist to monitor the child's ICP readings as a waveform on a monitor. Research continues about the use of hyperosmolar saline (hypertonic 3% saline) given via IV to shift water from intracellular to extracellular compartments, thus reducing cerebral edema and pressure. Research continues in the exploration of hypertonic saline versus mannitol in children with severe TBI and ICP, with hypertonic saline being more safe and effective (Fenn & Sierra, 2019).

Nursing Considerations for Traumatic Brain Injuries

Nursing considerations for TBIs include monitoring for very subtle changes in clinical presentation and then rapidly reporting them to the health-care team. Managing the airway is always the top nursing care priority for a child who presents with a traumatic head injury.

The parents will be in great distress, not knowing what the final outcome will be for their child. Upon discharge, the nursing staff must teach the family what clinical signs or symptoms to look for with increasing ICP and how to prevent further head trauma injuries. The child is typically admitted for observation and diagnostics, placed on NPO status until a thorough neurological evaluation is performed (swallowing, choking, and aspiration risks evaluated), and then treated as medically indicated for the specific injury. If the child is unconscious, you must maintain an NPO status to prevent aspiration, establish turning schedules to keep the child's skin free from pressure injury, provide suctioning prn, and provide other supportive nursing care as needed.

Treatments for TBIs include meticulous monitoring for symptoms of ICP; providing medications to reduce swelling of brain tissue, such as diuretics and corticosteroids; and offering anticonvulsants if warranted. Children may require a stay in the intensive care unit (ICU) on a cerebral pressure monitoring device such as subarachnoid bolts, intraventricular monitoring systems, or subdural monitoring systems.

OTHER NEUROLOGICAL DISORDERS

Although less common than brain injuries associated with trauma and injuries, children can present with other neurological disorders that require medical attention and nursing care. The following section describes those disorders that are not trauma-related but whose prevalence in children warrants an understanding of the condition, assessments, and required care.

Brain Tumors
Brain tumors are the most common solid malignancy during childhood with a frequency only second to leukemia. Tumors are classified according to their physical location and grade. Tumor locations include the supratentorial regions, the subtentorial region, the temporal lobe, and the posterior fossa. The most prevalent brain tumor in children under 7 years of age is the medulloblastoma. Cerebellar astrocytoma is the most common subtentorial tumor of childhood and has a 5-year survival rate of 90%. Brain tumors are graded as either low grade (localized) or higher grade (invasive; American Cancer Society, 2020).

Evaluating Brain Tumors
In general, the child with a brain tumor will present with signs and symptoms of ICP and with focal neurological signs that are associated with the size and location of the tumor. It is quite common that the child will have demonstrated behavioral or personality alterations for as long as weeks before the tumor is identified. These behaviors can include poor school performance, irritability, hyperactivity, forgetfulness, and lethargy. Many brain tumors cause nausea, vomiting, visual acuity changes, and headaches.

Interventions for Brain Tumors
Interventions for brain tumors are dependent on the size and location of the tumor and the age of the child. Typical treatment includes surgery, radiation, and chemotherapy. Complications of a tumor growing within the bony cranium include ICP, the compression of vital brain structures, hydrocephalus, brainstem herniation, and complications associated with the negative effects of irradiating the brain. These long-term effects include endocrine, intellectual, and motor deficits.

Nursing Considerations for Brain Tumors
Nursing considerations for a child with a brain tumor include providing a great deal of support for the family. A diagnosis of cancer causes fear, anxiety, sadness, and bewilderment. Families need information about the diagnosis, treatment, follow-up care, and long-term prognosis but are able to process the information only a little at a time. Repeat answers to their questions as many times as necessary.

Nursing care focuses on the observation and evaluation of changes in clinical presentation preoperatively and postoperatively. Follow all orders carefully for each neurological evaluation ordered. VSs should be taken frequently before and after brain surgery for tumor removal, and you should report signs of increased ICP.

Cancer treatment is often prolonged with untoward associated symptoms. Cancer treatment can cause nausea, hair loss, bone marrow suppression, neutropenia, pain, life-threatening infections, and emotional distress.

Patient Teaching Guidelines
If the child requires brain surgery to remove or debulk (surgically make smaller) the tumor, the child's postoperative clinical presentation may worsen at first and then improve as the cerebral edema decreases with healing. It is essential to prepare the family for this alarming, but expected, stage of healing.

Childhood Migraine Headaches
Children as young as infants can get the same types of severe headaches as adults. However, the symptoms associated with childhood headaches may present differently than adult symptoms because children frequently encounter bilateral pain, whereas adults experience unilateral pain. Children who are unable to describe the location and severity of the pain pose extra challenges in managing headaches. As the child grows, headaches may also evolve and present differently than they did during earlier periods. Because children engage in vigorous play and sports, it is imperative that significant head injuries be ruled out, such as those that cause intracranial bleeding and ICP.

Migraine headaches may cause nausea, vomiting, severe head pain, and sensitivity to sound and light. These headaches are associated with feelings of pulsation and throbbing; are sometimes relieved by sleep; and are often triggered by caffeine, menses, and stress.

Types of Childhood Migraine Headaches
Not all migraine headaches are the same. Children may present with one of the four types of childhood migraine headaches: chronic daily headaches, cluster headaches, tension headaches, and psychogenic headaches.

CHRONIC DAILY HEADACHES. Chronic daily headaches can cause symptoms similar to migraines but are much more frequent. If a child experiences headaches for more than 15 days per month for at least 3 consecutive months, then further diagnostics are warranted to rule out infection, abscess, or head injury.

CLUSTER HEADACHES. Cluster headaches are uncommon in school-aged children and are more common in adolescent males (Johns Hopkins Medicine, 2023). The sensory experience of cluster headaches can be described as "stabbing, sharp pain" unilaterally that can last anywhere from 15 minutes to as long as 3 hours. Children with cluster headaches often experience associated symptoms of agitation, congestion, runny nose, and teary eyes (Johns Hopkins Medicine, 2023).

TENSION HEADACHES. Causing a feeling of tightness around the head or on both sides of the child's head, tension headaches present as a dull ache rather than throbbing. Children with tension headaches often become more symptomatic with physical exercise and play. Tension headaches are differentiated by their pain presentation as well as a lack of nausea and vomiting, which are so often associated with migraines.

Sleep deprivation headaches are a type of tension headache associated with obese children who have sleep apnea or those with conditions that cause chronic hypoxia.

PSYCHOGENIC HEADACHES. Psychogenic headaches may be difficult to diagnose. They are associated with a mental health issue, such as conversion disorder, also called *functional neurological symptom disorder,* in which an individual experiences stress in physical symptoms that do not have a physical cause. Psychogenic headaches require treatment because pain is a subjective experience and requires professional assessments, interventions, and an evaluation of the effectiveness of the interventions.

Evaluating Childhood Headaches

Assessments for childhood headaches must include the following:

- A health history of previous headaches in younger years; a family history that indicates a genetic predisposition; and any neurological disorders, deficits, birth trauma, or vision disorders
- Risk factors such as sports that cause dehydration and previous head injuries
- A physical examination, including the location, severity, intensity, and description of pain, as well as associated symptoms such as nausea, vomiting, behavioral changes, photophobia, sound phobia, and congestion
- Assessment for any clinical signs of infection, including fever, a stiff neck, or a pertinent history of recent communicable diseases
- A head CT scan if the child demonstrates neurological symptoms such as seizures, pain upon rising in the morning, headache associated with vomiting, or any change in mental status such as personality, mood, or school performance

Interventions for Childhood Headaches

Interventions for childhood headaches depend on the type, severity, and associated disability. Treating any infections, especially chronic sinus infections, meningitis, or encephalitis, is paramount. If the child has experienced a significant head injury, then treatment may include hospitalization for observation and treatment of the injury. Stress can be a contributing cause of tension headaches. Eyesight should be checked because eye strain may contribute to the headache experience. If the child is experiencing bullying or relationship difficulties with peers, teachers, or parents, then referring the family for counseling may be warranted as part of a holistic approach to managing headaches. There are many medications currently being used to treat migraine headaches in childhood. The family will work with a pediatrician or pediatric neurologist to create a holistic treatment plan based on the location and severity of the headaches and the level of disability.

Nursing Considerations for Childhood Headaches

Headaches can be frustrating for both the child and the parent. Parents may be reluctant to offer young children pain medication for their headaches, and young children may be reluctant to take oral medications. It is important to take a holistic approach to identifying triggers and offering suggestions for symptom management.

The child's diet should be assessed because research has shown that foods and beverages that contain the preservative nitrate may be a trigger for headaches. Nitrates are found in hot dogs, cold cuts, bacon, and commercially prepared foods and food mixes. Although used to treat some headaches in adults, caffeine can be a trigger for headaches in children. Any foods or beverages that contain chocolate, as well as coffee, tea, and many sodas, may contribute to the child's headaches and should be avoided.

It is important to find meaningful and effective ways to help alleviate the child's symptoms, including prescribed medications, rest and relaxation, stimulation reduction, massage, warm or cold packs to the forehead, and other means of complementary therapy. Children may respond to sleep; resting in a dark and quiet room; NSAIDs; antiemetics; and the prescription headache medications sumatriptan succinate, isometheptene, and ergotamine. If the headaches continue, stronger medications, including propranolol, cyproheptadine, verapamil, valproate, and several of the antidepressants, may be used.

Cognitive Impairment

The term *cognitive impairment* (CI) refers to significant limitations in a child's intellectual functioning and adaptive behaviors. During the developmental period (birth to age 22), CI limits the child's social, conceptual, and adaptive skills. CI has replaced the older term *mental retardation.*

There are varying degrees of CI. Assessing a child's IQ, or intelligence quotient, identifies the degree of impairment:

- *Mild:* IQ of 50 to 55 and up to 70; 80% of those with CI. Considered educable to a mental age of 12 to 13 years old, mostly independent.
- *Moderate:* IQ of 35 to 40 and up to 50 to 55; 15% of those classified with CI. Most children with Down syndrome function at this level. Considered "trainable" to the mental age of an 8- to 10-year-old.
- *Severe:* IQ of 20 to 25 and up to 35 to 40. Considered the mental age of a toddler, this status requires complete custodial care for safety and activities of daily living (ADLs).
- *Profound:* IQ below 20 to 25. Considered having a mental age of an infant; requires complete care, supervision, and protection.

People with severe and profound CI comprise the remaining 5% of CI cases.

Evaluating Cognitive Impairment

The pediatric health-care team should focus on a child's developmental status and not chronological age. The team should determine the ability of a child with a CI to perform motor and psychosocial tasks. A true determination of the child's level of functioning is performed over time, and the child should have at least two testing periods.

Interventions for Cognitive Impairment

Interventions for a child with a CI start with ensuring that the child is safe and cared for. Using the Maslow hierarchy of needs, assist the family with basic support for the child's nutrition, safety, and socialization. Help the family make goals that are realistic for the child's level of functioning. Each goal should be broken down into distinct tasks that can be mastered over time with practice. Participating in ADLs, appropriate socializing, and safety precautions are all possible goals that the child can work on.

Nursing Considerations for Cognitive Impairment

One way to support a child with a CI and their family is to acknowledge successes as the child accomplishes goals. When a child with a moderate or severe CI masters a task such as oral hygiene or hand washing, the entire family should feel successful.

It is important that the pediatric health-care team encourage families of children with CIs to become active in national, state, regional, and local support organizations. The Special Olympics, the American Association on Intellectual and Developmental Disabilities (AAIDD), and county-run developmental centers are three examples of organizations that can provide support and assistance.

Hydrocephalus

Hydrocephalus is the buildup of too much CSF in the brain. This buildup of fluid can be caused by increased CSF production, decreased CSF reabsorption, or an obstructed flow of CSF within the ventricles and subarachnoid spaces of the brain. An obstructed flow of CSF is also called *noncommunicating hydrocephalus,* whereas impaired absorption of CSF is called *communicating hydrocephalus.* In the presence of tumors, structural abnormalities, trauma, or hemorrhage, noncommunicating hydrocephalus can develop, causing significant CNS symptoms and impairment. With scarring, hemorrhage, or the presence of congenital anomalies, communicating hydrocephalus can develop.

Evaluating Hydrocephalus

Assessments of suspected or actual hydrocephalus include frequent measurements of the circumference of the child's head. Take these measurements directly above the eyebrow, on the widest part of the child's head. Palpate the child's fontanel for the presence of a full and possibly tense bulge. In infants, the skull's suture lines may widen in the presence of increasing pressure, and the child's scalp veins may become distended and prominent, causing the appearance of venous engorgement (Fig. 27.11). Note the child's affect and mood, looking for a high-pitched cry, irritability, and/or lethargy. Also, observe for "sunset eyes," in which the white sclera is visible above and around the iris as the eyes appear to be looking down (Fig. 27.12). In severe hydrocephalus, the child may not have the neck and upper back strength to

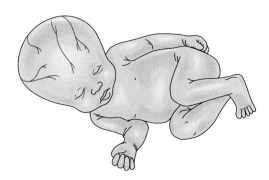

FIGURE 27.11 Distended vessels on an infant's scalp because of increased cerebral pressure.

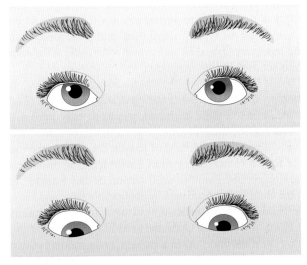

FIGURE 27.12 Sunset eyes related to ICP and hydrocephalus.

Ventriculoperitoneal (VP) Shunt

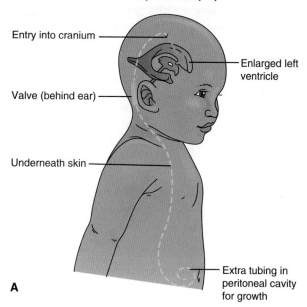

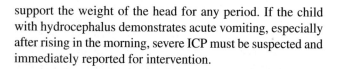

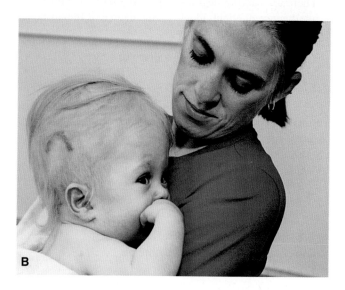

FIGURE 27.13 A and B, VP shunt.

support the weight of the head for any period. If the child with hydrocephalus demonstrates acute vomiting, especially after rising in the morning, severe ICP must be suspected and immediately reported for intervention.

Interventions for Hydrocephalus

The main intervention for hydrocephalus is the placement of a ventral-peritoneal (VP) shunt, which is placed surgically (Fig. 27.13). This shunt allows CSF to descend from the ventricle through the shunt tubing into the child's peritoneal cavity, where the fluid is absorbed and eliminated. The shunt must be monitored over time for malfunction. For example, the shunt may become blocked by biological material, or as the child grows and develops, the shunt may become too short for the child's size. The parents must be taught how to check for changes in clinical presentation associated with sudden increased ICP. They must also learn how to manually pump the shunt to ensure patency. This procedure is dependent on the type of shunt used, and postoperative and long-term care should be individualized based on the shunt manufacturer's recommendation.

Nursing Considerations for Hydrocephalus

Be aware that a child with hydrocephalus may have a CI or other associated neurological deficits. Children who have hydrocephalus because of shaken baby syndrome may have retinal hemorrhages and CI with learning disabilities (see Chapter 26). Families need support as they learn to care for the child whose head may be abnormally large and heavy. The child may need constant head support. For example, if the child sits in a high chair, the head may need to rest on a pillow; or if the child sits in a car seat, extra padding may be necessary to keep the head in a neutral central position.

Know how to manage an obstruction in the shunt and teach the family this management. Discuss signs and symptoms of infection with the family because the presence of the VP shunt places the child at risk for sepsis.

Increased Intracranial Pressure

Within the rigid cranial vault of the child's skull, any increased pressure can cause significant symptoms and injury. Increased ICP can result in the child's brain being herniated, which results in progressive deterioration of the brainstem and, without treatment, causes apnea and death. Health histories associated with ICP include head trauma, bleeding disorders, extensive fevers, and overhydration of a child with diabetic ketoacidosis (DKA) and syndrome of inappropriate antidiuretic hormone (SIADH). ICP that is caused by cerebral edema may be related to abscesses, meningitis, tumors, water intoxication, hypoxia, hydrocephalus, and other causes.

Evaluating Intracranial Pressure

Assessments of ICP include identifying associated clinical signs and symptoms of occipital headache, vomiting (projectile vomiting in older children), altered mental status, visual disturbances, and generalized neck pain. Continue to evaluate the child for hypertension, bradycardia, and bradypnea. A young child may demonstrate increased head circumference and a bulging anterior fontanel. Further assessments include the following:

- *Sunset eyes:* The white of the sclera is visible above the iris.
- *Posturing:* These can be decerebrate, indicating damage to the nerve pathway between the spinal cord and the brain, which is typically found with brainstem injuries,

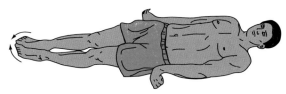

Abnormal Extension (decerebrate posturing)

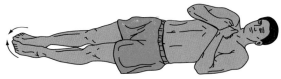

Abnormal Flexion (decorticate posturing)

FIGURE 27.14 Posturing with severe head injury: decerebrate and decorticate.

or decorticate, caused by a stroke, another anterior brain injury, or brain hemorrhages within the cerebral hemispheres (Fig. 27.14).

- *Seizures:* These may be generalized or focal.
- *Macewen sign:* A resonant "cracked pot" sound occurs when the child's suture lines are percussed (tapped). Enlarged bluish scalp veins are usually present as well.
- *Diplopia:* This refers to double vision.
- *Unequal pupils:* PERRLA (Pupils Equal, Round, and Reactive to Light and Accommodation) should be performed to evaluate for this condition.
- A sudden change in feeding habits is noted.
- Irritability, restlessness, and crying occur with holding or cuddling.

Interventions for Intracranial Pressure

Nurses should assist the team in an emergency response to increasing ICP. Immediate interventions for acute increased ICP include the following:

- Stabilizing the airway and administering CPR as needed
- Maintaining a patent airway
- Providing a source of oxygen to maintain stable oxygen saturations and ABGs
- Suctioning the child carefully and only if needed (suctioning can cause rebound increased ICP)
- Monitoring the child's pediatric GCS score; if the team determines the value is 8 or less, the child will need to be intubated STAT
- Elevating the HOB
- Treating the child's presenting seizure activities if needed
- Turning down the lights and providing an environment with low visual and auditory stimulation
- Preparing to assist the team in transferring the child to the highest level of care, such as the PICU
- Assisting in the rapid transfer to a diagnostic department, such as MRI or CT scanning
- Carefully managing the child's IV to maintain a portal for emergency medications such as diuretics and anticonvulsants
- Administering diuretics or corticosteroids, or both

Nursing Considerations for Intracranial Pressure

ICP can be life-threatening. Support the interdisciplinary team in stabilizing the child and then monitor the child for any sudden change in clinical status. Report any new symptoms or changes to existing symptoms immediately to prevent brain tissue anoxia and brain damage. The child may demonstrate signs of diabetes insipidus (DI) in which the child produces large quantities of very dilute urine with a low specific gravity, or signs of SIADH, in which the child's urine output (UOP) is grossly diminished.

Seizure Disorders

A *seizure* is a disruption of the electrical communication among the neurons and subsequent abnormal discharge of electrical activity within the child's brain. Recurrent seizures are commonly known as *epilepsy*. A seizure may also be called a *paroxysmal involuntary brain disturbance*. Seizures do not constitute a medical diagnosis but rather are a symptom of an underlying CNS injury or disorder, such as trauma, diabetes, hypoxia, or intercranial hemorrhage.

During a seizure, the child's brain either fires electrical stimulation between the neurons when it is not supposed to, or it does not fire when it should. The result is a disruption in the expected patterns of electrical current between the neurons, which leads to an excitatory or inhibitory mechanism and causes a seizure. The manifestations of the seizure may include a loss of consciousness, abnormal motor movements, behavioral abnormalities, autonomic dysfunction, and sensory disturbances.

The definition of a *seizure disorder* is when a child experiences an unprovoked seizure two or more times within a 24-hour period. Close to 40% of all childhood seizures are partial. Table 27.4 provides a description of types of seizures found in childhood. The cause of a seizure disorder is often unknown. Likewise, the cause of most neonatal and infant seizures remains unknown. Seizure disorders may have familial tendencies, may be associated with brain injuries, or may be caused by an infectious process. Full body seizures are called **grand mal seizures**. Common causes of seizures in pediatric patients include the following:

- Trauma
- Hemorrhage
- Brain malformations
- Genetic disorders
- Brain dysmaturity (small brain size and function related to fetal development)
- Infection, such as meningitis
- Fever
- Electrolyte abnormalities, especially related to sodium, and the presence of hyperglycemia or hypoglycemia
- Inborn errors of metabolism
- Imbalance of neurotransmitters
- Medication-related injuries or significant exposures (cocaine, chemotherapy, alcohol, lead, and tricyclic antidepressants)
- Structural CNS lesions

Table 27.4

Types of Childhood Seizures

Type of Seizure	Description	Characteristics	Treatment
Infantile spasms	Uncommon, generalized seizure presenting between 3 and 12 months of age; peaks at 4–8 months.	Sudden stiffening, then jerking; child flings arms out, bends body forward, and bends knees up; called *jackknife seizures*. Child may lose some motor skills after onset of diagnosis.	Treated with anticonvulsants and steroid therapy.
Simple partial seizure	Type of partial seizure only occurring in part of the child's brain. Symptoms depend on the location of electrical activity in the brain.	Child presents with clonic or tonic movements involving the extremities, neck, and face. May experience sensory sensations such as pain or numbness. Only lasts on average 10–25 seconds. Child experiencing simple partial seizure will remain conscious during the process with no postictal state. Some children verbalize during a simple partial seizure.	Treatment varies; may include anticonvulsant therapy based on the location within the brain and the severity of symptoms.
Complex partial seizure	Often starts with the motor activity associated with simple partial seizure and then progresses to other body sites with a loss of or altered state of consciousness.	Sometimes preceded by an aura, this common type of partial seizure does impair consciousness. In children, motor movements are complex and mimic purposes such as picking, pulling, or rubbing objects, or running in a repetitive nondirective way. In infants, the child will demonstrate chewing, lip smacking, salivation, and excessive swallowing movements.	Treatment consists of anticonvulsant therapy.
Grand mal or tonic-clonic seizure	A type of severe seizure that crosses over the brain's hemispheres and causes full-body neuromuscular seizure activity. This generalized dramatic seizure is associated with an aura, a loss of consciousness, a shrill and piercing loud cry, and tonic presentation followed by tonic-clonic movements of the entire body that alternate with the relaxation of muscles.	Child may experience pronounced saliva secretion, cyanosis because of apnea, and loss of bladder and sometimes bowel sphincter control. Will demonstrate a postictal state of deep sleep or may be semicomatose, in which the only response is to painful stimuli. This may last up to 2 hours with an average of 30 minutes. Child will be confused but will not recall seizure activity.	Airway must be supported after seizure activity. Do not force any object into the mouth to maintain airway during seizure (no tongue blades or oral airway insertion). Place the child in a side-lying position after the seizure activity stops to facilitate saliva drainage and allow the child's tongue to fall forward.
Absence seizure	Generalized seizure more often found in girls; tends to develop after the fifth year. Formally titled *petit mal seizure*.	Often identified in a classroom setting because the child suddenly "checks out" with blank stare, flickering eyelids, and lack of general body movements. May demonstrate facial twitches or myoclonic movements. Lasts approximately 30 seconds or less. Child may have many in one day. No postictal state.	Treatment consists of anticonvulsant therapy.

Table 27.4

Types of Childhood Seizures—cont'd

Type of Seizure	Description	Characteristics	Treatment
Myoclonic seizure	Type of generalized seizure involving the brain's motor complex.	Child will demonstrate sudden whole-body or limited body part massive jerking. Child may or may not lose consciousness. Often accompanies other forms of seizures.	Treated with anticonvulsant therapy.
Miscellaneous Seizures			
Febrile seizure	Type of generalized seizure associated with a rapid rise in core body temperature. Febrile seizures are considered age dependent and are rarely seen before 9 months of age or after the fifth birthday. They are the most common seizure noted during childhood, and they spontaneously remit without the use of specific anticonvulsant therapy. Incidence rate is 2%–5% of the population.	Previously healthy infant or young child presents with generalized seizure activity, often following bacterial or viral infections. Febrile seizures do not last more than 5 minutes, are generally not associated with brain damage, and are considered harmless for most children. Febrile seizures are not considered a seizure disorder, and the child may not be treated with long-term anticonvulsants unless the seizure is prolonged, focal, or recurs within 24 hours of the first one.	Treatment focuses on finding the source of the rapid rise in temperature and treating infection. Child should be monitored for repeated febrile seizures with every infection after first presentation. Child should receive antipyretic medications with first signs of infections to prevent further febrile seizures.
Status epilepticus (SE)	Defined as a continuous seizure that lasts longer than 30 minutes or the occurrence of serial seizures with no regained consciousness between. The most common form of seizures associated with SE are generalized tonic-clonic. The causes of SE include fever, sudden withdrawal of antiepileptic medication, electrolyte disturbance, hypoxia/ischemia, infection, or trauma. Considered a neurological emergency, a child in SE requires a finely orchestrated medical team approach to prevent the child's death.	Characterized by back-to-back seizure activity of clustered seizures in which the child does not regain consciousness or recover between seizures.	Children in SE need to be transferred to an intensive care environment for airway support and possible intubation if ventilation via bag valve mask is not successful. Diazepam or lorazepam should be administered immediately to manage the seizure activity. Treatment is life support and rapid administration of anticonvulsants to stop the continuing seizure activity. Oxygenation, stabilization of blood glucose, and stabilization of electrolytes should be aggressively managed to prevent morbidity and mortality.

Patient Teaching Guidelines

Parents are typically quite frightened when they learn that their child has had a febrile seizure. Therefore, it is important to teach them that this type of convulsive event is fairly common in childhood with an incidence rate of 2% to 5% of all children between 6 months and 5 years of age (CDC, 2020). Although simple (shorter duration) febrile seizures can be serious, they are not considered a seizure disorder and do not require anticonvulsant medications. Complex childhood febrile seizures (lasting longer than 15 minutes) place young children at risk for a diagnosis of epilepsy (Aslan, 2021).

Safety *Stat!*

Studies have shown a slightly higher risk of febrile seizures in children who received the measles, mumps, rubella (MMR) vaccine within the previous 5 to 12 days. That risk is slightly increased in children who receive the MMRV combination vaccine (MMR with varicella; CDC, 2020).

The degree of disability associated with a seizure disorder depends on the type of seizure and the location where the seizure originates within the child's brain. If the child experienced an anoxic event that prevented brain-tissue perfusion, the degree of disability may be mild to severe. Many children with seizure disorders also have accompanying brain injuries or insults. The degree of long-term disability depends on the cause and severity of the seizure disorder.

Evaluating Seizure Disorders

The child presenting with seizure activity should have a complete health history taken with associated risk factors identified. You should gather the following information from the family:

- Any family history of seizures or neurological impairments
- Complications associated with the prenatal, perinatal, and postnatal period
- Documented delays in the child's developmental motor milestones
- Exposure to environmental toxins, infectious diseases, or physical trauma, especially to the head
- A history of domestic abuse, child abuse, or any form of nonaccidental injury
- Age of child at the time of the first seizure

You should also gather the following information related to the presenting seizure event:

- Precipitating factors surrounding the seizure event or seizure disorder

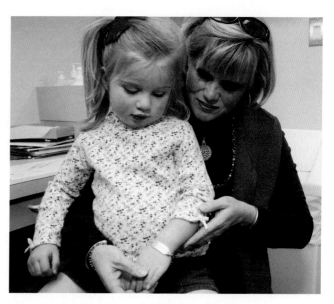

FIGURE 27.15 A child wearing a medical alert bracelet.

- Description of the child's clinical presentation during the seizure (helps to determine the possible type) such as grand mal or **myoclonic** (spasmodic jerky movements)
- The presence of an aura, a loss of consciousness, injury during seizure (head injury with a fall), and the **postictal** state
- Current medications, including past or current anticonvulsant therapies
- Compliance with the current medication regimen

Interventions for Seizure Disorders

The nursing care of a child with a seizure disorder begins by securing a safe environment. Note the child's mobility and the need for safety devices. Some children with a severe seizure disorder must wear helmets to keep their heads safe from injury when the seizure causes a fall. Maintain seizure precautions while the child is hospitalized. This includes padding the side rails, providing constant supervision while the child is ambulating in the halls or playing in the playroom, and maintaining safety while the child is being transported via gurney or wheelchair. Suction and oxygen should be available at all times.

If a child experiences a seizure, the child should be kept safe during the seizure activity. Do not try to stop or control the motor movements; do not try to place a tongue blade or any object in the child's mouth; and make sure to move objects that might cause bodily harm away from the child during the seizure. The child with a seizure disorder should wear a medical alert bracelet at all times (Fig. 27.15).

Adherence to the medication regimen is essential to prevent seizure activity. Families need to be taught the

- **WORD · BUILDING ·**

myoclonic: myo–muscle + clon–spasmodic contractions + ic–pertaining to

postictal: post–after + ict–a sudden attack + al–relating to

importance of exactly following the prescribed medication schedule and following up with monitoring routine serum blood levels of the anticonvulsant therapy to ensure therapeutic blood levels. The family should also be reminded that if the child becomes ill, vomits, or experiences any health deviation, they should report the symptoms to their primary health-care provider for guidance. GI illnesses, vomiting, and dehydration can all affect the anticonvulsant therapy. If a helmet is ordered for protection of the child with frequent **tonic-clonic seizures**, the family must be educated about having the child wear the helmet when awake. The family should conduct an evaluation of their home, remove furniture with sharp edges, and make any other home environment changes. Parents, caregivers, and teachers must be informed that sleepiness and slow reaction times may be generalized side effects of the child's seizure medications.

If a child's seizure disorder remains uncontrolled despite the use of various anticonvulsant therapies, surgery may be warranted to remove or surgically disrupt the area of brain tissue causing the electrical activity.

A cluster of seizures that are back to back is dangerous. This condition, called **status epilepticus (SE)**, can cause both significant injury and life-threatening hypoglycemia.

Research continues to provide innovations in seizure therapies. One technology being used to treat seizures is vagal nerve stimulation, which is a treatment to reduce the frequency and intensity of seizures by placing a small electric stimulator in the neck around the vagal nerve. While sending intermittent electrical signals to the brain, this technology interrupts a seizure that is just starting to develop. The vagal nerve stimulator is used for children who continue to have loss of consciousness during generalized or complex partial seizures when not controlled by medications.

Labs & Diagnostics

Tests for Seizure Disorders
Although there is no one test to diagnose childhood seizures, several diagnostics may be completed to put together what is referred to as a "constellation of information" to determine the type, location, and severity of the brain's abnormal electrical activity.

Laboratory Studies
• Serum electrolytes, including calcium levels and glucose levels, to rule out metabolic disorders, hypoglycemia, and hypocalcemia
• Anticonvulsant serum medication levels: These medications must be kept within a therapeutic range; low levels may cause seizures to occur, and high levels can lead to toxicity. Children metabolize anticonvulsant medications faster than adults do and therefore require larger doses per body weight and careful monitoring. Report immediately any serum subtherapeutic or toxic blood levels.

Common laboratory analyses of safe ranges are important to follow and any finding outside of a therapeutic range must be immediately reported.
Diagnostics Studies
• EEG to identify the location and type of seizure; this testing may be a 24-hour video monitoring EEG
• CT or MRI to rule out injury, brain tissue abnormalities, tumors, abscesses, and intracranial bleeds
• Skull x-rays if trauma is identified or suspected

Medication Facts

Cannabidiol oral solution, which is a pharmaceutical grade of cannabidiol oil, may be used by some parents as an intervention for refractory or persistent seizures.

Special Considerations for Seizure Disorders
There are several special considerations in managing seizures. These include recording seizure activity, providing anticonvulsant medications, and having the child with seizure disorders follow a **ketogenic** diet.

RECORDING SEIZURE ACTIVITY. One of the most important aspects of caring for a child with a seizure disorder is to teach and reinforce the need for the caregivers, guardians, or family members to document each seizure event. A log should be maintained for health-care professionals to review. For each seizure, the log should document the date; time; precipitating events; type of seizure activity, including motor movements; duration of the seizure; any associated events, such as loss of consciousness, bladder or bowel incontinence, nausea, or vomiting; and the postictal state, including periods of drowsiness and reports of headache.

KETOGENIC DIET. The **ketogenic diet** is a special diet that has been widely studied and provides relief from seizures for some children. First developed in the 1920s and further investigated in 1976, the ketogenic diet is a special high-fat, low-carbohydrate diet that is thought to help control seizures in some people who have a documented history of epilepsy. The term *ketogenic* means that the diet produces ketones within the body as fat is processed and broken down for energy. The theory behind the diet is that the process of ketone breakdown leads to a higher ketone blood level, thereby improving seizure control.

Most physicians who encourage the ketogenic diet do so when the patient has not had success in seizure control, even with several anticonvulsant therapies. The diet is offered as an

• WORD · BUILDING •
ketogenic: keto–ketone + genic–creating

adjunct therapy to children but is rarely suggested for adults. It helps to control seizures in certain cases but does not provide an immediate seizure-free status. The overall diet includes a 4:1 or 3:1 fat-to-protein ratio. Research has shown that children who begin and continue following a ketogenic diet can demonstrate between a 50% and 90% reduction in the number of their seizures. Of note, 30% of children with a seizure disorder have some drug-resistant epilepsy (DRE); a ketogenic diet is an alternative which successfully provides ketone bodies to the brain (Imdad et al., 2022). Conditions for which a ketogenic diet is suggested for seizure reduction include the following:

- Focal seizures
- Infantile spasms
- Dravet syndrome
- Doose syndrome
- Rett syndrome
- Glucose transporter 1 (GLUT-1) deficiency

Patient Teaching Guidelines

If a ketogenic diet is recommended for a child with a seizure disorder, be ready to provide the parents and the child with basic information and support while they implement the diet. Foods that are encouraged for consumption during the ketogenic diet include the following:

- Heavy whipping cream
- Butter
- Canola oil
- Olive oil
- Mayonnaise
- Coconut oil
- Bacon
- Peanut butter
- Sour cream
- Cheese

The child must not ingest carbohydrates. This includes fruits and starchy vegetables, breads, pasta, grains, and all sugars. For the diet to be effective in preventing seizures, the child must be 100% compliant. Families should work closely with a dietitian to learn about acceptable food selections and food restrictions. Because the diet is so restricted, the child will need to take vitamin and mineral supplements, including folic acid, vitamin D, calcium, and iron. Most ketogenic diets are initiated within a hospital environment over the course of 3 to 4 days to monitor the child's ketones and responses to the change in diet.

COMMON ANTICONVULSANT THERAPY. Common anticonvulsant therapy for long-term seizure management includes many medications. Table 27.5 provides examples of commonly used medications to control childhood seizures.

Table 27.5
Common Anticonvulsant Medications for Children

Medications:
Carbamazepine
Phenytoin
Valproate
Ethosuximide
ACTH
Clobazam
Diazepam nasal spray
Gabapentin
Lamotrigine
Levetiracetam
Topiramate

Some of these medications may be considered monotherapy (single medication therapy). Depending on the health-care provider's specific orders, medications are formulated in pills, others liquid, and some come as food sprinkles for ease in administration as needed by the child.

Common Side Effects:
Dizziness
Double vision
Grogginess
Nausea and vomiting
Skin rash (maybe severe such as Stevens-Johnson Syndrome)
Unsteady gait
Severe Side Effects:
Liver failure
Bone marrow failure

Sources: Children's Hospital of Philadelphia. (2022). *Seizure medications.* https://www.chop.edu/treatments/seizure-medications; Epilepsy Foundation. (2023). *Seizure medications with children.* Epilepsy Foundation. https://www.epilepsy.com/treatment/medicines/medications-children#Choosing-The-Best-Medication; Healthychildren.org. (2020). *Seizure medications for children and teens.* American Academy of Pediatrics. https://www.healthychildren.org/English/health-issues/conditions/seizures/Pages/Seizure-Medications-for-Children-and-Teens.aspx.

Safety *Stat!*

For status epilepticus, anticonvulsant therapy is for short-term emergency management and includes the following medications:

- Diazepam per rectum
- Phenobarbital
- Fosphenytoin

Nursing Considerations for Seizure Disorders

When teaching families about how to care for their child with a seizure disorder, provide the following information about anticonvulsant therapy:

- Adolescents must be seizure-free for 1 year to obtain their driver's license. They may be on anticonvulsant therapy to be eligible for a license.
- Parents must understand the importance of monitoring the therapeutic serum levels of anticonvulsant therapy.
- Teens should avoid alcohol because it reduces the threshold of seizures.

- Families should never abruptly stop administering anticonvulsant therapy to their child because doing so may cause seizures.
- Caregivers must understand the importance of medication administration; proper hydration; and promptly reporting any side effects, illness, or change in cognition or well-being.

Remind families to treat their child with a seizure disorder as they would any of their children. Children with chronic illnesses need play opportunities, social activities, outings, and school engagement. Any restrictions on sports activities, swimming, or physical education will be determined by the neurology team and are based on the type and severity of the seizures.

Key Points

- The two main divisions of the nervous system consist of the CNS and the PNS. Each of these two systems has unique functions that regulate body systems.
- The brain, which includes three protective membranes—dura mater, arachnoid membrane, and pia mater—provides the coordination of the entire nervous system.
- The child's age and developmental level provide guidance about how to evaluate functioning of the CNS. Although the CNS is one of the first systems to form during fetal development, it is actually one of the last to fully mature during childhood.
- Neurological disorders in childhood often require long medical treatment plans and care. The degree of disability and restoration of function depends on the location of the disorder, the amount of damage that has occurred, and the quality and timeliness of medical interventions.
- Children are at risk for several neurological disorders or injuries. CI, CP, seizure disorders, and lead poisoning are a few of these disorders. Identifying early signs and

symptoms of neurological impairment and expediting interventions maximize the potential for treatment and management. Children, especially adolescents, are at an increased risk of TBIs and SCIs.
- Insisting that children use protective equipment when playing sports, riding in a car, and playing at home or in parks is an important part of preventing head injuries and any lasting neurological deficits that may result.
- Families need a tremendous amount of support and education when they have a child with a neurological disorder. Many disorders carry a lifetime of care, and families need guidance to learn how to care for their child. They also need to receive information about support available from regional and national organizations.
- Preventing complications of many neurological disorders, such as cerebral edema, increased ICP, and contractions, is a priority. It is essential to establish a therapeutic relationship that supports collaboration and teaching and that provides emotional support.

Review Questions

1. A mother brings her toddler into the pediatric public health clinic stating that his "personality has changed." The mother states that the child has regressed developmentally and is, at times, hyperactive and very emotional. What cause of these changes should you suspect?
    1. Intentional child abuse with a possible head injury
    2. Early signs of an emotional or cognitive disturbance
    3. Meningitis or another brain infection
    4. Possible exposure to lead

2. A father calls the pediatric clinic stating that the local laboratory called to say that his 4-year-old child who has a seizure disorder had a serum blood level of phenobarbital of 52 mcg/mL. What should be the next action of the nurse receiving the call?

1. Ask the father to bring the child into the clinic for an appointment right away.
2. Ask the parents to take the child back to the laboratory for a second draw to recheck the value.
3. Tell the health-care provider the laboratory value and await instructions.
4. Tell the family to skip the next dose of the medication and then continue as ordered.

3. A nurse is teaching a community class about lead poisoning. To review the content, he asks the students to list examples of sources of lead. Which response requires clarification from the nurse?
    1. Root vegetables grown in contaminated soil
    2. Canned foods processed in other countries
    3. Pottery dishes where the protective glaze has worn off
    4. Lead pencils of all types

4. Which CN would be evaluated in a child who was in an MVA and now exhibits facial droop?
   1. CN III
   2. CN V
   3. CN VII
   4. CN XII

5. Which item is *not* considered a potential source of lead exposure to children?
   1. Glazed ceramics
   2. Treated building construction lumber
   3. Jewelry
   4. Imported cosmetics and particular remedies for health conditions

6. When reinforcing parental teaching about febrile seizures, what should you include?
   1. It is considered a seizure disorder and will require anticonvulsant therapy.
   2. It is associated strongly with genetic predisposition; all other siblings should be monitored.
   3. It relates to how rapidly the child's fever rises during an infectious process.
   4. It is considered a one-time event and requires no further medical attention or treatments.

7. What is the current CDC guideline for a serum lead level that shows lead exposure in children?
   1. 3.5 mcg/dL
   2. 10 mcg/dL
   3. 25 mcg/dL
   4. 50 mcg/dL

8. Which side effects are associated with the administration of the anticonvulsant therapy phenytoin?
   (Select all that apply.)
   1. Gum hyperplasia
   2. Ataxia
   3. Gastric distress
   4. Anemia
   5. Sedation
   6. Weight gain
   7. Nystagmus
   8. Hirsutism

9. Research has shown that foods and beverages that contain the preservative nitrate may be a trigger for headaches. Which food should a child whose headaches are triggered by nitrates avoid?
   1. Homemade applesauce
   2. Green leafy vegetables
   3. Aged cheeses (parmesan, cheddar)
   4. Hot dogs

10. The licensed vocational nurse (LVN) is working with a registered nurse (RN) who is giving care to a child suspected of having meningitis. Which symptom must the LVN immediately report to the RN?
    1. A headache described with a pain scale score of 4
    2. A sudden increase in thirst
    3. A change in energy level
    4. An abrupt eruption of a purplish rash or petechial rash

ANSWERS 1. 4; 2. 3; 3. 4; 4. 3; 5. 2; 6. 3; 7. 1; 8. 1, 2, 3, 4, 5, 7, 8; 9. 4; 10. 4

CRITICAL THINKING QUESTIONS

1. A 3-year-old child presents to the ED in postictal state after a generalized seizure. The parents report that the child has been fussy, hitting the side of her head with her fists, and intermittently crying. What do you suspect has occurred in this clinical situation? What priority nursing care should be initiated, and what short- and long-term teaching should be offered?

2. Discuss the components of a ketogenic diet and analyze the long-term consequences for the child.

3. Lead poisoning remains a serious national public health concern. How can nurses become involved in public health initiatives against lead poisoning in their communities?

Resources

For additional resources and information, including Postconference Questions and Activities, Answers, and References, visit www.FADavis.com.

 Student Study Guide

CHAPTER 28
Child With a Sensory Impairment

KEY TERMS

amblyopia (AM-blee-OH-pee-uh)
astigmatism (ass-TIG-muh-tizm)
cataract (KAT-uh-rakt)
cerumen (se-ROO-men)
color blindness (KUHL-uhr BLIND-ness)
conductive hearing loss (kon-DUK-tiv HEER-ing
   LOSS)
deafness (DEF-ness)
decibel (DESS-ih-bel)
enucleation (ee-NOO-klee-AY-shun)
esotropia (ESS-oh-TROH-pee-uh)
exotropia (EK-soh-TROH-pee-uh)
glaucoma (glaw-KOH-muh)
hard of hearing (HARD uv HEER-ing)
hyperopia (HYE-per-OH-pee-uh)
legal blindness (LEE-guhl BLIND-ness)
leukocoria (LOO-koh-KOR-ee-uh)
myopia (mye-OH-pee-uh)
nystagmus (niss-TAG-muss)
otitis media (oh-TYE-tiss MEE-dee-uh)
ototoxic (oh-toh-tahk-SIK)
refractive errors (ree-FRAK-tiv AIR-ruhz)
retinoblastoma (RET-ih-noh-blass-TOH-muh)
retinopathy of prematurity (ROP) (ret-in-OP-
   uh-thee uv PREE-muh-CHOO-rih-tee)
school vision (SKOOL VIZH-uhn)
strabismus (stra-BIZ-muss)

CHAPTER CONCEPTS

Growth and Development
Health Promotion
Safety
Sensory Perception

LEARNING OUTCOMES

1. Define the key terms.
2. Describe the most common causes of visual impairment during childhood and differentiate between the care of a child with eye trauma, eye disease, and eye tumor.
3. Analyze common reactions when a family is told that their infant or young child will have a sensory impairment.
4. Identify national organizations that provide support to families who have a child with a visual or hearing impairment.
5. Differentiate between blindness and visual impairment and between deafness and hard of hearing.
6. Describe the diagnostic examinations, assessments, treatments, and clinical outcomes of children with a confirmed diagnosis of retinoblastoma.
7. Discuss retinopathy of prematurity (ROP) and the care that can be provided to premature infants to reduce the possibility of developing this pathology.
8. Define the various visual impairments or visual disorders, including strabismus, amblyopia, and nystagmus.
9. Describe the various types and causes of congenital and acquired hearing impairments common to childhood.
10. Outline a plan of care for a child with a new diagnosis of hearing impairment and describe the new technologies available to assist a child with a hearing impairment.

CRITICAL THINKING

Scenario #1: **Lauren**, a 13-year-old girl, was attending a Fourth of July celebration with her family at their local community park. While there, a bystander lit a large firework that malfunctioned and sprayed Lauren's face with burning chemicals. She was taken to a local emergency department and received treatment for her facial wounds. Because of the extent of the burn on her eyes, she is required to wear bilateral eye dressings for no less than 3 weeks while her eyes heal. The only time the dressings are to be removed is during her ophthalmic evaluations by her pediatric eye specialist, who is monitoring her visual sensory impairment carefully, or by her parents if the dressing becomes wet or soiled. Lauren progresses from being very frightened that she could lose her vision to being

Continued

CRITICAL THINKING—cont'd

very angry at her dependence on her mother for her daily care, her loss of socialization throughout her summer vacation from school, and decreased visits from her peer group. She frequently expresses concern about the possibility of facial swelling.

Questions

1. Considering Lauren's developmental level, how would you expect her to react to her condition?
2. How might you assist the family in preparing a safe home for Lauren while she has the bilateral eye dressings that will be on for 3 weeks?

CONCEPTUAL CORNERSTONE

Sensory Perception and Growth and Development

Early identification of a visual or hearing impairment allows for interventions to be initiated that provide for speech development, socialization, growth and development, and academic success. Visual and hearing impairments that are not found early can cause delays in a child's development and create challenges in the school environment. Even a slight hearing loss creates the need for professional assistance, including speech therapy, academic accommodations, auditory training, and family involvement in continued screenings and life adaptation. Once an impairment is identified, there are numerous new procedures, technologies, and devices that can be used to improve the child's sensory function. National organizations now provide families with support and education. Nurses are instrumental in facilitating the relationships between health-care centers, academic settings, and national organizations.

Sensory impairments in childhood are a serious concern. Both visual and hearing impairments can have significant consequences on a child's cognitive, social, and emotional development; sense of well-being; and academic success. Early detection through screenings and prompt interventions will assist the child and family in adapting to a congenital or acquired sensory impairment.

Nurses are uniquely positioned to identify sensory impairments early. Nurses need to support and participate in national efforts to screen all early school-aged children for hearing and visual acuity and to help any affected child secure a referral for interventions and/or treatments. Nurses also have the opportunity to educate families about ways to prevent sensory impairments such as immunizations, injury prevention, and adherence to well-child checkups.

The incidence (new cases) and prevalence (existing cases) of sensory impairments are difficult to determine because they are not considered reportable conditions. Current estimates are that 14.9% of children in the United States have a hearing impairment that needs an intervention (Centers for Disease Control and Prevention [CDC], 2022a). The data on how many American children have a visual impairment vary widely, but estimates are 6.8% (CDC, 2022d). Worldwide, the leading cause of visual impairment throughout childhood varies; children in low-income countries tend to have childhood congenital cataracts, whereas children in middle income countries tend to have **retinopathy of prematurity** (**ROP**; World Health Organization [WHO], 2022). Globally, the lack of correctly fitting corrective lenses and uncorrected cataracts or refractive errors continue to impact children's vision (WHO, 2022).

Health Promotion

National School-Aged Child Screening Guidelines for Sensory Impairments

The following are commonly used guidelines for early detection of visual and hearing impairments:

- Vision and hearing screenings should be done within the first few months of entering public or private early childhood education, such as kindergarten, beginning at 4 years of age. Screenings should be conducted on any student new to a school from 4 years of age through 12th grade.
- Ideally, vision and hearing screenings are repeated in first, third, fifth, and seventh grades.
- Documentation should be collected on each child and should include the child's name, type of screening test done, date of screening, screener, and screening results.

Visual Screening

Visual screening tests should include the following:

- Distance acuity for both eyes (20/20, 20/30) with approved charts such as the Snellen "tumbling E," Snellen alphabet, or Sloan letter chart
- HOTV Crowded Test Set
- A muscle balance test, such as the Hirschberg corneal light reflex test or the cover–uncover test.

Hearing Screening

Hearing screening tests should include a pure tone sweep-check screen recorded for both ears conducted at an intensity level less than or equal to 25 decibels. The American Academy of Audiology publishes childhood hearing screening guidelines for early detection of hearing loss and reduction of loss of speech development (American Academy of Audiology, 2011). Recommendations are to screen populations of children at 3 years of age and no less than two more times during the school-age period (grades 1, 3, 5, and either grade 7 or 9). Children who fail pure tone, tympanometry, or otoacoustic emissions (OAE) screenings should be retested within 8 to 10 weeks. Infants who fail a hearing screening test (2–4 out of 1,000) should be retested in 1 month (DHCS, 2021).

Check with your state's Department of Health Services to find the screening guidelines that your state mandates for children at various ages.

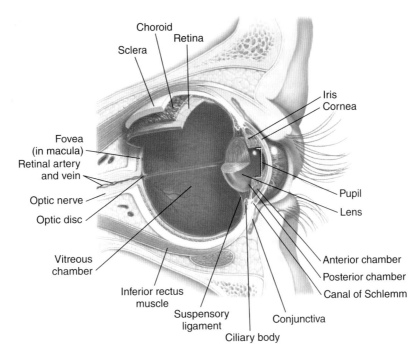

FIGURE 28.1 Anatomy of the human eye.

School screenings are highly effective in identifying children at risk for sensory impairments, although these screenings are limited to developing countries and are not administered worldwide.

Unfortunately, when a child experiences a sensory impairment, academic success is put at risk. Children in the classroom who are suffering visual impairments may report headaches and squint regularly during class. For example, nearsightedness, or myopia, has a profound effect on a child's ability to read material written on the board or projected on a screen.

Screening children for sensory impairment should be standardized across the nation. Yet, variances exist in screening settings, training of screening personnel, threshold of passing or failing a screening test, frequency of screenings, and referral of the child to an appropriate health-care provider. For children covered under a Medicaid health plan, screening for both vision and hearing should be done at each well-child checkup (Medicaid, 2022). Because of variations in screening services across childhood, nurses need to continue to be involved with the process of screening children for sensory impairments, and they need to rapidly report suspected deviations.

 THE DEVELOPMENT OF VISUAL ACUITY

The human eye develops during embryonic growth starting in the third week of life. As the fetus grows, the optic nerve extends from the growing neuroepithelium, as do the retina, iris, and ciliary body. Newborns have very poor vision, only recognizing light and dark, even though their eye anatomy is fully intact. Although it is true that 2 million nerve fibers connect the eyes to the brain, the newborn must learn how to process visual information. It is not until 3 months of life that an infant acquires the level of visual acuity needed to recognize a face. Nurses should encourage parents to hold their newborn close to their faces as part of the bonding process.

Structures of the Eye

The anatomy of the eye is very complex (Fig. 28.1). In general, the eye has three layers: the inner retina; the middle layer, which includes the iris, choroid, and ciliary body; and the outer sclera, including the cornea. There are two major chambers in the eye: the anterior chamber and the vitreous chamber. The anterior chamber is filled with a fluid called aqueous humor, and the vitreous chamber is filled with a fluid called vitreous humor. Communication between the eye and the brain takes place along the optic nerve.

 VISUAL IMPAIRMENT

Visual disturbances in young children are a common problem. The American Optometric Association (AOA, 2018) and The Vision Council (2023) estimated that 25% of all children have a visual disorder requiring screening and follow-up care, including glasses, and that only 15% of preschoolers and 7% of children starting first grade have had an eye examination (AOA, 2018). Unlike *visual disturbance*, the term *visual impairment* describes those disorders that most prescription lenses will not correct and that may require surgical interventions. Visual impairments during childhood can be either congenital or acquired. Congenital visual impairments include those associated with heredity, genetic anomalies, and maternal exposure to a toxin or infectious disease or early prematurity. Acquired visual impairments are associated with traumatic injury to the eyes, brain damage from anoxia, shaken baby syndrome, or a disease process that has an effect on the child's visual acuity.

Patient Teaching Guidelines

According to the AOA (n.d.), digital eye strain is a common problem. The heavy use of digital devices (cell phones, computer tablets, and e-readers) can lead to tired, itchy, and burning eyes; headaches; fatigue; blurred vision; head and neck pain; and loss of visual focus. Prolonged exposure has been associated with visual acuity risk and is called computer vision syndrome (CVS) or digital eyestrain (AOA, n.d.).

Teach patients and their parents or guardians the 20-20-20 rule: Take a 20-second break every 20 minutes and focus on something over 20 feet away. Other ways to lessen the negative effects of looking at a screen are to decrease any glare on the screen and to blink often to reduce dry eyes. The average child between 8 and 12 years of age spends 4 to 6 hours a day on TV and digital media, and teens spend as much as 9 hours a day (Academy of Child and Adolescent Psychiatry [AACAP], 2020). Guidelines for parents concerning screen time for children recommend *no* screen time for children under 18 months of age (unless it is educational programming or video chatting with an adult) and only 1 hour a day during the week and 3 hours a day on the weekends for older children (AACAP, 2020). No screen time should take place during family time or meals.

Team Works

Using Correct Terminology

It is important that the health-care team members use the correct terms when differentiating between visual impairment and blindness. The term *blindness* refers to a complete lack of visual sensory experience. *Visual impairment,* on the other hand, denotes that a child's vision is reduced or impaired but that some sensory experience is taking place. Similarly, the health-care team should differentiate between *deafness* and *hard of hearing*. When a child has **deafness**, the child does not process acoustic stimuli. The term **hard of hearing** denotes the ability to process some acoustic stimuli. The terms should not be used incorrectly, especially around families. When in doubt, confirm the child's past medical history.

Visual impairment in children can be caused by a genetic predisposition, prenatal exposure to a toxin or intrauterine infection, or postnatal conditions. Postnatal conditions include trauma, juvenile rheumatoid arthritis, albinism, any condition that affects the vasculature of the retina such as ROP, or sickle cell disease. Worldwide, vitamin A deficiency is the leading cause of preventable blindness and is associated with many other childhood morbidities (Imdad et al., 2022).

Trauma to the eye structures is a major concern in the pediatric population. Trauma to the eyes can be from vigorous play that causes an instrument such as a pencil or scissors to enter the eye, or it can be caused by a severe injury associated with fire, car accidents, exposure to chemicals, or exposure to prolonged sunlight. Corneal abrasions are one of the most common causes of mild trauma to the eye during childhood. See Box 28.1 for more about corneal abrasions.

Patient Teaching Guidelines

Protection of Sight

Sunlight can be very damaging to the eyes because of ultraviolet (UV) radiation. The most damaging exposure takes place when sunlight reflects off snow, water, pavement, or sand. Teach parents or guardians that children exposed to intense sunlight for long periods must wear sunglasses that block both UVA and UVB rays. Cumulative eye damage throughout childhood can have a lasting effect on vision because the human eye lens cannot repair itself. Moreover, the lens of a child's eye transmits approximately 70% more UV light than the lens of an adult eye. Appropriate sunglasses should be worn consistently from young childhood throughout the life span. Parents and caregivers serve as role models for the use of sun protection: sunscreen, sunglasses, and hats.

The most common type of visual disturbance leading to visual impairment is a **refractive error**. In a reactive error, the light rays bend as they pass through the lens and therefore do not fall directly onto the child's retina. A refractive error leaves a child either nearsighted because the

Box 28.1
Corneal Abrasions

Most corneal abrasions are caused by a foreign body on the eye. When a foreign body enters a child's eye structures, it causes considerable discomfort, resulting in the child rubbing or scratching around or on the eyes. Patching the eye for at least 24 hours to provide for comfort and the administration of sterile antimicrobial eyedrops may be warranted.

Table 28.1
Visual Impairments Found in Childhood

Impairment	*Description*
Amblyopia	Unilateral or bilateral decrease of best corrected vision in an otherwise healthy eye often because of asymmetric refractive error (deflection from a straight path or change in direction of light) or the presence of strabismus.
Astigmatism	A visual disorder where the refraction of a ray of light is spread over a diffuse area rather than sharply focused on the retina. This is because of a difference in the curvature of the cornea and lens of the eye.
Cataracts	An opacity (cloudy appearance) of the eye lens, often caused by trauma, aging, metabolic or endocrine disease, or the side effects of certain medications such as steroids.
Color blindness	An inability to distinguish certain colors or any colors at all.
Esotropia	Inward deviation of the eye laterally.
Exotropia	Outward deviation of the eye laterally.
Glaucoma	A group of eye diseases that leads to increased intraocular pressure and eventually the atrophy of the optic nerve.
Nystagmus	Involuntary back-and-forth movements of the eyes, most often noticeable when the patient gazes at rapidly moving or fixed objects.
Refractive error	A common eye disorder where the eye bends light and is unable to focus because of an abnormal shape of the eye.
Strabismus	Abnormal alignment of the eyes that interferes with binocular vision; both eyes do not properly align with each other (also called *cross-eye* or *wall-eye* in lay terms).

light rays fall in front of the retina (**myopia**), or farsighted because the light rays fall beyond the retina (**hyperopia**). Table 28.1 provides a list of common visual impairments found in children.

Assessments of Visual Acuity

Routine vision screening is an important part of a well-child visit, even when the child is an infant. Many visual abnormalities are treatable or correctable if they are discovered early and promptly. If left untreated, a child's visual impairment may lead to progressive visual loss and eventual blindness. It is important to screen early school-aged children so that a visual disorder or disturbance does not affect their scholastic performance.

The term *school vision* is used when a child is considered to be partially sighted with a measured or approximate visual acuity of 20/70 to 20/200. *Legal blindness* is a term used to note that a child's visual acuity is measured or approximated to be below 20/200 in the better eye, even with the best optical correction (American Foundation for the Blind, 2022).

Children should not only be routinely screened for visual acuity, but they should also be evaluated for strabismus, refractive errors, and **amblyopia** because these are the three visual impairments most commonly found in preschoolers (Prevent Blindness, 2023). If screening reveals a visual disturbance, it is essential to notify the child's parents or guardians, make a referral to a visual specialist, and ensure that the follow-up appointment is carried out.

Nurses participate in a variety of evaluations for visual acuity based on the setting in which they practice and the availability of equipment. The following list describes evaluations that are commonly used.

- *Unilateral cover test (infants or very young children):* Here an infant or young child is evaluated for the ability to follow an object when one eye is covered. A small toy can be used to entice the child to follow the object with their eyes. Each eye is then inspected. If an older infant or

· WORD · BUILDING ·
esotropia: eso–inward + trop–turning + ia–condition
exotropia: exo–outward + trop–turning + ia–condition
strabismus: strab–squinting + ismus–act of
hyperopia: hyper–excessive, beyond + op–eye + ia–condition

· WORD · BUILDING ·
amblyopia: ambly–dull + opia–condition of sight

young child becomes fussy during the examination, this may indicate frustration because the child cannot see the desired toy through the eye that is uncovered.

- *LEA symbol chart (ages 3 to 6, preschool):* This chart is used to check the visual acuity of children who do not yet know the alphabet. Visual acuity is screened with the child at a distance of 10 feet, using what is known as LEA symbols, which are common symbols that can be matched by this age group on a response card. The child either stands or sits and is instructed to match the symbols on a response card being shown.
- *Snellen test (age 6 through adolescence):* This form of visual testing uses a chart with numbers, letters, or figures. The child covers one eye, stands back 20 feet, and vocally names the letters, shapes, or figures to the testing personnel. The child typically starts with large letters, reads across to the end, and then reads the next line that is smaller. This continues until the child is unable to accurately read a line. Each line denotes a level of visual acuity.
- *Corneal light reflex test (early school-aged):* In this test, a light is directed toward the bridge of the nose. The child's light reflex is then examined for symmetry and to make sure the light shines in the same spot on both of the child's eyes. A misalignment is suspected if the light reflex is not symmetrical or is off-centered in both eyes.

Visual Impairment or Blindness in Infants

Identifying visual impairment in infants is more challenging than it is in an older child, who can demonstrate cues of squinting, eye-rubbing, or vocalizing difficulty focusing. Visual impairments in infants require a different set of assessment techniques. In young infants, certain disturbances of vision, such as ROP, cataracts, or glaucoma, have to be identified by inspection of the inner eye. In older infants, a child's inability to track an object that would normally be interesting to this developmental stage is suggestive of a visual impairment. For instance, if an infant does not track a colorful toy across visual fields or does not focus on the caregiver's face when close, an impairment should be suspected.

Eye Infections

Children are especially prone to eye infections. These infections can be viral or bacterial, and many are highly contagious. Two common infections are conjunctivitis and neonatorum eye infections.

Conjunctivitis

When a child presents with inflammation of the conjunctiva, conjunctivitis, or "pinkeye," must be ruled out. The conjunctiva is normally clear, smooth, and moist. If this lining, which covers both the eye and the underside of the lids, becomes inflamed, the eye should be evaluated for an infection, allergy, foreign body, or trauma. When the drainage is purulent, bacterial contamination must be suspected, and antibiotic eyedrops are ordered. A bacterial infection of the conjunctiva is highly contagious.

Nursing considerations include preventing the spread of the bacterial infection. Teaching should include how to cleanse the purulent drainage with a warm, moist cloth used only once and laundered in hot water. Proper hand washing followed by a "no touch" rule needs to be reinforced for both the caregiver and the child. When eyedrops are instilled, the tip of the medicine bottle should never touch the child's tissues because this will contaminate the medicine dropper and could lead to continued reinfection. If an antimicrobial ointment is ordered, the family should be taught to instill the ointment from the inner corner to the outer corner by dispensing a thin, even line into the lower eyelid.

Patient Teaching Guidelines

Care of a Child With Bacterial Conjunctivitis
Questions frequently asked by parents include the following:

1. *What are the most common causes of conjunctivitis in childhood?*
   Conjunctivitis is usually caused by infection or allergy. It is frequently referred to as *pinkeye* and is the most common acute eye disorder seen by pediatricians and pediatric nurse practitioners. Conjunctivitis may be viral or, more commonly, bacterial.
2. *What are the characteristics of an infectious conjunctivitis?*
   Typically, in bacterial conjunctivitis, the eye is very red and there is a sticky, light-colored discharge. The affected child is preschool-age and may also have an ear infection.
3. *Why does it matter if the cause is viral or bacterial?*
   Viral conjunctivitis does not require antimicrobial eyedrops or eye ointment treatment. The child should not receive prolonged periods of topical treatment if the cause is viral.
4. *What is the treatment for bacterial conjunctivitis?*
   The pediatrician or nurse practitioner will order antibiotic treatment to speed healing and kill the bacteria. Children can return to daycare centers and schools within 24 hours of treatment. The child should have both eyes treated even if only one eye appears red. Treatment with eyedrops is usually needed four times a day for no more than 5 days.
5. *What should I do at home for my child's bacterial conjunctivitis?*
   It is most important to finish all of the antibiotic eyedrop or ointment treatment. Make sure you wash your hands before and after applying the medication to the child's eyes. Remember, the infection is contagious. Applying warm, moist compresses to the child's eyes will help with the removal of the pus drainage and will feel soothing. Use a separate cloth for each eye and do

Patient Teaching Guidelines—cont'd

not reuse the cloth again without thoroughly washing it in hot water. Throw away any tissues the child uses, make sure that siblings or others in the home do not have contact with the cloths used for cleaning the infected eye, and wipe down counters and surfaces with a disinfectant cleaner. Encourage the child and everyone else in the family to wash their hands frequently.

6. *How do I apply the eyedrops or eye ointment?*
Applying eyedrops or ointment four times a day for up to 5 days can be a battle between you and your child. Try to get help from another adult. One adult holds the child and helps to lean the child's head back; the other adult opens the eyelid with one hand while instilling the medication with the other hand. The child will blink, sometimes excessively. Do not let the child rub the eyes after the instillation. Do not let the medication bottle tip touch the child's eyes because this may hurt and may contaminate the medication bottle. If possible, have the child lie down for a minute or two with the eyes closed. The entire medication dose must be completed unless instructed otherwise by the health-care provider.

Call your child's health-care provider IMMEDIATELY if you notice any of the following:

• The child's outer eyelids have become very red or swollen.
• The child reports that their vision has become blurred or changes in any way.
• The child has a fever, vomits, or starts acting very sick.

Safety *Stat!*

Contact Lenses and Eye Infections

If the child usually wears contact lenses, make sure that they wear glasses until the infection is gone and the health-care provider says it is safe to return to the use of the contacts. Do not allow the child to apply eye makeup. Throw away mascara if the child has used it during the infection.

Neonatorum Eye Infections

Also called *neonatal conjunctivitis* or *ophthalmia neonatorum*, this type of eye infection occurs as a newborn passes through the birth canal of a mother infected with either *Neisseria gonorrhoeae* or *Chlamydia trachomatis*. Treatment includes eyedrops containing erythromycin. It is imperative that you teach the family to cleanse the eyes of the infant with a clean cloth soaked in warm water. The cloth must not be reused, or reinfection may occur. If a neonatorum eye infection is left untreated, the infant may experience complete blindness.

Nursing Considerations for a Child With a Visual Impairment

Children of all ages who experience a congenital, a primary, or an acquired visual impairment need support and education. A traumatic event that leads to the sudden loss of vision affects the child both emotionally and developmentally. It is important to provide special care based on the cause of the visual impairment and the child's developmental needs. Children who suddenly lose their vision from a traumatic injury or accident need support when initially learning that they are going to be impaired. For the child who presents with significant eye trauma, a large health-care team may be assembled. This team may include the nursing supervisor; the hospital spiritual advisor; the child life specialist; and representatives from social services, child psychology, pediatric ophthalmology, and pediatric surgical services. These team members will be able to provide support to the child and family, rapid assessments, and interventions.

If a child is going home after eye surgery with bilateral eye dressings in place, the family should be instructed to create a safe home environment. Removing clutter, placing needed objects within reach of the child, providing verbal guidance for moving around the home, and supervising the child in activities of daily living are all important to secure safety.

Therapeutic Communication

Families who present to the pediatric health-care setting with a child who has just suffered a traumatic loss of vision or hearing need special support. The fear and anxiety associated with the potential loss of vision or hearing is profound, and each member of the family needs support. The health-care team can support the family in the following ways:

• Acknowledge each family member's feelings.
• Request backup from other members of the nursing staff in order to stay with the family.
• Provide presence; do not walk away unless necessary.
• Allow the parents to express their feelings, ask questions, and feel supported.

Evidence-Based Practice

A New Kind of Eye Patch

Eye patches and implants made from human placenta are being used to treat eye trauma and disease ranging from corneal abrasions to acute ocular burns. This serves as a new form of regenerative medicine. These dressings have been shown to reduce pain and promote wound healing. The innermost lining of the placenta (the amnion) contains growth factors, and a disc of this tissue is placed directly onto the damaged area of the eye. These patches can be

Continued

Evidence-Based Practice—cont'd

either grafts or temporary patches. Amniotic (placental) patches have been shown to increase tissue growth and promote new blood vessel formation.

Churchill, J. (2018). *Sight restored with placenta tissue.* American Academy of Ophthalmology. https://www.aao.org/eye-health/patient-stories -detail/jeff-workplace-chemical-burn; Klama-Baryła, A., Rojczyk, E., Kitala, D., Łabuś, W., Smętek, W., Wilemska-Kucharzewska, K., & Kucharzewski, M. (2020 April). Preparation of placental tissue transplants and their application in skin wound healing and chosen skin bullous diseases—Stevens-Johnson syndrome and toxic epidermal necrolysis treatment. *International Wound Journal, 17*(2), 491–507. https://doi.org /10.1111/iwj.13305; Nejad, A. R., Hamidieh, A. A., Amirkhani, M. A., & Sisakht, M. M. (2021). Update review on five top clinical applications of human amniotic membrane in regenerative medicine, *Placenta, 103,* 104–119. https://doi.org/10.1016/j.placenta.2020.10.026; Pogozhykh, O., Prokopyuk, V., Figueiredo, C., & Pogozhykh, D. (2018, January 18). Placenta and placental derivatives in regenerative therapies: Experimental studies, history, and prospects. *Stem Cells International,* 4837930. https://doi.org/10.1155/2018/4837930.

After recovering from eye surgery or treatments, a child may benefit from various assistive devices. There are six general forms of assistive devices available for a child with a visual impairment within a health-care setting:

- Signage and information presented about Braille
- Information and books in large print suitable for the individual child's need
- Audio recordings
- Computer speech output and speech recognition
- Computer screen readers that enlarge print
- Adaptive keyboards

DISORDERS OF THE EYE

During childhood, disorders of the eye are generally uncommon. Some, such as **retinoblastoma**, are very uncommon, whereas others, such as ROP, are becoming more common.

Retinoblastoma

When a child suffers from a cancerous tumor of the eye, **retinoblastoma** (a malignant tumor of the retina) must be ruled out. The retina is made up of nerve tissue that senses light as it comes through the lens, and then sends visual signals to the brain via the optic nerve. In approximately half of all cases of retinoblastoma, a gene mutation causes a tumor of the retina to grow in a child with no family history of eye cancer. Generally affecting children between the ages of 1 and 2 years, this cancer presents with a whitish glow when light falls on the retina of the affected eye. The phenomenon is known as **leukocoria**, also called cat's eye reflex. Other

· **WORD** · **BUILDING** ·

retinoblastoma: retino–retina + blast–sprout [immature cells] + oma–tumor

leukocoria: leuko–white + cor–pupil + ia–condition

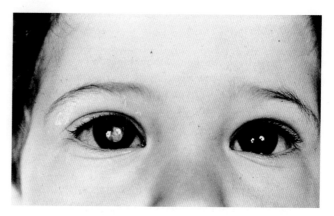

FIGURE 28.2 Retinoblastoma.

symptoms that the child may present with include double vision, "crossed eyes," misalignment, eye pain, redness, and overall visual impairment. Retinoblastoma may affect one or both eyes (Fig. 28.2).

Assessments for the presence of retinoblastoma include dilation of the pupil with an eye evaluation. A magnetic resonance image (MRI) or computed tomography (CT) scan will be ordered to evaluate for the presence of metastasis, especially around the bony orbit.

Treatment of retinoblastoma is dependent on the stage of the cancer. Treatment includes laser surgery or **cryotherapy** for small tumors. Radiation, chemotherapy, laser coagulation to seal off bleeding vessels, and possibly **enucleation** (eye removal) may be warranted for aggressive or larger tumors. If the tumor spreads to the bones around the eye or to the brain via the optic nerve, more aggressive therapy is needed to control the metastasis. As long as there is no evidence of the cancer spreading beyond the retina, the cure rate for early retinoblastoma is very high. In fact, 5-year survival rates are as high as 95%, depending on tumor invasiveness and metastasis (Cancer.net, 2019), with global survival rates ranging from 79% to 88% (Wong et al., 2022).

Retinopathy of Prematurity

First diagnosed in 1942, ROP is an eye disease of the premature infant with the potential of blindness. When an infant is born prematurely, the retina is not fully vascularized. At birth, the development of normal blood vessels stops, and abnormal vessels begin to proliferate. These abnormal retinal blood vessels branch excessively, are fragile, and are numerous. Because of the vessels' fragility, small hemorrhages may occur, leading to scarring. Sometimes, the vessels extend into the vitreous humor. The scarring process pulls the retina away from the basement membranes, resulting in impaired vision or blindness in the infant. Premature infants exposed to too much supplemental oxygen for too long are at risk for developing ROP, with infants born weighing less than

· **WORD** · **BUILDING** ·

cryotherapy: cryo–cold + therapy–treatment

1,250 g at the greatest risk. Approximately 1,400 to 1,500 premature infants, or 10% of 14,000 premature infants born annually, will develop ROP (Childrenshospital.org, 2025; National Eye Institute, 2022).

Assessment for the presence and severity of ROP begins with an eye examination, often performed in the neonatal intensive care unit (NICU). The examination determines the location of the disease within three zones: zone 1 extends from the center of the retina, and zones 2 and 3 extend around and out from zone 1. The examination also gauges the severity of the disease from stage 1 to stage 5. A child determined to be in stage 1 or 2 is not blind, but progression of the disease can occur.

Preventing ROP begins with the judicious use of supplemental oxygen and very careful monitoring of newborns receiving oxygen therapy. Using transcutaneous measurement devices and starting with low-flow oxygen therapy have been found to decrease the incidence and severity of ROP. Anemia, respiratory distress, and blood transfusions also contribute to the development of ROP.

Recent research has demonstrated that oxygen levels in excess of 40% are most concerning in the development of ROP. Furthermore, the absence of protective measures to reduce premature newborns' exposure to light also contributes to the development and severity of ROP. Careful administration of oxygen, early screening, and rapid interventions are required to reduce the incidence and severity of ROP. Although the cause of ROP is still not fully understood, the goal is to prevent the newborn from developing early ROP. A 52% reduction in ROP has been found when the pediatric team targets oxygen saturations between 70% and 96% (Owen & Hartnett, 2014).

Treatment for ROP consists of cryotherapy and laser treatments for zones 1 to 3. Scleral buckling (silicone banding of the eye to prevent the vitreous from pulling on the sclera) and vitrectomy (removal of the vitreous humor and replacement with saline so that scar tissue can be peeled back or removed) are also used. Vitrectomy is recommended for both of the infant's eyes whenever ROP is stage 3 or higher (American Association for Pediatric Ophthalmology and Strabismus [AAPOS], 2020).

In most infants with ROP, the disease spontaneously subsides. However, premature infants with severe forms of ROP may have complete and permanent blindness.

Patient Teaching Guidelines

National Organizations That Provide Support for Children With Visual Impairments

Part of the nurse's teaching for parents of children with visual impairments is to acquaint them with resources that are available to support them and their child. Families may find the following organizations helpful:

- *Lions Clubs International:* Information on free eyeglasses, regional and local visual screening tests (low cost or free)
- *National Association for Parents of Children With Visual Impairments:* Information on different visual disorders and pathologies
- *American Printing House for the Blind:* Information on providing written materials for the blind
- *American Council of the Blind:* Information for families with a blind child; resources and educational materials

---

 ## THE DEVELOPMENT OF HEARING

The sense of hearing begins during week 18 of gestation with intact hearing acuity achieved between weeks 22 and 23. The sounds of the mother's heart, digestion, blood flow, and other normal anatomical sounds are heard by the fetus. Research has shown that the fetus, starting at approximately 18 weeks' gestation, even with sounds muffled from amniotic fluid, demonstrates movement when exposed to sound; by weeks 27 to 29, the fetus responds to voices and noises (Shu, 2021).

Structures of the Ear

The human ear (Fig. 28.3) is anatomically somewhat simpler than the eye; it processes sound through six steps. Disease, damage, infection, or inflammation to any part of the internal ear can cause hearing impairment. The steps in the process of hearing are these:

1. Sound waves enter the outer ear and pass through the ear canal.
2. The eardrum vibrates and sends the vibrations to the three ear bones (malleus, incus, and stapes).
3. These bones change the sound vibrations to fluid vibrations in the cochlea of the inner ear.
4. A wave forms along the basilar membrane and travels inward, and the inner ear hair cells (sensory cells) then respond to the wave.
5. The tiny hairlike projections on top of the hair cells move in an up-and-down motion and hit the overlying structures. This process changes the motion into an electrical signal.
6. The electrical signal then is sent via the auditory nerve to the brain for processing and recognition.

 ## HEARING IMPAIRMENT

Hearing impairments, one of the most common disabilities in the nation, are categorized as any condition that interferes with the child's ability to receive auditory information from the environment or verbal communications taking place around them. The incidence of hearing impairments is estimated to be one to three out of every 1,000 well infants (CDC, 2022c). Causes of hearing loss include prematurity, high serum bilirubin levels requiring blood

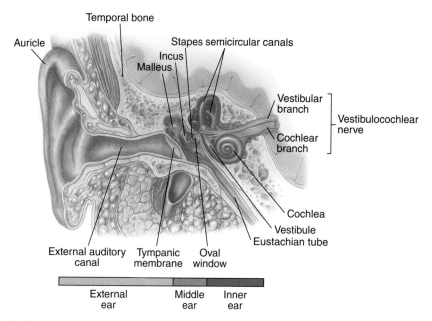

FIGURE 28.3 Structure of the human ear.

transfusion, **ototoxic** medications (both direct exposure and fetal exposure), meningitis, family history of hearing impairment, frequent **otitis media** (OM), and time spent in ICU settings.

Noise-induced hearing loss (NIHL) in childhood can be caused by exposure to loud noises, such as while hunting, snowmobiling, attending concerts, and listening to loud music with earbuds. Using noise-reduction devices such as earplugs and over-the-ear headphones rather than earbuds can help prevent NIHL (CDC, 2022b).

Patient Teaching Guidelines

Preventing Noise-Induced Hearing Loss

NIHL is the only type of hearing loss that can be prevented. Nurses must teach children and families prevention practices, such as:

- Knowing what noises can produce hearing impairments (loud and sustained)
- Wearing protective devices made to reduce sound, such as earplugs, earmuffs, and headphones
- Reducing exposure to loud and sustained sounds; stepping back and away from loud sounds such as amplifiers
- Preventing exposures to harmful sounds; being aware of potential sources
- Protecting the ears of children too young to protect their own ears
- Participating in hearing screening

· WORD · BUILDING ·

ototoxic: oto–ear + toxic–poisonous
otitis: ot–ear + itis–inflammation

Three Main Types of Hearing Impairment

Children can present with one of three distinct types of hearing loss: conductive, sensorineural, and combined. The following list describes the differences among the three.

- *Conductive hearing loss:* This condition interferes with the ability of the child to receive auditory communications from the child's environment; this occurs when the tympanic membrane cannot vibrate after sound passes through the ear canal. Cerumen buildup, OM, or foreign bodies can all be the causes of conductive hearing loss.
- *Sensorineural hearing loss:* This condition is directly related to damage to the auditory nerve or the cochlea. This condition may be congenital, such as with rubella syndrome, or acquired, such as exposure to ototoxic medications. The damage to the eighth cranial nerve causes the inner ear to malfunction.
- *Combined conductive/sensorineural hearing loss:* Also called *mixed hearing loss,* this condition involves the combination of conductive and sensorineural hearing loss.

Medication Facts

Exposure to ototoxic medications, such as the antibiotic category of aminoglycosides, can be a significant source of hearing impairments. When administering aminoglycosides, the pediatric health-care team must administer the medication within the safe dose range. Repeated blood tests of the serum levels of the antibiotic (peaks and troughs) help to ensure that the child is not exposed to toxic quantities of the medication. Other ototoxic medications include the chemotherapy medication cisplatin and certain IV diuretics, such as furosemide, when pushed too rapidly.

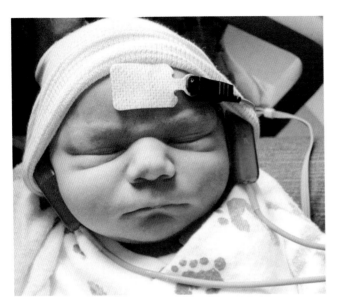

FIGURE 28.4 Newborn having a hearing screening test.

Sustained or repeated sounds of 85 decibels (the loudness of a snowblower) or above are likely to cause hearing damage. Older children who listen to music through earbuds at full volume are exposed to approximately 105 decibels, which damages the inner ear structures. The louder the sound in decibels, the shorter period is required to cause significant hearing damage. Earplugs or over-the-ear protective devices (earmuffs) should be worn during sustained exposure to loud sounds to prevent hearing damage.

New treatments for hearing loss may come from gene therapy. Research on the genes that are important to sensory hair cell development and the functions of these cells continues. In addition, researchers are investigating how to increase the protective properties of the inner ear cells (National Institute on Deafness and Other Communication Disorders [NIDCD], 2022).

Assessments of Hearing Impairment and Ear Structures

Hearing screening should begin early to promote optimal development for the infant (Fig. 28.4). Hearing impairments can interfere with a young child's ability to talk and can limit their interaction with others. Visual inspection and audiography should both be performed to rule out any hearing impairment.

Hearing acuity is often expressed in a unit of sound called a *decibel*. See Box 28.2 for a summary of the intensity of sounds as measured by decibels. If a child is unable to hear at a certain level of decibels, then they are considered hearing impaired up to that number.

• WORD • BUILDING •
decibel: deci–one tenth + bel–a unit of sound

Box 28.2
Sound Intensity Expressed as Decibels

0 = Softest sound a healthy, normal human ear can hear
10 = Sound of a heartbeat or the rustling of leaves
20 = Sound of a person whispering at 5 feet away
30–45 = Normal conversation between two people
60 = Noise found at a typical restaurant
70 = Noise found on a typical city street
80 = Sound of a loud radio played inside a room
90–100 = Sound of a passing train
105 = Sound of music through earbuds at full volume
120 = Sound of loud music (inside rock concert) or the sound of thunder
125 = Sound of sirens up close
140 = Sound of a jet plane taking off while standing nearby
150 = Sounds of firecrackers and firearms at close range
Greater than 140 decibels is the human pain threshold.

Visual assessment of a child's ears should begin during early well-child checkups during infancy. When visualizing the tympanic membrane of children under 3 years of age, the pinna should be pulled straight out and down. For children older than 3 years, the pinna should be pulled straight out and up. These positions allow for the maximal visualization of the eardrum.

Early infant behaviors indicating hearing impairment include the lack of a startle reflex to loud noises. If an infant does not turn their head to identify a noise, a hearing impairment should be suspected. For toddlers and preschoolers, a hearing impairment should be suspected if the child participates in gestures to communicate needs and has little or no speech or if speech is garbled and unintelligible. School-aged children and adolescents who sit closer than expected to speakers, turn the TV louder than others, or who demonstrate declining school performance and fewer social interactions should be worked up for an acquired hearing impairment.

Many states now require mandatory newborn hearing screening. Before a newborn is discharged from the hospital, a screening procedure takes place while the infant sleeps. Electrodes are placed on the neonate's scalp and mandible. Light sounds are transmitted via headphones, and brain electrical activity is assessed. If the newborn is not screened before discharge, screening can take place during a well-neonate visit.

Nursing Considerations for a Child With a Hearing Impairment

Pediatric nurses provide holistic care to a child with a hearing impairment. Providing technology that increases the child's acoustic processing and understanding of what is going on around them is very important. When prescribed, you should provide positive reinforcement for wearing hearing aids. Anticipatory guidance should include protecting the child from harm; caring for utilized hearing assistive devices; and promoting a normal childhood with play, socialization, and academics.

Patient Teaching Guidelines

It is imperative that children wear devices that are pre-scribed and made for them to enhance their sensory experiences. Wearing hearing aids at all times when awake and keeping a child's prescription glasses on enhances development and improves socialization and academic success.

DISORDERS OF THE EAR

Several disorders of the ear are common in pediatrics. Some disorders are congenital defects, and others are acquired. The following represent select common disorders of the ear found in children.

Buildup of Cerumen

Cerumen, or earwax, is a natural substance produced within the auditory canal to provide an antibacterial action. Cerumen can be produced in a variety of colors from golden, light yellow to a dark brown. Often quite viscous, earwax can build up in some children and be a contributing factor to hearing impairments. Upon inspection, a wall of earwax may be noted. The wax needs to be gently removed by irrigation with warm tap water or carefully removed with an earwax removal tool by a trained health-care professional.

Safety *Stat!*

Neither parents nor children should ever try to remove earwax by using any instrument, including pencils, sticks, or any sharp object, in the ear; this may perforate the tympanic membrane. The use of commercially made earwax removal devices remains controversial.

If a family seeks consultation for cerumen buildup, an over-the-counter (OTC) product for earwax removal may be successful in cleaning out simple accumulation. The family should be instructed to have the child lie down with the affected ear up, and then instill the prescribed number of drops per the product label. A cotton ball can be placed in the auricle of the ear to prevent rapid drainage of the medication. If an OTC medication is not successful in cleansing the ear, then a trained health-care professional should be notified and the child should be brought in for irrigation.

Otitis Media

Otitis media (OM) is a viral or bacterial infection that causes the buildup of inflammatory fluids or pus behind the tympanic membrane. OM is often accompanied by discomfort

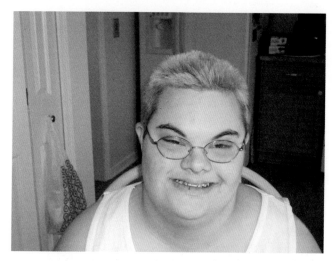

FIGURE 28.5 Children and adolescents with Down syndrome are more at risk for ear infections.

and is one of the most common childhood illnesses, with the greatest incidence between 6 and 36 months of age. The most common cause of conductive hearing loss is multiple episodes of OM. Young children have a greater slant in their eustachian tubes that can collect fluids and contribute to the development of OM. Parents need to understand that as their child grows, the angle and position of the eustachian tube will change, facilitating drainage and decreasing the repeated episodes of OM.

The pathology behind OM is a dysfunction within the eustachian tube. The eustachian tube is meant to provide drainage and ventilation of the middle ear. If a child is experiencing an upper respiratory infection, the eustachian tube becomes edematous and blocked. The trapped fluids act as a medium for bacterial growth and viral multiplication, and a middle ear infection develops. Children who are born with malformations of the head and neck are more susceptible to episodes of OM. Both dysfunction in the immune system of a child with Down syndrome (Fig. 28.5) and the abnormal anatomical structure of the child's face contribute to more frequent ear infections (Sacks & Wood, in Library.down -syndrome.org, 2023).

Infants who fall asleep with a bottle in the mouth can have a collection of fluids enter the eustachian tube and contribute to the development of OM.

Common causative organisms for OM include *Moraxella catarrhalis, Haemophilus influenzae,* and *Streptococcus pneumoniae.* OM with effusions is the buildup of fluid or pus behind the tympanic membrane. OM without effusions is the presence of inflammation within the inner ear without the presence of fluid or pus.

Signs of OM in an infant include irritability, pulling at ears, hitting the side of the head, diarrhea, vomiting, and fever; however, some children are asymptomatic. A confirmed diagnosis comes from visual inspection with an

CRITICAL THINKING

Scenario #2: You are teaching a well-child class for first-time parents and explaining that a lack of a complete set of childhood immunizations is associated with the development of one or more bouts of OM. The parents ask for more information.

Questions

1. Why would unvaccinated children experience more of these ear infections?
2. How would you educate the group of new parents about preventing OM?

otoscope to identify a red, bulging, and nonmobile tympanic membrane. Treatment for an ear infection may or may not include oral antibiotics. If the physician identifies the infection as being viral in nature, then the child's symptoms will be addressed, but no antimicrobial treatment will be offered.

Repeated OM may require surgical interventions. The placement of tympanostomy tubes through a procedure called a myringotomy can be performed in a day-surgery setting. The surgeon makes an incision into the eardrum and places a small tube. The tube allows the fluid to drain, reducing the pressure that is causing discomfort. Parents need to understand that the tubes will come out on their own; no surgical removal of the tubes is necessary. Typical preoperative care includes teaching the family about the operative process, anesthesia, and the reduction of symptoms after the fluids and pressure are released by the tubes. Postoperative care instructions include the signs and symptoms of ongoing infection, reporting of postoperative fevers, and

Medication Facts

Tinnitis, or the experience of abnormal sounds (humming, roaring, ringing, whistling, buzzing, and whooshing), can be caused by prolonged loud music exposure, smoking, and severe anemia. But it is also associated with ototoxic medications. Ototoxic medications can also cause balance and vestibular dysfunction. The six categories of ototoxic medications are as follows:

- Pain medications for select patients
- Antibiotics such as aminoglycosides
- Salicylates such as aspirin
- Loop diuretics such as furosemide
- Quinine
- Platinum-based chemotherapy

· WORD · BUILDING ·

otoscope: oto–ear + scope–instrument for viewing

understanding that the tubes will fall out on their own. Securing follow-up appointments after surgery is also an important part of teaching.

Nursing Considerations for Otitis Media

For children who have repeated episodes of OM that require tympanostomy tube placement, parents may need to be taught to use earplugs to prevent bath water or pool water from entering the ears.

A sudden relief of pain associated with OM may mean that the tympanic membrane has ruptured and the pressure buildup behind the eardrum has been relieved. You should assist the health-care provider to look in the auditory canal for drainage and carefully remove it.

One of the most important components of nursing education concerning OM is explaining to the parents that if the infection is bacterial, they must administer the entire dose of antibiotics. Some prescriptions are for 5 days, and others may be for 10 to 14 days of therapy.

If the health-care provider diagnoses the child with viral OM, then the parents need to understand that antibiotics will not be effective in treating the infection. Whether the OM is from a viral or a bacterial infection, children can be given an antipyretic and anti-inflammatory to reduce symptoms of pressure and discomfort.

You should teach families about the association of smoking and increased incidence of OM, the protective factor of breastfeeding, and the impact of reducing early introduction of formula on the reduction of cases of acute OM (Al-Nawaiseh et al., 2022).

OVERALL NURSING CONSIDERATIONS FOR A CHILD WITH A SENSORY IMPAIRMENT

The sudden onset of a child's sensory impairment may cause stress in the family's functioning. When a child loses hearing or sight or suffers from significant sensory loss, the family may experience a sense of loss about the child's productive future. It is important to determine the family's coping skills and ensure that there is a referral made to a mental health professional who can assist the family in coping. The child should never be socially isolated or kept from experiencing a healthy, stimulating childhood with socialization, cultural involvement, and play. Communication skills and self-help skills must be fostered, and parents need to be encouraged to "let go" and allow their child to develop independent skills.

Preventing a sensory impairment is the most important aspect of the nursing care of high-risk children. Teaching families and children of all ages how to protect their sensory organs should begin in early educational levels; reinforcement of information should continue throughout adolescence.

Patient Teaching Guidelines

Tympanoplasty

Tympanoplasty (ear-tube placement) is usually offered in an outpatient or short-stay surgery environment.

Preoperative Guidelines:

- Your child will be given anesthesia before the procedures and must not eat or drink after midnight the day before (but follow specific institutional policy). Any preoperative fevers, infections, cough, or respiratory infections must be reported to the surgical department. Any allergies the child may have should be reported.

In the immediate postoperative period, the child may experience:

- Mild pain in the ear and neck
- Drainage from the ear for 48 hours

Guidelines for home care after tube insertion include the following:

- Avoid getting water in the ear; be careful while bathing.
- No swimming until cleared by the surgical team.
- If the ear drains pus or if the drainage has an odor, report this finding to your health-care provider immediately.
- Follow instructions for using eardrops and complete the entire amount of the prescription as directed, even if the child feels better.
- Use acetaminophen for postoperative pain.
- Resume normal activities the day after surgery.
- If the tubes fall out or if there is increased discomfort in the ear, call your health-care provider.

Nursing Care Plan for the Child With a Sensory Impairment: Sudden Hearing Loss and Care in the Hospital

A 10-year-old boy has been admitted to the hospital for the drainage of bilateral abscesses adjacent to his tympanic membrane after several unsuccessful courses of antibiotics, including a course of an aminoglycoside antibiotic, which is known to be ototoxic. The child, now NPO (nothing by mouth) and awaiting surgery with his family, shows a noticeable hearing deficit. The child's physician makes a referral to a pediatric ears, nose, and throat (ENT) specialist.

Nursing Diagnosis: Sensory-perceptual alteration as evidenced by noticeable hearing deficit
Expected Outcome: The patient will regain some or all auditory function.

Intervention:	Rationale:
Immediately report patient's hearing loss to health-care provider.	*Aminoglycosides are a potentially ototoxic antibiotic medication, so the health-care provider will likely discontinue the medication and order a different one for the postoperative period.*

Nursing Diagnosis: Risk of injury related to decreased auditory cues of the environment
Expected Outcome: The patient's safety is maintained throughout the hospital stay.

Intervention:	Rationale:
You will identify safety issues for the child while he is in the hospital such as informing the child of the presence of a fire alarm.	*The child may not be able to hear hospital alarms.*

National organizations can assist the family in adapting to a child's sensory impairment and provide professional and peer support. These organizations include the following:

- National Federation of the Blind
- National Association for Visually Handicapped
- American Council of the Blind
- National Association for Parents of Children With Visual Impairments
- National Institute on Deafness and Other Communication Disorders (NIDCD)

Key Points

- Early identification of a visual or hearing impairment allows for interventions to be initiated that provide for speech development, socialization, and academic success.
- Nurses need to support and participate in national efforts to screen all early school-aged children for hearing and visual acuity and enable children to secure a referral for interventions and/or treatments.
- The most common cause of hearing impairment is conductive hearing loss, and it is associated with repeated cases of OM that lead to scarring.
- Routine vision screening is an important part of a well-child visit, even when the child is an infant. Many visual abnormalities are treatable or correctable if they are discovered early and promptly.
- Common reactions when a family is told that their infant or young child will have a sensory impairment include fear and anxiety. These reactions can be profound, and each member of the family needs interdisciplinary team support.
- Screening efforts are important during childhood so that visual and auditory impairments can be found early. Common vision screening techniques include the Snellen test, LEA symbols, and the unilateral cover test. Newborn hearing screening, which is mandated in many states, also allows for early identification of hearing impairments.
- Eye infections are common in children and include viral or bacterial conjunctivitis and ophthalmic neonatorum. Families need to learn specific care techniques to prevent the spread of eye infections.
- Retinoblastoma generally affects children between the ages of 1 and 2 years; this cancer presents with a whitish glow as light falls on the affected eye's retina.
- ROP is an eye disease of the premature infant. ROP causes a scarring process that pulls the retina away from the basement membranes, resulting in impaired vision or blindness. Excessive and prolonged supplemental oxygen use in premature babies and a birth weight of less than 1,250 g are associated with the development of ROP.
- A traumatic event that leads to the sudden loss of sensory processing affects the child both emotionally and developmentally. It is important to provide special care based on the cause of the impairment and the child's developmental needs.
- Children who suddenly lose their vision or hearing based on traumatic injury or accident need support when first learning that they are going to have a permanent impairment.

Review Questions

1. While inspecting the ears of a 2-year-old for possible OM, how should you pull the pinna for maximal visual evaluation of the tympanic membrane?
   1. Up and out
   2. Down and out
   3. Do not pull at all
   4. Straight out

2. What are the most common causes of ROP?
   1. Bright lights and prematurity
   2. Bright lights and oxygen therapy
   3. Oxygen therapy and loud noises
   4. Prematurity and oxygen therapy

3. What is the name of the visual appearance of the retina in a child with a confirmed retinoblastoma?
   1. Opacity reflex
   2. Cataract opacity
   3. Cat's eye reflex
   4. Cloudy reflex

4. While teaching new parents about the need to protect their premature infant's hearing in the NICU setting, which of the following would be included in the teaching session?
   1. Keep the noise level down to prevent the startle reflex.
   2. Keep the isolette covered with blankets to prevent exposure to sensory stimulation.
   3. Monitor the infant's temperature to check for a fever.
   4. Immediately notify a nurse if you hear your infant's IV or cardiorespiratory (CR) monitor's alarm.

5. What is one of the most effective means to prevent a hearing impairment during early childhood?
   1. Participate in school screenings for hearing deficits.
   2. Participate in well-child checkups throughout childhood.
   3. Ensure that the child has all immunizations.
   4. Ensure that the child completes the full prescription of antibiotics for OM.

6. Why do infants and young children have a higher risk for OM than older children do?
   1. Their genetic immune dysfunction
   2. The natural sugars that are present in milk, formula, and breast milk
   3. The anatomical location of the eustachian tubes
   4. The natural slant of the eustachian tube

7. The sticky natural substance that is found in the outer ear canal is called _____.

8. What are the most common pathological microbes associated with pediatric OM? (**Select all that apply.**)
   1. *M. catarrhalis*
   2. *H. influenza*
   3. *S. pneumoniae*
   4. *Corynebacterium diphtheriae*
   5. *Staphylococcus*

9. While reinforcing teaching to parents of young children, the licensed vocational nurse (LVN) describes the importance of completing all childhood immunizations. Which immunization is especially important in preventing OM?
   1. Pertussis vaccine
   2. PCV
   3. Rubella vaccine
   4. Mumps vaccine

10. The signs and symptoms of OM in an infant include which of the following? (**Select all that apply.**)
    1. Irritability
    2. Pulling at the ears
    3. Hitting the side of the head
    4. Diarrhea
    5. Vomiting
    6. Fever

ANSWERS 1. 2; 2. 4; 3. 4; 4. 1; 5. 3; 6. 4; 7. Cerumen; 8. 1, 2, 3; 9. 2; 10. 1, 2, 3, 4, 5, 6

CRITICAL THINKING QUESTIONS

1. What is the relationship between a young child not having their immunization requirements completed and the development of hearing impairment? Which childhood infectious or communicable diseases contribute to the risk for or actual development of a hearing impairment?
2. Fully immunized children are at less risk for repeated episodes of OM and the hearing impairment that may result from it. Given that fact, should childhood vaccinations be mandatory? Why or why not?
3. What are the controversies around the national recommendations concerning the prescription of antibiotics for a young child with OM?

Resources

For additional resources and information, including Postconference Questions and Activities, Answers, and References, visit www.FADavis.com.

Student Study Guide

CHAPTER 29
Child With a Mental Health Condition

KEY TERMS

addiction (uh-DIK-shun)
depression (dih-PRESH-uhn)
lethality of attempt (lee-THAL-ih-tee uv uh-TEMPT)
mental illness (MEN-tuhl IL-niss)
neuroleptic (NOO-ruh-LEP-tik)
neurotransmitter (NOO-roh-trans-MIT-uhr)
nonsuicide self-injury (NSSI) (NON-SOO-ih-syed SELF-IN-juh-ree)
schizophrenia (SKIT-suh-FREE-nee-uh)
suicidal gesture (soo-ih-SYE-duhl JESS-chur)
suicidal ideation (soo-ih-SYE-duhl eye-dee-AY-shun)
suicidal thinking (soo-ih-SYE-duhl THING-king)
suicide (SOO-ih-syed)
suicide attempt (SOO-ih-SYED uh-TEMPT)
tardive dyskinesia (TAR-div DIS-kih-NEE-zhuh)

CHAPTER CONCEPTS

Addiction
Cognition
Growth and Development
Mood and Affect
Safety
Self

LEARNING OUTCOMES

1. Define the key terms.
2. Describe current trends in the incidence and prevalence of mental health issues across the span of childhood.
3. Analyze the effect of a mental health diagnosis on the child's interactions with family, school, social networks, and society as a whole.
4. State the goals for therapeutic communication between you and the child and/or family during an acute phase of a mental health condition.
5. Describe commonly used evaluation tools for anxiety, depression, and mood disorders.
6. Analyze the effect of a diagnosis of attention deficit-hyperactivity disorder (ADHD) on a child's interaction with family and school.
7. Describe the clinical presentation and pharmacological management of schizophrenia in childhood.
8. Analyze the effect of bullying on a child's well-being and describe the relationship between bullying and childhood depression.
9. Describe the eating disorders of anorexia nervosa, bulimia, obesity, and binge eating without purging, and discuss the evaluation, clinical presentations, and therapeutic management of each.
10. Describe the types of suicide behaviors (gestures, attempts, and successful suicide) and identify the effects of suicide on those left behind.
11. Review the most common categories of medications for the management of a mental health diagnosis in childhood and state the common side effects and therapeutic ranges for each medication.
12. Analyze the development of substance abuse during childhood and identify the consequences and safety factors associated with substance abuse on the child's mental health, family interactions, social network, and school performance.

CRITICAL THINKING & CLINICAL JUDGMENT

You are part of the nursing team at a large after-school program in an urban educational facility and notice that the children attending since the COVID-19 pandemic are reporting more headaches, stomachaches, and generalized "not feeling well." As you care for these children,

Continued

CRITICAL THINKING & CLINICAL JUDGMENT—cont'd

you suspect their symptoms may be related to anxiety. One child you spoke with described how his family is not doing well because neither of his parents have found full-time employment since they lost their jobs in the restaurant industry, the family has experienced homelessness twice, and his aunt died of COVID. Realizing that the impact of the COVID pandemic has been widespread across the children who attend the after-school program, you research how prolonged isolation from quarantine, severe illnesses, fear, economic impact, and housing insecurity because of the pandemic can affect children's mental health.

Questions

1. Why do you suspect the children might be experiencing anxiety based on their physical symptoms?
2. How impactful has the pandemic been on children?
3. What can you do to assist the children who are expressing anxiety and the symptoms associated with anxiety?

CONCEPTUAL CORNERSTONE
Safety

Children who have been diagnosed with a mental health condition face several safety issues. For example, children with mood disorders such as depression and anxiety, or children and teens with eating disorders, are at risk for self-harm. Safety must be in the forefront of the minds of pediatric health-care team members. Any indication of self-harm or suicide risk must be taken seriously, and the child must be provided with a safe environment and immediate referral to a comprehensive psychological support program. Every suicide-related comment or any outward signs of self-harm such as cutting, participation in violence, or suicidal thoughts or attempts must be acted on immediately. Nurses caring for children and teens must also be aware of the phenomenon of **nonsuicide self-injury (NSSI)**. Nurses have the ethical and legal responsibility to provide safety to children with mental health issues; however, not every pediatric health-care setting is set up to provide for the needs of children with mental illness. Knowing what to screen for in all children, what to look for in high-risk children, and when to call for help are important aspects of maintaining safety and securing prompt interventions for children with mental health conditions and illnesses.

About 20% of children in the United States have some form of mental illness or mental health challenge. In any given year, more than 5 million children experience a mental illness that significantly interferes with the daily life of the child and the family. The term *mental illness* is inadequate, however, because significant physical factors can be associated with these disorders. Both heredity and brain chemistry are thought to be involved with the development of a childhood mental disorder.

Because children are naturally going through physical, emotional, and social growth and development, it is important to identify abilities and behaviors that are considered "normal" for the child's age. When ruling out a mental illness, health-care providers must first determine how the child copes with setbacks, adapts to change, and relates to others and the world within the context of developmental stage and age. Because there is not a known single cause of a mental illness, a combination of factors must be investigated. Parenting, family dynamics, heredity, stressors, biological chemistry, and psychological trauma are all common factors. Health-care professionals also need to determine if the behaviors being displayed are causing a significant disruption to the family's and child's life. Tests are then conducted to evaluate for mental illness. When identified early and treated with psychotherapy and medications, many children with a mental illness are able to live full, productive lives.

A significant study by the Centers for Disease Control and Prevention (CDC, 2024) looked at adverse childhood experiences (ACEs) and the impact of childhood trauma on future health, violence victimization, and risky behaviors. ACEs have been further linked to chronic health conditions, risky health behaviors, low life potential, and early death. Higher levels of depression, anxiety, **suicide**, sexually transmitted infections (STIs), substance abuse, and chronic illnesses such as diabetes and cancer have also been associated with ACEs. The longitudinal research findings propose that protective factors (supportive family environment, stable family relationships, access to health care and social services, and communities that support parents and help prevent abuse) can reduce the impact of childhood trauma across the life span.

Racial and ethnic discrimination have also had an impact on the prevalence of mental health issues in children. According to the CDC (2022c), children exposed to discrimination had higher rates of physical (37.8% vs. 27.1%) and mental health concerns (28.9% vs. 17.8%) than those not exposed.

One challenge for health-care professionals is to provide holistic care for a child who presents in an acute phase of a mental disorder. The team needs to quickly identify what the underlying mental diagnosis is, identify the severity of the child's presenting symptoms, intervene appropriately, and then secure follow-up with a mental health expert. Children may present to any health-care setting in an acute phase but will most likely present in an emergency department (ED) or clinic setting. A review of the child's history, medications currently prescribed, precipitating factors, and current mental state are all imperative and require a team approach.

• WORD • BUILDING •
suicide: sui–of oneself + cide–kill

Therapeutic Communication

Establishing rapport with a child who presents with an acute exacerbation of a mental illness or condition is a priority action. Finding strategies that work for the child's ability to communicate is challenging. Without appropriate therapeutic communication techniques, the team will have more challenges with evaluation, diagnosis, and treatment. Just taking vital signs, collecting specimens, administering medications, providing safety, and providing basic care can be challenging during an acute phase of a childhood mental illness.

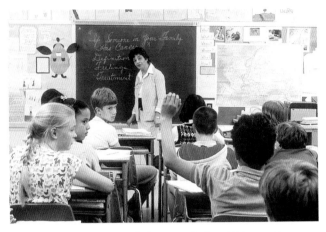

FIGURE 29.1 A structured classroom helps children with ADHD to learn. (Photo from the National Cancer Institute by Michael Anderson.)

Historically, most research in mental health issues has focused on the adult. Researchers are now investigating how factors associated with childhood development may have an effect on the child's mental health. Identifying emotional and behavioral problems across childhood is not an easy or straightforward process. Risk factors, hereditary influences, and medication effectiveness are central issues for continued research.

ATTENTION DEFICIT-HYPERACTIVITY DISORDER

Attention deficit-hyperactivity disorder (ADHD), a neurobehavioral psychiatric disorder, is one of the most common mental disorders diagnosed in both children and adolescents. ADHD persists to adulthood for up to 90% of those diagnosed (Pesantez, 2022; Sibley et al., 2021). So far, research has not been able to determine why the incidence of this disorder is steadily increasing. Children with ADHD have difficulty focusing on schoolwork and activities at home, controlling their behavior (impulsivity), paying attention, and relating to others. Approximately 9.8% of children between 3 and 17 years of age have ADHD, which equates to 6.0 million children (CDC, 2022c).

There continues to be no single test to accurately diagnose ADHD in children (CDC, 2022a). Brain-imaging technology has revealed that ADHD may be associated with how the brain is neurologically wired and physically structured. A significant developmental delay, as much as 3 years, in the frontal cortex is related to ADHD. The frontal cortex normally suppresses inappropriate actions, displays focused attention, and controls moment-by-moment memory. Research continues internationally to determine the intricacies of this disorder and the best treatments across the life span.

To maintain safety for the child with ADHD, members of the health-care team need to understand the types of ADHD so that they can anticipate a child's behavior. This is especially true when the team is attempting a medical procedure or trying to explain important topics to the child while in the clinic or hospital.

There are three main types of ADHD:

- *Predominantly inattentive:* It is challenging for the child to concentrate, finish a task, or follow conversations or academic instructions because they are easily distracted.
- *Predominantly hyperactive-impulsive:* The child struggles to sit still and keep their hands to themself; the child interrupts others frequently and fidgets, squirms, and may talk nonstop.
- *Combined presentation:* This includes behaviors listed in both of the preceding types.

Because ADHD often affects both school and home behaviors, children with this disorder need a combination of therapies. Management includes medications and tools to empower children, such as behavioral, social, educational, psychological, and life interventions (Mayo Clinic, 2021a). Further treatment includes medication with central nervous system (CNS) stimulants and nonstimulant medications (not rapid-acting but last 24 hours; Fig. 29.1).

Evaluating Attention Deficit-Hyperactivity Disorder

According to the *Diagnostic and Statistical Manual of Mental Disorders,* Fifth Edition, Text Revision *(DSM-5-TR),* for a child to be diagnosed with ADHD, they must exhibit a variety of symptoms including fidgeting, forgetfulness, and distraction (APA, 2022).

The preceding symptoms must be present for longer than 6 months' duration. The impairment must be present in at least two settings and must occur before the child's 12th birthday. In making the diagnosis of ADHD, serum lead levels should be checked and phenylketonuria (PKU) and other possible diagnoses should be ruled out (learning impairment, seizure disorder, learning disability, anxiety, poor nutrition over time, autism spectrum disorder (ASD), dyslexia, auditory processing disorder, heightened intelligence, and depression).

Children with ADHD often experience a host of negative feedback about their behaviors. They also often experience impatience from family, teachers, and others who interact with them. Parents need to be taught how to structure the child's day to increase routines and how to give clear instructions and set expectations. Social skills training includes group settings and can focus on problem-solving skills. Psychosocial treatments include behavior modification with positive reinforcements such as a token economy. The child receives a coin or marble to place in a jar for each desired behavior. Once the jar is filled, the child receives a prize or privilege. Token economies can be used for both the home and school environments.

Interventions for Attention Deficit-Hyperactivity Disorder

Many professionals offer parenting suggestions for raising children with ADHD. These include positive parenting, praise for task completion, promotion of creativity and talents, and well-defined life schedules. Interventions for ADHD are generally pharmaceutical in nature. Approximately 62% of children with ADHD are taking medications to help control the symptoms, 47% receive behavior therapy, and 32% receive both medication and behavioral therapy (CDC, 2022c). Alternative and complementary interventions for children with ADHD typically consist of structured and frequent exercise, but the standard of medical care is the use of medications to help the child focus and be successful in school. The following are common medications prescribed for children with ADHD:

- Methylphenidate
- Methylphenidate patch
- Amphetamine mixtures
- Lisdexamfetamine
- Dexmethylphenidate
- Guanfacine
- Atomoxetine

Nursing Considerations for Attention Deficit-Hyperactivity Disorder

Parents need support and education when they have a child with ADHD. When the child is in the hospital, the parents might find controlling the child's behaviors especially challenging because their routines and familiar processes are thrown off. Families should be given education about local and national support groups and organizations that specialize in locating resources and offering ideas for behavior modification. Nurses need patience when a child with ADHD is hospitalized because their symptoms can worsen, leading to mood swings and aggression.

Nurses need to check for the side effects associated with the use of psychostimulant therapy. These include decreased appetite, nervousness, insomnia, weight loss, tics, headaches, and stomachaches. Teach families not to allow their child to consume caffeine or decongestants and instruct them that ADHD medications should never be taken with monoamine oxidase inhibitors (MAOIs), a group of antidepressant medications. If the child is taking pemoline, liver function tests must be conducted because this medication is associated with life-threatening liver failure.

Patient Teaching Guidelines

Parents might express concern about administering medications to help control symptoms of ADHD. It is important to teach the family about the importance of the medications and the side effects. Parents should know that side effects of psychostimulant therapy include restlessness, headache, tremors, fever, blurred vision, and tachycardia. Concerns about these side effects should be addressed to the prescribing health-care provider.

Check if there is a complete multimodal approach to the child's care, including behavior modification; parental education and hands-on training; classroom accommodation; social skills training; and the family's active participation in local, regional, and national organizations.

AUTISM SPECTRUM DISORDER

ASD is a pervasive developmental disorder. The prevalence of ASD is thought to be 1 in 44 children, and autism is more common in boys than in girls with a ratio of 4 to 1 (CDC, 2022b). Research has demonstrated that there is no connection between autism and childhood immunizations (CDC, 2021).

The current definition of ASD encompasses conditions such as Rett syndrome (a brain, communication, motor and growth disorder) and Asperger syndrome (a milder form of autism). There is no known cause for autism, but it is known to exist from birth with early symptoms noted as early as late infancy. Genetics and environment most likely play roles in the development of autism (National Institute of Neurological Disorders, 2024). Autism consistently develops before the child is 30 months of age. The condition is characterized by a pervasive and severe impairment in the child's communication skills and social interactions and may be accompanied by repetitive and restrictive behaviors. The child will not relate comfortably with others and does not want to be touched, cuddled, or comforted by others.

Among children with ASD, 10% have a coexisting chromosomal or genetic condition such as Down syndrome, tuberous sclerosis, or Fragile X syndrome. Of those with ASD, 44% have above average intellect.

Evaluating Autism

The autism spectrum includes children with varying levels of disability from high-functioning "science nerds" to low-functioning nonverbal individuals. The child suspected of having autism should be tested for intelligence because

Safe and Effective Nursing Care

Tips to working with children on the autism spectrum in a health-care setting include the following:

- Minimize touch and explain to the child when touch is needed.
- Give the autistic child time to prepare for the next activity.
- Understand that autistic children may be withdrawn and quiet.
- Acknowledge that autistic children may have trouble with interpersonal relations, including avoiding eye contact and having unusual language disturbances.
- Stress to the parents that the autistic child might feel overwhelmed in a new environment.

many autistic children fall into a functional, cognitively impaired range on conventional psychological tests. An autistic child may present with some or all of the following symptoms and behaviors:

- Minimal interaction with others as well as being withdrawn and needing solitary play; may not respond to their name (Fig. 29.2)
- A desire for very limited touching, cuddling, or molding into the body (clinging or hugging closely or tightly) of their caregivers or family members
- A minimal display of anticipatory behaviors; the child does not respond to acknowledgment of others, such as a parent coming home from work and approaching the child
- Lack of anxiety in a young child when separated from the parent
- The use of peripheral vision instead of focused eye contact and the avoidance of direct eye contact
- Minimal meaningful speech; repetition of words heard over and over, a condition known as **echolalia**

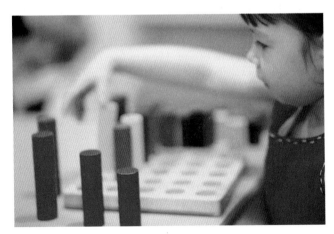

FIGURE 29.2 An autistic child often prefers to play alone.

- Pronoun reversal (mixing up grammar) and nonsensical rhyming
- Possible appearance of being deaf but, in actuality, not having a hearing impairment; may wander off and not hear others calling their name
- Lack of startle responses to some stimuli and heightened responses to others; overall, seeming to lack focus
- The performance of socially awkward or unacceptable self-stimulating behaviors (hand flapping, spinning in circles, striking or biting oneself) as well as repetitive and rhythmic motions such as rocking
- A display of distress and resistance to changes in daily routines
- A marked need for sameness and attachment to an object with tantrumlike rages if routines are disrupted

Interventions for Autism

There are no treatments or cures for autism. It is a lifelong neurological disorder. Therapy should begin at a young age and should focus on speech and language, parent bonding and training, and, if necessary, the securing of a special education classroom with knowledgeable and experienced teachers. Older children and adolescents should have behavioral therapy, psychotherapy, and cognitive therapy; and they may benefit from pharmacotherapy if the associated symptoms of anxiety, depression, or obsessive-compulsive disorder (OCD) are present.

Nursing Considerations for Autism

Nursing care of children with autism can be very challenging. In the hospital, autistic children may become very agitated because their routines are disrupted and they cannot understand their need to be hospitalized. Work with the child one-on-one, giving directions without rationales and minimizing touching to prevent emotional outbursts. The child's environment should be calm and nonstimulating. Be very supportive and empathetic to the parents, who may be distressed over their child's upset behaviors (meltdowns) during hospitalization.

Evidence-Based Practice

Caring for Children With Sensory-Processing Disorders
A visit to the ED can be overwhelming to any child; but to children with ASD, the noise, lights, and fast movements in an ED can be intolerable. Autistic children's distress at the sensory overload makes it much more difficult for health-care personnel to provide care. As a practice-improvement project, nurses in one ED set out to create a sensory-friendly ED. With input from community members and families and referring to current evidence, these nurses modified both the patient-care environment and the patient-flow process in their ED to better accommodate

Continued

• WORD • BUILDING •
echolalia: echo–repeat + lal–talk + ia–condition

Evidence-Based Practice—cont'd

children with ASD (Wood et al., 2019). To prevent what may become a traumatic experience, EDs can become certified autism centers as children with autism are disproportionally seen more frequently as compared with children without autism (International Board of Credentialing and Continuing Education Standards [IBCCES], 2022).

International Board of Credentialing and Continuing Education Standards. (2022). *Autism and the emergency department (ED): Why it's important.* https://ibcces.org/blog/2020/06/05/autism-and-the-emergency-department-ed-why-its-important; Wood, E. B., Halverson, A., Harrison, G., & Rosenkranz, A. (2019, January 21). Creating a sensory-friendly pediatric emergency department. *Journal of Emergency Nursing, 45*(4), 415–424. https://doi.org/10.1016/j.jen.2018.12.002

FEEDING AND EATING DISORDERS

Eating disorders are on the rise in both boys and girls. Eating disorders are serious and may be dangerous or even fatal if not identified early and medically treated. Often, eating disorders are associated with poor self-image, poor self-esteem, and very poor perception of physical self. The *DSM-5-TR* identifies six different types of feeding and eating disorders:

- Anorexia Nervosa (AN)
- Avoidant/Restrictive Food Intake Disorder (ARFID)
- Binge Eating Disorder (BED)
- Bulimia Nervosa (BN)
- Pica
- Rumination Disorder (RD)

Common Eating Disorders

The most common eating disorders are AN, BN, BED with or without purging, ARFID, RD, and pica. The symptoms vary among the various disorders, and there is overlap among them. Select disorders are presented next.

Anorexia Nervosa

The cause of AN is not known. Risk factors include negative self-image, problems eating during infancy, anxiety disorder, abundant focus on rules and achievements, and trying to be "perfect." Those who suffer from this eating disorder have a preoccupation with food, body shape, and weight (National Institute of Mental Health [NIMH], 2016).

AN includes the following main attributes. Children voluntarily refuse to maintain a normal body weight for their age, height, and size and weigh 85% or less of an expected normal weight. They have a tremendous fear of gaining weight, viewing themselves as "fat" even when being significantly underweight. They deny their condition, maintain a disturbingly poor body image, and do not recognize the seriousness of their condition. Girls will experience amenorrhea, the absence of at least three menstrual periods in a row.

Nursing Care Plan for the Adolescent With Anorexia Nervosa

Yvonne, age 14, is an honor student and a varsity athlete on the swim team. Yvonne's mother brings her to the clinic because Yvonne is "looking skinny" and "hasn't had a period in 4 months."

Despite the fact that she weighs only 75% of what would be expected for her age and height, Yvonne insists that she needs "to lose 5 more pounds."

Nursing Diagnosis: Imbalanced nutrition; less than the body's requirements
Expected Outcome: The patient will consume adequate calories on a daily basis to gain weight and have adequate growth by a designated date determined by the medical team.

Interventions:	Rationales:
An interdisciplinary team will meet in conference with family to explain goals of care and discuss the pathology and severity of the eating disorder.	*The patient and family need information to understand the severity of the eating disorder and the importance of following the plan of care.*
Nutritional services and a certified dietitian will construct a meal plan with increasing daily calories until adequate daily calorie consumption is attained.	*Calories need to be added gradually, and a maximum amount of nutrition needs to be present in a small amount of food.*
Nursing staff will ensure that the patient is consuming the recommended diet and not participating in self-induced vomiting after eating or excessive exercising.	*Patients with anorexia are extremely unwilling to gain weight. To mislead family and nursing staff, they may consume food at meals and purge afterward.*
Nursing staff will weigh the patient once weekly to monitor progress toward weight goal and will monitor for weighted materials in clothing to increase weight measured.	*Patients with anorexia are extremely unwilling to gain weight. To mislead family and nursing staff, they may place heavy objects in their pockets during weight checks.*
Nursing staff will work with the interdisciplinary team to develop a realistic behavior modification plan, including participation in counseling.	*Eating disorders are related to underlying emotional or psychological problems that require counseling interventions as well as dietary changes.*

Bulimia

Another common eating disorder is bulimia. The child with this disorder eats a huge number of calories and follows with purging behaviors of enemas, laxatives, diuretics, self-induced vomiting behaviors, extreme exercise, or a combination of these. Bulimia is characterized by an excessive appetite and insatiable eating, including sneaking and hiding food. *Bulimia* is defined as recurrent episodes of binge eating followed by guilt; humiliation; shame; and then self-induced vomiting, dieting, and exercise. The child will try to cover up or hide the behaviors associated with bulimia. Often the child or teen is of normal weight.

Binge Eating Disorder

BED is a very serious disorder in which the child or teen feels unable to stop eating. The child or teen consumes large amounts of food and calories, often rapidly, with associated feelings of being out of control, so that they cannot stop. Many who suffer from this disorder recognize that their behavior is out of control. The behavior may take place when the child or teen is alone and binge eats in secret. After the binge eating experience, the person feels disgusted with themself, ashamed of what they just did, and upset and guilty about not being able to stop. Complications include obesity; social isolation; problems with work and school; and the development of chronic illnesses such as type 2 diabetes, sleep apnea, and gastroesophageal reflux disease (GERD; Mayo Clinic, 2019b).

Avoidant/Restrictive Food Intake Disorder (ARFID)

Another type of eating disorder is the restricting type, in which the child participates in episodes of food restriction and severe calorie reduction. This disorder prevents food consumption outright.

Pica

When a child persistently consumes materials that are not food substances, the child is experiencing an eating disorder called *pica*. This disorder is more common in young children; about 10% of children under 6 have some pica behavior. To be diagnosed, a child must be at least 2 years of age. Developmental disability and cognitive impairment have been associated with the development of pica behaviors. Complications occur when the child eats dangerous substances such as paint chips, toxic plant materials, and sharp or hard objects. Ingesting large quantities of ice may cause iron deficiency. Medical conditions such as intestinal obstructions from nonfood items and anemia should be considered as complications of nonnutritive eating. Pica behavior must be present for no less than 30 days for pica to be considered a diagnosis (Nasser et al., 2022).

The pediatric health-care team must rule out any physiological pathologies before addressing the emotional component of pica. After lead poisoning, anemia, and parasites are evaluated for, treatment consists of behavioral modification through rewards and mild aversion therapy (Nasser et al., 2022).

Evaluating Eating Disorders

Suspicion of an eating disorder may arise from the child's physical status, clinical presentation, emotional state, and laboratory analysis. The following evaluations may be indicated and performed by the health-care team (Balasundaram & Santhanam, 2022; Mayo Clinic, 2018):

- Plot the child's weight and height on a national growth chart. If the child is significantly under or over the expected weight for height and sex, further evaluation is warranted.
- Draw metabolic panels to check for type 2 diabetes, lipid panels to check for elevated serum lipids, and electrolyte panels to determine if there are imbalances, including metabolic alkalosis from vomiting.
- If the child has engaged in pica, tests for lead or other toxins may be necessary, and a complete blood count (CBC) may be needed to test for anemia.
- Check blood pressure and cardiac function, including orthostatic blood pressures to detect true hypotension and electrocardiogram (ECG) to detect dysrhythmias associated with severe electrolyte imbalances.
- Inspect for evidence of malnutrition: thinning hair and hair loss, brittle fingernails, dry skin, enamel loss on teeth, amenorrhea, mood changes, bradycardia, hypothermia and cold intolerance, and loss of libido. The Russell sign, bite marks on fingers and knuckles, may be present from the child inducing vomiting.
- Inquire for use of laxatives, diuretics, enemas, and diet pills; report any use immediately to the health-care provider.
- Evaluate for sociocultural factors, such as preferences for being thin, and psychological factors, including impulsivity, pursuit of perfectionism, and a history of child sexual abuse.

Interventions for Eating Disorders

Similar to many of the mental health conditions found in childhood, treatment for eating disorders is considered multimodal and requires lengthy interventions. Psychotherapy is the mainstay of treatment and includes behavior modification. Medications such as antidepressants may be required to support the child. Other interventions are specific to the type of eating disorder being treated.

Nursing Considerations for Eating Disorders

You need to understand the anxiety associated with eating for a child with an eating disorder. These children may become angry, disruptive, and manipulative in order to avoid consuming calories, to binge in secret, or to eat their preferred nonfood substance. Make sure the child does not have an opportunity to purge (vomit) after meals or to engage in other harmful eating behaviors.

The nursing goals for children with eating disorders include securing a weight within 10% of expected for age and height; resolving underlying emotional and psychological problems; correcting malnutrition; preventing severe consequences such as type 2 diabetes, anemia, electrolyte imbalance, and cardiac dysfunction; and assisting with a treatment plan to restore the child's perception of health and healthy body image.

Left untreated, eating disorders can be fatal; therefore, it is imperative to identify and treat them early. Parents must be educated on the need to participate fully in therapy. Nurses can be instrumental in becoming involved with adolescent education and prevention through community action.

ANXIETY, MOOD DISORDERS, AND SCHIZOPHRENIA

Other types of mental illnesses can affect children, causing behaviors that impair all aspects of life including socialization, academics, preparation for adulthood, and intimate relationships. Disorders, such as anxiety, mood disorders, and **schizophrenia**, exist in adults as well.

Anxiety

Worrying, fearfulness, and feelings of anxiety are normal and regularly found throughout childhood. When the anxiety is no longer attached to a specific event, or when the feelings of anxiety become disabling for the child, then the anxiety is considered pathological and requires treatment. Infants experience a form of anxiety when they are only 7 to 8 months old. As they begin to understand that they are separated from their caregiver, they experience separation anxiety and then stranger anxiety. This is a normal and expected first experience of anxiety. If anxiety is experienced repeatedly throughout childhood and interferes with social, academic, and normal cognitive development, then the child should be evaluated.

Childhood anxiety disorders are becoming more common for children across all ages. Many people attribute this increase to stress in our society. Anxiety disorders can cause a child to feel overwhelmed and can be triggered by everyday activities such as going to school or facing homework and peer interactions. Feelings of irrational, persistent fear and worry take over the child's thinking and affect most aspects of the child's life.

Several subtypes of anxiety disorders exist within childhood:

1. *Separation anxiety disorder:* This disorder differs from the separation anxiety an infant commonly experiences in that the older child has unrealistic anxiety and persistent worry that harm will occur if separated from the primary caregiver. This includes resistance to attending school or social events or even going to sleep.

2. *Generalized anxiety:* With this disorder, children worry excessively about future events, competence, or previous behavior. Often, generalized anxiety is demonstrated through somatic (physical) reports and great difficulty relaxing.
3. *Panic disorders:* With panic disorders, children feel an overwhelming sense of worry and panic. They may present with physical symptoms of an increased heart rate, sweating, and increased blood pressure.
4. *Phobias:* Phobias are a type of anxiety that is experienced only under a specific condition that the child will try to avoid.
5. *Posttraumatic stress disorder (PTSD):* In this disorder, anxiety results from an external traumatic event that was perceived by the child or adolescent as very dangerous and/or life-threatening; intrusive and recurrent recollection of the event occurs, which causes the child extreme distress. This distress may be demonstrated through sleep disorders, sadness, and feelings of helplessness and vulnerability.
6. *Obsessive-compulsive disorder (OCD):* OCD is marked by a child's persistent repetitive thoughts, repetitive rituals, or repetitive movements that do not contribute to social acceptance with family, peers, and members of society.

Evaluating Anxiety Disorders

Nurses working with a team of health-care providers can provide assistance in conducting evaluations for anxiety disorders. Evaluations for anxiety disorders include the following:

- Biophysical evaluations of vital signs for tachycardia and tachypnea with shortness of breath
- Gastrointestinal (GI) symptoms of nausea and stomachache
- Neurological symptoms, such as headache and body pains
- Sleep disturbances; nightmares
- Poor school performance and decreased participation in age-appropriate activities
- Poor self-esteem
- Use of medications and alcohol to dull the sensations of anxiety

Interventions for Anxiety

Children need professional counseling to deal with an anxiety disorder. The goal is to increase their self-esteem and to teach them relaxation exercises and self-regulating interventions to address the feelings of anxiety. School-aged and older children may be able to conduct self-help exercises to reduce their anxiety. These include verbalization of feelings, exercise, deep breathing, visualizations, relaxation techniques, and problem-solving techniques. When moderate anxiety exists, the child needs a referral for cognitive-behavioral therapy (CBT) interventions. If the child has severe anxiety, therapy and possibly antianxiety medications are called for.

· WORD · BUILDING ·

schizophrenia: schizo–split + phren–mind, seat of emotion + ia–condition

Nursing Considerations for Anxiety

A child with an anxiety disorder who must be hospitalized may have a sudden increase in symptoms that warrant professional interventions. Child life specialists and staff pediatric psychologists should be called in to work with the anxious child. Anxiety causes suffering, and the child should be provided with care that reduces symptoms when they become ill.

Assist the anxious child by staying in close proximity, maintaining a calm and relaxed approach, and offering the child positive reinforcement for describing feelings. Young children may not be able to express themselves clearly but will respond to a calm environment and soothing support. Meditation, prayer, and alternative therapies can also be tried to assist with anxiety symptoms.

Patient Teaching Guidelines

Parents of children with anxiety disorders may look for alternative remedies to help their child. In fact, passion flower, theanine (an amino acid in green teas), and valerian have been reported to decrease the symptoms of anxiety (Mayo Clinic, 2024). Because dietary supplements are not regulated by the U.S. Food and Drug Administration (FDA), they are not extensively tested for safety and efficacy. The amount of the herb within a given supplement, the side effects, and health interactions or warnings may not be fully understood. Always inform patients and their families to check with their health-care provider before starting herbal remedies to avoid complications and unwanted interactions while taking other medications.

Mood Disorders

Bipolar Disorder

Bipolar disorder is characterized by alternating mania and depression, or a rapid cycling of mood. Children with the disorder may experience grandiose thoughts, pressured speech, extreme irritability, emotionality, distractibility, and high levels of activity, often at bedtime.

Treatment for bipolar disorder is lithium carbonate. This medication prevents or decreases the incidence of acute manic episodes. Therapeutic levels of this medication must be tracked by serum blood levels with the ideal level being 1 to 1.2 mEq/L for initial treatment followed by 0.5 to 0.8 mEq/L for maintenance. The most common side effects associated with the administration of lithium are fatigue, headache, impaired memory, ataxia, abdominal pain, dry mouth, and tremors. Once the medication is started, the therapeutic effects can take up to 5 to 7 days to occur.

Persistent Depressive Disorder

Persistent depressive disorder is characterized by periods of major depression and periods of what is considered normal mood lasting several days or several weeks. The feelings of depression, also called *dysphoria,* are less intense than a persistent major depression, but depression is classified as a chronic disorder. A genetic link is suspected with this disorder. Children may present with a preexisting disorder such as somatization disorder, anxiety disorder, or AN. Some children with this disorder will appear passive, dependent, and lonely, whereas others will be aggressive, angry, and negative. Because of the cyclic pattern of this disorder, children are at risk for developing substance abuse. Treatment consists of antidepressants.

Depression

Depression is not a state of sadness; it is a serious medical illness that affects young children and teens. The incidence of depression in children is increasing, and it is imperative that a nurse can identify symptoms, assist with a formal evaluation, and secure treatment. (Fig. 29.3). The highest rates of depression are reported in minority groups. Less than 25% of these children are receiving any treatment for depression. The best way to identify depression in children and teens is to regularly screen for the symptoms. The Depression Scale for Children takes only 3 to 5 minutes to administer and is considered quite sensitive in detecting depression.

The cause of depression in children is unknown. There may be an imbalance in brain chemistry, or it may be associated with another illness, substance abuse, or environmental influences. Stressful events such as a death, parental divorce, a move of the family, or severe illness may trigger depression. Depression also has a hereditary link. Childhood depression is not considered normal or associated with life's experiences. It is a medical diagnosis with severe symptoms and consequences that requires immediate medical attention. Early treatment may help avoid the depression getting worse, extending for a long period, or becoming a lifetime challenge.

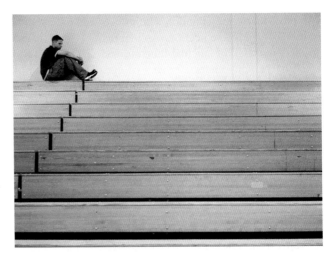

FIGURE 29.3 Children and adolescents experience depression.

A medical diagnosis of major depression in childhood occurs after the child has displayed symptoms nearly every day for 2 weeks or longer. The child feels hopeless, sad, and angry and demonstrates a loss of interest in activities usually enjoyed. It also includes impaired academic performance. Physical symptoms such as fatigue, sleep disturbances, appetite disturbances, muscle aches, and headaches may be present. Children may display frequent crying spells.

EVALUATING DEPRESSION. Childhood depression is complicated and requires professional training to appropriately diagnose and treat it. Many reliable and validated tools are available for professionals to use to confirm the diagnosis of depression across the developmental period. The following list indicates the most common symptoms displayed by different ages:

- *Preschool children* may demonstrate weight loss and a lack of interest in play normally expected of their age group.
- *School-aged children* may have trouble concentrating at school, paying attention, making decisions, and recalling information. School-aged children may be less confident in their academic performance and state that they "can't do anything right."
- *Adolescents* may demonstrate poor hygiene, stop communicating with their friends and family, and lose interest in teen life activities. Teens are at risk for suicidal thoughts. Depression is more common in girls than in boys.

INTERVENTIONS FOR DEPRESSION. If a child is diagnosed with a depression disorder, professional counseling is imperative and may be enough to treat the disorder. For more severe depression, the child will require professional counseling and antidepressant medications. Research supports continuing this combination of treatments for 2 years to reduce the risk of depression reoccurrence. Psychotherapy for children typically lasts between 8 and 20 sessions.

When a medication is ordered for a child with depression, you must know the common side effects and safety precautions for that medication. Antidepressants may cause an increased risk of suicidal thinking and behaviors when taken by patients under 25 years of age. The purpose of antidepressant medications is to help balance some of the natural chemicals (**neurotransmitters**) in the brain. Examples of commonly prescribed antidepressants include the following:

- Sertraline
- Escitalopram
- Fluoxetine
- Duloxetine
- Tricyclic antidepressants (referred to as *tricyclics*, or *TCAs*)

Safety *Stat!*

A child who is placed on an antidepressant must see a mental health specialist weekly for at least the first 4 weeks to evaluate for an increased risk of suicidal tendencies.

Labs & Diagnostics

Serum Levels of Psychiatric Medications

Several psychotropic medications must be maintained at a steady concentration in the blood. Monitoring the serum levels of these medications helps to ensure that the child is receiving an adequate, but not toxic, dose. Research shows that the most accurate monitoring of serum levels of psychotropic medications occurs when a child is being treated with only one medication, not multimedication treatments. After a serum level is ordered, check with the health-care team about when to administer the next dose. Watch for orders that change the child's doses in response to the serum medication levels.

Safety *Stat!*

Newer antidepressants have fewer side effects in children than do older medications. Side effects should still be monitored for and reported immediately to the prescribing health-care provider. Common side effects include nausea, headache, drowsiness or sleeplessness, agitation with jitters, constipation, dry mouth, and blurred vision.

MAOI antidepressants can cause a dangerous side effect if the child ingests a food or medication that contains tyramine. When a child ingests tyramine while on an MAOI, a sharp increase in blood pressure may occur, which has been associated with cerebral vascular accidents (strokes). Families must be taught that aged cheeses, cured meats, pickles, wine, and over-the-counter (OTC) decongestants contain tyramine.

CRITICAL THINKING

You are working in a pediatric clinic and take a call from a mother who reports that her teenaged son stopped taking his antidepressants suddenly when he "decided he felt so much better and did not need them." The mother is worried that her son made this decision on his own and is wondering if there is anything to worry about.

Question

1. What would you expect the registered nurse will say to the mother about the sudden stopping of antidepressant medications?

Medication Facts

Patients' families commonly ask about herbal remedies for depression. According to the Mayo Clinic's summary of St. John's wort (2021b), for some, taking this supplement may decrease the symptoms of mild depression, but it may also interact with many other medications. The St. John's wort plant and flower have been shown to help some types of depression in adults. In fact, St. John's wort is widely used internationally as a first-line herbal alternative for mild depression. For children with mild-to-moderate depression, more clinical trials are needed to determine the safety and effectiveness of this herbal substance. St. John's wort can interact with some medications, including medications for HIV, some chemotherapies, and organ transplant antirejection medications. Moreover, it can cause side effects that range from tremors, diarrhea, confusion, hypothermia, and muscle stiffness to death. Therefore, St. John's wort is not recommended for use in pediatric patients with depression (NCCIH, 2014).

NURSING CONSIDERATIONS FOR DEPRESSION. A child with depression needs astute nursing care. Monitor the child for social isolation, increasing symptoms with hospitalization, and the potential for self-harm. Engage the child life department to provide distraction and support for the child during your care. Ensure that the health-care team has a plan for the child and that the family is engaged in the care required. Administer the child's regular antidepressant medications on time, according to the child's regular schedule. Inquire if serum levels are required to monitor the appropriate blood serum levels.

Health Promotion

Sunscreen and Psychotherapeutic Medications
Several medications used to treat mental health disorders can make a child photosensitive (especially sensitive to sunlight). Children on the following medications should be protected from sun exposure:

- Chlorpromazine
- Fluphenazine
- Trifluoperazine
- Thioridazine
- Amitriptyline
- Nortriptyline
- Sertraline
- Fluoxetine

Protecting photosensitive skin includes the following measures:

- Limiting sun exposure
- Wearing adequate protective clothing when in the sun, even on cloudy days
- Wearing light-colored, lightweight, and loose-fitting clothes
- Wearing a brimmed hat
- Applying a sunscreen with at least an SPF 30 on a daily basis
- Choosing a waterproof or sport sunscreen if very active, sweating, or swimming

General guidelines for families of a child with depression include the following:

- Do not isolate the child. Keep the child associated with extended family members.
- Make sure that the child is seen by professionals who can help through counseling and medication.
- Make sure that the child takes the medicines that are ordered. Families should also know the common side effects to watch for.
- Know that as the depression is treated and the feelings lift, the child will have fewer negative feelings and better expectations for themselves.
- Encourage the child to set small goals to work on each day. This may include building a craft over time, increasing time spent on homework each day, or planting a garden.
- Provide healthy foods and snacks, and have family members be role models of good nutrition.
- Evaluate the child for medication and alcohol use because these substances are dangerous when taken with antidepressants.
- Provide activities that make the child feel good. Engaging in conversation or playing with the whole family may improve the child's feelings.
- Be aware that depressed children are often targets of bullying at school. School officials must be notified of all bullying episodes so that the child can be protected during treatment.
- Call the National Suicide Prevention Lifeline as soon as the child displays thoughts or actions of suicide.
- Do not give up on the child or yourself in caring for the child. Do not get discouraged and do not feel that you and your family are alone. Do not feel embarrassed—seek and secure help early.
- Talk about the depression as a family and seek clergy or traditional healers to provide support while receiving professional help as well.

Suicide in Childhood
Suicide is defined as death by taking one's own life. Suicide is the second leading cause of loss of life for children,

Box 29.1

Common Terms Associated With Suicide

Suicidal thinking: When a child or teen is thinking about suicide but has no plan; this is not uncommon; about 3% of the general teen population has reported suicidal thinking at one point in their development.

Suicidal ideation: Children and teens who have thought out a plan but have not carried out any behaviors toward suicide. An example would be a teen who is collecting pills but has not made a plan or a gesture toward taking their life.

Suicide attempt: Suicide attempts are very dangerous; the child or teen takes actual steps to ensure death. However, either the child is found by another person in time to secure emergency health care and resuscitation or is unsuccessful and lives through the attempt. Jumping off a high bridge, with full intention of death, but living through the jump and being rescued is one example.

Suicidal gesture: An attempt at suicide but without the means to take one's life; a nonfatal act of deliberately causing harm or injury to oneself. *This term is being phased out because it is seen as being dismissive.*

Lethality of attempt: This refers to the potential deadliness of a suicide attempt based on the patient's chosen method.

Suicide: This means death resulting from taking one's own life.

adolescents, and young adults ages 5 to 24 years of age (American Academy of Child and Adolescent Psychiatry, 2019).

Data from a 2017 comprehensive study by the American Foundation for Suicide Prevention (AFSP) estimate the suicide rate to be close to 14 per 100,000 deaths per year (AFSP, 2019), with boys outnumbering girls (81% vs. 19%). The three main causes of death associated with suicide are gunshot (50.57%); strangulation, suffocation, or hanging (27.72%); and poisoning (13.89%). Suicide attempts in children are far more common than lethal suicides, with up to 7% of children having at least one attempt to kill themselves between 9th and 12th grades. Almost twice as many female students attempt suicide than male students do. Out of every 300 suicide attempts in childhood, 1% are successful. There is a strong association between suicide and a major depressive disorder. In 10- to 24-year-olds in the United States, suicide is the second leading cause of teen death (CDC, 2022d).

Families experiencing marital difficulties, child abuse, or substance abuse are more likely to have an adolescent who is at risk of suicide. In addition, in one-third of adolescent suicide cases, a parent, sibling, or other first-degree family member has expressed suicidal thoughts, engaged in suicidal gestures, or has committed suicide. Box 29.1 contains several terms associated with suicidal thoughts and behaviors.

IDENTIFYING RISK FOR SUICIDE. Any threats of suicide must be taken seriously. The child's seriousness, impulsivity, desperation, and degree of premeditation should all be taken into account. With suicide threats, the precipitating event, if any,

should be identified. In addition, whether the child intended to be found and stopped or intended to have a serious injury or death should be determined.

Some hospital and clinic settings will automatically evaluate an older school-aged child or a teenager for suicidal thoughts. Check with your institution to see how to check for and document a child's suicidal thoughts.

INTERVENTIONS FOR SUICIDE. A child who shows evidence of suicidal thoughts or actions must be taken seriously, supervised constantly, and supported immediately. This may mean transporting the child to an inpatient hospital or psychiatric unit for further evaluations and treatments. Initial treatment may include medication to stabilize the child (Miller, 2022):

- Fluoxetine for children 8 years old and older
- Escitalopram for children 12 years old and older
- Sertraline
- Fluvoxamine
- Clomipramine

Safety *Stat!*

If a nurse suspects that a child is at risk for a suicide while in the hospital or if the child speaks about having suicidal thoughts while in the clinic, you must report this concern immediately and mobilize a team to provide safety. While hospitalized, the child will be placed on a suicide watch, and staff will be assigned to provide observation. Hospital and clinic rooms must be secured from any dangerous instrument or device that might be used for self-harm. Windows must be secured, either by design or by a lock that prevents opening. Constant supervision may be required for children with suicide risk, no matter what the clinical setting.

NURSING CONSIDERATIONS FOR SUICIDE. The nursing care of a child or teen with a suicide attempt requires immediate stabilization and hospitalization with round-the-clock observation. Both Child Protective Services and the police or other law enforcement department must be contacted. The child's home may be searched for weapons, medications, and access to medications. The following nursing care should be considered:

- Depending on the type of self-inflicted trauma, C-spine (cervical spine) stabilization, cardiorespiratory monitoring, or the collection of serum and/or urine toxicology screens may be needed.
- If the ingestion of a poisonous substance is suspected, the health-care team will need to contact the American Association of Poison Control Centers to discuss appropriate medical treatments. The child will require cardiorespiratory monitoring and support of the airway and circulatory system. A serum toxicology screen must be collected.
- Because most adolescents who attempt or are successful in committing suicide have a diagnosable psychiatric

illness, the child must be evaluated by a child mental health specialist for appropriate treatment (Healthyplace .com, 2019). You should ensure a timely consultation during early hospitalization.

Safe and Effective Nursing Care

Nonsuicide Self Injury

Nurses caring for children and teens need to be aware of the phenomenon of NSSIs. These injuries are not accompanied by suicidal ideation or intent but rather are ways of coping with anxiety. Examples of NSSI behaviors include:

- Burning
- Cutting
- Excessive rubbing to the point of skin excoriation
- Stabbing with various objects

Schizophrenia

Schizophrenia is a chronic, severe, and disabling psychiatric disorder characterized by delusion, hallucination, and disrupted thought disorder. The affected child appears to be in a chaotic state with paranoid delusions, **hebephrenia** (inappropriate silliness, laughter, and mannerisms or reduced expressions of emotion), alternating moods, aggressive behaviors, and social withdrawal. This severe, chronic, and debilitating mental illness affects 0.25% to 0.64% of the U.S. population, affecting 1.5 times more men than women. Most people are diagnosed between 16 and 30 years of age. If left untreated, schizophrenia is often severely disabling (NIMH, 2022).

The diagnosis of schizophrenia is typically made in the late teens to early 30s with symptoms being demonstrated earlier in males (NIMH, 2022). The patient experiences thinking that is completely out of touch with reality and may hear voices that are not there, see people who are not present, or suffer physical symptoms of "bugs crawling on the skin." Adolescents with schizophrenia may experience paranoia and feel as though people are plotting against them.

Evaluating Schizophrenia

Diagnosing schizophrenia in children is complicated and must be done by professionals who are experienced and trained in this area. Because of the severity of the disorder, evaluations include behavioral and emotional symptoms. Delusions, disordered thinking, disordered speech, hallucinations, and an impaired ability to function are all evaluated. If the child is young, early symptoms to evaluate for include late crawling and walking, delays in language development, and abnormal motor movements such as arm flapping and persistent rocking. Because there is so much overlap between these symptoms and those of ASD in a young child, it is essential that an experienced and well-trained health-care provider evaluate the child for an accurate diagnosis.

Interventions for Schizophrenia

There is no single treatment for schizophrenia, and treatment must continue throughout the individual's lifetime. The child may benefit from a **neuroleptic** medication to manage some of the symptoms of this disorder, such as hallucinations and psychotic delusions. Family involvement and a commitment to the child's medication regimen are imperative.

Safety *Stat!*

Suicide is a concern for people diagnosed with schizophrenia, and people with schizophrenia should be evaluated for self-harm (NIMH, 2022).

Nursing Considerations for Schizophrenia

Children with schizophrenia need strict follow-up to check for medication compliance and side effects. Neuroleptic medications can cause several side effects, including sedation, dry mouth, cramping, constipation, blurred vision, and difficulty urinating. When these medications are taken with tricyclic antidepressants, delirium, confusion, and poor attention may be side effects.

Safety *Stat!*

Tardive dyskinesia is a serious side effect of neuroleptic medications. With this condition, a person engages in involuntary twisting and writhing of the face, limbs, and trunk. Dyskinesia can develop in as many as 20% to 30% of patients treated long term with neuroleptics. These symptoms are reversible if they occur during the withdrawal or discontinuation of the medications but may not be reversible if they develop during medication therapy.

Another serious side effect of neuroleptic medications is neuroleptic malignant syndrome. This rare side effect is characterized by a "lead pipe" stiffness of the extremities and high fevers. For patient safety, it is imperative to regularly ask families about the development of early side effects.

OTHER TYPES OF MENTAL HEALTH DISORDERS

Similar to adults, children can have more than one mental health disorder at the same time. For example, children suffering from depression or anxiety may use medications to cope

---

- WORD - BUILDING -

hebephrenia: hebe–youth + phren–mind, seat of emotion + ia–condition

- WORD - BUILDING -

neuroleptic: neuro–nerve + leptic–seizing
dyskinesia: dys–abnormal + kines–movement + ia–condition

Table 29.1

Examples of Common Drugs and Medications Abused by Youth

Street Drugs	Prescription Medications
• Marijuana	• Barbiturates
• Cocaine	• Methamphetamine
• Crystal meth (methamphetamine)	• Cough and cold medicines: dextromethorphan
• Ecstasy	• Sleeping pills
• Heroin	• Antianxiety medications
• Acid (LSD)	• Fentanyl
• PCP (phencyclidine)	• Hydrocodone
• Mushrooms (psilocybin)	• Oxycodone
• Peyote plant (mescaline)	• Oxymorphone
• Nitrous oxide	• Hydromorphone
• Crack	• Meperidine
• Speed (ice)	• Diphenoxylate

• Gamma hydroxybutyrate (GHB; Xyrem)
• Bath salts
• Inhalants
  • Aerosols in household products
  • Pens, markers, glues
  • Cleaning fluids
	• Alprazolam
	• Diazepam
	• Dextroamphetamine
	• Methylphenidate
	• Amphetamine and dextroamphetamine
	• Ketamine
	• Benzodiazepines

Source: National Institute on Drug Abuse. (2020). *Commonly abused drugs charts.* https://www.drugabuse.gov/drugs-abuse/commonly-abused-drugs-charts

with their condition. Bullying is another type of disorder that has been directly linked to anxiety, depression, and suicide.

Substance Use Disorder

About 15% of children in the eighth grade report the use of at least one illicit drug in the prior 12 months. About 50% of adolescents report that they have been drunk or abused a drug within the last year. Some teens try illicit substances only a few times, and others develop cravings and urges that lead to abuse. The most commonly abused substances are tobacco, marijuana, alcohol, stimulants, crystal meth, hallucinogens, inhalants, prescription medications, opioids, heroin, cocaine, and "club drugs" (Therecoveryvillage.com, 2022). See Table 29.1 for a list of common medications currently being abused during childhood.

Children who live in homes where substance abuse is taking place are at a much higher risk for abusing drugs or alcohol themselves. Children who are experiencing depression or who do not feel valued by their parents are more likely to experiment with illicit substances and have a greater risk for abuse.

Feelings associated with substance abuse in children and adolescents include hopelessness, alienation, and depression. Injuries, accidents, unplanned pregnancy, violence, drowning, and suicide are also associated with substance abuse.

Patient Teaching Guidelines

Evaluating for Signs of Alcohol and Drug Use in Children and Teens

Parents need to be taught how to evaluate for substance use in their children. The following are behaviors or symptoms to be aware of:

- General changes in overall attitude
- Sudden personality changes that disrupt school attendance, grades, and extracurricular activities
- Sudden outbreaks of anger, aggression, nervousness, and jitteriness
- Increased secretiveness

- Engagement in a new social circle of friends who have no interest in meeting the family
- Withdrawal from responsibility
- Red eyes and reports of being overly tired
- Loss of interest in hobbies, activities, and sports previously engaged in
- Loss of interest in personal grooming, hygiene, and personal appearance to others
- Borrowing or stealing of money or objects to sell
- Association with known substance abusers
- Frequent trips to the bathroom, storage areas, basement, or other places where medications or alcohol could be stored

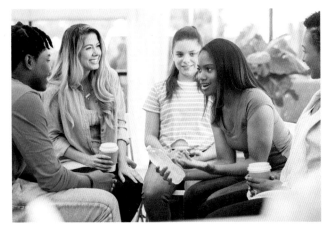

FIGURE 29.4 Teens can benefit from peer group therapy.

Evaluating Substance Use Disorder

Many young people use medications recreationally and do not consider it drug abuse. In fact, according to Robinson, Smith, and Saisan (2015), use does not always lead to abuse. What is important is not how much a person is using but whether the use is causing problems with a person's health, school work, home life, and relationships. A teen with a substance abuse problem may have physical signs (Box 29.2), such as needle marks, or may have affective signs, such as depression, guilt, shame, and medication-seeking behaviors. Other warning signs of substance abuse are worsening academic performance, problems with relationships at home, social isolation, and the presence of a family member who has or has had **addiction** problems (Robinson et al., 2015).

Interventions for Substance Use Disorder

Factors associated with treatment of a child with substance use disorder include the child's age, sex, values and culture, family factors, and the presence of a coexisting mental health disorder. Medications may be ordered to help treat the addiction. For instance, naltrexone may be given for alcohol or opioid dependency; bupropion may be given for marijuana or tobacco abuse; and methadone may be given for heroin addiction. After detoxification in either an outpatient or inpatient setting, treatment can include psychotherapy, behavior modification, CBT, and/or 12-step programs. Many children addicted to substances benefit from peer group therapy (Fig. 29.4).

Interventions and treatments for substance use disorder in children should account for three important considerations:

1. The child's physical needs must be met, including the symptoms of withdrawal.
2. The child's cognitive and emotional needs have been affected by the addiction.
3. The child's family dynamics will need repair if trust has been broken or the addiction has had severe consequences on family relationships. In general, children cannot stop the substance use without treatment and emotional support. Families must be aggressive in their interventions to help their child.

Nursing Considerations for Substance Use Disorder

Helping families secure professional interventions is key. Teach parents that if they suspect substance abuse, they should immediately contact their health-care provider to help find the right program and treatment for their child. Securing an educational advocate can provide assistance with navigating the child's or teen's school situation. Encourage parents to talk about the risks and dangers of illegal substances with their children; to communicate family values regarding substance use with their child or teen; and to set rules and consequences of breaking the family rules.

Teach parents never to leave prescription medications where children can find them. Prescription medications, such as acetaminophen and hydrocodone, diazepam, oxycodone, and even methylphenidate, can be abused. Some children even abuse OTC medications such as cough

---

Box 29.2

Physical Signs of Substance Abuse and Addiction in Children

Screening for physical signs of addiction should take place during well-child visits and any other health-care interactions. Nurses should screen for clinical signs and symptoms with each encounter.

- Physical signs of depression, such as being withdrawn
- Physical signs of abuse, violence, or injuries
- Pregnancy or STIs
- Nausea, vomiting, diarrhea, and other GI problems
- Insomnia and poor quality of sleep
- Sweating, shaking, and tremors
- Bloodshot eyes, pupil dilation or pupil constriction, and flushed face
- Poor personal grooming and body odor
- Poor oral hygiene and bad breath
- Impaired speech and coordination
- Lethargy, drowsiness, or inattentiveness

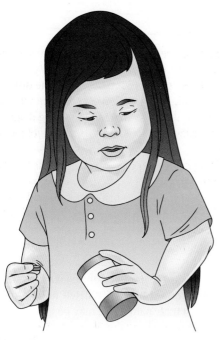

FIGURE 29.5 Child finding leftover narcotics.

syrup or cold pills. Medications should be locked away from children and their peers (Fig. 29.5).

Community-based organizations can be of vital assistance in supporting parents and family members and in making referrals for treatment of the addiction. Organizations that can provide education and support for families who have a child participating in substance abuse include the following:

1. Alcoholics Anonymous (AA) World Services
2. National Institute on Alcohol Abuse and Alcoholism (NIAAA): The Cool Spot
3. KidsHealth
4. National Institute on Drug Abuse (NIDA), NIH
5. Partnership for Drug-Free Kids

Bullying

Bullying is a national concern. Bullying takes many forms, including physical force and violence, spreading rumors about others, social exclusion, severe teasing, "ganging up" on others, and using social media to send insulting or obscene messages or pictures. Victims often display low self-esteem, loneliness, anxiety, depression, poor academic performance, and suicidal thoughts. Victims can experience poorer physical health, including headaches, sleeping problems, GI distress, and other inflammatory processes. Bullying is known to cause long-lasting emotional scars and lifelong memories. Children who witness bullying also suffer with fear, guilt, and distraction in schoolwork.

Bullying can begin as early as the later preschool period. Bullies may choose their victims at random, or they may persecute children who look different, such as those who are obese, are of small stature, or have unique features. Sometimes bullying victims have learning disabilities, developmental delays, or mental health issues.

Evaluating Bullying

Evaluating for bullying is important and may save lives. Try using questions such as: "Are there any kids at your school who tease you in a mean way?" or "Are there kids at your school who you really do not like? Why?" or "Have you been harassed on social media?"

Look for physical and emotional signs of bullying. Obvious signs of physical bullying can be cuts, bruises, black eyes, torn personal belongings, or damaged school supplies. Other signs may be extreme school aversion, frequent absences, symptoms of depression, somatic reports such as stomachaches, and poor school performance. Bullies choose victims who are less powerful than they are and who are "different" in some way from them.

Interventions for Bullying

Ideally, bullying should be stopped before a child is hurt or hurts themself. Interventions that school personnel can use during bullying events include the following:

- Stand between the children involved.
- Block eye contact between the bully and the victim.
- Do not try to sort out the facts at that moment; do not discuss the reasons at the time of the incident.
- Do not let bystanders walk away; they need to witness the intervention.
- State out loud the behaviors that you saw and heard.
- State clearly that bullying is against the rules and will not be tolerated.

Safety *Stat!*

Bullycide is a term used to describe a suicide directly related to bullying. Cyberbullying has superseded physical bullying as the reason for bullycidal behaviors. Bullycidal behavior is linked to persistent emotional pain and can be caused by peers or authority figures in a child's life. Living in constant confusion and terror and reliving embarrassing moments over and over again, the child or teen comes to see suicide as the only way out.

Nursing Considerations for Bullying

Under no circumstances can bullying be allowed within a health-care setting. Whether hospitalized in an acute care setting or a long-term facility, children must behave respectfully to each other. Any bullying witnessed within a health-care setting must be stopped and interventions implemented.

Nurses need to evaluate for bullying and know how to provide support and interventions. The health-care team, including child life services, can place a call to the school to describe the child's reported experiences, and a social worker should be notified. Requesting a referral for a child psychologist is appropriate. A child who has been bullied needs to be referred for help. Make sure that the family knows to contact the school authorities, who should have protocols for intervening in bullying.

Key Points

- The incidence and prevalence of ASD, ADHD, and depression and other mood disorders are increasing. An awareness of risk factors can assist health-care professionals to screen, identify issues, and intervene.
- A mental health issue has a serious effect on the child's interactions with family, school, social networks, and society as a whole and requires a holistic approach through counseling or therapy, medication, and follow-up care.
- Goals for therapeutic communication between you and the child and family during an acute phase of a mental health condition include establishing rapport, building trust, and communicating the importance of interventions to help the child cope and recover.
- Many professional evaluation tools exist to aid in diagnosing anxiety, depression, and other mood disorders. These tools are administered by mental health-care professionals, and the results guide treatments and therapy.
- ADHD has a serious negative effect on a child's interaction with family and school. Early identification and initiation of treatment can assist the child in demonstrating improved behavior in the classroom and greater achievements in academic performance.
- AN and BN have distinct patterns of behavior. Often associated with a child's poor self-image, poor self-esteem, and very poor perception of their physical self, the prevalence of these disorders in current society is increasing for both sexes. You need to understand the differences between the diagnoses and assist the team with interventions to prevent poor outcomes, including death. Other eating disorders that children may have include obesity and BED.
- There is no known cause for ASD, but it is known to exist from birth with early symptoms noted as early as late infancy. Genetics, irregular brain regions, and environment most likely play a role in the development of autism.
- Bullying can lead to depression, anxiety, and suicide. Bullying must be identified, and interventions must take place to provide for the child's safety and well-being. Bullying can manifest as threats of physical violence, actual violence, or emotional pain from ridicule, meanness, or social isolation.
- Nurses need to be able to identify the physical and affective signs of substance use disorder and addiction. Parents need to first acknowledge that their child has a substance abuse problem and seek information, help, and treatment for their child.

Review Questions

1. A teenage girl is seen in the pediatric clinic for a routine physical examination required for her to play high school sports. Her weight is plotted on a national growth chart and is within a normal range. Her mother expresses concern that her daughter may be experiencing an eating disorder. Which of the following could she be experiencing?
   1. AN
   2. ARFID
   3. BED
   4. Bulimia

2. You are teaching the family of a child who has just been placed on an MAOI antidepressant about tyramine. You know that the family understands the teaching when they identify which food as being safe for the child to eat?
   1. Aged cheese
   2. Pickles
   3. Red meats
   4. Dishes cooked with wine

3. Which of the following medications causes photosensitivity and an increased chance of severe sunburn?
   1. Lorazepam
   2. Doxycycline
   3. Lithium
   4. Chlorpromazine

4. Which is the highest-priority evaluation for a child admitted to the hospital for complications associated with substance abuse?
   1. Dynamics of family and parent interactions
   2. Child's social structure
   3. Thoughts of suicide
   4. Academic performance

5. A father brings his 30-month-old daughter into the pediatric clinic for a checkup. He explains that she has not begun to talk and watches a window ornament for long periods. He expresses concerns that his daughter may be autistic. What would be an appropriate question to ask this father?
   1. "Does your child cuddle up to you when you hold her?"
   2. "Does your child have an older sibling who 'talks' for her and shares her needs?"
   3. "Does your child attend a childcare facility where she may not be getting enough attention and play?"
   4. "Does your child have temper tantrums more than you would expect?"

6. Which treatment is the first-line antagonist for a suicide attempt with an overdose with acetaminophen?
   1. Acetylcysteine
   2. Activated charcoal
   3. Nasogastric lavage with 0.9% NS (normal saline)
   4. Baking soda

7. A teen who uses marijuana daily is admitted into a medication treatment facility. Which medication do you anticipate will be ordered for the teen?
   1. Naltrexone
   2. Bupropion
   3. Methadone
   4. Antabuse

8. Neuroleptics may be prescribed for a child with schizophrenia. Tardive dyskinesia is a serious side effect of neuroleptics and is characterized by which of the following?
   1. Twisting or writhing of the face, limbs, and trunk
   2. Grand mal seizures without loss of consciousness
   3. Copious salivation and drooling
   4. Fatigue and lethargy

9. You have been invited to give a presentation about bullying to staff working at a public health clinic. You would be correct in saying that bullying behaviors include which of the following? (Select all that apply.)
   1. Physical force
   2. Violence
   3. Spreading rumors
   4. Social exclusion
   5. Severe teasing
   6. Using social media to send insulting messages or pictures.

ANSWERS 1. 4; 2. 3; 3. 4; 4. 3; 5. 1; 6. 1; 7. 2; 8. 1; 9. 1, 2, 3, 4, 5, 6

CRITICAL THINKING QUESTIONS

1. A 12-year-old girl presents with syncope and severe abdominal pain. All diagnostic and laboratory tests come back negative. Her mother says that the girl is experiencing severe bullying in her school; she has very limited English language skills and has been targeted by a group of teen girls. Both the mother and the child are requesting to remain in the hospital until her symptoms improve. How would you go about referring her for counseling? What does this child need from you?

   Can a hospitalization provide this child an avenue for recovery and skill building? What are potential outcomes of a bullying situation that is not resolved at the school level?

2. Suicide is an important concern for children who have mental health issues, depression, and social isolation. How can a nurse assist with suicide-prevention education and early interventions when a child has been noted to be at risk for suicidal behaviors?

Resources

For additional resources and information, including Postconference Questions and Activities, Answers, and References, visit www.FADavis.com.

Student Study Guide

CHAPTER 30
Child With a Respiratory Condition

KEY TERMS

adventitious breath sounds (AD-ven-TISH-uhss BRETH SOWNDZ)
alveolar sacs (al-VEE-uh-luhr SAKS)
alveoli (al-VEE-uh-lee)
atelectasis (AT-el-EK-tuh-siss)
bronchodilation (BRONG-koh-dye-LAY-shun)
crepitus (KREP-it-us)
cyanosis (SYE-uh-NOH-siss)
hemoptysis (hee-MOP-tih-siss)
inhaler (in-HAYL-uhr)
laryngitis (LAR-in-JYE-tiss)
nasopharyngeal (NAY-zoh-fa-RIN-jee-uhl)
nebulizer (NEB-yoo-lye-zuhr)
pneumothorax (NOO-mo-THOR-aks)
rales (RAYLZ)
respiratory syncytial virus (RSV) (RESS-pih-ruh-TOR-ee sin-SISH-uhl VYE-russ)
rhonchi (RONG-kee)
stridor (STRYE-duhr)

CHAPTER CONCEPTS

Inflammation
Oxygenation
Perfusion
Safety

LEARNING OUTCOMES

1. Define the key terms.
2. Differentiate between the respiratory anatomy and physiology of a newborn and a child and those of an adult.
3. Describe the breathing patterns, adventitious breath sounds, and symptoms one may encounter in respiratory distress.
4. State the assessments conducted in the physical examination of an infant or child with a respiratory condition.
5. Describe the care required for a child with croup, including possible causative factors and developmental groups most vulnerable to this disease.
6. Discuss the various methods of intervention for a child with a respiratory condition, including the different oxygen delivery systems.
7. Compare and contrast the pathophysiology, diagnostic methods, and treatment for tonsillitis and epiglottitis.
8. Describe the pathophysiology of asthma, treatment protocols administered across childhood, and teaching required for the patient and family to minimize adverse effects.
9. Review the effect of respiratory diseases on a family and the teaching needs of the family to safely care for a child hospitalized for treatments or who is being cared for at home.

CRITICAL THINKING

Five-year-old **Heather** has been admitted to the pediatric unit of the hospital with severe asthma for her third inpatient visit within the last 12 months. Her father, who speaks only Cantonese, is her primary caregiver; her mother works long hours during the week. During Heather's last hospitalization, the family was given a prescription for a short-acting asthma rescue inhaler, a nonsteroidal anti-inflammatory inhaler, and antibiotics because her x-ray demonstrated a secondary pneumonia. Her father tells you that he was unable to fill all of the prescriptions because of limited family resources and chose to fill the antibiotic only. Heather received 6 hours of continuous nebulized albuterol in the emergency department (ED) and then was admitted for inhalation treatments every 2 hours.

Continued

CRITICAL THINKING—cont'd

Questions

1. What challenges do families often face in caring for a preschool child with severe asthma?
2. How will Heather's triggers be identified?
3. How could you assist the family with obtaining all necessary prescriptions for Heather?

CONCEPTUAL CORNERSTONE

Oxygenation

A child with a serious respiratory condition or infection will be at risk for ineffective gas exchange because of poor oxygenation. Acute respiratory illnesses such as bronchiolitis cause a young child to be significantly distressed. *Oxygenation* refers to the ability to take in sufficient amounts of oxygen to provide for the body's cellular demands. Without sufficient oxygenation and gas exchange, the child will become hypoxemic, hypoxic, and cyanotic. These three serious signs of inefficient oxygen intake and gas exchange can become life-threatening. Nurses must understand the symptoms associated with poor oxygenation and provide immediate relief through the administration of supplemental oxygen and medications that improve gas exchange.

Children who experience acute and chronic respiratory conditions require specially trained health-care personnel who are knowledgeable about the underlying pathophysiology and the treatments, equipment, and medications necessary to care for this pediatric subset. Diagnosis of these diseases relies on thorough history-taking and physical evaluation, making comprehension of these data essential. The possible severity of the illnesses may require practitioners with critical care backgrounds because routine symptoms can rapidly become life-threatening.

It is imperative for families of these patients to have a clear understanding of the disease process and treatment parameters. Often the child is cared for at home, either upon discharge from the hospital or if the symptoms do not warrant hospitalization.

THE DEVELOPMENT OF THE RESPIRATORY TRACT

Before birth, the fetus's lungs are not inflated but are filled with amniotic fluid. Oxygen and carbon dioxide are exchanged via the mother's circulation through the placenta and umbilical cord. When the newborn takes its first breath a few seconds after birth, oxygen flows into the lungs, starting inflation and reducing blood-flow resistance to the lung. Amniotic fluid drains, is suctioned, or absorbs. When the lungs begin the work of respiration, oxygen moves into the blood vessels, and carbon dioxide is exhaled.

Alveoli Development

The exchange of the gases oxygen and carbon dioxide occurs in microscopic sacs within the lung tissue called **alveolar sacs** or **alveoli** (plural). At full-term birth (40 weeks' gestation), the neonate has approximately 20 to 50 million alveoli. These gradually increase in number as the child grows, until reaching the total, adult amount of 300 million alveoli by the age of 8 years. As the number of alveoli increases, the alveolar surface area also increases, allowing the gas exchange to become more efficient and explaining the progressive slowing of the normal respiratory rate.

Anatomy of the Respiratory Tract of a Child Versus an Adult

The respiratory system (Fig. 30.1) takes in oxygen upon inspiration and expels carbon dioxide upon expiration.

A child's nose (Fig. 30.2) is relatively narrower than an adult's, causing it to become obstructed more easily. The nose contains no cilia (small hairs) to prevent the introduction of microorganisms to the lower airways, and the nose is richer in blood supply, which can cause an increase in inflammation. These factors can lead to mouth breathing and more difficulty breathing. The maxillary sinus is not well-developed until the age of 6, and the frontal sinus is not well-developed until the age of 12; this results in fewer incidences of sinusitis in children. The nasopharyngeal and palatine tonsils gradually develop between the ages of 1 and 10 years, at which point the tissue starts to shrink. In those years, the occurrence of tonsillitis is much more prevalent. The eustachian tube runs between the middle ear and the pharynx. It is wider and shorter than in the adult and acts similar to a conduit, bringing microorganisms from the pharynx to the middle ear, causing otitis media (OM). The throat is longer and narrower with soft cartilage that results in increased congestion, edema, obstruction, and difficulty breathing. The trachea and bronchi have soft cartilage, a smaller lumen, a lack of elastic tissue, and poor ciliary movement. The smaller number of alveoli in the lungs of young children causes more breathing difficulty and cyanosis; the lungs are less compliant than an adult's, causing the child to have to work harder to breathe. The pulmonary tissue is rich in vasculature, resulting in more inflammation.

 HEALTH HISTORY

Nurses should work with the health-care team to conduct a health history on a child who presents with a suspected respiratory condition. Important questions concerning the child's health and environment include the following:

• Chronic lung disease (CLD) in family members?
• Exposures to environmental toxins such as mold, pesticides, or pollution?
• Other acute or chronic health conditions experienced by the child?
• Respiratory conditions at birth?
• Smoking by family members or caregivers of the child?

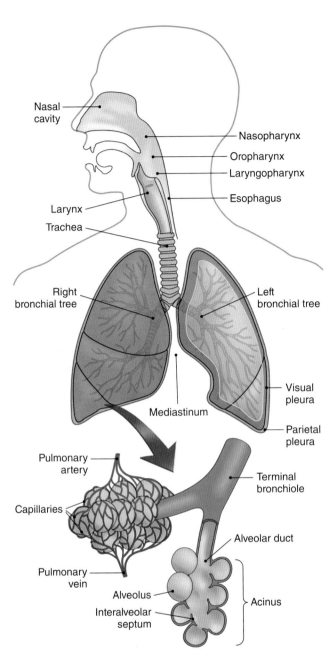

FIGURE 30.1 Respiratory system.

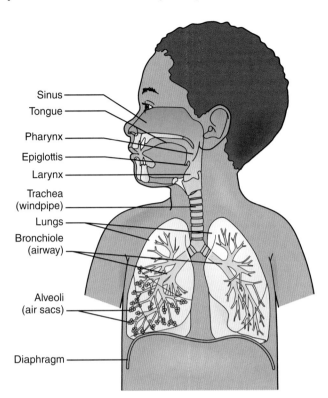

FIGURE 30.2 Respiratory structures of a child.

PHYSICAL EVALUATION

When encountering a child who presents with a respiratory condition, a thorough examination is warranted. A variety of techniques are used to understand and describe the child's respiratory condition.

General Respiratory Observations

The pediatric health-care team will want to be notified immediately if a child presents in respiratory distress. Any difficulty with ventilation or abnormal positioning to maximize air exchange should be reported immediately so that rapid interventions can take place. After viewing the child to check for distress, begin to evaluate the child's breath sounds.

Auscultation

Auscultation of the chest will serve to determine the characteristics of respiratory sounds, identify abnormal sounds, and evaluate vocal resonance. A pediatric stethoscope will help to localize abnormal sounds. The diaphragm of a pediatric stethoscope transmits high-pitched sounds more effectively. Auscultate the breath sounds over the entire chest, alternating between the two sides for comparison of the anterior and posterior. Breath sounds can best be heard when the child is at rest, but the deep breath taken between cries can be effective, too.

Percussion

Percussion evaluates the lungs' resonance and density. As with auscultation, a pattern of alternating sides will allow

---

Safety *Stat!*

Because the trachea and bronchi have soft cartilage, a smaller lumen (inside space), a lack of elastic tissue, and poor ciliary movement, these characteristics can work together to cause an increase in the occurrence of pediatric respiratory infections. The small lumen and poor ciliary movement also cause young children to have more difficulty clearing secretions. This places children at risk for the development of viral and bacterial infections caused by pooled secretions.

comparison. Indirect percussion is done by placing the middle finger of the nondominant hand in an intercostal space and tapping with the fingers of the other hand. Direct percussion involves tapping with the fingertips and is used for examining infants.

Olfaction

Olfaction is the sense of smell and the ability to distinguish different odors. This sense is easily altered in pediatric patients because they frequently have nasal congestion.

Palpation

Palpation is performed to evaluate chest movements, respiratory effort, abnormalities of the chest, and tactile fremitus. It is done with open palms and outstretched fingers. Placement of the palm on the chest can help determine the depth of retractions and the use of accessory respiratory muscles. Lightly touching the skin with the fingertips can locate **crepitus** (a crackling sound heard in the lungs) or subcutaneous emphysema, small pockets of air under the skin caused by trauma or fractures. *Tactile fremitus* is the vibration caused by talking or crying. Having the child repeat words while you alternate your hands over the chest and back aids in evaluating the quality of the vibrations.

Inspection

Inspecting the child's respiratory effort includes the respiratory rate, chest movements, signs of distress, and presentation of an emotional state such as anxiety. See Table 30.1 for a summary of expected respiratory rates per minute for children.

Chest Movements

Normal chest movement is bilaterally symmetric, rising and falling with inspiration and expiration. The chest movement of infants and young children is less pronounced than the abdominal movement. The abdomen rises as the chest does with inspiration. The diaphragm is the key respiratory muscle in all children younger than 6 years old.

Table 30.1
Pediatric Respiratory Rates per Minute

Age	Respiratory Rate per Minute
Birth–12 months	30–60
Toddler	20–30
Preschooler	20–25
6 years	20–25
9 years	17–22
12 years	17–22
Adolescent	15–20

Team Works
Breathing Patterns
It is imperative that all members of the pediatric health-care team can identify when a child demonstrates a change in respiratory pattern or displays respiratory distress. It is also important that each team member uses the same name of the breathing pattern so that there is no confusion (Fig. 30.3). The following list defines the most common abnormal breathing patterns:

- *Apnea:* A period of at least 20 seconds without breathing
- **Bradypnea:** A respiratory rate slower than normal (normal range depends on age)
- *Cheyne-Stokes breathing:* A cycle of respirations with rapid, deep breathing, followed by a gradual slowing of breathing, and finally a period of apnea
- *Hyperventilation:* Respirations that are deeper and more rapid than normal and result in a low carbon dioxide level
- *Hypoventilation:* Respirations that are more shallow and slower than normal and result in a high carbon dioxide level
- *Kussmaul's breathing:* Slow, deep, labored respirations, often caused by metabolic acidosis
- **Tachypnea:** A respiratory rate faster than normal (normal range depends on age)

Chest Configurations

An infant's chest is normally rounded: the lateral (side-to-side) diameter is approximately equal to the anteroposterior (front-to-back) diameter. This roundness should disappear by the age of 2, when the lateral diameter is greater than the anteroposterior diameter by 2:1. The following list defines chest configurations that are considered abnormal:

- *Barrel chest:* Chest is rounded in appearance; after the age of 2, the cause may be a chronic disease such as asthma or cystic fibrosis (CF).
- *Funnel chest* (pectus excavatum): Depression of the lower sternum, which causes a decrease in anteroposterior diameter; it is genetic in origin.
- *Pigeon chest* (pectus carinatum): The presence of a protuberant sternum, which causes an increase in the anteroposterior diameter; it is genetic in origin.

Signs of Respiratory Distress

A child who is experiencing difficulty breathing will look extremely anxious in response to hypoxia. A child who is in

• WORD • BUILDING •
bradypnea: brady–slow + pnea–breathing
tachypnea: tachy–rapid + pnea–breathing

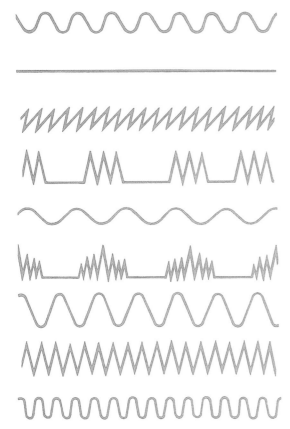

FIGURE 30.3 Normal and abnormal breathing patterns: eupnea, apnea, apneustic, Biot breathing, bradypnea, Cheyne-Stokes, hyperventilation, Kussmaul's breathing, and tachypnea.

respiratory distress will assume a position that will maximize the ability to draw air into the lungs:

- The *sniffing position* involves tilting the head back to maximize the effort to draw air into the lungs via the nose.
- In the *tripod position*, the child will sit or stand leaning forward with the arms resting on the knees. This increases the ability to use the thoracic and neck muscles to draw air into the lungs.

Safety *Stat!*

Any child who displays signs of respiratory distress needs to have the condition reported so they receive immediate interventions to help alleviate distress and increase oxygenation.

Evaluation of the Energy and Effort to Breathe

A child will show physical signs of increased effort to breathe. The following list describes the physical signs that a child will display when experiencing air hunger and trying to maximize oxygen intake:

- *Chest retractions:* The soft tissue of the chest shows a visible depression beneath the breastbone (substernal), above the collarbone (supraclavicular), between the ribs (intercostal), or beneath the ribcage (subcostal). The use of accessory muscles is an attempt to draw in more oxygen.
- *Use of accessory muscles:* A child under 6 years of age uses the diaphragm as the primary muscle for breathing. Use of the thoracic muscles for breathing indicates respiratory difficulty and may result in chest contractions. Therefore, the higher the level of the retractions, the greater the degree of respiratory distress the child is experiencing.

CRITICAL THINKING & CLINICAL JUDGMENT

Dashel, a 2-month-old infant, is brought to the public health community clinic with significant chest retractions and increased work of breathing. His older brother, 3-year-old Wessley, has been sick from a viral infection he caught in his preschool. Dashel presents with rhinorrhea, fever, and listlessness.

Questions

1. Why would Dashel be experiencing retractions?
2. What should you do when you observe Dashel's respiratory symptoms?

RESPIRATORY ABNORMALITIES

Children in respiratory distress often display abnormal clinical symptoms. These symptoms include signs of hypoxia and hypoxemia. *Hypoxia* describes a state of insufficient oxygen in general that can result in insufficient oxygen in the blood (hypoxemia). If you observe these symptoms, report the findings immediately to the health-care team.

Signs of Respiratory Distress

Several signs and symptoms may indicate that a child is not getting sufficient levels of oxygen. These signs and symptoms include the following:

- *Cyanosis:* Bluish coloring on the lips, around the mouth (circumoral), in the nailbeds, or pale or gray skin.
- *Diaphoresis:* Increased sweat, particularly on the head, while the skin is cool or clammy rather than warm to the touch; this may accompany tachypnea.
- *Head bobbing:* With insufficient oxygen levels, the infant thrusts the head forward with each inspiration; this is because of the neck muscles being too weak to hold the head stable with lung retractions.
- *Nasal flaring:* Nares open wider with each inspiration to draw more oxygen into the lungs.

Adventitious Breath Sounds

Abnormal breath sounds in a child are the same as in the adult. Common abnormal breath sounds, also called **adventitious breath sounds**, are found when a child has a condition that is interfering with normal oxygenation and ventilation. In young children, adventitious breath sounds are loud and may be heard without the use of a stethoscope.

- *Crackles/rales:* A high-pitched, intermittent sound caused by air passing through fluid in the lungs; it sounds similar to rubbing hair through one's fingers in front of the ear.
- *Grunting:* A grunting sound with each expiration may indicate the body's effort to improve oxygenation by trying to keep the alveoli open so that they are better able to fill with air.
- *Rhonchi:* A loud and low-pitched coarse or rattling sound often associated with mucus or secretions in the large airways.
- *Sibilant rhonchi:* A musical, hissing, or squeaking sound heard louder on expiration that is caused by bronchospasm or narrowing of the airways.
- *Sonorous rhonchi:* A coarse, snoring sound on inspiration or expiration that is caused by secretions causing a partial obstruction of the airways.
- *Stridor:* A high-pitched sound on inspiration usually accompanied by gasping in an attempt to draw in air past a severe airway obstruction. Stridor is considered a severe symptom.
- *Wheezing:* A whistling noise with inspiration and/or expiration that may be audible or only heard with auscultation; this may indicate that the airway is narrowed because of swelling, excessive secretions, and/or bronchoconstriction.

INTERVENTIONS FOR A CHILD WITH RESPIRATORY DIFFICULTIES

A child experiencing respiratory distress requires immediate support. Through interventions designed to reduce poor oxygenation and ineffective gas exchange, the pediatric health-care team can reduce the child's symptoms and improve the child's respiratory status. Emergency interventions to support the airway include oxygen delivery, suctioning, and airway management. Only oxygen delivery is discussed further here.

Emergency Interventions

The American Association of Pediatrics (AAP) established guidelines for emergency treatment in pediatric emergencies in their Pediatric Advanced Life Support (PALS) course. Included are supplemental oxygen therapy, airway management, foreign body (FB) aspiration, cardiopulmonary resuscitation (CPR), tracheostomy, endotracheal intubation, and mechanical ventilation.

Safety *Stat!*

Nurses, regardless of the clinical setting in which they practice, must be confident in their ability to respond to a child who presents with or develops respiratory distress. Knowing how to rapidly identify a child in distress, having the ability to select the most effective oxygen delivery system, and knowing how to support a child's compromised airway are some of the most important skills a nurse needs to master and practice on a regular basis.

OXYGEN THERAPY GUIDELINES

When a child presents with a respiratory condition, oxygen therapy is often prescribed. There are a variety of means to improve a child's oxygenation through supplemental oxygen (Fig. 30.4). The following list describes the most common interventions used to improve oxygen delivery:

1. *Oxygen hood:* A transparent plastic cylinder that encloses the neonate's head in a humidified, oxygen-rich

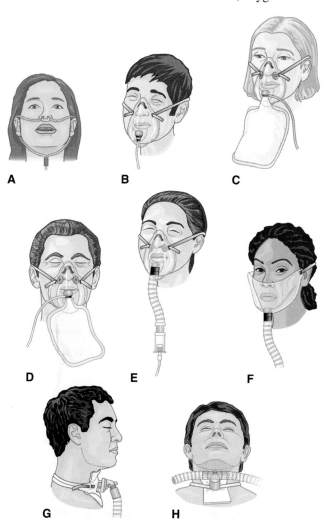

FIGURE 30.4 Various oxygen delivery systems. A, Nasal cannula. B, Simple face mask. C, Partial rebreathing mask. D, Nonrebreathing mask. E, Venturi mask. F, Face tent. G, Tracheostomy collar. H, T-piece.

environment. It allows freedom of movement and no attachment of a plastic apparatus to the face, which may induce crying and therefore increase oxygen consumption. It may produce cold stress, if unheated.

2. *Oxygen tent:* This device provides a transparent, plastic-enclosed, humidified, oxygen-rich environment for a pediatric patient too large for a hood.

3. *Blow-by oxygen:* This device consists of corrugated oxygen tubing that "blows" oxygen and/or nebulizer medication by an infant's mouth and nose, allowing inhalation without the attachment of a plastic apparatus to the face. This can be used by a family member with the child held on the lap or lying down.

4. *Nasal cannula:* This device consists of two soft, plastic prongs attached to oxygen tubing that allows low-flow oxygen to flow into the nasopharynx. It is contraindicated in nasal obstruction and is not recommended in neonates.

5. *Simple face mask:* This device includes a plastic reservoir system that fits over the mouth and nose, which is attached to oxygen tubing and fitted to the head with an elastic strap. Holes on either side of the mask allow exhaled carbon dioxide to be expelled from the mask. Possible aspiration of emesis is a consideration. It is not appropriate for neonates.

6. *Nonrebreather mask:* A plastic bag at the base of the mask provides an additional reservoir of oxygen. One-way valves on the reservoir bag and the side of the mask prevent expired carbon dioxide from mixing with the oxygen supply and prevent room air from entering the mask and diluting the oxygen concentration. This enables a higher concentration of oxygen to be delivered than with simpler devices. It is not appropriate for neonates.

7. *Venturi mask:* This device consists of a simple mask with a valve that allows a precise percentage of oxygen to be delivered rather than as measured by liter flow. It is not appropriate for neonates.

8. *High-flow nasal cannula:* A form of noninvasive oxygen support providing higher levels of airway pressure and removing nasopharyngeal dead space; this device provides humidification and heating with the advantage of minimal nasal trauma.

See Table 30.2 for information about oxygen delivery devices.

 INTERVENTIONS TO ASSIST A CHILD WITH RESPIRATORY DISTRESS

A child with respiratory distress may require supplemental oxygen as well as other interventions to ease the effort to breathe. Suctioning is a gold standard for young children with conditions that produce increased secretions; other interventions assist in the removal of secretions and aid in breathing. Medical equipment that provides key information on the status of the child's distress is also utilized.

Table 30.2
Oxygen Delivery Devices and Corresponding Oxygen Delivery

Device	Size for Children	Size for Infants
Nasal cannula	0.5–4 LPM	0.25–2 LPM
Simple mask	6–10 LPM	5–8 LPM
Partial rebreather	10–12 LPM	Varies depending on newborn or infant size
Venturi mask	Liter flow indicated for specific F_{IO_2} device	Liter flow indicated for specific F_{IO_2} devices
Nonrebreather mask	10–15 LPM	n/a
Aerosol	8–12 LPM	Depends on size and age of newborn or infant

Abbreviations: F_{IO_2}, fraction of inspired oxygen; LPM, liters per minute.

Chest Physiotherapy

This intervention involves the use of gentle percussion via cupped hands or a vibratory device to mobilize respiratory secretions to promote expectoration. This is followed by repositioning from side-to-side, with the head dependent, to optimize the drainage and expectoration of secretions.

Nasal Suctioning

This process involves gently extracting oropharyngeal and nasopharyngeal secretions by a suction catheter or a bulb syringe, as is age-appropriate. This may be preceded by flushing with minute amounts of normal saline to facilitate loosening and thinning of secretions.

Breathing Exercises

Expectoration of secretions and promotion of respiratory activity can be facilitated by having the child take a few deep breaths and then cough forcefully several times. This helps to mobilize secretions and optimize respirations by forcing the alveolar sacs to open and thus better fill with oxygen. The same effects can be obtained by the use of an incentive spirometer (IS), a plastic device that uses deep inspiration to exercise the lungs and airways.

Apnea Monitors

An apnea monitor is a device that can be sent home with an infant who has had one or more episodes of respiratory arrest, periods of apnea greater than 20 seconds, or an apparent life-threatening event (ALTE), also called a brief resolved unexplained event (BRUE; see Chapter 24). It is attached to the infant by chest electrodes or a belt and monitors dysrhythmias as well. Apnea monitors have not been proven to reduce mortality in sudden infant death syndrome (SIDS; see Chapter 18).

Oxygen Saturation Machines

Oximeters use fiberoptic science to measure the concentration of oxygen in the surface capillaries in the fingers, toes, or earlobes. They are a noninvasive method that measures the oxygen as a percentage.

 COMMON RESPIRATORY DISORDERS

Children, from infancy through adolescence, can be exposed to respiratory pathogens that cause common ailments. There are several common respiratory disorders or conditions frequently found in the childhood period.

Nasopharyngitis

Nasopharyngitis is otherwise known as the common cold. It is a viral infection caused by 1 of more than 200 viruses, but it is most commonly caused by a rhinovirus. Preschool and grade school children are the developmental groups most frequently affected by this infection. The symptoms may include coughing, sneezing, fever, nasal and upper airway congestion, sore throat, watery or itchy eyes, headache, and chills. Cold viruses spread from one person to another by the droplet method or direct contact.

Evaluations of Nasopharyngitis

The cold virus attaches itself to the lining of the nose and upper airway, causing the release of histamine, which causes swelling and congestion. Symptoms usually improve after 4 to 5 days and are gone by 10 days to 2 weeks.

Symptoms of nasopharyngitis are based on the severity of the inflammation located within the **nasopharyngeal** space. Feelings of pressure or fullness, congestion, coughing, sore throat, headache, and sinus pressure pain can all be experienced and should be checked.

Interventions for Nasopharyngitis

There is no test that detects the cold virus. However, a throat culture may be done to diagnose a possible bacterial infection, such as strep throat caused by one of the *Streptococcus* bacteria.

A child with a cold is more susceptible to bacterial infections such as sinusitis, OM (see Chapter 28), and strep throat. Antibiotic therapy may be used to treat the secondary infection. Otherwise, symptomatic treatment is given, such as antipyretics for fever, decongestants, analgesics for a sore throat or headache, antihistamines for itchy eyes, or a cough suppressant. Other methods of treatment may include increasing fluid intake to thin secretions, a cool-mist humidifier

for congestion, adequate rest, using a nasal aspirator to remove secretions from an infant, and avoiding exposing the child to secondhand smoke.

Nursing Considerations for Respiratory Infections

Because small children are more susceptible to viruses, family members need to be instructed in symptomatic treatment and preventing transmission of the virus through hand washing and covering their mouth and nose while coughing and sneezing. Many parents request antibiotics for a child with a cold and need education that this is not necessary unless there is a secondary bacterial infection as well. If the child is diagnosed with strep throat, adherence to oral antibiotic therapy is essential. The child may return to school 24 hours after the last fever and after the child has had a minimum of 24 hours of antibiotics.

Tonsillitis

Tonsillitis is an inflammation of the tonsils. The purpose of the tonsils is not known, but they are presumed to support the immune system. Increased numbers of bacteria are found in the tonsils, but this number decreases with age. Tonsillitis is usually caused by the bacteria *Staphylococcus aureus* and beta-hemolytic *Streptococcus*. The disease occurs more frequently in children under 6 years, and some experience it much more frequently than others.

Signs and Symptoms of Tonsillitis

The most common symptom of tonsillitis is throat pain exacerbated by swallowing. This may prevent the child from eating or drinking sufficiently or taking oral medications. Other complications can include adenoiditis, recurrent OM, middle ear fluid, peritonsillar abscess, and nasal obstruction with mouth breathing and snoring. Evaluation focuses on inspection of the throat, ears, and vital signs, especially an accurate temperature. A complete blood cell count (CBC) may be done to determine the degree of infection based on the white blood cell count (WBC) and to make sure that a prospective surgical patient has a sufficient red blood cell count (RBC).

Interventions for Tonsillitis

Treatment of a streptococcal tonsillitis usually includes some form of penicillin for 10 days. Tonsils must be removed after a peritonsillar abscess occurs, but otherwise the decision to perform a **tonsillectomy** depends on the frequency of infections and the child's age. Symptomatic treatment with liquid, oral acetaminophen for pain and fever is common. If the child requires hospitalization, intravenous (IV) acetaminophen may be given at the dose of 12.5 mg/kg for neonates or 15 mg/kg for infants through 12-year-olds.

• WORD • BUILDING •
nasopharyngeal: naso–nose + pharynge–pharynx + al–relating to

• WORD • BUILDING •
tonsillectomy: tonsill–tonsil + ectomy–surgical excision

Nursing Considerations for Tonsillitis

Your responsibility for a patient with tonsillitis includes symptom management, prevention of complications, preparation for surgery if indicated, and patient and family teaching. Pain and fever can be treated with over-the-counter (OTC) medications and sufficient fluid intake. Because swallowing is often painful, it is important to provide the child's favorite fluids, including ice cream and popsicles, which may prove soothing to an irritated throat. Fluid intake is also important to prevent dehydration, a more prevalent occurrence in the pediatric population. If a tonsillectomy is planned, you must ensure NPO (nothing by mouth) status, arrange for signed parental consent, and complete a preoperative checklist. The parents and the child should be informed, in an age-appropriate way, of each aspect of interventions and be allowed to ask questions.

Safety *Stat!*

A child in the postoperative period after a tonsillectomy must be monitored for frequent swallowing or throat clearing because this could indicate bleeding at the operative site.

Epiglottitis

The epiglottis is made of cartilage and is located at the base of the tongue. Epiglottitis is a serious, possibly life-threatening bacterial infection that causes inflammation and swelling of the throat. This swelling can cause breathing problems that may progress rapidly, triggering obstruction of the airway. Epiglottitis can become an emergency so quickly that the diagnosis itself necessitates immediate admission to a hospital. It is caused by either *Haemophilus influenzae* type B (Hib) or group A beta-hemolytic *streptococci* and primarily affects 2- to 8-year-olds.

Signs and Symptoms of Epiglottitis

The symptoms of epiglottitis may resemble the symptoms of an upper airway infection. These may include sudden onset of a severe sore throat, fever, hoarse voice, and a cough. Worsening symptoms may also involve drooling, no voice, leaning forward in the sitting position (tripod position), and keeping the mouth open (Fig. 30.5).

The diagnosis is usually made by physical examination and history of the symptoms. The child's health-care provider

---

Safety *Stat!*

Never use a tongue blade to visualize the throat of a child who presents with symptoms of epiglottitis. The use of a tongue blade on the infected tissue might result in further swelling and inflammation, potentially closing off the child's airway completely.

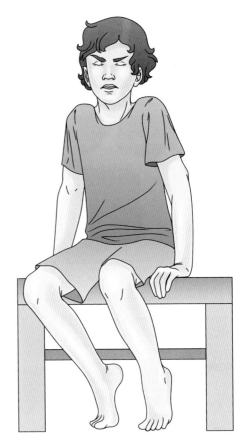

FIGURE 30.5 Child in a tripod position.

may also order a neck x-ray, an arterial blood gas (ABG), and a CBC. In extreme circumstances, a surgeon may perform a visualization of the airway in the operating room.

Interventions for Epiglottitis

In an emergency, the child's airway and breathing may be assisted with intubation and mechanical ventilation. Close monitoring of the breathing will determine when this is necessary. A health-care provider will start an IV line to administer antibiotics. In addition, they will give steroids to reduce and prevent swelling in the airway, and give IV fluids if the child is unable to swallow. Antibiotics for treatment of the infection include penicillins, cephalosporins, and sulfas.

Health Promotion

Hib vaccines are recommended for children at the ages of 2, 4, 6, and 15 to 18 months. Being fully vaccinated against Hib significantly decreases a child's risk of acquiring epiglottitis.

Nursing Considerations for Epiglottitis

Epiglottitis is a potentially critical condition that can be very frightening for the patient and family. It is your responsibility to explain all procedures and treatments and lend emotional

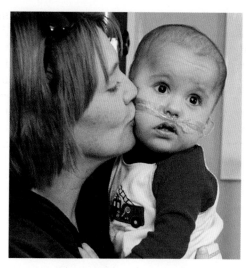

FIGURE 30.6 Child on oxygen therapy.

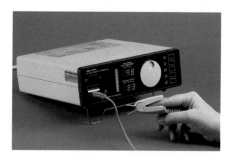

FIGURE 30.7 Pulse oximetry.

support. Monitor the patient's airway and breathing very closely and treat as needed; administer oxygen therapy, IV fluids, and medications (Fig. 30.6); and maintain the child on a pulse oximeter (Fig. 30.7).

Croup

Croup is a disease caused by a viral infection that causes swelling of the airway. This results in stridor upon inspiration. The most common virus that causes croup is the parainfluenza virus, but it can also be caused by **respiratory syncytial virus (RSV)**,

---

Learn to C.U.S.

You are assisting a pediatric nurse practitioner (NP) in caring for a toddler with suspected epiglottitis. The NP asks you to get a tongue blade to hold the child's tongue down to better visualize the airway structures and obtain a culture. You use the C.U.S. method of communication to express your concerns:

C: "I have a *concern* about your request.
U: I am *uncomfortable* using a tongue blade in the throat because this may cause complete obstruction.
S: I think we have a *safety* issue here."

---

influenza virus, measles, adenovirus, or enteroviruses. Infection occurs through direct contact with secretions, starts in the upper airway, and descends to the larynx. Croup is most common in infants and children aged 3 months to 5 years because their smaller airways occlude more easily with swelling. It affects boys more than girls and is seen more in winter.

Signs and Symptoms of Croup

The symptoms of croup are related to the presence of an infection and a swollen airway. The child may have a congested nose or throat, fever, **laryngitis**, and stridor. What may start out as a mild cough will progress to a harsh, "barking" cough that is the distinguishing feature of the disease. The symptoms are typically worse at night and usually improve within 3 to 7 days.

Croup is usually diagnosed via history and physical evaluation. Neck and chest x-rays (CXRs) may be done as well as a CBC to determine the extent of the infection. Pulse oximetry is a noninvasive method of measuring oxygen in the blood and can be monitored continuously, if need be.

Interventions for Croup

If the child's breathing is sufficiently compromised, hospitalization may be necessary. Breathing treatments with steroids and/or bronchodilators may be given to open the airway. Steroids may also be given by mouth or IV to reduce swelling in the airway. Treatment at home includes a cool-mist humidifier, encouragement of fluid intake, and bedrest to minimize respiratory effort.

Nursing Considerations for Croup

Croup is usually treated at home, and the family needs to know what to watch for to decide whether it is necessary to take the child to the doctor's office or ED. Clinical signs of respiratory distress include restlessness, increased respiratory rate, and difficulty breathing. If there is no cool-mist humidifier in the home, the same effect can be reached by taking the child outside in the cold, night air or into a bathroom with steam from a hot shower running.

Apnea

Apnea is a period of more than 20 seconds without any breathing. In pediatrics, most babies who experience apnea are premature (35 weeks' gestation or less). The apnea usually occurs during rapid eye movement (REM) sleep. The apnea may occur during the first week of life but is considered more serious when it occurs immediately after birth or after the second week of life. It is also more serious the longer it lasts, if the infant turns blue, or if it is accompanied by a slower heartbeat (bradycardia). Apnea accompanied by bradycardia is referred to as "As and Bs." Some possible causes of apnea are an immature central nervous system (CNS),

· WORD · BUILDING ·
laryngitis: laryng–larynx + itis–inflammation

airway blockage, bleeding or damage in the brain, infection, gastric reflux, metabolic abnormality, stimulation of reflexes such as hyperextension of the neck, or hyper- or hypothermia.

Signs of Apnea

A careful evaluation is important to determine whether there might be some cause for apnea other than prematurity. The health-care provider will perform a complete physical examination to rule out any physical disorders. They will perform blood tests such as a CBC and metabolic panel to check for infection, blood glucose abnormalities, electrolyte imbalance, or hyper- or hypocalcemia, and order chest and abdominal x-rays to check for anatomical abnormalities. An apnea study will be done to test breathing effort, heart rate, and oxygenation.

Interventions for Apnea

Periods of apnea can be stopped by stimulating the infant through massaging or patting the skin. Possible causes should be determined and treated to prevent further incidents. The breathing rate and patterns, as well as heart rate, will be closely monitored. Caffeine or theophylline may be given as CNS stimulants. A continuous positive airway pressure (CPAP) breathing machine may be used to keep the airway open through a continuous flow of oxygen.

Nursing Considerations for Apnea

Witnessing a child's apnea episodes can be very frightening for parents and other family members. Nurses need to explain what apnea is, how it can be treated, and the parameters that the infant must meet to be discharged. Parents' fears about a possible reoccurrence once the infant is discharged home must be addressed. If the infant will be using an apnea monitor once home, the family must be instructed in its use.

Asthma

Asthma is a chronic, inflammatory disease with symptoms triggered by exposure to substances causing an allergic reaction (allergens). Asthma symptoms are swelling and inflammation of the airway, tightening of the muscles around the airway, and increased mucus production. These symptoms result in a narrowing of the airway, making it more difficult to breathe. Causes of asthma are not entirely understood but may include a familial tendency for the disease, infections, a reaction to environmental substances, and exercise. Asthma is most commonly seen in children younger than age 5 years and children with a family history, allergies, and exposure to secondhand tobacco smoke.

Signs and Symptoms of Asthma

Symptoms of asthma may include coughing, either constantly or intermittently, but especially at nighttime. The child may report chest tightness, chest pain, or fatigue and may display anxiety. Shortness of breath (SOB) may occur, especially with increased activity. Wheezing, which sounds similar to whistling or a musical sound, may be heard with inspiration and/or expiration.

Asthma is diagnosed by physical examination, with particular attention paid to the existing symptoms and a history, including family history. Spirometry will measure and monitor oxygen levels, quantify the severity of the episode, and determine the effectiveness of treatment. Peak flow monitoring (PFM) measures the speed of the air exhaled to determine the severity of the patient's incapacity. A CXR will show consolidation in the lungs caused by infection or abnormalities of the airway passages. ABGs will show oxygenation and the ability to exhale carbon dioxide. A CBC will show the presence of infection in the WBC and the ability to transport oxygen on the hemoglobin (Hgb) molecule. Allergy tests may be done to try to determine possible causes of an exacerbation of the asthma.

Interventions for Asthma

Asthma therapy is intended to promote adequate oxygenation, improve the size of the airway, facilitate the removal of secretions, and alleviate anxiety. Supplemental oxygen may be given if oxygen levels are below normal. Steroids given orally or via IV and inhaled bronchodilators and breathing treatments reduce swelling and enlarge the airway to allow easier passage of air. Suctioning removes excess secretions from the airway, as does encouraging coughing. Increasing fluid intake helps to thin secretions. Sedation may be given for anxiety to facilitate treatment and procedures. Table 30.3 provides a list of common asthma medications, and Figure 30.8 depicts the most appropriate method to administer asthma medication inhalers.

Nursing Considerations for Asthma

It may be as frightening to be in the hospital as it is to have difficulty breathing for a child and family. Help to relieve this fear by providing calm explanations of procedures and treatments, making sure not to overwhelm the family with too much information. The child will most likely need to use an **inhaler** (a device used to breathe inhaled medications into the lungs) and a **nebulizer** (a device that aerates respiratory medications) at home. Therefore, the family, or the child if old enough, will need to be instructed in their use.

Many health-care providers caring for children with asthma provide written guidelines on how to respond to a child with asthma symptoms. The guidelines include a color-coded system to guide the parents of the child in interventions, depending on the child's daily peak flow.

Patient Teaching Guidelines

Color-Coded Zones for Asthma Evaluations and Interventions

Peak flow measurements are conducted on a device that measures how fast air is moved from the lungs. The color-coded areas on the device provide information similar to a signal on a traffic light, representing safe (green), caution (yellow), and danger (red) zones.

Continued

Table 30.3

Types of Asthma Medications

Category	Purpose	Medication Types
Long-term asthma control medications	Taken regularly to control chronic symptoms and prevent asthma attacks; the most important type of treatment for most people with asthma	• Inhaled corticosteroids • Leukotriene modifiers • Long-acting beta agonists (LABAs) • Theophylline • Combination inhalers that contain both a corticosteroid and a LABA
Quick-relief medications (rescue medications)	Taken as needed for rapid, short-term relief of symptoms; used to prevent or treat an asthma attack	• Short-acting beta agonists such as albuterol • Ipratropium • Oral and IV corticosteroids (for serious asthma attacks) • Racemic epinephrine
Medications for allergy-induced asthma	Taken regularly or as needed to reduce the body's sensitivity to a particular allergy-causing substance (allergen)	• Allergy shots (immunotherapy) • Omalizumab

Patient Teaching Guidelines—cont'd

Children over the age of 5 years are requested to perform peak flow measurements on a regular basis. Children with severe asthma are asked to perform peak flow measurements at least once or twice a day. The following peak flow findings indicate to the family what interventions are needed:

Green Zone:

- Peak flow measurements are between 80% and 100% of the child's personal best when not experiencing asthma symptoms.
- The child is instructed to take daily medications and participate in all normal activities.

Yellow Zone:

- Peak flow measurements are between 50% and 80% of the child's personal best when not experiencing asthma symptoms.
- The child experiencing asthma symptoms in the yellow zone is instructed to slow down, take their fast-acting inhaler now, and keep the inhaler available throughout the day.

Red Zone:

- Peak flow measurements are below 49% of the child's personal best when not experiencing asthma symptoms.
- The child is experiencing a severe asthma attack and should be seen by their health-care provider, be taken to the closest ED, or the parent should call 911. All medications should go with the child for evaluation.

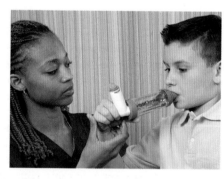

FIGURE 30.8 The appropriate method to administer asthma medication inhalers.

Health Promotion

Tips on Asthma Triggers and How to Reduce Triggers in the Home

1. Determine air quality for the day by checking the local weather report for mold, pollen, pollution, and high ozone levels; avoid or adjust physical activity and exercise on days of poor air quality.
2. Dust all hard surfaces throughout the home on a weekly basis using a damp cloth with soap.
3. Never smoke around a child, especially in the home or car.
4. Put dust covers on mattresses and pillows, and wash weekly.
5. Replace heating and cooling appliance filters on a regular basis.

Health Promotion—cont'd

6. Inspect the home every season for the buildup of mold, water leaks, and home damage caused by water to prevent exposure to various mold growths.
7. Vacuum carpet, floors, and any fabric-covered furniture on a weekly basis using a HEPA filter vacuum system that is cleaned after each use.
8. Check the home for pests, especially cockroach evidence, and seal all openings found along walls, plumbing openings, and cracks to prevent infestations. Keep the home clean and free of trash. Place screens on windows. Use insect traps (sticky tapes) instead of spraying pesticides.
9. Remove pets that have fur from the home and keep small caged animals (birds, lizards) in their clean cages as much as possible.
10. Know the child's triggers and monitor for their presence!

Adapted from Centers for Disease Control and Prevention. (2024). *Controlling Asthma.* https://www.cdc.gov/asthma/control/index.html; Indiana State Department of Health. (2014). *Top 10 ways to reduce asthma triggers at home.* http://www.in.gov/isdh/reports/breatheasyville/athome/toptenhome.html

Bronchiolitis

Bronchiolitis is a lower respiratory tract infection caused by a virus, most likely RSV, but can also be caused by the parainfluenza virus, rhinovirus, or adenovirus. Possible bacterial causes are mycoplasma pneumonia and chlamydia pneumonia. Bronchiolitis usually affects infants because of their immature immune systems and lack of cilia in their airways to block infections. The infection starts in the upper airways and then progresses to the lower airways, causing inflammation that obstructs breathing. Risk factors include winter season, male sex, secondhand smoke, bottle feeding, older siblings, and attendance in daycare.

Symptoms may include nasal or upper respiratory congestion, wheezing, cough, loss of appetite, increased crying, fever, and irritability. The infant may start breathing harder or faster than normal.

Evaluations of Bronchiolitis

Diagnosis is usually made by history taking and physical evaluation. A nasopharyngeal wash will be done to test for RSV or other viruses. To rule out other illnesses, other tests may be performed, such as a CXR, sputum culture, and blood cultures; a pulse oximeter will be used to monitor oxygen saturation levels.

Interventions for Bronchiolitis

Treatment of bronchiolitis is symptomatic and will depend on the specific symptoms displayed. Gentle bulb syringe aspiration of nasal oral secretions, antipyretics for fever, and nebulizer treatments with bronchodilators may be performed. In more severe cases, the infant may need to be hospitalized for IV therapy to treat dehydration, nasopharyngeal suctioning to clear secretions, and/or oxygen therapy for hypoxia or dyspnea. High-risk or premature infants may receive an immunization injection called palivizumab or respiratory syncytial immune globulin (RSV-IGIV) to prevent contracting the infection.

Safety Stat!

A young infant with RSV bronchiolitis may experience severe respiratory distress very suddenly. Rapid suctioning in both nares of the thick mucus produced by this condition may be enough to ease the infant's distress. Instilling saline drops right before suctioning may decrease the thickness of the mucus and allow more efficient suctioning.

Nursing Considerations for Bronchiolitis

If the infant is stable enough to be treated at home, the family will need instruction in caring for them. Encouraging fluids to thin secretions and to promote adequate hydration, giving nebulizer treatments for **bronchodilation** (a means of opening the airway), suctioning by bulb syringe, and other interventions may be ordered.

Bronchopulmonary Dysplasia

Bronchopulmonary dysplasia (BPD) or CLD is the term used for long-term respiratory problems in premature infants. BPD is caused by damage to the lungs from mechanical ventilation and prolonged oxygen treatment that causes scarring in the lung tissue. Specific causes may be underdeveloped alveoli, insufficient surfactant, the prolonged use of high-concentration oxygen, the pressure from a ventilator, suctioning, or the trauma of intubation. Risk factors are less than 34 weeks' gestation, less than 2,000 g (4 lb 6.5 oz) birth weight, respiratory distress syndrome, patent ductus arteriosus (PDA), White race, male sex, a family history of asthma, and chorioamnionitis (infected amniotic fluid). (See Chapter 17 for information on respiratory distress syndrome and Chapter 14 for more about the ductus arteriosus.)

Evaluations of Bronchopulmonary Dysplasia

The symptoms of BPD include respiratory distress, flaring nares, tachypnea, and chest retractions. Diagnosis is made when mechanical ventilation and/or oxygen is still necessary after a premature infant has reached the equivalent of 36 weeks' gestation. A CXR will show a spongy appearance of the lungs.

· **WORD · BUILDING ·**

bronchodilation: broncho–airway + dilat–expand, spread out + ion–action

Interventions for Bronchopulmonary Dysplasia

Treatment includes supplemental oxygen, mechanical ventilation until the lungs mature, bronchodilators and steroids to maximize airway clearance, fluid restriction and diuretics to diminish excessive fluid in the lungs, and good nutrition to promote healing and growth. Several months of mechanical ventilation may be required in the most severe cases. The infant may require home oxygen upon discharge from the hospital but will usually be weaned off it by the age of 1 year.

Nursing Considerations for Bronchopulmonary Dysplasia

Families with an infant on mechanical ventilation will need a great deal of support and teaching. They will have to learn about administering oxygen, breathing treatments, and medications at home. They also must be taught to guard against respiratory infections after discharge because the child is at higher risk. The possibility of rehospitalization must be considered.

Cystic Fibrosis

CF is an autosomal recessive genetic disorder caused by a mutation in the gene that regulates sweat, digestive enzymes, and mucus. The gene is called the cystic fibrosis transmembrane conductance regulator (CFTR; Cystic Fibrosis Foundation, 2022). The gene initiates excessive sodium absorption in the lungs, turning usually thin secretions to thickened secretions. Although similar changes occur in the gastrointestinal and reproductive systems, this chapter focuses on the effects of the disease on the respiratory system. There are approximately 40,000 adults and children with CF living in the United States (Cystic Fibrosis Foundation, 2022).

The thicker respiratory secretions of CF are harder for children to clear, which predisposes them to pneumonia. The bacteria *Pseudomonas aeruginosa* is the most prevalent cause of infection, followed by *S. aureus* and *H. influenzae*. Frequent infections may cause a chronic cough, wheezing, **hemoptysis** (blood in respiratory secretions or mucus), **atelectasis** (collapsed or airless lung) secondary to **pneumothorax** (a collection of air or gas in the pleural cavity), and apnea. The cough worsens in the morning or after exertion. Nasal polyps may form and may need to be surgically removed. A high rate of sinusitis may occur.

Signs and Symptoms of Cystic Fibrosis

CF can be diagnosed by genetic testing for the abnormal gene, either via a blood sample or buccal swab, but the sweat test for excessive sodium and chloride is the gold standard for diagnosis. A CXR will show consolidation from thick mucus and any chronic damage to the lungs, as will pulmonary function tests. A sputum culture and sensitivity will identify any bacterial source of an infection and antibiotics to treat the infection effectively.

Labs & Diagnostics

An infant with a sweat chloride test of greater than 60 mEq/L demonstrates a positive value for a diagnosis of CF.

Interventions for Cystic Fibrosis

Treatment is specific to the symptoms the child displays and focuses on decreasing their severity and progression. Physical therapy and exercise help to loosen secretions and induce coughing to expectorate them. Chest percussions do the same. Mucolytic agents break up secretions, causing them to become easier to remove. Nebulizer treatments provide medications directly to the lungs. Oral medications include pancreatic enzymes with each meal and snack and fat-soluble vitamins daily. In the most critical cases, bilateral lung transplantation or a heart–lung transplantation may be necessary.

Nursing Considerations for Cystic Fibrosis

Because CF is an autosomal recessive trait, the family may have questions about the risk of other children having the disease. A nurse not conversant with genetics will need to arrange a referral to an organization or person who can provide information. Family members will need to learn the importance of daily oral medications, how to provide nebulizer treatments and chest percussions, and the importance of ridding the lungs of sputum.

Mortality is a tender issue with families with a child with CF. Approximately 50% of those with CF are now at the age of 18 or older. Families need to understand that those with CF can expect to live healthy lives into their 40s, with some living beyond middle age (Cystic Fibrosis Foundation, 2022).

Foreign Body Aspiration

FB aspiration is one of the main causes of pediatric accidental deaths. It is most common in 1- to 3-year-olds but also occurs in children up to the age of 6. In the United States, FB aspiration causes about 3,000 deaths per year in children under the age of 3. Toddlers' developmental risk factors for aspiration include putting objects into their mouths, learning to walk and run, poor dentition, supervision by a sibling, and immature chewing and swallowing coordination. The aspirated FB lodges in a bronchus in 80% to 90% of all aspirations. The position of a young child's larynx also increases the susceptibility of aspiration. The items most commonly aspirated include small toys, beads, pins, vegetable matter, nuts, grapes, and round foods (Children's Hospital of Philadelphia, 2022).

· WORD · BUILDING ·

hemoptysis: hemo–blood + pty–spit + sis–process
atelectasis: atel–incomplete + ecta–expansion + sis–condition
pneumothorax: pneumo–air + thorax–thorax

After an FB is aspirated, there are three distinct clinical phases:

1. In phase one, the child may exhibit choking, gagging, coughing, hoarseness or aphonia, wheezing, stridor, and circumoral cyanosis. The possibility of death is very high.
2. The second phase is the asymptomatic period that can last up to several months after the aspiration, depending on the location, the amount of airway obstruction, and the aspirant.
3. The third phase shows renewed symptoms. Airway inflammation or infection from the FB may cause coughing, wheezing, fever, sputum production, and hemoptysis.

Signs of Foreign Body Aspiration

Diagnosis can be based on history and a focused physical evaluation. The health-care provide may order a chest or neck x-ray to help reveal the location of the FB or trapped air. A child also may present with adventitious breath sounds such as stridor and wheezing. The child should be checked for respiratory distress and adequate air exchange.

Interventions for Foreign Body Aspiration

If the young child is still able to breathe and cough, they should be closely monitored while attempts are made to spontaneously expel the FB. If there is apnea in an infant, back blows and chest thrusts are recommended by the AAP and the American Heart Association (AHA). Blind finger sweeps are not recommended because this might force the FB farther into the airway. Rigid bronchoscopy may be necessary for visualization of the airway and removal of the FB. After the object is removed, treatment is focused on the prevention of complications, including the prevention of infection, the reduction of swelling, and opening the airway. Antibiotics will be given for signs and symptoms of infection, such as increased mucus production with fever. Steroids and bronchodilators will be given to maintain the airway.

Nursing Considerations for Foreign Body Aspiration

Education is needed for the family to ensure that only developmentally appropriate foods are given to a child. After the FB is removed, further education will show what symptoms to observe for in a swollen or compromised airway. Instruction about discharge medications may be needed.

Nursing Care Plan for the Child With Foreign Body Obstruction

Tori, age 18 months, is brought to the ED by ambulance. Her mother reports that Tori was playing on the floor of the family home when she started gagging and coughing. The mother called 911 after the child was unable to cough anything out and became increasingly anxious and distressed. The emergency medical technician (EMT) reports that on the way to the hospital the child developed stridor and circumoral cyanosis.

Nursing Diagnosis: Ineffective airway clearance related to FB aspiration with choking
Expected Outcome: The patient is able to breathe without obstruction.

Intervention:	Rationale:
Maintain a patent airway.	*The airway must be cleared to allow for oxygenation and gas exchange.*

Nursing Diagnosis: Ineffective breathing pattern related to aspiration, obstruction, and choking
Expected Outcome: The patient breathes without adventitious breath sounds.

Intervention:	Rationale:
Position the patient for comfortable and effective breathing.	*The patient is likely to experience increased respiratory secretions and inflammation after aspirating an FB. Positioning the child with the head elevated will ease pooling of secretions and keep inflamed tissues as open as possible.*

Nursing Diagnosis: Impaired gas exchange related to the presence of FB and asphyxiation
Expected Outcome: The patient's oxygen saturation is within normal limits.

Intervention:	Rationale:
Administer oxygen as needed to promote effective gas exchange and adequate oxygen saturation.	*The child has been hypoxic because of FB aspiration. The body's carbon dioxide and oxygen levels need to be normalized, and the acid–base balance needs to be restored.*

Key Points

- There are distinct differences between the anatomy and physiology of a newborn and a child's respiratory system and that of an adult. These differences are important to understand in order to evaluate and interpret diagnostic data and to prevent complications. Differences include the size of the airways, respiratory rates, total tidal volumes, and others.
- Adventitious breath sounds during respiratory distress include stridor, rales, and rhonchi. You must be able to distinguish when a child is demonstrating an increased work of breathing, dyspnea, and respiratory distress to quickly intervene to reduce complications.
- The physical examination of an infant or a child with a respiratory condition is holistic and includes both the respiratory system and the cardiac system. Gas exchange and oxygenation are the two main concepts associated with the respiratory system. Evaluations of overall respiratory status include auscultation, palpation, olfaction, percussion, and inspection.
- Young children are particularly vulnerable to respiratory infections because of their limited immunity,

increasing social exposure to community-acquired infections, and their small airways and shorter tracheas. Young children can also have increased symptom severity and worse adventitious breath sounds. A child who is demonstrating SOB or respiratory distress requires immediate interventions, which may include bronchodilators, steroids, antibiotics, racemic epinephrine, oxygen, and fluids.
- Various oxygen delivery systems exist. These include infant crib tents, simple face masks, partial rebreather masks, nonrebreather masks, and ventilators. Each has a particular function and flow of oxygen.
- Epiglottitis is considered a respiratory emergency and requires experienced health-care team members to carefully manage the child's airway. Neither culture swabs nor a tongue blade should be used for examination or specimen collection because rebound inflammation can occur and occlude the child's airway. Epiglottitis is a severe condition that has a high mortality rate. Rapid diagnosis and antibiotics are required. Hib is often the bacterial culprit.

Review Questions

1. Two-week-old James has been admitted to the hospital with RSV. Which oxygen delivery system is most likely to be ordered for James?
   1. Nasal cannula
   2. Oxygen hood
   3. Nonrebreather mask
   4. Simple face mask

2. Which signs or symptoms may occur in a child with CF? **(Select all that apply.)**
   1. Wheezing
   2. Nasal polyps
   3. Hemoptysis
   4. Collapsed lung
   5. Apnea
   6. A barking cough

3. What sign or symptom is most worrisome in terms of degree of airway compromise?
   1. Fever
   2. Wheezing
   3. Cough
   4. Stridor

4. A 3-year-old presents to the ED with signs of respiratory distress. The child has epiglottitis associated with high fever, is apprehensive, and is drooling. Which intervention should be avoided?
   1. Listening to the child's lungs
   2. Checking the child's vital signs
   3. Weighing the child
   4. Inspecting the child's mouth and throat with a tongue blade

5. Which statement by the mother indicates understanding of your teaching related to a newborn?
   1. "I should expect my baby to breathe more slowly than I do."
   2. "I should use a blanket to cover my newborn when he sleeps."
   3. "I should give all of the pills in my baby's prescription to my baby even if the symptoms have gone away."
   4. "I should call my doctor if my newborn breathes fast while he's sleeping."

6. While the pediatric health-care team is teaching parents of a child who has just been diagnosed with CF, the mother asks if there was something she did to cause this illness. Which response from the team is correct?
   1. There is no known cause for the condition of CF.
   2. The development of CF is directly related to the child's immune system.
   3. CF is a trait passed on to the child by the father's genes exclusively.
   4. CF is an autosomal recessive trait from both parents' genes.

7. While being discharged from the pediatric clinic, the mother of a young child with strep throat asks when the child can return to preschool. Which response by the nurse is correct? **(Select all that apply.)**
   1. 24 hours after the last fever
   2. 24 hours after the first dose of oral antibiotics
   3. 24 hours after consuming 1 L of oral fluids
   4. 24 hours after the last reports of throat pain
   5. 24 hours after the last dose of pain medication

8. While at school, a school-aged child with a history of asthma develops feelings of a tight chest and cough. Which medication would the school nurse need to administer?
   1. Oral steroids
   2. Inhaled beta agonist
   3. Inhaled steroids
   4. Oral leukotriene modifiers

9. In a child who presents with RSV bronchiolitis, what treatments would the health-care team provide?
   1. Suctioning, oxygen, and rest
   2. Albuterol, oxygen, and steroids
   3. Racemic epinephrine, rest, and IV fluids
   4. Suctioning, steroids, and rest

ANSWERS 1. 2; 3. 4; 5. 3, 4, 4; 5. 4; 6. 4; 7. 1, 2; 8. 2; 9. 1

CRITICAL THINKING QUESTIONS

1. Your patient has a highly contagious respiratory infection. Explain the precautions that would be taken to prevent spreading the infection to other patients in the pediatric department.

2. What are the five methods of respiratory examination? Describe how to perform each one.

Resources

For additional resources and information, including Postconference Questions and Activities, Answers, and References, visit www.FADavis.com.

Student Study Guide

CHAPTER 31

Child With a Cardiac Condition

KEY TERMS

cardiovascular (KAR-dee-oh-VAS-kyoo-luhr)
hypoxemia (HYE-pok-SEE-mee-uh)
hypoxia (hye-POK-see-uh)
left-to-right blood flow shunt (LEFT-too-RITE BLUHD FLOH SHUNT)
oxygenation (OK-sih-jen-AY-shun)
perfusion (per-FYOO-zhun)
right-to-left blood flow shunt (RIGHT-too-LEFT BLUHD FLOH SHUNT)

CHAPTER CONCEPTS

Comfort
Communication
Family
Nutrition
Oxygenation
Perfusion
Safety

LEARNING OUTCOMES

1. Define the key terms.
2. Describe the overall anatomy and physiology of the cardiovascular system in the fetus, newborn, and child.
3. Differentiate between the most common congenital cardiac conditions found in infants and children.
4. Identify general relationships between cardiac and pulmonary functions.
5. Describe nursing observations and evaluations of the child who presents with a potential cardiac disorder.
6. Describe the nursing care of the child with a cardiovascular disorder.
7. Describe infectious sources of cardiac malfunction found in children.
8. Describe the educational needs of a child with a cardiac disorder and family using a developmentally appropriate approach.
9. Describe how to safely administer cardiac medications to a child, including the correct steps to administer medications, the evaluation of medication effects, and appropriate patient and/or parent teaching.

CRITICAL THINKING & CLINICAL JUDGMENT

Janisha, a 12-day-old and previously healthy infant girl, is brought to the emergency department (ED) by her parents. She exhibits irritability, difficulty breathing, poor appetite, sweating with feeds, and dusky (slightly bluish) lower extremities. The mother shares that her pregnancy and delivery were normal. When you examine Janisha, you note that she has a heart rate of 160 bpm, a respiratory rate of 44 breaths per minute, an axillary temperature of 98.2°F (36.8°C), a heart murmur, and a delayed capillary refill of 4 seconds. Her weight is 30 grams above her birth weight. After performing four-extremity blood pressure (BP) readings, you inform the pediatric health-care team that the baby has lower BPs and weaker pulses in her lower extremities than in her upper extremities.

Questions

1. Which examination findings are of particular concern and why?
2. Considering the examination findings, what should you do next?
3. Should you be concerned about the infant's poor feeding patterns?

The vast majority of children are born with healthy cardiovascular systems. Congenital (existing since birth) cardiovascular conditions are rare and complex, requiring a pediatric health-care team approach and a long period of follow-up and surveillance. Congenital conditions require a child to endure many diagnostic procedures, which are often followed by surgical repair. Acquired cardiovascular conditions are much more common across the developmental period. Whether a condition is congenital or acquired, you need a thorough understanding of the anatomy and physiology of the cardiovascular system. This includes fetal and newborn heart anatomy and physiology.

The heart's main function is to distribute oxygenated blood throughout the child's tissues. While learning the structures of circulation, it's a good idea to review the impact of adequate ventilation and subsequent oxygenation.

THE DEVELOPMENT OF THE CARDIOVASCULAR SYSTEM

To grasp the often-complex nature of cardiac conditions in children, it is important to start with an understanding of how the heart circulates blood and perfuses the tissues in the body in a child without cardiac disease. In the most basic of terms, the heart and blood vessels form a pump-driven circulation system. The heart contains specialized muscle, the myocardium, that is electrically sensitive. When the myocardium contracts in response to electrical impulses from natural pacemakers, it sends blood pulsing through the circulatory and pulmonary vascular system. The objective of the cardiac pump is to circulate oxygen-carrying blood out of the lungs to the body and return the deoxygenated blood from the body to the lungs. Key principles of cardiac function are as follows:

- The atria, ventricles, heart valves, and cardiac vessels are formed and begin primitive functioning around the eighth week of pregnancy.

· **WORD · BUILDING ·**
perfusion: per–through + fus–pour + ion–action

- The right atrium and ventricle circulate deoxygenated blood to the lungs. Then, the oxygenated blood cycles to the left atrium and ventricle to be pumped to the rest of the body.
- The precisely timed cardiac cycles of contraction (pumping) and relaxation (refilling) are driven by a complex electrical system of pacemaking nodes and myocardial (cardiac) muscle fibers located throughout the heart.
- Heart rate, pulses, capillary refill, and BP measurements provide essential, basic data about how well the heart can perfuse the tissues. Mental status and alertness and quantity of urine output can also be indicators of the cardiac output of blood to key organ systems. Signs of hypoperfusion that require immediate intervention and notification of health-care providers include:
  - Prolonged capillary refill time, greater than 3 seconds
  - Weak or absent pulses
  - Pale or cyanotic (bluish) skin color to the nailbeds, mucosa, and circumoral area (the area around the mouth)
  - Decreased mental status
  - Decreased urine output of less than 1 to 2 mL/kg/hour
  - Cool extremities
  - Tachycardia
  - Hypotension or near-normal BPs initially
  - An oxygen saturation of less than 90%
- Basic BP readings reflect the pressure during the cardiac contraction phase (systole) and relaxation phase (diastole).

· **WORD · BUILDING ·**
hypoxia: hyp–deficient + ox–oxygen + ia–condition
hypoxemia: hyp–deficient + ox–oxygen + em–blood + ia–condition
cardiovascular: cardio–heart + vascul–blood vessels + ar–relating to

Fluid and electrolyte balances are critical to monitor and manipulate in order to maintain optimal BPs and perfusion. A lack of adequate fluid in the cardiovascular space can lead to low BP and shock. On the other hand, fluid overload can lead to congestive heart conditions. Electrolytes such as sodium, potassium, and chloride, as well as other blood chemistries, are important in cardiac function.

Renal (kidney) function is an essential part of maintaining fluid and electrolyte balance. Urine output can indicate how effectively the heart is perfusing important organ systems because the kidneys are very sensitive to poor blood flow. The kidneys will slow down or stop making urine if they are not well-perfused.

Findings to immediately report to the health-care provider are decreased perfusion, unanticipated weight gain, an increased respiratory rate, and noncompliance with the medication plan. These evaluation findings can be signs of impending heart failure.

Fetal Cardiac Structures

Before birth, a fetus has blood flow pathways that allow the delivery of oxygen and nutrients to the baby without the use of the lungs (Fig. 31.1). Three shunts—the ductus arteriosus, the ductus venosus, and the foramen ovale—allow

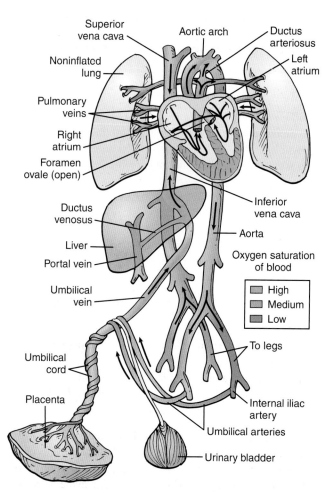

FIGURE 31.1 Fetal cardiac blood flow.

oxygenated blood to mix with deoxygenated blood. (Review fetal circulation in Chapters 4 and 14.) At delivery, the pathways change to allow increased blood flow to the infant's newly expanded lungs, and respiration begins.

Postnatal Blood Flow

Once delivery is complete and blood flow from the placenta stops, a brief period of change to extrauterine life occurs. This process is termed *transition.*

Typically, the majority of the transition process happens in a matter of minutes and continues through the first several months of life. This move from oxygenation via the maternal/placental route to the respiratory system is primarily dependent on the infant's ability to close the fetal shunts. Eventually, the fetal shunt structures seal shut and/or become ligaments (Table 31.1). Most shunts close spontaneously, but those that persist may require surgical repair.

Heart Rate and Blood Pressure

Heart rate and BP are related measurements of cardiac function. They vary according to the age of the child, with normal heart rate values decreasing with age and normal BP values increasing with age (Table 31.2). Be sure to check all vital signs accurately, including BP, heart rate, respiratory rate, temperature, and oxygen saturation. Measure BP annually in children and adolescents at 3 years of age or older. If there are health risks such as obesity, medications known to raise BP, renal disease, diabetes, and/or a history of aortic arch abnormalities, measure BP with every health-care encounter (Mattoo, 2023; Mayo Clinic, 2022). If a child is younger than 3 years old and has a history of preterm birth, congenital heart disease, solid-organ transplant, cancer, or other chronic illnesses known to increase BP or intracranial pressure, measure BP at every health-care encounter as well.

Electrical System of the Heart

The electrical conduction system of the heart regulates the precise timing of atrial and ventricular contractions.

1. Near the top of the right atrium is a small patch of tissue called the *sinoatrial (SA) node.* The SA node generates

Table 31.1
Comparison of Fetal and Postbirth Circulation

Fetal Circulation	*Postbirth Circulation*
Pulmonary Circulation • Decreased blood flow through the lungs	• Increased blood flow through the lungs
Systemic Circulation • Higher pressure in the right ventricle • Lower pressures in the left atrium, left ventricle, and aorta	• Decreased pressure in the right ventricle • Increased pressure in the left atrium, left ventricle, and aorta
Ductus Arteriosus • Allows blood to bypass the fluid-filled lungs by shunting blood from the pulmonary artery to the aorta	• Closes almost immediately after birth or may remain open or partially open for up to 15 hours after birth to allow increased blood flow to the lungs to permit oxygenation • May remain open if the lungs fail to expand • Anatomical obliteration within 1–3 months
Ductus Venosus • Shunts a portion of the left umbilical vein blood flow to the inferior vena cava, allowing blood to bypass the liver	• When the cord is clamped and umbilical blood flow is stopped, it closes completely by day 3 and forms a ligament
Foramen Ovale • An opening that allows blood to flow directly to the right atrium and bypass the lungs	• Functionally closes at birth when increased pressure in the left atrium and decreased pressure in the right atrium occur • Constant circulation leads to permanent closure within a few months
Umbilical Arteries • Carry deoxygenated blood from the hypogastric arteries to the placenta	• Blood flow disrupted when the umbilical cord is cut • Closed within hours of birth and permanently gone by 2–3 months
Umbilical Vein • Carries blood from the placenta, ductus venosus, and liver to the inferior vena cava	• Closed when the umbilical cord is cut and eventually forms a ligament

Sources: Krose, J. K., van Vonderen, J. J., Narayen, I. C., Walther, F. J., Hooper, S., & te Pas, A. B. (2016). The perfusion index of healthy term newborns during transition at birth. *European Journal of Pediatrics, 175*, 475–479. https://doi.org/10.1007/s00431-015-2650-1; Riviere, D., McKinlay, C. J. D., & Bloomfield, F. H. (2017). Adaptation for life after birth: A review of neonatal physiology. *Anesthesia and Intensive Care Medicine, 18*(2), 59–67. https://doi.org/10.1016/j.mpaic.2016.11.008

an electrical impulse about 60 to 100 times per minute. This impulse causes the atria to contract, pumping blood into the ventricles.

2. The electrical impulse continues to the atrioventricular (AV) node.
3. The impulse stops very briefly and then continues down the conduction pathways via the bundle of His into the ventricles, causing them to contract and send blood out to the body or to the lungs. The bundle of His provides electrical stimulation to both ventricles via the Purkinje fibers, found in the walls of the ventricles themselves.

Almost all heart tissue is capable of initiating an electrical impulse and a resulting contraction, in effect becoming the pacemaker. Arrhythmias (abnormal heartbeats) occur when:

• There is an interruption in the normal conduction pathway.
• The SA node generates an abnormal rhythm or rate.
• Another node (AV node) or tissue (the Purkinje fibers) becomes the primary pacemaker.

The heart's electrical impulses can be documented in a waveform shown on an ECG machine. The basic segments of the waveform reflect the timing of the contraction, relaxation, and rest (recharging) phases of the cardiac cycle as well as the valve function (Fig. 31.2).

Table 31.2

Normal Blood Pressures and Heart Rates for Children

Age	Systolic Blood Pressures	Diastolic Blood Pressures	Heart Rates
Premature	55–75 mm Hg	35–45 mm Hg	120–170 bpm
Neonate	50–75 mm Hg	30–45 mm Hg	120–160 bpm
Toddler	90–105 mm Hg	55–70 mm Hg	70–110 bpm
Preschooler	95–110 mm Hg	60–75 mm Hg	65–110 bpm
School-age	100–120 mm Hg	60–75 mm Hg	60–95 bpm
Adolescent	<120 mm Hg		55–100 bpm

Source: Adapted from Rudd, K., & Kocisko, D. (2023). *Pediatric nursing: The critical components of care* (3rd ed.). F. A. Davis. Copyright 2023.

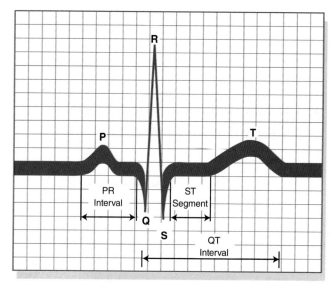

FIGURE 31.2 ECG waveform.

The first upward curve of the ECG tracing is the *P wave.* The P wave indicates that the SA node has fired an impulse and that the atria are contracting to pump blood into the ventricles. This is called a *sinus rhythm.* The next segment is the *PR interval.* This represents the AV conduction time. The steep upward spike, called the *QRS complex,* indicates that the ventricles are contracting, sending blood to the body and lungs. Next, there is a short upward segment called the *ST segment.* The ST segment reflects the time from the end of one ventricular contraction to the beginning of the rest period before the next contraction. The final upward notch is the *T wave.* The T wave indicates the resting period necessary for the heart to start the next beat.

Each segment of the ECG waveform has specific measurements that are considered normal. Variations in the timing or the shape of the different segments, or the speed of the overall heart rate, are analyzed by health-care providers as a diagnostic tool.

INTRODUCTION TO CARDIAC CONDITIONS

Children with heart disease are either born with the disorder or acquire it sometime after birth. Heart disease can affect the actual structures in the heart, and/or it can alter circulatory function. Cardiac conditions can adversely affect health through hypoxemia and impaired tissue perfusion caused by heart failure. These conditions are a leading cause of death from birth defects in the first year of life. Almost 1% of babies born in the United States, about 40,000 births annually, have congenital heart defects, making it the most common type of birth defect (Centers for Disease Control and Prevention [CDC], 2022b). Women who are obese, have diabetes, or smoke are at higher risk of having a baby with a heart defect (CDC, 2023).

To diagnose a cardiac condition in children, the pediatric health-care team works together to identify classic symptoms and clinical presentations. Table 31.3 provides an overview of types of congenital heart defects in children (CDC, 2022a).

Health History

A thorough health history of a child who presents with a cardiac condition, either congenital or acquired, is a priority nursing action. The history should include:

- Past medical history of the child, including the presence of known congenital anomalies and conditions associated with cardiac malformations, such as Down syndrome, fetal alcohol spectrum disorders (FASD), and Turner syndrome

Table 31.3
Types of Pediatric Congenital Heart Defects

Heart Defect	Description and Usual Shunt
Atrial septal defect (ASD)	A passage between the left atrium and right atrium that results in increased blood flow to the lungs (left-to-right shunt)
Ventricular septal defect (VSD)	A passage between the left and right ventricles that results in increased blood flow to the lungs (left-to-right shunt)
Pulmonary stenosis	Narrow pulmonary artery or valve that obstructs blood flow coming out of the ventricles
Aortic stenosis	A constriction at or around the aortic valve
Coarctation of aorta	A narrowing of the aorta at or around the location of the ductus arteriosus that obstructs blood flow out of the ventricles
Transposition of the great arteries (TGA)	The pulmonary artery is connected to the left ventricle versus the right ventricle, and the aorta is connected to the right ventricle versus the left ventricle (survival is dependent on PDA until surgical repair is done).
Hypoplastic left heart syndrome (HLHS)	Incomplete development of the aorta, aortic valve, left ventricle, and mitral valve. This necessitates the right ventricle circulating blood to the body as well as to the lungs.
Patent ductus arteriosus (PDA)	Occurs when the fetal shunt between the pulmonary artery and the aorta does not close and increases blood flow to the lungs (left-to-right shunt)
Tricuspid atresia	Complete obstruction of the tricuspid valve (right-to-left shunt)

- Maternal history associated with an increased risk of heart disease in children, including diabetes, rubella, obesity, alcohol use, smoking, and previous pregnancy losses
- Current and past medications, including over-the-counter products and holistic remedies
- Signs in infant: Cyanosis that worsens with activity or feeding; heart murmur; low weight for stature; diaphoresis (sweating); fatigue when feeding; and a weak, irritable cry
- Signs in older children: Decreased activity levels, dizziness or syncope, a thin build, and chest pain

Physical Evaluation

The child with heart disease can decompensate rapidly with only subtle signs of warning. It is very important that the members of the health-care team rapidly evaluate a child who is decompensating and act quickly to provide life-saving treatments. Children who receive cardiopulmonary resuscitation in a hospital setting have an approximately 54% chance of not surviving (Bimerew et al., 2021). Key observations for a child with a known cardiac condition include the following:

- Obtain a complete set of vital signs, including an oxygen saturation (pulse ox) reading and a pain score.
- Auscultate heart sounds. Develop the skills needed to identify heart sounds and to describe them accurately

when charting. Two typical heart sounds are the "lub-dub" for systolic-diastolic sounds; these sounds are labeled S_1 ("lub") and S_2 ("dub"). Abnormal heart sounds can be murmurs, which are sounds that result from turbulent blood flow in the heart. They have different characteristics, depending on the defect. These are the characteristics of the heart sounds that should be noted:

- *Location:* The anatomical location where the sound is best heard
- *Frequency:* Either a high pitch (best heard with the diaphragm of the stethoscope) or a low pitch (heard best with the stethoscope's bell)
- *Timing:* The time during systole, diastole, or both phases, during which the sound is heard
- *Intensity:* Loudness, which is graded on a scale of 1 to 6, which corresponds to from faint to very loud
- *Quality:* In charting, use descriptive terms such as *musical, click, swish, blowing, harsh,* and so on.
- *Duration:* Early, mid, late, or pan (across the whole sound); long or short
- *Radiation:* Other areas of the body where the heart sound may be heard
- Observe for signs of chronic hypoxemia, such as cyanosis, clubbing of fingers, poor weight gain, rapid respiration (tachypnea), dyspnea (labored breathing), and polycythemia (high RBC count).

- Monitor for signs of heart failure, such as tachycardia, heart murmurs (including extra heart sounds S_3 and S_4), cool extremities, weak pulses, sluggish capillary refill, anorexia, generalized paleness, mottling, fatigue, poor urine output, diaphoresis, cardiomegaly on chest x-ray, and poor growth (failure to thrive [FTT]).
- Look for signs of systemic venous congestion found in heart failure, such as peripheral edema, enlarged spleen and liver, neck vein distention (except in babies), and ascites (abdominal fluid collection).
- Observe for signs of pulmonary congestion associated with heart failure, such as exercise intolerance and recurrent respiratory infections. The health-care team must also investigate for tachypnea, stridor, grunting, nasal flaring, retractions (accessory muscle usage), and abnormal lung sounds such as crackles, which indicate extra fluid and dyspnea.
- Determine the social and cultural structure and support of the patient and their family members. Determine anxiety levels and developmental milestones reached to plan teaching and emotional support for the patient and the patient's family.

Labs & Diagnostics

Common Diagnostic Procedures and Laboratory Tests for Pediatric Cardiac Conditions
Common Diagnostic Procedures
- Electrocardiography (12-lead ECG)
- Chest radiography (x-ray)
- Echocardiogram ultrasound (echo)
- Cardiac catheterization

Common Laboratory Tests for Children With Cardiac Conditions
- Complete blood count (CBC) with differential
- C-reactive protein (CRP)
- Blood cultures
- Antistreptolysin-O (ASO) titer and throat culture, if *Streptococcus* infection suspected
- Hemoglobin (Hgb)
- Hematocrit (Hct)
- Serum electrolytes
- Arterial blood gas (ABG)
- **Erythrocyte** sedimentation rate (ESR)

GENERAL NURSING CARE OF THE CHILD WITH A CARDIAC CONDITION

Comprehensive nursing care that includes psychosocial, cultural, and emotional aspects, as well as physiological components, is key to optimizing the quality and length

- WORD - BUILDING -

erythrocyte: erythro–red + cyte–cell

of life for children who live with a cardiac condition. Preventing complications includes involving parents and caregivers in every phase of diagnosis, treatment, and recovery. The child's developmental stage and level should be taken into consideration so that the child can continue to develop and grow as expected cognitively and emotionally. The following aspects of nursing care will support a child with a known or suspected cardiac condition:

- Reduce fatigue and discomfort: Provide frequent rest breaks and small, frequent meals; cluster care to allow time between interventions; bathe as needed; and sooth and console the child to keep crying to a minimum, especially in the presence of cyanosis.
- Provide respite care for the parents, private time to hold their child, and a calm and soothing environment.
- Monitor daily weights and intake and output (I&O) to track nutritional and fluid status.
- Track vital signs, laboratory tests (including serum electrolytes), and renal function to evaluate for developing complications.
- Share developmentally appropriate resources and provide support for children and family to continue the child's growth and maturation.
- Administer prescribed medications and monitor for effect and untoward responses.
- Monitor the coping of the child and family, and provide culturally and spiritually appropriate care.
- Include interdisciplinary involvement with social services, child life specialists, and academic support for older children.
- Create a nursing care plan that reflects holistic care.

Safety *Stat!*

Obtaining accurate weights is essential! Weigh the child naked at the same time each day on the same scale. *Any change in weight must be reported right away.* Many cardiac conditions cause the child to hold fluids and gain water weight rather than experience actual growth. Several conditions could be causing an infant with a congenital heart defect not to grow and gain weight as expected and desired:

- The infant becomes fatigued during feedings and does not finish the nursing or bottle session.
- The cardiac condition is causing the child to become short of breath while eating, and therefore the child does not take in the full calories.
- The parents may be unaware of the child's calorie needs.
- The cardiac condition might be causing oxygenated blood to return to the lungs, causing fluids to build up. If the child has crackles or rales, the child might not be able to finish a meal because of shortness of breath.

SYSTEM-FOCUSED NURSING CARE

Because the cardiovascular system affects all the other body systems, a child with a heart disorder requires system-focused nursing care. Nursing care should be provided related to the pediatric patient's cardiac conduction, circulation, and perfusion:

- *Ensure fluid and electrolyte balance:*
  - Sodium restriction, if ordered
  - Fluid restriction, if ordered
  - Potassium supplementation, if indicated (may be contraindicated if child is taking angiotensin-converting enzyme [ACE] inhibitors)
- *Increase tissue oxygenation:*
  - Check the pulse oxygen saturation readings every 2 to 4 hours and prn.
  - Maintain clear airway by suctioning the child as needed.
  - Give humidified, cool oxygen by hood, mask, or nasal cannula as ordered.
- *Ensure adequate nutrition:*
  - Provide increased caloric density by offering an increased-calorie formula.
  - Supplement breastfeeding with a high-calorie formula or fortified breast milk.
  - Follow oral feeds with gavage (tube) feeding if the child is unable to take enough feeding for growth.
  - Allow rests with feedings, completing feeds within a half hour.
  - Position the infant in a semi-upright position.
  - If bottle feeding, consider a soft preemie or regular nipple with a cross-cut to allow a faster flow of milk with less effort.
  - Schedule small, frequent feedings. In infants, feed every 3 hours or consider continuous gavage feedings at night.
- *Decrease cardiac workload:*
  - Ensure bedrest and a low stimulation environment; keep lights low and noise level down.
  - Elevate the head of bed (semi-Fowler position at 45 degrees) or ensure that the infant is held upright; an infant or toddler car seat can be used to provide an elevated head of bed as well.
- *Teach the family about the care of the child according to the family's preferred method of learning:*
  - In-person presentation
  - Visual materials, which are printed
  - Visual materials via video
  - Demonstrate/return demonstration
  - Written materials (different languages may be required)
  - Online resources from professional and reputable organizations

CLINICAL JUDGMENT

You are caring for an infant patient who has been admitted for care for a congenital heart defect. You note that the patient's vital signs are showing tachycardia. Your first thought is that the child may need more oxygen and should be given supplemental oxygen to help reduce the unmet oxygenation demand causing the fast heart rate.

Questions

1. Should you place oxygen on the infant?
2. What might the infant patient experience if you give supplemental oxygen?

CARDIAC DISORDERS

Disorders of the cardiovascular system include both cyanotic and acyanotic heart defects (Figs. 31.3 and 31.4).

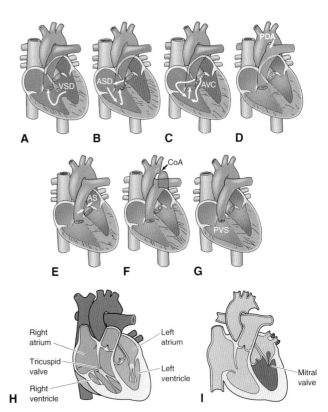

FIGURE 31.3 Select acyanotic heart defects. A, VSD: Opening between ventricles. B, ASD: Opening between atria. C, AV septal defect (AV canal): Low ASD continuous with high VSD and cleft of mitral and tricuspid valves. D, PDA: Fetal ductus does not close at birth. E, Aortic valve stenosis: Narrowing or stricture of the aortic valve. F, Coarctation of the aorta: Narrowing of the aorta at the insertion of the ductus arteriosus. G, Pulmonic valve stenosis: Narrowing of the entrance of the pulmonary artery. H, Tricuspid stenosis: Failure of the tricuspid valve to develop. I, Mitral stenosis: Failure of the mitral valve to develop.

Nursing Care Plan for a Child With a Congenital Heart Defect

Two-month-old Jamie has been brought by his parents to the ED straight from his well-child checkup. Jamie has gained only a few ounces since birth. His parents report that he appears to be exhausted and short of breath when he consumes less than half of a formula feeding. Jamie's nurse practitioner suspects that the infant has a previously undiagnosed heart defect, so she refers Jamie to a pediatric cardiologist. The cardiologist admits Jamie to the hospital for a complete cardiac workup.

Nursing Diagnosis: Decreased cardiac output related to cardiac malformations
Expected Outcome: The patient will experience improved cardiac output as evidenced by strong peripheral pulses, normal heart and respiratory rates, and less shortness of breath.

Interventions:	Rationale:
Observe the quality and strength of the heartbeat, peripheral pulses, skin color, and warmth.	*These interventions allow the nurse to monitor the perfusion and oxygenation of the child's tissues to determine if the condition is responding to treatment.*
Note the degree of cyanosis (mucous membranes, clubbing).	
Monitor signs of congestive heart failure (CHF; anxiety, tachycardia, tachypnea, shortness of breath, tired while feeding, periorbital edema, oliguria, and hepatomegaly).	

Nursing Diagnosis: Impaired gas exchange related to pulmonary congestion
Expected Outcome: The patient is able to maintain adequate oxygenation and ventilation.

Interventions:	Rationales:
Monitor the quality and rhythm of breathing.	*Infants can decompensate rapidly. Keen monitoring of status is essential for safety.*
Place the child in a car seat.	*Elevating the child's head by placing him in a car seat or holding him upright decreases the workload of the heart.*
Give oxygen as indicated.	*Supplemental oxygen will improve the child's low oxygen saturation because of impaired gas exchange.*

Nursing Diagnosis: Imbalanced nutrition: less than body requirements related to fatigue at mealtime and increased caloric needs
Expected Outcome: The patient gains weight appropriately.

Interventions:	Rationales:
Measure body weight each day with the same scales.	*It is essential to monitor for fluid retention and to distinguish growth from fluid retention.*
Record I&O correctly.	*Accurate I&Os help prevent fluid overload and monitor for kidney function.*
Give small portions of high-calorie formula frequently.	*Because feedings tire the infant, they need to ingest the maximum number of calories in a short time to allow for appropriate growth and development.*

Cyanotic Heart Defects

Cyanotic heart defects are a group of heart malformations or lesions that have **right-to-left blood flow shunts**. Right-to-left blood flow shunts refer to cardiovascular conduits through which blood flows abnormally from the right side of the heart, which usually perfuses the pulmonary circulation, to the left side of the heart, which usually perfuses the systemic circulation. Cyanotic heart defects produce some level of cyanosis; however, cyanosis may not be readily visible on assessment. Pulse oximetry, which measures oxygen saturation without a blood sample, is valuable. In fact, the routine use of pulse oximetry in newborn infants has been shown to significantly decrease newborn death rates because of congenital heart defects in states with

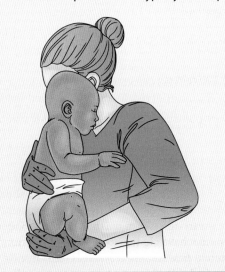

FIGURE 31.4 Select cyanotic heart defects. A, TOF: Includes VSD, pulmonic stenosis, overriding aorta, and right ventricular hypertrophy. B, Pulmonary atresia. C, Tricuspid atresia.

mandatory screening (Brigham and Women's Hospital, 2021). It is not unusual to confirm low oxygen saturations between 50% and 90% in infants with varying degrees of defect severity. Normal saturations typically are greater than 92%. Four characteristics that are found in cyanotic heart defects are:

- Defects that allow the mixing of oxygenated and deoxygenated blood
- An infant or a child who is ductal dependent (a neonate needs a patent ductus arteriosus [PDA] for survival in the initial period of life)
- Low pulmonary blood flow
- High pulmonary blood flow

Transposition of the Great Arteries

In transposition of the great arteries (TGA), the great vessels of the heart are anatomically switched. The pulmonary artery is connected to the left ventricle (vs. the right ventricle), and the aorta is connected to the right ventricle (vs. the left ventricle). The infant's survival is dependent on a PDA until surgical repair can be done. The signs and symptoms that are seen with this disorder include:

- Heart murmur
- Cyanosis that becomes severe in hours to days, as the PDA closes
- Heart failure
- Cardiomegaly (enlarged heart on chest x-ray)

A critical and life-preserving intervention includes the immediate administration of an IV drip of PGE1, which chemically maintains the patency of the ductus arteriosus.

Medication Facts

The action of PGE1 includes dilation of vessels and the inhibition of clotting. This allows a patent flow of blood through the ductus arteriosus and maintains perfusion before a surgical intervention is performed to reroute the blood flow and repair the PDA.

Tetralogy of Fallot

Tetralogy of Fallot (TOF) includes a set of four defects that result in mixed blood flow throughout the newborn's cardiovascular system. Without the mixed blood flow, the fetus would not have survived fetal development. This life-threatening condition requires a series of surgical repairs and can be diagnosed by ECG or cardiac catheterization, or both. The four defects that make up the diagnosis of TOF are:

- Ventricular septal defect (VSD)
- Pulmonary stenosis
- An overriding aorta
- Right ventricular **hypertrophy**

Signs and symptoms seen with the TOF defect are:

- Prominent heart murmur
- Growth retardation/FTT
- Polycythemia and clotting disorders
- Cyanosis (not affected by oxygen therapy), severe difficulty breathing, clubbed fingers, and acidosis

If oxygen saturations are very low, the cardiologist will consider ordering PGE1 to preserve the blood flow through the

Safety *Stat!*

Interventions for Tet Spells

- For Tet spells, also known as *hypercyanotic spells,* the immediate intervention is to have the child flex the knees to the chest to lower venous return. Have the child squat, or place an infant in a knee-to-chest position. You should call for assistance.
- Administer morphine to calm the child and slow tachypnea.
- Administer 100% oxygen, which easily dilates the pulmonary vessels, allowing more blood flow to the lungs, which in turn can help resolve the hypercyanotic spell.

· WORD · BUILDING ·

hypertrophy: hyper–excessive + trophy–growth

PDA and provide some oxygenated blood via mixing. Surgical repair for the TOF is completed when the child is about 6 months old. Long-term issues include pulmonary valve leaking, arrhythmias that necessitate a pacemaker, and periodic evaluation via ECG, a Holter monitor, or an exercise stress test.

Hypoplastic Left Heart Syndrome

Hypoplastic left heart syndrome (HLHS) is a severe, complex heart condition that consists of incomplete development of the aorta, the aortic valve, the left ventricle, and the mitral valve. The condition necessitates that the right ventricle compensate by circulating blood to the body as well as to the lungs. Signs and symptoms of HLHS include:

- Weak pulses to all extremities
- Low pulse oximetry readings that do not increase with the administration of oxygen
- Critical, life-threatening hypotension and shock when the ductus arteriosus closes

If possible, plans are made to deliver the infant in a high-level care facility that can provide aggressive treatment immediately. Surgical repair must be staged in three steps to be completed by 3 years of age. Heart transplantation is also considered because of multiple long-term concerns such as blood clot formation, rapid fatigue with exercise, arrhythmias that necessitate pacemaker placement, and cardiac failure.

Tricuspid Atresia

This heart condition is a complete obstruction of the tricuspid valve that results in a right-to-left shunt. There is an absence of the right atrium to the right ventricle. A three-part, staged surgical repair is required. These children present with:

- Severe cyanosis a few hours after delivery that worsens as the ductus arteriosus closes
- Heart failure
- Growth retardation/FTT

As with other ductal-dependent cardiac malformations, PGE1 is indicated to keep the blood flow through the ductus arteriosus. These infants are often placed on a ventilator very soon after birth. This defect is severe, and children with it are critically ill and are at risk for arrhythmias and sudden death. Cardiac transplantation is considered an option if a donor heart is available for an infant.

Acyanotic Heart Defects

This group of heart malformations or lesions is comprised of those that have a **left-to-right blood flow shunt** (blood flows from the left side of the heart, which usually perfuses the systemic circulation, to the right side of the heart, which usually perfuses the pulmonary circulation). Acyanotic heart defects rarely produce initial cyanosis but can leave the body undersupplied with blood flow. The defects in this group can flood the lungs with excess blood flow, leading to CHF.

Patent Ductus Arteriosus

PDA is a defect that occurs when the fetal shunt between the pulmonary artery and the aorta does not close. The defect causes increased blood flow to the lungs in a left-to-right shunting pattern. Premature infants are especially susceptible to PDAs. A PDA can be asymptomatic. If symptoms are present, the signs and symptoms of this disorder are:

- Labile (fluctuating) oxygen saturations and BPs as the PDA intermittently opens and closes
- Systolic heart murmur (sounds similar to a machine hum)
- Wide pulse pressure (the difference between the systolic and diastolic BPs)
- Bounding pulses
- An active chest wall to the left of the sternum above the heart

The PDA can be closed surgically, but efforts are usually made to support the infant until the PDA closes spontaneously or an attempt is made to chemically close it with a course of indomethacin, which inhibits prostaglandins and promotes constriction of the ductus arteriosus.

Ventricular Septal Defect

VSDs are the most common congenital heart defects, according to the American Heart Association (2022). This defect is a passage between the left and right ventricles that results in increased blood flow to the lungs, resulting in a left-to-right shunt, which can lead to CHF. The signs and symptoms associated with a VSD are:

- Possibly no obvious signs and symptoms, if the defect is very small
- Heart failure
- FTT
- A delayed, harsh, loud murmur usually not heard until pulmonary pressures decrease between 4 and 8 weeks of age

Treatment for CHF that results from a VSD can include diuretic therapy to decrease fluid in the lungs and digoxin to strengthen the contractions of the heart. Symptomatic VSDs require surgical closure of the defect.

Atrial Septal Defect

An atrial septal defect (ASD) is comprised of a passage between the left and right atria that results in increased blood flow to the lungs, creating a left-to-right shunt. The ASD can be a residual opening remaining from the foramen ovale fetal shunt. Signs and symptoms of an ASD are:

- Possibly no obvious signs and symptoms
- A harsh, loud murmur
- Potential for an enlarged right atrium
- Mild CHF

If the defect is large or symptomatic, then surgical repair is needed. In some cases, minimally invasive repairs can be accomplished during a cardiac catheterization.

Aortic Stenosis

This malformation consists of a constriction (narrowing) at or around the aortic valve. If the aortic valve is constricted, then the left ventricle must pump harder to eject blood out into the body. An aortic stenosis is associated with the following signs and symptoms:

- Heart murmur
- Chest pain; weak, thready pulses; intolerance to exercise; hypotension; syncope; and dizziness
- An enlarged left ventricle

A 12-lead ECG may be normal but the defect is seen on cardiac ultrasound. Exercise stress tests give information about the severity of the restriction and the reduced tolerance to activity. Repair can be done through a cardiac catheterization procedure in which the constricted valve is dilated. If the catheterization is not successful in restoring normal aortic blood flow, open heart surgery with possible valve replacement is needed. If the valve is replaced, antibiotic prophylaxis will be necessary.

Pulmonary Stenosis

Pulmonary stenosis consists of a narrow pulmonary artery or valve that obstructs the blood flow coming out of the right ventricle. This condition necessitates surgical repair. ECG tracings are normal. Diagnosis is best made by ECG, and cardiac catheterization will be considered to measure the degree of stenosis. Signs and symptoms of pulmonary stenosis are:

- Systolic heart murmur, often with a "click" quality
- Cyanosis, which is apparent when narrowing is severe
- Intolerance to exercise
- Enlargement of the right ventricle

During cardiac catheterization, the stenotic valve may be dilated (widened) to relieve the obstruction. If the defect is too complex, open heart surgical repair will be necessary.

Coarctation of the Aorta

Coarctation consists of a narrowing of the aorta at or around the location of the ductus arteriosus that obstructs blood flow out of the left ventricle. Diagnosis is made by ECG. Pulse oximetry can be very useful to help detect a coarctation because of the tendency for higher oxygen saturations in the upper limbs than in the lower extremities. More than a 3% difference between upper and lower extremity saturations is cause for further investigation. Often, infants who are diagnosed with a coarctation were discharged home within a few days of birth only to be readmitted within a few weeks of life. Those infants begin to have difficulty breathing and eating, have an increased heart rate, and may show signs of congestive heart disease because of the natural closing of the PDA. The PDA can mask the effects of the reduced blood flow

distal to the coarctation. When the ductus arteriosus begins to close, the infant can become extremely ill very quickly. Depending on the severity and location of the defect, surgical repair may be indicated. Signs and symptoms of this condition are:

- Heart murmur to the left sternal border area
- Tachycardia
- An enlarged heart evidenced on chest x-ray
- Tachypnea, particularly with feeding or crying
- Difficulty eating, because of shortness of breath from extra blood flow to lungs, and fatigue
- Weak or absent lower extremity pulses, which result from decreased cardiac output
- Lower BPs to the lower extremities than to the upper limbs
- Possible development of CHF as the PDA closes
- Hepatomegaly from fluid overload associated with CHF
- Vertigo, headaches, and leg pain
- Increased oxygen saturation and BPs in the upper extremities as compared with the lower extremities
- Low weight or slow weight gain because of inability to finish feeds

Safety Stat!

To detect coarctation of the aorta, take BPs on all four extremities. If the pressure is higher in the upper extremities than in the lower extremities, this finding must be reported immediately.

PGE1, which causes vasodilation of the ductus arteriosus and allows it to temporarily remain open, may be indicated to reduce the development of heart failure. Postoperative complications may include renal damage, which results from clamping the descending aorta during surgery. Prophylaxis with antibiotics may be needed if aortic valve malformations are diagnosed.

Safety Stat!

Hypertension is also a common complication associated with coarctation of the aorta and may necessitate antihypertensive therapy. Meticulous monitoring of BPs is important. Do not take a BP when an infant or young child is crying; this will not provide an accurate measurement.

Congestive Heart Failure

CHF is a major complication of cardiac disease. Generally, if CHF develops before 1 year of age, it is because of a congenital defect. If it develops after 1 year of age, it is most likely from an acquired cause.

Evaluating Congestive Heart Failure

Undetected or untreated CHF leads to death, so strong evaluation skills and early detection are key. The cardinal signs of CHF include:

- Tachycardia
- **Cardiomegaly**
- Tachypnea
- **Hepatomegaly**

Interventions for Congestive Heart Failure

Treatment of CHF is focused on improving cardiac output. Treatment includes the following:

- Preventing, when possible, congenital heart defects by minimizing maternal risk factors such as obesity, diabetes, and smoking
- Reducing cardiac workload
- Using diuretics to treat symptoms of fluid overload
- Supporting nutrition for maximal growth and development
- Providing cardiac surgery to repair the defect if it is progressing

Medications can be used to manage the symptoms of CHF. Medications include digoxin to strengthen the contractions of the heart and diuretics such as furosemide (potassium wasting) or chlorothiazide (potassium sparing) to increase urine output and reduce fluid overload. An ACE inhibitor, such as captopril or enalapril, may be used to reduce the systemic resistance (afterload) that the heart must pump against.

Nursing Considerations for Congestive Heart Failure

Nursing considerations for a child with CHF include:

- Close monitoring of fluid and electrolyte levels, including a check of heart sounds, the presence of swelling, and lung sounds (crackles or rales), all of which indicate increased lung congestion
- Observing for worsening CHF despite the current treatment plan
- Reducing the cardiac workload
- Providing supplemental oxygen as ordered
- Meticulous observations of daily weights

Some children with CHF, especially if the failure is from cardiomyopathy or congenital heart disease, require cardiac transplantation. The nursing interventions for cardiac transplantation include:

- Maintaining a plan of care according to the health-care provider's order for pharmacological support, fluid and electrolyte management, and infection control
- Preparing for surgery and providing postoperative care
- Providing the child and family with developmentally appropriate and culturally and spiritually sensitive support
- Providing instructions on maintaining the essential medication regimen posttransplant
- Instructing the patient and family regarding signs and symptoms of organ rejection

Rheumatic Fever

Rheumatic fever is an inflammatory disease that affects children from 6 to 12 years of age. Rheumatic fever can occur after a throat infection or scarlet fever caused by *Streptococcus*. If a child is only partially treated or untreated for these infections, rheumatic fever can result. The disease can cause permanent damage to heart valves; adequate treatment requires long-term antibiotic therapy.

Evaluating Rheumatic Fever

Presenting signs and symptoms of rheumatic fever include:

- A recent history of a respiratory infection
- Throat pain
- Nontender nodules under the skin over bony prominences
- A pink, flat, nonitching rash on the trunk and the surfaces of the extremities next to the body that appears and disappears rapidly
- Enlarged joints that have painful swelling, indicating inflammatory changes; intermittent periods of pain that resolve without treatment and return to a different joint
- Cardiac changes, including an enlarged heart, tachycardia, changes in heart rhythm, a new heart murmur, chest pain, and faint heart sounds

---

Patient Teaching Guidelines

Digoxin Administration Guidelines for Parents Giving Home Medications

- Take the child's pulse for a full minute before giving a digoxin dose. The cardiologist will determine the minimal heart rate for administration. Call the health-care provider before giving any medication if the heart rate is lower that the minimal specified rate.
- Administer digoxin every 12 hours.
- Watch closely for signs of digoxin toxicity or overdose. Notify the health-care provider immediately if any of the following signs are noted:
  - Decreased heart rate
  - Nausea and vomiting
  - Loss of appetite
- If a dose is missed, do not give an extra dose or increase the dose.
- If the dose is vomited, do not repeat.
- Give water after the dose to prevent tooth decay.
- Keep digoxin in a locked cabinet and in the original package.

- WORD - BUILDING -

cardiomegaly: cardio–heart + megaly–abnormal enlargement
hepatomegaly: hepato–liver + megaly–abnormal enlargement

- Fever
- Fatigue
- Poor appetite
- Intolerance to activity
- Neurological changes, including chorea (involuntary, unpredictable muscle movements of the face, arms, and/or legs)
- Irritability, behavioral issues, and decreased ability to concentrate

Interventions for Rheumatic Fever

Rheumatic fever can be prevented by completing antibiotic treatment for streptococcal throat infections and scarlet fever. Management of the disease includes:

- Laboratory tests, including throat cultures and blood samples for an elevated or rising serum ASO titer, an elevated CRP level, and an ESR that reveals a response to inflammation
- 12-lead ECG
- Long-term treatment with penicillin or erythromycin

Patient Teaching Guidelines

Parents need to understand the importance of long-term oral antibiotic therapy for rheumatic fever. Treatment can last from 5 to 18 years of age.

Nursing Considerations for Rheumatic Fever

Nursing considerations for the care of a child with rheumatic fever include:

- Assisting with procedures
- Providing developmentally appropriate patient education regarding treatments and disease management
- Reassuring the patient and family about the self-limiting nature of the chorea symptoms
- Monitoring the heart rate, rhythm changes, and the presence of murmurs for cardiac decompensation
- Preparing for a surgical valve replacement and postoperative care
- Providing patient and family education regarding medical follow-up care
- Administering antibiotic therapy
- Providing patient and family education about completing the antibiotic therapy regimen as well as adhering to long-term medication, prophylactic antibiotics before dental work, and follow-up appointments every 5 years

Kawasaki Disease

Kawasaki disease is an inflammatory disease that affects the skin, mucous membranes, blood vessels, and lymph nodes. The disease occurs mainly in male children of Asian descent who are younger than 6 years of age. However, the condition can affect children of all ages and races. The cause of Kawasaki disease is unknown, but there may be an association with a viral or an autoimmune factor. Most children recover completely but will need medical follow-up to monitor for progressing intravascular inflammation. Inflammation of the coronary arteries (blood vessels that supply the heart muscle itself) and aneurysms can result from the inflammation and cause significant complications. Healing and recovery from Kawasaki disease may take weeks.

Evaluating Kawasaki Disease

Signs and symptoms of this disease include:

- A high, persistent fever of 102°F (38.9°C) to 104°F (40°C) that lasts 5 days or longer and that may not respond to antipyretics such as acetaminophen or ibuprofen
- Extremely red and swollen eyes without drainage
- Skin and mucous membrane changes such as red membranes in the mouth; dry, cracked, red lips; a bright-red tongue (strawberry tongue) with a white coating; red and peeling skin on the genitalia, hands, and soles of the feet; and flat rashes on the trunk
- Joint changes, including painful, swollen hands and feet on both sides of the body
- Swollen lymph nodes (or sometimes only a solitary node) in the neck
- Potentially associated symptoms of irritability, cough, runny nose, diarrhea, vomiting, and abdominal pain

Interventions for Kawasaki Disease

Treatment for Kawasaki disease involves the immediate administration of IV gamma globulin. Significant improvement is usually seen within 24 hours. Aspirin therapy, glucocorticoids, and cyclosporin are also used (Sundel, 2023).

Safety Stat!

In general, children should not be given aspirin because of its association with Reye syndrome. Kawasaki disease is one of the only conditions in which a child receives aspirin therapy.

Nursing Considerations for Kawasaki Disease

Care for a child who presents with Kawasaki disease includes the following:

- Monitoring for signs of developing coronary artery inflammation, **myocarditis**, **pericarditis**, meningitis, and arthritis
- Administration and maintenance of intravenous gamma immunoglobulin (IVIG) therapy

· WORD · BUILDING ·
myocarditis: myo–muscle + card–heart + itis–inflammation
pericarditis: peri–around + card–heart + itis–inflammation

- Pain management
- Developmentally appropriate patient and family teaching related to Kawasaki disease and treatment
- Administration of high-dose aspirin therapy for anti-inflammatory and blood-thinning action

If Kawasaki disease is recognized and treated early, children can recover fully from it; however, a small number do die from the disease, and some develop coronary artery disease anyway. Because of this, follow-up care with an ECG every 1 to 2 years is recommended.

Safety *Stat!*

Children who have been diagnosed with Kawasaki disease need to have scheduled follow-up appointments. Parents need to understand the importance of these subsequent appointments to monitor heart function.

Subacute Bacterial Endocarditis

Subacute bacterial endocarditis (SBE) is an infection in the lining of the heart. Early diagnosis, while the symptoms are subtle and relatively mild (subacute), is important in order to prevent severe disease. The cause of bacterial **endocarditis** is turbulent blood flow or other factors that damage the lining of the heart. Circulating bacteria, inflammatory cells, and clots adhere to the damaged area and proliferate. A few strains of *Streptococcus* and *Staphylococcus* are common infectious organisms.

Evaluating Subacute Bacterial Endocarditis

Risk factors for SBE include the following:

- Congenital cyanotic heart disease
- The presence of central venous catheters
- IV medication use
- Residual postoperative defect or cardiac catheterization
- Rheumatic fever (*Streptococcus* infection)

Interventions for Subacute Bacterial Endocarditis

If the infection is caught early and the bacterium is sensitive to treatment by penicillin, then the cure rate

· WORD · BUILDING ·

endocarditis: endo–inside + card–heart + itis–inflammation

is almost 100%. If diagnosed late or if the bacterium is not sensitive to treatment by penicillin, the mortality rate from SBE is up to 25%. This makes preventive measures in susceptible children a high priority. Preventive antibiotic therapy before invasive procedures and dental work is essential.

The primary symptoms of SBE are flu-like symptoms that last more than 2 weeks, and this condition is more common in those with heart defects. In contrast, *acute* bacterial endocarditis is more common in those with a normal heart configuration. Patients with acute bacterial endocarditis typically present with the following symptoms, which last fewer than 2 weeks:

- Fever
- Fatigue, sweats, chills, loss of appetite, joint pain, confusion, headache, malaise, and cough
- May have a positive history of IV medication use

Nursing Considerations for Subacute Bacterial Endocarditis

Nursing considerations for children at risk for SBE are:

- Administering IV antibiotics for about 8 weeks to treat SBE
- Providing developmentally appropriate patient and family teaching about antibiotic prophylaxis for dental procedures and surgical procedures that involve the respiratory and gastrointestinal mucosa
- Providing patient and family teaching about the signs and symptoms of SBE and the need to contact the health-care provider immediately if SBE is suspected

Safety *Stat!*

Parents need to understand that prophylactic oral antibiotic therapy is essential before the child undergoes any dental procedures. The family must contact their pediatric health-care provider ahead of time to ensure that a prescription for antibiotics can be obtained, filled, and administered before any dental cleaning or procedures take place. A new prescription should be requested before each dental procedure.

Key Points

- Overall, the development of a pediatric cardiac anomaly is rare.
- There is a direct relationship between the pulmonary system and the cardiovascular system. Without an effectively functioning heart, the oxygenation process carried out by the lungs will not be effectively distributed.
- Congenital heart defects are categorized into two large groups: those that produce cyanosis (right-to-left shunting) and those that do not produce cyanosis (acyanotic, left-to-right shunting).
- Children can present with infectious processes within the cardiovascular system. These include Kawasaki disease, SBE, and rheumatic fever.
- CHF is a major complication of cardiac disease. Generally, if CHF develops before 1 year of age, it is because of a congenital defect. If CHF develops after 1 year of age, the etiology is most likely from an acquired cause.
- The cardinal signs of CHF in children with cardiac conditions include tachycardia, cardiomegaly, tachypnea, and hepatomegaly.
- Educating parents about the care of their child with a cardiac infection or anomaly is very important to maintain safety. Correct medication administration, adequate caloric intake, and prevention of infections are all important areas of nursing education.
- A holistic approach to nursing care, with awareness of the developmental tasks and emotional and social needs of the child and family, will positively impact the quality of life for patients with heart disease.

Review Questions

1. A 22-month-old child squats intermittently when walking. She is irritable, cyanotic, and appears listless. What is the most likely cardiac malformation the child has?
   1. Tricuspid atresia
   2. TGA
   3. TOF
   4. Pulmonary stenosis

2. Oxygenated blood mixes in the fetal heart through a shunt between the pulmonary artery and the aorta. What is the name of the shunt?
   1. Pulmonic-aortic shunt
   2. Ductus arteriosus
   3. Ductus venosus
   4. Foramen ovale

3. Which of these pregnant women is at higher risk of having a baby with a congenital heart defect? (**Select all that apply.**)
   1. Kamala, who is 30 years old and has chronic hypertension
   2. Raquel, who is 19 and has anorexia
   3. Lori, who is 25 and has diabetes
   4. Ashleigh, who is 34 and has renal disease
   5. Yolanda, who is 28 and smokes cigarettes

4. Which of these cardiac conditions found in children arises from malformations in the fetal development of the heart?
   1. Rheumatic heart disease
   2. CHF
   3. TGA
   4. Hypoxemia

5. A 7-year-old boy has returned from a cardiac catheterization. Which postoperative interventions should you plan to provide? (**Select all that apply.**)
   1. Check pulses for symmetry and strength.
   2. Ensure continuous cardiac monitoring and pulse oximetry to monitor for dysrhythmias, bradycardia, hypotension, hypoxia, and hypoxemia.
   3. Maintain the affected extremity in a flat position for 4 to 8 hours to prevent postprocedure bleeding.
   4. Check for a history of a reaction to contrast medium or allergy to iodine.
   5. Monitor I&O closely for sufficient urinary output, dehydration, or hypovolemia.
   6. Determine the pain level using a developmentally appropriate tool for the age of the child.

6. A term newborn is diagnosed with TGA. Which priority nursing intervention should be instituted immediately?
   1. Administering an ECG
   2. Providing oxygen via nasal cannula at 2 liters per minute
   3. Preparing for intubation and placement on a ventilator
   4. Establishing IV access and initiating a PGE1 drip

7. When you are looking at an ECG strip, the P wave indicates that which of the following areas in the heart has fired an electrical impulse?
   1. Purkinje fibers
   2. AV node
   3. Bundle of His
   4. SA node

8. Pediatric heart failure is most common in infants with congenital heart disease but can present in older children because of which condition?
   1. Myocarditis
   2. Excessive exercise and a thin body frame
   3. Rhinovirus infections
   4. Severe nausea and vomiting

9. Coarctation of the aorta causes the infant to struggle to feed because of shortness of breath. What causes the infant's shortness of breath?
   1. The infant's lungs are unable to ventilate and provide the body with oxygen.
   2. Oxygenated and deoxygenated blood are mixing in the infant's heart.
   3. The infant's tissues are not receiving adequate oxygen because of constricted blood flow.
   4. The infant's lungs are not receiving adequate perfusion to allow for gas exchange.

10. Sam, a licensed vocational nurse (LVN), sees that it is time for his 5-year-old patient's digoxin. How should Sam prepare to administer this medication? (**Select all that apply.**)
    1. Confirm that the dose on hand matches the ordered dose.
    2. Use two identifiers to confirm that the correct patient is receiving the medication.
    3. Take the patient's temperature.
    4. Take the child's pulse for 1 full minute.
    5. Ask the patient if she wants to take the medicine.

ANSWERS 1. 3; 2. 2; 3. 3, 5; 4. 3, 5; 1, 2, 3, 5; 6. 4; 7. 4; 8. 1; 9. 3; 10. 1, 2, 4

CRITICAL THINKING QUESTIONS

1. Describe the effects on cardiac output and pulmonary blood flow of neonatal cardiac left-to-right shunting and of right-to-left shunting. What symptoms are associated with each type of shunting?
2. Explain indications of adequate tissue perfusion that reflect good cardiac function and compare these with signs and symptoms of poor tissue perfusion.
3. A 5-year-old previously healthy boy is seen in the pediatrician's office with irritability; extremely red eyes; dry, cracked, red lips; red palms and soles of his feet; joint pain; and fever for a week. His heart rate is 118 bpm, and his BP is 116/80 mm Hg. What diagnosis could be made, and what nursing care should take priority?

Resources

For additional resources and information, including Postconference Questions and Activities, Answers, and References, visit www.FADavis.com.

 Student Study Guide

CHAPTER 32
Child With a Metabolic Condition

KEY TERMS

acanthosis nigricans (ak-an-THOH-siss NYE-grik-anz)
acromegaly (AK-roh-MEG-uh-lee)
Cushing syndrome (KUSH-ing SIN-drohm)
diabetes insipidus (DI) (DYE-uh-BEET-eez in-SIP-ih-duss)
diabetes mellitus (DM) (DYE-uh-BEET-eez MEL-ih-tuss)
diabetic ketoacidosis (DKA) (dye-uh-BET-ik KEE-toh-ASS-ih-DOH-siss)
exophthalmos (EKS-off-THAL-muhs)
gigantism (jye-GAN-tizm)
glucagon (GLOO-kuh-gon)
goiter (GOY-tuhr)
Graves disease (GRAYVZ dih-ZEEZ)
Kussmaul's respirations (KOOS-mowlz RES-pih-RAY-shunz)
lipodystrophy (LIP-oh-DISS-truh-fee)
polydipsia (POL-ee-DIP-see-uh)
polyphagia (POL-ee-FAY-jee-uh)
polyuria (POL-ee-YOO-ree-uh)

CHAPTER CONCEPTS

Growth and Development
Reproduction and Sexuality
Metabolism
Professionalism
Stress and Coping

LEARNING OUTCOMES

1. Define the key terms.
2. Identify the functions of the endocrine glands and the hormones secreted by each.
3. Discuss the location of each of the following endocrine glands: pituitary, thyroid, parathyroid, adrenal, pancreas, testes, and ovaries.
4. Analyze the effect of a metabolic disorder across the life span of a child including alterations in growth and development.
5. Review the complications associated with hyposecretion or hypersecretion of the various endocrine glands.
6. Differentiate the pathology between type 1 diabetes mellitus (T1D; formerly *insulin-dependent DM*) and type 2 diabetes mellitus (T2D; formerly *noninsulin-dependent DM*).
7. Identify the various inborn errors of metabolism (IEM) including the evaluations, treatments, and nursing care associated with each.
8. Discuss the need for long-term care and follow-up for children who are diagnosed with a metabolic disorder.
9. State the conditions associated with the development of syndrome of inappropriate antidiuretic hormone (SIADH).
10. Explain the need for rapid identification of metabolic disorders during childhood to provide treatment that delivers appropriate support for growth, metabolism, and nutrition for child health and development.

CRITICAL THINKING

Scenario #1: Four-year-old **Ivonne** is brought to the community hospital emergency department (ED) by her father. The father explains to the health-care staff that the child has been very tired lately. She is "always thirsty and hungry" and has begun to wet her pants lately even though she is potty trained. The child presents with dark circles under her eyes and appears very thin. After completing a health history and initial examination, the health-care team orders a set of laboratory tests including a comprehensive metabolic panel and urinalysis. The urine comes back positive for ketones, and the child's

Continued

CRITICAL THINKING—cont'd

blood glucose level is 423 g/dL. The team admits the child into the pediatric unit with an initial diagnosis of type 1 diabetes (T1D) and requests a consult with a pediatric endocrinologist. The following day, as the father is learning how to check the child's blood glucose level, the child cries and fights with him about having her finger poked. You sit down with Ivonne and her father to teach them and help her understand what is happening.

Questions

1. Why does the health-care team suspect T1D and not T2D?
2. What concerns do you have about Ivonne resisting finger sticks for blood glucose testing, and how can you assist with teaching Ivonne and model proper technique for her father?
3. What teaching does the father need from the pediatric health-care team?

CONCEPTUAL CORNERSTONE
Metabolism

Metabolism is a very complex concept. The human body relies on a fine balance of hormones in very small amounts to be accurately secreted from 10 endocrine glands. When hormones are balanced, the child should grow and develop as expected, experience puberty as expected, and be able to reproduce. When the balance is off and there is hyposecretion or hypersecretion of hormones, endocrine dysfunction occurs, and pathological conditions can develop. Complications can include disruptions in growth, energy, storage of glucose, fluid balance, responses to stressful stimuli, sodium and electrolyte balance, and sexual development. Medical science now provides evaluation techniques, laboratory evaluations, and medical treatments that have moved the field of endocrinology to advanced levels. Nurses work with health-care teams to assist families in adjusting to hormone imbalances and endocrine dysfunctions.

THE ENDOCRINE GLANDS

The metabolic system is made up of the endocrine glands, including the pituitary gland, thyroid gland, parathyroid gland, adrenal gland, pancreas, ovaries, and testes. Endocrine glands not covered in this chapter are the thymus and pineal glands (Fig. 32.1).

There are three functional units in each part of the endocrine system: (1) the gland in which the hormone, the chemical messenger, is produced; (2) the target cell where the chemical messenger acts; and (3) the transport system through which the chemical messenger travels. Each gland

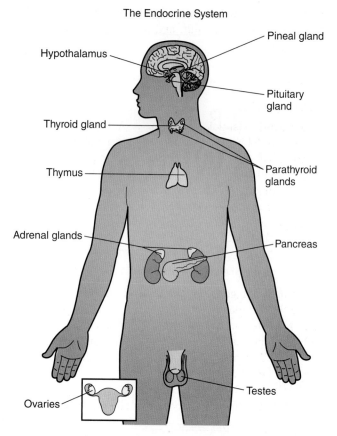

FIGURE 32.1 The endocrine system.

secretes small amounts of its hormone into the bloodstream, which delivers the hormone that then influences the action of distant cells.

An integral system of feedback regulates the production and secretion of hormones based on the body's long-term needs, such as growth, or short-term needs, such as fluid balance.

Pituitary

The pituitary gland is considered the master gland of the endocrine system. The pituitary is a round, pea-size gland located in the brain; it is attached to the hypothalamus. The pituitary has an anterior and a posterior lobe. The anterior lobe controls the release of the other hormones from the endocrine glands located throughout the body. The pituitary secretes several hormones, each with an essential purpose.

Thyroid

The thyroid gland is a reddish-brown soft mass with right and left lobes. It is located in the neck, between the sides of the cricoid and thyroid cartilage at the sixth tracheal cartilage just posterior to the larynx. The thyroid gland secretes triiodothyronine (T_3), thyroxine (T_4), and calcitonin. Thyroid hormones help regulate blood calcium concentrations and the processing of protein, fat, and carbohydrates (CHO). The thyroid gland plays a major role in regulating the basal metabolic rate; it influences body temperature, appetite, heart rate, cardiac output, and the utilization of oxygen and carbon dioxide.

> ### Safety *Stat!*
>
> Desmopressin (antidiuretic hormone [ADH]) is administered to children with hemophilia or other bleeding disorders to induce release of natural clotting factors. When administering desmopressin, do not allow the child to drink fluids for up to 6 hours afterward. The child may experience overhydration and the dilution of serum electrolytes.

Parathyroid

As its name suggests, the parathyroid gland is located next to the thyroid gland. The main function of the parathyroid is to regulate and maintain calcium levels. The gland also influences potassium, phosphate, and magnesium levels in the body. The parathyroid gland secretes the parathyroid hormone (PTH). If it produces too much PTH, hyperparathyroidism and hypocalcemia occur. If it produces too little PTH, hypoparathyroidism occurs, leading to hypercalcemia.

Adrenal

The adrenal glands, located superior to the kidneys, are responsible for the production and release of substances called mineralocorticoids. The adrenal glands also produce the three sex hormones: progesterone, estrogen, and androgens (such as testosterone). The sex hormones regulate the child's sexual maturity. The medulla of the adrenal gland produces epinephrine (adrenalin) and norepinephrine that affect the child's stress response as well as the glucocorticoids cortisol and corticosteroid. If the adrenal glands produce too much adrenalin, the child may experience tachycardia, tremors, restlessness, hypertension, and nausea/vomiting. If they produce too little adrenalin, the child may experience weakness, dry lips and skin, feeding difficulties, and vomiting. Older children with adrenal insufficiency may experience dizziness, muscle weakness, weight loss, and poor appetite.

Pancreas

The pancreas is an organ that has many functions. The endocrine portion of the pancreas secretes the hormone insulin from the β (beta) cells located in the islets of Langerhans; it also secretes the hormone **glucagon** from the α (alpha) cells. Glucagon is stored in the liver and is used to regulate blood glucose levels should the child experience hypoglycemia. Damage to the α and β cells results in poor control of blood glucose. α and β cells have these functions:

- *α cells:* The α cells produce and secrete glucagon, which increases blood glucose. Glucagon is considered an antagonist to the hormone insulin.

- *β cells:* The β cells produce and secrete insulin, which promotes glucose, protein, and fatty acid transport into cells. β-cell secretions promote the movement of potassium and phosphate ions across cell membranes, carrying glucose molecules into cells.

Ovaries

The ovaries are the female gonads and are responsible for reproduction and sexual maturity. Located in the pelvis below and behind the fallopian tubes, the ovaries are the size of large almonds. These gonads secrete progesterone and estrogen. Estrogen stimulates overall RNA and protein synthesis, pubic and axillary hair growth, breast development during puberty and pregnancy, and pelvic enlargement. It also promotes the epiphyseal closure of bones. Estrogen causes fluid retention by influencing the action of the renal tubules to absorb more water and sodium, whereas progesterone helps prepare the uterus for implantation of a fertilized ovum. During pregnancy, progesterone helps to calm the uterine smooth muscle, preventing premature contractions.

Testes

The testes are the male gonads and are responsible for reproduction and sexual maturity. The testes secrete testosterone, which stimulates the production of spermatozoa, the epiphyseal closure of bones, muscle development, body hair growth, and the enlargement of external genitalia. Located in the scrotum, the testes have ducts that emerge from the top of the gland and attach to the epididymis.

COMMON ENDOCRINE GLAND DISORDERS

When a gland experiences dysfunction, the body's metabolic status is interrupted. Even small disruptions in hormones secreted by the various glands can have a large effect on the child's homeostatic state. Therefore, it is vital that you identify a metabolic dysfunction as soon as possible so that treatment can begin.

Syndrome of Inappropriate Antidiuretic Hormone

The overproduction and excretion of ADH from the posterior pituitary results in the kidneys absorbing more water, decreased urine output, and increased fluid retention. The child's fluid volume expands in the vessels, and the extra fluid results in hyponatremia, the condition of diluted sodium concentrations within the blood. When a child experiences shaken baby syndrome (SBS), head trauma, a brain tumor, brain surgery, or an infection of the brain, they are at risk for developing syndrome of inappropriate antidiuretic hormone (SIADH). The fluid retention from SIADH can contribute to increased intracranial pressure, a dangerous condition that can be fatal.

Diagnosing Syndrome of Inappropriate Antidiuretic Hormone

The clinical symptoms of SIADH are those of hyponatremia, including weakness, confusion, and anorexia. Acute SIADH also presents with symptoms of fluid overload and decreased urine output. Checking urine specific gravity may be required to identify the development of SIADH.

Interventions for Syndrome of Inappropriate Antidiuretic Hormone

Interventions for SIADH are aimed at controlling fluid retention and balancing low serum sodium levels. Treatments for SIADH include the following:

- Fluid restriction
- The administration of IV solutions; isotonic or hypertonic
- IV administrations of diuretics, usually furosemide

Nursing Considerations for Syndrome of Inappropriate Antidiuretic Hormone

Be aware of the risk of developing SIADH. Any signs of fluid retention, reduced urine output, or changes in the child's neurological status should be reported to the appropriate health-care provider. Identify symptoms of dilutional hyponatremia such as weakness and confusion. It is important that you can distinguish between SIADH and **diabetes insipidus (DI)**. DI is the opposite of SIADH. In DI, less ADH is produced and secreted, and the child's urine has a very low specific gravity. DI causes the child to produce copious urine.

Deficient Anterior Pituitary Hormone: Pituitary Dwarfism

Pituitary dwarfism occurs early in fetal development, when the growing fetus's pituitary does not secrete adequate growth hormone. The cause of dwarfism is unknown but may be related to lesions or trauma. A child born with pituitary dwarfism will demonstrate normal body proportions but have a shorter overall stature. A child deficient in growth hormone typically demonstrates a growth pattern of less than 2 inches annually until the preschool period, when delayed growth becomes even more apparent. Young children with dwarfism may appear to be overweight. When growth hormone deficiency (GHD) is suspected, the health-care provider will analyze the child's bone age (an x-ray of the wrists), blood serum level of growth hormone, and previous measurements on growth charts.

Diagnosing Pituitary Dwarfism

As the child grows, they will appear younger than their age. Intelligence is normal with dwarfism, and the child displays an expected mental age and cognitive processing. The child with dwarfism will have a delayed but normal development of puberty. Evaluations include both a laboratory evaluation of GHD and radiographic evaluation of bone age.

Interventions for Pituitary Dwarfism

Dwarfism is not a condition that requires treatment. Once diagnosed with GHD, the child can be given injections of human growth hormone. Some children will respond to this treatment, and others will not. The earlier the treatments are started, the greater chance of response. Children should be supported to embrace their size and be given positive reinforcement for their accomplishments.

Nursing Considerations for Pituitary Dwarfism

Nursing care of the child with pituitary dwarfism includes a thorough check for dental anomalies because the child's jaw may have growth retardation. This delay leads to challenges in the eruption of the permanent teeth. The child and family may need emotional support to help cope with the challenges of dwarfism. You should provide information about local and national support groups and information about dwarf-related growth patterns. (Further information can be found at the Human Growth Foundation and the MAGIC Foundation.)

Therapeutic Communication

Parents of children with GHDs may be very stressed and emotional. You should provide therapeutic communication that allows the family to share their feelings and fears. Acknowledge the parents' fears and worries and reassure them that their child will be followed closely but will grow, develop, and thrive.

Hypersecretion of Anterior Pituitary Hormone: Gigantism

Gigantism is a condition of accelerated linear bone growth that results from the excessive production and secretion of insulinlike growth factor (IGF-1). The clinical presentation of this hypersecretion may be gigantism (large overall size) or **acromegaly** (unusually long extremities). The cause of gigantism may be pituitary hyperplasia or a pituitary tumor. Acromegaly is a severe condition that is often diagnosed late and has cerebrovascular, respiratory, and cardiovascular complications. Bone malignancies are also associated with this condition.

Diagnosing Gigantism

If the hypersecretion of IGF-1 occurs after the child's epiphyseal growth plates have sealed, then the condition may manifest as enlarged hands, feet, jaw, tongue, and nose. The child may also present with thickening of the skin on the body and

· WORD · BUILDING ·

acromegaly: acro–extremity + megaly–abnormal enlargement

coarseness of the facial features. The condition is complex and is also associated with the following:

- Mild to moderate obesity
- Visual changes
- Soft-tissue hypertrophy
- Peripheral neuropathies, such as carpal tunnel syndrome
- Osteoarthritis
- Endocrinopathies
- Headaches
- Oily skin and acne
- Excessive sweating

Interventions for Gigantism

After laboratory studies are conducted to identify the presence of excess IGF-1, other tests may be done, including magnetic resonance imaging (MRI) to evaluate the pituitary gland for tumors and x-rays to evaluate the severity of skeletal malformation. There is no single treatment for gigantism or for the complication of acromegaly. Surgical interventions for pituitary tumors may be required, and research continues on medications for growth hormone excess.

Nursing Considerations for Gigantism

Nursing care of the child with gigantism includes psychological support for possible altered body image. The child will be larger than peers, or may have certain body parts that are unusually large. As the child enters the preteen and teenage years, extra support is needed to cope with looking different from other children.

Hyposecretion of Thyroid Gland Hormones: Hypothyroidism

A child's basal metabolism rate is regulated by the hormones secreted by the thyroid gland. To function properly, the thyroid depends on a consistent source of dietary iodine and tyrosine. Hypothyroidism, insufficient production of thyroid hormones, can be congenital and can be caused by a spontaneous gene mutation. Children whose diets or drinking water are deficient in iodine are at risk for developing hypothyroidism. Hypothyroidism may also be caused by decreased gland development over childhood or from medications that suppress the production of thyroid hormones. Congenital hypothyroidism occurs in approximately 1:4,000 live births and is two times more common in girls. This condition leads to cognitive impairment if not identified and treated early.

Diagnosing Hypothyroidism

The child should be evaluated for an enlarged tongue; short, thick neck; short stature; and possible hypotonia. For acquired hypothyroidism, the child should be evaluated for the presence of a **goiter** (an enlargement of the thyroid gland) as well as for signs and symptoms of a slowed metabolic rate, including:

- Hypothermic skin temperatures
- Slow pulse

- Easy weight gain
- Decreased appetite
- Constipation
- Unexpected tiredness and fatigue
- Delayed mental processing
- Decreased perspiration on exertion

Routine neonatal screening for hypothyroidism is required in all states. The optimal time for screening is between 2 and 6 days of life via a heel stick. Testing done earlier than this is problematic because it may demonstrate a falsely high thyroid-stimulating hormone (TSH) level. There is a natural increase in TSH shortly after birth. If the T_4 level is found to be decreased, then the child's TSH level should be drawn. A T_4 level under 3 mcg/100 mL and a TSH level greater than 40 mcg/100 mL are considered indicative of primary hypothyroidism.

Interventions for Hypothyroidism

Treatment for hypothyroidism includes following the child's T_3 and T_4 blood levels and appropriately administering T_4 and thyroid hormones as replacement for low blood levels. The child should receive adequate vitamin D as part of the treatment.

Nursing Considerations for Hypothyroidism

Nursing care for the child with hypothyroidism should focus on teaching the family that medication compliance for life is essential and that regular checkups and blood levels are important for the child's care. The child will be placed on a thyroid hormone replacement therapy such as levothyroxine. These medications can be crushed and placed in a small amount of formula, food, or water, preferably 1 hour before feeding. Infants should not be given soy formula, iron supplements, or calcium supplements with levothyroxine replacement therapy because these substances reduce the total amount of the medication absorbed into the bloodstream (Mayo Clinic, 2022).

Hypersecretion of Thyroid Gland Hormone: Hyperthyroidism

When thyroid hormone levels are above normal, the child will be diagnosed with hyperthyroidism. One form of hyperthyroidism is an autoimmune condition called *Graves disease*. The highest incidence of Graves disease is found in adolescent girls, but it may be found in young children if their mother has Graves disease. The female-to-male ratio for the development of Graves disease is 4:1.

Diagnosing Hyperthyroidism

Diagnosis of hyperthyroidism includes screening for T_3 and T_4 blood serum levels. Clinical signs and symptoms include tremor, muscle weakness, nervousness, irritability, fatigue, weight loss, diarrhea, excessive perspiration, and protrusion of the eyeballs called *exophthalmos*. The child may present with a nontender enlarged thyroid gland called a *goiter*. Many children experience heat intolerance, sweating, and weight loss despite increased appetite.

Interventions for Hyperthyroidism

Medications for hyperthyroidism decrease and limit the secretion of thyroid hormone. Medications include propylthiouracil or methimazole. If the child demonstrates a "thyroid storm," which is a state of excessively high levels of thyroid hormone, administration of a β-adrenergic blocking agent such as propranolol may be required to reduce the symptoms of adrenergic hyperresponsiveness.

Nursing Considerations for Hyperthyroidism

Nursing care includes teaching the family that the child may display an inability to stay seated at school, a short attention span, and problems with academic success. The family needs to understand that medication therapy will be required for the rest of the child's life. Because of the child's increased metabolism, the family should be encouraged to provide five meals a day that are high in protein and calories. Body weight should be monitored on a regular basis. If the child has gastrointestinal symptoms such as cramping and frequent defecation, supportive care should be presented. If the child's condition is severe and there is eye protrusion, the family must be taught how to instill moistening drops into the conjunctiva.

Safety *Stat!*

If a child with hyperthyroidism demonstrates significant eye protrusion, the family must be taught how to safely prevent eye injury. The eyes must be kept moist, and the child needs to wear protective eyewear and sunglasses.

Hyperfunction of the Adrenal Gland: Cushing Syndrome

Cushing syndrome occurs when there is an overproduction and a hypersecretion of adrenal hormones, leading to a prolonged exposure to corticoid hormones. High levels of cortisol are produced, which result in a decreased secretion of adrenocorticotropic hormone (ACTH). Cushing syndrome is often associated with tumor growth in the adrenal gland or with the excessive or prolonged use of corticosteroids for the management of inflammatory illnesses.

Diagnosing Cushing Syndrome

The patient with hyperfunction of the adrenal gland will demonstrate symptoms such as these:

- Central obesity (adipose tissue on the chest, face, and abdomen)
- Decreased glucose tolerance
- Poor wound healing
- Muscle weakness and atrophy from increased glucogenesis
- Easy bruising
- Osteoporosis
- Acne
- Hirsutism (male-pattern hair growth in females)
- Hypertension
- Mood disorder
- Decreased linear growth

Interventions for Cushing Syndrome

If Cushing syndrome is related to the chronic use of steroid hormones, a gradual tapering down and discontinuing of the medication may improve the syndrome. Surgery may be required if an adrenal tumor is causing the syndrome. Before the child or teen has surgery, the medical team may prescribe medications that inhibit cortisol production along with medications that help to reduce the side effects of high blood pressure (BP) and high blood glucose.

Nursing Considerations for Cushing Syndrome

Nursing care includes ensuring that there is an order for slowly tapering corticosteroids if the child is on these medications. Fast withdrawal or abrupt discontinuation of corticosteroids results in Cushing syndrome. Be aware of the need to support the child's immune function and monitor the child for the development of infections. Families need to understand that mood swings are expected with the hypersecretion of ACTH and that the mood disorder may last weeks to months after treatment is discontinued.

DIABETES MELLITUS

The metabolic system is associated with several complex and costly disease processes including diabetes mellitus. The two common pathologies are type 1 diabetes (T1D) and type 2 diabetes (T2D). Currently, nearly half of all American adults have diabetes or prediabetes. More than 37 million American children and adults currently have diabetes, accounting for 11.3% of the nation's population (CDC, 2022b).

Type 1 Diabetes Mellitus

Previously called *juvenile diabetes* or sometimes referred to as *insulin-dependent diabetes,* type 1 **diabetes mellitus (DM; T1D)** is a chronic metabolic disorder marked by **hyperglycemia**. In T1D, the body produces no insulin. Insulin, the hormone produced by the β cells, allows glucose to enter cells for energy, growth, and all types of cellular function. Insulin is essential for life. T1D may be further categorized as immune-mediated (autoimmune process damaging

· WORD · BUILDING ·

hyperglycemia: hyper–excessive + glyc–sugar + em–blood + ia–condition

the pancreas) or idiopathic type 1 (rare with known identified cause; Johns Hopkins Medicine, 2023).

T1D requires the child to take daily and lifelong injections or to use an insulin pump. Most commonly diagnosed between 10 and 14 years of age, T1D can be diagnosed anytime between infancy and young adulthood. The incidence of T1D in children from birth to 19 years of age is approximately 25% (CDC, 2022a).

Approximately 20% of T1D cases have a genetic association, but other causes include an autoimmune response or environmental factors, such as exposure to a significant viral infection. After an upper respiratory illness, for example, autoantibodies may begin to attack the β cells of the pancreas. These autoantibodies can be present as long as 9 years before the clinical symptoms of T1D start. Starved for glucose, the child's body breaks down fat for energy, forming ketones. The presence of ketones denotes metabolic acidosis.

Often the diagnosis of T1D occurs when the child first presents with **diabetic ketoacidosis (DKA)**. DKA is a dangerous toxic state that requires intensive care. As fats are converted to energy, the liver produces ketones. Ketones accumulate in the body, spilling into urine, and cause a metabolic acidotic state. The child's body attempts to compensate by excreting more carbon dioxide through deeper and faster respirations called *Kussmaul's respirations*. As the body loses its ability to compensate, the child experiences severe dehydration, severe acute kidney injury, and eventually coma and death. In the pediatric intensive care unit (PICU), the child's serum potassium levels, pH, Po_2, Pco_2, and blood urea nitrogen (BUN) are all followed closely to evaluate the management of DKA. Children typically present with very high blood glucose levels when they have developed DKA. A minimal level would be greater than 200 mg/dL, but most of the time the child presents with blood sugars much higher.

Safety *Stat!*

Hypoglycemia (excessively low blood sugar) is dangerous and can lead to lethargy, coma, and death. In 2022, the Endocrine Society published an urgent position paper describing the three levels of severe hypoglycemia:

Level One: A glucose level of less than 70 mg/dL but greater than 54 mg/dL

Level Two: A glucose level of less than 3 mmol/L (less than 54 mg/dL) that denotes a serious clinical status requiring rapid glucose intake (Know your institution's policy on interventions.)

Level Three: A glucose level producing severe cognitive impairment needing immediate external recovery assistance (Endocrine Society, 2022)

Diagnosing Type 1 Diabetes Mellitus

Evaluations of T1D are multifocal and include a variety of clinical presentations within different body systems. You need to check all body systems if T1D is suspected:

- Excessive blood glucose leading to **glycosuria** (occurs when blood glucose levels exceed the renal threshold of 160 mg/dL)
- Elevated 8-hour fasting blood glucose levels
- Osmotic diuresis with the presence of high blood glucose, leading to large amounts of urine, dehydration, hypotension, and eventual kidney shutdown
- Excessive hunger (**polyphagia**), increased and excessive thirst (**polydipsia**), and excessive urination (**polyuria**)
- Thin appearance; may look malnourished and report feeling fatigued
- Fruity breath
- Dry and flushed skin
- Blurred vision
- Yeast infections in females
- Confusion

A diagnosis of T1D consists of one serum blood plasma glucose level of greater than 200 mg/dL or two blood plasma glucose levels of greater than 126 mg/dL. A child with diabetes who is experiencing an illness or stress can have hyperglycemia and may need to have their insulin temporarily adjusted.

Interventions for Type 1 Diabetes Mellitus

The first priority is to evaluate for and treat DKA. This requires stabilizing the child's acidotic metabolic state and normalizing serum electrolytes. Typically, a child with DKA presents to the ED and then is rapidly transferred to the PICU for close monitoring and treatment. The child is treated with normal saline boluses for dehydration correction and IV insulin drips (continuous infusion) until the blood glucose level reaches 250 to 300 mg/dL. At that time, the IV fluid is switched to D51/2NS to prevent hypoglycemia rebound. The insulin infusion (insulin drip) is titrated to prevent the blood glucose level from dropping more than 50 mg/dL per hour. IV fluid therapy is conducted according to institutional protocol, which must be strictly followed.

After stabilization, the child is weaned from IV insulin to subcutaneous injections before being transferred to the pediatric unit for intensive family teaching about managing diabetes. Under no circumstances should the child receive IV solutions with potassium until the child's urine output is well established. Adding potassium supplementation to

---

· **WORD** · **BUILDING** ·

glycosuria: glycos–sugar + ur–urine + ia–condition
polyphagia: poly–much + phag–eat + ia–condition
polydipsia: poly–much + dips–thirst + ia–condition
polyuria: poly–much + ur–urine + ia–condition

the IV puts the child with an existing electrolyte imbalance at risk for **hyperkalemia** and possible heart dysrhythmias. Specific care protocols exist at each health-care institution to rapidly guide the health-care team in treating a child's DKA state.

Nursing Considerations for Type 1 Diabetes Mellitus

After stabilizing the child with DKA, the next priority is to engage the family in the child's care by having them check the child's blood glucose and draw up the insulin. Teaching should begin right away and must include all members of the child's family.

Medication Facts

Typical Insulins

- Lispro is a rapid-acting, clear insulin with an onset of 5 to 15 minutes, a peak of 30 to 90 minutes, and a duration of less than 4 hours.
- Regular insulin is a short-acting, clear insulin with an onset of 30 minutes, a peak of 2 to 3 hours, and a duration of 6 to 8 hours.
- Neutral protamine Hagedorn (NPH) is an intermediate-acting, cloudy insulin with an onset of 1 to 2 hours, a peak of 6 to 12 hours, and a duration of 18 to 26 hours.
- Glargine is a long-acting, clear insulin used for basal needs only with an onset of 4 to 6 hours, a peak of 14 to 24 hours, and a duration of 28 to 36 hours.

Patient Teaching Guidelines

Mixing and Administering Insulins

1. Draw up the clear insulin in an insulin syringe first, and then draw up the cloudy insulin so that the clear insulin does not appear contaminated with the cloudy insulin if any enters the clear insulin vial during preparation.
2. Do not shake insulin vials. Instead, gently rotate the vial in your hand and treat it carefully. The amino acid chains can break with vigorous handling.
3. Rotate the child's injection sites to prevent **lipodystrophy** (a change in subcutaneous fat under the skin; either atrophy or hypertrophy). Include the child in the process of selecting sites.
4. To avoid hypoglycemia (excessively low blood sugar), make sure that the child has eaten before the injected

insulin peaks. This is especially important if the treatment plan includes a rapid-acting insulin such as lispro.
5. Call the child's health-care provider to adjust the dose of insulin if the child is sick, stressed, starting a new exercise plan, or experiencing a growth spurt. More or less insulin may be required.
6. Insulins may be given by a specific insulin syringe and needle, an insulin pen with adjustable quantities for injection, or a subcutaneous insulin pump.
7. Do not mix rapid-acting insulin lispro into the same syringe with long-acting insulin glargine.

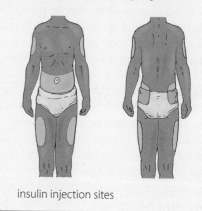

insulin injection sites

Nursing care for a child with a new diagnosis of T1D consists of these interventions:

- In the early stages of diagnosis and care, the child must have blood glucose checked four times each day with a home blood glucose monitor (Fig. 32.2).
- The pediatric endocrinologist will follow the child's case closely for several weeks after the initial diagnosis and will adjust the child's rapid-acting and long-acting

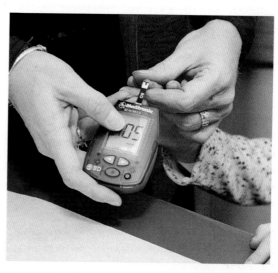

FIGURE 32.2 Blood glucose monitor for home use.

- WORD · BUILDING ·

hyperkalemia: hyper–excessive + kal–potassium + em–blood + ia–condition

lipodystrophy: lipo–fat + dys–abnormal + trophy–growth

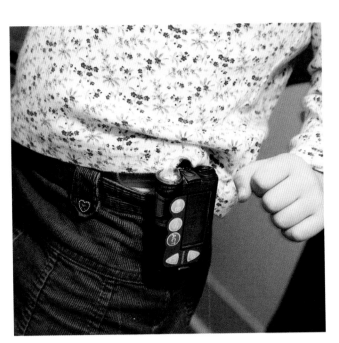

FIGURE 32.3 Insulin pump worn by a child.

insulins for the best control. Meticulous documentation by the nursing staff of all blood glucose checks and insulin administration, including the site, is essential.

- CHO counting for all meals and snacks is now the universal gold standard. CHO counting should begin immediately and should involve the child and family in food selection as well as in calculating the total CHOs per meal or snack. The child's rapid-acting insulin will be calculated based on the total amount of CHOs the child anticipates eating and is typically one unit of rapid-acting insulin for every 15 to 30 g of CHO (Determined by endocrinologist and can vary).
- Insulin pumps may be used after the child's diabetes is well-controlled with injections (Fig. 32.3).
- Long-term blood sugar control and compliance with treatment are monitored by testing blood levels of hemoglobin A1c (HbA1c). This laboratory value measures the average amounts of blood glucose over 90 days with the goal being an HbA1c level related to the child's age.

Labs & Diagnostics

Understanding Hemoglobin A1c

HbA1c is a measure of glycosylated hemoglobin. It is used to determine a person's overall blood glucose level during the previous 90 days.

Target HbA1c level for all ages of pediatric patients is <7.5%. Two A1c tests of 6.5% or higher on two different blood draws indicates that the child has diabetes (Mayo Clinic, 2023).

CHO counting is an important tool to determine how much insulin a child will need to take and is a means of reducing spikes in blood glucose. Almost 100% of CHOs consumed rapidly become blood glucose.

Most children should have a goal of 45 g to 60 g of CHOs per meal, which is to be determined by the endocrinologist. Families must be taught to read food labels and predetermine how many CHOs the child is likely to consume. The following list provides some examples of the CHOs in typical food servings:

- One fruit serving = 15 g of CHO
- One milk serving = 12 g of CHO
- One starch (bread, pasta, cereal) serving = 15 g of CHO
- One vegetable (nonstarchy) = 5 g of CHO

Teaching is the most important part of caring for a child with diabetes. It is important for families to understand that both hypoglycemia and hyperglycemia are concerns. You should teach the family how to recognize values that are associated with each, what causes the values, and what the symptoms are for each. Table 32.1 provides information about what is important for families to understand about hypoglycemia and hyperglycemia.

The child should always wear a medical alert bracelet so that if hypoglycemia or hyperglycemia occurs, the condition can be identified and help can be summoned quickly.

Hospitalized patients are at risk for severe hypoglycemia in any of the following conditions:

- NPO (nothing by mouth) status
- Reduced oral intake because of illness or surgery
- Discontinuation of enteral feedings
- Insulin given before the meal followed by lack of oral intake or delay in arrival of food
- Rapid transport before the child has a chance to finish the meal, leaving too much insulin circulating
- Sudden reduction in oral or IV corticosteroid therapy

Safety Stat!

Treatment for hypoglycemia includes the following steps:

- Rapidly administer 15 to 20 g of a fast-absorbing CHO (fruit juice).
- Retake the child's blood glucose within 15 minutes.
- Give a second dose of CHOs if needed.
- Monitor the child's vital signs.
- Keep the child quiet and supervise constantly until the blood glucose level is stable.
- If the child has a decreased level of consciousness, give dextrose 50% via IV and follow up with IV glucagon if ordered.

Table 32.1

Characteristics of Hyperglycemia and Hypoglycemia

	Hyperglycemia	*Hypoglycemia*
Blood Glucose Range	Greater than 200–250 mg/dL	Less than 70 mg/dL
Blood pH	Greater than 7.2	Normal
Causes	Not producing enough insulin Having insulin resistance Injecting too little insulin	Eating too little; eating later than usual; taking more exercise than usual; being ill, injured, or stressed; having a medication interaction
Symptoms	Fatigue Flushed appearance to skin Dry skin Dehydration Polyuria Polyphagia Ketones in urine Dark-colored urine	Pale Diaphoresis (sweating) Confusion Slow thinking Decreased level of consciousness Tremors Poor coordination Dizziness Weakness Nervousness Irrational behavior/personality change Blurred vision
Interventions	Give rapid-acting insulin such as Lispro, as ordered. Provide fluids. Do not add potassium until urine output is restored.	Give a fast-acting source of CHO such as 4 ounces of orange juice or apple juice, a small gel tube of cake icing, or an over-the-counter glucose product made for a child with diabetes.

Complications of T1D should be discussed and include the following:

- A life expectancy shortened by up to one-third
- Nephropathy (kidney disease) as the primary cause of death
- Comorbidities that include renal failure, premature atherosclerosis, heart disease, and stroke
- Retinopathy, which commonly develops sometime during the life span
- Poor wound healing that requires specialists to intervene

Families need to understand that diabetes is a labor-intensive and lifelong chronic illness that is best managed by competent family members at home with the support of a specialized health-care team.

Type 2 Diabetes Mellitus

T2D, formerly called *adult onset diabetes* or *noninsulin dependent DM,* is typically seen in overweight and obese children and is more common than T1D. This disease process is assuming epidemic proportions because of soaring childhood obesity rates across the nation. The majority of children with T2D have a genetic predisposition to the disease. Environmental factors related to T2D include moving from a low incidence area to a higher incidence area, being in colder climates, and being exposed to viral infections (American Diabetes Association, 2017). T2D is now predicted to be the biggest cause of morbidity (disease) and mortality (death) for the next generation of adults. Unlike T1D, T2D is caused by insulin resistance. The liver, adipose tissue, and muscle tissue become less sensitive to the insulin that is produced. T2D is diagnosed via laboratory analysis of hyperglycemia.

Diagnosing Type 2 Diabetes Mellitus

The following may be observed when a child presents with T2D:

- Hyperglycemia as indicated by elevated levels of blood glucose in finger sticks or laboratory values. This may be confirmed by fasting plasma glucose (FPG), a 2-hour plasma glucose test (2-h PG), or an elevated HbA1c (glycosylated hemoglobin).
- Darkened and thickened skin pigmentation, called **acanthosis nigricans**, around the base of the neck at the flexural area

Nursing Care Plan for the Juvenile With Type 1 Diabetes

Eleven-year-old José is brought to the ED by his concerned parents. They report that their son has been reporting nausea since yesterday and vomited "a few times" during the night. They wonder if José's unquenchable thirst and frequent urination this past week are related to his "stomach flu." Flushed in the face, José is breathing deeply and rapidly, allowing you to detect a fruity odor to his breath. The ED nurse does a finger stick to check José's blood glucose level; it is 475 mg/dL.

Nursing Diagnosis: Fluid volume deficit related to excessive urination because of hyperglycemia
Expected Outcome: Patient will remain normovolemic as evidenced by urinary output greater than 30 mL/hr, normal skin turgor, good capillary refill, normal BP, palpable peripheral pulses, and blood glucose levels between 70 and 200 mg/dL.

Intervention:	Rationales:
Monitor fluid and electrolyte balance to prevent dehydration and complications such as decreased sodium, potassium, calcium, and magnesium.	Excess blood glucose can cause nausea and vomiting, resulting in electrolyte imbalances. These electrolyte deficiencies can lead to further complications and cardiac arrhythmias.
Administer medications as appropriate: insulin, IV fluids, electrolyte replacement, and antiemetics.	Medications will be given to lower the blood glucose level to prevent further production of ketones, fluids will be given to correct hypovolemia, and antiemetics may be given to manage symptoms of vomiting.

Nursing Diagnosis: Risk for injury
Expected Outcome: The patient will not experience any falls while in the hospital.

Intervention:	Rationales:
Prevent injury and falls; transport patient to PICU in a wheelchair; assist with ambulation.	Fatigue, weakness, and confusion are common in DKA because of electrolyte imbalances and the cells' inability to access circulating glucose to produce energy.

Nursing Diagnosis: Knowledge deficit related to newly diagnosed T1D
Expected Outcome: Before discharge, the patient and his family will verbalize understanding of T1D and the plan of care and will demonstrate the skills needed to manage the patient's care at home.

Interventions:	Rationales:
Patient and family will receive nutrition and lifestyle education from a diabetes educator.	Educating patients and families to manage T1D helps prevent future episodes of DKA.
Patient and family will be taught how to check blood sugars and administer insulin and identify the warning signs of hyper- and hypoglycemia.	Knowing the warning signs/symptoms of DKA allows the patient and family to take steps to reverse it.
Follow-up care will be scheduled before discharge.	The patient and family will have greater success managing T1D if they are followed closely by their health-care provider, especially when newly diagnosed.

- Hypertension
- Sleep apnea
- Hyperlipidemia

Interventions for Type 2 Diabetes Mellitus

The first-line treatment for T2D consists of exercise and weight loss. If these are unsuccessful, oral hypoglycemic medications are prescribed, and insulin may be required if blood glucose levels are unable to be controlled by oral medication.

Nursing Considerations for Type 2 Diabetes Mellitus

Nursing considerations for T2D in childhood include supporting the child and educating all members of the family about the disease process. Teach the family about the importance of lifestyle changes to prevent periods of hyperglycemia. It is important that families understand that weight management and blood glucose control both assist with reducing the chance of the child developing serious complications associated with diabetes.

Patient Teaching Guidelines

Home Health Care Instructions for Children of All Ages With a New Diagnosis of Diabetes

Before discharge, the child's family must be able to verbalize understanding of the child's medical condition and to successfully demonstrate the skills they will need to safely care for the child at home.

Medication Information

1. Keep an accurate list of the child's medications, including trade and generic names.
2. Understand timing of medications in relation to meals and bedtime and the action of each of the insulins ordered for the child.
3. Interpret insulin dosing based on CHO counting and sliding scale coverage (insulin coverage that changes based on the child's routine blood glucose level).
4. Prepare to give the injection by washing hands with soap and water and drying thoroughly.
5. Double-check the expiration date of the vial of insulin, then draw up insulins using the proper syringe, and double-check the level drawn up by holding the syringe at eye level.
6. Prepare the injection site by using an alcohol prep pad and allowing the alcohol to completely dry.
7. Inject the insulin at either a 45- or 90-degree angle (based on the injection site and the amount of subcutaneous adipose).
8. Check the expiration date of the insulin and store it safely.
9. Dispose of lancets and syringes safely.

Monitoring Glucose

1. Wash the child's hands before the finger stick blood glucose check.
2. Use the glucometer that the family will have at home.
3. Keep a log of all blood glucose values for the pediatric endocrinologist to monitor.
4. Devices are available that provide glucose monitoring without finger sticks. These devices—either noninvasive (scanner) or minimally invasive—are placed subcutaneously and monitor either interstitial fluid glucose or blood glucose. Some types not only measure the child's real-time blood glucose level but also administer insulin for immediate correction. Results can be sent to a smartphone and/or to the health-care provider for monitoring. Many of these devices may not be approved for use by children at this time.

High and Low Blood Glucose Values

1. Recognize the signs and symptoms of low and high blood glucose levels.
2. Retest the child's blood glucose if the level is greater than 240 mg/dL.
3. Test the child's urine for ketones if the measured glucose level is greater than 300 mg/dL.

Supplies

1. Keep supplies safe at home and out of the reach of younger children.
2. Keep a "to-go" supply kit when traveling.
3. Keep a checklist of needed supplies for home health care (lancets, syringes, test strips if needed, insulin(s), alcohol pads, ketone slips, and a source of CHO if the child is hypoglycemic).

When to Call for Professional Help

1. Two blood glucose levels of less than 70 mg/dL or greater than 300 mg/dL
2. Low blood glucose levels that require glucagon
3. Any level of ketones found in the urine

Emergency telephone numbers should be posted by the home phone (if there is one) and loaded in the parents' smartphones.

CRITICAL THINKING

Scenario #2: You have been assigned to a home visit with **Ronnie**, a teen with developmental delay and a known diagnosis of T1D. Ronnie's mother states she wants Ronnie to start an exercise program but asks how that might affect the teen's blood glucose.

Questions

1. What blood glucose shift can happen when a child starts to exercise?
2. What should you explain to the mother about her concerns?

Evidence-Based Practice

All Carbohydrates Are Not Equal

T2D is predicted to be the seventh leading cause of mortality by 2030, according to the World Health Organization (WHO). This spike in diabetes diagnoses correlates with the development of high-fructose corn syrup (HFCS) in the 1960s and the subsequent widespread use of HFCS in most processed foods. In their review of 150 human and animal studies on the effects of fructose metabolism, Ang and Yu (2018) and Wood (2021) found that consumption of fructose, especially HFCS, is one determining factor in the development of obesity, insulin resistance, metabolic syndrome, and T2D. Some studies also linked fructose consumption with hypertension. Limiting consumption of fructose to 25 to 40 g daily "is the best solution to prevent these metabolic diseases."

Ang, B. R. G., & Yu, G. F. (2018). The role of fructose in type 2 diabetes and other metabolic diseases. *Journal of Nutrition and Food Sciences, 8*, 659. https://doi.org/10.4172/2155-9600.1000659

Wood, T. (2021). *Both sucrose and high fructose corn syrup linked to increased health risks.* https://www.ucdavis.edu/health/news/both-sucrose-and-high-fructose-corn-syrup-linked-increased-health-risks

INBORN ERRORS OF METABOLISM

Inborn errors of metabolism (IEM) are a large class of rare genetic diseases caused by altered biochemistry. IEM prevent the body from properly and effectively turning food consumed into an energy source. These alterations are usually caused by defects in specific proteins (enzymes) that break down and metabolize food sources, some of which have toxic effects as they accumulate.

IEM are autosomal recessive genetic disorders. This means that a child with one of these disorders must have inherited the gene for it from both parents. The incidence of IEM is 1 out of 2,500 births in the United States (Jeanmonod et al., 2024). It is essential to identify symptoms of the pathology as early as possible and make dietary changes to prevent complications. Without early intervention, developmental disorders such as hypothyroidism, growth failure, failure to thrive (FTT), delayed puberty, ambiguous genitalia, and sensory impairments can result. Psychological disorders such as depression and psychosis can also occur. In addition, severe neurological deficits, such as developmental delay, poor muscle tone, and seizure disorders, can be caused by the accumulation of toxic by-products in the body (Jeanmonod et al., 2022).

Types of Inborn Errors of Metabolism

There are more than 100 IEM for which testing can be performed. The four IEM that are most commonly encountered are:

- *Phenylketonuria (PKU):* PKU is marked by an inability to metabolize phenylalanine. The liver has a deficient amount of the enzyme phenylalanine hydroxylase, which normally breaks down phenylalanine into tyrosine. Phenylalanine is an essential amino acid found in most natural sources of protein. The buildup of phenylalanine over time causes brain damage. The child will also demonstrate a musty-smelling urine. Decreased levels of tyrosine cause a deficiency of the pigment melanin. Most children with PKU are blonde and have blue eyes. Their fair skin is prone to the development of eczema and photosensitivity. Testing for PKU should take place after the newborn is 24 hours old and has ingested some protein via breast milk or formula.

- *Galactosemia:* This defect is caused by deficiency of the enzyme that breaks down galactose, a sugar found in all dairy products and many infant formulas. This deficiency can result in liver failure, renal tubular damage, and cataracts.

- *Maple syrup urine disease (MSUD):* MSUD is caused by a deficiency of decarboxylase, an enzyme that breaks down several amino acids. Without decarboxylase, the child may experience altered tonicity and seizures. The child will demonstrate a maple syrup odor to their urine.

- *Hereditary fructose intolerance:* Hereditary fructose intolerance is caused by the deficiency of the protein enzyme aldolase B, which is needed to break down the natural fruit sugar, fructose. When fruit juices or other foods containing fructose are ingested, individuals with hereditary fructose intolerance may experience nausea, bloating, abdominal pain, diarrhea, vomiting, and low blood sugar. Continued ingestion of fructose may result in seizures, coma, and ultimately death from liver and kidney failure.

Diagnosing Inborn Errors of Metabolism

IEM are diagnosed through newborn blood screening panels, which should take place after the first 24 hours of feedings in the immediate neonatal period (Fig. 32.4). All newborns should be screened to identify biological markers. Rapid, accurate testing reduces morbidity and mortality rates in newborns. Most infants with IEM will show symptoms within a few weeks of life. In older infants, FTT, lethargy, and neurological toxicity will be seen.

If the child was born at home or was discharged early from the hospital, it is important to obtain a newborn screening specimen as soon as possible. This analysis can be done by having a home health-care nurse draw the newborn's blood or by having the child seen in a pediatric clinic. Symptoms to watch for include:

- *PKU:* Elevated phenylalanine in the blood. Key indicators will be a musty body odor, poor weight gain, and delayed growth.

- *Galactosemia:* Infants present with feeding difficulties, lethargy, poor weight gain, jaundice, liver damage, and bleeding. Galactosemia leads to life-threatening complications in just a few days after birth.

- *MSUD:* Infants present with a distinctive sweet odor of the urine, vomiting, poor feeding, lethargy, seizures, and developmental delay.

Interventions for Inborn Errors of Metabolism

In general, interventions for IEM should start as soon as the child is diagnosed. The child might present in metabolic acidosis, which will need to be immediately corrected with

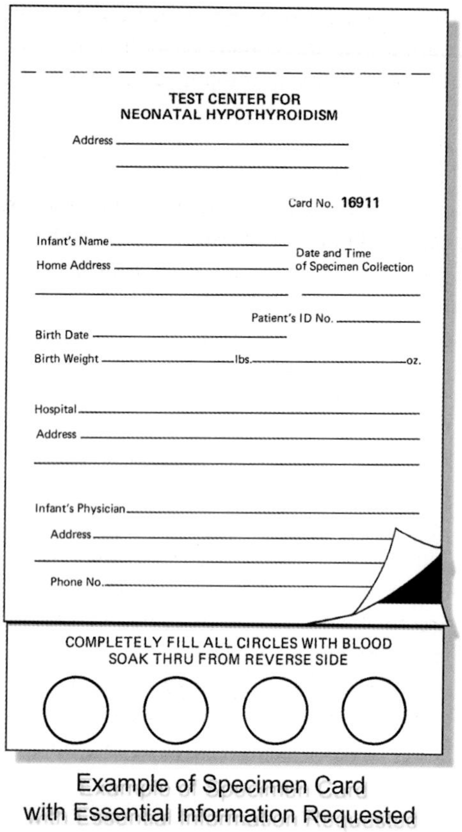

```
- - - - - - - - - - - - - - - -

        TEST CENTER FOR
    NEONATAL HYPOTHYROIDISM

   Address _____
          _____

                    Card No. 16911

   Infant's Name _____
   Home Address _____    Date and Time
                                    of Specimen Collection
                                    _____

                    Patient's ID No. _____
   Birth Date _____
   Birth Weight _____ lbs. _____ oz.

   Hospital _____
   Address _____

   Infant's Physician _____
   Address _____
          _____

   Phone No. _____

   COMPLETELY FILL ALL CIRCLES WITH BLOOD
     SOAK THRU FROM REVERSE SIDE

      ( )    ( )    ( )    ( )
```

Example of Specimen Card
with Essential Information Requested

FIGURE 32.4 PKU test specimen card.

sodium bicarbonate. If the child presents with seizures, anti-convulsants will need to be administered. The gold standard for treating IEM is through dietary therapy; enzyme replacement; and, when applicable, organ transplantation. Treatment with medical foods (i.e., metabolic formulas) is considered a successful intervention for the prevention of disability or death (Berry et al., 2020). Specific treatments for common IEM include:

- *PKU:* Eliminate dietary phenylalanine. High-protein foods such as milk, eggs, meat, beans, and nuts should be reduced or avoided. If infant formula is used, a formula with an enzymatic hydrolysate of casein is used. Children must avoid eggs, flour, fish, legumes, nuts, breads, cheese, poultry, meats, and other foods that contain phenylalanine.
- *Galactosemia:* Eliminate dietary galactose (not lactose). Galactose makes up approximately 50% of the sugars found in milk. Most infants with galactosemia cannot tolerate human or animal milk or any form of foods that contain galactose. Soy-based, lactose-free, or meat-based formula such as Nutramigen must be administered.
- *MSUD:* Restrict branched-chain amino acids in the diet, which are found in high-protein foods.

Key Points

- The functions of the endocrine glands and the hormones secreted by each one are essential for growth and development, sexual reproduction, metabolism, fluid balance, and the body's response to stress stimuli.
- The effects of a metabolic disorder include alterations in growth and development. Many disorders have devastating effects, such as neurological consequences, and therefore must be identified early and rapidly so that treatments can be initiated.
- Conditions associated with hyposecretion of the various endocrine glands include hypothyroidism and T1D. Diseases of hypersecretion of endocrine glands include hyperthyroidism (Graves disease), hyperadrenal activity (Cushing syndrome), and hypoglycemia.

- T1D and T2D differ in clinical presentation, but both require hypoglycemic medications to control glucose levels.
- IEM are autosomal recessive genetic disorders and cause multiple conditions of altered biochemistry, including abnormal enzyme accumulation of a reactant, some with toxic effects.
- Children with metabolic disorders need long-term care and follow-up to evaluate for complications; possible learning disabilities and challenges; and compliance with diets, medications, and treatments. Most metabolic disorders are followed by laboratory analysis, which provides information to the pediatric health-care team on needed care, education, and encouragement.

Review Questions

1. In SIADH, the amount of ADH being produced decreases. What would you expect to observe in the patient with SIADH?
   1. Polyuria
   2. Oliguria
   3. Polydipsia
   4. Increased appetite

2. The endocrine system is responsible for which of these body functions? **(Select all that apply.)**
   1. Regulating the child's metabolism
   2. Growth
   3. Fluid and electrolyte balance
   4. Digestive processes
   5. Stress response
   6. Sexual reproduction

3. A father brings his 13-year-old son to the pediatric clinic and states that he is concerned that the teen has minimal body hair and a high voice. What is your most appropriate response?
   1. "Your son will need a visit to the laboratory for a venipuncture."
   2. "Your son is very delayed in puberty and will need testosterone injections."
   3. "There is no concern at this time. Teens progress through puberty at various times."
   4. "A computed tomography (CT) scan of the brain to evaluate his pituitary gland will be ordered for your son."

4. An infant was born 36 hours ago. Laboratory tests have just been ordered for the neonatal screenings, including hypothyroidism. Why is this not the optimal time to test the infant's thyroid level?
   1. The baby is becoming active and will therefore be difficult to draw via a heel stick.
   2. The baby needs to ingest protein first before the laboratory tests are drawn.
   3. After 24 hours, there is a natural rise in the TSH.
   4. T_4 levels fluctuate the first week of an infant's life.

5. Which of the following are initial symptoms of a new diagnosis of T1D? **(Select all that apply.)**
   1. Fruity, sweet odor on breath
   2. Sudden weight loss
   3. Extreme thirst
   4. Frequent urination
   5. Increased appetite

6. A 17-year-old boy asks you why he has to learn how to inject insulin rather than just take a pill the way his grandmother does for her diabetes. What is your best response?
   1. "Your grandmother's diabetes has improved, so she moved from injections to pills."
   2. "You will be able to take pills also as you grow older and manage your blood sugars well."
   3. "You have a different type of diabetes that needs to be controlled by insulin injections."
   4. "Let's ask the doctor if you can take pills while you are in school and take injections at home."

7. The parents of a 10-year-old boy diagnosed with T2D ask you what aspects of their son's diabetes management he should be involved in. Which response is correct? **(Select all that apply.)**
   1. CHO counting
   2. Meal planning
   3. Choosing after-school activities to increase exercise
   4. Recording blood sugar test results in a log
   5. Testing blood sugar at home as ordered

8. Aliyah, age 16, was diagnosed with T2D 3 months ago and was instructed by her nurse practitioner (NP) to eat fewer CHOs, lose weight, and exercise more. Today, she is following up with her NP. What is the most accurate way for the NP to determine Aliyah's compliance with the diet and exercise regimen?
   1. Reviewing Aliyah's blood glucose testing log
   2. Asking Aliyah how she thinks she's doing
   3. Drawing blood for a fasting glucose level
   4. Drawing blood for an HbA1c level

9. You are discussing the best way to continue playing on the football team with a 16-year-old high school junior with T1D. What should you instruct the teen to do before exercising?
   1. Take an additional three units of fast-acting insulin.
   2. Eat a high-CHO snack to ensure an increase of calories.
   3. Drink two 8-ounce bottles of electrolyte sports drink.
   4. Eat a high-protein snack of cheese, crackers, and turkey slices.

10. You are teaching an 11-year-old about rotating injection sites for her insulin. Which response by the patient indicates that she understands the reason for rotating injection sites?
    1. "Using the same site increases the risk for infection there."
    2. "Using the same site can cause scar tissue that leads to reduced absorption of the insulin."
    3. "Using the same site can cause the insulin to act more rapidly than it should."
    4. "Using the same site can lead to changes in the fat under the skin."

ANSWERS 1. 2; 2. 1, 2, 3, 5; 6. 3; 4, 3; 5. 1, 3, 4; 6. 3; 7. 1, 2, 3, 4, 5; 8. 4; 9. 4; 10. 4

CRITICAL THINKING QUESTIONS

1. Children who present with head trauma are at risk for SIADH. When this occurs, the child is at risk for fluid overload and increased intracranial pressure. What nursing observations are required to identify the clinical presentation of SIADH, and what precautions should be taken to provide safe nursing care for these children?

2. Families often ask questions about the differences in growth and maturity that they see in their teen children's friends compared with their child. With the diversity in growth, body hair distribution, sexual maturity, and voice maturation, devise an appropriate response to concerns expressed.

3. A teenager with diabetes can have problems adhering to a diet of counted CHOs. What are the current recommendations for helping a teen with diabetes control blood glucose levels? Can the teenager go a little "crazy" with the diet once in a while, such as at a birthday party?

Resources

For additional resources and information, including Postconference Questions and Activities, Answers, and References, visit www.FADavis.com.

 Student Study Guide

CHAPTER 33
Child With a Musculoskeletal Condition

KEY TERMS

compartment syndrome (kom-PART-ment SIN-drohm)

developmental dysplasia/dislocation of the hip (DDH) (formerly congenital hip dysplasia) (dee-VEL-uhp-MENT-uhl diss-PLAY-zhuh)

epiphyseal plates (EP-ih-FIZ-ee-uhl PLAYTS)

juvenile idiopathic arthritis (JIA) (formerly juvenile rheumatoid arthritis [JRA]) (JOO-vuh-NYEL ID-ee-uh-PATH-ik arth-RYE-tiss)

kyphosis (kye-FOH-siss)

lordosis (lor-DOH-siss)

osteomyelitis (OSS-tee-oh-MYE-uh-LYE-tiss)

pressure injuries (PRESH-uhr IN-juh-reez)

scoliosis (SKOH-lee-OH-siss)

traction (TRAK-shun)

CHAPTER CONCEPTS

Comfort
Infection
Inflammation
Mobility
Nutrition
Perfusion
Teaching and Learning

LEARNING OUTCOMES

1. Define the key terms.
2. Describe the normal anatomy and physiology of the musculoskeletal system throughout childhood.
3. Describe nursing care of a child with a musculoskeletal disorder related to the developmental stage the child is in.
4. Critique holistic assessments conducted to rule out a musculoskeletal disorder in childhood.
5. Identify various childhood injuries that lead to traumatic musculoskeletal injuries or disorders.
6. Differentiate the laboratory values that are used to identify and monitor disease progression for a child with a musculoskeletal disorder.
7. Describe the various bone fractures potentially experienced in childhood and the associated traction and/or therapy used for each.
8. Discuss the principles behind traction and the psycho-socialbiological needs of a child who is required to undergo time in traction.
9. Analyze various childhood disease processes of the musculoskeletal system such as congenital clubfoot, juvenile idiopathic arthritis (JIA), scoliosis, and muscular dystrophy.
10. Describe safety concerns while caring for a child in traction.

CRITICAL THINKING

Noah, a 14-year-old, suffers a compound fracture of his left tibia and fibula while playing football. The wound was immediately stabilized by paramedics on the field but was considered to be a serious "dirty" or contaminated wound because considerable amounts of dirt were introduced into the open wound site during the injury. Paramedics irrigated the wound with 0.9% normal saline, and the teen was immediately placed on broad-spectrum antibiotics upon arriving at the emergency department (ED). The wound required three surgical debridements before the placement of metal hardware to stabilize the fractured bones. Noah has been in the hospital for 3 weeks because of the nature of the complicated wound when you are assigned to his unit.

Continued

CRITICAL THINKING—cont'd

Questions

1. Considering his developmental stage, what pain evaluation tool is best to use with Noah?
2. What complication should you be aware of during the healing process?
3. What signs and symptoms would indicate a complication?

CONCEPTUAL CORNERSTONE

Teaching and Learning

One of the most important concepts related to the musculoskeletal system and associated disorders during childhood is teaching and learning. Families need teaching and anticipatory guidance from infancy through adolescence concerning the prevention of significant injury and trauma. Fractured bones, soft tissue injuries, and associated conditions are common during childhood. Teaching about protective pads, helmets, sports safety, motor vehicle safety, pedestrian safety, and more must start during young childhood and continue through adolescence. Nutrition is also an important part of teaching and learning concerning the musculoskeletal system. Children need adequate calcium, vitamins, and protein to maintain musculoskeletal health. Many congenital and acquired disorders of the musculoskeletal system require a family to learn about the care of the child and how to anticipate complications. Surgery, casting, and immobility all require significant and holistic pediatric health-care team teaching to prevent complications and maximize the healing process.

Active children are very prone to injuries of the musculoskeletal system. Providing supervision during play for young children, insisting on appropriate guidelines and protective equipment throughout childhood, and intervening promptly after injury are all important aspects of care. Children most prone to injuries are those who are obese, who are risk-takers, who are inadequately supervised by adults, and who participate in sports activities before they have acquired the appropriate motor skills and coordination.

THE DEVELOPMENT OF THE MUSCULOSKELETAL SYSTEM

The musculoskeletal system develops in utero and is structurally intact at birth. All of the bones are present at birth but consist more of cartilage than of bone material. This allows the infant to be flexible during the birthing process. The other components of the musculoskeletal system include bone marrow, where blood cell production (hematopoiesis) occurs; joints; and muscles. The musculoskeletal system's interrelated functions include body structure, protection, blood cell production, mobility, and movement.

Bones

The musculoskeletal system comprises two distinct components: skeletal muscles and skeletal bones. The skeletal system grows and develops across childhood. Bones grow in length in the **epiphyseal plates** (the "growth plate" of long bones). When the epiphyseal plates close, growth stops. Children who have bone injuries heal in approximately half the time it takes for adults with similar injuries to heal because children's bones are still growing. Children's injured bones tend to heal faster than those of adults because children's bones are still growing and children's bone remodels (strengthening and reshaping), which leads to complete healing (Nationwidechildrens.org, n.d.). The closer the fracture is to the growth plate, the faster the fracture heals (Nationwidechildrens.org, n.d.). According to kidshealth.org (2023), most bone injuries heal well with full resumption of activities. Long bones are the sites of most orthopedic musculoskeletal disorders and fractures.

Children's rapid growth and active status requires nutrition that supports the musculoskeletal system. A child's nutrition affects the ability of the child's bones to grow at expected rates and to heal after injury. Table 33.1 outlines pediatric daily nutritional requirements for muscle and bone health throughout childhood.

Blood Cell Production

Blood cells are produced in the marrow of long bones. Red blood cells (RBCs), white blood cells (WBCs), and megakaryocyte cells that produce platelets for clotting are all formed within this marrow. A double protective layer of connective tissue called the *periosteum,* rich with nerves and blood vessels, covers the long bones. A child's nutrition affects the bones' ability in and effectiveness at producing the blood cells in the long bone's marrow. Iron, vitamins B_{12} and folate, and protein are required for adequate production of bone marrow cells.

Joints

Joints are another component of the musculoskeletal system. A *joint* is a location where two or more bones join together for structure and function. The function of joints is to provide either a fixed attachment of bones or to provide mobility. The cranial sutures or the symphysis pubis are fixed joints; the hip joint, with its structure of a ball and socket, provides mobility. There are three major categories of joints:

1. *Synovial joints* are between long bones and provide motion.
2. *Fibrous joints,* such as those between cranial sutures, are fixed joints.
3. *Cartilaginous joints* provide cartilage cushions; for example, the symphysis pubis, rib attachments, and vertebral discs. They are fixed joints.

Table 33.1

Daily Nutrients for Bone Health During Childhood

Developmental Stage	Protein Requirements	Calcium Requirements	Vitamin D Requirements	Vitamin C Requirements	Iron Requirements
Infancy	Newborn: 2.4 g/kg/day Infant: 1.75 g/kg/day	500 mg	400 IU	25 mg	11 mg
Toddlerhood	13–15 g	500 mg	600 IU	15 mg	7 mg
Preschool-Aged	19–21 g	800 mg	600 IU	25 mg	10 mg
Early School-Aged (ages 6–10)	34 g	1,300–1,500 mg	600 IU	45 mg	8 mg
Later School-Aged (ages 11–13)	35 g	1,300 mg	200 IU	45–50 mg	8–10 mg
Adolescence	45–52 g	1,300–1,500 mg	200 IU	60–75 mg	11–15 mg (Teen girls may require more based on menstrual cycles and heaviness of flow.)

Sources: Agriculture and Consumer Protection Agency, FAO Corporate Document Repository. (2014). *Energy and protein needs of infants, children and adolescents.* http://www.fao.org/docrep/003/AA040E/AA040E07.htm; Healthychildren.org. (2019). *Children and broken bones.* https://www.healthychildren.org/English/health-issues/injuries-emergencies/Pages/Children-And-Broken-Bones.aspx.

Muscles

The striated muscles provide voluntary contraction and relaxation at the command of the central nervous system. The muscles that provide the mobility of the musculoskeletal system are attached to the bones by tendons. Ligaments either hold bones to each other at the site of the joint, or they provide an attachment of organs to bones. Unlike tendons, ligaments are nonelastic; yet similar to tendons they have a small blood supply and require long periods for healing after an injury.

 COMMON CHILDHOOD INJURIES

Two common types of childhood injuries within the musculoskeletal system are soft tissue injuries and fractures.

Soft Tissue Injuries

A *soft tissue injury* is an injury within the musculoskeletal system that does not include the child's bones. A *strain* is an injury from the excessive use of a muscle or tendon, such as trauma from a forcible stretch or violent contraction. A *sprain* is a painful trauma to ligaments that ranges from a pull to a tear.

A *dislocation* is a temporary displacement of a bone from its normal position. Dislocation occurs between long bones when joints are not limber. Shoulder dislocation occurs when the shoulder joint capsule, which has limited muscle padding for protection and only the rotator cuff for ligament support, becomes stretched and then dislocates.

A *contusion* is a bruise or bruising of a musculoskeletal structure, such as a "bruised bone." Contusions occur when there is an impact injury and the tissues tear, leading to hemorrhages in soft tissue, resulting in a significantly ecchymotic (bruised) and tender area. With a collision type of impact, the contusions can be so significant that the child becomes temporarily disabled with the trauma, bleeding, pain, and swelling.

When a child experiences a soft tissue injury, parents, coaches, caregivers, and health-care providers can apply the interventions that make up the RICE mnemonic to foster a more rapid healing process (Fig. 33.1):

- *R = Rest* the limb to prevent further trauma or injury. Especially with active young children, providing rest will slow down the child and prevent the child's activity from causing more harm.
- *I = Ice* the site of the injury with careful consideration to application intervals that will not cause tissue damage from the intense cold. Ice should be applied for no longer than 10 to 15 minutes at a time with 30 to 60 minutes between applications. A towel or layer of cloth should be

placed between the ice and the skin. Ice should be used for only 36 to 48 hours after the initial time of the injury.

- C = *Compress* the site with bandages, such as ACE bandages, to help prevent swelling through edema and to provide support and immobilization of the injured site.
- E = *Elevate* the injured limb to prevent edema buildup and drain existing edema.

Fractures

A *fracture* is an injury directly to bone material. Fractures are common during childhood, and the two most common fractures are clavicular (collarbone) and greenstick fractures. Athletic injuries and falls from a distance are common causes of pediatric clavicular fractures. Infants with cephalopelvic disproportion (who have a larger head and body than the mother's pelvic size can withstand) are also at risk for these fractures.

Greenstick fractures are fractures of the long bones caused by a side bend of the bone, which leads to a

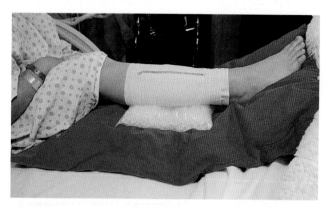

FIGURE 33.1 Application of RICE.

fracture on the tension side of the bend. There are many types of fractures, including transverse, spiral, oblique, greenstick, comminuted, and compression (Fig. 33.2). Box 33.1 provides a list of common fracture types seen in children.

Box 33.1

Common Types of Fractures in Children

1. *Bend fracture:* A child's bone may bend up to 45 degrees without breaking. The consequences of this bending include slow straightening, some degree of deformity, and possible slow healing.
2. *Buckle fracture:* Also called *torus,* this fracture consists of a raised projection.
3. *Greenstick fracture:* This fracture is considered incomplete and will extend only partially through the affected bone.
4. *Comminuted fracture:* This is a fracture in which the bone is splintered or broken into pieces.
5. *Complete fracture:* This is a fracture that splits the bone into two pieces.
6. *Growth plate fracture:* When the fracture is within or extends through a growth plate, called the *physis,* the child may suffer bone growth deformities, including shorter limb lengths. Growth plate fractures are also called *impacted fractures.*
7. *Complicated fracture:* This is a fracture in which the fractured bone impairs, damages, or complicates the function of another body part or organ, such as a rib fracture that extends into lung tissue.
8. *Compound or open fracture:* This is a fracture that is so severe that the bone extends through the muscles, fat, and tissues, protruding through to the skin's surface.
9. *Spiral fracture:* This is a fracture that follows a helical line along and around the course of a long bone; may be associated with child abuse injuries.

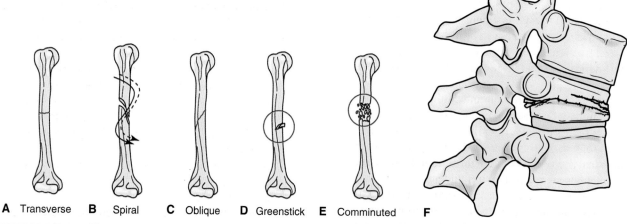

A Transverse   **B** Spiral   **C** Oblique   **D** Greenstick   **E** Comminuted   **F**

FIGURE 33.2 Types of fractures: A, Transverse: Line crosses the shaft at a 90-degree angle. B, Spiral: A diagonal line coils around the bone; caused by a twisting force. C, Oblique: A diagonal line across the bone. D, Greenstick: Bone is bent but not broken; more common in children. E, Comminuted: Three or more fracture fragments. F, Compression: Bone becomes wider and flatter; usually seen in the spine.

CHILDHOOD SCREENING FOR MUSCULOSKELETAL CONDITIONS

Screening children for musculoskeletal disorders should begin in early childhood. During well-child checkups, the health-care provider should ask parents about any injuries or evidence of trauma. The child should be evaluated for normal gait, full range of movement, and pain or discomfort in the joints. School-aged children should be evaluated for the development of **scoliosis** (lateral curvature of the spine). Screening children is important because orthopedic anomalies, disorders, or injuries may interfere with development within the musculoskeletal system, affect the functioning of other organs, and prevent the child from participating in sports activities and social events.

Health Promotion

Children across all developmental periods should be evaluated for the risk, development, or presence of being overweight or obese. Being overweight or obese causes a child to be more prone to musculoskeletal injuries.

While evaluating a child with a skeletal injury, child abuse must be ruled out. With an estimated 25% of all fractures in children 3 years old and younger found to be caused by child abuse, it is imperative that the pediatric health-care team be aware of this possibility. Fractures of certain bones warrant greater suspicion of abuse. For instance, a rib fracture in a child has the highest probability of abuse (71%); children under 3 presenting with rib fractures should be evaluated for child abuse (Mitchell et al., 2021). The probability that a child's humeral fracture was caused by abuse is 48% (Kemp et al., 2008). The probability of abuse for a child aged birth to 18 months with a femoral fracture is 95% (Mitchell et al., 2021). An incongruence between the reported history of the child's injury by the parent and the injury the child presents with is cause to suspect abuse. However, distinguishing intentional fractures from unintentional fractures can be a challenge.

Spiral fractures are of particular concern. A spiral fracture injury (helical line along and around the course of a long bone) caused by childhood play activities is rare. A clinical finding of a spiral fracture warrants further child abuse evaluations. Multiple fractures in various stages of healing should also raise high suspicion of child abuse. In addition, infants who present with femur, midshaft, metaphyseal, humerus, radius-ulna, and tibia-fibula fractures should raise suspicion; these fractures are not a common finding in this age group.

The medical team may order a variety of diagnostic examinations and laboratory values to determine any other possible cause of the fracture, such as bone disease, calcium deficiencies, or underlying pathologies. If abuse is confirmed, the child's case must be referred to the local Child Protection Services (see Chapter 26).

General Evaluations of Musculoskeletal Deviations

The pediatric health-care provider should conduct a thorough holistic evaluation of the child's site of pain, injury, or potential disorder. The following list provides a guideline for this evaluation:

- Evaluate function in the affected part:
  - Determine the child's ability to perform range of motion (ROM) of the affected body part, the child's ability to perform fine and gross motor movements, the amount of weight the child can bear on the affected limb, whether or not the injury or affected area is bilateral, and the presence of inflammation and pain.
  - Palpate the bone and joints under question for warmth, alignment, and any abnormal nodules, lumps, or unusual findings.
  - Evaluate the child's affected limb for muscle tone, the degree of weakness, the presence of deep tendon reflexes, the quality of pulses, and the presence of abnormal sensations.
- Evaluate the child's body size and weight in relation to the deficit, disorder, or injury and plot the measurements on a standardized growth chart.
- Evaluate the child's autonomy of movement, ambulation, and independence in terms of mobility and fine or gross motor skills.
- Request a final summary of the child's x-ray regarding the amount of ossification and the presence of a fracture or other injury.
- Check the child's laboratory studies related to the musculoskeletal system for the presence of deficiencies.

Labs & Diagnostics

Tests Related to the Musculoskeletal System During Childhood

Blood Tests for Bone and Muscle Health:

- *Complete blood cell count (CBC):* Used to determine the degree of anemia associated with a significant bleed after a musculoskeletal trauma
- *Elevated WBC:* Used to determine the presence of infection in conditions such as **osteomyelitis** (inflammation of the bone tissue and the marrow caused by an infection)
- *Erythrocyte sedimentation rate (ESR):* Indicates the presence of prolonged inflammation and may be elevated in the presence of Ewing sarcoma
- *C-reactive protein (CRP):* A protein produced by the liver that becomes elevated in the blood plasma in the presence of inflammation
- *Bacterial cultures:* Cultures drawn from the blood to determine the particular organism causing infection in conditions such as osteomyelitis

Continued

Labs & Diagnostics—cont'd

- *Rheumatoid factor (RF):* An antibody present in 10% of children with juvenile idiopathic arthritis (JIA), formerly known as juvenile rheumatoid arthritis (JRA)
- *Antinuclear antibodies (ANA):* A serum test that may indicate the presence of JIA

Diagnostic Tests for Bone and Muscle Injuries, Disorders, or Diseases:

- *Prenatal ultrasound:* An evaluation for the presence of musculoskeletal disorders, such as congenital clubfoot
- *Radiograph:* An x-ray or other image used to check for the location and severity of fractures
- *Periodic radiograph:* An x-ray or other image used to determine the effectiveness of treatments and the rate of bone healing
- *Computed tomography (CT) scan:* Imaging used to determine the presence and extent of injury, infection, tumors, nodules, bleeding, and inflammation
- *Bone scan:* An imaging test used to determine the presence of tumors, nodules, abscesses, and overall bone health
- *Salter-Harris fracture classification system:* A system used to identify the severity of growth plate injuries; graded between I and V
- *Bone scintigraphy:* A nuclear scanning test used to evaluate bone images through a radioactive isotope injected into the body to illuminate injury, disease, or a condition
- *Magnetic resonance imaging (MRI):* Medical imaging used to visualize the exact location and severity of an injury
- *Arthrography:* X-ray imaging done under general anesthesia that allows determination of the best position of the femoral head for healing

Box 33.2

Ten Consequences of Immobilization During Childhood

The following are concerns you should keep in mind while caring for a child who must undergo a prolonged bedrest for immobilization of a musculoskeletal injury or disorder:

1. Bone demineralization and the release of calcium into the blood (the condition mimics osteoporosis); hypercalcemia and the potential for development of kidney stones (renal calculi)
2. Decreased joint mobility and the potential for the development of joint contractures
3. A decrease in muscle mass called *disuse atrophy,* which is a decrease in the size, endurance, and strength of muscle tissue
4. An accumulation of respiratory secretions, which leads to the potential of respiratory infections
5. The development of a weak cough as abdominal, back, and respiratory muscle strength diminishes
6. A decreased rate in metabolism with a reduced overall daily caloric intake
7. The development of orthostatic hypotension from venous pooling that leads to syncope/dizziness
8. Decreased cerebral blood flow
9. The development of feeding issues (caused by eating supine), decreased appetite, and constipation
10. Decreased circulation of blood to the skin, reducing healing, and promoting skin breakdown and the development of pressure injuries

Interventions for Orthopedic Injuries

Immobilization, casts, braces, and **traction** (a therapy used to help in the healing process of a fracture, often using two lines of pull for extension and stabilization) are considered the cornerstones of treatment for orthopedic injuries and fractures.

A child with a musculoskeletal injury often requires the injury to be immobilized so that healing of the affected fracture, degenerative disease, bone infection, or spinal cord disorder can be promoted. Because immobilization is the complete opposite of the natural state of movement and exploration of a child, it is considered a stressful event and may have lasting consequences on the child's developmental process. Immobilization works by resting the affected site, decreasing muscle spasms that may interfere with healing, providing an opportunity for traction, and promoting bone growth. Box 33.2 provides information about 10 of the potential negative consequences of immobilization.

Casts

Children who experience common simple fractures are often placed in a cast and sent home for recovery. After radiographic confirmation that the fracture is present, where it is, and its severity, a child may be casted in an outpatient or emergency setting. Casting materials may be plaster or synthetic. Synthetic casts are typically made out of a polyester-cotton tape or a knitted fiberglass tape permeated with a resin made of polyurethane. While the material is drying or setting, you should handle the cast with only the palm of the hand because finger manipulation may cause indentation. The area inferior or distal to the affected site must be checked for neurological, sensory, and circulatory status. The family should be taught how to evaluate the child's affected limb, check for cast integrity, and be taught when to report a change in status (Fig. 33.3). If the fingers, toes, or skin below the cast are pale, cool, and without pulse, you should report this finding immediately so that the chance of injury can be diminished.

A severe complication of a bone fracture is the development of **compartment syndrome**. This syndrome occurs when the traumatic injury causes pressure to build up in a confined space, such as in the rigid fascia surrounding the muscles. Muscle tissue bundles are surrounded by a sheath of connective tissue that does not adapt to increasing pressure. If a bleed occurs or there is a buildup of inflammatory

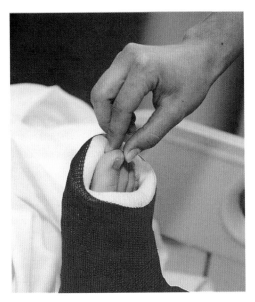

FIGURE 33.3 The nurse checks for CRT.

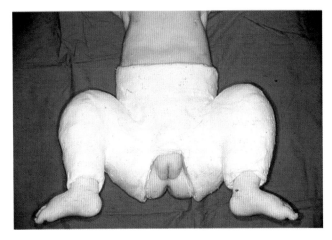

FIGURE 33.5 Child in a spica cast.

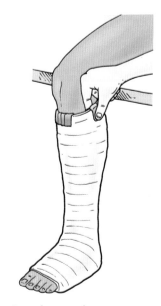

FIGURE 33.4 Petaling of a cast edge.

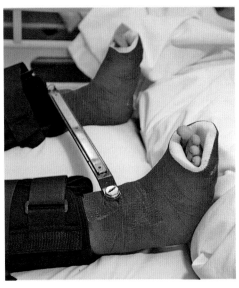

FIGURE 33.6 A cast is applied to the affected extremity to keep it immobile while healing.

fluids, the pressure building up within the muscles can lead to ischemia and necrosis, causing severe tissue damage. If a child who is casted reports increasing feelings of pain and pressure, the situation should be reported immediately so the cast can be removed to check for pressure and tissue damage and recasted. Tight dressings, tight casts, bleeding episodes, inflammatory fluid buildup, burns, trauma, and surgical procedures all place a child at risk for severe tissue damage from compartment syndrome.

A cast should be snug but free of irritation, and the cast material should be kept free of moisture. The application of tape in a petaling design (Fig. 33.4) helps to reduce irritation around the cast edges; in addition, many casts have cushioning within the casting material. Because infants grow so rapidly, a cast may have to be removed and recasted to account

for limb lengthening. This will be influenced by how long the cast must remain for healing.

There are a variety of types of casts used for fractures or injuries during childhood (Figs. 33.5 and 33.6). Spica casts, for example, are used for infants and toddlers to provide stability and immobility during bone healing.

Patient Teaching Guidelines

Care of an Infant With a Hip Spica Cast for Developmental Dysplasia/Dislocation of the Hip

For a child with a cast, teach the family:

• While the cast is drying, use only the palms of the hands to turn or lift a child. Never use fingers, which can indent the cast.

Continued

- After application of the cast, maintain taped petals to prevent the cast edges from causing skin irritation or breakdown.
- Keep the cast dry at all times. Wrap the cast during bathing with plastic and tape.
- In children with severe skeletal injuries that require surgical interventions, check for circulation, color, sensation, movement, and temperature. To prevent injury, teach the family to report any changes to their health-care provider immediately.
- Never pick up the child via the crossbar between the abducted legs because this could lead to breakage of the cast and the need to recast.
- For young children, use a disposable diaper under the edges of the cast to prevent the cast from getting wet or soiled.
- When transporting a child with a spica cast in the car, a special car seat is required that allows the child room for leg abduction while sitting in an upright position.

Braces

Braces are appliances used to assist a child with mobility and posture. Braces are individually made for each child's size, height, and need and are constructed of leather, metal hinges, and/or plastic shells. For instance, a child with scoliosis may wear a thoracic-lumbar-sacral-orthotic (TLSO) brace to help the lateral curvature of the spine realign during the adolescent growth period.

Parents and health-care professionals of a child wearing a brace should perform the following routine evaluations:

- Skin integrity around the site of the brace should be checked. For instance, a child in a TLSO brace for scoliosis should have the skin around the superior and inferior brace edge checked for skin breakdown or irritation.
- Proper fit should be determined as the child grows.
- Any reports of discomfort or pain experienced while in a brace should be reported.

Traction

The use of traction during childhood has three distinct purposes. First, traction is used to provide a realignment of a body part after injury or surgery. Second, it is used to decrease muscle spasms through pulling, stretching, and fatiguing the muscles during the healing process. Third, it is used to provide immobilization of the fracture site during the healing process. Traction has three components:

1. *Forward force,* which is conducted by the child's pulling their body forward
2. *Countertraction,* which is a backward pull accomplished by the use of weights (sandbags or waterbags) typically over the side or the end of the hospital bed

3. *Friction,* which is provided by the child's body weight lying on the sheets, helping to keep the child's body in alignment and countertraction in place

All three components of traction are necessary to heal a significant fracture in a child who is immobile for a period of time.

There are two types of traction: skin traction and skeletal traction. Skin traction is provided by bandages wrapped around the injured limb and providing a pull on the skin during traction. Skeletal traction provides a direct pull on the skeleton and includes the surgical placement of metal hardware, such as pins, wires, bolts, and rods. Care must be taken to observe for inflammation and infection at the sites of the metal hardware used to maintain skeletal traction. Nurses must plan to provide wound care to the sites of the pins.

During traction, it is the health-care provider's responsibility to ensure that the child stays in alignment. This can be challenging because children are in constant motion. The child should be checked frequently for centering on the bed and alignment with the traction, and the weight should hang freely over the side of the bed. Traction weights found on the floor should be reported because further injury to the site may have occurred. If the child requires realignment or needs to be readjusted, the weights should be left freely hanging. During traction, the use of the weight should never be interrupted, such as by placing the weights on the bed for transport. The child's family needs to understand the type and function of traction so that they can assist in caring for the child, maintaining traction, and reporting problems.

For both skin and skeletal traction, a thorough skin examination is warranted because the child is at risk for impaired skin integrity. A child in traction should have slight changes in position on a regular basis to prevent the development of **pressure injuries**. Also referred to as *decubitus ulcers or pressure ulcers,* pressure injuries are skin wounds that result from impaired circulation or inadequate perfusion from pressure. Position changes and turning schedules should be every 2 hours and should be documented. For skeletal traction, the pin site should be checked for problems with healing, such as the presence of drainage, pus, or redness not associated with healing. Check for neurovascular integrity by checking circulation, color, sensation, movement, and touch.

Nurses use the mnemonic CCSMT when checking the neurovascular integrity of a patient in traction.

- *C = Circulation* should be checked by pressing on the skin and observing for capillary refill time (CRT). CRT should be brisk in a healthy child without preexisting cardiovascular disease.
- *C = Color* should be checked. Look for any deviation, such as pale or blue skin.
- *S = Sensation* should be checked by asking the child if they are experiencing any abnormal feelings of buzzing, burning, or tingling. These may indicate nerve regeneration or nerve damage.

- M = *Movement* should be checked by asking the child if they can wiggle toes or fingers or move the extremity below the site of injury.
- T = *Touch* should be checked by asking the child if they can feel the presence of the caregiver's fingers on the skin below the site of the injury.

Nurses also use the mnemonic of the five Ps to ensure that the injured site is receiving adequate perfusion and is not ischemic:

- P = Pain
- P = Pallor
- P = Pulselessness
- P = **Paresthesia**
- P = Paralysis

CRITICAL THINKING & CLINICAL JUDGMENT

A young school-aged child calls for a nurse to come to his hospital bedside. When you arrive in his room, you note that he is in obvious pain with pale, sweaty skin and shaking movements. He is 12 hours post-op for a significant fracture of the tibia and fibula. As you examine him, you use the CCSMT mnemonic and find that the color of the skin inferior to the site of the fracture is quite pale.

Questions

1. What could be the cause of the child experiencing these symptoms?
2. What would you do next in the immediate care of this child?

For skin traction, the edges of the bandages should be checked for skin breakdown. If the child is required to use a bedpan and urinal, the skin should be checked for breakdown related to the presence of urine and/or feces. It is imperative that a child in traction receive frequent skin care, meticulous hygiene after toileting, and daily sponge baths.

TYPES OF TRACTION. Various types of traction are used to stabilize the bone and fracture sites for healing and to maintain the position of healing. The following are some types of traction used in childhood bone injuries:

- *Buck extension:* Buck extension is a type of skin traction applied to the child's leg in a fully extended position. This traction is used for shorter term periods of immobilization and healing. With complete stabilization, the child may be able to turn to a side-lying position.
- *90/90 traction:* This is a type of skeletal traction in which the child's lower leg is supported by a sling or a boot

- WORD - BUILDING -

paresthesia: par–abnormal, irregular + esthes–sensation + ia–condition

while the distal section of the fracture is pinned or wired. 90/90 traction allows the child more movement of the central part of the body, thus facilitating greater movement for toileting, hygiene, skin-integrity checks, and play (Fig. 33.7).

- *Bryant traction:* Bryant traction is the only skin traction available for a child aged 2 or younger with a lower-extremity fracture. Bryant traction allows the child to provide their own countertraction by lifting the buttocks up and off the crib or by dangling the legs in the air with the traction pulling up and over the end side of the crib (Fig. 33.8). The legs are straight, and the body is in a 90-degree angle toward the ceiling. Although only one leg may be affected, both legs are suspended in the same way.
- *Ilizarov external fixator:* Using a system of telescoping rods, pins, and wires, the Ilizarov device promotes limb lengthening by consistently and gently providing tension to lengthen bone tissue (Hosny, 2020). After an osteotomy is performed in surgery, the device provides tension to grow new bone tissue by acting similar to a new growth

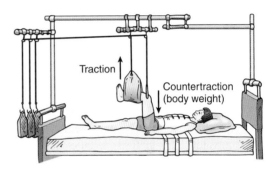

FIGURE 33.7 The 90/90 femoral traction is most commonly used to treat femur fractures and complicated femur fractures.

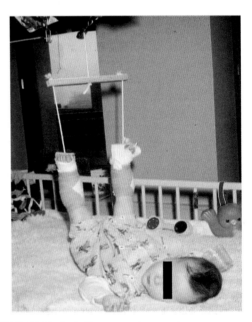

FIGURE 33.8 A baby in Bryant traction.

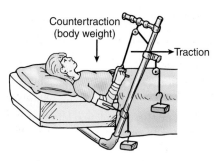

FIGURE 33.9 Dunlop traction is used in the treatment of a supracondylar fracture of the humerus.

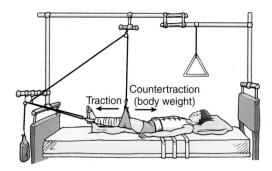

FIGURE 33.10 A child in Russell traction (with trapeze).

plate. Distraction, or pulling of the traction, allows for new blood vessels to develop in the longitudinal direction and encourages neovascularization (new vessels) in bone and soft tissue (Hosny, 2020). The device, brought to the United States by a Russian scientist, also allows for the correction of rotational or angular defects and immobilization for childhood bone fractures. These devices can be as small as thumb-size or as large as is needed for a lower extremity. Special care is given to preventing infection at the various pin sites. Because of the length of time required to benefit from wearing the device, families must be taught how to provide aseptic pin care.

• Other traction setups used in children include Dunlop's and Russell's (Figs. 33.9 and 33.10).

Safety *Stat!*

Neither the health-care team nor the family should ever disrupt the line or pull of traction or the weight of the sandbags because the site might become reinjured.

HAZARDS AND COMPLICATIONS OF LONG-TERM TRACTION.
While caring for a child with traction, all members of the pediatric health-care team must be observant for complications. Maintaining safety for the child in traction is the highest priority. Children may require extended lengths of time in traction, which inherently puts the child at risk for several concerns.

• *Skin breakdown:* Prevent skin breakdown by checking frequently to provide early identification. Cleanse the skin frequently. Provide meticulous skin care after each toileting episode, removing all urine and feces. Use a mirror to observe for the development of redness or pressure injury formation when the child is lying supine. Check the bed for small toys, such as crayons, jacks, and Legos, because the child may have decreased skin sensation while on prolonged bedrest and may not know that there is an object against their skin. A small object underneath the child can cause a pressure injury. Use standard tools to determine the severity of any confirmed redness or skin breakdown. Implement and document a rigorous turning schedule to make sure that pressure injuries are not forming.

• *Constipation:* Prevent constipation by providing adequate fluids and a fiber-rich diet. Be creative in how the fiber content of the diet is increased. Involve the family and provide favorite and familiar fruits and vegetables, smoothies, or fiber additives.

• *Boredom and decreased stimulation:* Prevent regression and behavior problems from boredom by eliciting assistance from members of the child life staff and the volunteer staff to provide a program of developmental stimulation. Provide activities, music, homework, arts, socialization, and reading to stimulate the child on a regular basis. Find stimulating activities that are appropriate for the child's developmental stage.

• *Pain:* Determine the child's pain level by using a valid, age-appropriate pain assessment tool such as the Wong-Baker FACES pain rating scale, Oucher scale, or numerical scale.

• *Respiratory congestion and complications:* Prevent the buildup of pulmonary secretions from prolonged bedrest during traction by using an incentive spirometer. Other breathing exercises that children enjoy include blowing games, such as blowing bubbles and keeping a cotton ball in the air by blowing through a straw.

• *Bone health:* For a child in traction, it is imperative to maintain a diet rich in protein and vitamins for bone health and bone healing. Nutritional disorders, vitamin or protein deficiencies, and failure to thrive (FTT) can all affect a child's bone health and the ability of bones to heal.

Patient Teaching Guidelines

Parents must understand the importance of play and stimulation for their child. The child should be provided activities, creative art projects, and learning opportunities appropriate for their developmental stage.

Patient Teaching Guidelines—cont'd

- *Toddlers* may experience great stress by not being able to move, so activities should maximize their ability to move, provided safety is maintained. Tossing a large soft ball, playing with building blocks in bed on the overbed table, and playing with large trucks or dolls are recommended.
- *Preschoolers* will need a variety of art projects, and games that include make-believe are often well accepted.
- *School-aged children* will benefit from board games, cards, and appropriate media. School-aged children must be given the opportunity to feel industrious and complete their homework.
- *Teenagers* will want intellectually stimulating and peer-focused games as well as appropriate screen time with video games and social media. Homework must continue in this age group.

 COMMON MUSCULOSKELETAL DISORDERS: CONGENITAL DISORDERS

Children may present with congenital or acquired disorders within the musculoskeletal system. Congenital disorders are those that exist from birth. These conditions are found in the early infancy period, or they may not surface until the child is older and ambulatory. Acquired disorders may be caused by traumatic injuries.

Clubfoot

Congenital clubfoot *(talipes equinovarus)* is a deformity of the foot that causes the heel to turn inward and the entire foot to be in a plantar flexion (downward position) and a rigid adduction. The condition may be identified in utero via a prenatal ultrasound. This condition is typically unilateral but may be found bilaterally (Fig. 33.11).

Nursing Care Plan for a Child in Traction

Danny, age 18 months, darted into the street and was hit by a car. Evaluation in the ED reveals that Danny sustained a simple fracture of the right femur but no other major injuries. Danny is admitted to the pediatric unit for placement in Bryant's traction as he recovers.

Nursing Diagnosis: Risk for constipation related to prolonged bedrest and decreased fluid intake
Expected Outcome: The patient will not develop constipation while at prolonged bedrest during traction.

Interventions:	Rationales:
Provide a variety of favorite fluids to ensure adequate hydration.	*Adequate fluid intake promotes regular elimination.*
Engage the dietary office and nutritionist to plan a diet that will provide high fiber via fruits and vegetables.	*Increased fiber intake promotes regular elimination.*

Nursing Diagnosis: Risk for impaired skin integrity related to pressure points of traction
Expected Outcome: The patient will not develop pressure injuries while in traction during hospitalization.

Interventions:	Rationales:
Provide meticulous skin care, thoroughly removing urine, feces, and sweat.	*Keeping skin clean and dry helps to maintain skin integrity.*
Use a mirror to thoroughly examine the skin of the buttocks, back, and shoulders for pressure injury.	*It is essential both to maintain traction on the leg and to monitor for pressure injuries. Using a mirror allows the nurse to visualize the skin that is in near-constant contact with the bedding.*

Nursing Diagnosis: Risk for ineffective coping related to prolonged bedrest
Expected Outcome: The child will engage daily in social activities and appropriate play activities for the developmental stage.

Intervention:	Rationale:
Consult with child life specialists, and encourage parents to bring some of the child's favorite toys from home; invite hospital volunteers to read to and play with the child.	*Prolonged bedrest can have negative emotional and psychological as well as physical effects on a child. Providing age-appropriate play and activities alleviates boredom and promotes normal development.*

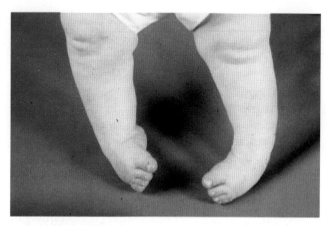

FIGURE 33.11 Congenital clubfoot.

Diagnosing Clubfoot

At birth, the delivery team notes the deformity during the initial newborn assessment. The deformity is identified, and the parents are provided support and education concerning the treatment plan for nonsurgical correction.

Interventions for Clubfoot

The infant will undergo a series of casting procedures to stretch and move the deformity into alignment. Serial casting is performed because the young infant grows rapidly and the deformity moves into place. It is not uncommon to have the child's foot recasted every 2 weeks.

Patient Teaching Guidelines

Parents of a child with a clubfoot may have concerns about bringing their infant back to the casting clinic at frequent intervals for the removal of a cast and the application of the next one. Explain to the family members that because the infant is rapidly growing in length and weight, serial casting is the safest way to ensure that the cast will be effective and not cause pressure.

Nursing Considerations for Clubfoot

Clubfoot is a painless disorder, so the infant does not suffer. The goal is to correct the disorder as much as possible before the older infant begins to bear weight in standing and attempting to walk. Families will need support because they may feel anxiety and despair that their newborn is not "perfect." Reassure the family that the condition will start to be treated within days to weeks of birth.

Developmental Dysplasia/Dislocation of the Hip

Developmental dysplasia/dislocation of the hip (DDH), formerly known as congenital hip **dysplasia**, is a spectrum of

• **WORD** • **BUILDING** •

dysplasia: dys–abnormal + plas–growth, formation + ia–condition

anatomical abnormalities of the hip joint and is the most common congenital musculoskeletal disorder in infants and children. During a well-child assessment of a newborn, evidence of an abnormally shallow acetabulum of the hip is noted, and the femoral head may move slightly or have a significant "slip" out of the socket. The hip joint is unstable and requires intervention. Risk factors for hip dysplasia are related to both the environment and genetic factors including breech presentation, large birth weight, multiples, oligohydramnios (low levels of amniotic fluid during fetal development), female sex, first-born children, and family history of ligament laxity. Although more than one factor may contribute to the development of DDH, fetal responses to a mother's pregnancy hormones is considered an environmental factor (Stanford Children's Health, 2023). The incidence of this condition is up to 34 per 1,000 live births.

Diagnosing Developmental Dysplasia/Dislocation of the Hip

Physical examinations performed on a newborn to confirm the presence of a shallow hip socket and the slipping of the femoral head within the acetabulum include the following:

• *Ortolani and Barlow maneuvers* (see Chapter 15).
• *Shortened leg on the affected side:* The caregiver lays the child supine with the knees bent up, checking for an apparent shortening of the femur; the affected hip demonstrates a lower knee.
• *Asymmetrical skinfolds in the gluteus:* During evaluation of the newborn, there is asymmetry of the skinfolds on the affected hip (Fig. 33.12).

Interventions for Developmental Dysplasia/Dislocation of the Hip

After DDH is confirmed via radiographic examination, the severity of the shallowness of the acetabulum is determined. Immediate treatment is started to stop the progression of the deformity. In young infants (younger than 6 months old), the femoral head is placed into the acetabulum, and the child is splinted in a flexed 90 degrees and abducted position, using one of a variety of abduction devices, such as the popular soft brace called the Pavlik harness (Fig. 33.13). This device holds the ball portion of the joint firmly in the hip socket. Use of an abduction device must continue for up to 6 months. Parent education is vital, and frequent evaluations with strap length adjustments are warranted because the infant is experiencing rapid growth. Older children will require abduction orthotics or open reduction surgical procedures.

Nursing Considerations for Developmental Dysplasia/Dislocation of the Hip

Early newborn screening is an essential aspect to early identification of DDH. With screening of all newborns, early identification and rapid placement of an abduction device will allow up to a 95% cure rate without the need for surgical interventions. Encourage families to go to the website of the International Hip Dysplasia Institute for more information about treatments and care.

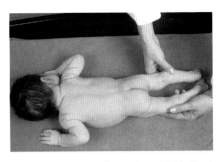

FIGURE 33.12 Inspecting an infant's gluteal folds for developmental dysplasia/dislocation of the hip.

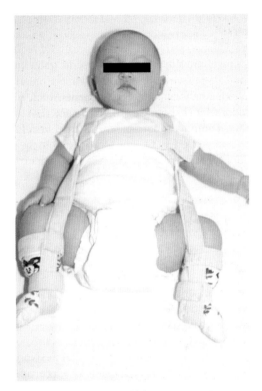

FIGURE 33.13 An infant in a Pavlik harness.

Patient Teaching Guidelines

Parental education is essential because the family must understand the importance of 24-hour-a-day use of the abduction harness. Diapering an infant and young child in an abduction harness is challenging and teaching via demonstration and return demonstration is ideal.

The family also needs to understand how to check for the integrity of the abduction device and what complications are associated with a poor fit, slipping of the straps, or a loss of skin integrity under the strap contact sites. Evaluations that need attention include straps that are not snug enough to keep the infant in an abducted position (knees up and out); straps that easily fall away from their required position; and

skin that is red, raw, or open. It is important to keep a layer of cotton under the straps to prevent skin chafing and skin sores from developing. If these complications are found, the family should report them to their health-care provider for assistance and skin care treatments.

For older children with DDH, immobilization using traction or surgical interventions to produce a reduction may be needed. The surgical procedure of an osteotomy has an aim of reconstructing an acetabulum with a shallow angle so that the femoral head stays in place. A period in postsurgical casting may also be needed.

Duchenne's Muscular Dystrophy

Duchenne's muscular dystrophy (Duchenne's MD), also referred to as *pseudohypertrophic muscular dystrophy,* or dystrophinopathies, is one of a group of 30 genetic diseases that cause progressive weakness and degeneration of skeletal muscles. Duchenne's MD is the most common form found in childhood, occurring in approximately 1 out of every 3,500 male births and typically diagnosed between the ages of 3 and 5 years (Muscular Dystrophy Association, 2023). This progressive disorder of the voluntary neuromuscular system is X-linked and therefore is almost exclusively a male-dominated disorder. The protein dystrophin, produced in skeletal muscle, is greatly reduced by a mutation in the gene that encodes dystrophin. This reduction in or absence of dystrophin causes the muscle cells to become fragile and damage easily.

Diagnosing Duchenne's Muscular Dystrophy

Around the third to fourth year of life, soon after the child begins to walk, the child presents with progressive muscle weakness that produces difficulty in performing normal activities. First symptoms include difficulty in running, skipping, climbing stairs, or riding a tricycle or bicycle. Then, the child demonstrates a waddling gait (because of weakness of pelvic muscles) and difficulty in rising from a squatting or sitting position on the floor, referred to as the Gowers sign. As time progresses and the muscles are infiltrated with fatty tissue, the child's muscles feel firm or, as some describe, "woody" on palpation. As the disease progresses, the skeletal (voluntary) muscles become affected, including the shoulder muscle groups. During the later stages of the disease, the child's muscles experience profound dystrophy. Gait becomes impossible, and the child may progress to respiratory failure from wasting of the thoracic and diaphragm muscles. Mortality is associated with respiratory disease, failure, and arrest and disease of the muscles of the heart (cardiomyopathy), typically in the teen years (Muscular Dystrophy Association, 2023).

To confirm the diagnosis, blood and urine tests are performed. Serum aldolase, creatinine kinase, and myoglobin are measured for abnormally high levels. Serum electrophoresis is performed to determine how much of various proteins is present in the child's DNA. Muscle biopsies are also conducted to monitor the child's presentation of symptoms by determining the severity of nerve disease, muscle wasting disease, inflammation, and overall myopathy.

Interventions for Duchenne's Muscular Dystrophy

Research continues in the use of corticosteroids and gene therapy through clinical trials. The child and family are supported through the slow declining process. Care is focused on promoting optimal functioning as long as possible, treating respiratory infections early, and delaying the debilitating process for as long as possible using positive-pressure ventilation, tracheostomy, and mechanical ventilation. Family-centered care supports and empowers the family by including them in all treatment discussions, treatment plans, and end-of-life care. Solicit the assistance of occupational therapists to help the child with the progressive weakness.

Nursing Considerations for Duchenne's Muscular Dystrophy

Care of a child with Duchenne's MD should focus on three areas: injury prevention, normal growth and development, and the preservation of self-help skills, such as activities of daily living (ADL). Be prepared to provide emotional support, spiritual support, and therapeutic communication. Evaluate the child and family for symptoms of social isolation, depression, stress, and anger and evaluate overall quality of life.

Research continues in the areas of gene replacement therapy to investigate if the defective dystrophin gene can be replaced with a more functional gene. Cell-based therapies are also being investigated to promote the production of critical proteins, such as dystrophin, by specific muscle cells.

Encourage families to seek state-of-the-science information and support from national organizations such as the Muscular Dystrophy Family Foundation, the Muscular Dystrophy Association, and Parent Project Muscular Dystrophy (PPMD).

Osteogenesis Imperfecta

A very uncommon disorder with devastating consequences, *osteogenesis imperfecta (OI)* is an autosomal dominant, heterogeneous disease. This disease is commonly known as "brittle bone disease" because the child suffers from fractures and skeletal deformity. In fact, this disorder may be so severe that the infant does not survive the birthing process. The child's entire life is affected by this disorder with a decrease in life expectancy, an expectation of multiple fractures, and the use of a wheelchair for mobility.

Children with OI have a defect in the genes that produce the precursor of collagen. Without healthy collagen, the major component of bone, the bone is fragile and susceptible to faulty mineralization, fractures, and very abnormal growth, which leads to deformities. The child may present with a bluish discoloration of the eye sclera, hearing loss, joint laxity (looseness or increased flexibility), and poor structure of the bones that support the child's teeth.

Diagnosing Osteogenesis Imperfecta

Prenatal screening typically is not performed for this rare disorder, so early identification is by death in utero or a newborn suffering several fractures during the birthing process. If prenatal diagnostics are performed and the disease is identified in utero, then the infant must be born by cesarean section for the greatest chance of safety and survival.

Interventions for Osteogenesis Imperfecta

OI cannot be treated medically. The child and family are offered supportive care and genetic counseling. Research continues in the area of bone marrow transplantation. Goals of supportive care are to reduce the possibility of further fractures, prevent the development of contractures, promote safety, and reduce injury.

Nursing Considerations for Osteogenesis Imperfecta

Newborns, infants, and young children with OI require special handling to prevent injury. Very specific guidelines must be followed about restricting activities while promoting play, socialization, education, and development. Much education is required for family members to understand the severity of the disease. Families should be encouraged to find further education and support by seeking guidance from the national organizations for OI, including The National Organization for Rare Diseases and the Osteogenesis Imperfecta Foundation.

COMMON MUSCULOSKELETAL DISORDERS: ACQUIRED DISORDERS

Legg-Calve-Perthes Disease

A child who presents with an aseptic necrosis of the femoral head is diagnosed with Legg-Calve-Perthes disease. The child is typically between the ages of 2 and 12 upon diagnosis, which is confirmed via radiography or a CT scan. The pathophysiology of the disorder remains unknown, but the basis of the problem stems from a disrupted circulation pattern to the tissues of the femoral head. Occurring over a period of several months to years, there is a slow disruption to the blood supply to the tissues, including the femoral head, the acetabulum, and the growth plate (epiphysis).

Diagnosing Legg-Calve-Perthes Disease

The disorder is typically observed in the older child; preschool-aged and school-aged children may present with a limp hip joint, discomfort, or hip joint stiffness, especially after joint manipulation. The child may or may not have a history of a trauma in the area.

Interventions for Legg-Calve-Perthes Disease

The child is put on rest because activity may further exacerbate the disorder by causing microfractures to the femoral head's epiphysis. Traction, bracing, and surgical interventions may all be warranted to restore hip ROM and assist with the revascularization of the affected area. Treatments are most effective for children younger than age 10; older children may develop a significant degenerative arthritis without treatment.

Nursing Considerations for Legg-Calve-Perthes Disease

Be aware that treatment for this disorder is a lengthy process. Families need support when the treatment plan calls for long periods of reduced activity for healing. Working with the child's school personnel to adapt a physical education and play program will assist with the adherence needed for appropriate healing.

Slipped Capital Femoral Epiphysis

Also known as a *coxa vara,* a slipped capital femoral epiphysis occurs as a spontaneous displacement of the most proximal epiphysis of the femoral head in an inferior and a posterior direction. Because it occurs most commonly during an active accelerated growth episode, the child presents with either a sudden or a progressive slip of the functional joint, causing a hip disability, a limp, and reports of hip pain.

Diagnosing Slipped Capital Femoral Epiphysis

Considered to be idiopathic, a slipped capital femoral epiphysis is confirmed via radiography and ruling out endocrine, hormonal, and renal dysfunction, or disorders. An obese child is at a greater risk for this disorder. Radiographs will demonstrate the presence of a displacement of the femoral head, an abnormally wide femoral growth plate, and a "slipping" of the femoral neck within the acetabulum, causing trauma on the blood vessels feeding the epiphysis.

Interventions for Slipped Capital Femoral Epiphysis

Slipped capital femoral epiphysis requires a 100% non–weight-bearing status, bedrest, and surgical intervention of the placement of metal pins or metal screws to correct the deformity.

Nursing Considerations for Slipped Capital Femoral Epiphysis

The most important aspect of assisting the child toward a cure is early identification and reporting of the symptoms of this disorder so that immediate bedrest, immobilization, non–weight-bearing status, and surgical interventions can be initiated.

Scoliosis

Scoliosis, abnormal curvature of the spine, is typically not identified until a child is 10 years of age or older and is considered idiopathic in most cases. The disorder involves three distinct vertebral presentations: a lateral curvature of the spine, a thoracic hypokyphosis (upper posterior rib protrusion), and a degree of spinal rotation that causes the apparent rib asymmetry so often noted in a screening assessment. Rarely reporting pain, the child will typically present in a preadolescent growth spurt with a report of improperly fitting clothing or one shoulder being higher than the other.

Scoliosis affects approximately 2% to 3% of the population (American Association of Neurological Surgeons, 2023).

Two other conditions that an adolescent may present with are **kyphosis** and **lordosis**. It is important to distinguish these conditions from scoliosis:

- *Kyphosis:* A condition of exaggerated angulation of the posterior curvature of the thoracic (upper) spine; in lay language, kyphosis is also referred to as "humpback" or "hunchback" in nature.
- *Lordosis:* A condition of anterior convexity of the lumbar spine.

Diagnosing Scoliosis

Children should participate in schoolwide screenings or scoliosis screenings during well-child checkups. Typically, the most common and rapid early identification is made by simply having the child lean forward at the hips while the screening personnel visually inspects the child for a rib hump deformity. Once identified, scoliosis is then further evaluated to rule out pathology of other diseases or accompanied disorders (Fig. 33.14).

Scoliosis is then checked for the degree of deformity, which will determine the treatment plan. Bracing and exercise is the preferred method of treating mild spinal curves while the child is experiencing a growth spurt. Bracing is never considered curative because, without the growth spurt, the brace could not guide the spine into alignment as the skeleton is maturing. Surgical interventions are required when the spinal lateral curvature is greater than 40 degrees. Up to 23% of those with idiopathic scoliosis present with

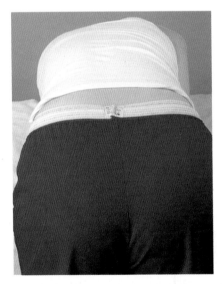

FIGURE 33.14 Assessment of scoliosis includes having the child bend forward to see the unevenness of the ribs.

• WORD • BUILDING •

kyphosis: kyph–humpback + osis–condition
lordosis: lord–curving forward + osis–condition

back pain at diagnosis (American Association of Neurological Surgeons, 2023).

Interventions for Scoliosis

Bracing is conducted by individualizing an apparatus that is well-fitted and worn 23 hours a day. A popular brace constructed of leather and metal is called the *Milwaukee Brace* or *CTLSO* (cervical-thoracic-lumbar-sacral orthosis). TLSO are large, plastic, snug-fitting braces that extend from the underarm down to below the waist. These braces are also constructed individually for each child and are worn for the entire length of the predicted adolescent growth spurt. They may be required to be worn for 2 to 3 years to be effective.

Surgical procedures for severe lateral curvatures require straightening and realignment using internally fixated metal rods, wires, and/or pins with or without spinal bony fusion. The surgical procedure requires an extensive hospitalization stay that includes monitoring the child closely for pain and neurological integrity, log-rolling the child while changing positions until mobilization is reestablished, and preventing a postoperative spinal injury.

Considerable pain is expected from the surgical manipulation of bone and tissue trauma occurring with surgical procedures. Therefore, narcotic pain control measures should be administered around the clock, not just prn, and should be accompanied by muscle relaxers for spasms to assist the child in mobility and surgical recovery.

Patient Teaching Guidelines

If a patient-controlled analgesia (PCA) machine will be used for postoperative pain control in a child having scoliosis surgery, teach the child to use the machine before surgery, when learning can take place without the distraction of the pain experience.

Nursing Considerations for Scoliosis

The prepubescent and adolescent child is often concerned with body image. Not only does having scoliosis cause the child distress, but the bracing and orthotics required can lead to difficulties with adherence to the treatment plan. Consistently remind the teen that if the brace is not worn during the greatest growth spurt, the scoliosis may progress, causing further body image concerns.

Postoperative care of the child undergoing surgical correction for significant scoliosis requires meticulous nursing care focused on safety. This care consists of keeping the child medicated for pain, free of injury, flat on the back, and carefully log-rolled. Request assistance from at least one other caregiver and/or a physical therapist (PT) to prevent injury. A PT can be instrumental in motivating and supporting a child in adhering to the treatment plan as well as in providing safe tips for early mobility (as early as the day after surgery).

Juvenile Idiopathic Arthritis

Juvenile idiopathic arthritis (JIA) is a group of idiopathic chronic inflammatory joint diseases that first manifest during the early childhood period. The disorder may be linked to an autoimmune dysfunction after an exposure to a viral or bacterial infection followed by an acute attack on the joint tissue by the immune system. The exact cause remains unknown for most of the subtypes. The rheumatic process leads to the destruction of the child's synovial tissue layers, which line the joints and secrete a lubricating material for ease of joint motion. The chronic nature of the disease leads to very painful joint destruction and fibrosis of the joint cartilage. Joints appear enlarged and abnormally shaped. They may feel warm during periods of inflammation exacerbation.

Diagnosing Juvenile Idiopathic Arthritis

The child with JIA may present with any combination of the following: painful, stiff, and swollen joints; fatigue; recurrent fevers; skin rashes in some cases; limp without injury; and warmth over joint areas. Confirmation of the disease is by laboratory assay and clinical presentation. Laboratory values include an elevated ESR, leukocytosis, possible positive ANA test, low hemoglobin and hematocrit levels, and elevated CRP levels. MRI may be ordered as well as bone marrow aspiration and joint fluid collection. Clinical presentation includes the onset of the disease before the child's 16th birthday and the presence of inflammation in more than one joint that lasts for at least 6 weeks. JIA may be difficult to diagnosis.

Interventions for Juvenile Idiopathic Arthritis

After confirmation and ruling out of other conditions, interventions are initiated rapidly. Because there is no cure for JIA, the plan of treatment consists of decreasing inflammation, reducing pain, and preventing severe joint erosion and joint dysfunction from the acute inflammatory process. The child's ROM and normal growth patterns should be supported both during an acute exacerbation and during periods of decreased inflammatory processes. A team approach should be used to provide the child with physical, social, educational, emotional, and spiritual support. Box 33.3 provides information about the classifications of medications used to treat JIA.

Physical management includes working with an occupational therapist and a PT at regular intervals to improve muscle strength and ROM. Other management measures include splinting, pain reduction, and mastery of self-care and independence.

Nursing Considerations for Juvenile Idiopathic Arthritis

Nursing care consists of education about the disease and the prevention and management of discomfort. Teach the child and family to balance rest and activity, support normal growth

---

• **WORD** • **BUILDING** •

idiopathic: idio–self-produced, unknown + path–disease + ic–pertaining to

Medication Classifications Used to Treat Juvenile Idiopathic Arthritis

- *NSAIDs:* NSAIDs can reduce inflammation and relieve pain. These are over-the-counter medications and include naproxen sodium, ibuprofen, and others. Side effects include gastrointestinal (GI) distress, gastric ulcers, tinnitus, higher levels of bruising, bleeding into the stomach, fatigue, and liver damage.
- *Steroids:* Medications in the corticosteroid category relieve pain and reduce inflammation by slowing the damage occurring to the joint tissues. Examples of steroids include prednisone and methylprednisolone. Serious side effects can occur and include thinning of the bones, weight gain with a round face, cataracts, diabetes, and easy bruising.
- *Immunosuppressants:* This classification of medications includes azathioprine, cyclophosphamide, and cyclosporine. The most concerning side effect of immunosuppressants is their effect on the immune system, which is an increased susceptibility to infection.
- *Disease-modifying antirheumatic drugs (DMARDs):* Methotrexate, hydroxychloroquine, minocycline, and leflunomide are examples of DMARDs and are known to cause bone marrow suppression, severe lung diseases, and liver tissue damage.
- *Tumor necrosis factor-α (TNF-α):* This factor, naturally produced in the body, is administered to produce an anti-inflammatory process that helps to reduce painful joints, swollen joints, morning stiffness, and overall pain.

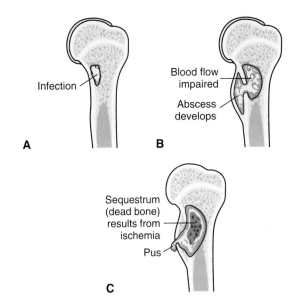

FIGURE 33.15 Sequence of osteomyelitis development. A, Infection begins. B, Blood flow is blocked in the arc of infection and an abscess with pus forms. C, Bone dies within the infection site and pus continues to form.

and development, and facilitate adherence to treatment plans including frequent outpatient visits. Help the child find what level of joint pain is acceptable using a developmentally appropriate pain scale and then provide pain-relief measures with the acceptable level of discomfort as stated by the child as the goal.

Osteomyelitis

Children under the age of 10 years are at the greatest risk for the development of **osteomyelitis**. This bone infection is caused by trauma or injury or migrates from an infection found elsewhere in the body. The causative organism of osteomyelitis varies by age: neonates present with group B streptococci, infants can present with *Escherichia coli,* and older children may present with *Salmonella, Staphylococcus aureus,* and *Neisseria gonorrhoeae.* Puncture wounds, otitis media infections, dental abscesses, pyelonephritis, open fractures, and contamination from surgical procedures can all lead to the development of osteomyelitis in childhood.

Osteomyelitis develops as the causative organism is trapped in the vasculature of the bone, causing inflammation, edema, and vascular congestion (Fig. 33.15). The inflammation and growing infection destroy bone tissue, causing great discomfort. In young infants, the infection may cross from the bone vasculature into the joint space, spreading the infection.

Diagnosing Osteomyelitis

Osteomyelitis should be suspected when a child presents with a history of a puncture wound or infection that now produces pain, warmth at the site, guarding, refusal to use the extremity, fever, and leukocytosis. Isolating and identifying the causative agent is imperative to identify the correct antibiotic. Cultures of aspirated fluids, serum blood cultures, or sinus drainage through the skin should all be collected and sent to the laboratory for antibiotic susceptibility testing. Evaluating for risk factors for osteomyelitis can help with the differential diagnosis. Risk factors include puncture with a foreign body, bone trauma or injury, immunosuppression, and malnutrition.

Treatments for Osteomyelitis

After cultures are collected, empiric antibiotics are started immediately with the most likely coverage for the suspected organism. Immediately upon return of the culture findings, the antibiotics are adjusted to cover the exact microbe. Because of the enclosed bony structure of the skeleton, antibiotics are often required for a period of 3 to 4 weeks. A child may benefit from the use of a peripherally inserted central catheter (PICC line) instead of sequential peripheral IVs. If antibiotics are not effective, surgical interventions to remove the infection may be required.

Nursing Considerations for Osteomyelitis

Nursing concerns focus on the accuracy of antibiotic administration and the control of discomfort. Febrile states should be reported and antipyretics administered. If an open wound is present, such as with an osteomyelitis-related surgical wound or a puncture site, standard precautions should be used to prevent cross-contamination to other patients. Children can experience poor appetite and poor oral intake; you should monitor for appropriate caloric and fluid intake to promote healing.

• **WORD · BUILDING** ·

osteomyelitis: osteo–bone + myel–marrow + itis–inflammation

Key Points

- The musculoskeletal system exists from birth and contains two distinct components: skeletal muscles and skeletal bones. The skeletal system grows and develops across childhood. Bone growth in length occurs in the cartilage area of the bones called the epiphyseal plates; when the epiphyseal plates close, growth stops.
- RBCs, WBCs, and megakaryocyte cells that produce platelets are formed within the bone marrow. A double protective layer of connective tissue, called the *periosteum,* which is rich with nerves and blood vessels, covers the long bones.
- A child's nutrition affects the bones' ability and effectiveness in production of blood cells in the long bone's marrow. Iron, vitamins B_{12} and folate, and protein are required for adequate production of bone marrow cells (Mayo Clinic, 2015).
- Common musculoskeletal injuries in childhood include strains, sprains, contusions, and fractures of various types.
- Laboratory values that are used to identify and monitor disease progression for a child with a musculoskeletal disorder include CBC, ESR, blood cultures, RF, and ANA.

- Bone fractures experienced in childhood may require immobilization, casting, or traction therapy. Traction uses lines of pull to immobilize, provide stability, and create tension on the fractured site. Examples of traction include Bryant traction, Buck extension, cervical, 90/90 traction, Ilizarov device, and Russell traction.
- Children undergoing immobilization and/or traction for an extended period require interdisciplinary care that includes physical therapy, occupational therapy, the support of child life specialists, and the dietary office. The child's developmental level should be considered as holistic interventions and play are created.
- Congenital childhood disease processes of the musculoskeletal system include congenital clubfoot, DDH, OI, and Duchenne's MD.
- Acquired childhood disease processes of the musculoskeletal system include Legg-Calve-Perthes disease, slipped capital femoral epiphysis, scoliosis, and JIA.
- Maintaining a safe environment is imperative while caring for a child in traction. Complications such as discomfort, constipation, skin breakdown and pressure injuries, and boredom should be anticipated and addressed.

Review Questions

1. Which of these risk factors are associated with the development of osteomyelitis? **(Select all that apply.)**
   1. Foreign body
   2. Bone injury
   3. Female sex
   4. Immunosuppression
   5. Malnutrition
   6. Infancy

2. You are caring for a young boy admitted to rule out fracture of the femur. While the child has been transported off the unit for an x-ray of his affected limb, the parents state that they are leaving the unit for the night to care for their other children and will be back in the early morning to visit before work. What is your best response?
   1. "That is fine; we will see you in the morning."
   2. "I will tell your son what your plans are for you so that he understands why you are not here."
   3. "I think it would benefit your son if you wait to say good night to him before you leave and explain when you will return."
   4. "I will call a member of child life to come and sit and play with your son so that he is not in distress."

3. Before surgery, what is the priority nursing care for an adolescent with scoliosis?
   1. Teaching the parents how to use an age-appropriate numerical pain scale
   2. Discussing with the child how to use a PCA machine

   3. Verbalizing what an "advancing diet" will be, starting from NPO and progressing to a regular diet
   4. Determining the child's knowledge base of the pathology of severe scoliosis

4. You have been notified that you will be admitting to the pediatric floor a child with complications associated with Legg-Calve-Perthes disease. In preparing for the admission, you know that this diagnosis is congenital and involves:
   1. Bilateral phalanges
   2. A slipped femoral head
   3. The entire vertebral column
   4. The head of the femur

5. While checking a child who is in a spica cast, you perform frequent checks to the interior aspects of the affected casted limb. Which of the following are checked? **(Select all that apply.)**
   1. Circulation
   2. Color
   3. Movement
   4. Touch
   5. Sensation
   6. Strength

6. What percent of fractures for children under 3 years old are suspected to be caused by child abuse?
    1. 15%
    2. 25%
    3. 40%
    4. 100%

7. A school-aged child sustained a soft tissue injury while playing soccer. What do you suggest the parents do immediately? (**Select all that apply.**)
    1. Apply ice to the site of the injury.
    2. Have the child lie down or sit down and rest the injured extremity.
    3. Offer the child an appointment to see an orthopedist.
    4. Apply compression to the site to reduce the chance of swelling.
    5. Administer an opioid pain medication to immediately control pain.
    6. Elevate the extremity.

8. The parents of a child with a new diagnosis of JIA ask why the child has so much pain. What would be a correct response from you?
    1. "Adherence to anti-inflammatory medications will reduce overall pain."
    2. "The pain is directly related to the child's developmental stage; the older the child, the more pain the diagnosis will cause."
    3. "The severe pain is related to immobility because the child will hold the affected joint still for an extended period."

4. "This disease destroys the joint tissues that normally lubricate the joint and make motion smooth and pain-free."

9. What is the highest priority in caring for a child with a newly placed spica cast?
    1. Report any changes in discomfort.
    2. Report any changes in circulation, sensation, and movement.
    3. Confirm parents' understanding of the purpose and care of the cast.
    4. Determine if the fracture was caused by intentional injury.

10. Laboratory values that are used to identify and monitor disease progression for a child with a musculoskeletal disorder include which of the following? (**Select all that apply.**)
    1. CBC
    2. ESR
    3. Potassium
    4. RF
    5. ANA
    6. Serum protein levels
    7. Blood cultures

ANSWERS 1. 1, 2, 4, 5; 2. 3; 3. 2, 4; 4. 5; 1, 2, 3, 4, 5; 6. 2; 7. 1, 2, 4, 6; 8. 4; 9. 2; 10. 1, 2, 4, 5, 6

CRITICAL THINKING QUESTIONS

1. What are various holistic interventions that a nurse can provide to a child who is experiencing prolonged bedrest in traction? Which departments or professionals can provide support, distraction, play, and assistance in preventing common side effects or untoward reactions to the experience of prolonged traction?

2. How should the health-care team initiate care and treatment for a child with a confirmed spiral fracture? What might be a suspected cause of the injury? What steps would be taken to rule out intentional injury on a child who presents with a spiral fracture?

3. How could a nurse intervene for a family whose early school-aged child refuses to eat fruits and vegetables during a prolonged hospitalization for a significant femur fracture that requires 6 to 8 weeks of bedrest with traction? What are ways to prevent skin breakdown and constipation for this child? Develop a care plan for this child to prevent complications.

Resources

For additional resources and information, including Postconference Questions and Activities, Answers, and References, visit www.FADavis.com.

Student Study Guide

CHAPTER 34
Child With a Gastrointestinal Condition

KEY TERMS

Clostridioides difficile (C. difficile) (klos-trid′ē-oy-d′ēz dee-fih-SEEL)
Crohn disease (KROHN dih-ZEEZ)
emesis (EM-uh-siss)
encopresis (EN-ko-PRE-sus)
fistula (FISS-tyoo-luh)
gastroenteritis (GAS-troh-EN-tuh-RYE-tiss)
gluten intolerance (GLOO-tuhn in-TOL-uh-rents)
intussusception (IN-tuh-suh-SEP-shun)
rumination (RU-min-A-shun)
Salmonella **food poisoning** (SAL-muh-NEL-uh FOOD POY-zuh-ning)

CHAPTER CONCEPTS

Comfort
Elimination
Growth and Development
Nutrition

LEARNING OUTCOMES

1. Define the key terms.
2. Explain the growth and development of the gastrointestinal (GI) tract from the newborn period through adolescence.
3. Describe the components of a health history for a child who presents with a GI disorder.
4. Describe assessment techniques when caring for a child who presents with dehydration, vomiting, diarrhea, constipation, or abdominal pain.
5. Describe the pathophysiology and clinical presentation of intestinal infections such as *Clostridioides difficile (C. difficile)*, viral gastroenteritis such as rotavirus, and parasitic infections in the GI tract.
6. Identify data that would need to be reported immediately associated with various congenital or acquired GI abnormalities.
7. State common diagnostic tests used to rule out specific GI infections or disorders.
8. Describe the care of a child who has been hospitalized for surgery to correct a congenital or acquired GI disorder including perioperative assessments, symptom management, and diet progression.
9. Describe the teaching needs of a family whose child presents with an infectious GI disorder. Include providing safety to others to prevent cross-contamination through effective communication, use of infection control measures, and evidence-based practices to control spread.

CRITICAL THINKING

Gabriel, an 8-year-old, has been admitted to the pediatric unit of the hospital with a new diagnosis of Crohn disease. The child has been losing weight over the last 6 months, and his growth chart reveals that his weight is in the 25th percentile. He has had a history of slightly bloody watery stools off and on over the last 3 months and was seen by his community-based pediatrician on several occasions. Today he is admitted for an upper GI series by radiology; a nutrition consultation; and infusion of a new IV medication, infliximab (Remicade). Gabriel was placed on an oral anti-inflammatory 4 weeks ago but continues to report abdominal pain, bloating, flatulence, and continuing bloody stools. You are on the pediatric unit today and caring for Gabriel.

Continued

CRITICAL THINKING—cont'd

Questions

1. What symptom would you look for in an 8-year-old with the diagnosis of Crohn disease?
2. While you are speaking with the family, his parents ask what foods he should avoid. How would you answer their question, keeping in mind what foods might not be tolerated by a child with Crohn disease?
3. What side effects of immunosuppressant medications, such as infliximab (Remicade), should you observe for?

CONCEPTUAL CORNERSTONE

Elimination

The primary responsibility of the gastrointestinal (GI) system is to digest and absorb foods and fluids and provide for elimination of waste. Congenital, acquired, and infectious GI conditions affect the elimination process. These conditions can be serious in the pediatric population because of the potential rapid loss of fluids and electrolytes, acid-base imbalances, and poor nutritional intake that may affect growth and development. During the absorption, digestion, and elimination process, the GI system is exposed to infectious pathogens. Acute and chronic abdominal pain is often associated with GI conditions. Children can present with abdominal pain that can be nonspecific with no identifiable pathology or etiology. Children can also present with acute abdominal pain that represents serious conditions such as acute appendicitis, severe food poisoning, or intussusception. You must evaluate the child's overall elimination process, fluid balance, and discomfort and report the findings.

GI conditions may present as either acute disorders caused by bacteria, parasites, or viruses, or they may present as congenital or acquired structural disorders. These conditions may cause inflammatory responses and/or problems with motility of the GI tract. Some disorders present with constipation and others with diarrhea. The term *gastroenteritis* is defined as an inflammatory process that occurs in the stomach, small intestine, or large intestine. Clinical signs and symptoms include nausea, vomiting, anorexia, abdominal distention, abdominal pain, and diarrhea. It is imperative that you observe the degree of dehydration and report the severity of the child's condition promptly.

THE DEVELOPMENT OF GASTROINTESTINAL ABNORMALITIES

Many GI disorders can be traced to the child's fetal development. The disorder may or may not be first detected during the newborn period. As the child grows and matures, the disorder may appear with the introduction of solid foods and the further advancement of the child's diet. A thorough health history should include questions about the child's food habits, known food allergies, the use of vitamins or supplements, cultural practices concerning food and eating, bowel habits, and at least a 3-day intake history. An investigation concerning any symptoms associated with daily nutritional practices should include questions concerning the child's ingestion, digestion, absorption, and elimination.

Maturity of the Gastrointestinal Tract in Infancy

Neonates are born with what is considered a sterile gut. So how does the infant acquire the intestinal bacteria essential to the process of digestion and elimination and to fighting disease-producing microbes? Normal exposure to the environment, including the mother's breast tissue, introduces the microbes that make up the digestive system's normal flora. Vitamin K cannot be processed without the presence of this normal flora; thus, newborns receive a shot of vitamin K to assist with the production of clotting factors.

The newborn has only a small stomach capacity of approximately 15 to 20 mL. As the infant grows quickly during their first year of life, so does the volume capacity of the child's stomach. By the end of the second week of life, the newborn's stomach capacity expands to 90 mL.

Safety *Stat!*

It is imperative to know the volume capacity of the stomach during the newborn period because overfeeding can lead to distress, bloating, distention, and regurgitation of breast milk or formula.

HEALTH HISTORY

You should take a thorough health history of a child who presents with either an acute GI disorder or a structural GI disorder. Components of this health history should include the following:

- Food habits, including the typical daily intake of foods consumed, daily calories consumed, the estimated amount of fluids consumed daily, and levels of appetite

---

Safety *Stat!*

Many GI disorders and infections cause the child to experience significant diarrhea. Diarrhea can lead to loss of body fluids rapidly if the stool loss is continuous. The loss of fluids from the intestinal tract can lead a child to experience mild, moderate, or severe dehydration.

· WORD · BUILDING ·

gastroenteritis: gastro–stomach + enter–intestines + itis–inflammation

- Elimination habits and patterns
- Problems associated with each step of the digestive/elimination process, including refusal, dysphagia, evidence of heartburn, delayed stomach emptying, spitting up, wet burps or regurgitation of food, abdominal pain, abnormal stooling patterns, and excessive flatulence
- Past medical history related to the GI system, including illnesses, injuries, accidents, surgeries, and significant family history

PHYSICAL ASSESSMENT

The nurse assists with the physical assessment of the child and prepares by placing the child in a comfortable supine position. Young children do not tolerate GI assessments as well as older children. If tickling is a problem, place the child's hand on the abdomen and then gently place your hand over the child's hand. Have the child slowly pull their hand away; this will reduce the sensation of tickling. The following are included in a GI assessment and should be conducted in this order:

1. Measure weight and height.
2. Ask about bowel elimination routine and last bowel movement, including normal frequency and consistency.
3. Determine the hydration status, including mucous membrane moisture, turgor, the presence or absence of tears, and peripheral pulses.
4. Inspect the abdomen for contour, rashes, lesions, asymmetry, masses, and pulsations.
5. Inspect the mouth for dentition, tooth decay, and oral lesions or infections such as yeast infections (fungus called *Candida albicans*).
6. Palpate light and deep, and observe for rebound tenderness.
7. If the child has been having an itchy anus, inspect the site for sores, lesions, and excoriation. Follow protocol to obtain worms and/or eggs at the site. You should evaluate the presence of GI tract parasite infections. These infections include helminths (worms), cestodes (tapeworms), and trematodes (flatworms) that cannot multiply in the human body, as well as various single cell protozoan parasites (*Giardia, Entamoeba,* and *Cryptosporidium*) that multiply readily.

While evaluating a child's abdomen, you should follow a specific order to prevent the child from refusing or guarding their abdomen if pain or discomfort is elicited: Start with auscultation, proceed to percussion, and then perform light to deep palpation. Further evaluations may be needed and include laboratory evaluation and further diagnostic testing. All abnormal findings should be reported immediately.

Labs & Diagnostics

Common Diagnostic Tests Performed for Gastrointestinal Function

- Laboratory tests
  - *Chemistry panels:* Demonstrate the blood levels of electrolytes that are affected by fluid loss, dehydration, persistent diarrhea, and persistent vomiting.
  - *Complete blood cell count (CBC):* Demonstrates the level of anemia by showing the hematocrit and hemoglobin levels; anemia can be caused by nutritional deficiencies, GI bleeds, and chronic inflammatory processes. White blood cell (WBC) count is monitored as evidence of infectious processes.
  - *Liver profiles:* Demonstrate the involvement of the liver in inflammatory processes and other liver-related pathologies.
  - *Lipid profiles:* Demonstrate the levels of triglycerides and lipids in the blood.
  - *Erythrocyte sedimentation rate (ESR):* Demonstrates the level of inflammatory chemicals found in the blood. Elevated ESR can denote the severity of the inflammatory bowel process.
  - *Thyroid function:* Demonstrates the functioning of the thyroid gland, which helps to regulate metabolism. This test consists of thyroid hormones including triiodothyronine (T_3), which affects most physiological processes such as metabolism and digestion.
  - *C-reactive proteins (CRP):* Demonstrates the presence and severity of inflammation. Different from ESR, the CRP represents a substance produced by the liver in response to inflammation caused by macrophages and interleukin secretion.
  - *Fecal fat collection (72 hour):* Collecting a timed sample of feces for fecal fat can demonstrate how the body is processing dietary fat. Elevated findings are indicative of the bowel mucosa being unable to process, break down, and prepare for the digestion of oral fats.
  - *Stool examination:* Microscopic evaluation can demonstrate the presence of ova and parasites, and for culture. Stool for occult blood is often tested for bleeding disorders and inflammatory processes. Stool should be inspected for the presence of worms such as helminths and evidence of parasites.
- Diagnostic tests
  - Bowel and abdominal radiograph
  - Abdominal and pelvic ultrasound
  - Upper GI series
  - Barium enema
  - Rectal biopsy
  - **Rectosigmoidoscopy**

· WORD · BUILDING ·

rectosigmoidoscopy: recto–rectum + sigmoido–sigmoid colon + scopy–examination

COMMON GASTROINTESTINAL DISORDERS

Children present to health-care providers with a variety of mild to severe GI disorders. These disorders can affect the consumption of fluids and can also affect nutrition, digestion, and elimination. The following sections describe common GI disorders found across childhood.

Vomiting

Vomiting, or *emesis*, is defined as the forceful expulsion or emptying of stomach contents caused by either a GI disorder or by a non-GI disorder, such as increased intracranial pressure, food allergies or intolerances, the ingestion of a toxic substance, or the administration of chemotherapy. GI disorders that cause a child to vomit include reverse peristalsis from a pyloric sphincter blockage, esophageal reflux, overdistention from increased intake, or severe gastroenteritis. The vomiting experience is controlled by the emetic center of the medulla, called the *chemoreceptor trigger zone*. Antiemetic medications effective in preventing or reducing nausea and vomiting work by influencing this center.

You must identify if the child is experiencing true emesis or wet burps. Wet burps or the simple spitting up of undigested breast milk, formula, or food is caused by an increase in pressure in the stomach, especially immediately following a forceful burp. True vomiting is characterized by rapid expulsion of most or all of the stomach contents. Vomiting is a well-coordinated and well-defined process, unlike spit-up, which is passive.

Evaluating Vomiting and Associated Symptoms

Vomiting is a common pediatric experience and is associated with many conditions. The following list provides guidance on the evaluation of vomiting in children:

- Differentiate vomiting from wet burps or simple spitting up in the infant.
- Determine the frequency, consistency, and precipitating factors.
- Identify the characteristics of the vomit, such as the presence of blood, bile, mucus, or undigested foods, which may indicate slow gastric emptying.
- Determine if the vomiting is associated with fever, diarrhea, or headaches.
- Observe the abdomen for the presence of distention, pain, and bowel sounds.
- Measure the girth of the abdomen using a clean paper measuring tape, placing the tape directly over the child's umbilicus.
- Evaluate the child's overall nutritional status, feeding schedule, and any other associated factors.

• WORD · BUILDING ·
emesis: eme–vomit + sis–process

- During infancy, ask about the feeding position and the quantity of food taken in. If the child is fed formula, identify the type used and the recipe for mixing it.
- Check for metabolic alkalosis, which results from large losses of acid-rich stomach contents.
- Check for clinical signs of dehydration such as skin turgor, a low moisture level of the mucous membranes, thirst, and tachycardia.
- Check for conditions that produce vomiting, such as the presence of an associated infectious illness.
- Check the child's psychological status because emotions and rising adrenaline levels with stress both may trigger the chemoreceptor trigger zone.
- Ask about the experience of projectile vomiting, which is associated with pyloric stenosis.
- Check the child for self-induced vomiting or rumination. **Rumination** is a process of regurgitating into the mouth and chewing stomach contents. Rumination can be voluntary or involuntary, such as when stomach contents are regurgitated because of involuntary contraction of the abdominal muscles.

INTRACTABLE NAUSEA AND VOMITING. When a child is experiencing intractable symptoms, such as vomiting, even with the use of antiemetics, it is important to assist the team in ruling out other severe conditions. Pyloric stenosis, obstructions, tumors, foreign bodies, and the ingestion of poisonous materials should be considered.

Interventions for Vomiting

When a child is experiencing vomiting, safety is imperative. Children with decreased consciousness may be at risk for aspiration of the vomit into their pulmonary system. The following guidelines provide tips on how to keep a vomiting child safe:

- Place the child on NPO (nothing by mouth) status and maintain until there has been no vomiting for 12 to 24 hours.
- Ensure safety for the child by preventing the aspiration of stomach contents: Place the child in an upright position and maintain a patent airway.
- Ensure the presence of suction, either wall suction or a bulb syringe.
- Introduce fluids, such as an oral electrolyte solution, first; progress the diet as tolerated. Young children tolerate an oral solution such as Pedialyte, and older children do well with low-sugar, noncarbonated beverages. Introduce one tablespoon of fluid at a time (breast milk, diluted broth, electrolyte solution or ice chips, not juice) every 15 minutes.
- Withhold medications or, if essential, give in a rectal or parenteral form.
- Record intake and output (I&O) exactly and monitor the stool status for possible accompanied diarrhea.
- Instigate good oral hygiene after vomiting.
- Medicate for nausea.

Medication Facts

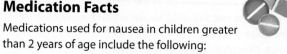

Medications used for nausea in children greater than 2 years of age include the following:

- Promethazine, an H1 receptor blocker and antihistamine
- Prochlorperazine, a weak dopamine receptor blocker suppressing the chemo receptor zone (CRZ)
- Metoclopramide, a dopamine receptor antagonist
- Ondansetron, a select serotonin (S-HT3) receptor blocker

Nursing Considerations for Vomiting

The child who has had an extended period of vomiting should be monitored for dehydration, aspiration, sore throat, and weight loss. Persistent vomiting can be detrimental to the child's teeth, and oral hygiene should be provided after each vomiting episode.

Gastroesophageal Reflux

The return of stomach contents through the esophagus can be caused by a poorly developed or an incompetent cardiac sphincter. Premature infants and children with conditions that cause decreased muscle tone are especially prone to the development of gastroesophageal reflux (GER), also called *gastroesophageal reflux disease (GERD)*. The acidity of stomach contents causes the child to experience pain and, in severe cases with repeated exposure, can cause the esophagus to erode. Symptoms appear immediately after the child consumes food as levels of stomach acid increase. If a child with GERD aspirates the acidic stomach contents, they are at risk for developing pneumonia. Most cases of reflux resolve by 1 year of age, but complicated cases will need surgical interventions.

Diagnosing Gastroesophageal Reflux

The child with a confirmed diagnosis of GER should be assessed for severity and esophageal tissue damage from the stomach acid reflux. Important assessment considerations include the following:

- The child's GER behaviors in relation to eating/feeding patterns
- The onset of GER in relation to the child's positioning
- The pH of the stomach contents
- Coexisting weight loss or failure to thrive (FTT)
- Severity of discomfort in the chest area, described as inconsolable crying in infancy or adultlike patterns of heartburn seen in older children

Prepare the child for diagnostic assessment procedures, including barium swallow or an upper GI series of x-rays.

Interventions for Gastroesophageal Reflux

A child with GER needs to be supported to prevent complications. The following list addresses the most important aspects of care:

- Place the child in an upright position before, during, and after feedings. This can be done by holding the child in the lap, placing the child in a car seat, propping the child upright with pillows, or placing the child in an infant bouncy seat.
- Provide small meals, feed slowly, and check for tolerance.
- Burp frequently to prevent a buildup of swallowed air.
- Administer ordered GERD medications as directed, at least 30 minutes before eating.
- Pharmacology may include medications that reduce the amount of stomach acid produced, delay stomach emptying, and increase gastric peristalsis. The prevention of esophagitis is imperative to reduce the child's discomfort.
- If the child is an infant, work with the nutritionist to determine the feasibility of thickening the formula. This may require an alternative nipple because thicker formula may not flow through a traditional nipple. Thicker formula can become a safety hazard and should not be done unless the child has been assessed by a nutritionist or a speech therapist has evaluated the child's swallowing reflex.

Nissen's fundoplication surgery may be required for a child with persistent and severe GERD that leads to growth problems and esophageal tissue damage from stomach acid. This surgical procedure creates a lower esophageal sphincter that significantly reduces the reflux of stomach acid into the esophagus. The surgical procedure includes creating an antireflux valve made up of a portion of the fundus of the stomach, thus creating a high-pressure zone. This requires more pressure to cause reflux.

Nursing Considerations for Gastroesophageal Reflux

GERD is not only uncomfortable; it can lead to serious medical issues. Frequent regurgitation of acidic stomach contents places the child at risk for developing esophageal erosion and scar tissue that can lead to strictures or narrowed lumen. It is imperative that GERD is identified early, differentiated from other pain such as indigestion or more severe problems such as heart pain, and treated with pharmacological and nonpharmacological interventions such as positioning after eating and sleeping positions with the head of the bed elevated.

Diarrhea

Diarrhea is an increased frequency and decreased consistency of stool. Excess water enters the bowel because of osmotic pull, an electrolyte imbalance, poor water absorption with an inflammatory process, or increased peristalsis. Diarrhea has several possible causes, including infectious processes, food allergies, exposure to toxins, or malabsorption conditions. It is a common outcome of many childhood illnesses, including both GI and respiratory disorders, and may accompany the administration of antibiotic therapy. Great caution should be taken to check for the development of metabolic acidosis with extended periods of diarrhea; with excessive stool loss, there is a loss of bicarbonate, an alkaline substance used by the body to neutralize stomach acid.

Dehydration is also associated with stool loss. Monitoring a child during periods of diarrhea is important to determine overall fluid loss. Careful evaluation of I&O allows the nurse to determine if a child will need further fluids either orally, if the child can, or via IV. Report any change of condition rapidly to prevent complications of dehydration. Diarrhea can cause severe fluid loss that progresses to electrolyte imbalances, hypovolemic shock, and even death in the pediatric patient. See Table 34.1 for information about levels of dehydration.

Evaluating Diarrhea

Assist the health-care team by providing meticulous and accurate measurements of the child's stool output. Make sure that there is a diaper scale handy, or place a "top hat" in the toilet or commode to measure accurate stool losses. All abnormal findings should be reported immediately.

Safety Stat!

When a child presents with diarrhea, immediately place the child on contact precautions to prevent the possible spread of infection to other patients, family, and the health-care team. If *Clostridioides difficile (C. difficile)* is suspected, place the child on expanded contact precautions requiring hand washing, not the use of sanitizing hand gel.

- Measure the overall stool loss and the duration of symptoms.
- Measure the overall I&O, evaluating for significant imbalances.
- Check the color and consistency of the stool.
- Weigh the patient daily.
- Evaluate pain and cramping.
- Check for the presence of frank or occult blood in the stool.
- Determine the relationship of diarrhea stooling with feeds.
- Check the skin integrity around the anus.
- Check the patient's hydration status (Table 34.2).
- Listen to bowel sounds, and palpate the abdomen for masses and distention.
- Check for the presence of accompanying fever.
- Check for the presence of causative factors such as stress, inflammatory bowel disease, food sensitivities or intolerances, allergies, and medications.

Interventions for Diarrhea

Diarrhea can cause significant discomfort for a child, regardless of the child's age. Not only should the following list of interventions for diarrhea be followed, but special attention to the child's anal skin integrity should be given because copious diarrhea can lead to skin breakdown and further discomfort. Consider asking the health-care provider to order a soothing and protective cream.

1. Place the child on NPO status for bowel rest until fluids are ordered and can be tolerated.
2. Begin oral rehydration fluids; for infants, administer an electrolyte solution as ordered.

Table 34.1
Levels of Dehydration

Levels of Dehydration	Estimated Weight Loss	Clinical Presentation
Mild	Up to 5%	Dry mucous membranes, elevated pulse, capillary refill at 2 sec, slightly increased thirst, urine specific gravity over 1.020
Moderate	Up to 10%	Irritability, great thirst, mild orthostatic blood pressure (BP), capillary refill between 2 and 4 sec, decreased tears, oliguria, moderate thirst, increasing urine specific gravity
Severe	10%–15% or more	Extreme thirst, tachycardia, orthostatic BP, sunken anterior fontanel, anuria, lethargy to comatose state in infants

Table 34.2

Types of Dehydration

Type of Dehydration	Signs and Symptoms	Causes	Treatments
Isotonic, in which water and sodium losses are proportional (serum sodium is normal, between 130–150 mEq/L)	Decreased urine production, fatigue, tachycardia, and headaches	Severe vomiting and diarrhea, sweating, hemorrhage, slower significant bleeds, and gastroenteritis	IV boluses of normal saline solution (0.9%) or, if tolerated, oral rehydration with oral electrolyte solutions such as Pedialyte
Hypotonic, in which serum sodium levels are below expected values (serum sodium is low, less than 130 mEq/L)	Mainly neurological signs such as lethargy, headaches, confusion, coma, and death	Addison's disease, cystic fibrosis, loop diuretic overuse, overhydration with plain water, and heat stroke	IV boluses of normal saline (0.9%) or infusions of lactated Ringer's solution with dextrose; may be supplemented with oral electrolytes to assist with correction
Hypertonic, in which there is a greater water loss than sodium loss (serum sodium is high, more than 150 mEq/L)	Very dry mouth, restlessness, severe thirst, fatigue, lack of tears, and doughy skin texture	Not drinking enough fluids, medications that cause increased urination (polyuria), fevers, sweating too much, or consuming seawater	IV boluses of ½ normal saline (0.45%) or, if tolerated, oral rehydration with diluted oral electrolyte solutions

3. Avoid fruit juices or any fluids with concentrated sugars.
4. Introduce foods slowly and monitor for tolerance.
5. Resume a well-balanced diet (may need to be bland) within 24 hours if tolerated.
6. Administer antidiarrheals, antiprotozoals, or antibiotics as ordered.
7. Cleanse the diaper area carefully, especially the rectal area, after each stool to prevent breakdown. Apply topical ointments for protection and soothing. Do not use commercial baby wipes because these may contain alcohol, which causes further skin breakdown.

CLINICAL JUDGMENT

You are a home health-care nurse caring for a child with complex health-care needs and find your school-age patient has significant diarrhea. Observing the child's environment and home health-care orders, you see that the child is on two enteric formulas that infuse into her percutaneous endoscopic gastrostomy (PEG) tube, as well as oral intake of a regular diet as tolerated. Her mother asks if her daughter should fast for a few days to "rest her system."

Question

1. How should you respond to the mother's question?

Nursing Considerations for Diarrhea

When the cause of a child's diarrhea is unknown, contact precautions should be initiated. If there is suspicion of *C. difficile,* then expanded contact precautions and enteric precautions should be initiated and strict hand washing should be enforced. *C. difficile* is not inactivated by alcohol-based hand sanitizers; 20-second hand washing is required to prevent the spread.

Health Promotion

Food Poisoning

Families need education regarding the prevention of serious GI illness from food that is contaminated by infectious pathogens. Teaching families about safe food preparation, appropriate disinfection of kitchen surfaces, and hand washing before and after handling food will help reduce the incidence of food poisoning.

Salmonella **food poisoning** is a fairly common GI illness. This illness is caused by *Salmonella* bacilli that produce a range of reactions from mild gastroenteritis to fatal food poisoning. The incubation period is approximately 6 to 72 hours (but can be a week) after ingestion (Centers for Disease Control and Prevention [CDC], 2023). There are more than 1,400 species of *Salmonella* bacilli. Safe food handling, cleaning food preparation surfaces, cooking food thoroughly, and hand washing all help to reduce the incidence of this infection.

Constipation

Constipation is an increased consistency (hard and dry) and decreased amount of stool when compared with the child's normal and expected stooling pattern. Constipation is the most common report during childhood, with a prevalence of up to 30% of children and a factor in 1 out of every 20 office visits (Borowitz, 2022; National Institute of Diabetes and Digestive and Kidney Diseases, 2018). Although children each have unique stooling patterns, including some who do not stool every day, constipation is considered an abnormal state of dry, hard, and infrequent stooling. Constipation may be associated with straining, but the presence of straining does not mean that the child is constipated.

Symptoms of constipation include the following:

• Fewer than three bowel movements per week
• Hard, dry, and difficult-to-pass stools
• Large-in-diameter stools
• Painful-to-pass stools
• Associated abdominal pain
• Blood on the outer surface of stool
• Traces of liquid stool on underwear

Childhood constipation can be categorized as either acute or chronic. Acute, or infrequent and resolvable, constipation can be associated with a diet low in liquids, which leads to a decreased amount of fluid in the GI system, producing hard, drier stools. Often, increasing fluids and providing a high-fiber diet rich in fruits and vegetables is all that is needed for a child with infrequent constipation. Sometimes changes in a child's routine, presence of stressors, hot weather, long travel experiences, and starting school are associated with constipation. In addition, too-early toilet training can lead to rebellion and holding of stools. With food jags, children may eat large amounts of one food. If the favorite food is low in fiber, such as macaroni and cheese, constipation may follow.

With chronic constipation, interventions are needed to produce a normal stooling pattern. Chronic constipation is fairly common and may relate to poor fluid intake, decreased activity levels, or poor nutrition. Question the child's medical history because anatomical malformations or digestion disorders are associated with chronic constipation. The family should seek health care if the following develops:

• Fever
• Vomiting
• Distended abdomen
• Anal fissures (small painful tissue tears at anus)
• Rectal prolapse

Patient Teaching Guidelines

Chronic Constipation

The family of a child with chronic constipation needs education and support to help their child regain or establish a regular evacuation pattern.

• The child will need an organized, planned toileting routine supported by the family and the family's lifestyle.
• Suppositories, enemas, and possibly GoLYTELY (a polyethylene glycol electrolyte solution) may be needed to empty the child's bowel as the toileting routine is initiated.
• Increasing the child's daily intake of fiber and fluids is an important addition to the toileting routine.
• A timer can be used to encourage the child to stay on the toilet for a predetermined time twice a day to get a routine established; usually 5 to 10 minutes, depending on the child's age, is sufficient.
• Positive reinforcement, counseling, and education should all be part of the bowel retraining routine.

Evaluating Constipation

Although constipation usually requires only home interventions, you should check for the frequency of, precipitating factors related to, and the severity of a child's constipation. Whether the constipation is situational or chronically experienced should be differentiated.

• Note the frequency of passing hard, dry, and infrequent stools. Ask how long the situation has been present.
• Ask for a sample of the stool and perform the guaiac test for the presence of frank or occult (hidden) blood.
• Measure the patient's abdominal girth and document it daily (Fig. 34.1).
• Determine the level of pain during stooling and any accompanying abdominal pain.
• Inspect the child's perirectal area for the presence of rashes, inflammation, bleeding, and fissures on the anal area.
• Question the child and caregiver about the child's reluctance to use the toilet in public, at friends' homes, at the family home, or at school. Determine if the child is demonstrating the withholding of stooling for a length of time.

Interventions for Constipation

Interventions for constipation range from simply modifying the child's diet with fluids and fiber to requiring daily

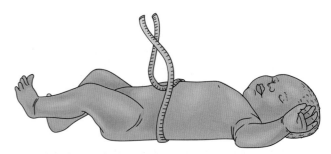

FIGURE 34.1 Measurement of abdominal circumference.

medications that soften stool or increase peristalsis. A regular pattern should be established using the least invasive measures first. Adding fresh fruits and vegetables to a child's diet when these foods have been limited or absent may be enough to produce a regular stool pattern.

- Teach the family to add fiber to the child's diet with each meal (fruits, vegetables, beans, whole grain cereals, breads, and pastas).
- Promote physical activity.
- Create a consistent toileting routine.
- Provide an opportunity for the child to try new high-fiber foods such as prunes or other dried or fresh fruit that they may not have tried before.
- Provide stool softeners, such as glycerin suppositories, oral mineral oil, or docusate sodium.
- If appropriate, add a small amount of corn syrup to the infant's formula to increase the osmotic load and help liquefy hard stools (discuss with the health-care provider before initiating this intervention).
- Lubricate the anal area to allow easier passage of hard stools.
- If appropriate, digitally remove the stool very gently.
- Remind the child to heed urges and not delay stooling.
- Encourage a squat position to pass stool. Considered a natural position that improves elimination, the position can be improved by having a short stool set in front of the toilet on which to place the child's feet, elevating the knees.

Nursing Considerations for Constipation

If these interventions are not successful in treating a child's constipation, it may be appropriate to discuss with the health-care provider the initiation of prescribed laxatives. Unlike stool softeners that provide lubrication via increased water to the stool, laxatives increase peristalsis and increase water to the stool.

If a child presents with chronic constipation, it is important to refer the child for further workup. The child may have an obstructive condition, **encopresis** (Box 34.1), or another diagnosis that requires in-depth diagnostics and careful follow-up.

Cleft Lip and Cleft Palate

Other conditions that can cause GI problems are cleft lip and cleft palate. Cleft lip occurs during fetal development in approximately the seventh week of gestational growth. In this condition, the tissues of the upper lip fail to fuse completely. Clefts may be partial or complete and unilateral or bilateral (Fig. 34.2). Cleft lip is more common in boys than in girls. One serious complication of cleft lip is the risk of aspiration during feedings or with wet burps because there is incomplete closure of the mouth. Effectiveness of the child's sucking ability must be determined, and a feeding device may be needed to ensure adequate nutritional intake. Children with unrepaired cleft lip and cleft palate may experience

Box 34.1

Case Study

A Preschooler With Encopresis

Encopresis is a form of chronic constipation that requires a bowel retraining routine. A preschool boy presents with frequent incontinence of stool during the late afternoon. The mother reports that the child has "dirty" underwear every day and every few days will produce a large stool in his pants with the child seemingly not aware or bothered by the presence of the stool and the smell of feces. The parents finally bring the child in after hiding their concerns from friends and family for almost a year. The child is shy and cautious in his interactions. Diet history demonstrates a well-rounded, age-appropriate diet complete with fruits and vegetables.

After an emotional discussion with the pediatrician, a diagnosis of encopresis is made. Recommendations included a commercially prepared enema on day one followed by time on the toilet reading books for no less than 10 minutes three times a day. The child was to produce at least a "half cup" of stool per day. The family was to not punish the child in any way for accidents, and they were to find ways of identifying and decreasing stress in the child's life. Dietary modifications included increased oral fluid consumption, more fresh fruits, and a high-fiber cereal daily. After 6 weeks of the program, the child's encopretic episodes decreased, and the family reported much less distress.

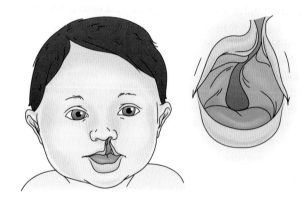

FIGURE 34.2 Infant with cleft lip and cleft palate.

FTT from reduced oral intake and poor suck. They are at increased risk of aspirating food into the airway and are more likely to develop ear infections (Stanford Children's Health Care, 2023).

Cleft palate occurs during the 9th and 10th weeks of fetal development. Cleft palate is twice as common in girls than in boys. The severity of the incomplete fusion of the bone and tissue of the upper jaw and the palate will determine the complexity of the long-term care. In severe cases, not only are the soft and hard palates involved but portions of the maxilla as well. Aspiration is common, and the child with cleft palate is at risk for more frequent respiratory infections and bouts of otitis media. Natural defenses against bacterial infections are decreased with the increased open spaces in the oral cavity.

The surgical repair of cleft lip usually takes place when the infant is at least 10 weeks of age and weighs 4.5 kilograms. Surgical repair of cleft palate is much more complex, may take serial surgeries for extensive fusions, and will not take place until the infant is older than 10 months and weaned from the bottle.

Diagnosing Cleft Lip and Palate

Initial diagnosis for cleft lip and/or cleft palate takes place in utero during routine ultrasound evaluations of the fetus. If the condition was not noted during prenatal care, then the condition(s) should be evaluated during the immediate postbirth examination. The following list provides guidance for evaluating for the presence and severity of cleft lip and/or cleft palate:

- Observe the infant for respiratory distress during feedings.
- Check for the infant's ability to produce a complete and quality suck and swallow, and for the presence of an airtight seal around the nipple.
- Check for the development of abdominal distention during feedings and burp the baby frequently.
- Check for bonding issues and provide support during the early newborn period.

Interventions for Cleft Lip and Palate

Interventions for cleft lip and palate include preoperative and postoperative interventions. Cleft lip repair may be performed at 3 to 6 months of age. Cleft palate will take place at approximately 9 to 18 months of age because it is a more complex procedure. The palate needs three layers of closure: the inner nasal lining, middle layer of muscle and fascia, and oral mucosa. In some cases, a bone graft is used. After surgery, a portion of the cleft palate may be left open to allow for jaw, mouth, and palate growth.

PREOPERATIVE INTERVENTIONS. Preoperative interventions include the following:

- The infant should be fed smaller, more frequent feedings slowly in an upright position; care should be given to avoid aspiration with feedings.
- Feedings should be stopped frequently to provide thorough burping and to prevent wet burps that are associated with aspiration.
- Provide preoperative interventions to improve the infant's nutrition: a cleft lip nipple with a palate flap (Fig. 34.3), medicine droppers, syringe feedings, or manual compression of the nipple.
- Request gavage feedings if nipple feedings do not demonstrate a successful growth pattern and weight gain.
- Administer a small amount of sterile water to the infant after feedings to remove residual formula or breast milk from the open palate area; sterile water reduces bacterial growth.
- Provide emotional support and education to the family to improve bonding and to increase holding and touching.

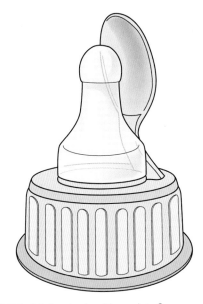

FIGURE 34.3 A cleft lip nipple with a palate flap.

- Provide the family with preoperative education about the surgical procedure for cleft lip (**cheiloplasty**) and/or cleft palate (**staphylorrhaphy**) and the postoperative care they can anticipate.

POSTOPERATIVE INTERVENTIONS. Postoperative interventions include the following:

- Maintain an airway free of secretions and monitor for edema or any narrowing that places the infant at risk for airway compromise; monitor for distress, cyanosis, tachycardia, or restlessness.
- Monitor for postoperative infections; no oral temperatures should be taken after surgery to prevent tissue damage.
- Treat pain promptly and thoroughly; reevaluate at regular intervals and provide distraction/diversion.
- Prevent trauma to the suture line by avoiding crying, and use padded arm restraints to prevent rubbing of butterfly closures or fine sutures.
- Introduce feedings cautiously and monitor for dysphagia.
- After cleft lip repair (Fig. 34.4) on an older infant, care must be taken to prevent trauma to the suture line; only soft toys should be offered, and any item that is pointed or stick-shaped should be avoided.
- To prevent further trauma, no straws or suction devices should be used.
- Clean the suture line carefully after feedings and as needed to keep the site clean.
- Do not brush the child's teeth after palate surgery until ordered (at least 2 weeks).
- As needed, medicate for associated nasal congestion.

· WORD · BUILDING ·

cheiloplasty: cheilo–lip + plasty–surgical repair
staphylorrhaphy: staphylo–palate + rrhaphy–surgical repair

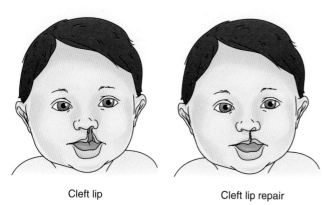

Cleft lip   Cleft lip repair

FIGURE 34.4 A young infant with corrected cleft lip.

Be aware that the corrected cleft lip or palate rarely leads to poor self-esteem or poor self-image. With new surgical procedures, suture lines are barely visible and typically do not cause emotional distress to patients of either sex. However, uncorrected cleft palate places the child at risk, and families must be evaluated for the competency of care during feedings when the newborn is discharged home before surgery. Long-term follow-up is imperative for cleft palate care, and families should be offered professional counseling if warranted during the period of waiting until the surgery is performed. Dental and orthodontic follow-up care is imperative because faulty dentition is a potential complication of surgical correction of cleft palate. Nursing diagnoses for a child with cleft lip and/or palate can be found in Box 34.2. Using nursing diagnoses can help you determine priority goals and interventions for safe care of children after surgery.

Safe and Effective Nursing Care

When caring for children in the postoperative period after surgery to correct cleft palate, use the acronym ESSR:

Enlarged nipple,
Stimulate sucking by rubbing the nipple on the lower lip,
Swallow, and
Rest after each swallow to allow for complete swallowing (Hogan & White, 2003).

Do not allow the infant to rub the suture line. Position the child supine or side lying to prevent injury to the surgical site (Pediatric Plastic Surgery Institute, 2024). Explain to the family that blood drainage is normal after surgical intervention.

Esophageal Atresia

The word *atresia* refers to an anatomical abnormality where a passageway terminates. An atresia is a pathological closure of the passageway where a normal anatomical opening should be. An esophageal atresia (EA) is an abnormal termination of the esophagus, alone or in association with other congenital defects. The presence of the esophageal blind pouch at the proximal end of the esophagus prevents the passage of breast milk, formula, or any fluids. Food does not enter the stomach, and the newborn is at risk for aspiration of the fluids from the pouch, dehydration, and starvation. The health-care team must differentiate between an EA and a tracheoesophageal fistula (TEF; Fig. 34.5), another anatomical abnormality discussed later.

Diagnosing Esophageal Atresia

An infant may present with respiratory distress after the first introduction of breast milk or formula. If the anatomical anomaly allows for the passage of oral fluids, the child might become acutely distressed as the fluids pass into the infant's lungs. Evaluation of EA and TEF includes checking for the following:

- The presence of excessive oral secretions
- Coughing, choking, and respiratory distress
- Possible intermittent cyanosis associated with fluid intake or excessive oral secretions
- The presence of an esophageal/tracheal fistula as well as the presence of tracheal irritation from the infant's gastric acid passing from the esophagus into the trachea

Interventions for Esophageal Atresia

If an EA is suspected, you should immediately report the findings to the pediatric health-care team and stop any further feedings. You should also:

1. Maintain NPO status until a PEG tube is passed for feeds.
2. Suction frequently to prevent aspiration and periods of respiratory distress.
3. Prepare the child for surgery to repair the anatomical defect.

· **WORD** · **BUILDING** ·
atresia: a–without + tres–perforation + ia–condition

Box 34.2

Nursing Diagnoses for Cleft Lip and Palate

- Risk for infection related to decreased infection-fighting potential
- Risk for injury related to aspiration potential
- Breastfeeding ineffective related to lip or palate integrity alteration
- Altered nutrition less than body requirements related to poor oral intake
- Infant feeding pattern ineffective related to unrepaired congenital defect
- Knowledge deficit related to congenital defect
- Pain related to surgical procedure and postoperative period
- Home maintenance impaired related to required complicated feeding procedures in preoperative period to prevent aspiration, FTT, and other feeding complications
- Parenting at risk for impairment because of bonding issues

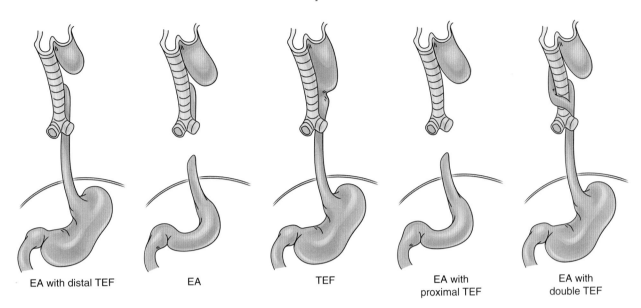

EA with distal TEF   EA   TEF   EA with proximal TEF   EA with double TEF

FIGURE 34.5 Illustration of EA and TEF.

Nursing Considerations for Esophageal Atresia

Feed infants suspected of having an anatomical defect a very small amount of fluids for the first feed to check for the presence of these anatomical defects. If a newborn tolerates a small amount of sterile water, then further feedings or breastfeeding can be initiated.

Tracheoesophageal Fistula

Infants with a confirmed TEF are born with an abnormal opening, called a *fistula*, between the trachea and the esophagus. There are many combinations of defects that can be present, and syndromes should be ruled out. Cardiac defects may accompany the presence of structural anomalies. After feeding, the newborn suffers tracheal irritation as the stomach acid enters the trachea, causing inflammation and discomfort.

Diagnosing Tracheoesophageal Fistula

Perform a rapid and thorough evaluation of a child's airway, paying special attention to the child's swallow and choking. Check for the following:

1. Coughing, choking, and intermittent cyanosis caused by food passing through the fistula into the trachea
2. The presence of abdominal distention from air entering the stomach from the fistula
3. Pain or discomfort from the gastric acids refluxing across the fistula

Interventions for Tracheoesophageal Fistula

Once TEF is suspected, you should assist the pediatric health-care team to prepare the child for surgical interventions. The team will request the following:

1. Maintain an NPO status until diagnostic examinations are completed and a definitive diagnosis is reached.

2. Maintain a patent airway for the infant and have suction available at all times.
3. Prepare for surgery to reconstruct a patent trachea and esophagus without the presence of the abnormal fistula opening.

Nursing Considerations for Tracheoesophageal Fistula

Parents will need to be reassured and educated about the impending surgical procedure to repair the fistula. Explain that the surgery involves removing the TEF and then the reattaching of the ends of the esophagus. In certain situations, more than one surgery may be required. Expect the child to be on gastrostomy tube feedings until they are well healed.

Pyloric Stenosis

When the circular muscle that surrounds the pyloric valve grows, it narrows the valve opening (stenosis) and blocks gastric emptying. Hypertrophy and hyperplasia of this muscle are progressive, and symptoms of gastric distention appear over time. Pyloric stenosis is identified with classic episodes of projectile vomiting, the clinical finding of an olive-shaped mass during palpation (Fig. 34.6), and visible peristaltic waves on the infant's abdomen. The cause of the disorder is unknown. Infant males are affected five times more often than females, and White children are at greatest risk. A surgical procedure called a *pyloromyotomy* is required and entails a small incision on the abdomen to split the hypertrophied tissue.

Diagnosis of Pyloric Stenosis

Parents are typically the first to identify that the infant has a significant deviation in the ability to pass food from the stomach to the intestines, noting the frequency and force

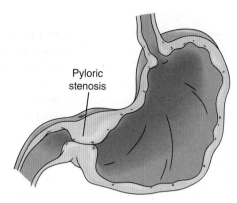

FIGURE 34.6 Pyloric stenosis.

of the infant's vomiting episodes. To narrow down the suspected cause of the vomiting, the following should be noted:

1. Progressively worsening projectile vomiting of nonbilious vomit in a previously healthy and thriving infant
2. Palpable, olive-shaped mass located in the infant's upper right abdominal quadrant
3. Clinical signs of dehydration, including decreased urinary output (UOP), decreased tears, poor turgor, sunken fontanels, and metabolic alkalosis from excessive vomiting

The child may resume feeds after projectile vomiting subsides.

Interventions for Pyloric Stenosis

Once pyloric stenosis is identified via palpation and diagnostics tests, the child will need to be prepared for surgery. A pyloromyotomy is a surgical cut through the outside layer of the pyloric muscle, allowing the inner lumen to bulge out and therefore open a channel for the passage of food to the duodenum. Guidelines for the child include the following:

1. Maintain an NPO status before pyloromyotomy surgery and prepare the family for postoperative care.
2. Before surgery, try to position the child on the right side to help prevent aspiration of vomitus.
3. After surgery, maintain nasogastric tube (NGT) patency, flush the tube as needed, and monitor strict I&O.
4. Correct any electrolyte imbalance.
5. Introduce clear fluids slowly and cautiously as ordered during the early postoperative period (usually within 6 to 8 hours after surgery).

Nursing Considerations for Pyloric Stenosis

Infants may present to the health-care facility with FTT and moderate to severe dehydration. Parents and caregivers may not have recognized the severity of the vomiting. Check the child for distress and report immediately any changes of clinical status.

Hirschsprung Disease

When a newborn does not stool within days of life or when a child presents with poor passage of stool, infrequent explosions of stool, or ribbonlike stool, congenital

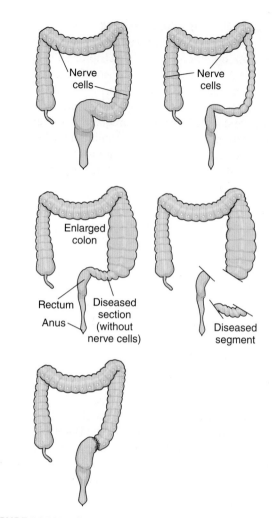

FIGURE 34.7 Hirschsprung disease.

aganglionic megacolon, or Hirschsprung disease, is suspected (Fig. 34.7). Considered a megacolon disorder, this diagnosis is characterized by the absence of neurological tissue, called *ganglia cells,* to migrate to the lower colon, delaying and blocking stool. The ganglia cells are part of what is known as the enteric nervous system (ENS) made up of over 500 million nerve cells. This condition is also called *congenital aganglionosis* and most commonly affects the rectosigmoid region of the child's bowel. The incidence is four times more common in males than in females. Other risk factors for Hirschsprung disease include having a sibling with the disease and having other inherited conditions such as congenital heart disease or Down syndrome (Mayo Clinic, 2021).

Symptoms are associated with the inability of the aganglionic segment of colon tissue to produce peristaltic waves because of the lack of innervation (nerve supply). This causes an accumulation of stool. A serious consequence of untreated Hirschsprung is perforation of the colon and infection called enterocolitis (Zhu et al., 2022). Most cases of this perforation and infection were found at the proximal ganglionic (nerves present) segment (Zhu et al., 2022).

Diagnosing Hirschsprung Disease

This condition is usually diagnosed during early infancy. As many as 80% of children with Hirschsprung disease have symptoms within 6 weeks of life (Boston Children's Hospital, 2023). If children have a short segment of colon affected, symptoms may not be severe enough to present for months to years. If a child has a history of infrequent stools, explosive stools, or stools that are thin and ribbonlike, a further assessment is warranted. The most common findings that lead the pediatric health-care team to suspect Hirschsprung disease include the following:

- Failure of a newborn to pass meconium stool within the first 48 hours of life, followed by subsequent chronic constipation
- Gradual onset of vomiting
- Evidence of FTT in the infant with possible hypoproteinemia and anemia
- Vomiting, constipation, episodic and explosive stooling, diarrhea, and abdominal distention and distress
- Reluctance to ingest feedings and loss of appetite
- Fatigue

Interventions for Hirschsprung Disease

Care for the child with Hirschsprung's disease requires surgical intervention to remove the segment of bowel that does not have nerves and is causing the lack of peristalsis. The child will have diagnostics to confirm the disorder, including a tissue biopsy to identify the lack of nerves in the distal colon. Interventions for a child in the perioperative experience include the following:

- In the preoperative period, monitor the child's stooling pattern and the characteristics of the stool passed.
- Prepare the family for the surgical procedure, including the possibility of a temporary placement of a colostomy (for non–pull-through surgical procedures).
- If an anal pull-through is performed, monitor for bleeding, edema, unusual drainage, fever, or any unexpected alteration in skin integrity.
- Postoperatively, provide meticulous skin care, antibiotics, pain control, and teaching/support for the family as they learn stoma care.
- After the return of bowel sounds and the passage of confirmed flatus, introduce feedings slowly and monitor for tolerance.

Nursing Considerations for Hirschsprung Disease

During the preoperative period, as the child prepares for the surgical removal of the portion of the lower bowel that is aganglionic, you should monitor for symptoms of electrolyte imbalances and dehydration. During the extended postoperative period, the family will need education and support to care for the temporary colostomy at home. Well-fitted colostomy appliances are required to reduce the chance of distressing leaks. Parents need to learn how to evaluate their child with a colostomy for complications of skin breakdown, obstruction, and emotional distress.

Intussusception

Intussusception is an acute GI condition that is characterized by invagination, or telescoping, of one bowel segment into the other (Fig. 34.8). The most common site of the telescoping of the bowel is the ileocecal valve. Most commonly lacking an identified cause, intussusception has been associated with hyperactive peristalsis, intestinal polyps, or an abnormal bowel lining. Unfortunately, this condition can recur and may lead to peritonitis. The child, typically between 6 and 24 months of age, presents in acute abdominal pain, guarding the abdomen and drawing the knees up toward the chest. Intussusception can become a life-threatening condition if the bowel becomes ischemic and necrotic from the edema and inflammation associated with the invagination. If the ischemic bowel segment becomes gangrenous, the child will need immediate surgery with a temporary colostomy.

Diagnosing Intussusception

The nurse assists the health-care team in checking for the presence of this condition. The common evaluations associated with intussusception include the following:

- Acute abdominal pain in a previously well child without previous GI symptoms
- Passage of red, blood-tinged stool referred to as *red currant jelly stool*
- Abdominal distention and tenderness
- Possible passage of bile-stained vomitus

Interventions for Intussusception

The pediatric health-care team will need to provide rapid interventions for a child who presents with an intussusception. Immediate reduction of the invagination is required

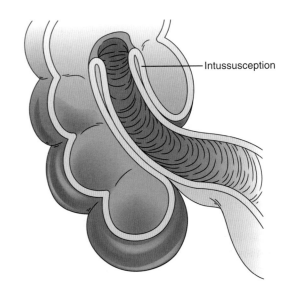

FIGURE 34.8 Intussusception.

· **WORD** · **BUILDING** ·
intussusception: intus–within + suscep–receive + tion–action

to prevent severe tissue inflammation, injury, hypoxia, and death to the tissues.

1. A barium enema or water-soluble contrast enema will be performed to reduce the invaginated or telescoped bowel. In addition, air pressure may be used to confirm and then reduce the telescoped bowel.
2. Prepare the child and family for surgery if the enema is not successful.

Nursing Considerations for Intussusception

The family will need to be taught that the condition can re-cur and that immediate care must be sought to prevent complications. The family should state which symptoms should be monitored for so that they are confident about when to report the condition and come directly to the emergency department (ED).

Imperforate Anus

An imperforate anus is a congenital condition in which the child is born without an anal opening. Therefore, the child does not pass meconium or any stool substance. You should identify this condition during the newborn's first evaluation and immediately report the condition for consideration of surgery. The infant should be kept NPO until a complete evaluation is performed. New procedures allow for the re-construction of the anal opening with active nerves by means of transplantation of nerve tissue.

Appendicitis

Appendicitis is the inflammation and often infection of the small lymphoid tissue called the *vermiform appendix*. The appendix is a tube-shaped blind sac located at the end of the intestinal cecum. If the lumen of the appendix becomes obstructed, usually by hard fecal material, parasites, or in-fectious bacteria, then the appendix becomes inflamed with the accumulation of mucus and subsequent distention. As the pressure increases, there is a higher risk of rupture. If the tis-sue becomes edematous or ischemic, which leads to perfora-tion, the child is then at risk for sepsis and peritonitis.

The average range is 5 to 20 years, but the most com-mon age of onset of appendicitis is 10 years old (Nemours KidsHealth, 2023). It is considered the most common cause of emergency abdominal surgery. It is imperative that a child be assessed rapidly by health-care providers if appendicitis is suspected. Although rare, death can occur because of sepsis from peritonitis.

Diagnosing Appendicitis

Appendicitis can mimic other abdominal conditions and therefore careful evaluations to confirm this condition must be made. If appendicitis is suspected, no deep palpations should be conducted to prevent serious complications and increased pain. The pediatric health-care team will conduct diagnostic examinations and monitor laboratory values to check for infection. The following should also be assessed:

- Progressive lower-right abdominal pain with associated nausea, vomiting, chills, and fever
- Elevated WBC count on laboratory evaluation
- Positive ultrasound findings of an enlarged or distended appendix
- A sudden stop of persistent and progressive abdominal pain, which should be reported immediately because it may mean that perforation or rupture has occurred

Interventions for Appendicitis

Once confirmed, a diagnosis of appendicitis will need to be treated. Immediate surgery is warranted for children whose appendix has ruptured. Newer interventions include treat-ing a milder, nonruptured appendicitis with nonsurgical means, including IV antibiotics and IV fluids. The follow-ing list should be considered when preparing a family for interventions:

- Prepare the child and family for a surgical appendectomy.
- Maintain NPO during evaluations and the preoperative period.
- Place the child in the semi-Fowler position; this is often the position of comfort.
- Postoperatively, monitor the child for pain, bleeding, or wound infection.
- During the postoperative period of recovery for a child with a ruptured appendix, anticipate slower healing, more pain, and the need for an NGT and possible surgical drainage device.

Nursing Considerations for Appendicitis

Anticipate a difference in the postoperative period between children who experience appendicitis with rupture and those who experience it without rupture. When a child is postoperative without rupture, the child should follow an uncomplicated postoperative period with early ambulation and restoration of oral fluids with a rapidly progressive diet. Recovery is more complicated for children following a rup-tured appendix. Children may require days of antibiotics, experience much more pain, and resume ambulation later. Maintain close observation during the postoperative period for possible complications from the rupture, including ob-structions, sepsis, and hazards of longer periods of postop-erative bedrest.

The assessment of peritonitis associated with appendici-tis rupture includes a high fever; a greatly increased WBC count; severe abdominal pain; the absence of bowel sounds; a rigid, boardlike abdomen; and the possible development of shock and death.

Inflammatory Bowel Syndromes: Ulcerative Colitis and Crohn Disease

The most common pediatric inflammatory bowel diseases are ulcerative colitis and **Crohn disease**. The cause of either diagnosis is unknown but may be linked to dietary intake, infectious processes, or genetic causes. The human leukocyte antigen B27 (HLA-B27) and inflammatory bowel disease may be linked. Early in the child's disease experience, the two diseases look very similar and share similar clinical presentations and symptoms. The differentiation of the diseases requires careful consideration as both are characterized by remissions and exacerbations.

Ulcerative colitis is slightly more prevalent than Crohn disease with a peak incidence age range of 15 to 20 years old. One-third of children with ulcerative colitis have a family history of the disorder (Crohn's & Colitis Foundation, 2022).

Ulcerative Colitis

Ulcerative colitis primarily affects the colon and rectum in the large intestine with continuous lesions involving the superficial mucosa (Crohn's & Colitis Foundation, 2022). The bowel will demonstrate what is termed a "lead pipe" visual appearance as the bowel's muscle tissue hypertrophies with deposited fat and fibrous tissues.

DIAGNOSING ULCERATIVE COLITIS. A child with ulcerative colitis may have very mild or very severe symptoms. The following list of assessments is used for all children, regardless of the severity of their disease:

- Copious, frequent bloody stools, ranging from 3 to 20 per day
- After defecation, relief of abdominal pain
- Significant weight loss that usually occurs over just a few months' time
- Anemia, electrolyte imbalances, and an increased ESR
- Fever, tachycardia, pallor, and fatigue
- The presence of "extraintestinal symptoms," including joint tenderness, arthritis, and skin rashes

Diagnostics include a Hematest of stools, colonoscopy, barium enema, and biopsies.

INTERVENTIONS FOR ULCERATIVE COLITIS. Interventions for inflammatory bowel conditions will vary depending on the severity of the disease and include the following:

- Pharmacological interventions are initiated to reduce the inflammation and to support the child's nutrition; they include antidiarrheals, anti-inflammatories, and analgesics.
- Modifications in the child's diet will be needed to help control the diarrhea.
- In severe exacerbations, the child will require IV parenteral nutrition, IV steroidal anti-inflammatories, and the correction of acidosis and anemia.
- In 23% to 45% of ulcerative colitis cases, the child will require surgery to remove the diseased bowel segment (Crohn's & Colitis Foundation, 2022).

Crohn Disease

As with ulcerative colitis, Crohn disease also causes ulcerations along the mucosal lining of the bowel but may affect any part of the alimentary tract from the child's mouth to the anus. Unlike ulcerative colitis, the lesions in Crohn disease are called "skip" lesions because they are discontinuous with healthy bowel segments between lesions (Crohn's & Colitis Foundation, 2022). Crohn disease is known to cause fistulas, fissures, and thickened intestinal walls with 50% of cases resulting in granulomas.

DIAGNOSING CROHN DISEASE. A child with Crohn disease may have very mild or very severe symptoms. The child may have remissions and exacerbations of the inflammation in the bowel. The following list of assessments is used for all children, regardless of the severity of their disease:

- Diarrhea with frank or occult blood
- Moderate to severe cramping abdominal pain
- Weight loss with eventual growth retardation from nutritional deficiencies and electrolyte imbalances
- Abscess formation and perianal fissures and fistulas
- Extraintestinal manifestations of finger clubbing, arthritis, and amenorrhea and delayed sexual development

INTERVENTIONS FOR CROHN DISEASE. Interventions for Crohn disease include the following:

- Pharmacological interventions are similar to those for ulcerative colitis. Pharmacological interventions are initiated to reduce the inflammation and to support the child's nutrition; they include antidiarrheals, anti-inflammatories, and analgesics. A step-up approach is preferred. Medications for Crohn disease include:
  - *Mild:* 5-aminosalicylic acid (5-ASA), antibiotic therapy
  - *Moderate:* Corticosteroids (prednisone), infliximab (Remicade)
  - *Severe:* Immunomodulatory medications (5-ASA), antitumor necrosis factor (anti-TNF), 6-mercaptopurine, and/or methotrexate (chemotherapeutic medications)
- Nutritional deficiencies should be corrected. Iron supplements are given if anemic from an inflamed intestinal wall, which prevents iron absorption.
(Crohn's & Colitis Foundation, 2022)

Medication Facts

Infliximab

Indicated for active moderate-to-severe Crohn disease, infliximab (Remicade) neutralizes and prevents the activity of tumor necrosis factor-α, resulting in antiproliferative and anti-inflammatory activities. Nursing considerations during infusion include paying special attention to the child's reactions, such as fever, chills, pruritus, and urticaria, especially with the first and second infusions. Children can develop severe infections during the course of treatment, necessitating cessation of further treatment. Monitor for signs and symptoms of severe infections, including fever, sweats, cough, dyspnea, malaise, and weight loss.

Nursing Considerations for Inflammatory Bowel Diseases

Monitor the daily weight and fluid status of a child with an inflammatory bowel disease to identify disease progression and therapy responses. Promote the positive oral intake of fluids and foods that can be tolerated. For abdominal pain, provide distraction, diversion, heating pads, frequent position changes, and, when needed, narcotic pain relief. Maintain skin integrity when a child is having an acute exacerbation of diarrheal episodes. When diarrhea is under control, slowly introduce low-residue, high-protein, high-calorie, and bland foods.

Be aware of the potential complications associated with inflammatory bowel diseases. Perforation, sepsis, hemorrhage, and obstructions should all be carefully monitored. With ulcerative colitis, it is imperative that families continue to bring their child in for follow-up visits because there is a 20% risk of colon cancer after the first 10 years. Surgical treatments are required if a child is not responsive to pharmacological interventions. Either an ileostomy or a colostomy may be performed. With education, guidance, and support, the child with an inflammatory bowel disease who has had surgery to remove the diseased portion of bowel can expect to live an active and engaged life (Crohn's & Colitis Foundation, 2022).

Celiac Disease

Celiac disease is the inability to fully digest the glutenin or gliadin protein components of certain grains. Lacking the necessary enzyme in their intestinal mucosal cells, the child experiences atrophy of the villi located in the proximal small intestine, leading to a decrease in intestinal absorption. The accumulation of the undigested amino acid glutamine is toxic to the child's intestinal lining, and chronic diarrhea results. The child may experience weight loss, foul-smelling stools, and increased flatulence. This is also called **gluten intolerance**, or *gluten-sensitive enteropathy*. The child with celiac disease is unable to tolerate food products that contain rye, wheat, oat, and barley glutens. Most infants will be symptomatic approximately 2 to 4 months after the introduction of foods that contain gluten. Some children do not present with symptoms until after 5 years old. Although the cause is unknown, celiac disease is suspected to have an environmental influence. The child will require lifelong dietary modification to prevent even the smallest exposure to glutens. Iron, folic acids, and fat-soluble vitamins are all malabsorbed because of the inflammatory effect celiac disease has on the proximal small intestine.

Diagnosing Celiac Disease

The assessment of celiac disease includes the following:

- Flare-ups and celiac crises associated with a precipitating event, such as gluten ingestion, infections, prolonged fasting, or exposure to anticholinergic medications, which will present as acute abdominal pain, severe diarrhea, electrolyte imbalances, and possible metabolic acidosis

- The passage of steatorrhea or greasy, bulky, and very malodorous stools that appear frothy and full of fat
- Organic FTT, including weight loss or lack of gain, muscle wasting, and anemia
- Anorexia and abdominal pain, which are common

Anticipate laboratory studies of antigliadin antibodies (IgG and IgA) and a 72-hour quantitative fecal fat study. Also anticipate sending the child for a biopsy of the jejunum to check for a flat mucosal surface with hyperplasia.

Interventions for Celiac Disease

Interventions for celiac disease include the following:

- Instruct the parents of the patient to provide the child with a gluten-free diet.
- Correct any electrolyte disturbances.
- Restore fluids if the child presents with dehydration from diarrhea, tachycardia, poor skin turgor, and elevated urine specific gravity.

Nursing Considerations for Celiac Disease

Reinforce the importance of following a gluten-free diet, including a restriction of breads, pasta, and snacks that contain rye, wheat, oats, or barley. Many commercially prepared frozen food items and desirable childhood snacks contain gluten, and families must become astute at reading and analyzing food labels. Unrestricted food items include eggs, fish, poultry, pork, beef, dairy, fruits, vegetables, rice, and cornmeal. With the increasing incidence of celiac disease in the general population, many wheat-alternative breads and cereals are now available. The growing awareness of the disease is also prompting grocery stores and restaurants to provide gluten-free food and menu choices.

Support is available for families from the American Celiac Society, the Gluten Intolerance Group, and the Celiac Disease Foundation. Written instructions should be provided for families and follow-up is imperative to determine a child's risk for episodes of celiac crises. Research has shown that measuring celiac disease–related antibodies is one way to closely predict a child's clinical outcomes and monitor long-term compliance with a gluten-free diet. As a child's antibody levels decrease, health-care professionals can be more confident that the child's diet is free of glutens (Petroff et al., 2018). Antibodies currently being tested include antitissue transglutaminase (tTG) antibodies, deamidated gliadin peptide (DGP) antibodies, and endomysial antibodies (EMA; National Institute of Diabetes and Digestive and Kidney Diseases, 2019).

Necrotizing Enterocolitis

Necrotizing enterocolitis (NEC) is an inflammatory disease of the intestinal tract that occurs primarily in premature infants or sick full-term infants. This condition is marked by varying degrees of dead or necrotic tissue in either the

· WORD · BUILDING ·

enterocolitis: entero–intestines + col–colon + itis–inflammation

Nursing Care Plan for the Child With Celiac Disease

Annika, an 8-year-old, has a history of intermittent severe abdominal cramping pain and "stinky farts." At today's office visit, the pediatrician is reviewing Annika's diagnostic laboratory work with the family. Annika tested positive for high levels of antigliadin antibodies, and her level of fecal fat was high as well. Based on her history of symptoms and these laboratory results, the pediatrician diagnoses Annika with celiac disease.

Nursing Diagnosis: Acute pain related to inflamed GI mucosa as evidenced by bloating and cramping
Expected Outcome: The patient will demonstrate a 0 or a 1 on a subjective or objective pediatric pain scale.

Intervention:	Rationale:
The child will be placed on clear liquids for 24 hours to allow the digestive system to rest and to pass gluten-containing foods from the system.	*The inflamed GI mucosa needs to rest. Clear liquids are easy to digest and will not irritate the already irritated tissues.*

Nursing Diagnosis: Knowledge deficit related to necessary dietary changes
Expected Outcome: The family will describe at least five meals that offer gluten-free items that are appropriate for the child's developmental stage.

Intervention:	Rationale:
Teach the child and family to avoid food products containing wheat, rye, oats, or barley. Engage them in reading labels of foods they enjoy to look for these ingredients. Identify gluten-free alternatives to the patient's favorite foods.	*Celiac disease has no cure. The only way to control the patient's symptoms is for her to avoid all sources of gluten. Following a strictly gluten-free meal plan will allow her to avoid abdominal pain and bloating and will promote healthy growth and development.*

transmural or mucosal segments of the intestines. This life-threatening condition requires nursing and medical care in an intensive care environment. Several factors are involved in the development of NEC, including bacterial or viral infections, intestinal ischemia, and immaturity of the gut, which all lead to a damaged bowel with ischemia that develops into necrosis.

Diagnosing Necrotizing Enterocolitis

The assessment of NEC includes the following:

- A history of prematurity, maternal preeclampsia or hemorrhage, umbilical catheters, cocaine exposure, sepsis, or asphyxia
- Free peritoneal gas and bowel inflammation that demonstrates dilated loops and thickening of the bowel

The onset of NEC typically occurs in three stages:

1. *Stage 1:* Marked by fluctuating temperatures, hypoglycemia, abdominal distention, heme-positive stools, poor perfusion, lethargy, and recurrent apnea/bradycardia
2. *Stage 2:* Marked by the items in stage 1 plus severe distention, grossly bloody stools, extreme abdominal tenderness, and absent bowel sounds
3. *Stage 3:* Marked by the evidence of the beginning of septic shock, including the deterioration of vital signs,

metabolic acidosis, severe edema of the abdominal wall, and disseminated intravascular coagulation (DIC)

Interventions for Necrotizing Enterocolitis

Interventions for NEC include the following:

- The child will require IV antibiotics, vascular support, and IV feedings in an intensive care environment.
- An ostomy may be required to remove the necrotic tissue and allow the bowel to rest and heal.

Nursing Considerations for Necrotizing Enterocolitis

NEC is a life-threatening disease with a long healing time. Associated with mortality, this condition requires an astute, high level of intensive care. Parents will need emotional support while their newborn or young infant is critically ill and will need to be taught how to care for the infant's ostomy.

Enteral Feeding

In pediatrics, there are many reasons a child may need to receive enteral feedings. These include congenital intestinal function disorders; oral malformations; conditions that cause dysphagia; FTT, which requires additional calories; and neurological disorders that disrupt adequate calorie consumption. Caloric need will be determined by a nutritionist

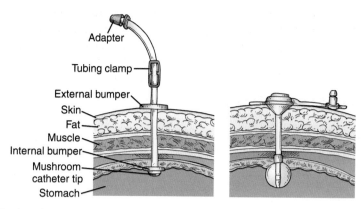

FIGURE 34.9 Types of enteral feeding devices.

working with the health-care team to ensure weight maintenance or weight gain. Daily weights, hydration, adequate stooling, and tolerance of the feedings will determine if the procedure is successful.

There are several means of administering enteral feedings to children. The placement of an NGT, or nasojejunal tube placed below the pyloric valve into the small intestine, is the primary means to administer nutrition for short-term requirements. If a child needs enteral feedings for an extended time, a gastrostomy tube (called a PEG tube) may be placed surgically, extending from the external abdominal wall to the stomach. When the gastrostomy tube is at the skin level, it is often referred to as a "button" (Fig. 34.9).

Children with incompetent cardiac sphincters, neurological impairment, inadequate cough, or poor motor control may be at risk for aspiration of the tube-feeding solution and should be monitored closely for signs of aspiration pneumonia. The prevention of aspiration pneumonia can be accomplished by positioning a child in an upright position and checking for the amount of residual formula still present within the child's stomach before starting the feeds. Follow orders meticulously to check for remaining, or residual, stomach contents and hold feeds if the amount exceeds recommendations. Typically, the health-care provider will order how frequently to check residual and how much residual will be allowed before the administration of an NGT feeding. For instance, if an older infant has more than 30 mL of residual feed in the stomach before starting the next bolus feed, the feeding may be held for an hour or more to allow the stomach to empty. To prevent electrolyte imbalances, always return the aspirated stomach content during residual checking.

Safety *Stat!*

The determination of residual feed in a newborn, an infant, or a young child's stomach helps to prevent overfeeding, which may result in vomiting and the potential aspiration of vomitus.

Patient Teaching Guidelines

Family Education for the Administration of Enteral Feeds Via a Nasogastric Tube

Teach parents or caregivers how to care for their child with a feeding tube from the beginning of therapy. The involvement of family in the care of the child's tube and feeding will empower the family to care for their child. Instruct the family in all aspects of the process, including how to appropriately mix the feeding solution, safely administer the solution, and monitor for untoward effects such as bloating, diarrhea, constipation, or vomiting.

1. Interpret the order for the feeding procedure.
2. Wash hands to prevent contamination of the feeds.
3. Mix feeding powder correctly with clean water for a correct amount of feed (may be continuous or bolus feeds).
4. Attach the feeding bag to the connecting tubing (some products come commercially attached).
5. Position the child in a safe, upright position, if able.
6. Check the placement of the feeding tube.
7. Check for the presence of residual feeding solution in the stomach by slowly aspirating stomach contents.
8. Flush tubing with 3 to 10 mL of clean water to ensure that the entire tube is patent.
9. Double-check the setup from the bag to the tubing to the child's nares to ensure that there are no kinks or knots.
10. Slowly start feeds to ensure tolerance.
11. Monitor the child for potential or actual aspiration pneumonia (observe for coughing, vomiting, signs of distress, or a change in condition).
12. When feeding is complete, remove the tubing from the NGT in the child.
13. Clean the bag and the tube with tap water and save them for the next feeding.
14. Change the bag and the tubing at ordered intervals to prevent contamination or problems with feeding solution buildup and clogging.

Your responsibility with enteral feedings encompasses the accuracy of the procedure, clinical improvement, and safety. The following information provides nursing care checklists for pre-, intra-, and postenteral feedings.

- Prefeeding
  1. Ensure a complete order, including the feeding solution type, the amount to be administered, the time period for administration (either bolus or continuous), the frequency and length of time of the feeds required, the quantity of residual allowed before feedings are held, and whether or not the child's medications may be administered via the feeding tube.
  2. Obtain feeding solution and ensure that the formula has not expired. Mix formula with ordered fluids if in a powder form. Double-check the accuracy of the mixture because too-dilute feeding solutions may cause weight loss over time if the child does not receive the ordered calories, and solutions that are too concentrated may lead to diarrhea or stomach distress.
  3. Set up equipment and ensure that the tubing and bag are clean. The tubing and bag should be changed every 24 hours.
     a. NGTs stiffen when left in place for a long period. Make sure that there is no presence of irritation of the skin around the nares caused by this process.
     b. If inserting the tube for the feed, make sure that the wire stylet used for inserting the tube has been removed.
- Intrafeeding
  1. Confirm placement by attaching a small syringe to the end of the NGT and aspirating for stomach contents.
  2. Ensure patency by flushing the tube with 3 to 5 mL of clean water. Do not force the flush if resistance is encountered because this could damage the tubing or cause perforation.
  3. Begin feeds and monitor for tolerance and aspiration. The infusion may be delivered by gravity or by pump.
  4. Continue feeds as ordered, either bolus or continuous.
  5. If the child is an infant, provide nonnutritive sucking during the infusion. This has been noted to decrease restlessness, improve weight gain, increase states of alertness during feeds, and assist parents with learning infant feeding cues such as oral readiness (Harding et al., 2014; Selekman & Jakubik, 2007).
- Postfeeding
  1. When the infusion is complete, disconnect the tubing and flush the NGT/GT well with 3 to 10 mL of water, depending on the age of the child. Use smaller amounts for infants.
  2. Determine the child's tolerance and monitor for distention, abdominal discomfort, and diarrhea.

Safety *Stat!*

Do not leave NGT/GT feeds hanging for an extended period. Feeds left at room temperature for more than 4 hours are at risk for the development of bacterial contamination. Follow institutional policy and procedure closely. Refrigerate dated formulas or open cans used for feeding.

Key Points

- The development of the neonate's GI system goes through a series of steps, including progressing from a sterile gut environment to having an intestinal lining that is colonized with active bacteria. This process is essential for healthy digestion.
- A nurse can expect to encounter a wide variety of GI disorders across childhood. Most take astute evaluations and rapid interventions because the child may be at risk for severe fluid loss and subsequent dehydration, electrolyte imbalances, acid-base imbalances, and nutritional disorders.
- Acute GI infections require contact precautions to prevent the rapid spread of the disease to others. If *C. difficile* is suspected or confirmed, the pediatric health-care staff must initiate expanded contact precautions that include hand washing with soap and water. Alcohol-based hand gel is not sufficient in inactivating *C. difficile*.
- Chronic bowel diseases require a team approach with engaged follow-up care and continued teaching. Because of the relationship between nutrition, fluid balance, and chronic bowel diseases, families need education for their child's care and support for ongoing follow-up care. Many chronic bowel diseases are marked with exacerbations and remissions, so families need to recognize when health-care interventions are required.
- Celiac disease is caused by gluten intolerance. With the increasing incidence of this chronic condition, pediatric team members need updated information to provide education about the dietary restrictions of foods that contain wheat, oats, rye, and barley.
- Offering emotional support for children with colostomies or ileostomies can positively influence the experience of a chronic GI disorder, especially for school-aged children and adolescents who have body-image concerns.

Review Questions

1. A 7-year-old girl was admitted to the hospital for increasing lower-right quadrant abdominal pain with an admitting diagnosis of suspected appendicitis. Although her admission pain score was rated as a 9 to 10 on a numerical scale, she suddenly says her pain has subsided. What should be your next action?
   1. Report to the charge nurse that the child's pain is suddenly gone.
   2. Anticipate immediate surgery.
   3. Allow her to rest comfortably.
   4. Provide her choice of oral fluids.

2. Clinical findings associated with moderate dehydration demonstrate the severity of a child's condition. Which findings denote moderate dehydration? (**Select all that apply.**)
   1. Rapid pulse
   2. Dry mucous membranes
   3. Moderate thirst
   4. Normal fontanel
   5. 10% body weight loss
   6. Greater than 3-sec capillary refill

3. While helping a family make menu choices for their child with a new diagnosis of celiac disease, which food choices would you support them ordering?
   1. Corn tortillas with melted cheese and a fruit salad
   2. Turkey sandwich on rye bread with a side of sliced apples
   3. Chili with Texas ten-grain toast and watermelon slices
   4. Spaghetti with meat sauce and grapes

4. An infant returns from surgery to correct Hirschsprung disease. Which intervention should you avoid?
   1. Introducing fluids when bowel sounds are definitively identified
   2. Positioning the infant supine
   3. Taking the temperature rectally
   4. Providing a quiet environment to heal

5. A child is admitted to the hospital with intussusception. What form and color of stool did the parents report their child having?
   1. Ribbonlike brown stool in normal quantity
   2. Watery, light brown stool in large quantity
   3. Thick, greenish stool
   4. Scant stool appearing similar to red jelly

6. To help prevent diarrhea for a child taking oral antibiotics, what should you expect to also give?
   1. Pedialyte oral boluses
   2. A high-fiber diet
   3. Macrobiotic granules
   4. An NPO status and bowel rest

7. Which symptoms are indicative of pyloric stenosis? (**Select all that apply.**)
   1. Severe abdominal pain
   2. Projectile vomiting
   3. Bilious vomiting
   4. FTT
   5. Lower intestinal cramping

8. A young child presents to the ED with moderate dehydration associated with 5 days of vomiting. Clinical signs and symptoms of which condition would you expect to see?
   1. Metabolic acidosis
   2. Metabolic alkalosis
   3. Respiratory acidosis
   4. Respiratory alkalosis

9. A nurse is caring for a school-aged child with FTT associated with cystic fibrosis who requires nasogastric feedings. How might you safely check for the correct placement of the NGT before initiating the child's first nutritional feeding? (**Select all that apply.**)
   1. Demonstration of a high pH level in the NGT aspirate
   2. Aspiration of stomach contents
   3. Sound of air passing in the stomach via 5 cc of air through the tube
   4. Symptoms of coughing with flushing
   5. Placement of the end of a tube in a cup of water showing bubbling
   6. Radiography

10. Which of the following signs would be expected in a young diapered toddler with an intestinal parasite?
    1. Nausea and vomiting
    2. Frequent diarrhea
    3. Persistent anal itching
    4. Perineal rash with satellite lesions

ANSWERS 1. 2; 2. 1, 2, 3; 3. 1; 4. 3; 5. 4; 6. 3; 7. 2, 4; 8. 2; 9. 2, 3, 5, 6; 10. 3

CRITICAL THINKING QUESTIONS

1. When a child presents to the ED in severe dehydration from intractable vomiting, what is the most accurate method of determining the child's severity of dehydration if the health-care team does not have a baseline weight?

2. Describe the very best protective practices and isolation techniques that a nurse can use if they are taking care of a toddler with *C. difficile* diarrhea.

3. If a child with severe lower-right quadrant pain and a mildly distended abdomen presents to the ED to rule out appendicitis and suddenly has a cessation of pain, what could this mean and what should the nursing team do as a priority form of care?

Resources

For additional resources and information, including Postconference Questions and Activities, Answers, and References, visit www.FADavis.com.

 Student Study Guide

CHAPTER 35
Child With a Genitourinary Condition

KEY TERMS

acidosis (ASS-ih-DOH-siss)

alkalosis (AL-kuh-LOH-siss)

ascites (ass-EYE-teez)

diurnal incontinence (dye-ERN-uhl in-KON-tih-nents)

epispadias (EP-ih-SPAY-dee-us)

fluid maintenance calculation (FLOO-id MAYN-tuh-nents KAL-kyoo-LAY-shun)

glomerulonephritis (gloh-MAIR-yoo-loh-nef-RYE-tiss)

hemolytic uremic syndrome (HUS) (HEE-muh-LIT-ik yoo-REE-mik SIN-drohm)

hyponatremia (HYE-poh-nay-TREE-mee-uh)

hypospadias (HYE-poh-SPAY-dee-us)

intersex conditions (IN-ter-seks kon-DIH-shunz)

mesoderm (MEZ-oh-derm)

nephrotic syndrome/nephrosis (nef-ROT-ik SIN-drohm/nef-ROH-siss)

nocturnal incontinence (nok-TER-nuhl in-KON-tih-nents)

CHAPTER CONCEPTS

Elimination
Fluid and Electrolytes

LEARNING OUTCOMES

1. Define the key terms.
2. Describe how a child's renal system affects fluid and electrolyte status as well as acid-base balance.
3. Describe the clinical presentation of dehydration across childhood and plan of nursing care for a child in a dehydrated state.
4. Analyze the common causes of a urinary tract infection (UTI) and discuss the risk factors associated with each age group.
5. Differentiate between glomerulonephritis and nephrotic syndrome in relation to assessments, medical treatments, and nursing care for each.
6. Describe various forms of congenital anomalies of the genitourinary (GU) tract.
7. Present a nursing care plan for a child with enuresis.
8. Describe various means to collect urine specimens for children of various ages.
9. Calculate fluid maintenance requirements for children of various weights in kilograms to safely maintain fluid status and prevent fluid overload.

CRITICAL THINKING

John, a 4-year-old, is admitted to the pediatric unit with a diagnosis of minimal change nephrotic syndrome. He is started on high-dose corticosteroids and remains hospitalized in guarded condition, where you are a member of his care team. John's weight on admission was 19.27 kg (42.5 pounds), and his height was 104 cm (41 in.). Physical examination revealed edema of his eyelids and face. Massive edema was also present in his extremities and scrotum. He appeared to have ascites. John's skin was pale and warm to touch and shiny in appearance. His vital signs were within normal limits.

Urine analysis reveals 4+ proteinuria and a specific gravity (SG) of 1.030. His urine is dark and frothy in appearance. John's urinary output for 24 hours is 500 mL. His serum albumin level is 1.5 g/100 mL, his hematocrit is within normal range for his age at 13.8 g/dL, and his serum sodium is 132 mEq/L. The child's blood

Continued

CRITICAL THINKING—cont'd

urea nitrogen (BUN) and creatinine are 11.6 mg/dL and 0.86 mg/dL, respectively.

Questions

1. What are three main clinical concerns you will want to check for related to the child's primary medical diagnosis of minimal change nephrotic syndrome?
2. You are giving the child medications and a meal tray. What is the rationale for providing prednisone (Rayos) and a low salt diet?
3. You are discussing the medication with the child's mother. What are the side effects of long-term corticosteroid therapy in children that you would explain to the mother?

CONCEPTUAL CORNERSTONE

Elimination

The urinary system is responsible for the removal of waste products from the blood and the formation of urine. Disturbances in the system can lead to an increased level of BUN and creatinine in the blood and, ultimately, without treatment, renal failure. Through the elimination process, the urinary system influences the regulation of the body's fluid and electrolyte balance. The kidneys respond to dehydration and hypotension with decreased urine output (UOP).

A child with an infection of the urinary system, such as a bladder infection or kidney infection (**pyelonephritis**), often experiences pain and discomfort. Providing both pharmaceutical and nonpharmaceutical pain-reducing interventions is a primary nursing function. Report any concern with the process of urinary elimination, such as changes in quantity, color, clarity, and any symptoms experienced by the child. Meticulous care of children with complex urinary elimination conditions such as glomerulonephritis and nephritic syndrome requires teamwork and astute assessments.

The urinary system consists of the two kidneys, two ureters, one urinary bladder, and one urethra. The genitals are the reproductive organs: the prostate gland, testicles, and epididymis in men; and the uterus, fallopian tubes, ovaries, vagina, external genitalia, and perineum in women. (See Chapter 4 for more information about the reproductive system.) Because of their proximity to each other and their common embryological origin, the urinary and reproductive systems are often considered together and referred to as the genitourinary (GU) system.

Essential for life, the GU system provides a means to process and eliminate waste products from the blood, regulate body fluids, regulate acid-base balance, and reproduce. During childhood, the GU system matures. In infancy, the child is poorly able to regulate fluid balance, concentrate wastes into urine, and eliminate waste by-products of metabolism. As the child grows, this system becomes more efficient. In the presence of urinary disease or disorder, the child may experience fluid retention, hypertension, and the build-up of waste products in the blood, called *uremia*.

Disorders of the GU system are common during childhood. Approximately 1.2 million children develop a urinary tract infection (UTI) each year in the United States. According to Devarajan (2020), approximately 3.9 per 1,000 hospitalized children will experience an acute kidney injury such as **hemolytic uremic syndrome (HUS)** or **glomerulonephritis**. Annually, renal dialysis will be required for 4,500 children, and 2,000 infants will die because of diseases of the urinary system. Although many GU disorders are present at birth, acquired disorders are common enough to warrant an understanding of signs and symptoms of infections, strictures, renal failure, and reproductive complications. The GU system is complex, and many children with chronic disorders will have several specialists caring for them during the management of their disease. These can include pediatric urologists, pediatric nephrologists, pediatric surgeons, geneticists, transplant surgeons, pediatric nutritionists, social workers, and neurodevelopmental specialists.

Some disorders found during childhood are associated with kidney damage; others are associated with obstructions or blockages that prevent the elimination of urine from the bladder; and others are associated specifically with the male GU tract. Box 35.1 outlines examples of disorders associated with kidney damage.

Safety *Stat!*

A male child or teen who presents in acute pain in the testicle area may be experiencing testicular torsion. This is an acute condition of the spermatic cord becoming twisted, which requires a surgical procedure to prevent damage to the tissues. Symptoms include sudden and severe pain, swelling, nausea, vomiting, and a lump in the scrotal sac.

· WORD · BUILDING ·

pyelonephritis: pyelo–pelvis + nephr–kidney + itis–inflammation

· WORD · BUILDING ·

hemolytic: hemo–blood + lyt–lysis, destruction + ic–pertaining to

uremic: ur–urine + em–blood + ic–pertaining to

glomerulonephritis: glomerulo–glomerulus + nephr–kidney + itis–inflammation

Box 35.1

Disorders Associated With Kidney Damage

- *Glomerulonephritis:* A form of kidney inflammation (nephritis) in which lesions are found in the glomeruli; noted for occurring after a *Streptococcus* infection
- *HUS:* A life-threatening, acute condition of microangiopathic hemolytic anemia, thrombocytopenia, and acute nephropathy; often caused by eating contaminated raw or rare hamburger or other meats or contaminated produce
- *Chronic and recurring UTIs:* UTIs that recur after treatment was completed; may be the same or a different microbe causing the infection
- *Hydronephrosis:* An obstruction of urinary outflow by any means, including kidney stones or bladder outlet obstruction
- *Polycystic kidney disease:* Any of several hereditary conditions where numerous fluid-filled cysts are found throughout the kidney and possibly other organs

Disorders associated with blockage of the elimination of urine from the bladder:

- *Neurogenic bladder:* Nerve damage resulting in abnormal retention or leaking of urine from the bladder
- *VUR:* Refluxing of urine up into the ureters before or after urination
- *Ureterocele:* Condition of a cystlike dilation of tissue near a ureteral opening into the urinary bladder caused by a congenital stenosis of the ureteral orifice
- *Megaureter:* Condition of an abnormally large ureteral lumen

Disorders associated with males only:

- *Hypospadias:* Abnormal positioning of the urinary meatus in various areas of the penis or base of the penis
- *Undescended testes:* Congenital disorder regarding lack of normal descending of the testes into the scrotum
- *Cryptorchidism:* Absent or ectopic testes; failure of one or both testes to descend from the inguinal canal into the scrotum
- *Testicular torsion:* Sudden twisting of the testicle structures (processus vaginalis around the spermatic cord) leading to intense pain and damage if not surgically repaired; considered a surgical emergency
- *Micropenis:* Congenital disorder of an abnormally small penis
- *Priapism:* Unrelenting erection associated with sickle cell anemia; a large clot in the vessels of the shaft of the penis
- *Male hydrocele:* Fluid collections within the scrotal sac

THE DEVELOPMENT OF THE GENITOURINARY SYSTEM

The development of the urinary system begins during the 11th to the 12th week of fetal development. By the 13th week of fetal development, the kidneys are producing urine. Early **mesoderm** tissues (the middle embryonic germ layer) give rise to the structures that then form the reproductive organs

and the kidney. The newborn's immature kidneys produce larger quantities of urine than in the later developmental stages and produce urine that has a lower SG. This is because the immature kidney is less efficient at concentrating waste products. As the infant develops, the GU system matures and becomes effective in the process of removing waste products from the blood and forming urine.

RENAL FUNCTION

The function of the kidneys is fivefold and is essential for homeostasis. One function is to *eliminate liquid waste products* from the blood into the form of urine. This process of detoxification of the blood is essential for life. The kidneys also *produce erythropoietin* when the body is experiencing a state of hypoxia to stimulate the bone marrow to produce more red blood cells (RBCs). The kidneys *produce renin,* a powerful chemical that stimulates the production of angiotensin I, which then stimulates the production of angiotensin II, causing the peripheral vasculature to constrict in response to low total fluid volume. Angiotensin II also promotes the secretion of aldosterone, whose function is to promote reabsorption of water and sodium by the kidneys to raise blood pressure in response to low circulating volumes. The final responsibilities of the kidneys are to *regulate fluids and electrolytes* and to *regulate acid-base balance.*

The body water percentage in infants is approximately 75% to 80%, whereas the body water percentage of teenagers is close to that of adults, approximately 55% to 65%. A premature infant's percentage of water is closer to 90%. The extracellular fluid percentage in a child is much higher than the extracellular fluid of adults—42% to 45% versus 20%. The infant cannot conserve a source of body water as well as an adult and has less reserve than an adult to pull from the intracellular space. The infant has an extracellular fluid turnover rate of close to 50% per day, whereas adults have only a 20% daily fluid turnover rate. The higher extracellular fluid percentage and the higher turnover rate leave the infant at greater risk for dehydration. As the body grows and matures, adipose and solid body structures influence the total body water and reduce volume. Infants also have a larger total body surface area to body weight as compared with adults, causing greater fluid losses.

The child's renal immaturity affects the efficacy of the kidney's function. Developmental differences in children influence not only fluid and electrolyte balance, but also the process of waste elimination.

Safety *Stat!*

- Young children have a slower glomerular filtration rate (GFR). This slower rate leaves them more vulnerable to the effects of medications and toxins.

· WORD · BUILDING ·

mesoderm: meso–middle + derm–skin

Metabolism

Young children have a higher metabolism than adults to provide energy for rapid growth. Their metabolism rate is approximately two to three times higher than that of an adult. This higher rate requires more water to remove the greater quantity of waste products associated with a higher metabolism. Because of higher respiration, heart, and peristaltic rates, the young child experiences more insensible water loss. Insensible fluids are lost normally through the pulmonary (breathing), cutaneous (evaporation, sweating), and gastrointestinal (GI; fecal) systems. If the child is experiencing a greater caloric expenditure, such as during high fevers, the insensible fluid loss is even greater. (A child will experience about 30 mL of insensible fluid loss for each degree of temperature above 38°C [100.4°F]).

Body Electrolytes

The electrolyte levels in the body have a major role in maintaining homeostasis. With fluid overload or severe dehydration, electrolyte imbalances occur, leading to potential pathology. Sodium, potassium, magnesium, phosphorus, and calcium all play integral roles in maintaining fluid balance, supporting neuromuscular activity, stimulating bone growth, and regulating the acid-base balance. Children become symptomatic when electrolyte imbalances are present, and treatment by replacement therapy may be required.

Sodium

Water follows the movement of sodium. Therefore, as sodium crosses back and forth between cell walls, it highly influences the distribution of body water. Sodium is the principal cation of the child's extracellular fluid and provides the body's osmolarity (fluid movement). Hypernatremia can be caused by excessive loss of body water that is greater than a loss of body sodium. It can also be caused by improperly mixed infant formulas, ingestion of seawater, or excessive salt intake. **Hyponatremia**, which is a decreased concentration of sodium in the bloodstream, can be caused by using diuretics, vomiting, diarrhea, burns, third spacing, tap-water enemas, and an excessive intake of parenteral fluids, also known as *IV fluids*.

Potassium

Potassium plays a large role in neuromuscular excitability. Cardiac conduction depends on normal serum levels of potassium. Potassium is the principal cation of intracellular fluid and therefore is the major determinant of cell membrane resting potential. Hyperkalemia can be caused by an excessive intake of parenteral potassium or by an impaired renal excretory mechanism. Hypokalemia is very serious because potassium regulates skeletal, smooth, and cardiac muscles. Hypokalemia results in electrocardiography changes.

Magnesium

Nerve and muscle activity also depend on a normal serum level of magnesium. Tetany, seizures, and tremors are associated with low serum magnesium. Hypomagnesemia can be caused by several malabsorption syndromes, hypoparathyroidism, prolonged IV therapy, diuretic use, and hypercalcemia. Hypermagnesemia is rarely observed and is directly related to decreased renal function or the overconsumption of magnesium-containing laxatives, IV fluids, antacids, or enemas.

Phosphorus

Phosphorus has two major roles: (1) to interact with calcium to provide adequate bone growth and (2) to assist in the production of energy for a child's rapid metabolism. A dysfunction of serum phosphorus can be demonstrated with the use of several cytotoxic (chemotherapy) medications.

Calcium

Serum calcium regulates cell membrane permeability, supports the clotting cascade, and determines bone and teeth health. Hypocalcemia is associated with vitamin D deficiency, malabsorption disorders, or nutritional deficiency. Hypercalcemia is associated with vitamin D intoxication,

· WORD · BUILDING ·

hyponatremia: hypo–deficient + natr–sodium + em–blood + ia–condition

ongoing states of immobilization, malignancies, and the excessive use of thiazide diuretics.

Acid-Base Balance and Renal Regulation

The kidneys have a significant role to play in acid-base balance. If a child presents with metabolic or respiratory **acidosis** (elevated acidity in the blood) or **alkalosis** (reduced acidity in the blood), the respiratory system will be the first to contribute to achieving a state of homeostasis. This is done by either blowing off excess carbon dioxide (CO_2) to help correct acidosis, or by retaining CO_2 to help correct alkalosis. The renal system will also assist in the regulation of the acid-base imbalance but takes considerably longer to upregulate than the respiratory system. The renal system will either retain bicarbonate (HCO_3; for acidosis), or will release HCO_3 (for alkalosis).

FLUID MAINTENANCE REQUIREMENTS

Monitoring for adequate fluid intake is an important role of the nurse. Young children who are ill may not ingest enough fluids orally to maintain fluid balance. Fever, infection, diarrhea, and vomiting all contribute to extra fluid losses. Therefore, the nurse calculates the child's daily fluid maintenance requirements and provides care with this in mind.

Fluid requirements can be conceptualized in three ways:

1. The child may need fluid maintenance to provide what is needed for a balanced fluid level.
2. The child may need fluid deficit replacement, after a significant bleed, for example.
3. The child may need fluid replacement for ongoing fluid losses, such as diarrhea, gastric fluid loss, or burn-associated fluid losses.

Some medical conditions such as pediatric cardiac disease, cancer, or burns may influence the daily fluid maintenance needs. In such cases, the health-care provider may write an order to either give more or less than the basic fluid maintenance calculation. For example, an order may state "provide one-half maintenance" if the child is at risk for fluid overload.

Information about **fluid maintenance calculation**, which is a calculation used in pediatrics to determine the daily maintenance of fluids that should be consumed or administered, is found in Chapter 23. To calculate more or less than maintenance, divide the total amount of fluid due for the 24-hour period by 2 for "half times maintenance," or double the total amount of fluid required for "two times maintenance."

Water Intoxication

Childhood deaths have been associated with the intake of large amounts of free water. The medical diagnosis associated with overhydration of water is called *water intoxication.* Children who have severe mental illness, low cognitive function, or pathologies associated with extreme thirst should be monitored for appropriate free water intake. Fatal water intoxication causes pleural effusions and acute dilutional hyponatremia leading to confusion, seizures, coma, then death. Fatal water intoxication can also be caused by forced water intake as a form of child abuse or excessive administration of hypotonic fluids.

CRITICAL THINKING & CLINICAL JUDGMENT

You are a home health-care nurse and have been assigned to visit a family as part of a program to provide more support for new parents. While visiting the family, you see the mother feeding a bottle of sterile water to her 2-week-old newborn.

Questions

1. What is your concern for the newborn?
2. What teaching should you provide to the mother?

Urine Output

As children grow and are better able to concentrate their waste products, the number of times they void their urine each day decreases. To determine an infant or a young child's intake and output (I&O), weigh the child's diaper on a scale in grams (Fig. 35.1). One gram of urine is considered 1 mL

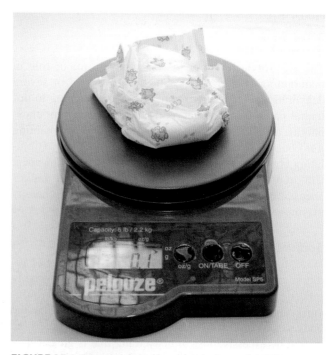

FIGURE 35.1 Example of a scale to weigh diapers for I&O.

of urine. Subtract the weight of a dry diaper from the total weight of the urine and diaper together to account for the urine alone. The following denote the average UOP for different age groups:

- Newborns produce approximately 10 mL/hour.
- Infants produce approximately 5 to 10 mL/hour.
- Toddlers and preschool children produce approximately 15 to 20 mL/hour.
- School-aged children produce approximately 10 to 25 mL/hour.
- Adolescents, similar to adults, produce approximately 40 to 80 mL/hour.

Many conditions require an assessment of a child's urine. Make sure that the specimen is collected in an accurate manner because some tests, such as a urine culture, require sterile technique, and others are clean-catch methods. Box 35.2 provides information about collecting urine. See Figure 35.2 for a photograph of an infant with a uro-bag in place.

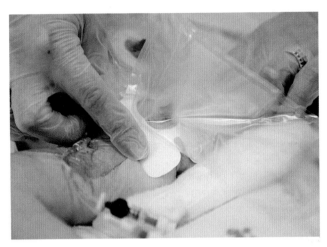

FIGURE 35.2 The nurse must be able to collect urine specimens in a bag that fits over the perineum in females or over the penis in males.

Box 35.2

Urine Specimen Collection

Clean Catch: Cotton Balls Placed in Diaper
- Not suitable for a sterile specimen for culture and sensitivity but adequate for SG, pH, presence of blood and ketones
- Must obtain adequate volume to squeeze specimen into specimen container
- Do not use unless diaper is free of any stool.
- Cleanse the child's perineum well before placing cotton balls to obtain specimen.

Clean Catch: Uro-Bag: Female
- Placed on the labia majora under the diaper to catch the urine specimen

Clean Catch: Uro-Bag: Male
- Cut to fit, the bag is placed over the penis and testicles to catch the urine specimen

Clean Catch: Midstream Sample
- For older children sitting on the toilet or commode, urine is caught in specimen container as the child voids, midstream.

Sterile Sample: In and Out Catheterization
- When an indwelling catheter is not required, this sterile procedure passes a small catheter into the child's bladder to obtain a sterile specimen, typically for culture and sensitivity.

Sterile Sample: Indwelling Catheterization
- When a child has an indwelling catheter in place, a sterile syringe and needle are inserted in a cleansed rubber port located along the collection tubing to obtain a sterile specimen.

Labs & Diagnostics

Tests for Genitourinary Disorders

Urinalysis
- Checks for presence of blood, glucose, ketones, and protein, and measures pH
- Conducted via dipstick (laboratory paper strip placed in child's urine for rapid diagnosis)
- Blood, glucose, ketones, and protein are substances not normally found in the child's urine; considered abnormal finding.

Urine Culture and Sensitivity
- Collected for culture of bacteria or other infectious organisms
- Placed in a culture tube and held in the laboratory
- Specimen is checked over time for growth
- Sensitivity of the bacteria grown out in the specimen is checked to match appropriate and effective antibiotic therapy (such as for a UTI).

Specific Gravity
- SG is checked via machine to determine the concentration of urine.
- Normal values are 1.010 to 1.030.
- The lower the number, the more dilute the urine; water has an SG of 1.000.

IV Pyelogram
- This checks the renal pelvic structures by radiography (x-ray) following the administration of an IV injected contrast material (dye).

Voiding Cystourethrogram
- The voiding cystourethrogram (VCUG) checks the bladder and surrounding structures during the process of voiding after the administration of contrast material (dye), which is instilled into the child's bladder.
- VCUG determines the presence of reflux or strictures.

Continued

Labs & Diagnostics—cont'd

Blood Urea Nitrogen

- BUN checks the index of the GFR.
- BUN is a waste product of protein metabolism excreted via the kidneys.
- Normal values fluctuate with the child's age but are approximately 10 to 20 mg/dL.

Blood Creatinine

- This checks the kidney function by measuring the waste product of energy metabolism from muscle.
- Normal values fluctuate with the child's age but are approximately 0.2 to 2 mg/dL.

Creatinine Clearance

- This is considered the best measure of kidney function in the child.
- Creatinine is the end product of energy metabolism from muscle.
- It is collected over a period, such as 24 hours, and the specimen is kept refrigerated.

DEHYDRATION

When a child's fluid intake is significantly reduced or there is a condition present that causes a loss of water and electrolytes, the child is at risk for developing dehydration. In very young children, severe dehydration can be life-threatening. Severe diarrhea, intractable vomiting, and prolonged diaphoresis (sweating) can all cause a significant fluid imbalance by causing greater loss than intake. Hypovolemia ensues, followed by circulatory collapse and shock if not corrected in a timely manner. There are three types of dehydration, each of which needs unique corrective mechanisms (see Table 34.2).

Evaluating Dehydration

Checking a child for dehydration is imperative. The following guidelines can help:

- Strictly measure and record I&O to monitor progression or management, including an hourly inspection of stool, urine, and vomit.
- Note the SG and color of the child's urine.
- Determine the severity of dehydration (see Table 34.1).
- Obtain a daily weight to compare with baseline.
- Note and report any of these signs and symptoms:
  - Dry skin and poor tissue turgor
  - Dry mucous membranes
  - Sunken fontanels and sunken eye sockets
  - Pale skin and poor perfusion; delayed capillary refill and hypotension
  - Decreased body temperature, rapid pulse, and tachypnea
  - Lethargy, weak cry, and poor muscle tone

Interventions for Dehydration

Interventions for mild, moderate, or severe dehydration include oral fluid replacement if tolerated. Mild dehydration may be corrected with 30 to 50 mL of fluid per kilogram of weight; moderate dehydration may be corrected with 60 to 90 mL of fluid per kilogram of weight. When severe dehydration or moderate dehydration with the inability to take in PO fluids is present, the child will require an IV placement for normal saline boluses (typically 20 mL/kg, repeated as needed) followed by at least the equivalent of a child's fluid maintenance calculation. Severe dehydration may need as much as 100 mL/kg of normal saline to correct it.

Nursing Considerations for Dehydration

Children who are hospitalized with dehydration are typically quite sick and require close monitoring. If a child cannot tolerate PO (oral) fluid replacement therapy, IV therapy should not be delayed. If the cardiovascular system is affected and the child demonstrates symptoms of poor perfusion, they may be moved to a pediatric intensive care unit (PICU) for closer monitoring. For a child with dehydration seen in a clinic setting, the health-care provider will need to determine if the child can be rehydrated with oral rehydration fluids or should be sent to an emergency department for IV fluids.

Patient Teaching Guidelines

Oral Rehydration

If the dehydration is mild, the parents may be told to start the child on oral rehydration as tolerated. They should provide commercial electrolyte solutions such as Pedialyte to infants and young children. It is acceptable to dilute the electrolyte solutions with water or to add a small amount of juice just to flavor the water, but not in young infancy. Parents should not try to rehydrate an older child with soda or sugary drinks because this will contribute to dehydration. Milk should also not be used to rehydrate children.

Safe and Effective Nursing Care

The Dehydrated Child

It is important to think holistically and treat symptoms of discomfort, fever, and fatigue. For example, the child with intractable vomiting should be provided mouth care with lemon/glycerin swabs. Closely monitor the child for any changes in clinical status, including changes in vital signs and mental status. Any change in mental status should be reported immediately because this may be a critical sign. For accurate daily weights, use the same scale and weigh the child without clothes or diaper on. If the child is an infant, provide a pacifier to allow sucking stimulation while receiving IV fluids.

COMMON GENITOURINARY DISORDERS

Across the developmental period, children can present with a variety of GU infections and disorders. Some infections are influenced by age, such as *Escherichia coli* infections in diapered infants and young children who are toilet training. Nurses who are versed in common GU disorders and infections can assist the pediatric team in early and rapid diagnosis, preventing complications such as scarring, strictures, or infertility in the adolescent period or adulthood.

Urinary Tract Infections

UTIs are one of the most common childhood infections for which parents seek medical attention for their child. Infant males have more UTIs than infant females because of the presence of bacteria in uncircumcised infants. Past infancy, girls are more likely to develop UTIs because of their short urethra, which allows bacteria to migrate up the urinary tract. Most commonly caused by bacteria, a UTI can be located in three areas:

1. Bladder = cystitis
2. Urethra = urethritis
3. Kidney = pyelonephritis

UTIs can be caused by urine refluxing back into the ureters during or after urination, incomplete bladder emptying, or inadequate cleansing of the perineum after stooling. Diapered infants and toilet-training toddlers are at greatest risk for UTI from stool entering into the urethra. Diagnosis occurs when there are greater than or equal to 5×10^4 colonies of bacteria per mL of urine.

Diagnosing Urinary Tract Infections

Because UTIs are so common in young children, you must keep this in mind when interacting with families who are seeking care for children with fevers. The child with a suspected UTI should be checked for the following:

- Frequency, urgency, and pain (dysuria) associated with urination (although infants may not show symptoms of dysuria, only fever)
- Odor of urine
- Color and clarity of the urine, noting the presence of RBCs and white blood cells (WBCs)
- Fever (especially in infancy period)
- Dehydration
- Hematuria and low pH

Labs & Diagnostics

Urinalysis
The key information provided by a urinalysis is the following: appearance, SG, pH, odor, glucose, protein, ketones, RBCs, WBCs, casts, nitrites, and leukocyte esterase.

- Lethargy and poor feeding
- Abdominal, pelvic, or flank pain
- History of previous UTIs

Interventions for Urinary Tract Infections

Interventions for UTIs range from increasing oral fluid intake to IV antibiotics. Early identification can prevent complications such as urosepsis, a life-threatening condition in immunocompromised children in which bacteria enter the bloodstream from the urinary tract. Interventions include:

- Providing favorite PO fluids or maintaining a patent IV for fluid replacement and fluid therapy to help wash out the bacteria from the bladder
- Increasing fluid consumption to more than 100 mL/kg/day
- Treating fever and discomfort
- Providing education on proper personal hygiene after toileting (for girls, wiping front to back only)
- Teaching all family members how to clean female genitalia after stooling to ensure that any fecal material is removed from the outer and inner labia
- Administering antimicrobials as ordered, including cephalosporins, sulfonamides, amoxicillin, or nitrofurantoin

---

Medication Facts

Antibiotics Used for Urinary Tract Infections
Antibiotics commonly used for the treatment of UTIs in children include the following:

- Amoxicillin (first line medication but associated with *E. coli* resistance)
- Ampicillin
- Cephalexin
- Cefixime
- Cefprozil
- Gentamicin
- Trimethoprim/sulfamethoxazole (highest cure rate)
- Amoxicillin/clavulanate

Patient Teaching Guidelines

Teaching Families About the Child's Personal Hygiene
UTIs are very common in young children. A large number of infants and children will be brought in for medical care for symptoms associated with UTI. Nurses should teach prevention activities to decrease the incidence.

- Hand washing to prevent infection
  - Parents need to teach their children to wash their hands after every time they use the bathroom. If soap and water are not available, hand sanitizers should be used.

Continued

Patient Teaching Guidelines—cont'd

Children should wash their hands after playing outside, in playgrounds, or at parks. Children should also wash their hands before and after helping to prepare foods, especially raw foods.

- Hand washing can be presented as a fun game to young children. Singing the ABCs, "Twinkle, Twinkle Little Star," or another short song while washing encourages the child to spend the time needed to be thorough.
- Girls wiping front to back
  - Because females have a shorter urethra than males, they are particularly vulnerable to UTIs.
  - Young girls must be taught how to wipe their perineum from front to back, not back to front, to prevent the contamination of stool into their urinary meatus. This contamination is a common source of UTI.
  - Reinforcing this process is important. Young girls need reminders on a regular basis.
- Position for urination
  - Most young girls void with their legs together. This leaves them prone to urine refluxing into their vaginas, which can lead to vulvitis, vulvovaginitis, and infection. Girls should be taught to relax during urination and not strain or rush (Cincinnati Children's Hospital, 2021).
- Diaper cleanup of stool
  - Parents and caregivers need to wash their hands before changing a child's diaper if they have been handling contaminated substances.
  - Parents and caregivers need to carefully remove all stool from a young child's perineum after each stooling.
  - Parents and caregivers should not delay in changing diapers with stool.
- Irritants
  - Avoid irritants; children should not sit in tubs with strong bubble bath soaps or sit in water with shampoo residue (Cincinnati Children's Hospital, 2021).

Health Promotion

Preventing Urinary Tract Infections and Sexually Transmitted Infections in Sexually Active Teens

The development of UTIs and sexually transmitted infections (STIs) in sexually active teens is fairly common. You should teach the following information to teens of both sexes:

- Urinate before and after sexual intercourse. An empty bladder before sex reduces the friction associated with the development of bladder inflammation. The act of urinating flushes the urethra and helps to cleanse bacteria out from the opening of the meatus.

- If participating in anal intercourse, take precautions to conduct personal hygiene immediately after sex to cleanse the perineum of bacteria harbored in the rectum. Vaginal intercourse immediately after anal intercourse increases the chances of contracting infections.
- Seek health care for painful urination, blood in the urine, fevers and chills, discharge from the genitalia, or cloudy urine.
- Use a fresh latex condom for each act of intercourse. Do not use condoms past their expiration date.
- Seek medical attention for known contact with an infected sexual partner, even if no symptoms are present.

The following information is also important to pass along:

- Genital warts can be prevented by preexposure immunization against human papillomavirus (HPV).
- Hepatitis A and B can be prevented via preexposure immunization.
- With prompt identification and treatment, curative therapy is available for bacterial STIs. Viral STIs, such as herpes and HIV, can be managed but not cured.
- Interactions with health-care professionals about birth control, STI treatment, and related care are confidential.

Nursing Considerations for Urinary Tract Infections

When there is a history of UTI, it is important to teach the family prevention techniques, including the avoidance of strong detergents, soaps, bubble bath, or bath salts that may contribute to inflammation. In addition, the family should be aware that UTIs in childhood are associated with chronic and severe constipation (American Academy of Pediatrics, 2023; Cincinnati Children's Hospital, 2021). Promoting regular elimination with adequate fluids and a high-fiber diet can also help to prevent UTIs. When the child is on antibiotics, you should explain the possibility of side effects such as diarrhea, rash, nausea, vomiting, abdominal pain, photosensitivity, and flatulence. Functional constipation in pediatrics is now a known risk factor for the development of UTIs and for the development of pyelonephritis (Axelgaard et al., 2023).

Enuresis

Enuresis is a condition of voiding dysfunction. **Nocturnal incontinence**, the most common form, is the occurrence of involuntary voiding at night (bed wetting) after the child has completed toilet training. **Diurnal incontinence** is daytime incontinence and is mostly associated with a condition called *unstable bladder*. Although girls typically acquire bladder control at a younger age than boys, the overall occurrence of this condition is as high as 20% of children older than 5 years. Treatment is typically not offered until after the age of 6 in both genders because this condition is very common.

Diagnosing Enuresis

Determining the cause and severity of enuresis starts with a thorough medical examination and health history. Causes of urinary incontinence during childhood may be related to:

- Unstable (uninhibited) bladder
- Holding on to urine or infrequent daytime voiding
- Cystitis
- Neurogenic bladder
- Bladder outlet obstruction
- Sphincter abnormality
- Trauma
- Overflow incontinence
- Iatrogenic causes

Interventions for Enuresis

Interventions for enuresis in children 5 years of age and younger involve reassuring the parents that the condition is typically self-limiting and that the child should not be punished or scolded for the accidents. For young children, fluids should be restricted after the evening meal, and the child should be reminded to void before going to bed. Research has demonstrated a direct link between nocturnal incontinence and severe snoring (Gomez Rincon et al., 2022). If the parents report snoring, a referral to an ear, nose, and throat (ENT) physician should be offered. An adenoidectomy may help cure some cases of nocturnal incontinence. For older children, active treatment consists first of motivation with activities such as a star chart and rewards. Older children may benefit from the use of an alarm that detects wetness via electrodes in the linen or underwear. Medications can be used to manage enuresis but are not considered curative. Desmopressin acetate, a synthetic form of an antidiuretic hormone, reduces urine production at night. Anticholinergic therapy with oxybutynin chloride may help during the daytime.

Nursing Considerations for Enuresis

Nursing considerations for childhood enuresis include role modeling empathy for the parents and demonstrating a non-judgmental, nonpunitive attitude toward the child. For parents of children younger than 5 years, reinforce the need to provide emotional support, fluid restrictions in the evening, and bedtime voiding. For older children, support the parents in initiating a plan of motivation with rewards. The child should never be scolded, belittled, or made to feel bad by caregivers or parents; they are already at risk for peer humiliation and teasing. Often, simple steps to reduce the need to void at night are enough to assist the child and family with the stress of a child experiencing enuresis.

Nephrotic Syndrome/Nephrosis

Nephrotic syndrome/nephrosis is characterized by the development of pores along the final filtration membrane of the kidney and subsequent loss of serum proteins. Most cases of

· WORD · BUILDING ·

nephrosis: nephr–kidney + osis–condition

nephrotic syndrome during childhood are considered idiopathic, meaning no known cause is found, with a good overall prognosis. There are two main categories of nephrotic syndrome with subcategories:

- Primary childhood nephrotic syndrome
  - Also called *minimal-change nephrotic syndrome,* the pathology is associated with relapses throughout childhood. Relapses are associated with poorer clinical outcomes and higher mortality rates. It is more commonly found in boys than girls. Diagnosis is confirmed by physical examination, urine testing, blood testing, kidney ultrasound, and kidney biopsy.
- Secondary nephrotic syndrome caused by common diseases or conditions
  - Diabetes
  - Hepatitis
  - Lupus
  - Henoch-Schonlein purpura
  - Mercury exposure
  - Lithium toxicity
  - Certain medications such as aspirin

The cardinal symptoms of nephrotic syndrome are fourfold (Fig. 35.3):

1. *Severe proteinuria:* Severe loss of protein through porous nature of the final urine filtration membrane, the glomeruli, into the urine
2. *Severe hypoproteinemia* (also called *hypoalbuminemia*): Severely low levels of protein left in the serum, leading to generalized edema, especially noted in the abdomen **(ascites)**
3. *Hyperlipidemia:* Elevated serum total cholesterol, triglycerides, and total lipids
4. *Edema*

Diagnosing Nephrotic Syndrome/Nephrosis

Because of the complexity of diagnosing nephrotic syndrome, you must be able to identify significant clinical signs and report changes in clinical status to the pediatric health-care team. Signs of nephrotic syndrome include the following:

- Fatigue
- Decreased appetite (anorexia)
- Fluid accumulation (edema)
- Weight gain with abdominal swelling
- Golden-yellow, foamy urine (may be blood in urine)
- Diarrhea
- Loss of appetite
- High blood pressure

Interventions for Nephrotic Syndrome/Nephrosis

Treatment is generally supportive. Conduct daily weights at the same time of day and on the same scale. Treat fluid retention with diuretics, and manage hypertension. Administer corticosteroids to decrease the size of the pores through

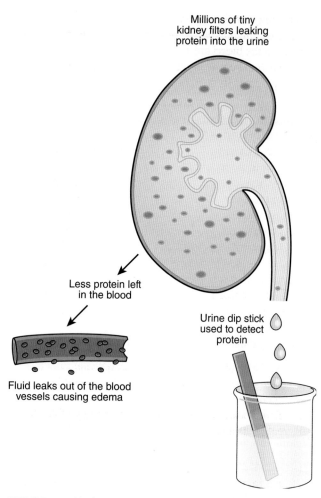

Millions of tiny kidney filters leaking protein into the urine

Less protein left in the blood

Fluid leaks out of the blood vessels causing edema

Urine dip stick used to detect protein

FIGURE 35.3 Nephrotic syndrome.

which proteins are lost. When the level of serum proteins is very low, the child may require IV administration of albumin. A nutritionist will follow the child and initiate a low-salt, high-protein diet. In severe cases, immunosuppressive therapy may be required.

Safety *Stat!*

When a child is on high-dose corticosteroids for a lengthy time period, you must watch for signs of hypertension, hyperglycemia, immunosuppression, poor wound healing, emotional lability, height delays, and excessive hunger. All symptoms associated with long-term corticosteroid use must be reported.

Nursing Considerations for Nephrotic Syndrome/Nephrosis

Nursing considerations for a child with nephrotic syndrome include emotional support for the entire family. The edematous appearance of the child can frighten the parents, who need support to process and understand the pathology of the disease. Monitor vital signs and daily weights carefully and report any changes to the health-care team. Protect the child's skin because edema causes the skin to become vulnerable to breakdown. Provide a low-sodium diet to minimize edema. Monitor for problems with skin integrity, GI distress, poor nutrition, and fatigue. Teach families to look for symptoms of a relapse after the child is discharged. These symptoms include the appearance of albumin in the child's urine (frothy, golden-colored, and viscous) as well as changes in the child's weight, fatigue level, and appetite.

Patient Teaching Guidelines

Low-Sodium Diet
A low-salt diet may be ordered for a child who presents with nephrotic syndrome in order to decrease the fluid retention and third spacing related to hypoalbuminemia. Reducing sodium prevents fluid effusions in the lungs, decreases fluid retention, and reduces the leakage of fluids from the intravascular space to the extravascular space.

Complications associated with a diagnosis of nephrotic syndrome include:

- Infection caused by loss of proteins used to build infection-fighting cells
- High blood cholesterol caused by the increased production of lipids in the liver
- Blood clots caused by the loss of proteins in the urine, causing greater risk of developing clots

---

Medication Facts

Medications for Nephrotic Syndrome
Medications used in the care of a child with nephrotic syndrome include the following:

- Diuretics for fluid overload
- Antibiotics if peritonitis occurs
- Corticosteroids for the reduction of the size of the pores on the glomeruli
- 25% albumin infusions to reduce edema and replace lost albumin (Rudd & Kocisko, 2023)

If a child does not respond to treatment, then medications that reduce the production of antibodies that damage kidney tissue may be ordered. These include:

- Mycophenolate
- Cyclophosphamide
- Tacrolimus

Acute Glomerulonephritis

When a child experiences disease of the kidney's glomeruli, a condition called *acute glomerulonephritis (AGN)* may occur. The glomeruli are small structures of the kidney that contain the blood vessels and the collection tubules, called *nephrons,* where urine is filtered from the blood. Glomerulonephritis (also called *poststreptococcal glomerulonephritis*) follows a severe infection such as a strep infection. The larger immune/antigen complexes used to fight the infection become clogged in the nephrons, causing inflammation and impairment of the kidney's ability to filter urine. Streptococcal infections, inflammatory diseases of the arteries, and genetic predispositions are the most common causes of AGN. Glomerulonephritis may present 1 week to 10 days after a strep throat or strep upper respiratory infection that was not treated. This disease primarily affects school-aged children and is rare in children under the age of 2. This condition lasts a brief time, and the kidneys usually recover.

Diagnosing Acute Glomerulonephritis

A child with AGN will present with classic symptoms that identify the disorder. Different from nephrotic syndrome in that serum proteins are not lost, AGN has clinical symptoms that represent kidney injury as the final filtration membrane becomes clogged with antibody/antigen molecules.

Assessments of AGN include the following:

- Dark brown (tea-colored) urine
- Low overall UOP
- Fatigue and lethargy
- High blood pressure
- Edema
- Sore throat
- Rash on buttocks and legs
- Joint pain
- Headache
- Increased breathing effort
- Seizures

Diagnostic evaluation for AGN includes throat, blood, and urine cultures to identify the presence of a streptococcal infection; urinalysis; chest x-ray for pulmonary congestion; renal ultrasound; and possibly renal biopsy. Laboratory findings that are suggestive of the pathology of AGN include:

- Mildly to moderately elevated BUN and creatinine
- Elevated antistreptolysin-O titer (ASO)
- Elevated anti-DNase B titer
- Elevated erythrocyte sedimentation rate (ESR)
- Depressed complement C3 and complement C4 levels

Interventions for Acute Glomerulonephritis

Interventions for AGN involve preventing fluid overload and the buildup of further waste product (urea). These interventions occur through the following:

- Administering diuretics
- Correcting electrolyte imbalances
- Treating the strep infection with antibiotics

- Managing associated hypertension
- Administering phosphate binders to reduce mineral phosphates in the blood
- Dialysis for short-term management of the buildup of waste products in the blood

Nursing Considerations for Acute Glomerulonephritis

Nursing considerations for a child who presents with AGN include rapid interventions to prevent significant glomerular injury. Rapidly identify any history of an infection anywhere in the body and report this significant information to the primary health-care provider. For instance, a typical latency period for AGN after an episode of acute pharyngitis is 7 to 10 days; whereas, for a streptococcal skin infection, the latency period can be much longer, lasting up to 6 weeks.

Keep in mind that AGN affects multiple systems. Headaches, GI disturbances, malaise, hypertension, and rapid weight gain are all associated with the disease and need meticulous nursing care.

Nursing diagnoses associated with AGN include:

- Excess fluid volume related to impaired renal function
- Impaired urinary elimination related to glomerular dysfunction
- Deficient knowledge regarding the pathology of AGN and its treatments and management

Hemolytic Uremic Syndrome

HUS is a rare and potentially lethal form of kidney failure in children who have developed an infection such as *E. coli,* especially Shiga toxin-producing *E. coli* (STEC) *infections strain 0157:H7.* This strain infects the digestive tract, producing toxins that enter the child's bloodstream and destroy RBCs. Outbreaks of HUS are more common in the summer and are closely associated with the consumption of inadequately cooked meats; unpasteurized dairy products or juices; and contaminated swimming pools, water parks, daycare facilities, and fast food restaurants. HUS can also be associated with certain medications and conditions such as a weakened immune system (Mayo Clinic, 2023). It is most commonly seen in young children under 5 years of age in the United States (Mayo Clinic, 2023). Care team members can expect to identify microangiopathic hemolytic anemia, severe thrombocytopenia, and acute kidney injury. Children who present with HUS and are experiencing seizures have a poor prognosis. Other rare causes of HUS include medication-induced hereditary syndromes, pregnancy-associated syndromes such as HELLP syndrome or preeclampsia (see Chapter 8), or malignancies.

Diagnosing Hemolytic Uremic Syndrome

A young child with HUS may present with vomiting, severe abdominal pain, and watery or bloody diarrhea. The child will appear quite ill, pale, fatigued, and dehydrated and may demonstrate unexplained, small bruises visible only in the lining of the mouth. Because of the damaged RBCs, the very small blood vessels of the kidneys become clogged. Because the kidneys are no longer able to eliminate waste products, uremia develops, and the child experiences fluid retention. High blood pressure and edema lead to the need for dialysis.

Interventions for Hemolytic Uremic Syndrome

The child with HUS often requires a PICU stay. There is no known cure for HUS. The child's symptoms of initial dehydration followed by fluid retention will be treated, as will electrolyte disturbances, anemia, and discomfort. IV nutrition and antihypertensives may be required. Mortality in HUS is increased with dehydrated patients; therefore, IV fluids should be initiated right after diagnosis is confirmed (Ardissino et al., 2016).

Antibiotics will be administered although this treatment does not decrease the duration of GI symptoms (bloody diarrhea). Platelet infusions may be required for associated low platelet counts. Dialysis is required for BUN levels greater than or equal to 80 mg/dL. Prevention starts with public health measures to reduce exposure to *E. coli* and teaching families to thoroughly wash fruits and vegetables.

Nursing Considerations for Hemolytic Uremic Syndrome

The family experiences stress and anxiety not knowing what is wrong with their child and will be concerned about the high level of care required right after a confirmed diagnosis. Providing emotional support while answering all questions will be important to the well-being of the family. Because of the severity of the diagnosis, family members will be fearful of the potential of poor outcomes or the threat of death.

Nurses should observe for complications associated with HUS. These complications include kidney failure, high blood pressure, seizures, and clotting disturbances (Mayo Clinic, 2023).

Teach families about safe food preparation and washing of fruits and vegetables to prevent HUS. Part of anticipatory guidance for new parents is to remind them that adequate and safe food preparation reduces the likelihood of contamination and illness.

Congenital Genitourinary Anomalies

Many GU disorders are present from birth (congenital). It is important to know the child's birth history and any surgical or nonsurgical procedures that were conducted to remedy the anomaly. Congenital anomalies can cause obstructions, strictures, an absence of anatomy, abnormal openings, or a delay in and/or inefficient urinary elimination, including urine reflux. One of the most common GU anomalies is vesicoureteral reflux (VUR; Box 35.3).

Exstrophy of the Bladder

Exstrophy of the bladder is a condition in which the lower portion of the abdominal wall and the anterior bladder wall are both missing, causing the child to be born with an exposed, or open, bladder on the abdomen. Occurring more

---

Box 35.3

Congenital Anomalies of the Genitourinary System: Vesicoureteral Reflux

VUR is a condition in which urine flows back from the bladder into the ureters and often up into the kidneys during or after urination. Damage to the kidney structures occurs because of scarring from recurrent UTIs. VUR is more common in young girls than young boys. However, as children grow, VUR is more common in boys because there is more pressure when voiding. The most common symptoms are urgency, dribbling of urine, UTI, and eventually kidney damage (such as the presence of an abdominal mass from a severely swollen kidney) and hypertension. Identification of the disorder is by renal ultrasound and voiding cystourethrogram (VCUG). VUR is graded on a scale of 1 to 5. If the child's reflux is graded 1 to 3, they may need no therapy and the condition will eventually resolve on its own. For 4 to 5, the child may require surgical interventions such as a flap-valve apparatus to prevent the reverse of flow. If the child has had several UTIs, the scarred ureter and/or kidney tissue may need to be removed.

---

frequently in boys than in girls, this condition appears as a red mass and demonstrates a continuous drainage of urine. The newborn's skin may become excoriated, and the condition requires surgical repair soon after birth.

Diagnosing Congenital Genitourinary Anomalies

Checking newborns for the presence of a congenital anomaly is part of routine well-newborn nursing care. Visual inspection of the external genitalia, as well as inspection of the first urine elimination, are important in the early identification of a GU anomaly. Palpation should be conducted as part of the initial assessment.

Interventions for Congenital Genitourinary Anomalies

Many congenital GU anomalies require surgical interventions. Depending on the severity of the condition, the pediatric surgical team may wait until the infant is less vulnerable to the complications of anesthesia or until the family feels that the child's psychosocial development may be affected by the anomaly. For instance, if a newborn boy is born with **hypospadias** (an abnormal opening on the glans penis for the elimination of urine; Fig. 35.4), surgery may be conducted before the child has concerns with body image. **Epispadias** is a congenital condition in which the meatus, the opening of the urethra, is located on the dorsum (top) of the penis.

Nursing Considerations for Congenital Genitourinary Anomalies

Infants and young toddlers will not recognize that they have a congenital anomaly. Be available to answer the family's questions concerning the child's anatomy and physiology related to the GU system, including any abnormalities. If the surgical correction can wait until the child is older, the family may feel strongly that the procedure should take place before

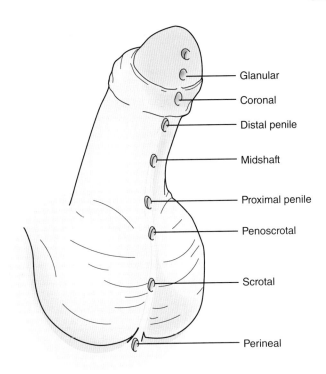

Glanular

Coronal

Distal penile

Midshaft

Proximal penile

Penoscrotal

Scrotal

Perineal

FIGURE 35.4 Locations where hypospadias may occur.

the child recognizes that they are different from other children. The decision about when the surgical procedure takes place may or may not be up to the parents' preferences. If it is, the parents should be supported in their decision and given anticipatory guidance about body-image concerns for each of the developmental stages of childhood.

Genetic or Congenital Reproductive System Differences

Sometimes, an infant is born with a genetic or congenital reproductive system difference. Although these conditions require assessments and diagnostic examinations, not all of them require treatment. Genetic or congenital reproductive system differences include intersex conditions, Turner syndrome, and Klinefelter syndrome.

Intersex Conditions

Intersex conditions are a variety of conditions that contribute to the development of physical sex characteristics that are atypical. The external genitalia, internal reproductive organs, sex chromosomes, or sex hormones may be affected. Found in approximately 1:2,000 live births, some intersex conditions, such as ambiguous genitalia, are apparent at birth. Others are less apparent. For example, a child born with XX chromosomes and congenital adrenal hyperplasia has genitals that look thoroughly male. On the other hand, a girl born with XY chromosomes and complete androgen insensitivity syndrome has genitals that appear typically female (American Psychological Association [APA], 2019).

Turner Syndrome

Turner syndrome exists when a girl is born with only one X chromosome. This condition results in short stature and underdeveloped gonads (sex organs). The condition may not be recognized at birth but may be demonstrated later during childhood. Characteristics include a webbed neck, widely spaced nipples, a small mandible, epicanthal folds, a broad chest, and delayed sexual maturation during adolescence. Turner syndrome does not affect intellectual development. Management may include growth hormone therapy. Women with Turner syndrome will likely have fertility issues.

Klinefelter Syndrome

Klinefelter syndrome occurs when a boy is born with an extra X chromosome (XXY), producing a child who is relatively tall with incomplete secondary sex development. Most are infertile with azoospermia (an absence of sperm) and small testes. The condition is often not noted until adolescence, when puberty is absent. Klinefelter syndrome is associated with learning disabilities, immaturity and impulsivity, and anxiety. Nearly half of men with Klinefelter syndrome develop metabolic syndrome. Management includes long-acting supplemental testosterone therapy (Los & Ford, 2023).

Acquired Reproductive System Disorders

The term *acquired reproductive system disorders* refers to conditions that develop after birth as compared with primary disorders that are present since birth. Foreign bodies in the vagina, inflammatory conditions such as pediatric vulvovaginitis, adhesions, and STIs are examples of acquired conditions.

Foreign Objects in the Vagina

When a child presents with a foreign object in the vagina, the health-care team will conduct an initial assessment for sexual abuse. However, the presence of a foreign object is not diagnostic of abuse. Some young children place small toys or items in their ears, nose, rectum, or vagina. Considering the age and developmental stage of the child, the pediatric health-care team should rule out the presence of a mental health problem. Manual removal of the item is attempted.

Pediatric Vulvovaginitis

Vulvitis, or vulvar inflammation, is often associated with vaginitis from candidiasis (fungal) infections. Young, prepubertal girls lack protective pubic hair and labial fat pads, and are therefore more susceptible to trauma and irritation. Chemicals in many soaps and commonly used bubble-bath substances may also cause irritation and sensitivity to the vulvar skin and tissues.

Labial Adhesions

Labial adhesions may arise from several causes. These include scarring from surgical procedures, complications from female genital mutilation (FGM) practiced in some cultures, insufficient wiping after toileting, and scarring from chemical or thermal burns.

Sexually Transmitted Infections

Infections passed from person to person during intimate genital contact or sexual intercourse are called *STIs*. The adolescent population has the highest risk for acquiring an STI and the

Nursing Care Plan for the Child With Klinefelter Syndrome

During a back-to-school checkup for Jason, age 14, his parents ask the pediatrician why Jason hasn't yet started growing body hair the way the other boys his age have done. The doctor conducts a thorough assessment and notes that Jason is tall for his age, lacks body and facial hair, and has smaller than normal testicles. In addition, Jason looks and acts younger than a typical 14-year-old boy. The doctor says he will need to draw laboratory tests for genetic testing, but that he is fairly certain that Jason has Klinefelter syndrome.

Nursing Diagnosis: Growth and development altered, as evidenced by delayed secondary sex characteristics
Expected Outcome: The patient will develop secondary sex characteristics appropriate to his gender.

Intervention:	Rationale:
Long-acting testosterone therapy will be administered.	*Replacing the absent or low-level male hormones will allow the patient to look more similar to his peers, a high-priority concern for an adolescent.*

Nursing Diagnosis: Risk for ineffective coping related to diagnosis of a genetic difference that affects reproduction
Expected Outcome: The patient and family will communicate their feelings about the diagnosis in a healthy way.

Intervention:	Rationale:
Refer the patient and family to counseling so that they can share their concerns and fears about Jason and his future.	*Both the patient and his family will likely have questions and fears about how his diagnosis will affect his future health and relationships. A counselor can help them verbalize and work through these questions and fears in a healthy way.*

Nursing Diagnosis: Knowledge deficit related to diagnosis of a rare genetic condition
Expected Outcome: The patient and family will verbalize understanding of what Klinefelter syndrome is and what effects it could have on the patient's health.

Intervention:	Rationale:
Teach the family about Klinefelter syndrome and offer them information about organizations such as the American Association for Klinefelter Syndrome Information and Support (AAKSIS).	*Because Klinefelter syndrome is rare, the patient and family will need basic medical information about what it is and what it affects. They will also have many nonmedical questions that would be better answered by other people with the condition.*

highest rates of STIs in the general population. Adolescents who have unprotected sex with an infected individual, are younger than age 15, and who inject drugs are at the highest risk.

Be prepared to ask questions about a teen's health history, sexual history, use of birth control (especially condom use), and the presence of symptoms of STIs. Assessments should be holistic and include a history and a physical examination, including inspection, palpation, and olfaction, and should be conducted with respect and privacy in mind. See Table 3.2 for a list of STIs and their signs and symptoms, diagnosis, and treatment.

Safety *Stat!*

Except for infants who experience maternal-child transmission, an STI diagnosed in a prepubertal child warrants screening for sexual abuse.

Safety *Stat!*

The early identification and treatment of STIs are imperative. If left untreated, some infections can cause scarring of tissues, leading to difficulty becoming pregnant or to infertility.

Safety *Stat!*

It is essential to talk to sexually active teenagers about using condoms correctly to prevent STIs and pregnancy. Teens must understand that condom use lowers the risk of both STI transmission and pregnancy. However, it is not 100% effective at preventing either, and teens need to understand this fact.

Key Points

- The GU system is a complex system composed of the kidneys, ureters, bladder, urethra, and reproductive organs.
- The kidneys have many important functions, including filtering water and solutes from the blood, and reabsorbing needed water, protein, electrolytes, glucose, and amino acids while allowing unwanted or unneeded substances to be excreted as urine.
- The kidneys regulate the acid-base system, which maintains homeostasis. The kidneys further produce and secrete renin and erythropoietin hormones.
- Cardinal signs of a GU system dysfunction include fluid retention, fluid loss, dehydration, and electrolyte disturbances.

- Children can present with acquired GU disorders such as UTI, nephrotic syndrome, and glomerulonephritis; or they can present with complications associated with congenital GU disorders.
- Many congenital GU disorders require meticulous follow-up care and surgeries.
- Your role is to support a team effort in early identification, treatment, and follow-up care needed to assist a family whose child has a GU dysfunction.
- Education is required to prevent infections of the GU system.

Review Questions

1. A young child hospitalized with nephrotic syndrome needs to consume adequate nutrition. The nurse has orders for which type of diet?
   1. Low-sodium, low-protein
   2. High-sodium, high-protein
   3. Low-potassium, low-sodium
   4. Low-sodium, high-protein

2. A teenager admitted with acute kidney injury is depressed and angry over her condition. The nurse spends time with the teen, reinforcing the need for continued social interactions and family support. Which activity would be best for this child?
   1. Playing movies and video games in her room
   2. Attending an arts and crafts program in the playroom
   3. Ambulating the halls of the hospital for mild exercise
   4. Interacting on social media on a laptop in her room

3. Glomerulonephritis is marked by the deposition of immune complexes in the tiny tubules of the kidney. Which situation would contribute to the development of this disease?
   1. A 1-year-old infant with bilateral ear infections
   2. A 3-year-old child, just entering preschool, with high fevers
   3. A 7-year-old with croup
   4. An 11-year-old with vulvitis

4. An infant presents to the urgent care clinic with tachycardia, no tears, sunken fontanels, and a serum sodium level of 139 mEq/L. Which type of dehydration is mostly likely occurring?
   1. Osmotic dehydration
   2. Hypotonic dehydration
   3. Hypertonic dehydration
   4. Isotonic dehydration

5. When reviewing the laboratory findings for a child hospitalized for a third relapse of nephrotic syndrome, which laboratory results would be expected?
   1. Hypoalbuminemia and proteinuria
   2. Proteinuria and hyponatremia
   3. Hypoalbuminemia and hypernatremia
   4. Hypoalbuminemia and negative proteinuria

6. A newborn has been diagnosed with undescended testes. What information does the health-care team need to communicate to the parents at this time?
   1. Surgery is a safe option to bring the testicles down into the scrotal sac.
   2. Manual manipulation, although producing discomfort, is an option.
   3. No interventions are conducted at this time, and the child will be reassessed at 1 year.
   4. During circumcision, the neonatologist can perform a small procedure.

7. A teenage boy is brought into the hospital in severe pain to be tested for testicular torsion. He had been working out in the weight room at his high school. The parents express concern about their son's ability to be fertile after the procedure. What is the best explanation for the health-care team to give the parents?
   1. With a delay in treatment, the son may be infertile because of tissue ischemia.
   2. With prompt surgical correction, the teen should be fertile.
   3. Because of the removal of the testicles during surgery, infertility is an assumption.
   4. Without experiencing a relapse, the teen should remain fertile.

ANSWERS 1. 4; 2. 4; 3. 2; 4. 4; 5. 1; 6. 3; 7. 2

CRITICAL THINKING QUESTIONS

1. An 11-year-old female child presents to the urgent care clinic with a significant perineal rash with itching and the sensation of burning on her labia. She also reports a history of dysuria. Her father states that she bathes in bubble baths every day. What would your health history include? What key examinations would you conduct to further investigate this situation and clinical presentation? How would you conduct them?

2. A mother calls the pediatric telephone-triage line stating that her 8-year-old son has been wetting his bed every night for the last 3 weeks. She is concerned about his social life because he is preparing to attend a 2-week summer camp shortly. What questions would you ask for the history? What follow-up would you recommend, if any?

3. A child is currently admitted for her fourth bout of nephrotic syndrome. What are your nursing care concerns for this child and her family?

Resources

For additional resources and information, including Postconference Questions and Activities, Answers, and References, visit www.FADavis.com.

Student Study Guide

CHAPTER 36
Child With a Skin Condition

KEY TERMS

contactant (kon-TAK-tent)
dermatological (DER-muh-toh-LOJ-ih-kuhl)
exanthem (eg-ZAN-them)
Lund-Browder classification tool (LUHND-BROW-duhr KLAS-ih-fih-KAY-shun TOOL)
macular rash (MAK-yoo-luhr RASH)
papular rash (PAP-yoo-luhr RASH)
poison ivy
poison oak
poisonous sumac (POY-zuhn-uhs SOO-mak)
pustule (PUHSS-tyool)
rule of nines (ROOL uv NYENZ)
urticaria (ER-tih-KAIR-ee-uh)
vesicle (VESS-ih-kuhl)
vitiligo (vit-ih-LYE-goh)
wheal (WEEL)

CHAPTER CONCEPTS

Growth and Development
Infection
Inflammation
Safety
Tissue Integrity

LEARNING OUTCOMES

1. Define the key terms.
2. Review the special needs of a newborn's and young infant's skin.
3. Determine best practices to manage the symptoms of skin disorders across childhood.
4. Differentiate among various rashes common during childhood.
5. Describe the care of children with a first-, second-, or third-degree burn.
6. Describe skin disorders that can be considered evidence of child abuse.
7. Review personal protective equipment (PPE) that should be used to prevent the spread of various childhood skin infections.
8. Discuss the short- and long-term consequences of body piercing and tattooing.
9. Create a teaching plan for new parents to learn how to prevent burns during childhood, including electrical, immersive, contact, and heat burns.

CRITICAL THINKING & CLINICAL JUDGMENT

The father of **Kat**, an 11-month-old infant, brings her to the public health clinic for a "growing, red, wet rash on her elbows and right face in the cheek area." The father tells you that the child has been fussy lately, waking up during the night every 1 to 2 hours in tears, and sweating during long crying episodes. The rash appears to be raised; bright, beefy red; moist in the center; oval shaped in all three locations; and about 3 to 5 cm wide and 5 to 6 cm in length. You observe Kat's discomfort and itching and report it to the health-care team.

Questions

1. Based on Kat's signs and symptoms, what do you suspect is the cause?
2. What can you do in the short term to relieve her discomfort?

CONCEPTUAL CORNERSTONE
Growth and Development

Skin, the largest organ of the body, has particular developmental aspects. Newborns are very susceptible to skin injury, and their skin absorbs medications readily. Infants can experience a variety of rashes, including contact dermatitis and candidiasis. Infants are particularly susceptible to food allergies with a skin component because of their expanding diets during the second 6 months of life. Rashes associated with medications are also common throughout childhood. Toddlers and preschoolers, who are exposed to more social environments, are particularly susceptible to communicable diseases and infections that may have distinct rashes (measles, roseola, skin *Streptococcus* and *Staphylococcus* infections). School-aged children may experience burns from a variety of causes. Adolescents can experience a variety of skin conditions, from infections to burns to acne. Take a developmental approach to providing anticipatory guidance to families concerning skin issues. Prevention of skin breakdown, rashes, infections, and pressure injuries is of primary importance to children across the developmental period if particularly vulnerable. Vulnerable children include those with immobility issues, immunosuppression, malnutrition, poor hygiene, severe developmental delays, and genetic predispositions.

The skin is composed of layers. The epidermis is the tough outer layer of the skin, and the dermis is the highly vascular inner layer that provides support. The skin also includes a layer of subcutaneous fat. The accessory structures of the skin include sebaceous glands that provide sebum for the follicles of the hair, sweat glands that provide thermoregulation, nails for structure and the safety of the fingers, and hair. The skin itself is very sensitive to temperature, touch, pain, and pressure. In addition to defending the body from the invasion of infectious organisms, the skin also protects the underlying tissues, organs, and vasculature from injury. Via pores, the skin helps the body to excrete salt and water. A major function of the skin is to synthesize vitamin D.

Common skin disorders found in childhood are classified as chemical, allergic, or microbial.

Chemical
- Contact with chemicals
- Medication reactions

Allergic
- Food allergies (citrus, strawberries, mango, papayas, wheat, and others)
- Skin allergies to a variety of causes

Microbial
- Fungal skin infections
- Viral skin infections
- Parasitic skin infections (bites, mites)

Rashes (**exanthems**) are very commonly associated with many childhood disorders and infections. Rashes lead to mild, moderate, and severe discomfort with pruritus (itching) and can be caused by a variety of culprits, including allergies, chemicals, and microbes.

If a child's rash is of viral origin, do not give aspirin to the child for symptom management because of the correlation between aspirin and the development of Reye syndrome (see Chapter 27).

Wheals are round, elevated skin lesions, often temporary, that look white in the center and are surrounded by red inflammation. Wheals are often seen with insect bites and urticaria. The pediatric team may have to treat wheals for itching with an antihistamine topical cream or oral or IV antihistamine.

SKIN AND CHILDHOOD

Quality nursing care across the life span begins with excellent skin care in the newborn period. Skin breakdown, no matter the age of the patient, is now one measure by which hospitals evaluate their effectiveness. Tools such as the Braden Q scale allow nurses to check and measure skin integrity. Although older adults are at greater risk for skin breakdown, injury, and delayed healing, pediatric patients can have skin problems, too. Therefore, a complete assessment of all skin surfaces is imperative. In pediatrics, the causes of skin problems may be classified as follows:

- Pressure injuries caused by frictional forces
- Moisture, associated with prolonged exposure to urine and feces
- Childhood activity
- Infectious agents (scabies, fungus, warts [also called molluscum contagiosum or verruca], pediculosis, *Staphylococcus, Streptococcus,* poison oak, poison ivy, poisonous sumac)

Common areas of skin breakdown in adults are the sacrum, heels, and coccyx. In children, skin breakdown is prevalent on the occipital area, nose, buttocks, groin, back, chest, face, and ears.

Skin breakdown is staged by the following descriptions:

- *Stage I:* Nonblanchable erythema with skin intact
- *Stage II:* Partial-thickness tissue loss appearing as a superficial ulcer that involves the layers of the epidermis or dermis, or both
- *Stage III:* Full-thickness tissue loss appearing as a deeper ulcer that involves the subcutaneous tissue and extends down to, but not through, the fascia
- *Stage IV:* Full-thickness tissue loss with damage, destruction, or necrosis of underlying supporting structures, bone, and muscle; extending sinus tracts may be present

Safety *Stat!*

Newborn skin is very thin. All topical medications should be assumed to be absorbed systemically. Apply topical medications exactly as ordered and in a very thin layer.

Neonatal Skin

All newborns should have 100% of their skin inspected shortly after birth for any unusual or common skin conditions or marks. Having this baseline will help the health-care team identify any deviations from the child's normal skin presentation. (For more about skin conditions of the newborn and caring for newborns' skin, see Chapter 15.)

Infant Skin

The skin of young children is more sensitive and thinner than that of older children and adults. Young infants bruise easily, and their skin is more reactive and sensitive to a variety of factors. Because an infant's epidermis is loosely bound to the dermis, the child is susceptible to poor adherence of the tissue layers and has a greater chance of lesions and blisters when the skin is inflamed. Health-care team members should be diligent about interventions to keep the newborn's and infant's skin intact. For example, paper tape should be used rather than adhesive tape, which can cause tears when being removed. Assessment of a child's skin should include the following considerations:

1. Check rashes (Fig. 36.1):
   - *Macular rash:* A flat rash with circumscribed boundaries and color changes
   - *Papular rash:* A raised, solid lesion with circumscribed boundaries and color changes
   - *Vesicle:* A rash with small, raised, clear, fluid-filled lesions with circumscribed boundaries
   - Note the distribution, size, shape, color, warmth, severity of the rash, and whether or not it has exudate
2. Note any discomfort, tenderness, or pruritus. Pruritus can be severe enough to disrupt a child's quality and length of sleep.

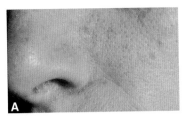
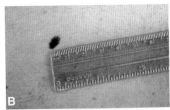
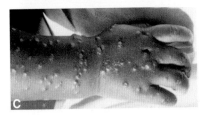

FIGURE 36.1 Lesions associated with various rashes. A, Macule. B, Papule. C, Vesicle.

3. Check for the presence of hives, also called *urticaria*, which commonly accompany symptoms of allergies or allergic reactions.
4. Check the child's hair shafts for evidence of infection, pus, or nits (lice eggs).
5. Ask about the child's recent travel history, family history of skin conditions, and any associated systemic pathologies or illness, such as exposure to communicable diseases.
6. Explore the child's reported history of allergies to topical applications, foods, or environmental substances.
7. Ask about an infant's recent exposure to new foods (citrus, protein, or formula).
8. Explore the child's recent skin exposure to soaps, detergents, lotions, medications, or any other **contactants** (substances that cause an allergic or sensitivity response when exposed to the skin).

SPECIAL CONSIDERATIONS FOR SKIN DISORDERS

Children are vulnerable to a variety of skin disorders and, because of their age, they have special considerations associated with wounds, rashes, and infections. Depending on their age or developmental level, children may have trouble describing their sensations, keeping their hands and fingernails away from a lesion or wound, keeping their hands clean, and preventing the spread of **dermatological** (pertaining to the study of the skin) infections from others. Children need parental assistance to manage rashes, lesions, infections, and their associated symptoms and to prevent their spread.

If a young child has a surgical wound, they will need to have it covered securely to prevent skin irritation or wound damage because of picking or manipulating the dressing, sutures, or staples. Managing wound healing is a nursing responsibility because children will not be able to verbalize the presence of drainage or a change in the appearance or integrity of a wound. Nurses and caregivers must pay special attention to wound management, wound healing, and preventing the spread of infection if the wound becomes contaminated. It's a team effort to keep infants from scratching wounds and toddlers from pulling off dressings.

Aggravation of Skin Disorders

Heat often irritates a rash, producing greater symptoms of discomfort. Most rashes are soothed with the application of cool compresses, cool water baths, or cool water rinses. Do not apply warm packs to a child's lesions during hospitalization unless specifically ordered to do so. Warm packs may be applied to promote healing if the child has an infectious rash such as pustules, cellulitis, or severe urticaria. Contact precautions should be used when caring for children with skin conditions in which warm packs are used.

The symptoms of discomfort associated with severe and persistent itching require nursing interventions. Children

· **WORD** · **BUILDING** ·
dermatological: dermato–skin + logic–study of + al–pertaining to

may benefit from baking soda paste applications, calamine lotion, oatmeal paste applications, or an oral antipruritic such as antihistamines. The child should be offered sources of playful distraction appropriate to their developmental stage. Exposing the site of the discomfort to air may be beneficial. Neither baby powder nor cornstarch should ever be applied to a rash because they may promote fungal or bacterial growth. Many young children experience worsened symptoms when commercially prepared baby wipes are used on sensitive skin because these wipes may contain alcohol.

Preventing scratching takes creative interventions. Young infants may benefit from having their hands covered with clean socks to prevent scratching. Older infants may benefit from the use of pediatric soft full or half arm restraints, sometimes called "no-no's."

Heat Rash

Heat rash, also called "prickly heat" or miliaria, is a non-contagious common phenomenon during childhood. Associated with dressing young children too warmly or exposure to high heat and humidity, this condition causes blocked sweat ducts. Heat rash can happen to children of any age in very hot weather. The blisters are most common on the neck, chest, and shoulders and are itchy or "prickly" in nature. The blocked sweat glands, which lead to the bright red rash, can be treated at home. Common treatments include:

- Oatmeal baths or topical application of an oatmeal paste
- Cold compresses
- Sandalwood powder paste
- Baking soda paste
- Aloe vera application
- Wearing of loose clothes
- Two to three quick cool baths daily
- Avoiding oils or lotions on the skin

Severe cases may require topical treatments of calamine lotion, 1% hydrocortisone, or topical antihistamines.

Safety Stat!

Administering antihistamines to infants and young children can be dangerous. Do not administer oral or topical antihistamines to infants or young children without an order, and double-check medication calculations carefully to make sure that the correct amount is administered. Oral antihistamines can cause severe sedation and death if given in inaccurate doses to infants or small children.

Wound Healing

Normally, the skin provides a protective barrier to the body. When a child develops a lesion or wound, the barrier does not function properly. Healthy children's skin heals rapidly, provided they are well nourished, well hydrated, kept clean, and are given nursing care that promotes healing. Factors that delay wound healing are associated with dry wound bases, nutritional deficiencies, issues with circulation, chronic illnesses, and infection.

- *Dry wound base environments:* The health-care team should take measures to ensure that the base of the child's wound is moist but free of pus or exudates. Dry wound bases delay healing. Wet to dry dressing changes may be required to keep the wound base moist.
- *Nutritional deficiencies:* The health-care team should consult with dietary staff to ensure that the patient is receiving adequate vitamins A, C, and B_1 as well as protein and zinc, all of which contribute to healthy skin and wound healing.
- *Issues with circulation:* Pressure injuries, poor vascular circulation, and smoking can contribute to poor circulation, leading to a reduced supply of oxygen, fluids, and nutrients to the wound site.
- *Chronic illnesses:* Children who have preexisting chronic illnesses such as diabetes, severe anemia, sickle cell disease, or issues with peripheral vascular disease may experience delayed wound healing. Chronic mental health issues, chronic stress, and chronic anxiety may also contribute to delayed wound healing through poor self-care and poor hygiene. Stress hormones negatively influence wound healing.
- *Infection:* Children with wounds are at risk for secondary infections within the primary wound. Fecal contamination and strep or staph infections can all cause a secondary infection. The presence of infection, whether primary or secondary, itself delays wound healing. The presence of pus, microbial invasion, and inflammatory fluids related to the infection all delay the epithelial wound base from healing. Many bacteria release toxins that are damaging to healing tissues, and the presence of bacterial infections can increase moisture that delays healing.
- *Medications:* Some medications, such as immunosuppressants, corticosteroids, chemotherapies, anticoagulants, and NSAIDs, inhibit wound healing (Almadani et al., 2021; Guo et al., 2023).

Medication Facts

Wounds should not be treated with full strength chemicals such as povidone iodine or hydrogen peroxide because these solutions are cytotoxic (preventing new growth of healing tissues) to children's wound healing.

Preventing the Spread of Infection

The health-care team should make a rapid decision about the use of personal protective equipment (PPE) during patient contact. Determine if contact isolation is warranted for anyone exposed to the child's skin, secretions, or personal belongings. It is better and safer to place a child immediately on contact precautions, even before a diagnosis, than to wait and risk exposure of family, visitors, and other health-care team members.

Health Promotion

Hand washing equipment should be accessible to all and signs should be posted to remind staff, families, visitors, and patients to wash hands frequently.

If the child attends day care or school, it is important to determine if the child's skin condition warrants isolation from other children. Most childcare providers have a list of conditions that require the child to stay at home until the rash or infection is considered no longer contagious. For instance, a child who contracts the varicella-zoster virus (chicken pox) will need to stay home until the vesicle skin lesions are completely scabbed over and free of any oozing secretions. Check with the Centers for Disease Control and Prevention (CDC) for information about isolation precautions and care guidelines to prevent the spread of an infectious skin disorder.

Clothing Suggestions During Skin Disorders

Families should be encouraged to dress the child with a skin disorder in loose, comfortably fitting, cotton clothing. Clothing that is too tight or that is made from synthetic materials may intensify the itching and discomfort experienced by the child. Clothing that wicks perspiration and secretions away from the rash or lesions may be helpful. Encourage the family to be careful with soiled clothing and bedding; they should wash it separately from the rest of the family laundry.

 COMMON SKIN DISORDERS

It is very common to encounter children with skin conditions. Children can experience a variety of acquired skin conditions or have a secondary skin infection superimposed on an existing wound. Skin conditions can have developmental influences such as infants in diapers, children new to preschool classrooms with close contact, and school-aged children exposed to *Streptococcus* and *Staphylococcus.*

Nurses must use meticulous precautions when handling children who have communicable skin lesions and infections. While in the health-care environment, children with known infections and those with infections in which the microbe has not yet been identified should be placed on contact precautions (gloves, gown). Families need to be reminded to wash their hands, wear gloves if indicated, and assist the team in preventing the spread of an infectious skin condition to others within the hospital or clinic setting. See Box 36.1 for common medications used for children's skin conditions and Box 36.2 for a list of common skin conditions in childhood, their clinical presentations, and common treatments.

Box 36.1
Pharmacology for Common Pediatric Skin Lesions or Disorders

Topical Applications:
Anesthetics
Antibacterial
Antifungal
Antihistamines
Antipruritics
Antiviral
Tar preparations
Topical steroids (hydrocortisone creams or triamcinolone)
Zinc oxide creams

Oral Medications:
Antibiotics
Antifungals
Antihistamines

Contact Dermatitis: Diaper Rash

Contact dermatitis is a common ailment of young children who are diapered. Contact dermatitis is related to the moist, warm environment inside the diaper. Soaps, detergents, bubble baths, wool, tight clothes or diapers, and clothing dyes can cause this uncomfortable condition. When the child passes stool or urinates in the diaper, the condition is further irritated by the acidity of the excrement or by the formation of ammonia from the urine within the diaper.

Evaluating Contact Dermatitis

Assessments of contact dermatitis include the following (Fig. 36.2):

- Characteristic bright-red maculopapular rash within the area of contact between the skin and diaper
- Contiguous rash boundaries without satellite lesions that are classic for yeast infections
- Weeping of the skin rash
- Irritability or inconsolability of the infant, especially during diaper changes

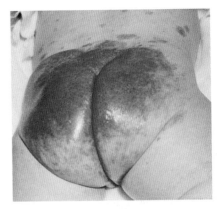

FIGURE 36.2 Infant with contact dermatitis.

Box 36.2

Common Childhood Rashes or Skin Conditions

- *Lyme disease:* This is the most common tick-spread illness in North America and Europe. The organism is spread by deer tick bites and may be difficult to diagnose without a blood test because many children do not display the signs and symptoms of a Lyme disease rash (bulls eye rash). The rash appears in association with fever, joint pains, mild sore throat, and a cough and presents as a target with concentric circles of red next to clear areas.

- *Rocky Mountain spotted fever (RMSF):* RMSF is a rash caused by tick bites where bacteria are harbored in the tick's salivary glands. More common in the southeastern United States than in the Rocky Mountains, this rash appears as blanchable red spots on the wrists and ankles, spreading centrally toward the trunk. Later, the red rash will become raised and will have a nonblanching center.

- *Petechiae:* This is not a rash but rather a collection of small red or purplish flat lesions that do not fade when blanched and are caused by small broken capillaries in the skin. The presence of petechiae is associated with a viral illness or very low platelet levels.

- *Meningococcemia:* This is a life-threatening meningococcal sepsis caused by the bacterial invasion of the blood by *Neisseria meningitidis.* The rash appears as red or purple blotchy areas all over the child's body. Rapid administration of IV antibiotics is required to save the child's life.

- *Kawasaki disease:* This disease usually affects male children under 6 years of age. Without treatment, there can be serious effects on the child's heart. The child appears very ill, has high fevers, red eyes, red tongue (strawberry tongue), cracked lips, and a rash with macules; papules appear very bright on the hands and soles of the feet.

- *Hemangioma:* A type of benign tumor of the skin that presents as a birthmark with a vascular abnormality. Also called a *port wine stain,* a *strawberry hemangioma,* or a *salmon patch,* a hemangioma can be a small single lesion or large, multisite lesion. When an infant is first born, the hemangioma may be invisible or very faint. As the infant grows, the lesion grows rapidly and deepens in color. Over time, the child's lesion may become smaller and fainter. If involution is to take place, it may take several years. Treatment may include steroids, embolization of the blood vessels by the injection of a material that blocks blood flow, laser treatments, or surgical removal. If a child's hemangioma is causing breathing problems, bleeds regularly, impairs vision, or causes growth disturbances, it will require more aggressive medical and/or surgical treatments.

- *Warts:* Caused by the papillomavirus, warts are also known as *verruca.* Warts are typically roundish, elevated, firm papules. Treatment is focused on local destruction with curettage, cryotherapy with liquid nitrogen, or application of a caustic solution. Warts in children can appear suddenly and disappear on their own without treatment.

- *Styes:* A localized infection and swelling of the glands of the eyelid. Styes typically present with inflammation followed by a raised tender lesion that may secrete purulent drainage. Pain, edema, inflammation, and conjunctivitis are common signs and symptoms. Treatment is focused on draining the stye. Warm packs to the area (a clean dressing or small towel must be used each time) several times a day for up to a week might be necessary to clear the stye.

- *Candidiasis:* Very common during infancy and early toddlerhood, *Candida albicans* is a form of yeast (fungus) that causes severe diaper rashes. This fungus causes a bright-red and very uncomfortable rash with satellite lesions and grows readily in warm moist areas such as skinfolds. Cutaneous yeast infections require the application of an antifungal cream until clear.

- *Herpes simplex:* Herpes simplex is divided into two general categories: Type 1 produces "cold sores" in the mouth, whereas Type 2 causes genital lesions (although lesions also can be found on the cornea and face). Symptoms include a tingling, itching, then burning sensation on the skin, followed by an eruption of vesicles most often located directly on mucocutaneous junctions such as the lips, nose, and genitalia. The herpes virus is contagious and is managed, but not cured, with topical, oral, or IV acyclovir.

- *Frostbite:* A term used to denote severe tissue damage from freezing temperature or direct contact with frozen material. Two pathologies occur with frostbite; the intracellular fluids freeze within the tissues, and the cold temperatures cause tissue damage that then blocks the blood supply. The frostbitten tissues are usually numb until treatment is initiated, then the tissue becomes very painful. Treatment includes total body warming, hydration with warm fluids, and immersion of the affected body part in warm to tepid water. In extreme tissue damage, debridement or amputation may be needed.

Interventions for Contact Dermatitis

Interventions for contact dermatitis include keeping the skin under the diaper area clean and dry by changing the diaper immediately after soiling. Wash the skin very gently with a mild soap and water, and apply a layer of vitamins A and D ointment or a zinc oxide–based ointment after cleansing. Expose the skin to air. A severe rash may require the application of topical hydrocortisone 1% creme.

Nursing Considerations for Contact Dermatitis

The health-care team will determine if a child's severe diaper rash is from contact with an allergen or a substance that the child reacts to, or if the rash is yeast (Fig. 36.3).

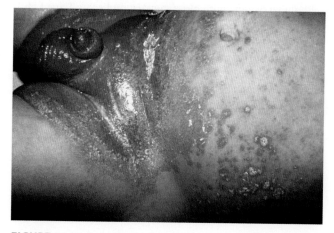

FIGURE 36.3 Infant with the fungal infection candidiasis.

Patient Teaching Guidelines

Preventing and Treating Severe Diaper Rash for Infants and Toddlers

Prevention

1. Thoroughly wash and dry the soiled skin and surrounding area with each diaper change.
2. Change the infant's or toddler's diaper as quickly as possible after soiling.
3. Cleanse the skinfolds, labia, and scrotum carefully after each bowel movement.
4. Apply a thin layer of skin protective ointment such as a zinc oxide–based cream.
5. Remove foods from the diet that have been associated with diaper rash (strawberries; mango; citrus fruits such as oranges, lemons, limes, and grapefruits).
6. Use only cotton diapers or diapers with minimal synthetic material.
7. Use commercial diaper cleansing cloths sparingly because they may contain alcohol or other chemicals that cause drying of the skin. It is best to use a soft washcloth and water.
8. Do not clothe the child in materials that contain aggravating dyes, harsh materials, or chemicals.
9. Use only mild soaps on the skin of young children to prevent chemical rashes.
10. Do not launder the infant's clothes or cloth diapers with highly scented detergents or with fabric softeners because this may irritate skin.

Treatment

1. Promptly begin a regimen of quality skin care, including at least twice-daily washing of the affected area and application of recommended or prescribed medications. Follow medication application instructions carefully to prevent an overdose of topical medications that may be absorbed systemically through an infant's thin skin. Washing with mild soap and water and a soft washcloth allows for all layers of medications, creams, and excrement to be removed completely to enhance skin healing.
2. Allow the affected area to be in open air to help dry and heal the skin.
3. Manage discomfort with acetaminophen or ibuprofen if the child is over 6 months of age. NEVER give a child aspirin.
4. Wash hands thoroughly before and after caring for a child with diaper rash to prevent secondary infections or transmission of the infectious agent to others.
5. Do not use plastic diaper covers; prevent the plastic diaper lining from contacting the rash.
6. Provide foods that increase the stool pH (more alkaline) such as fruits and vegetables and reduce fish, grains, and eggs.

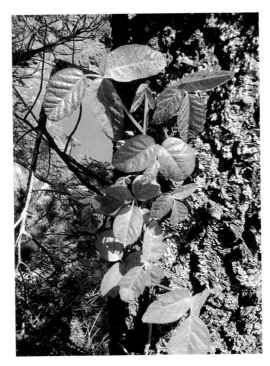

FIGURE 36.4 Poison oak.

Poison Oak, Poison Ivy, and Poisonous Sumac

Children who are exposed to the oily sap of **poison oak, poison ivy,** or **poisonous sumac** can experience a delayed reaction (Fig. 36.4). This reaction is a hypersensitivity response of the immune system by the T cells. If the child has not been exposed previously, the delayed reaction is between 5 and 25 days after exposure. If the child has had a previous exposure, the response is noted within 1 to 2 days. The lesions found on the skin are not the source of cross-contamination or further spread. The inadequate removal of all of the oily sap is what causes more lesions. Animals, especially family dogs, are a source of poison ivy, poison oak, or poisonous sumac sap because they carry the plant's oils to humans and shared environmental surfaces.

CLINICAL JUDGMENT

You are working in an urgent care center and caring for a young child whose father was burning vegetation, including poison ivy, that he had pulled up the day before. During the burn, the child was playing outdoors. The child was exposed to the smoke of the fire and is now having respiratory distress.

Questions

1. Why would playing near burning poison ivy lead to respiratory distress?
2. How should you educate the father to prevent future exposures?

Evaluating Poison Ivy, Poison Oak, and Poisonous Sumac

Poison ivy sap (also called urushiol) causes severe pruritus and itching, localized streaks of redness that extend from the site of exposure, and vesicles that break open and form crusts. Vesicles form in 24 to 72 hours after exposure and are very uncomfortable. If a child also presents with respiratory symptoms, they may have inhaled urushiol smoke from burning leaves and branches. For a child in severe respiratory distress, the family should call 911 or go directly to the emergency department.

Interventions for Poison Ivy, Poison Oak, or Poisonous Sumac

A child who has a significant rash caused by contact with urushiol oil needs treatment to prevent discomfort from constant itching and irritation. Interventions for the rash caused by poison ivy include:

- Washing the skin carefully to remove all plant oils (urushiol oil can stay active for many years in protected areas, such as the underside of a lawn mower; Food and Drug Administration [FDA], 2021)
- Washing the entire surface of the skin and scalp carefully to prevent exposing other skin surfaces or family members to the urushiol oil (Poison ivy does not spread under the skin; only the plant's oil causes and spreads the rash.)
- Preventing the child from touching other body parts until a thorough cleansing has been completed
- Washing the child's clothing or any material the child touched before cleansing
- Thoroughly cleaning car upholstery and seatbelts that may have been exposed to urushiol oil
- Drying the skin carefully and then applying calamine lotion in two or three layers, letting each layer dry between applications
- Administering topical or oral antihistamines if ordered

Nursing Consideration for Poison Ivy, Poison Oak, or Poisonous Sumac

Nurses can be instrumental in teaching the public about poison ivy prevention and treatment. Posting a photograph for the public to view in areas where poison ivy grows and where children play can help identify how the plant leaves look.

Patient Teaching Guidelines

Families need to know that there are actually three plants that produce urushiol oil. Poison oak usually has three-leaf clusters, but some varieties have five, seven, or nine per cluster. It is mostly found in the Southeast or West Coast. Poisonous sumac is a shrub found only in wet climates. All parts of the shrub contain toxic urushiol, not just the leaves. Poison ivy (generally a vine but can be a shrub) has three-leaf clusters.

Families need to know that poison ivy rashes are not contagious, but the oils can be transmitted to others (FDA, 2021).

Cellulitis

Cellulitis is a deep bacterial infection of the skin. Several layers of skin can be affected, including the epidermis, dermis, and connective tissues. A child may present with acute inflammation of the skin associated with a history of recent trauma, puncture wounds, sinusitis, impetigo, or otitis media. The infectious agent causes intense redness because of the enzyme factors that break down the skin's network of fibrin. These factors are an immune response designed to contain the spread of the infection.

Usually found on the face, eye orbit, arms, and legs, cellulitis can begin and spread quite rapidly. The three most common infectious agents are group A beta-hemolytic streptococci, *Streptococcus pneumonia*, and *Staphylococcus aureus*. Some children respond to oral antibiotics at home; those with more extensive infections require hospitalization for IV antibiotic therapy. Complications of cellulitis include meningitis, glomerulonephritis, and septic arthritis.

Evaluating Cellulitis

Assessments of cellulitis include both inspection and palpation. Cellulitis can be superficial, or it can cause a swelling of the affected area. Assessments include the following:

- Warmth, edema, tenderness around the affected site, and pitting edema over the affected site
- Possible presence of red "streaking" lines that extend from the site
- Febrile state and the presentation of appearing ill (headache, chills, weakness)
- Enlarged regional lymph nodes
- Elevated white blood cell (WBC) count
- Risk factors, such as having an immunocompromised state or diabetes

Interventions for Cellulitis

Interventions for cellulitis include the following:

- A broad-spectrum oral antibiotic therapy for 8 to 10 days if cellulitis is contained and the infection is responsive within 2 days of therapy (Oxacillin, sulfamethoxazole, or amoxicillin are commonly used oral antibiotics.)
- IV antibiotic therapy if the cellulitis is extensive or invades structures such as the eye socket with periorbital cellulitis (Nafcillin, dicloxacillin, or ceftriaxone are common IV antibiotics.)
- Warm packs, which can be soothing and can help reduce associated edema
- Nonocclusive dressings, which may be applied if the skin around the area is torn, ruptured, or oozing

Nursing Considerations for Cellulitis

When a child presents with cellulitis, contact precautions should be initiated. Blood cultures may or may not be collected. The severity of the infection, the cause of a puncture wound, and the presence of a fever from an associated systemic infection are indications that a blood culture may be needed.

Eczema

Considered an autoimmune pruritic superficial inflammatory skin disorder, eczema, sometimes called *atopic dermatitis,* is associated with a hereditary allergic tendency. Eczema is part of a trio of conditions called *atopy.* Atopy is a hypersensitivity reaction from immunoglobulin E (IgE)-mediated reactions and is associated with asthma, eczema, and allergic rhinitis (hay fever). Up to 15% of American children have eczema (National Eczema Association, 2023) and the incidence is increasing.

Eczema can present as a reaction to stress, as atopic dermatitis, or as an allergic reaction. Infant eczema appears on the face first with raised, red papules that then spread to the scalp and arms. The characteristic lesions appear raised, red, and with weeping vesicles. The condition is associated with chronic relapsing pruritic lesions and may resolve by the time the child reaches adulthood. Most children with eczema present with severe itching (pruritus), and the majority of diagnoses (80%) occur between infancy and 6 years of life (National Eczema Association, 2023). Commonly, both parents of a child with this disorder have a history of contact dermatitis, asthma, and hay fever. There is no laboratory or diagnostic test for eczema (Fig. 36.5).

Triggers associated with childhood eczema exacerbations include the following:

- Certain foods, such as dairy
- Winter months
- Saliva (such as from teething)
- Allergens, such as dust mites, general dust, pollen, and pet dander
- Dry skin
- Sweating and heat
- Infections

(National Eczema Association, 2019)

Eczema in a toddler appears as intense pruritus with a rash similar to the presentation of eczema in an infant. Some children may have continuous eczema from infancy through toddlerhood, whereas others experience the onset in toddlerhood.

Adolescent eczema often appears as lichenification (large, dry plaques or thickened lesions) typically on the face, neck, back, feet, fingers, toes, and dorsal aspects of the hands.

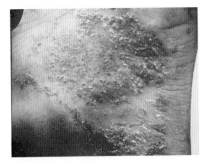

FIGURE 36.5 Child with eczema.

Evaluating Eczema

Observations for eczema include the following:

- The child's history of allergies and atopy (eczema, rhinitis, and asthma together)
- Red, scaling papules and vesicles with layers of crusting with severe itching
- Common warm and moist locations, such as the popliteal and antecubital spaces
- Other common locations, such as the scalp, cheeks, wrists, neck, hands, and groin
- The presence of lichenification, which is indicative of chronic inflammation and which appears as thickened, deep lines
- The presence of sleep disturbances

Children in various ages present with specific eczema symptoms:

- Young infants present with a red and weepy rash on their cheeks, forehead, scalp, and face.
- Older infants present with a red rash or yellow crusted rash on their elbows and knees, as they are learning to crawl and be mobile.
- Toddlers typically have eczema rashes on their elbow and knee folds, ankles, hands, eyelids, and mouth.
- School-aged children may present with eczema on their hands and folds of skin (elbows and knees; National Eczema Association, 2023).

Interventions for Eczema

Treatments and care for a child with eczema need to be individualized for each child. Depending on the developmental level of the child, treatments will be implemented to decrease itching, provide symptom management, prevent infections, and minimize exacerbations. Overall, treatments include:

- Preventing secondary infections from persistent scratching and the resulting introduction of bacteria; keeping the child's fingernails trimmed short
- Showering or bathing after sweating and then immediately applying a thin layer of over-the-counter (OTC) emollient cream or lotion that is dye-free and without perfume or fragrance
- Avoiding bubble bath concentrations or bath oils
- Applying a thin layer of steroid creams to the affected areas
- Applying or administering immunomodulators as ordered (topical cyclosporin, methotrexate, interferon gamma, leukotriene inhibitors, or IV immunoglobulins)
- Avoiding contact with wool, synthetics, or any fabrics that cause sweating and further itching
- Avoiding harsh or highly scented detergents and soaps or lotions
- Avoiding wearing tight or constrictive clothing
- Preventing access to the rash (The child should not be able to lick, chew, or scratch the inflamed tissues. Soft gauze wraps may be needed to prevent the child from having access to the afflicted areas.)

- Never scrubbing the inflamed site or washing in hot water; washing with warm water at least once daily and patting dry

In eczema resistant to these treatments, phototherapy (broadband ultraviolet B [BB-UVB] waves) may be used (American Academy of Dermatology, 2024).

Nursing Considerations for Eczema

Families will need teaching concerning the care of a young child with eczema. Education must include the prevention of skin scarring at the affected site by preventing secondary infections. The family should try to identify if any foods cause exacerbations of their child's eczema and avoid any known allergens. Common allergens are pets, environmental allergens, and contact allergens. The family should be taught to avoid prolonged sun exposure and to apply sunscreen to prevent sunburns, which will highly irritate the site. Oral antihistamines and anti-inflammatory medications may be required if the pruritus is so intense that the child is experiencing sleep deprivation.

Safety Stat!

Families interested in trying alternative or OTC eczema treatments should speak to a dermatologist before applying any of these to their children's skin. Some OTC "cures" have been shown to be toxic to infants and young children. These products are not regulated by the FDA. Alternative treatments that remove healthy foods from young children's diets are not based on empirical research. These, too, should be discussed with a professional before implementing.

Thrush

Thrush is caused by the yeastlike fungus *Candida albicans,* which is normally found in the vagina and the gastrointestinal tract and along the entire surface of the skin. The fungus proliferates in warm, moist areas and is common along the skinfolds of obese persons. Thrush can also develop when a child is on oral antibiotic therapy. Chronic conditions such as hyperglycemia can also predispose a child to a *C. albicans* infection.

Evaluating Thrush

Assessments include the following:

- Reports signs of itching, burning, and irritation
- White plaques along the inside of the mouth with a bright-red surface underlying the white patches
- Red and moist skin lesions that often present in characteristic "satellite" lesions, especially found in the perineum area, and that extend away from the center of the large fungal lesion

Interventions for Thrush

Interventions for thrush should be started immediately upon identifying the classic symptoms of a skin or mouth yeast infection so that treatment can be started before the infection spreads. Interventions for infections with *C. albicans* include the following:

- Topical application of a thin layer of antifungal cream on the skin
- A second application of antifungal cream with a healing skin ointment (Aquaphor, Desitin) to the lesions to prevent body secretions from contributing further to the inflammation
- Administration of oral antifungal suspensions if the child presents with oral thrush
- Cool water or Burow solution soaks with clean, soft, cotton cloths
- Loose-fitting cotton clothing
- Exposing the lesions to air

Nursing Considerations for Thrush

Many children with significant oral thrush have a change in their sense of taste. Some children will not want to eat during a thrush infection, and the medication may take a few to several days to treat the infection. Warning families of this potential side effect of the infection and discussing possible alternative food choices, such as fruit smoothies, may be of assistance.

Cutaneous Fungal Infections: Ringworm

The term *tina* refers to a cutaneous (skin) infection with a fungus. A skin infection with fungus is very common in school-aged children and is acquired through close personal contact and, on occasion, contact with infected pets. The term *ringworm* can be very misleading to families because cutaneous ringworm infections are not caused by "worms" (Fig. 36.6).

There are several types of ringworm infections named according to the location of the infection:

- Tinea capitis involves the scalp and hair.
- Tinea pedis is the medical name of athlete's foot.
- Tinea unguium is a fingernail or toenail fungal infection.
- Tinea cruris is "jock itch," a common and noncontagious fungal infection in young athletes.

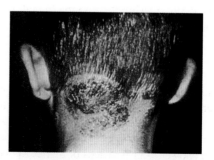

FIGURE 36.6 Child with ringworm.

- Tinea corporis is a fungal infection involving the groin, extremities, and trunk.
- Tinea versicolor is a fungal infection of the skin, characterized by darker and lighter varied patches on the child's back or chest, which causes uneven tanning. This condition is most commonly found in adolescence.

Evaluating Cutaneous Fungal Infections

Assessments for cutaneous fungal infections include the following:

- *Tinea capitis:* Patchy hair loss with an area of scaling on the scalp
- *Tinea pedis:* Intense itching between the child's toes with a characteristic erythematous rash that may include painful fissures that weep
- *Tinea cruris:* After sweating, itching in the child's groin skinfolds with a characteristic red rash
- *Tinea corporis:* Cutaneous lesions that are ring-shaped and can be found as one lesion or many; characteristics are annular, scaling, erythematous, sharply marginated, indurated lesions with hyperkeratotic borders. The center of the ring may be clear or pink, and the ring of the rash may consist of vesicles.

Interventions for Cutaneous Fungal Infections

Interventions for the various cutaneous fungal infections include the following:

- *Tinea capitis:* Applying a thin layer of topical antifungal medication as ordered, using antifungal shampoos, and cleaning all potentially contaminated home and personal objects to prevent reinfection
- *Tinea pedis:* Applying a thin layer of topical antifungal medication as ordered, antifungal powder, or antifungal spray to feet and between toes; having the child wear sandals in locker rooms and public showers
- *Tinea cruris:* Applying a thin layer of topical antifungal medication as ordered to the affected area, changing underwear frequently when sweaty, and showering immediately after exercise. Advise patients or the patients' parents not to store damp athletic clothes in a gym bag for any length of time because it contributes to fungal growth.
- *Tinea corporis:* Applying a thin layer of topical antifungal medication as ordered to both the lesion and the skin around the circular lesion because the fungal infection spreads outward from the angular shape

Nursing Considerations for Cutaneous Fungus Infections

Adolescents who participate in sports where pads or helmets are worn are at an increased risk for fungal infections. This age group should receive written information about how to cleanse sports pads on a regular basis and should be encouraged to shower after practices or games to decrease the chance of contamination or transmission.

Scabies

When a child presents with severe itching and characteristic red lines with bright-red patchy lesions, scabies must be suspected. Very contagious, a scabies infestation is acquired by having close body/skin contact with an infested individual. Scabies mites are tiny insects that burrow deeply into the skin; females lay their eggs along the burrowing tract. Males die after mating. Females lay approximately one to three eggs per day, and the eggs hatch every 30 days. After hatching, the larvae travel to the skin surface. Intense itching occurs because of movement, mite secretions, ova, and feces. The incubation period is considered 1 to 2 months after contact with an infested person.

Evaluating Scabies

Assessments of a scabies infestation include identifying classic clinical signs of red streaks where the mite burrows superficially under the skin and lays her eggs as well as severe itching. Specific assessments for a scabies infestation include the following:

- Intense itching that becomes worse at night, often interrupting a child's healthy sleeping pattern
- Skin "burrows" that appear linear, *S*-shaped, or curved and that run along the superficial skin on the extremities, neck, legs, or trunk with a characteristic rash of macules, papules, and bright-red erythema (may be 1 to 10 cm in length; Fig. 36.7)
- Rashes that intensify between the child's fingers, wrists, buttocks, knees, elbows, and genitals
- The presence of rash and "burrows" on other members of the family
- Skin scrapings from burrow tract marks that reveal mites, ova, and feces under microscopic evaluation

Interventions for Scabies Infestation

Interventions for a scabies infestation include treating the child and possibly other family members and cleaning the surfaces and bedding that the child comes in contact with. Treatment for scabies includes the following:

- Apply a thin layer of scabicide, such as permethrin cream; it is washed off after 8 to 10 hours (follow the instructions on the medication's package insert).
- The child may require scabicide to be applied on the entire body from the chin down to between the toes.
- The entire family may require treatment: Each member must have skin surfaces assessed, or the infestation will continue within the family.

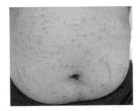

FIGURE 36.7 Classic rash on the abdomen caused by scabies.

Nursing Considerations for Scabies

Although treatments are essential to rid a child of scabies, treatment must include the environment where the child lives and plays. The following guidelines should be discussed with the family to stress the importance of treating the child's living surroundings:

- Washing all clothing, linen, and blankets in a hot water cycle; washing sheets and clothes daily until all family members are free of mite infestation
- Vacuuming furniture, floors, carpets, and car interiors carefully
- Storing nonwashable items in a tightly closed plastic bag for 3 to 4 weeks
- Notifying the child's school about infestation and following the school district's requirements
- Understanding that the characteristic red burrow lesions may be present for 2 to 3 weeks after treatment as the epidermis heals
- Teaching the family that poor hygiene or unsanitary living conditions are not associated with a scabies infestation
- Teaching the family not to share clothing, towels, bedding, or any personal hygiene items

Impetigo

Impetigo should be considered when a child develops a superficial infection of the skin that appears most commonly on the face and extremities and is often demonstrated as round, oozing lesions (Fig. 36.8). Impetigo is a highly contagious superficial rash caused most commonly by group A beta-hemolytic streptococci. When an infection is identified as being caused by the microbe *S. aureus*, it is often called *bullous impetigo*. The bacteria are usually carried in the child's nares and are passed between children by contact with sporting equipment, shared toiletries, toys, towels, or books. Impetigo accounts for more than 10% of all childhood rashes. The lesions can be spread over the body by the child's scratching and passing the bacteria on their infected fingernails and hands. This infection is very common in the toddler and preschool period.

Evaluating Impetigo

Differentiating one rash from another can be a challenge for the pediatric health-care team. Some lesions, such as impetigo, can mimic other infections. Assessment of impetigo includes the following:

- Macular rash that progresses to a papular rash and then to a vesicular rash, followed by a **pustule** (a small, raised skin lesion protruding above the skin line and filled with pus)
- Vesicles that rupture and ooze a honey-colored liquid
- Oozing lesions that are topped by honey-colored crusts
- Mild regional swollen lymph nodes
- Feeling of burning and itching
- History of exposure to biting and stinging insects
- Others in the house affected with similar rashes

Interventions for Impetigo

Medication therapy includes topical and/or oral antibiotics. Common topical antibiotics include bacitracin ointment or mupirocin ointment. Oral antibiotic therapy can include cephalosporins or erythromycin. The full course of antibiotics must be completed. After 48 hours of antibiotic therapy, the child is no longer considered contagious and, if approved, may return to school or day care.

Nursing Considerations for Impetigo

Nursing considerations for impetigo include soaking the lesions and then gently washing the site with warm compresses to remove the layers of crusts. The compresses or cloths should be immediately washed or discarded to prevent the spread of the bacteria to others. The child's nails should be cut short. Young children may need to have their hands covered to prevent scratching or digging at the lesions. If possible, lesions should be covered to prevent

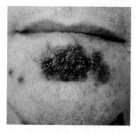

FIGURE 36.8 Teenager with impetigo.

the spread of bacteria. All members of the family should use separate linens, towels, and washcloths. Good hand washing techniques will reduce the chance of spreading the bacterial infection.

Labs & Diagnostics

Diagnostic Tests for Skin Disorders

- *Skin biopsies:* An invasive procedure that can produce discomfort, a skin biopsy is performed to obtain a small quantity of tissue for analysis. Because of the invasive nature of a skin biopsy, informed consent must be obtained from the parent or legal guardian before the procedure is performed. It is best to obtain a skin sample in the treatment room; the discomfort potential should prevent the procedure from occurring in the child's bed (safety zone). Request an order for a topical anesthetic before the procedure and apply within a time frame that allows for a maximal anesthetic property.
- *Skin scraping:* A noninvasive procedure in which a sterile instrument or applicator is used to obtain epithelial cells for microscopic examination within a laboratory
- *Skin cultures:* A noninvasive diagnostic procedure using a sterile applicator to identify the presence and type of bacteria, fungus, or virus within a lesion. This should be performed with a gentle swiping gesture and quickly capped off and sent to the laboratory to prevent cross-contamination. Adhere to institutional policy because some culture applicators have color-coded designations for viral (may be green) versus bacterial (may be red) samples.

Lice

Lice infestations are common during childhood. Lice are highly communicable parasites that are spread via combs, brushes, linens, coats, hooded jackets, play clothes, and hats. Lice can infest a couch, a bed, or car upholstery and therefore pose a communicable risk to others quite readily.

Lice do not fly or jump; rather, they need direct contact with another head of hair. The adult female louse lays her eggs at the very base of the hair shaft and secures each egg sac, or nit, onto the base of the hair shaft. Only via direct contact does the adult louse leave the primary host and infest a new host.

The adult female louse can lay hundreds of eggs during her 30-day lifetime. Adult lice live for only 48 hours away from a host on which to feed. The adult louse has six legs and ranges in color from tan to black. The nits hatch every 10 to 14 days and can stay alive for 8 to 10 days away from a host. Lice are considered parasites because they feed on human blood. As a child scratches their scalp intensely, scabs form, which attract the feeding lice.

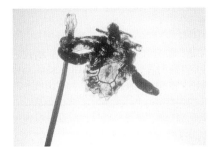

FIGURE 36.9 Adult louse and nit on a child's hair shaft.

Symptoms of a lice infestation are intense itching from three sources: the crawling behaviors, feeding behaviors, and waste products of adult lice. When a child demonstrates intense itching of the head, lice should be suspected (Fig. 36.9).

Evaluating Lice

Assessments of lice infestation include looking carefully for nits, empty egg sacs, and live adults on the move in several places on the child's scalp. Assessments should include the following:

- The presence of adult lice in the hair that may demonstrate rapid movement during assessment
- The presence of nits in the child's hair, which are typically 1 to 2 mm in diameter
- How long the child has been infested, which is determined by the distance between the scalp and the nits (Adult female lice lay their eggs next to the scalp so that the newly hatched larvae can begin to eat immediately. The farther away the nit is from the scalp, the longer the child has been infested.)
- The severity of the symptoms associated with the lice infestation
- The emotional effect of the infestation on the child's well-being

Interventions for Lice

The treatment for lice is threefold:

1. The hair must be treated with a pediculicide.
2. Each nit (egg sac) must be removed meticulously, one by one, with great care and patience.
3. The child's environment must be treated. Combs and brushes must be replaced or washed with hot water. Linens and clothes also must be washed in hot water. Car upholstery must be treated, and carpets must be thoroughly vacuumed. All stuffed toys and items that cannot be washed must be placed in a tightly sealed plastic bag for 2 weeks to make sure that the nits die.
4. The child's school or day care should be notified concerning the presence of lice.

Nursing Considerations for Lice

Because lice infestations are so common during childhood, there is plenty of opportunity to influence the education and knowledge of families, schools, and other institutions that children attend. Classrooms should not have coat racks where multiple clothes are hung on top of each other, and children need to be reminded not to share hats or hooded jackets. Children should have personal items kept in separate compartments, such as plastic tubs with lids that are marked with each child's name. Children must be reminded that although they want to share personal items with their friends, they should not do so to prevent lice infestations.

Acne

Because of increased hormones and sebaceous gland activity, adolescents are especially at risk for acne, a skin condition associated with clogged pores. The increased circulation of androgens in both sexes is the main cause of acne during teenage years. Normal bacteria found on the skin can contribute to the development of acne as the bacteria break down fatty acids and leave waste products. Most teenagers experience some degree of acne, and some cases are quite severe, requiring special skin care and medical treatment. A severe case of acne is called *acne vulgaris*.

The pathophysiology of acne involves the clogging of the narrow channel of the sebaceous gland with sebum at the base of a hair follicle. The trapped sebum is a medium for bacterial growth. As the bacteria multiply, the hair follicles

Nursing Care Plan for the Child With Head Lice

A mother brings her 3-year-old son straight to the pediatric clinic from his day care. She tells you that the day-care provider found lice on one of the children and now all the children must be checked. On observation, the 3-year-old is vigorously scratching the sides of his head behind his ears. After donning gloves, you part the child's hair, discover lice nits at the base of several hair shafts, and point these out to the mother. The mother is visibly upset and states, "We are clean people. Only dirty people have lice!"

Nursing Diagnoses: Risk for impaired skin integrity related to scratching, risk for infection related to scratching, risk for ineffective individual coping (mother), knowledge deficit as evidenced by mother's statement that "only dirty people have lice"

Expected Outcomes: The patient will be free from active lice infestation and will avoid skin infections. The patient's mother will verbalize understanding of lice transmission and list ways to prevent future reinfestation.

Intervention:	Rationale:
Teach the mother how to use OTC pediculicide shampoo and to use a nit comb to remove lice and nits from hair.	*Some pediculicide shampoos kill only adult lice and nymphs, so nits (eggs) must be manually removed.*
Observe skin for signs of infection. Ensure patient's nails are trimmed and clean.	*Vigorous scratching can excoriate skin and lead to skin infections. Scratching to relieve itching is a normal response and often is done during sleep. Make sure that nails are trimmed and clean to reduce likelihood of infection.*
Address the mother's emotional distress.	*Reassure the mother that anyone can have lice and provide guidance on how to cope. Try to help her view the situation as a medical condition and avoid scolding or punishing the child.*
Provide education for the patient's mother on ways to completely treat the infestation.	*The caregiver must understand that treatment of head lice is a multifaceted process that takes time and effort including:* • *Reapplying pediculicide shampoo within 7 to 10 days to ensure that all newly hatched lice and nymphs have been removed* • *Washing the child's bed linens, towels, and clothes separately in hot water* • *Vacuuming carpets, rugs, furniture, and mattresses to remove lice that may be hiding there* • *Sealing items that cannot be washed, such as toys or stuffed animals, in a plastic bag for 2 weeks to kill any remaining lice or nymphs*

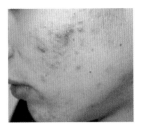

FIGURE 36.10 Teenage boy with comedones.

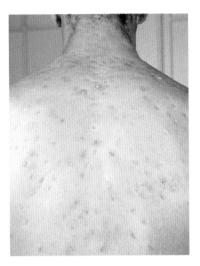

FIGURE 36.11 Teenager with inflammatory acne with pustules.

become infected; they expand into comedones (classic white pimples). Noninflammatory blackheads (open comedones) are also common and are caused by the comedo (the singular of *comedones*) being exposed to air; the color changes as the trapped material oxidizes.

Common bacteria associated with acne include *Propionibacterium acnes* and *Staphylococcus epidermidis*.

Evaluating Acne

Assessment of acne includes noting the presence of clogged pores as well as comedones (Figs. 36.10 and 36.11). It is important to look for physical scarring and to determine the emotional effects of the child's or teen's acne on their self-esteem and self-perception.

Interventions for Acne

Care for a child with acne should begin with an honest conversation about how the child currently cares for their skin followed by teaching of an appropriate skin care regimen. Good skin care and OTC topical medications that contain benzoyl peroxide and/or salicylic acid may be sufficient to treat mild acne. Otherwise, a health-care provider may prescribe oral antibiotics or other medications.

Nursing Considerations for Acne

Teenagers need to be reminded that acne is not caused by greasy foods or chocolate, emotions, or poor hygiene. Certain

lanolin-based face and body products, excessive sweating, menstrual cycles, and unclean athletic or safety helmets can all exacerbate an existing acne condition.

Medication Facts

If isotretinoin is ordered for a teenage girl with severe acne, you and the patient need to have a serious conversation about pregnancy and birth control. Whereas isotretinoin is a very effective treatment for acne, it is also highly teratogenic; that is, it causes severe birth defects in a developing fetus. In fact, most health-care providers routinely require female patients to have a negative pregnancy test before starting isotretinoin. A sexually active teenage girl must be taught to use two methods of birth control for no less than 1 month before treatment begins to no less than 1 month after treatment is complete.

Patient Teaching Guidelines

Skin Care for the Teenager With Acne

1. Wash the face twice a day with a mild soap and warm, not hot, water.
2. During a severe flare-up, use a cleansing product that contains 2% salicylic acid.
3. Do not reuse washcloths; use a clean cloth for each wash to prevent the spread of bacteria.
4. Dry the face gently and carefully.
5. Apply a thin layer of an antiacne cream, such as topical benzoyl peroxide.
6. Apply a very warm cloth to a pimple that is full of pus to promote drainage.
7. Keep hands away from the face. Never "pop" or squeeze either closed or open comedones because this can cause inflammation, infection, and scarring.
8. Consult a health-care provider for oral antibiotics or other medications if there is no improvement after 2 months of following a strict daily skin care routine.

Vitiligo

Vitiligo is a condition of depigmentation, or loss of natural skin color, that has no known cause (Fig. 36.12). This condition is found worldwide at a rate of 0.1% to 2% of the population and is characterized by a progressive, acquired absence of melanocytes in the skin. Vitiligo may cause significant disfigurement and emotional distress. Not only can the skin become affected, but the hair may become white, and eye color may be lost. The condition may affect the inside of the mouth and nose and the genitals. Most children, teens, and adults with vitiligo report having no symptoms other than pigment loss, whereas a few report itching and

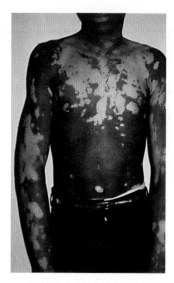

FIGURE 36.12 A young man with vitiligo.

slight pain. Segmental vitiligo affects only one segment of the body, such as one arm, leg, or section of the face, and stops after a year or so of progression. Nonsegmental vitiligo is more common, appears on both sides of the body, and progresses with expansion of pigment loss throughout one's life (American Academy of Dermatology, 2022).

Although there is no cure, nurses caring for children and teens with vitiligo should provide families with information on current treatments and cosmetic enhancements, if children are experiencing emotional distress. Narrowband ultraviolet B monotherapy, immunosuppressants, topical steroids, and cosmetic camouflage may provide help with the condition. Surgical procedures for vitiligo are still under study and include blister roof grafting; cultured and noncultured cellular transplantation; and, most effective thus far, split thickness skin grafts (Mulekar & Isedeh, 2013). Repigmentation by noncultured epidermal melanocyte cell grafting procedures has been successful with more than 68% improvement (Rodrigues et al., 2017) and clinical trials continue investigating cell-to-cell networks between melanocytes, keratinocytes, and immune cells that impact the inflammation and reduced repigmentation caused by vitiligo (University of California Irvine [UCI] School of Medicine, 2022).

Childhood Burns

Burns are a very real threat to children, being the fifth most common cause of childhood accidental death (Johns Hopkins Medicine, 2023a). Burn injuries can range from very mild redness and tenderness to massive tissue injury that causes life-threatening complications. The majority of children hospitalized under 4 years of age are admitted for burns, with 75% of these cases being preventable (Johns Hopkins Medicine, 2023a).

Because most burns occur in children younger than 5 years old, parents need to evaluate the home environment for potential sources of burns. Water heaters must be set at or below 48.9°C (120°F); matches, lighters, and candles should be placed out of children's reach; front burners on the stovetop should not be used; hot outdoor grills and barbecue equipment must be kept out of reach; and flammable chemicals and liquids should be stored in locked cabinets.

Childhood burns may be accidental or may be the result of intentional child abuse. Glove or sock burns, cigarette burns, or burns associated with a hot object are indications of child abuse (see Fig. 26.1). Glove or sock burns are immersion burns, which occur when a child's hand or foot is held in very hot water, leaving a burn mark where a sock or glove would be worn.

Burns can be classified into five categories:

Electrical: Burns caused by electrical currents passing through the body; extent depends on strength and duration of current

Thermal: Burns caused by contact, such as from hot metal in ovens or scalding hot water (also called heat burns)

Chemical: Burns caused by exposure to highly caustic chemicals, such as battery acids

Radioactive: Burns caused by ionizing radiation or exposure to prolonged fluoroscopy procedures

Immersive: Burns associated with a body part immersed in scalding hot water. Hot water causes third-degree (also called full-thickness) burns in:

- 1 sec at 68.9°C (156°F)
- 2 sec at 65°C (149°F)
- 5 sec at 60°C (140°F)
- 15 sec at 56.1°C (133°F)

(Burn Foundation of America, 2015; Toon et al., 2011)

Evaluating Childhood Burns

When a child is burned, the health-care team determines the percentage of the body burned using a scale such as the **rule of nines** (an assessment tool that estimates the extent of a burn, used in late adolescence and adulthood) or the **Lund-Browder classification tool** (an assessment tool that estimates the percentage of body surface area [BSA] burned; Fig. 36.13). Assessment tools have proven to be effective in accurately determining the size and severity of a child's burn. The final percentage is then used to calculate the child's fluid resuscitation needs and the subsequent wound interventions necessary to promote healing. Minor burns are partial- or full-thickness burns that extend to less than 10% of the child's total BSA. Major burns are full-thickness burns that constitute greater than 10% of the child's BSA, that involve the respiratory tract, and/or that include associated fractures or soft-tissue injuries.

Evaluation of burns includes using a classification system that addresses both the depth and the degree of the burn (Table 36.1). Box 36.3 provides the most common nursing diagnoses for children with burns.

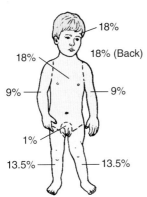

18%

18% (Back)

18%

9%   9%

1%

13.5%   13.5%

Percentages in a Child

FIGURE 36.13 The modified rule of nines: BSA chart for estimating the percentage of the body burned.

Table 36.1

Classifications of Burns

Burn Degree	Signs and Symptoms
First-degree burn (partial-thickness burn)	• Affects the epidermal layer only • Painful, dry, edematous skin appearing red • Appears as a sunburn; skin will peel off within 5 to 10 days • Damaged tissue heals within 3 to 7 days without evidence of scarring
Second-degree burn (partial-thickness burn)	• Extends through the epidermis into the dermis • Edematous with weeping of moisture • Very painful • Heals at various speeds depending on size and location • May require grafting
Third-degree burn (full-thickness burn)	• Extends through the epidermis, dermis, subcutaneous fat, and structures • Leathery dead tissue appears dry and pale • Does not blanch because it is avascular • Most without pain • Heals at various speeds depending on size, complications, secondary infections, and grafting success
Fourth-degree burn (full-thickness burn)	• Extends below the dermis and underlying structures to or through the bone

Team Works

A team approach is needed to provide a thorough assessment of a child who has experienced a burn.

1. Start with the child's airway and proceed through the steps of cardiopulmonary resuscitation (CPR) as needed.
2. Inspect the child's lips and mouth for evidence of soot and smoke. Heat and smoke can cause serious upper and lower airway damage. The child may need supplemental oxygen, airway support, and even intubation. A child with a significant burn or smoke exposure may have rapid pulmonary edema.
3. Evaluate the child for symptoms of shock.
4. Evaluate the child for **hypovolemia**.
5. Determine the child's level of pain.
6. Evaluate for a fluid shift from intravascular to interstitial compartments, and check for wound weeping.
7. Evaluate for renal function and urine output.
8. Determine the level of consciousness (LOC).
9. Evaluate for infection at a burn site after the first 24 hours, which is when infectious organisms have had time to multiply and invade wounds.

Patient Teaching Guidelines

Each developmental stage and associated age range has a type of burn associated with it. Give parents anticipatory guidance and share burn-prevention strategies.

Infants: Sunburns, hot liquids spilled on the skin, standing infants pulling down hot cups of liquid, and death by home fires. Always test foods and fluids for level of heat before giving them to a child. Never hold an infant while drinking hot liquids.

Toddlers: Contact with hot liquids, hot water in baths, pulling down hot pans or pots of liquid on the stove, and

Continued

• WORD • BUILDING •

hypovolemia: hypo–deficient, decreased + vol–volume + em–blood + ia–condition

Patient Teaching Guidelines—cont'd

electrical burns. Keep pot and pan handles turned to the back of the stove. Keep toddlers out of the "traffic pattern" in kitchens to prevent spilling hot liquids while they play.

Preschoolers: Same items as toddlers, plus playing with matches.

School-aged children: Experimenting with fire, chemical burns, electrical burns, and firecrackers. Teach school-aged children how to cook only when they are developmentally ready.

Adolescents: Experimenting with fire, fireworks, or electricity.

Most burns that occur with boys take place outside, and most burns with girls take place within the home. Scalding burns are the number one cause of burns in children and account for 17% of burn hospitalizations (CDC, 2016).

Interventions for Childhood Burns

Stop the burning process by removing the source of the burn. Care for a burn wound by applying cool water (never ice because this may damage tissues further) and/or applying a cool, moist, clean cloth to prevent heat loss. Apply topical medications to promote healing and provide protection (bacitracin ointment or mafenide cream). Elevate the burned body part and administer medication as needed for pain.

Treatment for burns includes an immediate stabilization of the child with special consideration to the child's airway and ventilation, fluid status, prevention of infection, and symptoms. With exposure to smoke and heat, the child's airway may be significantly compromised, which requires CPR. Immediate and longer-term treatment needs include the following:

1. Start by providing immediate CPR, using techniques from the American Heart Association, including an age-appropriate CAB (compressions, airway, breathing) technique; maintain a patent airway following CPR and Pediatric Advanced Life Support (PALS) as needed.
2. Stop the burning process by removing the source of the burn.
3. Treat shock through fluid resuscitation therapy.
4. Use sterile technique at all times.
5. Relieve pain, including using morphine for major burns.

Health Promotion

Preventing Sunburn in Children

Children are exposed to a large amount of sun. In fact, 80% to 90% of total lifetime sun damage occurs before a person's 18th birthday (Cleveland Clinic, 2023; DermRF, 2015).

Repeated sunburns that blister the skin place a child at greater risk later in life for the development of the aggressive skin cancer *melanoma*. Repeated sun exposure also places that child at risk for damage of the cornea. *The sun emits three types of ultraviolet (UV) rays:*

1. UVA causes damage to the connective tissues and is the greatest risk for the development of skin cancer.
2. UVB penetrates the child's skin less deeply.
3. UVC does not cause increased risk because it is absorbed by the atmosphere (Johns Hopkins Medicine, 2023b).

Parents and caregivers must be educated about the need to protect a child's skin. Lifelong skin protection should be encouraged. From late preschool on, the young child should be encouraged to take part in their skin protection.

- Avoid sun exposure between 10 a.m. and 4 p.m.
- Wear protective clothing and a wide-brimmed hat. Adopt the "no hat, no play" rule for outdoor play (Jindal et al., 2020).
- Wear sunscreen with at least a 30 SPF and reapply after swimming, exercising, and sweating.
- Do not allow an infant younger than 1 year of age to have any significant sun exposure.
- Do not apply sunscreen to infants younger than 6 months of age; their skin is thin, and the chemicals in sunscreen are readily absorbed.
- Children with pale skin are at greater risk of sun damage and require more protection.

Nursing Considerations for Childhood Burns

The most important nursing consideration for burns is prevention. Prevention must be focused on providing information about the cause of burns for each developmental period. Anticipatory guidance for each developmental period must include family education on burn prevention.

Patient Teaching Guidelines

Preventing and Treating Minor Burns
Burn Prevention
Infants:

- Do not drink hot liquids around an infant, especially if holding an infant.
- Test the temperature of baby foods that have been microwaved before offering them to an infant.
- Do not microwave formula or breast milk; use a hot water bath or bottle warmer away from the child.
- Do not apply hot packs to an infant's skin because this is a source of significant burns.
- Test the temperature of a bath before placing the infant into the water.

Continued

Patient Teaching Guidelines—cont'd

Toddlers:

- Set water heaters to 48.9°C (120°F) or less.
- Test all bath water before allowing the child to climb into it.
- Do not allow toddlers around the stove, oven, or outdoor grill when cooking.
- Do not use front burners on the stove and turn pan handles away from the front of the stove.

Preschoolers:

- Keep all matches and lighters away from young children.
- Do not allow preschoolers to help light fires or candles.
- Keep burning candles out of reach of preschoolers.
- Do not allow a preschool child to cook unsupervised.
- Teach preschoolers burn-prevention safety through developmentally appropriate play.
- Lock up all flammable chemicals and liquids.
- Clean the garage frequently, disposing of soiled rags exposed to flammable substances.

School-Aged Children:

- Communicate family rules around burn prevention and frequently reinforce fire safety.
- Do not allow a school-aged child to cook unsupervised.
- Include the child in home fire-safety inspections, such as having the child check the batteries in smoke detectors.
- Never allow children to use firecrackers or fireworks without direct adult involvement, guidance, and constant supervision.

Adolescents:

- Teach teens regarding safety concerns around flammable chemicals and liquids.
- Teach teens about fire safety around cars and gas stations.
- Give positive reinforcement for safe behaviors.

Treatment of Minor Burns

- Prevent further burning. Take the child out of the sun and prevent subsequent sun exposure until fully healed.
- Place cool washcloths on the skin.
- Dry by patting gently with a clean cloth.
- Apply a thick layer of burn cream with a topical anesthetic.
- Wear only loose cotton clothing over the burn.
- Do not allow the child to pull off sloughing tissue.

Tattoos and Piercings

Body modifications in the form of tattoos and piercings are popular among people of all ages. Although laws and regulations vary slightly from state to state, tattooing a child under the age of 18 is illegal without a parent's permission. Adolescents, who are still developing critical thinking skills, are at risk for not understanding the long-term consequences of tattooing. Regardless of laws, some teens may be driven to find illegal sources of tattooing, or they may have peers provide tattooing.

Every part of the skin on the body can be pierced or tattooed. The concern of the health-care team is to prevent infection after the piercing or tattooing has taken place. The healing process for piercings is directly related to the location. If a child has pierced ears, it may take up to 1 month for the piercing to heal. If the child has a navel piercing, the healing process may take upwards of a year to heal because of moisture, clothing irritation, or adipose layers of the stomach.

Evaluating of Tattoos and Piercings

Piercing sites should be checked for warmth, redness, pus, heat, and discomfort. If infection is suspected, a bacterial and fungal skin-culture swab may be warranted. The site should be thoroughly cleansed with hydrogen peroxide, and a thin layer of antimicrobial cream should be applied. In the presence of an infection at the piercing site, the jewelry should not be removed during the treatment because this may cause an abscess to form. An allergic reaction to metals should be suspected if the rash or irritation does not heal with a regular skin care regimen. In this case, the jewelry should be removed in order for the allergic rash or lesion to heal. The child should take note of the particular metal that caused the allergy to avoid wearing any other jewelry of this type of metal.

Interventions for Tattoos and Piercings

Tattoo sites should be inspected for redness, pus or sanguineous discharge, heat, swelling, and discomfort. The tattoo site should be cleansed with mild soap and water daily. Solutions with hydrogen peroxide or alcohol should not be used because they may interfere with healing. A thin layer of antimicrobial ointment can be applied for the first few days to prevent infection and prevent scab formation. A child with a new tattoo should not swim, soak in baths, or use a hot tub until the skin of the tattoo is completely healed. Sunblock lotion or cream should always be applied to a tattoo.

Know your state laws and provide appropriate information for teenagers interested in having a tattoo. Nurses can be very influential in the decision-making process for teens. If a teen is planning on getting a tattoo, they need to know the laws, risks, and long-term consequences of tattooing.

Nursing Considerations for Tattoos and Piercings

A major nursing concern is preventing or treating infections associated with a new tattoo or piercing. Teaching appropriate piercing care is also important to prevent future infection. Teens should be cautioned to use only tattoo artists or body piercers who are licensed to perform these body modifications and to look for evidence that a tattoo shop or piercing studio has passed a state department of health inspection. Complications associated with tattooing include cutaneous localized as well as general inflammatory eruptions, allergic contact dermatitis, lichenoid granulomatous reactions, infections at the site (5% occurrence), and infectious endocarditis (Juhas & English, 2013; Khunger et al., 2017; Storm, 2023). Further infectious diseases associated with tattooing performed without sterile technique and sterile equipment include:

- HIV
- Hepatitis B virus
- Hepatitis C virus
- *Mycobacterium haemophilum*
- *Mycobacterium tuberculosis*

The potential negative long-term effect of tattoos placed during childhood or young adulthood might include regret. Tattoos placed on areas of the body that are hard to conceal (face, neck, lower arms, and hands) may affect future career opportunities and may cause permanent discoloration, even with tattoo removal. Removing tattoos can be expensive and challenging depending on the size of the tattoo and the darkness of the ink used to color the design. Surgical removal, laser technology, or skin grafting may be required.

Patient Teaching Guidelines

Removing Tattoos

Tattoo removal is most commonly done by laser therapy. The newest techniques can remove colors that were previously difficult to remove. Multilaser removal equipment allows the body to flush the ink into the circulatory system for safe removal. Pregnant and breastfeeding mothers should not be treated by laser tattoo removal. According to the FDA, some tattoo removal creams on the market contain acids and can cause significant rashes or permanent scarring. Salabrasion, or salt rubs for tattoo removal, also can cause infection or leave permanent skin damage.

Key Points

- The skin of newborns and young infants is fragile, and special care should be given in providing nursing care. Newborns rapidly absorb topical medications.
- A variety of rashes can be found during childhood. Being able to describe the size, depth, type, and look of lesions is an important nursing consideration. Differentiating among macules, papules, wheals, pustules, vesicles, and other lesions is a nursing standard of practice.
- Some skin disorders are evidence of child abuse. Being able to differentiate accidental burn marks from suspected child abuse burns such as sock burns, glove burns, and cigarette burns is important. Cigarette burns can mimic the look of impetigo. Burns with multiple degrees and thicknesses, as well as splash marks, need to be differentiated from immersion burns or intentional burns, such as sock or glove burns.
- Part of anticipatory guidance is implementing a teaching plan for new parents on how to prevent burns during childhood, including electrical, immersive, contact, and heat burns. Provide information about setting the home water heater to 48.9°C (120°F), keeping all pots on back burners with handles pointing away from the front of the stove, never drinking hot liquids while holding children, and keeping heaters or outdoor grilling equipment safely away from all children.
- PPE should be consistently used to prevent the spread of various childhood skin infections. You must be able to quickly implement contact precautions to prevent the spread of viral, bacterial, and fungal skin infections. Hand washing equipment and signs should be made available for staff, families, visitors, and patients to use frequently.
- Body piercing and tattooing have short- and long-term consequences. Site infection, contraction of infectious diseases, regret, social shunning, and poor self-esteem are all possible consequences.

Review Questions

1. What causes the extending bright-red streaks associated with scabies?
   1. The scratching of the child's fingernails
   2. The spreading of the infectious bacteria
   3. The burrowing of egg-laying mites
   4. The enzymes released by the immune system

2. How should parents be taught to bathe their infant who has severe eczema?
   1. Soap and cool water twice daily during an exacerbation
   2. Warm water only once a day with gentle pat drying
   3. Bath water as hot as the child can tolerate to soothe the skin
   4. Cold water soaks at least three times a day with air drying

3. A nurse is providing teaching to the parents of a young child with a fungal diaper rash. You know that more instruction needs to be provided when the parents make which statement?
   1. "We will bathe the child in warm water with added hydrogen peroxide to treat the rash."
   2. "We will bathe the child's skin to remove all layers of medication, diaper cream, and urine at least once a day."
   3. "We will provide some diaper-free time to allow the skin to be exposed to air every day."
   4. "We will assess for extending satellite lesions and will report if they are not improving."

4. A toddler with a severe pruritic rash has an order for diphenhydramine. The dose is 0.5 milligram per kilogram of weight by mouth every 6 hours as needed. The child weighs 22.5 pounds. How much diphenhydramine will you administer in one dose? _____

5. A new preschool teacher calls the pediatric clinic for guidelines on how to care for a child who presents with a large impetigo lesion. What is the most important action to prevent the spread of the infection?
   1. Keep the lesion covered with a large adhesive bandage.
   2. Teach the child and family good hand washing techniques.
   3. Cover the wound with a thick layer of zinc oxide to prevent the spread.
   4. Tell the family they will need to keep the child at home until the lesion is healed.

6. A mother of a 10-year-old boy asks about the warts located on several of the fingers on her son's right hand. What is your best response?
   1. Warts are precancerous lesions that need to be surgically removed by a physician.
   2. Warts are benign, not contagious, and will not spread anywhere else on your son's body.
   3. Warts are caused by a variety of infectious organisms including fungi, viruses, and bacteria.
   4. Warts are caused by the papillomavirus, can spread to other body parts and other people, and are treated with acids or freezing nitrogen.

7. Why are parents and caregivers instructed not to give aspirin to a child who presents with a rash caused by a viral agent?
   1. To prevent masking a fever
   2. To prevent the potentially serious risk of Reye syndrome
   3. To prevent the child from developing Kawasaki disease
   4. To encourage the child's fever to provide a natural pyrogenic effect that kills viruses

8. A licensed vocational nurse (LVN) is assisting in a class for new parents about injury prevention. What details are correct to include in the LVN's discussion of second-degree burns? (**Select all that apply.**)
   1. Extend through the epidermis into the dermis
   2. Edematous with weeping of moisture
   3. Very painful
   4. Extend through the epidermis
   5. Heal at various speeds depending on size and location
   6. Possibly require grafting

9. _____ is an autoimmune disorder that typically presents as a red rash that is not communicable to others.

10. A father is preparing to bathe his toddler when his cell phone rings. Turning to grab the phone, the father is momentarily distracted. The toddler climbs into the tub of scalding water and screams. What is the priority intervention?
    1. Run cold water over the child.
    2. Remove the child from the scalding water.
    3. Call 911.
    4. Check the child's airway.

ANSWERS 1. 3; 2. 3; 3. 1; 4. 5.1 mg; 5. 2; 6. 4; 7. 2; 8. 1, 2, 3, 5, 6; 9. Eczema; 10. 2

CRITICAL THINKING QUESTIONS

1. Children with mobility issues and challenges are at risk for the development of pressure injuries. What illnesses, disease processes, or pathologies place children at risk? How are pressure injuries evaluated during childhood? Are the tools the same for children as for adults?

2. How do skin differences in very young children influence their nursing care?

3. What are the social, financial, and educational ramifications, if any, of teenagers having visible tattoos? What are your thoughts about health-care personnel having visible tattoos?

Resources

For additional resources and information, including Postconference Questions and Activities, Answers, and References, visit www.FADavis.com.

Student Study Guide

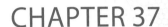

CHAPTER 37
Child With a Communicable Disease

KEY TERMS

antigen (AN-tih-jen)
communicable (kom-YOO-nik-uh-buhl)
epidemic (EP-ih-DEM-ik)
immunity (im-YOO-nih-tee)
incubation period (ING-kyoo-BAY-shun
   PEE-ree-uhd)
personal protective equipment (PPE)
   (PER-suh-nuhl pruh-TEK-tiv ih-KWIP-ment)
toxoid (TOK-soyd)

CHAPTER CONCEPTS

Growth and Development
Infection
Safety

LEARNING OUTCOMES

1. Define the key terms.
2. Describe the purpose of vaccines and childhood immunizations and discuss the most common infections for which children are immunized.
3. Describe the purpose and use of various PPE used to prevent the spread of infection within health-care environments.
4. Differentiate among the various types of isolation techniques, including standard precautions, airborne precautions, contact precautions, droplet precautions, and reverse (also called *protective*) precautions.
5. Describe the most commonly encountered childhood infectious diseases and describe the transmission, incubation, common symptoms, and treatments or supportive therapy for each.
6. Describe the communicable diseases that are of international concern.
7. Describe basic safety precautions for preventing the spread of childhood communicable diseases.

CRITICAL THINKING

Scenario #1: **Philip** reports to his second-grade teacher with fever, nausea, and a severe sore throat. He says that he has been feeling sick for 2 or 3 days, but today is the worst he has felt. You are working with the school nurse, and the decision was made to have the child picked up from school by his father. After a visit to Philip's pediatrician, his father receives a call later in the day that the rapid *Streptococcus* A test has returned positive. Philip is to start on oral antibiotics immediately. The father notifies Philip's teacher and the school nurse, and you contact parents of all children in the class according to the school's policy. Philip stays home from school for 3 days and then returns to the classroom on day four.

Questions

1. What are the classic symptoms of *Streptococcus* A (strep) throat?
2. What are the common antibiotics given to treat this condition?
3. Why is there a protocol for you to notify parents of the child's fellow classmates?
4. What are the guidelines that you must teach to the parents about oral antibiotic therapy for *Streptococcus* A?

659

CONCEPTUAL CORNERSTONE
Infection

Children with communicable illnesses are at risk for spreading their infections to others. Young children do not have the knowledge, skill, and capacity to prevent the spread of infections by controlling body fluids such as mucus, saliva, and stool. Infants easily transmit infections by placing their wet fingers into another's mouth, and toddlers do not have the capacity to learn infection-control measures without consistent teaching. Preschool children share their items readily with their peers, transmitting infectious pathogens, and school-aged children do not always participate in good hand washing techniques at school and after school. Nurses have the responsibility to provide parents with information on infection-control measures so that other members of the child's family and community do not acquire infections. Anticipatory guidance is a means to share information with parents concerning when and how to teach secretion control (sneezing into sleeve, using tissues, washing hands frequently and independently). The concept of infection control includes measures implemented by health-care institutions and behaviors performed by health-care team members, parents, and children. The two most important aspects of infection control are hand washing and the use of **personal protective equipment (PPE)**, which is equipment that is made available to health-care professionals to prevent the spread of infections or diseases. PPE includes goggles, face shields, masks, gowns, and gloves.

One significant challenge of pediatric nursing is that young children may not be able to tell a parent, nurse, or health-care provider what is wrong or to describe in depth what their symptoms are. The nurse's and health-care team's observation, recognition, and prompt treatment can make the difference in length and severity of a childhood illness. For example, symptoms such as decreased oral intake, diarrhea, abdominal pain, sore throat, rash, itching, and low-grade fever can indicate any number of childhood illnesses. Children with **communicable** (capable of being transmitted from one individual to another) diseases often present with secondary conditions such as dehydration from prolonged poor oral intake or a lengthy bout of diarrhea. Sometimes the child will present in a critical state of sepsis and require immediate lifesaving interventions. It is imperative that nurses be familiar with the most commonly encountered childhood communicable diseases so that containment, prevention of spread, rapid treatment, and prevention of complications can take place.

Many childhood illnesses, such as polio or smallpox, are no longer common because of vaccination programs and effective treatments (World Health Organization, 2021). Ironically, the effectiveness of vaccines in eradicating or reducing the incidence of illness may cause parents to falsely believe that they do not need to immunize for these serious, sometimes fatal, diseases. Learning and staying current about childhood illness, infections, communicable diseases, vaccines/immunizations, and treatments is a very critical part of being an effective advocate for pediatric patients.

Many governmental and medical school websites provide annual updates on childhood communicable diseases. Use these websites to update your clinical practice by learning about current infections, care trends, and infection-control measures associated with the infections. For instance, when COVID-19 became a pandemic, the Centers for Disease Control and Prevention (CDC) provided infection control guidelines based on the most current information on the prevention of transmission of COVID-19. These resources can be used for quick reference as well as for family or community teaching. The resources also provide guidance on local or national reporting mandates. Only a few childhood communicable diseases, such as pertussis, tuberculosis (TB), and measles, are followed for **epidemic** and endemic patterns. *Epidemic* refers to an infectious disease or condition that attacks many people at the same time in the same geographical area; *endemic* refers to a disease that occurs continuously or in expected cycles in a population with a certain number of cases expected for a given period.

Health-care personnel who work with children are at risk for contracting communicable diseases simply because having close contact with body secretions is part of caring for children. Therefore, using PPE is mandatory when caring for a child with a communicable disease.

Information on what to wear and how to implement infection-control measures can be found in each health-care institution's policies and procedure manuals. When a child is hospitalized for complications associated with a communicable disease, post a sign on the patient's door to alert team members, family members, and visitors of the necessary precautions to take. Never post the child's diagnosis because that would breech patient confidentiality and privacy rules (Health Insurance Portability and Accountability Act [HIPAA]).

There are instances where health-care team members who are exposed to infectious diseases may have to take medication. For example, a team provided emergency care for a young child with the pneumonic version of the Bubonic plague, requiring the child to be hospitalized. All health-care professionals who encountered the infected child and who were exposed to the child's respiratory secretions before donning PPE masks had to take oral antibiotics to prevent infection.

The local public health department dictates how the condition will be treated and the medications required. Upon notification of an unusual microbe, such as the pneumonic version of the Bubonic plague, or upon notification of one of the mandatory reportable infectious conditions, such as measles or pertussis, the public health department works with the medical team of the clinic or hospital and provides

· WORD · BUILDING ·

epidemic: epi–upon + dem–people + ic–pertaining to

guidelines about preventable staff antibiotic use (CDC, 2022d; United States National Library of Medicine, 2019). The interdisciplinary health-care staff caring for a child and family who presents with a reportable communicable disease must rapidly communicate to the local public health department concerning the illness. See the following list for current examples of reportable diseases:

- Anthrax
- Botulism
- Chicken pox
- Chlamydia
- Cryptosporidiosis
- Diphtheria
- Gonorrhea
- Hepatitis A, B, and C
- Listeriosis
- Lyme disease
- Malaria
- Measles
- Meningococcal disease
- Mumps
- Pertussis
- Plague
- Rabies
- Rubella
- Salmonellosis
- Severe acute respiratory syndrome (SARS)
- Smallpox
- Tetanus
- Toxic shock syndrome
- TB
- Vancomycin resistant *Staphylococcus aureus*
- Yellow fever

Safe and Effective Nursing Care

Members of the pediatric health-care team must be knowledgeable about the use of PPE for specific isolation measures, which will help to prevent the spread of disease. The level of protection is dependent on how an infectious organism is transmitted and the anticipated contact and exposure of staff.

- *Standard precautions:* Hand washing, gloves, gowns, masks, eye protection, and facial shields as needed
- *Airborne precautions:* Private room with door closed, hand washing, masks, gowns, gloves, eye protection, and facial shields as needed
- *Droplet precautions:* Private room or room with patient with same organism, hand washing, mask if within 3 feet of patient, gown, gloves, and eye shielding as needed
- *Contact precautions:* Hand washing, gown, and gloves; may also be called *enteric contact precautions* when the microbe is present in the stool

- *Expanded contact precautions:* Hand washing only, no alcohol-based hand gels; gown and gloves
- *Protective precautions:* Also called *reverse precautions* or *neutropenic precautions;* the patient is protected from communicable diseases by a positive-pressure room. Here as the door opens, air is pushed out toward the hallway to prevent airborne or droplet-transmitted microbes from entering the child's room.

Most signage is now standardized to list what PPE is required and has pictures or illustrations of what is required. Gloves, masks, and gowns should be available for staff, family, and visitors to use, and precautions should be enforced.

 ## VACCINES

Immunity refers to the body's ability to develop antibodies against specific bacteria, viruses, and toxins that can prevent future illness from exposure to the same antigen. An **antigen** is a foreign substance such as bacteria, viruses, toxins, and foreign proteins that stimulates the formation of antibodies and therefore provides immunity.

The effectiveness and duration of immunity depends on the strength of the immune response as well as the type of organism. Immunity to disease can be active or acquired. Active immunity results from the development of antibodies or sensitized T lymphocytes after being exposed to an invading organism. Acquired immunity is obtained by either exposure to a bacterium, virus, or toxin sufficient to stimulate an immune response by the body, or stimulating the body's immune response through vaccination or immunization. Passive immunity is the temporary immunity acquired by transfusing immune globulins or antitoxins either artificially from another human or from an animal that has been actively immunized against an antigen, or naturally from the mother to the fetus via the placenta.

Patient Teaching Guidelines

How Immunizations Work to Fight Infections During Childhood

- A weakened form of the germ that causes disease is injected into a child's body via a needle and syringe. Sometimes the vaccine is made up of just part of the germ but enough to activate the child's immune response.
- The child's body then produces antibodies in large numbers that can fight off the infection.
- Antibodies, a type of protein, are a part of the child's immune system. When the immune system recognizes

Continued

· WORD · BUILDING ·

antigen: anti–against + gen–producer

Patient Teaching Guidelines—cont'd

germs have entered the body, these small proteins attach themselves to the germ and kill it.

- If a fully immunized child is exposed to the germ that causes disease, they will have sufficient antibodies to fight off the germ so that the disease does not occur.
- Not all childhood vaccines provide lifetime protection against disease. Some need to be given again in adulthood.
- Virtually all childhood diseases can be prevented by the completion of an immunization schedule (Table 37.1).

Safety *Stat!*

If a health-care provider suspects that a child is having a reaction to an immunization, the provider must call for help while ensuring that the child is never left alone. Allergic reactions, although rare, can be life-threatening because they can cause anaphylaxis (bronchial constriction, throat swelling, and hypotension). If an allergic reaction occurs, it does not necessarily prevent the child from receiving other vaccines. Once the substance in the vaccine that caused the reaction is identified, a vaccine that does not contain that substance will be administered.

Table 37.1
Commonly Administered Immunizations

Vaccine Type	Schedule	Type	Common Side Effects	Serious Rare Reactions
Hepatitis B	Three doses: Birth–2 months, 1–4 months, 6–18 months	Inactivated virus	Low-grade fever, soreness at site of injection (administered in the vastus lateralis muscle)	Serious allergic reactions, high fevers
MMR: measles, mumps, and rubella	Two doses: 12–15 months, 4–6 years	Live virus	Fever, mild rash, swelling of the neck or cheeks, temporary stiffness and pain in joints, temporary low platelets	Seizures, serious allergic reactions, deafness, permanent brain damage
DTaP: diphtheria (*C. diphtheriae*), tetanus (*Clostridium tetani*), and acellular pertussis	Five doses: 2 months; 4 months; 6 months; 15–18 months; booster 4–6 years	Inactivated virus	Injection site reactions, nonstop crying for longer than 3 hours, tiredness, vomiting, low-grade fever	Seizure, fever greater than 40.6°C (105°F); any tetanus-containing vaccine can, in very rare instances, cause Guillain-Barré syndrome.
Varicella	Two doses, one at 12–15 months and one at 4–6 years	Live virus	Fever, mild rash, and swelling of injection site	Seizures, lowered consciousness, permanent brain damage
Pneumococcal conjugate	Prevnar: Four doses at 2 months, 4 months, 6 months, and 15 months. One catch-up dose can be given through age 5 if any doses were missed.	Polysaccharide conjugate vaccine	Drowsiness, loss of appetite, redness or tenderness at the injection site	Life-threatening allergic reactions (very rare)
Haemophilus influenzae type B (Hib)	Four doses: 2 months, 4 months, 6 months, and 15 months	Polysaccharide conjugate vaccine	25% of children experience redness, swelling, and pain at injection site; 5% may experience a moderate to high fever.	None known
Influenza	Annually from infancy through old age	Inactivated virus	Soreness, swelling and redness at injection site, fever, body aches, fatigue, headache	Severe allergic reactions, Guillain-Barré syndrome (rare)

Children's immunizations or vaccines are scheduled to protect them from infections they may be exposed to. Immunization schedules are updated as new data become available. To keep up with the latest guidelines and recommendations, check the CDC. It is important to know the type of vaccine being given to understand what side effects may occur and to provide education to caregivers.

Types of Vaccines

There are several types of immunizations available with more than 30 types of vaccines and **toxoids** (substances that are chemically modified to retain their antigen properties but are no longer considered poisonous) licensed for use in the United States. The main types of vaccines are described in Box 37.1.

Box 37.1

Types of Vaccines

- *Polysaccharide conjugate vaccine:* Uses sugars from the bacteria and bonds them to portions of another germ. This type of vaccine does not contain live viruses and does not contain the whole microbe, so it will not cause the infection or disease.
- *Live (attenuated) virus vaccine:* This type of vaccine uses the whole virus, which has been manipulated in the laboratory in several ways to produce a weakened strain. These viruses mimic the natural virus so closely that the body can produce antibodies to provide immunity to the actual disease. The main benefit of a live virus vaccine is the strength of the immunity it produces. It is often effective with just one dose. The main deterrent to this type of vaccine is its ability, on rare occasions, to actually cause the disease because it is a live virus. This is particularly important to note in immunocompromised patients. Examples of this type of vaccine are MMR, varicella, rotavirus, oral polio, and the nasal flu vaccines.
- *Whole (inactive) virus vaccine:* This type of vaccine contains the whole, killed organism, which retains the surface and internal structures that are strong stimulants to the immune system. The virus is killed, or inactivated, by heat, phenol, formalin, or thimerosal. This kind of vaccine is effective, but there is the possibility of an allergic reaction. This type of vaccine requires multiple doses to be given initially to produce sufficient immunity, and it often requires booster doses to maintain immunity. Examples of this type of vaccine are anthrax, cholera, whooping cough, rabies, inactivated polio, and typhoid.
- *Recombinant vaccine:* A newer form of vaccine-recombinant technology, this vaccine produces a genetically altered organism. It contains some manufactured proteins that match the germ's proteins closely, which stimulate the immune response in the body. These vaccines do not contain any part of the original germ, so they do not have the risk of causing the disease. Examples of this type of vaccine are pneumococcal pneumonia and *Haemophilus influenzae*.

Toxoids

Toxoids operate somewhat differently than other vaccines. Instead of producing antibodies against the organism itself, toxoids produce antibodies against toxins secreted by the organism.

To make the toxoid vaccine, bacteria are grown in large amounts. The toxin they produce is inactivated by chemical, heat, or other treatments, producing a toxoid that can be given as a vaccination. After vaccination, the body produces antibodies that will inactivate the bacterial toxin in the case of future exposure. This is the type of immunization used for diphtheria and tetanus.

Common Immunizations

Whenever a child is seen by the health-care team, immunizations should be discussed because adherence to the recommended schedule is important. Parents must be encouraged to keep track of each child's immunization document because this is needed for entrance into school. Table 37.1 provides a list of commonly administered immunizations. Be aware that immunization schedules may change. Both the CDC and the National Institutes of Health (NIH) provide information on the most current recommendations. Schedules exist for catching up if a child has missed doses. Missed doses of immunizations can be caused by the child having a severe infection at the time of the vaccine being due, an immunosuppressive illness, or a new immigration status, among other reasons.

Known Concerns About Vaccines

Over the last several decades, individuals and organizations have expressed concerns over the increasing number of required or recommended childhood vaccines and their potential side effects. While nurses celebrate vaccines for their lifesaving qualities, some social media, print, and internet sources circulate frightening theories and rumors. It is imperative that nurses be prepared to calmly and respectfully discuss vaccination concerns shared by family members (Box 37.2).

Reporting Immunization Reactions

Severe reactions to vaccines are rare but sometimes do occur with childhood immunizations. Serious reactions should be reported through the Vaccine Adverse Event Reporting System (VAERS), a national vaccine safety surveillance program run by the CDC and the Food and Drug Administration (FDA). Check with the local public health department to find out which reactions are mandated to be reported.

 COMMON COMMUNICABLE DISORDERS

Children are susceptible to many infectious diseases, some of which will be mild and others that require hospitalization. Influenza, for example, can present as a mild infection with an uncomplicated course of illness, or it can be fatal. The child's health status at the time of becoming infected with a communicable illness will influence how the child

· **WORD** · **BUILDING** ·
toxoid: tox–poison + oid–resembling

Box 37.2

Parental Concerns About Childhood Vaccines and Immunizations

Thimerosal

Thimerosal is a water-soluble, crystalline powder used as an antiseptic that was used as a preservative in immunizations. Thimerosal is no longer used with the exception of some influenza vaccines. Concerns emerged because thimerosal is mercury-based and has been connected to minor reactions. Current science has not found a link between thimerosal and autism or any other serious harm. Families can ask for influenza shots that do not contain thimerosal.

Aluminum

Aluminum is added to many vaccines to improve their effectiveness. Combination vaccines may increase the amount of aluminum in a vaccine to make it optimally effective. It is unclear and insufficiently studied to determine how much aluminum may be toxic to infants and children and what effect it may have.

Guillain-Barré Syndrome

This disorder is an autoimmune reaction in which the immune system attacks the nervous system, causing temporary paralysis that usually lasts a few weeks and can require intensive care. The most common vaccines that Guillain-Barré has been associated with are tetanus-containing vaccines and meningococcal vaccine, although it has been associated with other vaccines, including influenza. Parents need to understand that this is a rare complication and having a tetanus, meningococcal, or severe flu infection has much greater and more common risks.

Encephalitis/Encephalopathy

Encephalitis is inflammation and swelling of the brain. In rare cases, infants will develop this condition postimmunization and have a high fever and intense screaming alternating with lethargy. The symptoms can last up to a few days. In a small number of cases, encephalitis can progress to encephalopathy, a form of brain injury that causes permanent damage. This is associated with the old DTaP vaccine, the MMR vaccine, and tetanus-containing vaccines.

Hypotonic/Hyporesponsive Episodes

Hypotonic/hyporesponsive episodes (HHE) are rare, sometimes serious reactions associated with pertussis-containing (DTaP)

vaccinations. This reaction causes a sudden onset of hypotonia. The episode can last a few minutes to hours, and it occurs in children younger than 2 years of age. The reaction can sometimes require cardiopulmonary resuscitation (CPR). Frequently, children are hospitalized after an episode for observation even if symptoms have subsided.

Autism

The medical and scientific community is clear: *There is no link between immunizations and autism.* Yet questions remain among the public and parents, largely based on a research article published in 1998 in the medical journal *The Lancet,* which has since retracted the article. The lead author of the article, Andrew Wakefield, and his colleagues proposed the theory that the MMR vaccine might cause autism, based on their very small and deeply flawed study. It was later revealed that Wakefield's study was an elaborate fraud, and he lost his medical license. At least 20 epidemiological studies have been conducted that show no correlation between autism, the MMR vaccine, or thimerosal used in the vaccine.

Seizures

Seizure activity is a rare reaction that some children have experienced after vaccination. Generally, seizures are considered to be secondary to fever. Febrile seizures are generally self-limiting and do not result in future health problems.

Autoimmune Reactions

Autoimmune reactions have been reported with some vaccines; these are an overreaction of the immune system to some component of the vaccine. Reported vaccine-associated autoimmune diseases have been rheumatoid arthritis, thyroid disease, diabetes, and multiple sclerosis.

Religious Objections

Some religious faiths teach that medical procedures and treatments must be refused, limited, or delayed until prayer or clergy are consulted.

---

presents and is treated. If a child has an underlying chronic illness such as asthma or cystic fibrosis, or a condition that causes immunosuppression, they may be more vulnerable to infections and require special consideration.

Patient Teaching Guidelines

If the parents of a child hospitalized with a communicable illness express concerns about immunizations, or if they have refused or delayed their child's immunizations, the health-care team must provide additional teaching to parents before discharge. Information the team should share includes the following:

- Educating the family about the importance of a complete immunization program for all children to prevent childhood diseases such as the one that the child is being treated for
- Providing written information on the immunization schedule and on each immunization being administered
- Teaching them that there are catch-up schedules that can start right away
- Educating them about each of the diseases/infections and their complications
- Scheduling a follow-up appointment for after discharge so that they can be seen right away by a pediatrician who will implement a catch-up immunization schedule

Influenza: The "Flu"

Influenza is a yearly occurring viral infection that occurs in the winter and has significant mortality and morbidity worldwide, particularly in the very young, older adults, and immunocompromised patients. There are several strains of the virus with a different strain dominating each year. This makes developing the yearly vaccine challenging. Each year the flu shot is developed based on genetic sequencing research that indicates which strains will be most prevalent during the upcoming year (CDC, 2022c).

The flu can last for several days, and patients can become quite ill. Dehydration is a major complication of the illness, resulting from high fevers, nausea, vomiting, and diarrhea.

Severe muscle aches and pains are common with influenza. Superimposed bacterial infections, such as pneumonia, are complicating factors that can compromise patients further and require antibiotics and hospitalization. School-aged children have the highest flu infection rate in the population and may be hospitalized because of the complications of this virus. Influenza requires droplet precautions. If a child has an aerosol-generating procedure, airborne precautions may be used. The **incubation period**, which is the time interval between exposure to a communicable disease or infection and the presentation of the first symptoms, is between 24 and 72 hours.

Diagnosing Influenza

Common flu symptoms include the following:

- *Generalized symptoms:* Rapid onset of fever, chills, conjunctivitis, headache, malaise, muscle pain (myalgia), and sudden onset of rigor.
- *Respiratory symptoms:* Inflammation of the larynx and trachea, cough, sore throat, nasal congestion, and retrosternal pain are associated with the flu. Children often develop croup, pneumonia, and bronchitis as secondary conditions.
- *Gastrointestinal symptoms:* Vomiting, abdominal pain, and diarrhea with secondary dehydration can occur with the flu and require fluid replacement therapy.
- *Central nervous system (CNS) symptoms:* Headache and dizziness can occur with the flu, requiring pain medications and bedrest.

Safety *Stat!*

When a child presents with flu-like symptoms (cough, fever, body aches) in any clinical setting, the child and family should be placed away from others, and a mask should be placed on the child. Preventing the spread of influenza to vulnerable sick children is a nursing imperative. Droplet and contact precautions should be implemented right away. For H1N1 (very serious) strains of the flu, an N95 mask is required.

Interventions for Influenza

The only medication that is currently approved for treating influenza in young children is oseltamivir phosphate. This medication can be administered to children as young as 1 year old. The capsules can be opened and mixed with a small amount of thick, sweet liquid, such as chocolate syrup. The medication should be started within 48 hours of symptom onset. After 48 hours, the medication has not been found to be as effective (CDC, n.d.-a). Although antiviral medications come in oral, inhaled, and intravenous forms, only inhaled zanamivir is approved for children 7 and older (CDC, n.d.-b).

Nursing Considerations for Influenza

Supportive treatment for influenza is geared toward maintaining adequate hydration and controlling fever. Young children are at risk for febrile seizures because the flu can cause rapid increases in body temperature. Therefore, temperature control is particularly important in this patient population.

It is not uncommon to hear people say, "I don't get the flu shot—it gives me the flu." The standard flu vaccine or "flu shot" is an inactivated influenza vaccine that contains only killed viruses, so it cannot give someone the flu. Antibodies that protect against the illness are produced at about 2 weeks after the vaccination. During this time, someone who received the flu shot can be exposed to the flu virus and become infected. Some people experience aches and pains after an injection, but these symptoms are mild in comparison with the actual flu symptoms and usually subside in 1 to 2 days. If a person has an allergy to eggs, that allergy might cause a reaction because most flu vaccines are produced in an egg product. Current research suggests that each month after a flu shot, flu antibodies are reduced by approximately 7% (CDC, 2022b; Ferdinands et al., 2017).

One type of influenza vaccine is an intranasal spray that uses a live attenuated (weakened) influenza virus. These immunizations can give some children adverse side effects that include fever, malaise, muscle pain, and other generalized symptoms.

Flu vaccines are recommended for anyone older than 6 months. Vaccinations are usually started in the fall and contain three viral strains that are likely to be prevalent in the coming winter. Three strains of influenza viruses are common: influenza B viruses, influenza A H1N1 viruses, and influenza A H3N2 viruses. The yearly flu vaccine is made by using one strain of flu virus from each type.

Measles

Measles is a very contagious respiratory illness caused by the rubeola virus and spread by infected airborne droplets that are expelled when someone coughs or sneezes. A person is contagious from 4 days before the rash starts until 4 days after the rash appears. The virus is most often spread when one first gets ill before it is diagnosed. Once exposed, a person displays symptoms within 8 to 12 days. Once a person contracts the illness and recovers, they are considered to have lifelong immunity.

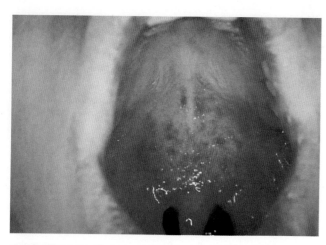

FIGURE 37.1 Koplik spots.

FIGURE 37.2 Rash caused by rubeola (measles) virus.

Diagnosing the Measles

Once contracted, the measles cause fever, a generalized red rash, red eyes (conjunctivitis), runny nose, cough, and general malaise. The development of bluish spots on the buccal mucosa (Koplik spots) is unique to this disease (Figs. 37.1 and 37.2).

Interventions for the Measles

There are no interventions or treatments for a child who has a measles infection. The viral infection will last about 4 to 5 days with a spreading rash and high fevers. The child may require extra fluids and support for fevers and itching.

Postexposure vaccinations may help children who are not yet fully vaccinated against the measles, provided the immunization is administered within 72 hours of exposure to the measles virus. The infection may still develop after the incubation period, but it is often milder with fewer symptoms and a shorter course of infection.

Members of high-risk populations such as pregnant women or children with immune dysfunction diseases may require IV immunoglobulins (antibodies) to prevent serious complications.

Vitamin A is also known to reduce the symptoms and severity of the infection for those who have low vitamin A levels, especially for children who are malnourished or for those children who are at higher risk for complications. In such children, two doses of 200,000 IU of vitamin A during the toddler developmental period were found to reduce mortality by 83% to 87% (Cochrane.org, 2023; Oregon State University Linus Pauling Institute, 2019).

Nursing Considerations for the Measles

Cases of the measles can be mild to severe. Mild cases of the illness produce self-limiting symptoms that can be treated at home supportively by reducing the fever, maintaining hydration, and getting rest. In children, this illness is over within about a 2-week time period.

Moderate cases of this illness can involve secondary ear infections, pneumonia, and high fevers. These cases will require antibiotics and possibly hospitalization, depending on the severity. The child usually recovers without complications.

Serious cases of measles are rare but can involve complications in the brain tissue called *encephalitis* or *encephalopathy*. Pneumonia and respiratory infection can be serious and require hospitalization and intensive care. Very rarely (1 to 2 per 1,000 cases), measles can cause death.

Patient Teaching Guidelines

Caring for a Child Whose Communicable Disease Causes a Rash

Family members can provide comfort for a child who has a significant rash associated with a childhood communicable disease, such as the measles or varicella. Ideas for making a child more comfortable and less symptomatic include the following:

- Dress the child in only cotton clothing, no synthetics.
- Dress the child in loose-fitting, lightweight clothing.
- Keep the rash covered from the sun.
- Keep the skin cool and dry.
- Provide cool baths or cool compresses on the rash; try oatmeal baths.
- Do not allow the child to scratch the rash lesions; cover the hands of infants or young toddlers; apply infant mittens if needed.
- Use mild soaps when bathing the child.
- Prevent the child from becoming sweaty.
- Change the child's bed linens daily.
- Administer oral antihistamines if needed to prevent scratching.
- Apply calamine lotion for topical relief.

Mumps

Mumps, also known as *viral parotitis,* is a virus that only affects humans and causes illness that can last from several

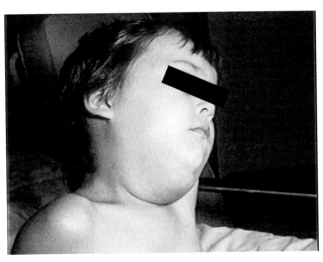

FIGURE 37.3 Child with a mumps infection.

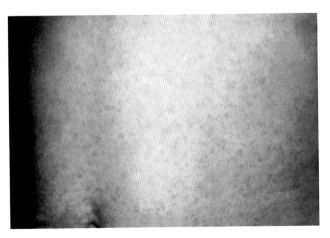

FIGURE 37.4 Rubella.

days to several weeks. Any child who has neither had mumps nor received a vaccination is susceptible. Before the development of the vaccine in 1967, mumps was a common illness in the United States. With routine vaccination, fewer than 300 cases of mumps are reported each year.

Mumps is spread by respiratory droplets, frequently through the coughing and sneezing of an infected person. The usual incubation period is 16 to 18 days; it is contagious from 7 days before to 5 days after salivary gland swelling begins. The illness usually affects children 5 to 9 years old but can infect adolescents and adults.

Diagnosing the Mumps

The characteristic symptom of mumps, salivary gland inflammation (also known as *parotitis*), causes swelling of the glands, cheeks, and jaw. The swelling can be unilateral or bilateral, and it can last for 1 to 10 days (Fig. 37.3). The fever that accompanies the acute phase of the illness can range up to 40°C (104°F) for 1 to 6 days. Mumps typically starts with a few days of fever, headache, muscle aches, tiredness, and loss of appetite and is followed by swelling of salivary glands. Diagnosis is usually made after observation of symptoms or a known mumps exposure. Although serological tests are available for definitive diagnosis, the mumps virus can be isolated from throat washings, urine, cerebrospinal fluid (CSF), and other body fluids.

Interventions for the Mumps

Treatment of mumps is supportive and includes analgesics/antipyretics, fluids, rest, scrotal elevation, and ice packs, all focusing on symptom relief. Complicated cases may require hospitalization. Respiratory isolation precautions should be implemented, and the child should be kept from school or day care until all manifestations of the symptoms have subsided, about 9 days after parotid swelling.

Nursing Considerations for the Mumps

Mumps is usually a mild disease but can have complications. Inflammation of the testicles (epididymitis) in males

who have reached puberty is the most common complication. Fertility issues are often a concern but are rare. Females may experience inflammation of the ovaries and/or the breast. Other rare complications that have been reported are meningitis and **encephalitis**. At one time, when mumps was more prevalent, deafness was a significant complication but is now rarely reported (Clason, 2019).

Rubella: German Measles

Rubella is an airborne virus spread by coughing and sneezing or by contact with nasopharyngeal secretions, urine, blood, or stool of those infected. Rubella causes a fever and rash for 2 to 3 days. The symptoms are usually considered mild in comparison with other illnesses and often are unrecognized. At times, a child may have body and joint aches, but rubella does not usually cause severe illness in a child who is otherwise healthy. Rubella is considered a highly infectious viral disease among children who are not immunized. Children can be infectious up to 10 days before the appearance of the rubella rash.

Diagnosing Rubella

Children with rubella will present with a 1- to 2-day history of not feeling well, mild fevers, and a sore throat. The child may present with a maculopapular rash that typically begins on the child's forehead or face and progresses downward to the rest of the body (Fig. 37.4).

Interventions for Rubella

Treatment for rubella is usually symptomatic for an individual who has the disease and includes medication for fever and aches, fluids, and rest.

Nursing Considerations for Rubella

The primary risk of rubella, and therefore the primary reason for vaccination, involves women who contract this illness

· **WORD · BUILDING ·**
encephalitis: encephal–brain + itis–inflammation

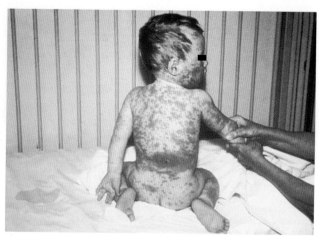

FIGURE 37.5 Roseola rash.

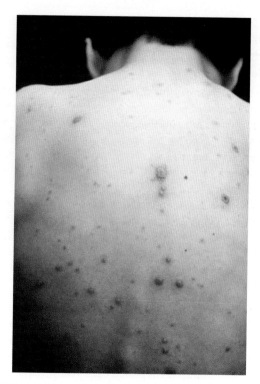

FIGURE 37.6 Lesions caused by varicella infection.

while pregnant. Exposure to rubella, particularly during the first 12 weeks of pregnancy, can cause serious birth defects such as heart problems, hearing and vision loss, brain damage, and liver or spleen damage. Acquiring a rubella infection during pregnancy can also cause a miscarriage or premature delivery. The vaccine for rubella is usually given with measles and mumps in the form of the measles, mumps, rubella (MMR) vaccine.

Roseola

Roseola, also known as *exanthem subitum* or human herpesvirus type 6b (HHV-6b), is a viral infection caused by the HHV-6 pathogen. The transmission of the virus is by saliva of an infected person. The approximate incubation period for roseola is 10 days. Roseola typically presents with low-grade fevers and fussiness for 1 to 2 days, followed by a sudden elevated fever. The classic roseola rash starts after the last fever (sometimes the day of the last fever); it begins on the child's face and then progresses downward (Fig. 37.5).

Diagnosing Roseola

Diagnosis of viral roseola is based on the identification of the classic rash. The roseola rash is red, pink, and papular in nature. Checking for a recent history of fevers will also assist in the diagnosis.

Interventions for Roseola

There are no treatments for roseola. Supportive care includes antipyretics such as acetaminophen or ibuprofen, rest, and hydration.

Nursing Considerations for Roseola

The greatest concern with a child who develops a roseola infection is the spike in temperatures. Rapid high temperatures are associated with febrile seizures.

Varicella: Chicken Pox

Varicella, also called *chicken pox,* is a common childhood illness that is highly contagious. Varicella is an airborne

virus that is spread through coughing, sneezing, and direct contact with infected lesions. Once someone is infected with the varicella virus, the organism lies dormant and resides within the nerves of the body. The infection can recur in adulthood in the form of shingles, which is an outbreak along nerve tracts that causes significant pain and discomfort.

Diagnosing Varicella

The illness begins with fever, malaise, poor appetite, and lesions, often on the chest or back (Fig. 37.6). The lesions then spread to the body and extremities distally. An individual with varicella begins to be contagious 1 to 2 days before the rash appears. On the second day of illness, the rash lesions turn to blisters and begin to itch; new lesions will continue to develop. By the third day of illness, the blisters crust over. The cycle of new lesions, blisters, and crusting affects the entire body, including the face and extremities, and continues throughout the course of the illness, about 5 days. At the point when all lesions crust over and the child is no longer febrile, they are considered to no longer be contagious. Once someone recovers from a primary varicella infection, they usually have immunity for life.

Varicella used to be a very common illness in the United States with about 3.5 million reported cases of this disease each year. It is estimated that vaccination programs have decreased the incidence of the illness by about 75% (CDC, 2022a).

The CDC recommends two doses of chicken pox vaccine for children: the first dose at 12 to 15 months and a second dose at 4 to 6 years. The vaccine will provide up to 98% immunity of contracting a varicella infection.

Interventions for Varicella

There is no treatment for varicella. Children will need supportive care including fluids, rest, and isolation to prevent the spread to those not vaccinated, pregnant women, or young children who are not fully immunized. Immunocompromised children, such as those receiving high-dose steroids or those being treated for cancer, may be given the varicella zoster–specific immunoglobulins known as *VZIG*.

Moderate cases of varicella can involve a secondary bacterial infection of the lesions and be more painful, sometimes leaving a scar. Acyclovir, an antiviral medication, is sometimes used in older children and adults within 72 hours of developing a rash to help control the severity of the illness and prevent fever. Acyclovir can limit the outbreak of lesions and the accompanying uncomfortable itching, thus reducing the likelihood of secondary infections.

Safety *Stat!*

Rare but serious complications of varicella can include pneumonia, septicemia, toxic shock syndrome, septic arthritis, encephalitis, hemorrhagic conditions, and death.

Nursing Considerations for Varicella

Severe complications from chicken pox for healthy individuals are rare, but chicken pox can be life-threatening to patients who are immunocompromised or who have HIV/AIDS. Use appropriate PPE and infection-control measures when caring for a child with confirmed or suspected varicella infection. Initiate contact and airborne precautions: wash hands before entering the child's room, again before care, after care, and again after removing PPE. Wear a mask, gloves, and gown at all times when providing care. Careful removal of the soiled PPE is warranted, and used items should be placed in a biological infectious waste container with a tight lid.

CRITICAL THINKING

Scenario #2: You are working in a public health center, and the grandfather of an older infant boy with varicella is preparing to take him home. He says that if his grandson's temperature goes up, he'll give him some aspirin because it helps reduce fevers.

Question

1. Is teaching necessary in this situation? If so, why?

Safety *Stat!*

Serious complications can occur in pregnant women who are infected with varicella in the first 20 weeks of pregnancy. Approximately 2% of women infected in this period of gestation will have children born with congenital varicella syndrome. This can result in scarring of the skin; abnormalities in the limbs, brain, and eyes; and low birth weight. If a woman develops a varicella rash from 5 days before to 2 days after delivery, the newborn will be at risk for neonatal varicella. Without immediate antiviral treatment, up to 30% of such newborns may develop severe neonatal varicella infection, which can be life-threatening (Mayo Clinic, 2019).

Varicella outbreaks in settings such as childcare centers, schools, and hospitals can last as long as 4 to 5 months. Outbreaks are monitored by public health departments and the CDC. Outbreaks in community settings can result in significant loss of school for children and work for parents. In hospital settings, varicella identification is a major focus of infectious disease departments because of the vulnerability of hospitalized patients who are immunocompromised.

Polio

Polio is a virus that caused worldwide epidemics in the 20th century and was prevalent in the United States as recently as the 1950s. Polio still exists, with 22 new cases reported in 2017. However, before the development of the vaccine, each year in the United States thousands of people died, and an estimated 35,000 people were crippled by the disease.

Diagnosing Polio

The main assessments for polio are the onset of abrupt symptoms of a cold followed by low-grade fevers. Paralysis can present within 3 days, but this depends on the degree of nerve tissue involvement (Fig. 37.7).

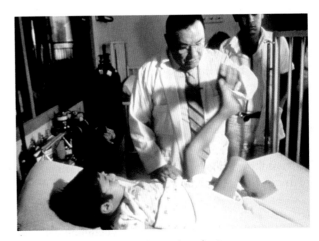

FIGURE 37.7 Paralysis caused by polio infection.

Interventions for Polio

There is no treatment for polio. Once infected, the child will need to be supported through the paralysis. Mechanical ventilation may be required if the paralysis extends to the trunk and compromises the child's ventilation. Aggressive physical therapy may be ordered to improve the associated muscular **hypotonia** with the paralysis.

Nursing Considerations for Polio

The majority of children and adults infected with the polio virus may never show symptoms or develop the disease, but they may act as carriers and spread the virus.

Because of vaccination programs, polio is no longer prevalent in the United States. Vaccination is recommended for children under the age of 5. Two types of vaccines protect against polio: the inactivated polio vaccine (IPV) and the oral polio vaccine (OPV). In the United States and other countries where the disease has been eradicated, IPV is given in a four-dose series.

Haemophilus Influenzae Type B

Haemophilus influenzae type B (Hib) is a bacterium that causes meningitis, blood infections, bone infections, epiglottitis, and pneumonia. These illnesses can be life-threatening and require immediate medical intervention, hospitalization, and antibiotic treatment; intensive care can sometimes be required. Before the development of the Hib vaccine, there were about 20,000 cases of serious infections reported in the United States each year.

Diagnosing Haemophilus Influenzae Type B

Transmission occurs in children through nasopharyngeal droplets or respiratory droplets. Mild cases often start with cold symptoms that sometimes progress to fever, ear infections, and respiratory infections such as bronchitis or pneumonia and often can be treated with antibiotics.

An infant or child with a moderate case of Hib infection can present as quite ill. Common presentations include respiratory symptoms in addition to secondary infections. The child may appear lethargic and ill, show signs of increased work of breathing and labored respiration, and have signs of mild to moderate dehydration from fever and poor oral intake.

Interventions for Haemophilus Influenzae Type B

Because Hib is caused by bacteria, the child will be treated with antibiotic therapy. A child may be admitted to the hospital for hydration, antibiotics, and monitoring.

Nursing Considerations for Haemophilus Influenzae Type B

Long term, meningitis can cause hearing loss, learning disorders, and/or nerve injury. Epiglottitis can rapidly occlude the child's airway. The classic presentation of epiglottitis includes drooling, dystonia, and dysphagia with the child appearing quite toxic and in a tripod position to maximize ventilation. The child needs immediate emergency care, airway support, and rapid antibiotics to avoid death.

Safety *Stat!*

A child who presents with symptoms of epiglottitis should never have any type of throat assessment such as a visual inspection with a tongue blade. Touching the site can result in rapid swelling and total occlusion of the child's airway.

Since the development and widespread administration of the Hib vaccine in the 1980s, reported cases of serious Hib have decreased to 0.08 per 100,000 children. Parents need to understand that between 3% and 6% of cases in children are fatal. Those who survive Hib meningitis have long-term neurological problems. This vaccine is considered safe and has few side effects. Considering the serious illnesses that can arise from Hib infection and the few side effects associated with the vaccine, this vaccine is recommended for all infants.

Pneumococcus

Pneumococcus, also known as *Streptococcus pneumoniae*, is a bacterium that can cause several illnesses such as ear infections, serious respiratory infections such as pneumonia, and meningitis. Blood tests are used to identify *S. pneumoniae*; then oral or IV antibiotics can be given. Severe pneumococcal disease affects mainly infants and children under the age of 5 years. These young patients can present with symptoms of meningitis or sepsis and will require treatment with aggressive antibiotics; often they require pediatric intensive care unit (PICU) stays. Infections of this type have a 20% to 30% mortality rate with complications that include brain damage and hearing loss in some children.

Diagnosing Pneumococcus

Early symptoms of pneumococcus are similar to cold symptoms and may progress to ear infections, bronchitis, or pneumonia.

Interventions for Pneumococcus

Mild cases are treated on an outpatient basis with antibiotics. In more severe cases, the child may appear lethargic and have increased respiratory distress. Severe cases should be treated in the hospital with IV antibiotics, monitoring, and nursing care.

Nursing Considerations for Pneumococcus

The pneumococcus vaccine is limited in effectiveness because it does not cover all the dozens of strains of pneumococcus that exist—only the most common strains (typically

• WORD • BUILDING •

hypotonia: hypo–deficient + ton–tone, tension + ia–condition

22 to 23 strains at a time). Many emerging strains of pneumococcus are resistant to antibiotics and may not be covered by current vaccines. The National Foundation for Infectious Diseases (NFID, 2022) reports that approximately 2,000 cases of severe (sometimes fatal) infection occur annually in the United States (blood infection, meningitis).

Approximately 50% of children vaccinated with pneumococcal conjugate vaccine (PCV) report local and systemic side effects, and 80% experience fussiness. Fevers are found in 5% of children after the vaccine. Severe reactions including pneumonia, chest cold, and gastroenteritis have been reported during vaccine trials; however, these may have been unrelated to the vaccine (CDC, 2017).

Patient Teaching Guidelines

Caring for a Child With Strep Throat

Parents of young children need to know how to recognize strep throat and must understand its treatment.

Symptoms include:

- Severe sore throat, often with rapid onset
- Red, raw, swollen throat tissue with white spots
- High fever
- Low energy
- Swollen lymph nodes in the neck
- Not wanting to swallow; pain with swallowing

Treatment considerations are as follows:

- Antibiotics will be prescribed after a rapid strep test or throat culture comes back positive for *Streptococcus* A.
- The child must finish the entire course of oral antibiotics to prevent the development of resistant strains of bacteria and to make sure that the infection is completely treated.

It is essential to notify the child's school or day care of the child's diagnosis as soon as possible. Strep infections have a rapid incubation period (24 to 72 hours) and are easily transmitted to other children in a classroom or childcare setting via respiratory secretions.

Nursing Care Plan for the Child With Otitis Media Caused by Pneumococcus Bacteria

Ten-month-old Kylie is brought to an urgent care clinic by her teen parents, who are visibly upset. The parents report that the infant has been fussy and irritable for 2 days, and today she started pulling on her ears. Kylie is running a fever of 38.9°C (102°F), and her throat is red. The health-care provider diagnoses the infant with bilateral otitis media (OM) and infected sore throat most likely from pneumococcus.

Nursing Diagnosis: Acute pain as evidenced by fussiness and tugging at ears
Expected Outcome: The patient will experience relief from pain as evidenced by not pulling the ears and decreased crying episodes.

Intervention:	Rationale:
Determine level of pain with the FLACC pain scale.	*Initial pain evaluation gives the nurse a baseline to determine the effect of medication.*
Administer an antipyretic/analgesic (acetaminophen or ibuprofen).	*An antipyretic/analgesic will both ease the patient's pain and bring down her fever.*
Position the patient for comfort, sitting up in a parent's arms or lying on the side of the unaffected ear.	*Lying flat or on the side of the affected ear can cause more swelling and fluid accumulation in the eustachian tube, resulting in increased pain.*

Nursing Diagnosis: Knowledge deficit related to treating infection in children
Expected Outcomes: The patient will remain free from further infection and complications from OM. The parents will verbalize understanding of necessary interventions to prevent and treat common infections in their child.

Intervention:	Rationale:
Teach parents to administer all the prescribed antibiotics.	*To fully treat the infection and prevent antibiotic resistance, a full 10-day course of antibiotics is usually required.*
Teach parents how to prevent future infections and complications.	*Keeping the child away from tobacco smoke, practicing good hand hygiene, and not giving the child a bottle or sippy cup while lying down will help to lower the child's risk for future ear infections.*

Diphtheria

Diphtheria is a serious throat infection caused by *Corynebacterium diphtheriae* bacterium. The bacterium secretes a toxin that irritates the respiratory tract, causing severe coughing and breathing difficulty. Diphtheria is spread by respiratory droplets from coughing and sneezing and is contagious 2 weeks after the development of symptoms.

Diagnosing Diphtheria

Symptoms of diphtheria start as a sore throat and develop into a visible white coating on the tonsils or in the nose. This coating is referred to as a *pseudomembranous coating.*

Safety *Stat!*

In moderate to severe cases of diphtheria, the pseudomembranous coating on the tonsils or in the nose becomes so thick that it becomes difficult for the child to breathe. This can lead to swelling, swollen neck glands, and airway obstruction.

Interventions for Diphtheria

With the development of the diphtheria vaccine, new cases of this illness have dropped from about 200,000 cases per year in the 20th century to two cases per year. Although rare now in the United States, early symptoms should be known and identified rapidly (Anderson et al., 2021). The vaccine for diphtheria is part of the DTaP vaccination (diphtheria, tetanus, and acellular pertussis). Vaccination does not provide lifetime immunity, and boosters are needed every 10 years to maintain immunity (CDC, 2022e).

Nursing Considerations for Diphtheria

Diphtheria is a serious infection. The child with a diagnosis of diphtheria must be treated immediately with both antibiotics and an antitoxin that will neutralize the diphtheria toxin spreading in the child's body. The toxin can cause heart arrhythmias or heart failure and can lead to nerve damage and paralysis. This illness can be fatal for as many as one in five children under the age of 5.

Tetanus

The tetanus infection is caused by a toxin secreted by the bacterium *Clostridium tetani*. Tetanus enters the body through punctures from rusty metal, dirty needles, open wounds, or a break in the skin exposed to contaminated surfaces. The tetanus toxin then spreads and begins to bind to the neurons of the CNS, gradually causing paralysis throughout the body. Left untreated, the illness can be fatal. The incubation period for tetanus is usually about 7 to 8 days with a range of 3 to 21 days. Once tetanus binds to nerve cells and symptoms begin, there is no cure.

Diagnosing Tetanus

Tetanus is often called *lockjaw* because the stiffness usually starts with the jaw muscles and spreads to the neck, causing

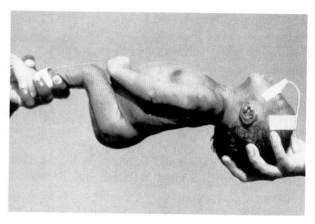

FIGURE 37.8 Tetanus infection.

swallowing difficulty. Within 24 to 48 hours, rigidity and spasms may develop and spread to the trunk and extremities. The child's neck and back become stiff and arched, the abdominal wall becomes rigid, and the severity of the muscle contractions can cause fractures of the spine and long bones (Fig. 37.8). Other symptoms can include fever, tachycardia, high blood pressure, sweating, and cardiac arrhythmias.

Interventions for Tetanus

The treatment for a contaminating injury includes the following:

1. Immediate cleansing of the wound with clean water and a disinfectant
2. Immediate medical attention to prevent the toxin from developing and spreading
3. Antibiotics to kill the bacteria
4. Tetanus immune globulin (TIG) shot to neutralize any toxin that is free-floating and not bound to nerve cells
5. Evaluation of previous immunizations: A person who has received a series of tetanus vaccinations and has received a booster shot within 5 years will already have antibodies and should be protected from developing the disease.

The vaccine for tetanus is part of the DTaP vaccination. Vaccination does not provide lifetime immunity, and boosters are needed every 10 years to maintain immunity (CDC, 2022e).

Nursing Considerations for Tetanus

Because of widespread vaccination against this disease, the incidence of tetanus in the United States has only been 30 cases a year, occurring mostly in adults who have never been vaccinated or did not get boosters (CDC, 2022e).

Pertussis: Whooping Cough

Pertussis is a common, serious, and very contagious bacterial infection of the upper respiratory tract, which is especially concerning in infants. The disease is spread by being in close contact with someone coughing and sneezing and can be spread by parents, siblings, and caregivers. Children at greatest risk for serious illness from pertussis are infants younger than 6 months.

The bacteria that cause pertussis secrete a toxin that severely irritates and damages the lining of the throat and lungs. Initially, the symptoms resemble those of a cold, including runny nose, congestion, and sneezing. After 1 to 2 weeks, the patient has repeated, violent, prolonged coughing fits that can last up to 30 to 60 seconds. The severity of the coughing spells makes it difficult to inhale, and inhalation only occurs when the respiratory tract has been emptied of air. The characteristic "whooping" sound is the result of trying to inhale through the glottis, which is irritated from the coughing spells and narrowed by spasm and secretions. The patient has an impaired ability to clear secretions because of damage to the cilia of the lungs. Thick, tenacious secretions obstruct the bronchi and bronchioles of the lungs, often leading to atelectasis and pneumonia. The incubation period for pertussis is 7 to 10 days, and onset usually occurs 6 to 20 days after exposure.

Diagnosing Pertussis

Although at first the symptoms of the illness may be mild with dry cough, within 2 weeks the cough often progresses to the coughing spells characteristic of the disease, which then continue to increase in severity and frequency. With the severe coughing episodes, cyanosis can occur, the eyes can roll back, and the level of consciousness can change. Seizures and, in rare cases, encephalopathy have been associated with the illness.

Interventions for Pertussis

Hydration and nutrition are important considerations in treating these patients and are particularly important because children, particularly infants, are highly susceptible to dehydration. Postcoughing emesis is common with pertussis infections, and oral intake is often difficult because of coughing episodes and difficulty breathing.

Although many cases of pertussis can be treated at home, hospitalization is often required when an infant demonstrates apnea, respiratory compromise, and neurological impairment secondary to anoxic episodes. Airway maintenance and adequate hydration and nutrition are priorities in treatment. Infants with pertussis can be very ill and sometimes require extended periods of hospitalization.

Nursing Considerations for Pertussis

Pertussis outbreaks peak every 3 to 5 years in the United States. Pertussis education and immunization programs are geared to increase awareness of the prevalence and seriousness of the disease. In young infants, particularly those younger than 6 months old, whooping cough can be life-threatening. The vaccine for pertussis is part of the DTaP vaccination. Vaccination does not provide lifetime immunity, and boosters are needed every 10 years to maintain immunity (CDC, 2022e).

Therapeutic Communication

Pertussis infections in young children and infants are very frightening for parents. The characteristic cough is traumatic for the child and scary to witness for the parents. It is important to be supportive and therapeutic in all interactions with the family. This is especially important if the young child was underimmunized or not immunized fully or was infected by an older sibling who was underimmunized or not immunized. Parents and siblings may feel guilty for causing the child's distress. The family will require teaching about the importance of childhood immunizations, but during the course of the acute illness and hospitalization, the parents need support.

Hepatitis A

Hepatitis A is a virus that affects the liver, causing temporary inflammation. The virus is transmitted by stool or blood and is often the result of contaminated objects put in the mouth, poor hand hygiene and food handling, and contaminated water. The infection can easily be transmitted in restaurants and homes if there are poor hand washing and hygiene practices.

Community outbreaks of hepatitis A can be common because it is most contagious 1 week before symptoms begin. A vaccine for Hep A is available.

Diagnosing Hepatitis A

Approximately 4 weeks after exposure, an exposed person starts to feel ill. The severity of the disease varies depending on the age of the infected person. Most children under the age of 6 often do not show symptoms; of those who do, the symptoms resemble mild intestinal flu symptoms. Children 6 to 12 years often feel ill but have what are considered mild symptoms. Older children and adults can have severe symptoms that resemble food poisoning or gastroenteritis, lasting up to a few weeks.

Moderate cases of hepatitis A in children can involve abdominal pain, vomiting, diarrhea, and dehydration for several days.

Interventions for Hepatitis A

In cases characterized by abdominal pain, diarrhea, and dehydration, hospitalization for antinausea and antidiarrhea medication, as well as IV rehydration, may be needed. In an outbreak of hepatitis A, preventive measures can be taken. Both children and adults can be given an infusion of IV immunoglobulin (IVIG) within 2 weeks of exposure; this has an 85% chance of preventing the development of the disease.

Nursing Considerations for Hepatitis A

Many families may not be familiar with hepatitis A. Because the virus is transmitted easily via stool, blood, contaminated objects, food, and water, it is important to teach and reinforce learning about hand hygiene. Parents should be aware of community breakouts of hepatitis A and should perform strict hand hygiene when taking children to visit family in long-term care facilities, hospitals, or other health-care settings where stool and blood are handled.

Hepatitis B

Hepatitis B is a blood/body fluid-borne virus transmitted through sexual activity; use of contaminated IV drug needles, tattoo needles, health-care–related needle sticks; human bites; or at birth when a baby is exposed to contaminated blood and body fluids. Household contacts of those living with someone with chronic hepatitis B virus (HBV) places the child at risk. HBV is virulent and can survive outside a person on a razor or toothbrush for up to 1 week. There is a three-injection vaccine series for Hep B. (Worldwide, up to four injections may be required.) Hepatitis infections in infants are serious.

Diagnosing Hepatitis B

Symptoms of hepatitis B in teens and adults are nausea, vomiting, abdominal pain, diarrhea, fatigue, fever, loss of appetite, joint pain, dark urine, clay-colored stools, and jaundice. Symptom onset occurs within 90 days of exposure. The clinical presentation of hepatitis B for infants (none or few symptoms) and children under 5 (poor appetite, fatigue, joint and muscle pain, jaundice) is quite different. Children may be asymptomatic.

Interventions for Hepatitis B

When a patient is diagnosed with hepatitis B, antiviral medications such as interferon alfa-2b, lamivudine, or tenofovir disoproxil fumarate may be administered (MedlinePlus, 2022). Close monitoring of a child with chronic HBV is important to evaluate for liver damage and possible liver cancer. Postexposure HBV vaccine given within 12 hours of exposure can help prevent HBV infection (Kodani & Schillie, 2020).

Nursing Considerations for Hepatitis B

About 25% of infants infected with hepatitis B develop liver cancer or liver failure later in childhood and sometimes require a liver transplant. Children who acquire hepatitis B later in childhood, during the toddler or preschool years, often become chronically infected. The long-term outlook for these children is poor and often results in chronic illness and liver failure (Kodani & Schillie, 2020).

Rotavirus

Rotavirus is an intestinal virus that is extremely contagious and transmitted through stool, saliva, and poor hand washing and hygiene practices. Rotavirus infections are most common in the fall and winter seasons and are a frequent cause of illness and hospitalization in young infants and children. Rotavirus is resistant to disinfectant solutions and antibacterial hand soaps. This virus is easily spread in day-care centers, where frequent diaper changes occur and children share toys and food.

Diagnosing Rotavirus

Initial symptoms of rotavirus are similar to gastroenteritis and involve fever, vomiting, and diarrhea. The diarrhea can last more than a few days, up to a few weeks in some cases, and can be more frequent and foul smelling. Infants and young children are at risk for dehydration because of fluid loss from vomiting and severe, prolonged diarrhea.

Interventions for Rotavirus

Treatment involves antinausea medication, rehydration, and sometimes treatment with probiotic powder to decrease diarrhea by increasing the number of "good" intestinal bacteria.

Medication Facts

Zinc deficiency has been found to be associated with immune system impairment and greater severity of serious infectious childhood diseases. In childhood communicable or infectious diseases that have associated diarrhea, zinc supplementation has shown to greatly shorten the duration. Zinc supplementation has also been shown to prevent pneumonia in children between 2 months and 5 years of age (Lassi et al., 2016).

Nursing Considerations for Rotavirus

The rotavirus vaccine is a liquid given by mouth. Depending on the brand, it can be given in a two- or three-dose series at 2, 4, and 6 months with at least 1 month between doses. The vaccine contains whole, live viruses that multiply in the intestines and cause a mild case of the illness to stimulate the body's immune system. A primary point of education with this vaccine is to teach the parents and caregivers that the live virus can be expelled in the diapers up to 15 days after the first dose. It is unclear how contagious postvaccine stools can be, but careful hand washing and hygiene precautions are imperative to prevent transmission of the disease to other children and family members.

Common side effects of the vaccine include fever, vomiting, and diarrhea in 10% of children and poor feeding in 25% of children. Severe reactions to the vaccine include seizure (see Chapter 27), Kawasaki disease (see Chapter 31), and intussusception (see Chapter 34; CDC, 2019).

Human Papillomavirus

Human papillomavirus (HPV) is spread through unprotected sex. There are 40 strains of the virus, and it often goes undetected because there are often no visible signs. Both women and men can carry the virus, and without immunization most sexually active women and men will have come into contact with the virus by their 20s and can act as carriers. Most HPV infections clear on their own; however, when they do not, health problems such as genital warts and various cancers can develop (CDC, 2019). HPV is associated not only with cervical cancer, but also with anal, head, and neck cancer in males; genital warts across the life span; and, rarely, the presence of warts in the airway of infants and children (American Academy of Pediatrics, 2019).

Diagnosing Human Papillomavirus

During birth, an infant can be exposed to HPV infection from a mother with cervical HPV. Newborns can become ill very quickly with high fever and seizures and may become lethargic. HPV infection in newborns can be very severe (CDC, 2019) and can lead to infant death.

Interventions for Human Papillomavirus

There is no treatment for HPV. However, there are ways to manage the complications and problems that arise from having an HPV infection, including treatment for genital or anal warts, treatment for abnormal Pap smears in teen girls, and surgery for warts that grow into the throat or airway structures (CDC, 2024g).

Nursing Considerations for Human Papillomavirus

Nurses have the opportunity to teach preteens and teens how to keep from getting or to stop the spread of HPV infections. First, all girls and boys at age 11 or 12 should get the HPV vaccine (CDC, 2021). The vaccine can be given in either a two or three shot series. The HPV vaccine does not protect against all strains of HPV, only the most common ones. Common side effects from the vaccine include injection site reactions, headache, fatigue, muscle aches, and joint pain. Second, sexually active teenagers should be taught to use condoms to decrease the likelihood of infection. Finally, sexually active girls need to understand that a regular Pap test (see Chapter 3) can detect if the cervix has precancerous lesions because of HPV (Mayo Clinic, 2015).

COVID-19

COVID-19 (SARS-CoV-2) caused the 2019 to 2023 pandemic. A SARS developed as the viral pandemic spread across the world. The disease has caused clinical manifestations ranging from the symptoms of a common cold to severe diseases including severe acute respiratory distress syndrome (ARDS). Health-care institutions were strained to provide care to patients across the life span. Nurses must have a full understanding of the properties of the pathogen, the characteristics of the infection, the transmission of the virus, the process of vaccine development and guidelines, and the best practices for protecting themselves and others from its spread.

Causative Agent

The COVID-19 virus is an RNA strain of the large family Coronaviridae, which has been causing frequent respiratory infections such as the common cold for decades. The common cold, the Middle East respiratory syndrome (MERS), and the SARS infections all form the family Coronaviridae.

The COVID-19 virus enters the host cell through a spike (S) protein binding to what is known as the angiotensin-converting enzyme 2 (ACE2), a membrane-bound aminopeptidase found to be highly expressed in human lung tissue. This pathological process is the basis for the invasion of alveolar epithelial cells, resulting in severe respiratory disease and symptoms. Patients with certain comorbidities such as lung disease (i.e., chronic obstructive pulmonary disease [COPD], smokers), cardiovascular disease, hypertension, diabetes, and immune dysfunction including cancer patients and transplant recipients have been proven to be most susceptible to the severity and lethality of the disease, as well as being linked to increased ICU admissions. This is because of the role that ACE2 plays in the healthy function of the lungs, heart, and immune system.

Diagnosis of COVID-19

COVID-19 has been shown to have a varied presentation; most cases have been mild with a minority of cases in adults progressing to a severe level of disease with a death rate of approximately 2%. Death rates from COVID-19 in children are still being studied. Symptoms typically appear within 2 to 14 days after one has been exposed to the virus. Mild COVID-19 infections seem to be confined to the large conducting airways, and severe COVID-19 disease progresses to the small airways, or those responsible for CO_2–O_2 gas exchange. The majority of infections are considered mild in nature. Confirmation of COVID-19 is done by taking either a molecular or antigen swab from mucus or saliva from the nose or mouth (CDC, 2024b).

Nursing Considerations

Symptoms include fever, cough, fatigue, headache, sore throat, new loss of smell or taste, shortness of breath, congestion and sometimes nausea, vomiting, and diarrhea (CDC, 2024a). The term "long-term" or "long" or "postacute sequelae" COVID is the experience of the longer-term health conditions associated with a COVID-19 infection. These symptoms include fatigue, lung symptoms, mental health conditions, pain, and others (Mayo Clinic, 2022).

Interventions for COVID-19

There are now several COVID-19 vaccines available and approved for infants and children (CDC, 2024c; CDC, 2024d). See the CDC website for this most current information. Two messenger RNA (mRNA) vaccines are currently available in the United States, one developed by Pfizer/BioNTech (BNT162b2) and one by Moderna (mRNA-1273). In these two vaccines, the injected mRNA material carries instructions to make the SARS-CoV-2 "spike" protein—the spiked projections on the surface of macrophages that then attract antibodies to fight the infection. These are not live virus vaccines, and the mRNA "message" degrades within the cell. The third type of vaccine is the recombinant replication-incompetent adenovirus serotype "26" whose genetic material converts to a messenger to promote the production of spike protein antigens.

Nursing Considerations for COVID-19

Nurses can be instrumental in teaching families about how to prevent COVID-19 infections and decreasing the spread of the infection. Reinforcing handwashing, infection avoidance and basic hygiene can reduce the spread. Testing five days after exposure (without symptoms) or testing when symptoms start is very important in family decision making concerning attending school, social activities, and childcare facilities. COVID-19 infections continue to be concerning when children have pre-existing conditions (chronic lung disease, asthma, obesity, immunocompromised conditions and sickle cell disease) (CDC, 2024e).

NONIMMUNIZABLE COMMUNICABLE ILLNESSES

Many infectious diseases do not have an associated childhood immunization. These infections are of particular concern because there is no way to prevent them. Pediatric health-care providers must identify risk factors, common clinical presentations, and symptoms, and then determine best treatment options and nursing care.

Children are particularly vulnerable to the development of communicable illnesses. During infancy and early childhood, the child's immune system is maturing. As the child is exposed to infectious materials, the child's immune system begins to produce immunoglobulins that provide protection. The younger the child, the more vulnerable they are to the development of diseases and illnesses because the child has fewer circulating immunoglobulins. Nasopharyngitis (the common cold), croup, and epiglottitis are discussed in Chapter 30.

Respiratory Syncytial Virus

Respiratory syncytial virus (RSV) is the most common cause of respiratory illness and lower respiratory tract infections in infants and children and is a major cause of bronchiolitis, croup, and pediatric pneumonia. RSV in the adult population often causes cold symptoms. The effect on infants and children can be far more significant. At particular risk for severe respiratory complications from RSV infection are infants, especially premature infants. A RSV vaccination is now available for infants and children. See the most current CDC guidelines for the administration of the vaccine across the lifespan (https://www.cdc.gov/vaccines/schedules/downloads/child/0-18yrs-child-combined-schedule.pdf).

Causative Agent

RSV occurs regularly, most often between winter and early spring with a peak between January and March. It is estimated that 50% of children will be infected with RSV within their first year of life during the winter months. By the age of 3, almost 100% of children will have had RSV at least one time and often more than once. Children can get repeated infections from RSV because the body does not develop immunity even after having the illness. However, repeated infections within a year are often milder. RSV is transmitted by direct airborne exposure to large droplets. The virus is shed profusely and may survive for 4 to 7 hours on skin and surfaces, despite routine infection control. The most effective prevention of transmission of RSV is implementing hand washing, protective gear, and infection-control precautions. Because droplet precautions are required when within 3 feet of the symptomatic child, gown, gloves, and mask are required to be worn.

Clinical Presentation

RSV is a virus that initially produces symptoms in the nasopharyngeal passage and then spreads to the lower respiratory tract. Inflammation of small airways and sloughing and necrosis of the bronchiolar epithelium occur once the virus migrates to the lower respiratory tract. The increased mucus production and significant inflammatory response often cause narrowing and plugging of the small airways, resulting in atelectasis and airway obstruction. Symptoms initially begin as increased nasal secretions but then progress to increased congestion, coughing, paroxysmal coughing spells, and inability to clear secretions. Infants—under 6 months in particular—can present in moderate to severe respiratory distress with increased work of breathing, decreased oxygen saturation, and fatigue that leads to the inability to clear secretions.

Treatment

Hospitalization is often required for infants with severe respiratory distress to provide supplemental oxygen, suction secretions, provide hydration, and monitor respiratory status for distress.

Parvovirus B19 and Fifth Disease *(Erythema Infectiosum)*

Parvovirus B19 is a common viral infection that is associated with several clinical diseases. The most common of these diseases is fifth disease, also known as *erythema infectiosum*. The incubation period for this disease is 4 to 14 days but can range up to 20 days. Parvovirus B19 is spread through respiratory droplets during coughing and sneezing. The virus can also be spread through blood and blood products. The most contagious period is when there are mild signs of a cold, but the rash and joint pain have not yet appeared.

Causative Agent

Fifth disease is caused by parvovirus B19.

Clinical Presentation

This infection is asymptomatic in about 20% of cases. In those who are symptomatic, the initial symptoms are often a mild and benign fever, runny nose, and headache and upper respiratory symptoms. The symptoms mimic so many other illnesses that it is often undiagnosed. However, there is a distinguishing rash that occurs in three phases. The initial face rash is referred to as a "slapped cheek" appearance and is characteristic of this disease (Fig. 37.9). It is followed a few days later by a rash that often spreads to the trunk and

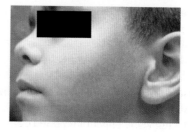

FIGURE 37.9 Fifth disease.

extremities. There is usually itching and joint pain with the rash. When the rash fades, it often appears as a classic lace-like pattern. The rash usually fades in about 3 weeks. The third stage of the rash may continue for weeks or months and may recur in response to environmental stimuli such as sunlight, heat, exercise, and stress.

Treatment

Parvovirus usually resolves on its own without specific treatment. Intervention in this illness is symptomatic and supportive. Medications to relieve fever, headache, and joint pain are often given. NSAIDs are often used. Topical medications to control itching and antihistamines are also used. Rest and fluids are encouraged.

Mononucleosis

Caused by Epstein-Barr virus (EBV), infectious mononucleosis is frequently referred to as the "kissing disease" because the virus is primarily spread through saliva.

Causative Agent

Mononucleosis is caused by EBV, a virus of the herpes family.

Clinical Presentation

Many people exposed to infectious mononucleosis do not develop illness. The virus can exist in a latent state, and someone with the virus not exhibiting illness can be a carrier. The illness primarily affects older children, adolescents, and young adults. Adolescents and young adults who are infected with EBV contract infectious mononucleosis 35% to 50% of the time. The incubation period for this illness can be 4 to 6 weeks after exposure. Symptoms can develop suddenly or come on slowly. The acute phase of the illness can last 2 to 4 weeks. Fatigue is common with this illness and may persist for months after the acute illness has passed. The characteristic signs of mononucleosis are fever, sore throat, and swollen lymph nodes (lymphadenopathy). The initial signs of the illness, usually fever, chills, loss of appetite, and malaise, are quickly followed by lymph node enlargement, splenomegaly, and tonsillopharyngitis with exudates. The lymph nodes can be enlarged for several days to a period of several weeks.

Treatment

Most patients recover from infectious mononucleosis with symptomatic and supportive treatment. Rest, fluids, and NSAIDs for fever and pain are recommended for symptom management. Corticosteroids may be used in severe cases of swollen and enlarged lymph nodes that may occlude the airway or cases that produce neurological or cardiac complications.

Lyme Disease

Lyme disease is the most common vector-borne disease in the United States and one that has received much publicity. States with the highest number of reported cases include New England, New York, New Jersey, Pennsylvania, Minnesota,

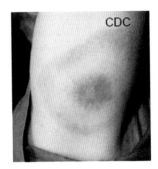

FIGURE 37.10 Lyme disease rash.

and Wisconsin. Ticks must become engorged with blood before they can transfer the infecting organism to a host. This can take 48 to 72 hours. Therefore, inspecting for and removing ticks after walking in wooded areas is the first line of defense in the prevention of illness.

Causative Agent

Lyme disease is caused by a spirochete, *Borrelia burgdorferi*, a bacterium transmitted by the deer tick.

Clinical Presentation

Lyme disease is an inflammatory illness that can affect joints and the nervous system. Clinically, there are two different stages to the illness:

Early stage: The early stage of the disease is 7 to 14 days after the initial bite. A localized rash, called *erythema migrans,* originates at the site of the bite and expands as a solid red rash or as a central spot surrounded by a ringed red rash (resembles a bull's-eye; Fig. 37.10). This rash then spreads to multiple areas of the skin. This usually occurs soon after the initial bite. Other symptoms include joint pain, headaches, fatigue, fever, chills, facial palsy, and a stiff and aching neck with swollen lymph glands.

Late disseminated disease: This phase of Lyme disease can occur months after the initial infection and usually involves arthritis (pain and swelling) of large joints. Swelling can last 1 week up to several weeks. In this phase of illness, there can be neurological involvement: disorientation, confusion, inability to concentrate, and aseptic meningitis. Numbness of the hands and feet is often present. Fatigue and joint and muscle pain can persist for weeks or months after treatment has been completed for acute illness.

Treatment

When caught and treated early, Lyme disease has a very good prognosis for children. Treatment is supportive, as well as the administration of amoxicillin or ceftriaxone antibiotics.

Rocky Mountain Spotted Fever

Rocky Mountain spotted fever (RMSF) is also known as tick-borne typhus. The infection can occur via a bite from the Rocky Mountain wood tick or the dog tick. It is the second most common tick-borne illness in the United States. Despite its name, the disease is prevalent in the southeastern

United States. Over 50% of cases are diagnosed from April to September in states such as Delaware, Maryland, Virginia, West Virginia, North Carolina, Missouri, and Oklahoma. As with other tick-transmitted diseases, the tick has to engorge with blood before transferring the infectious bacteria, so surveillance and removal of ticks is the best prevention of the illness. The organism multiplies in the endothelium and smooth muscles, causing damage to cells and blood vessels, resulting in occlusion of small blood vessels. Coagulopathies develop and disseminated intravascular coagulation (DIC) has been associated with the illness. The incubation period for RMSF is usually 5 to 7 days.

Causative Agent

RMSF is a bacterial illness caused by *Rickettsia rickettsii*. RMSF is a serious, sometimes fatal, disease if not treated correctly in the first 8 days of illness.

Clinical Presentation

Initial symptoms are often headache, malaise, and muscle pain. The symptoms of RMSF often worsen with the abrupt onset of chills and fever. Other symptoms may involve a rash 2 to 5 days after the fever. This begins as maculopapular rash but within 1 to 3 days becomes hemorrhagic. Other symptoms of RMSF include headache, nausea and vomiting, abdominal pain, muscle pain, loss of appetite, and reddened eyes.

The damage caused by the organism also affects the skin, CNS, heart, lungs, liver, and kidney, as well as larger blood vessels as they become occluded. Vascular occlusion leads to necrosis and gangrene of digits and areas of distal perfusion.

Treatment

RMSF can be treated with antibiotics. Tetracycline, doxycycline, and chloramphenicol are the most frequently used medications. Prognosis is relatively good in patients who are treated within 4 days of the onset of symptoms. Treatment of RMSF often requires hospitalization and time-intensive care for treatment of DIC and other multisystem complications of the illness.

Southern Tick-Associated Rash Illness

One of the newest tick-borne diseases identified in the United States is southern tick-associated rash illness (STARI).

Causative Agent

The tick responsible for transmission is the lone star tick. The lone star tick is common in southern states as well as on the East Coast up to Maine.

Clinical Presentation

The symptoms of the disease are similar to those observed in Lyme disease, although the infectious organism responsible for the illness is not known.

Treatment

STARI responds well to a treatment program similar to one used to treat Lyme disease.

Patient Teaching Guidelines

Tick Prevention and Removal

Families who live in areas where ticks are prevalent need to be taught how to prevent being bitten by ticks and how to safely remove any ticks that do bite them.

Tick Prevention

Several protective measures are recommended to prevent being bitten and infected by ticks. These measures should be used in areas where grass, trees, or brush grow:

- Wear long pants.
- Tuck pant legs into socks so that ticks cannot get inside pant legs.
- Wear a long-sleeved shirt and tuck it inside the pants.
- Spray insecticide containing permethrin on boots and clothing.
- Apply insect repellent containing DEET on your skin and reapply every few hours.
- Inspect for ticks, particularly in hair and on creased areas of the body where ticks may hide.

Tick Removal

If preventing a tick bite is not successful, the following measures are recommended to remove the tick:

- Use fine-tipped tweezers to grasp the tick as close to the skin's surface as possible.
- Pull upward with steady, even pressure. Do not twist or jerk the tick; this can cause the mouthparts to break off and remain in the skin. If this happens, remove the mouthparts with clean tweezers.

Tuberculosis

TB is a highly contagious bacterial infection spread through coughing, sneezing, singing, or heavy breathing. The droplets can remain suspended in the air for hours, and masks and respiratory isolation precautions are needed to prevent transmission. Pediatric TB is particularly challenging to diagnose because the clinical presentation differs from that of adults in significant ways. TB occurs most frequently in children younger than 5 and older than 10 years of age.

About 50% of infants and children have no physical findings and are diagnosed only when traced through an adult who is suspected to have TB. Older children and adolescents show signs and symptoms resembling those of adults, such as fever, night sweats, anorexia, and decreased activity. Infants will often show signs of failure to thrive (FTT) or poor weight gain. Children younger than 5 years old make up 60% to 75% of pediatric cases of TB in the United States.

Not everyone infected with TB is symptomatic or develops the disease. When infants and young children contract TB, they are more likely to develop TB disease and develop life-threatening forms of the illness such as disseminated TB and TB meningitis.

Causative Agent

TB is caused by the bacterium *Mycobacterium tuberculosis*. A single sneeze can release up to 40,000 droplets. Each one of these droplets may transmit the disease because the infectious dose of TB is very low.

Clinical Presentation

Once in the body, the organism multiplies and creates an inflammatory exudate. The bacilli are then carried through the local lymphatic system to the nearest group of lymph nodes. The incubation period between the introduction of the bacilli and the development of delayed hypersensitivity is usually 3 to 12 weeks. Changes to the lung happen mostly at a microscopic level; it can become "calcified" and walled off. Some children will have a febrile illness, mild cough, and respiratory symptoms for 1 to 3 weeks when the hypersensitivity first develops. Other symptoms of a TB infection include weight loss, lethargy, FTT, night sweats, and prolonged fevers.

Treatment

After confirmation of a TB infection by positive skin test, sputum analysis, chest x-ray, identification of associated symptoms, and/or a positive TB blood test, the child is treated for 6 to 9 months with one of several anti-TB medications such as the isoniazid-rifapentine regimen. The CDC website has the most current information on treating TB in children.

Cytomegalovirus

Cytomegalovirus (CMV) is a common viral infection, although most with an infection will not know they have the virus because of the lack of symptoms associated with it. Some health-care providers call a CMV infection a silent infection because rarely does one show clinical signs or symptoms. Once infected, the body retains the virus for life. If a child becomes immunocompromised (e.g., cancer, HIV, weakened immune system, transplant recipients) then the concern is that the child will develop a CMV infection.

Causative Agent

CMV is a virus that is spread through blood, saliva, semen, urine, breast milk, and body fluids. A fetus can acquire CMV through transmission during pregnancy. Newborns will not show CMV (i.e., it is undetected) until they are 2 to 3 weeks old.

Clinical Presentation

There is no clinical presentation associated with CMV unless the child is immunocompromised. If immunocompromised, CMV infections can be severe.

Treatment

There is no treatment or cure known for a CMV infection. If immunocompromised, the child should be treated with immunoglobulin to decrease the chance of a CMV infection.

HIV

The vast majority of children who are infected with HIV become so via pregnancy, childbirth, or exposure to breast milk of an infected adult. Testing newborns for HIV is not accurate because antibody tests reflect maternal antibodies for up to 18 months.

Causative Agent

HIV is a lentivirus that replicates via RNA strands. The HIV virus spreads through the body via fluids and affects specific immune cells.

Clinical Presentation

Clinical presentation of HIV is based on the development of associated conditions, infections, and cancers that are caused by the immunocompromised state of the HIV-infected child. Signs and symptoms of HIV infection in the pediatric population include severe fungal (thrush), bacterial (severe OM, pneumonias), or viral infections (CMV retinitis, zoster infections). Wasting syndromes, FTT, and delayed developmental and motor milestones are not uncommon.

Treatment

There is no cure for HIV. HIV-associated infections are treated as needed. Antiretroviral medications are administered based on the child's CD4 cell count. Monitoring a child's immune status is done by regular analysis of the CD4 T lymphocyte cell count. Nephrotic toxicity and CNS toxicity are both concerns with HIV antiretroviral medications.

Clostridioides Difficile

C. difficile is a bacterium that causes severe inflammation of the colon called *colitis*. It is very easy to transmit the bacteria to others who touch contaminated surfaces or items touched by the child. This includes food trays, bed or crib rails, toilets and bathroom fixtures, doorknobs, vital-sign equipment, and toys. Diapered young children are at particular risk for transmitting the bacteria to others. Health-care providers who do not participate in strict hand washing techniques or who have contaminated uniforms can easily pass the bacteria to other patients.

Causative Agent

C. difficile is a spore-forming, gram-positive, anaerobic bacillus that produces two endotoxins: toxin A and toxin B.

Clinical Presentation

A child with a *C. difficile* infection might present with a history of copious watery diarrhea with or without blood. Fever, abdominal pain, cramps, or tenderness is common; loss of appetite, nausea, and vomiting can all occur. Diseases that can result from a *C. difficile* infection include toxic megacolon, sepsis, pseudomembranous colitis (PMC), and, rarely, death (CDC, 2024f; Mayo Clinic, n.d.).

Treatment

Antibiotics are administered to treat a *C. difficile* infection. According to the CDC (2021), one in six patients will present with the infection again approximately 2 to 8 weeks after the initial infection. All staff providing care for the child must ensure meticulous hand washing. House cleaning staff must make sure that all contact areas are cleansed for *C. difficile* per protocol. Some institutions require "expanded contact precautions" for *C. difficile* because the bacterium is resistant to alcohol-based hand gels and some cleaning products.

Key Points

- Children are at risk for developing common infections such as the cold virus, RSV, and strep throat. Other less commonly encountered childhood infectious diseases, such as measles, mumps, and pertussis, place children at risk for severe complications.
- Childhood immunizations are an important and life-saving part of a comprehensive health-promotion and disease-prevention program for children.
- There is no medication or immunization that is completely without risks and side effects. The best a pediatric health-care professional can do is rely on available medical research and continue to study the efficacy and safety of vaccines.
- Using reputable online sources such as the CDC and the NIH to find information about childhood vaccines is an important part of being an informed nurse. Learning about both illnesses that have vaccines and those that do not is important for rapid identification of infectious processes, treatments, and infection-control procedures.
- Childhood infectious diseases prevented by a complete vaccine schedule include varicella, measles, mumps, rubella, polio, hepatitis B, diphtheria, pertussis, tetanus, pneumococcus, hepatitis A, Hib, and rotavirus.
- Because immunization schedules change according to public need, it is important to review the recommended schedule of childhood immunizations on a regular basis.
- Immunizations can pose a slight risk, but the risks of contracting vaccine-preventable illnesses are significantly larger. Many illnesses, such as polio and smallpox, are no longer common because of vaccination programs. The effectiveness of vaccines in eradicating or reducing the incidence of illness may cause parents to falsely believe that they do not need to immunize for these serious, sometimes fatal diseases.
- Even vaccine-preventable illnesses that are not typically fatal can have severe consequences. Outbreaks of measles or chicken pox can be a health emergency in institutions such as hospitals or with vulnerable populations such as pregnant women or immunocompromised children.
- Outbreaks in schools may result in extended absences from school and activities and may require parents to take time from work to care for children who need to stay at home.
- Health-care professionals working with children with diagnosed or suspected childhood infectious diseases must use PPE, infection-control precautions, and isolation as needed. Infection-control precautions include standard, airborne, droplet, contact, expanded contact, and protective precaution, which is also referred to as reverse or *neutropenic precautions.*
- Severe reactions are rare but sometimes do occur with childhood immunizations. It is important that nurses and health-care providers understand the need to report serious reactions to the VAERS.

Review Questions

1. You are explaining to new parents how vaccines increase a child's antibodies to protect them from infection if the child is exposed to a communicable disease. How should you describe the effectiveness of childhood vaccines?
   1. They are considered 100% effective in protecting children across the developmental period.
   2. They are only effective if started in infancy and the entire immunization schedule is followed exactly as recommended.
   3. They cannot be "caught up" if doses are missed.
   4. They are useful in the prevention of childhood communicable diseases, but they are not always 100% effective.

2. What is one difference between *enteric contact precautions* and *contact precautions?*
   1. Enteric precautions refer to PPE and behaviors used to prevent the spread of diarrhea.
   2. Contact precautions are used exclusively for diapered infants who present with diarrhea.
   3. There is no difference between contact precautions and enteric precautions.
   4. Contact precautions are used when there is a likelihood of infection transmission through direct or indirect contact with a patient or their care items.

3. The father of a child who has been admitted for IV antibiotics for methicillin-resistant *Staphylococcus aureus* (MRSA)–positive pneumonia asks you what the term *incubation period* means. What is your best response?
   1. "The incubation period relates to the severity of the illness presented by the child."
   2. "The incubation period is the time between exposure to the infection and the first symptoms."
   3. "The incubation period is the process of growing the child's blood culture sample."
   4. "The incubation period is the time between first exposure and recovery."

4. A 6-month-old infant is due for the last dose of hepatitis B vaccine. Which site should you select for administering the injection?
   1. Abdomen
   2. Deltoid
   3. Gluteal region
   4. Vastus lateralis

5. A nurse is reviewing the immunization record of a 9-month-old with the parents. Which immunizations would you expect to see listed?
   1. Hepatitis B series only
   2. MMR, DTaP, and PCV
   3. MMR, hepatitis B, and Hib
   4. Hepatitis B, DTaP, Hib, IPV, and PCV

6. You are preparing to give a flu shot to a toddler. When you ask the parents if their child has any allergies, they tell you that he is allergic to eggs. What action should you take next?
   1. Administer the flu shot.
   2. Inform the parents that the child cannot receive any more childhood immunizations.
   3. Document the allergy in the child's chart and administer the flu shot.
   4. Ask the health-care provider if the child can receive the intranasal flu vaccine.

7. Although there is no treatment for an HPV infection, there are treatments for complications associated with HPV. What are some of the complications of HPV? **(Select all that apply.)**
   1. Genital warts
   2. Abnormal Pap smears
   3. Encephalopathy
   4. Liver cancer
   5. Hepatitis

8. Attending kindergarten is an important milestone for a young child. Which immunizations, if all prior immunizations are complete, would be needed for a 5-year-old attending kindergarten?
   1. MMR, IPV, and DTP
   2. Hib and DTP
   3. Hepatitis B
   4. Pertussis vaccine

9. _____ _____ is obtained in two ways: (1) by exposure to a bacterium, virus, or toxin sufficient to stimulate an immune response by the body, or (2) by stimulating the body's immune response through vaccination or immunization.

10. The parents of 1-year-old DeShawn bring him to the clinic for a well-child visit. When it is time for their son to receive his scheduled immunizations, the parents refuse, stating, "We don't want him exposed to any more thimerosal." Which response by the nurse is most appropriate?
    1. "Don't believe fake news. It's safer to get vaccines than to get these diseases."
    2. "I understand your concern. I don't immunize my children either."
    3. "In fact, studies show that thimerosal is safe at low levels, but we do have thimerosal-free vaccines that we can give your child."
    4. "Clearly you don't love your son if you won't protect him from serious illnesses."

ANSWERS 1. 4; 2. 4; 3. 2; 4. 4; 5. 4; 6. 4; 7. 1, 2, 4; 8. 1; 9. Active immunity; 10. 3

CRITICAL THINKING QUESTIONS

1. How are school-aged children exposed to communicable diseases?
2. What behaviors of preschool children make them at particular risk for communicable diseases? What are common communicable childhood infections and diseases during the early school-aged child's developmental period?
3. Using the principles of anticipatory guidance, list common means parents can take to reduce the spread of communicable diseases and infections in their children.

Resources

For additional resources and information, including Postconference Questions and Activities, Answers, and References, visit www.FADavis.com.

Student Study Guide

CHAPTER 38
Child With an Oncological or Hematological Condition

KEY TERMS

hemophilia (HEE-muh-FIL-ee-uh)
induction phase (in-DUK-shun FAY-ze)
leukemia (loo-KEE-mee-uh)
maintenance therapy (MAYN-tuh-nents THER-uh-pee)
neutropenia (NOO-troh-PEE-nee-uh)
petechiae (pee-TEE-kee-ee)
purpura (PER-pyoo-ruh)
sickle cell anemia (SCA) (SIK-uhl CELL an-NEE-mee-uh)
stomatitis (STOH-muh-TYE-tiss)
thrombocytopenia (THROM-buh-SYE-tuh-PEE-nee-uh)
vaso-occlusive episode (VAY-zoh-uh-KLOO-siv EP-ih-sohd)

CHAPTER CONCEPTS

Cellular Regulation
Comfort
Communication
Growth and Development
Health Promotion
Infection
Safety

LEARNING OUTCOMES

1. Define the key terms.
2. Describe the characteristics of childhood cancer, including the pathology of solid and blood/lymphatic-based malignancies.
3. Describe the composition and function of the components of blood and relate each function to the pathology of hematological and oncological diseases.
4. Analyze the pathology of anemias and relate types of anemia with an anemic child's clinical presentation.
5. Identify the assessments conducted for a child who presents with iron-deficiency anemia and sickle cell anemia (SCA) and describe the required medical and nursing care for each.
6. Identify the developmentally appropriate pain scales used for a child during a sickle cell episode (crisis) and review effective pain control measures.
7. Describe the nursing care required for a child who is receiving a blood product transfusion: packed red blood cells (PRBCs) and platelets.
8. Differentiate the types and pathology of hyperbilirubinemia as well as medical care and nursing care for an infant with hyperbilirubinemia.
9. Describe the pathology of immune thrombocytopenia and treatment protocols administered across childhood.
10. Identify the most common forms of hemophilia and describe the teaching needs of families to administer emergency treatments for a child experiencing a bleeding episode.
11. Describe the effect of childhood cancer on the functioning and teaching needs of the family caring for a child who is hospitalized for treatments or is home in a neutropenic state.
12. Analyze the issues of safety associated with a child with an oncology disorder, including error reduction, protection from infection, and safe implementation of care.

CRITICAL THINKING

Two-year-old **Maya** has been admitted to the pediatric intensive care unit (PICU) for blood transfusions for severe anemia. Her presenting hemoglobin is 4.1 g/dL. She saw her pediatrician the day before admission for fatigue and pale skin color. The pediatrician drew her laboratory values and determined the severity of her clinical presentation. She was sent to the hospital for a direct admit to the PICU for transfusion therapy and nutrition education. She receives two transfusions: The first is 6 mL/kg of packed red blood cells (PRBCs), and the second is 10 mL/kg of PRBCs. She receives her transfusions over a course of 6 hours and then demonstrates a rise in hemoglobin to 7.3 g/dL. The cause of her anemia is determined to be nutritionally based as she continued to take bottles of whole milk throughout the day and evening. Her parents meet with the dietitian for a long session of teaching on iron-rich foods. Maya is given a discharge prescription for oral iron supplements and will be followed up by her pediatrician.

You see Maya in the pediatrician's office 1 month later and observe symptoms of continued anemia, which could be related to lack of adherence to the oral iron prescription. The child was found to have a close to normal hemoglobin at this follow-up appointment.

Questions

1. How can you recognize the signs of lack of adherence to supplemental iron medication for anemia?
2. What information should be included in teaching the family about administering oral iron supplements?

CONCEPTUAL CORNERSTONE

Cellular Regulation

Cellular regulation is different for cancer cells than it is for noncancerous cells. Cancer cells do not stop dividing, do not have contact inhibition, and do not perform the original function of the cell. There are 250 different types of childhood cancers in two major categories: solid tumors and bloodborne malignancies. The experience of abnormal cellular regulation leading to the development of cancer causes a variety of symptoms. Nursing care measures include using developmentally appropriate pain-evaluation tools, providing pharmaceutical and nonpharmaceutical symptom management, and reevaluating the success of symptom control measures.

Nursing care of children who have an oncological disease (cancer) or a hematological disease (anemia or other blood disease) requires a specific body of knowledge and skill set. The diagnosis of a hematological/oncological condition carries with it the potential for great emotional distress for each member of the family; yet, the majority of childhood cancers are curable. Rapid diagnosis and timely therapy help to ensure an optimal chance of a cure. A thorough search for metastatic disease most often precedes biopsies of suspicious lesions. Histological evaluation of suspected cancer cells allows for the selection of the most appropriate therapies.

Families experiencing either a new diagnosis or providing ongoing care to a child with a hematological/oncological condition must learn specific skills to care for their children to prevent what can be life-threatening side effects of treatment or complications of the disease process. This chapter reviews the foundations of care required to manage childhood cancer, anemias, and hyperbilirubinemia.

INTRODUCTION TO HEMATOLOGICAL CONDITIONS

Caring for a child diagnosed with a blood disorder requires knowledge of the normal composition and function of blood. The capacity of the blood to carry oxygen, fluids, and nutrients, and to collect and transport waste products, becomes interrupted when a child has a condition of the hematological system. Reviewing the normal physiology of the blood system and the function of each component allows you to understand and expect the clinical presentation of the child.

THE DEVELOPMENT OF THE HEMATOLOGICAL SYSTEM

The hematological system begins to develop early in fetal development and continues to mature throughout early childhood. This section reviews the essential cellular components of the blood and the fluid portion that provides nutrients and fluids to the body.

The Composition and Function of Blood

The plasma portion of the blood is made up of about 10% solutes and 90% water. The main plasma solutes are proteins and electrolytes. These proteins include circulating antibodies, albumin, fibrinogen, globulins, and clotting factors. The cellular elements of blood are the white blood cells (WBCs), the red blood cells (RBCs), and the thrombocytes, which produce platelets. All of the formed elements of the blood are thought to originate from the primitive cells called *stem cells.*

Blood is formed in the hematopoietic system found within the bone marrow (myeloid tissue) and lymphatic system (Fig. 38.1). The lymphatic system consists of several components, including the lymphatic vessels, which carry lymph fluid, and the lymphoid solid structures of the lymph nodes. The solid structures include the spleen, the thymus, and the tonsils.

Blood contains RBCs, called *erythrocytes,* and WBCs, which include neutrophils, eosinophils, basophils, T lymphocytes, and B-lymphocytic plasma cells. All of these cells have distinct functions to assist in the maintenance of homeostasis

Cells of the Immune System

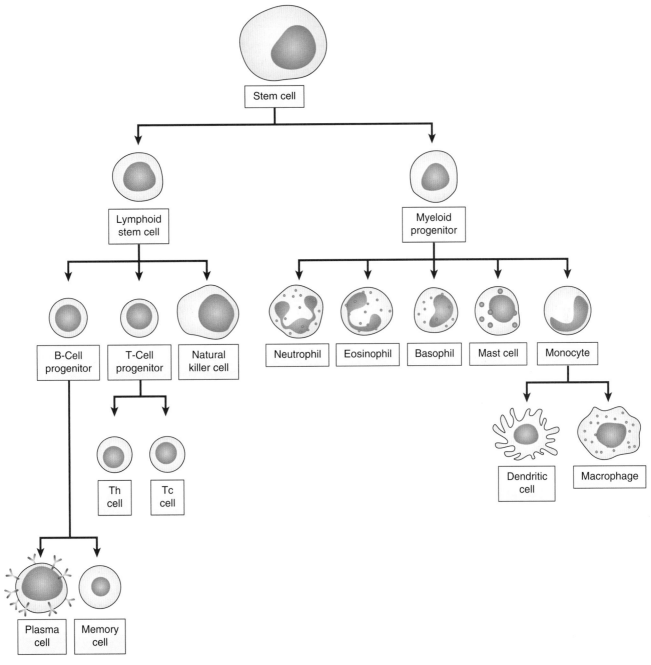

FIGURE 38.1 Bone marrow cells.

within the child's hematological system. See Table 38.1 for information on a complete blood cell count (CBC).

The functions of the components of blood are as follows:

- *Oxygenation:* RBCs contain hemoglobin molecules that attach and release oxygen. Transporting oxygen to all tissues of the body is essential for cellular metabolism. When a child presents with anemia, the transportation and release of oxygen throughout the body is compromised.
- *Cellular nutrition:* Blood plasma carries all the essential nutrients for cellular metabolism. Disruptions in the

volume of blood diminish the body's ability to distribute proteins, vitamins, electrolytes, water, and nutrients.
- *Excretion of wastes:* Cellular waste products are collected by the blood and transported to the liver for processing and to the kidneys for excretion.
- *Maintenance of acid-base balance:* The vascular system carries bicarbonate concentrated from the kidneys to assist in the balance of pH in the blood.
- *Regulation of body temperature:* Blood circulating through the vascular system distributes heat and helps to maintain a normal body temperature.

Table 38.1

Interpreting a Complete Blood Cell Count With a Manual Differential

Cell Component	Function	Expected Values
WBC	Infection-fighting cell	1–23 months: 6.1–17.5 $\times$ 10^3/microL 2–10 years: 4.5–13.5 $\times$ 10^3/microL
RBC	Oxygen-carrying capacity	3–6 months: 3.81–5.61 $\times$ 10^6/microL 7 months–15 years: 3.81–5.21 $\times$ 10^3/microL
Hemoglobin	Molecule to attach oxygen	3–6 months: 11.7–16.3 g/dL 7 months–15 years: 10.3–14.3 g/dL
Hematocrit	Percentage of RBCs in blood	3–6 months: 35%–49% 7 months–15 years: 31%–43%
Reticulocytes	Newly formed RBCs	3.8–5.5 million/mL or 0.5%–2.5% of total number of RBCs
Mean corpuscular volume (MCV)	Average volume or size of RBC	Range from 80 to 95 fL
Mean corpuscular hemoglobin (MCH)	Average hemoglobin level per cell	Divide hemoglobin by number of RBCs
Segmented neutrophils	Mature infection-fighting cell	15%–32% across childhood
Bands	Immature infection-fighting cell	5%–16% across childhood
Lymphocytes	Immunoglobulin production/delayed hypersensitive reaction	26%–76%
Absolute neutrophil count (ANC)	Determines ability to fight infection	1,500 to 8,000/microL

- *Defense against foreign antigens:* Blood provides the distribution of immune cells and immunoglobulins to areas of the body experiencing infection.
- *Transport of hormones:* Hormones manufactured in the endocrine glands throughout the body are transported to target cells by circulating blood.

Red Blood Cells

An RBC lives about 120 days. After that time, the cell grows old and its membranes become fragile and rupture. The hemoglobin found within the RBC is then broken down into two components: (1) hemosiderin (iron), which is recycled, and (2) bilirubin, which must be processed and excreted in bile. When the body is in a status of reduced oxygen (hypoxia), a chemical message is sent to the kidneys signaling them to produce the hormone erythropoietin. This hormone regulates the production of new RBCs, called *reticulocytes,* in the bone marrow. The main purpose of the RBC is to carry oxygen to the cells of the body. Effective oxygen transport depends on having an adequate number of circulating RBCs as well as having sufficient hemoglobin within each RBC. Testing the blood's hemoglobin level provides a measurement of the amount of this protein, which transports and distributes oxygen to tissues. A hematocrit test measures the percentage of circulating RBCs within the blood and gives a clinical picture of the severity of certain anemias. The percentage of the child's hematocrit is about three times that of the total concentration of hemoglobin (in g/dL).

White Blood Cells

WBCs fight infection. Neutrophils, the most prolific of the WBCs, are considered the primary defense in bacterial infections. After killing the bacteria, the neutrophils then consume (phagocytize) them and transport the bacterial cell components to be eliminated. Monocytes are large phagocytic cells involved with an early inflammatory reaction. Lymphocytes produce antibodies and a delayed hypersensitivity response. There are two types of lymphocytes: (1) the T cells, which must mature in the thymus gland and then circulate to become sensitized to specific antigens, and (2) the B cells, whose main function is to synthesize and secrete antibodies in response to specific antigens. Some T cells are called "killer" (cytotoxic) cells because they have the unique ability to produce chemical compounds that are lethal to microbes. Other T cells are called "helper" cells because they activate other cells to trigger an immune response. T cells have a very significant role in the body's fight against the presence of cancer cells.

Thrombocytes

Thrombocytes, also called platelets, are very small pieces of megakaryocyte cell wall membrane that assist with clotting. Platelets adhere to the lining of blood vessels to form clots (a type of plug) to manage bleeding. Additionally, platelets have two unique properties: (1) They secrete chemicals that attract other platelets to the damaged cellular site, and (2) they secrete serotonin, a substance that causes vasoconstriction to prevent further bleeding at the site of injury.

COMMON HEMATOLOGICAL ABNORMALITIES AND DISORDERS

Anemias

Anemias are defined as conditions or diseases that reduce the total circulating hemoglobin within the blood. Anemias minimize the body's ability to circulate oxygen to all tissues, including organs and muscles. Reduced oxygen levels cause complications in growth, cellular repair, and overall homeostasis. Anemia can be categorized in six ways:

1. Impaired production of hemoglobin or impaired or decreased production of RBCs
2. Nutritional deficiency that impairs the production of RBCs
3. Metabolic condition that causes disturbances of RBC production, including nutritional disorders
4. Increased destruction of RBCs
5. Impaired or decreased rate of production of the hormone erythropoietin
6. Excessive blood loss

Clinical manifestations of anemia depend on the cause of the anemia and its severity. The following are clinical signs and symptoms of anemia:

- *Changes in behavior:* Irritability, fatigue, and reduced play
- *Skin:* Pallor, ulcers, and **petechiae** (very small hemorrhagic purplish spots found on the child's skin when the child's platelets are also low), ecchymoses (bruising), and jaundice rashes
- *Cardiopulmonary:* Dizziness, dyspnea, edema, and palpitations
- *Gastrointestinal:* Bleeding, diarrhea, vomiting, anorexia, and melena
- *Genitourinary:* Urinary frequency and hematuria
- *Nervous system:* Syncope, paresthesia, seizures, decreased mental concentration, and loss of consciousness
- *Musculoskeletal system:* Cramps, muscle pain, weakness, numbness, discoloration, and swelling
- *Endocrine:* Polyphagia, polydipsia, polyuria, and temperature intolerance
- *Eyes, ears, nose, mouth, and head:* Diplopia, visual blurring, cataracts, sclera jaundice, tinnitus, vertigo, epistaxis,

stomatitis (inflammation of the mouth, often painful), bleeding gums, buccal mucosa ulcerations, and texture changes on tongue

Diagnosing Anemias

Children who present with signs and symptoms of anemia need to have a thorough assessment performed. The following list notes aspects that should direct the physical assessment of the child:

- Diet history, especially questions about the diversity of food intake and the quantity of milk consumed daily
- General performance status, concentration, level of mental activity, reports of weakness, exercise and play intolerance
- General appearance, including height, weight, and rate of physical growth
- Blood values, including a CBC with differentiation of cell lines and peripheral smear to identify abnormal cell morphology
- RBC indices such as mean corpuscular volume (MCV), mean corpuscular hemoglobin concentrate (MCHC), and ABO and Rh typing.
- Urine, emesis, and stool checks for blood
- Skin pallor from tissue hypoxia
- Jaundice and color of nailbeds, mucous membranes
- Vital signs (VS), checking for an increased heart rate (HR), respiratory rate (RR), increased pulsations, heart murmurs, and an evaluation of orthostatic hypotension

Interventions for Anemias

Nursing care of the child with anemia includes protecting the child from injury. The child may require oxygen therapy if anemia is severe, and the hypoxia is causing difficulty in breathing. The child will need a quiet environment with choices of quiet play activities that promote social, physical, and cognitive development. The child will need to have structured rest periods and naps if developmentally appropriate. The health-care provider should notify a nutritionist and make a referral for a dietary assessment and a family teaching session and for the development of a nutritional plan. The child may require blood transfusions if anemia is severe. The family will need education about the need for oxygen therapy and the need for the child to save energy and decrease fatigue. The family will also need to understand the frequency of phlebotomy to check the status of the child's anemia and the care, benefits, and risks associated with transfusion therapy.

Medical care depends on the type and cause of the anemia. The child may require several medical interventions, including iron therapy, oxygen therapy, transfusion therapy, and frequent follow-up appointments.

· **WORD** · **BUILDING** ·
stomatitis: stomat–mouth + itis–inflammation

Further laboratory assessments and diagnostic studies for anemia may include:

- *Direct Coombs test* for the presence of antibodies attached to the RBC that cause hemolysis (breakdown of RBCs)
- *Ferritin* to assess the major iron storage protein (will be decreased in iron-deficiency anemia)
- *Serum iron* to measure the amount of iron bound to transferrin
- *Lead levels* to determine if the cause of the anemia is related to lead poisoning
- *Osmotic fragility,* which is associated with hereditary spherocytosis
- *Hemoglobin electrophoresis* to determine which specific type of hemoglobin is reduced, if the child has a hemoglobinopathy

Iron-Deficiency Anemia

Iron-deficiency anemia is the most common form of anemia affecting children in the United States. The incidence of iron-deficiency anemia worldwide is as high as 30% to 40%; in the United States, 20% of older infants and toddlers have anemia, with 50% of those having iron-deficiency anemia. Left untreated, iron deficiency can strongly affect a child's growth and development (Health Research Funding, 2019; Mayo Clinic, 2022).

Maternal iron stores are depleted in the infant by 6 months of age. At that time, the infant must have sufficient iron intake from their nutritional means in order to avoid becoming deficient. Risk factors for iron-deficiency anemia include the introduction of solid foods to an infant before the recommended age of 6 months, the introduction of cow's milk before the child's first birthday, or the excessive consumption of cow's milk during the early childhood period. Overconsumption of milk (more than 24 ounces of cow, goat, or soy) causes the young child to feel full and refuse to eat a well-balanced, iron-rich diet, leading to anemia. Cow's milk is low in iron, is not a complete protein for humans, and can cause microscopic bleeds within the intestinal lining of infants, all contributing to anemia (Health Guidance for Better Health, 2018; Mayo Clinic, 2022).

Safety *Stat!*

Preterm infants are also at risk for developing iron-deficiency anemia. Loss of as little as 1 to 7 mL of blood per day through chronic gastrointestinal (GI) bleeding can lead to anemia in this population. An infant with iron-deficiency anemia will display microcytic anemia or small, pale RBCs.

Diagnosing Iron-Deficiency Anemia

A child with iron-deficiency anemia will display the symptoms listed in the general discussion of anemias.

Laboratory tests are used to assess and confirm a diagnosis of iron-deficiency anemia:

- Decreased hemoglobin
- Decreased hematocrit
- Decreased serum iron concentration
- Decreased MCV
- Decreased MCHC

Interventions for Iron-Deficiency Anemia

Iron-deficiency anemia is corrected by diet; the oral intake of iron supplements; and, if needed in moderate cases, intramuscular (IM) injections of iron. Severe cases of iron-deficiency anemia in which the child is symptomatic with fatigue, shortness of breath, and tachycardia require blood transfusions. Although mild iron deficiency may be treated with oral iron supplementation, this therapy requires weeks to months to correct the anemic state. If a child taking oral iron has issues with compliance or adherence to the regimen, IV administration of iron sucrose may be required.

Medication Facts

Iron sucrose IV infusions may be required if a child has difficulty adhering to lengthy oral iron regimens or has difficulty absorbing iron. IV iron sucrose administration results in significant increases of hemoglobin, MCV, serum iron, % iron saturation, and ferritin (Kaneva et al., 2017; Lepus et al., 2022).

Nursing Considerations for Iron-Deficiency Anemia

Caring for a child with iron-deficiency anemia takes a team approach. Families need to learn about the physiology and pathology of anemia and commit to treatment and prevention. The team should work together in explaining all aspects of care required, taking into consideration the best teaching approach that works for each family. The following list includes important points to consider when taking care of an anemic child:

- Teaching the family to make sure that the young child rinses their mouth after taking oral iron preparations because the medication can stain the child's teeth
- Teaching families that oral elemental iron should be taken with a source of vitamin C, such as a small amount of orange juice, to improve absorption, and should be taken either 1 hour before or 2 hours after ingesting milk products or antacids
- Teaching families that supplemental oral iron can cause the child to become constipated and produce dark stools
- Educating the family to prevent relapses of iron-deficiency anemia by encouraging well-balanced meals
- Referring the family to a nutritionist
- Assessing for contributing factors such as a low economic status of the family

Sickle Cell Anemia

Sickle cell anemia (SCA) is one type of sickle cell disease that causes a child to have abnormal, sickle-shaped hemoglobin S (HbS). Occurring in one out of every 365 live births of African American babies in the United States (Centers for Disease Control and Prevention [CDC], 2022b), this condition is marked by chronic hemolytic anemia and vaso-occlusion. These two outcomes cause pain and fatigue and affect the child's quality of life.

When a child with SCA experiences a trigger, the bone marrow produces rigid, sickle-shaped RBCs, which increase blood viscosity and cause tissue hypoxia because of the obstructed blood flow. Symptoms of the disorder appear after 4 to 6 months of age; before this time, the young infant has the presence of fetal hemoglobin. If the child does not present with SCA as an infant, they will during toddlerhood or preschool during an episode of infection such as in the GI or respiratory tract.

Triggers that cause a sickling episode include either an increased demand for oxygen, such as emotional distress, infection, or pain, or a decreased demand for oxygen, such as pulmonary infections. Children who travel to high altitudes, where there is less oxygen, can also experience sickle cell episodes. Sickle cell episodes cause the child severe pain, often requiring narcotic pain control measures.

Risk factors for the development of SCA include being of African descent. SCA is an autosomal recessive genetic disorder in which the normal hemoglobin A (HbA) is either partially or completely replaced with HbS.

There are four common types of SCA crises, or episodes. Each can cause significant pain and may be life-threatening.

- *Vaso-occlusive crisis:* This type of SCA crisis lasts up to 6 days and presents with severe pain in the joints; bones; and abdomen and with swollen joints, feet, and hands. The child may experience visual disturbances.
- *Aplastic anemia crisis:* This is a form of extreme anemia caused by the severe destruction and lack of production of the child's RBCs.
- *Sequestration crisis:* This type of SCA crisis is caused by large quantities of blood that collect and pool in the child's spleen and liver, causing tachycardia, weakness, and dyspnea. It may lead to shock as the vascular volume of the child's blood decreases.
- *Hyperhemolytic crisis:* This type of SCA crisis is caused by an increasing rate of RBC destruction, which leads to severe anemia and a state of jaundice.

Newborn screening is imperative for the early identification of children with SCA. Once a child is diagnosed with SCA, teaching must be initiated with the parents to prevent, as much as possible, the triggers that lead to painful SCA episodes (crises).

Diagnosing Sickle Cell Anemia

The health-care team should evaluate each body system, including respiratory, cardiac, musculoskeletal, skin, and neurological/mental status. Laboratory values, such as a CBC, a percentage of sickled cells, fluid status, and electrolytes, are all evaluated on a regular basis, especially during an SCA episode.

Laboratory tests include:

- CBC
- Sickledex (sickle cell index or sickle solubility test) to screen for the presence of HbS
- Hemoglobin electrophoresis to separate the various forms of hemoglobin, thus providing a definitive diagnosis

Nursing evaluations of a child with SCA include meticulous evaluation of pain scores on a consistent, validated pain scale appropriate to the child's age (Wong-Baker FACES or numerical scale). Children experiencing a pain episode must be managed with pain medications that provide comfort during a painful crisis situation.

Interventions for Sickle Cell Anemia

Children experiencing an SCA crisis need specific treatments to improve their status rapidly. Interventions for a child experiencing a **vaso-occlusive episode** (an SCA crisis with a large number of sickled cells produced) include pain control, hydration, oxygenation if needed, and rest. Blood transfusions may be warranted to improve oxygen delivery to cells. Exchange transfusions may be needed to reduce the circulating numbers of sickle cells. Nursing care includes monitoring intake and output (I&O) and providing adequate oral fluids and nutrition when able to tolerate. Many children find comfort in warm packs placed on swollen and painful joints. Oral penicillin is ordered to provide prophylaxis against infections. If a child presents with a fever or any evidence of infection, antibiotics will be ordered.

Nursing Considerations for Sickle Cell Anemia

Because SCA is a chronic, lifelong disorder, the child requires nursing care that promotes independence, self-care to prevent dehydration and infections, and family involvement to provide support to a child who suffers periodic SCA episodes (Fig. 38.2). Because many children require hospitalizations for SCA episodes, it is important to provide care that promotes early identification of potential complications and rapid treatments that minimize the lengths of stay. You should assist the pediatric health-care team in identifying the following clinical manifestations of a child with SCA during an episode:

- Reports of pain, especially in joints where rigid sickle cells form clots, leading to hypoxia
- Abdominal pain, nausea, vomiting, and anorexia
- Shortness of breath
- Fatigue
- Tachycardia
- Jaundice
- Muscle weakness
- Lethargy
- Irritability
- Impaired healing
- Priapism (prolonged and painful erections because of the presence of viscous blood/clots in the penis)

Emotional support is very important for both the child and the family. Knowing that painful episodes are a lifelong reality may cause distress, fear, and depression. Encouraging the family to meet with social services, spiritual care providers,

and counseling services may help them to cope with the disease. Fatigue can also cause a child and their family distress. Refer to Box 38.1 for information about factors concerning fatigue in SCA.

Other nursing concerns surrounding the care of a child with SCA include:

- Maintaining skin integrity to prevent infections
- Teaching the child and family to avoid taking aspirin
- Teaching relaxation techniques
- Providing the adolescent with a behavioral contract to adhere to medical treatments, nursing care, self-care, and health promotion
- Providing family education and emotional support

Box 38.1

Biobehavioral Factors of Fatigue in Sickle Cell Anemia

SCA, a disease of global concern, produces a significant level of fatigue during vaso-occlusive episodes. Although pain is the symptom most frequently associated with this disease, acute and chronic episodes of fatigue affect the patient's quality of life, decreasing their sense of well-being. Nurses can assist the child with SCA by teaching the child and family to prevent or decrease factors that contribute to fatigue. According to Ameringer and Smith (2011), many factors contribute to fatigue. By applying their findings to nursing care, one can provide education and assistance to improve understanding and reduce the impact of fatigue:

- *Hypoxemia:* Inflammation and hypoxemia are two key processes of SCA. Hypoxemia is found to be associated with fatigue. Preventing situations in which there is an increased oxygen demand will reduce the severity of hypoxemia-related fatigue. Teaching families about preventing infections will reduce the severity of hypoxemia.
- *Anemia:* Hemoglobin levels should be maintained. Families must be taught to maintain regular health-care visits so that the child's CBC will be monitored for increasing anemia and the need for transfusion therapy. Families must learn to follow serial CBC results.
- *Hyperviscosity of blood:* Dehydration should be prevented because it leads to an increased viscosity, or thickness, of the blood. Teach the family to provide adequate hydration on a daily basis, especially in hot seasons and with physical exercise.
- *Elevated inflammatory cytokines:* A child in a SCA episode will demonstrate elevated cytokines, which contribute to the experience of fatigue. Families need to be taught to increase rest and provide hydration. Promote adequate sleep because inflammation associated with SCA contributes to the child's fatigue experience.
- *Stress:* A child's experience with a chronic illness such as SCA is associated with stress. Linked with fatigue, stress produces an increased release of cortisol, which then causes an increase in cytokines, producing more fatigue. Families need to be taught to identify stressors in a child's life and to make efforts to decrease perceived stressful situations or events.

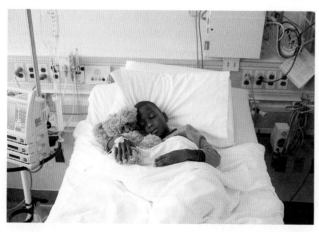

FIGURE 38.2 A child receiving treatment for sickle cell anemia (SCA).

Hyperbilirubinemia

Hyperbilirubinemia is a condition of the neonate in which there is an increase in the breakdown of RBCs that release bilirubin. The child presents with jaundice from lipid-soluble unconjugated or indirect bilirubin accumulating in the tissues. Unlike unconjugated bilirubin, conjugated bilirubin is water-soluble and is typically excreted through the infant's urine and bile. For a complete discussion of hyperbilirubinemia, see Chapter 17.

Immune Thrombocytopenia

Immune thrombocytopenia (also known as idiopathic thrombocytopenia purpura [ITP]) is an acquired hemorrhagic disorder in which the child's total number of circulating platelets is severely reduced. The child will present with bruising, bleeding, or injury, most commonly presenting between 2 and 6 years. The disorder may be acute or chronic, and the cause is unknown. Current theory is that the child is experiencing an autoimmune phenomenon. Immune thrombocytopenia often follows an acute viral infection such as an upper respiratory infection or an experience of a childhood communicable disease, such as varicella or the measles. An antiplatelet antibody is produced in the spleen, which rapidly and severely reduces the production of platelets, leading to bleeding into the tissues, called *purpura*. Petechiae (tiny, pinpoint bruises) are seen on the child's skin, and the child might present with hematuria and/or blood in the stools. Upon presentation, the child's platelet count is usually under 20,000/microL. A bone marrow aspiration may be performed to rule out other disorders, such as an oncological diagnosis of **leukemia** (malignancy of the bone marrow's WBCs).

Thrombocytopenia is a decrease in the quantitative number of circulating platelets in the blood, resulting in a count of lower than 100,000/microL. This disorder requires the implementation of and strict adherence to bleeding precautions:

- Frequently observing for bruising, petechiae, and bleeding from gums, rectum, and nose
- Regularly checking for hematuria and occult or frank blood in the stool
- Meticulously monitoring for changes in the mental status or any change in the neurological system for symptoms of intracranial bleeds from low platelet count

Diagnosing Immune Thrombocytopenia

Assessments for immune thrombocytopenia include the following:

- Bruising and bleeding into the tissues (purpura)
- Petechiae or pinpoint bruising
- Bleeding of the mucous membranes
- Blood found in the child's urine or stool

• **WORD** • **BUILDING** •

hyperbilirubinemia: hyper–excessive + bilirubin–bilirubin + em–blood + ia–condition

bilirubin: bili–bile + rub–red + in–chemical compound

thrombocytopenia: thrombo–coagulation + cyto–cell + pen–lack + ia–condition

leukemia: leuk–white + em–blood + ia–condition

Laboratory tests for immune thrombocytopenia include the following:

- CBC and platelet counts, on a regular basis. You should report drops in the child's overall platelet count or when the count falls below 20,000/mm^3.
- Coagulation studies.
- Bone marrow biopsy may be ordered to rule out leukemia or other severe conditions.

Interventions for Immune Thrombocytopenia

Treatment for immune thrombocytopenia includes the administration of oral or IV corticosteroids. The administration of IV immunoglobulins (IVIG) is considered if the child does not demonstrate improvement. The administration of anti-D antibody in one dose for children with RhD-positive blood types may also be ordered but only for those children with no mucosal bleeding, no infections, and a normal WBC count. Infusions of donor platelets are not considered generally helpful but may be considered in cases of immune thrombocytopenia that have life-threatening bleeding.

Nursing Considerations for Immune Thrombocytopenia

Nursing considerations for immune thrombocytopenia include the following:

- Because the child is at risk for bleeding, the child should be carefully monitored for signs of internal bleeding. These signs include headache, stomachaches, painful joints, and hematuria.
- Family members should be taught to maintain a safe environment for the child and to choose quiet play activities such as coloring, painting, reading, puzzles, clay work, or crafts.
- Nursing care includes teaching families about maintaining safety until treatment allows a rise in the circulating platelet counts. You will administer IVIG for a goal of a rapid rise in platelets, and prednisone to decrease the formation

Medication Facts

The administration of IVIG requires meticulous dosage calculation and medication administration. The IVIG solution comes in a glass bottle that requires the use of vented IV tubing. Premedications may be ordered to prevent reactions. The health-care team should work closely with the pharmacy to determine the rate and total volume required based on the child's height and weight. Calculations should be double-checked by two nurses. Infusions should start slowly to check for untoward reactions and then should be increased every 15 minutes after repeated VS. Monitor the child for hypotension, fever, and urticaria. All assessments should be carefully documented, and any change of condition during the infusion or after completion should be reported immediately.

of antiplatelet antibodies. New treatments include the administration of anti-D antibody (one dose) before the administration of prednisone. Children may be hospitalized for the time required to elevate the platelets. This provides safety and monitoring for the onset of bleeds.

Hemophilia

Hemophilia A and B, the most common forms of this disorder, are both X-linked recessive disorders in which the child has an impaired ability to control bleeding. Lack of clotting factors results in extended bleeding times. Typically, the disorder is manifested in infancy as the child begins teething, sitting up, or crawling. The young child presents with unusual bruising with only minor falls or bumps. Hemophilia is categorized as mild or severe, depending on the amount of clotting factor (in percentages) that is present. Mild hemophilia may be seen when the child has 48% of their expected level of clotting factors.

About 80% of all hemophilia cases are type A hemophilia, in which the child has a deficiency in factor VIII. Less common is type B hemophilia, in which the child has a deficiency in factor IX. Factor IX deficiency is also referred to as *Christmas disease.*

Diagnosing Hemophilia

Assessments for a child with hemophilia include the following:

- Active bleeding or excessive bleeding with minor cuts
- Reports of joint pain and stiffness
- Impaired mobility
- Bleeding in the mouth or gums from teething
- Presentation of hematuria
- History of tarry stools
- History of epistaxis (nosebleeds)

Laboratory tests for hemophilia include the following:

- Prolonged partial thromboplastin time (PT)
- Factor-specific assays to determine the type of clotting deficiency
- DNA testing to identify traits in female family members

Patient Teaching Guidelines

Patients and their families may not understand why only female family members require DNA testing for the presence of the hemophilia gene mutation. Nurses can reinforce the teaching of health-care providers by explaining that **hemophilia** is a rare bleeding disorder that is passed down from parents who either have the disease or are carriers of it.

Humans have 22 pairs of chromosomes in addition to the sex chromosomes (X and Y). Men have X-Y sex chromosomes, and women have X-X sex chromosomes. Boys inherit the X chromosome from their mother and Y chromosome from their father. Girls inherit one X chromosome from each parent.

Congenital hemophilia is linked to the X chromosome and therefore predominantly affects males who receive an abnormal X chromosome from their mother. The mother who carries the hemophilia gene can pass on either her normal or abnormal X chromosome to her children. Fathers with hemophilia have only the abnormal X chromosome that they pass on to all of their daughters, who become carriers. In very rare circumstances, a daughter can be born with hemophilia by having an affected father and carrier mother (CDC, 2022a).

Interventions for Hemophilia

Treatment for hemophilia includes rapid administration of the clotting factor in which the child is deficient. Nurses need to teach families how to store and administer factors via IV. Corticosteroids may be used to treat complications associated with bleeding, such as chronic synovitis, **hemarthrosis**, or hematuria. DDAVP (1-deamino [8-D-arginine] vasopressin) is often prescribed before scheduled dental or surgical procedures.

Nursing Considerations for Hemophilia

Nursing care for a child with hemophilia is complex and must be holistic in nature. Nursing concerns include:

- Avoiding taking temperatures rectally or administering any medications via rectal suppository
- Avoiding skin puncture procedures or subcutaneous, IM, or intradermal (ID) medications
- Applying pressure for no less than 5 minutes directly over the site of any required injections, needlesticks, or venipuncture
- Monitoring stool, urine, and nasogastric fluids for frank or occult blood
- Teaching the family to provide safety and prevent any injuries that may lead to a bleed, including discussing with the family the need for the child to play only low-impact, low-contact sports
- Teaching the family to monitor for bleeds, including symptoms such as headache or changes in HR
- Teaching the family to administer factor replacement therapy via a rapidly placed butterfly IV needle, typically into the antecubital space
- Coordinating comprehensive care and follow-up for the family, including referring the family to a social worker and physical therapist

---

• WORD • BUILDING •

hemophilia: hemo–blood + phil–tendency toward + ia–condition

• WORD • BUILDING •

hemarthrosis: hem–blood + arthr–joint + osis–condition

- Teaching families that the child's risk of exposure to infectious diseases is now minimized with the production of replacement factors via recombinant products

CLINICAL JUDGMENT

You are assisting a school nurse at an elementary school, and one of the students has hemophilia. You were just notified that the student tripped in the cafeteria and hit his head.

Question

1. What should you do next?

Thalassemia Major

Thalassemia major is one of a group of inherited hypochromic (pale color of the RBCs) and microcytotic anemias that vary in terms of severity. This condition produces a hemolytic anemia, causing severe weakness. Transfusions are required to extend life expectancy. If thalassemia major is left untreated, a child can experience growth impairment; delayed or absent puberty; and cardiac complications, including intractable arrhythmias and chronic congestive heart failure. Without transfusions, the child's bone marrow tries to compensate by expanding. Hypertrophy then occurs, leading to thin bones prone to pathological fractures. Thalassemia major is found in populations throughout the Mediterranean, India, and the Middle East.

Nursing Care Plan for Care of a Child With Hemophilia

Jesse, a 13-month-old boy, started walking recently. His parents bring him to his pediatrician's office because they are concerned about the bruises he develops from the normal falls or bumps that happen to newly mobile toddlers. On examination, the child is irritable, and his legs, arms, and forehead are covered with ecchymoses in various stages of healing. The pediatrician asks if there is any family history of hemophilia. Jesse's mother states that her deceased maternal uncle had it, but she doesn't know much more than that. The pediatrician orders a STAT CBC with differential and tests for clotting factors.

Nursing Diagnosis: Risk of injury related to hemophilia bleeding disorder
Expected Outcome: The patient will experience minimal injury from internal bleeding.

Intervention:	Rationale:
Check patient for signs of internal bleeding in addition to obvious cuts, scrapes, or bruises.	*Patients often experience deep bruising from minimal contact or minor injuries. The deep bruising may lead to bleeding into joint spaces (swollen joints) and vital organs.*
Observe patient for evidence of pain.	*Younger children do not know how to express pain and exhibit symptoms through guarding or irritability and fussiness.*

Nursing Diagnosis: Risk for altered growth and development
Expected Outcomes: The patient will grow and develop as normally as possible.

Intervention:	Rationale:
Administer replacement clotting factors as necessary.	*Replacement of clotting factors is the primary treatment for hemophilia; other supplements, antibodies, and antifibrinolytics may be required.*

Nursing Diagnosis: Knowledge deficit related to new diagnosis of hemophilia
Expected Outcome: The parents verbalize ways to maintain a safe home environment for their son.

Intervention:	Rationale:
Teach the family to provide for a safe home environment by • Minimizing clutter to prevent tripping and falls • Padding corners of furniture • Dressing the child in extra clothes for padding • Using child safety gates to prevent falls down stairs • Using only soft toothbrushes • Selecting daily activities that are low risk for injury • Avoiding aspirin and aspirin-containing medications • Observing for signs and symptoms of bleeding, including tenderness, pain, swelling, warmth, tingling, and decreased mobility of joint or extremity	*Because there is no cure for hemophilia, the best way to avoid complications from the disease is to prevent bleeding episodes. The family, and Jesse when he gets older, must take every precaution to avoid cuts, scrapes, bumps, and bruises.*

Diagnosing Thalassemia Major

Assessments for a child with thalassemia major include the following:

- Anemia, with abnormally small (microcytic) cells
- Fatigue
- Pallor

Interventions for Thalassemia Major

Interventions for a child with thalassemia major are limited. This condition does not have a cure. Interventions to maintain adequate perfusion include:

- Regular transfusions to keep the hemoglobin level above 10 g/dL
- If possible, bone marrow transplantation

Nursing Considerations for Thalassemia Major

Nursing considerations for a child undergoing treatment for thalassemia major are related to the frequency of transfusions required. Nursing care includes:

- Monitoring for transfusion reactions related to the consequences of multiple transfusions
- Understanding that repetitive transfusions can lead to iron overload, which requires treatments to remove stored iron
- Educating the family about the severity of the disease, including educating them about the need for lifelong transfusions

 TRANSFUSION THERAPY

Blood-product support is often a cornerstone of both hematology and oncology therapy. Many treatments to cure cancer produce periods of severe chemotherapy-induced anemia. RBC deficiency can result from the side effects of medications, an increased loss, or decreased production. Children with SCA require blood-product support to optimize the recovery of a sickle cell episode (crisis). The indication for blood-product therapy is to restore volume, minimize bleeding, correct coagulopathies, replace plasma proteins, or improve the child's oxygen-carrying capacity. The standard treatment for severe anemia is the administration of 10 to 15 mL/kg of leukocyte-reduced, irradiated PRBCs to obtain at least 6 to 8 g/dL of hemoglobin posttransfusion.

Blood-Product Therapies

The administration of blood products may be required for a child with a severe anemia. The most commonly administered blood product is PRBC, in which most of the serum and WBCs have been removed. Each blood product is different and has unique properties. Transfused products and considerations for each are listed next:

- *Whole blood:* Rarely given because of the chance of severe reactions, whole blood is transfused for traumas in which massive volume is lost or sometimes used for blood-exchange transfusions. Child and donor blood must be matched for ABO and Rh-compatibility.
- *PRBCs:* These are most commonly used for the improvement of oxygen-carrying capacity. For every 10 to 15 mL/kg transfused, the expected rise in hemoglobin is 3 g/dL. Transfusion time should be 3 hours per single transfusion. Filters are required.
- *Platelets:* These are transfused when a child's platelet count is below 20,000/mm³ or if there is evidence of bleeding. Single-donor infusions are preferred because they decrease the exposure to foreign proteins. A single unit should raise the overall platelet count by 10,000/mm³. Although cross-matching is not required, ABO and Rh-compatible platelets are preferred. The length of the transfusion is as fast as the child can tolerate it.
- *Granulocytes:* These transfusions are rarely performed because of the chances of severe reactions and are saved for children who are experiencing severe neutropenia with documented and resistant infections. Single-donor granulocytes are required.
- *Fresh-frozen plasma:* This is transfused to provide a source of stable coagulation factors such as fibrinogen and factors II, V, VII, IX, X, and XI. Cryoprecipitate is made from fresh-frozen plasma to produce a product that is high in factors.

Safety *Stat!*

A whole blood transfusion causes more side effects than a transfusion of PRBCs because all of the components of the blood are transfused. These components can cause a variety of side effects from mild to life-threatening. Whole blood is rarely transfused, and its use is limited to extreme and time-sensitive life-threatening emergencies.

Because of the potential frequency of transfusion therapy for children with hematological or oncological conditions, it is important to provide blood products with the following special preparations:

- Irradiated blood products to prevent graft-versus-host disease (GVHD)
- Leukocyte-depleted products for all children with cancer or those who experience repeated febrile reactions
- Cytomegalovirus (CMV)-negative components; ensuring that transfused products are not infected by this virus diminishes the potential of the child becoming infected.

Potential Complications of Transfusion Therapy

Children receiving transfusion therapies need to be carefully monitored for side effects and complications. Immediately respond to and report any suspected or actual adverse reaction to transfusion therapy. Various side effects, their complications, and treatments for each are listed next:

- *Febrile responses* are manifested by chills, flushing, headache, chest pain, muscle pain, and elevated temperatures. Acetaminophen (Tylenol) is given to prevent or treat febrile reactions.
- *Urticaria responses* produce hives and itching. Diphenhydramine (Benadryl) is given to reduce this reaction. Without treatment, the child may experience wheezing, dyspnea, and respiratory distress.
- *Hemolytic responses* can occur when alloimmunization has taken place. In alloimmunization, the more transfusions the child is exposed to, the greater numbers of antibodies are formed against the transfused foreign proteins. Matching the recipient to the donor decreases the severity of alloimmunization, thus reducing the chances of increasingly severe hemolytic reactions.
- *Septic shock* can occur on the rare occasions when the transfused product is contaminated with a type of bacteria that flourishes in cold temperatures such as cold product storage. This type of microbe is called a *psychrophile*. Other infections can be transmitted via blood products. Currently hepatitis B and C, HIV Types 1 and 2, Human T-Lymphotrophic Virus Types I and II, *Treponema pallidum (syphilis),* West Nile virus, and *Trypanosoma cruzi (Chagas disease)* are all tested for in each unit of donated blood (Food and Drug Administration [FDA], 2023).
- *Circulatory overload* can occur when the total volume of the transfused unit adds volume to the child's vascular space. Transfusions can affect the total vascular volume, potentially causing symptoms of circulatory overload. Symptoms of circulatory overload include hypotension, bradycardia or tachycardia, and cyanosis.

Safety Stat!

Alloimmunization (the production of antibodies against the blood product) is a reaction to transfused foreign protein antigens and is often manifested by fevers. These antigens are found on all components of blood. If alloimmunization takes place, leukocyte depletion of the transfused product is essential. For example, leukocyte-depleted PRBCs would be required for a child who has been exposed previously to transfused products that then lead to alloimmunization.

Nursing Care for Transfusion Therapy

Nurses caring for children must know their institution's policies concerning the administration of blood products. In some states, only the registered nurse (RN) is allowed to spike a unit of blood, hang the blood, and monitor the patient's condition and response. In other states, licensed vocational nurses (LVNs) can evaluate the patient during a transfusion and take VSs. The following steps, in order, provide guidance for the transfusion of blood products.

1. Review the child's previous transfusion history to anticipate a potential transfusion reaction.
2. Evaluate the child's laboratory values to confirm the need for a transfusion.
3. Ensure that a blood-product transfusion consent is signed and in the chart.
4. Determine the child's pretransfusion status, including VS and lung sounds.
5. Determine the need to administer a premedication such as acetaminophen or diphenhydramine.
6. Verify the physician's precise transfusion order for the type of product and special processing (CMV-negative, irradiated, or leukocyte-depleted components), premedications, filters, and rate/volume. Blood may be ordered as a dose, such as 10 to 15 mL/kg of PRBCs.
7. Before spiking and hanging the bag, double-check with a second RN at the bedside that the correct patient and unit are present by verifying:
   - The patient's name
   - The patient's medical record number
   - The patient's date of birth
   - Type of product ordered
   - Special processing or handling
   - Rh type
   - Blood group
   - Expiration date
   - Unit number
   - Lot number (if provided)
8. Hang the unit only with a 0.9% sterile normal saline IV bag.
9. Monitor the child throughout the transfusion, carefully following institutional policy. The child should be carefully monitored for the first 15 minutes with the nurse staying at the bedside with the child, and VS checks should be done because this is the time period when 90% of all transfusion reactions occur.
10. If a transfusion reaction is suspected, you must stop the transfusion, then send the tubing, transfused product bag, and normal saline bag all together to the blood bank.
11. Document thoroughly all aspects of the transfusion.

Safety Stat!

The two medications that members of the pediatric health-care team should have immediate access to if a transfusion reaction is suspected are diphenhydramine and epinephrine.

Safe and Effective Nursing Care

The Importance of the Health History and Physical Assessment

It is imperative that the health-care team know whether or not a child has received blood products before. As a child is exposed to the foreign proteins found in each transfused product, the child's immune system produces antibodies against these foreign proteins. The more antibodies are present, the greater the chance the child will have a blood transfusion reaction and therefore require transfusion premedications such as antipyretics, antihistamines, and possibly steroidal anti-inflammatories.

Before any transfusion, you should assist the team in conducting a thorough physical evaluation of the child. In addition to VS, lung sounds should be evaluated because transfused products may cause fluids to shift.

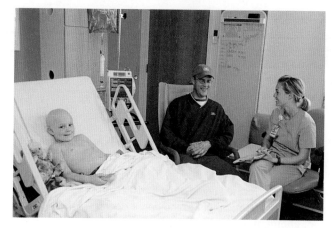

FIGURE 38.3 Child with an oncology diagnosis. Many parents maintain a bedside vigil to support their child during treatment for cancer.

COMMON ONCOLOGICAL DISORDERS

The overall prognosis of childhood cancer depends on the tumor type (histology), the extent of the cancer at the time of diagnosis, the rapidity of treatment, and the effectiveness of the therapy. The majority of childhood cancers are curable; therefore, the oncology team that provides care to the child with cancer and their family has a treatment goal of curing that cancer. Rapid diagnosis and rapid initiation of appropriate therapy optimize the chances of a child having a complete cure.

There are more than 250 types of childhood cancer, each with a particular clinical presentation and treatment plan. Childhood cancer is considered rare with less than 1% of all cancers across the life span occurring in children. The incidence of childhood cancer is less than 1% with only 11,000 new cases of childhood cancer being diagnosed per year in the United States. Although cancer remains the leading cause of death from disease in childhood, the cure rate of all childhood cancers combined now is 85% for children to 86% for teenagers (Cancer.Net, 2023).

See Box 38.2 for a summary of common types of cancer found in children.

No single cause of childhood cancer has been identified. The development of cancer is complex and multifaceted (Fig. 38.3). Attributing the development of a cancer diagnosis solely to genetics or to the environment is misleading. The concept of "ecogenetics" or "multifactorial etiology" is more acceptable because it addresses the *combination* of exposure to toxic environmental carcinogenic substances with variations in genetic factors.

At the cellular level, cancer has unique genetic properties that allow the indiscriminate growth of abnormal cells. The properties of cancer cells include the following:

- An inactivation of the tumor-suppressor genes that, under normal circumstances, would shut down the cell during abnormal growth.

- A process occurs in which proto-oncogenes (genes that help regulate growth) convert to oncogenes, which promote abnormal cellular growth.
- The process of apoptosis (programmed cell death) is not functioning; when an abnormal cell that is damaged does not die, it leads to the growth and spread of tumor cells.
- Chromosome translocation occurs, leading to new cancer genes.

Specific childhood cancers, such as retinoblastoma, are thought to develop according to a *two-hit model*. This model suggests that two mutations are needed for cancer to develop.

Leukemia is the most common form of malignant cancer found in children. Solid tumors of the central nervous system (CNS), such as brain tumors, are those most commonly found in childhood. Some childhood cancers are unique to the pediatric population and are rarely found in adults. These cancers include neuroblastoma, Wilms tumor, retinoblastoma, Ewing sarcoma, and osteosarcoma. The most significant improvement of clinical outcomes for children with cancer has been the implementation of chemotherapy protocols with combination medication therapies and the improvements of supportive care and nursing care. Preventing medication errors, complications, and severe symptoms, as well as providing safe, holistic care, are the most important aspects of pediatric oncology nursing. Specialized knowledge is required to provide effective and safe care to children with cancers. Nurses should seek national and institutional certification in chemotherapy administration, biotherapy administration, the care of central lines, and safety promotion such as chemotherapy-spill cleanup.

Diagnosis of Childhood Cancers

A child with cancer will present either with vague symptoms that do not respond to traditional therapies or with symptoms that are suggestive of cancer. Vague symptoms may include prolonged fevers, the inability to heal a wound, chronic

Box 38.2
Childhood Cancers

Aplastic Anemia

A disorder of the bone marrow, aplastic anemia is characterized by the depletion of all marrow elements. The production of marrow cells is decreased or completely lacking, which results in acute pancytopenia or the severe reduction of thrombocytes, which produce platelets, RBCs, and WBCs. Severe aplastic anemia presents with a granulocyte count of fewer than 500/mm³, a platelet count of fewer than 20,000/microL, and a reticulocyte count of fewer than 1%. This type of cancer can be caused by medications, chemicals, radiation, or viruses. The overall prognosis of this condition is poor but improving, with up to 80% of children under 20 having a 5-year survival rate (St. Jude Children's Research Hospital, 2023a). Long-term survival is up to 90% if the child receives a successful bone marrow transplant. Medical treatment is bone marrow transplantation or immunotherapy, such as cyclosporine, if a compatible match is not found (St. Jude Children's Research Hospital, 2023a).

Hodgkin's Lymphoma

Hodgkin's lymphoma accounts for only 5% of all childhood cancers. This disease is a malignant proliferation of lymphocytes. Hodgkin's lymphoma presents as painless, firm adenopathy (swollen lymph nodes) of the cervical or supraclavicular nodes. Treatment consists of multidrug chemotherapy with supplemental radiation in some cases.

Non-Hodgkin's Lymphoma

Non-Hodgkin's lymphoma is a disease of malignant proliferation of T or B lymphocytes. Children often present with an intrathoracic tumor (mediastinal mass) and dyspnea, chest pain, pleural effusions, and dysphagia. Treatment consists of surgical excision of the tumors and multidrug chemotherapy regimens.

Neuroblastoma

A common tumor of neurological tissue, neuroblastoma appears most commonly along the sympathetic nervous system tissues. Most are located in the child's abdomen and are often discovered as a mass or multiple masses on plain radiographic imaging. Treatment consists of surgery, radiation therapy, and chemotherapy.

Nephroblastoma (Wilms Tumors)

Wilms tumors are malignancies of the kidneys in which metastasis is rare. The child with an encapsulated kidney tumor will have a better prognosis. The median age of diagnosis is 3 years old, and the most frequent presenting sign is an abdominal mass. Treatment consists of surgical removal of the affected kidney followed by multidrug chemotherapy.

Osteogenic Sarcoma

Osteogenic sarcoma, the most common pediatric bone cancer, is a tumor found in the diaphysis of a child's long bone, such as the femur, ulna, proximal humerus, ileum, or radius, or in a flat bone such as the skull, spine, or pelvis. Often the child presents with a pathological fracture as an initial symptom. As many as 15%–20% of children will present with metastasis (spread) of the cancer cells, typically to the lungs. The clinical course follows a sequence. First, the tumor cells replace destroyed normal bone. Then, the abnormal growth penetrates the bone cortex and extends via radiating spindles. Finally, the tumor extends along the bone marrow cavity through the veins and to the lungs. The peak age of diagnosis is 10 years, and the survival rate is 70%–75%. Treatment consists of surgery followed by chemotherapy. Limb salvage is not always an option (St. Jude Children's Research Hospital, 2019).

Retinoblastoma

Retinoblastoma presents in a child's eye as a chalky, white intraocular tumor, often with a calcified and necrotic foci. Originating from the posterior side of the retina, the retinoblastoma may present with metastasis spreading to the optic nerve and beyond. A parent may seek health care based on the finding of a peculiar look to the child's eye, "cat's eye reflex," more formally known as *leukocoria*. Treatment consists of cryotherapy (freezing therapy), radiation, focused laser therapy, chemotherapy, stem cell transplant, and/or enucleation (removal) of the affected eye. This tumor has an excellent prognosis and a 97% survival rate (St. Jude Children's Research Hospital, 2023b).

---

fatigue, recurring otitis media, or pain. Symptoms that may suggest the presence of a diagnosis of childhood cancer are included in Box 38.3.

Invasive diagnostic procedures are conducted to confirm or rule out the presence of cancer and to determine its exact location, to identify its histology, and to stage the severity of the cancer. Diagnostic procedures include bone marrow biopsies, lumbar punctures, and surgical procedures for cancer staging or tumor debulking. Further diagnostic studies include computed tomography (CT) scans with contrast and phlebotomy.

The six forms of therapy for childhood cancer are summarized in Box 38.4. Each treatment has been developed with the goal of achieving remission and long-term survival.

Psychosocial Aspects of Childhood Cancer

The diagnosis of cancer in a child is a powerful, life-changing event for the entire family. Fear fills the hearts of those who are close to the family, and resources are needed to support the well-being of the family structure. Family members may express shock, anger, guilt, and disbelief early in the child's diagnosis and throughout treatment.

A complete assessment of a family with a child recently diagnosed with cancer should be done by a multidisciplinary team of specialists. Coping strategies should be identified and supported. A child life specialist should immediately become involved, providing support, engagement, play, and education for the child and their siblings. It is important to help the family meet its basic needs, including education,

Box 38.3

Symptoms Suggestive of Pediatric Cancers

- Significant weight loss
- Recurring febrile states
- Chronic fatigue or malaise
- Presence of petechiae or abnormal bruising or bleeding
- Night sweats
- Prolonged pharyngitis
- Lymphadenopathy
- Abdominal discomfort, masses, and distention
- Headaches and vomiting episodes in the morning
- Cat's eye reflex (see discussion on retinoblastoma)
- Pancytopenia
- Chronic drainage from the ears
- Mobility issues such as limping, arthralgia, or guarding of musculoskeletal structures
- Rectal or abnormal vaginal bleeding
- Significant bone pain
- Visual disturbances
- Periorbital ecchymosis

transportation, and language-interpretation services, as well as sleeping, eating, and work/school routines. Great fear about finances and medical coverage may be expressed early in the diagnosis. Financial stressors may be addressed by having a pediatric oncology social worker attend to the family's concerns. The farther away the family lives from the medical center where the child receives treatment, the more they must pay for transportation, meals, tolls, lodging, and vehicle maintenance.

Oncology team members should explain each step of the treatment process and the care requirements for each day. Because of emotional stress, family members may need to have the same topic explained repeatedly to understand complex treatment information.

The family's culture and spirituality may play important roles in the care of the child with cancer and in the communication patterns with family members. Whenever possible and safe, families should be encouraged to implement their cultural or religious practices to provide support to the child. A determination of cultural or religious/spiritual practices should be conducted early in the treatment process so that

Box 38.4

Treatments for Childhood Cancers

Chemotherapy

The majority of chemotherapeutic medications act on the division or multiplication of cancer cells. Unfortunately, the properties of chemotherapy that work effectively on killing cancer cells also affect normal, healthy cells. Side effects include severe nausea and vomiting, myelosuppression, renal impairment, liver function abnormalities, ototoxicity, cardiac toxicity, hypotension, pulmonary fibrosis, peripheral neuropathy, paralytic ileus, mood changes, growth retardation, hyperglycemia, and, rarely, allergic reactions. These unpleasant side effects must be managed by meticulous prevention, evaluations, and rapid interventions.

Surgery

Surgery is indicated for a child with cancer to diagnose, stage, resect, debulk, debride, or provide relief of mechanical obstruction. Surgery is almost always performed under general anesthesia. As much as possible, the child with cancer needs to be prepared for the surgery by having adequate hydration, nutrition, platelets and clotting factors, RBCs, and an adequate WBC count to provide healing to the surgical site.

Radiation Therapy

Radiation therapy involves the application of high-energy particles or radiation waves to treat cancer cells by preventing replication. The goal is to spare those adjacent healthy cells found around the site of the cancer. A total dose of radiation is calculated and then divided into serial radiation therapy sessions. Radiation is used to treat specific types of childhood cancer that are responsive to this type of treatment. Side effects can occur with radiation therapy and include many systems. Common side effects include GI distress, dysphagia, headache, nausea and vomiting, prolonged fatigue, liver tenderness, skin reactions, and pneumonitis.

Biotherapy/Immunotherapy

Several forms of biological response modifiers are used to help treat childhood cancer. Categories of biotherapy include monoclonal antibodies, cytokines, and investigational substances such as synthetic lipophilics, which have been shown to eradicate osteosarcoma lung metastasis. Side effects of biotherapies include potential allergic reactions, hypotension, headaches, rigors, fever and chills, and flu-like syndromes. The latest cancer treatments for children with relapsed cancers are medications tailor-made to target the tumor's expressed proteins and CAR T-cell therapy (chimeric antigen receptor or CAR), which is genetically engineered to attack cancerous cells.

Bone Marrow Transplantation

Hematopoietic stem cell transplantation is used with certain cancers to replace a child's damaged, absent, or diseased stem cells. Healthy stem cells from donors (allogenic) are harvested, treated, and infused into the child's circulatory system. The child and donor are matched as closely as possible for the best clinical outcomes. Allogenic stem cells harvested from the child may be used in certain circumstances for complete removal of residual tumor cells.

Gene Therapy

Focusing on the cause of the cancer, gene therapy has been investigated to help treat damaged cells. This type of therapy includes the transfer or insertion of new genes into the genome of a cell via a transportation carrier called a *vector*. Vectors are either viruses or nonviral substances such as chemicals. Gene therapy is not conducted on reproductive cells, so that the inserted genes are not passed on to future generations.

family wishes can be provided for. Decision-making, consent procedures, disease definitions, disease and prognosis disclosure, nutrition, hygiene, grieving practices, perspectives on medications, and the use of alternative or complementary practices may all be culturally influenced or bound. Recognizing cultural differences and providing support are paramount for successful cancer treatment and follow-up care.

Evidence-Based Practice

How Therapeutic Are Therapy Animals?

Researchers set out to measure the effects of animal-assisted intervention on the stress, anxiety, and quality of life for children diagnosed with cancer and their parents. Newly diagnosed patients were randomized to receive standard cancer care plus visits from a therapy dog (intervention group) or standard cancer care alone (control). Levels of stress, anxiety, and quality of life were measured over 4 months using self-report inventory instruments and evaluations of blood pressure and HR. Children in both groups experienced a reduction in anxiety, whereas parents in only the intervention group showed significantly decreased stress. Over time, no significant differences between groups were observed, leading researchers to suggest that animal-assisted interventions may provide benefits for parents and families during the initial stages of cancer treatment.

McCullough, A., Ruehrdanz, A., Jenkins, M. A., Gilmer, M. J., Olson, J., Pawar, A., Holley, L., Sierra-Rivera, S., Linder, D. E., Pichette, D., Grossman, N. J., Hellman, C., Guérin, N. A., & O'Haire, M. E. (2018). Measuring the effects of an animal-assisted intervention for pediatric oncology patients and their parents: A multisite randomized controlled trial. *Journal of Pediatric Oncology Nursing, 35*(3), 159–177. https:// doi .org/10.1177/1043454217748586

Safe and Effective Nursing Care

Providing care to children with oncology diagnoses includes caring for children receiving chemotherapy. Therefore, it is imperative that nurses protect themselves from exposure to chemotherapeutic agents. Wearing the appropriate self-protective equipment to prevent exposure, knowing which container is safe for chemotherapy waste, and knowing how to clean up a spill of chemotherapeutic medications are all care imperatives (Fig. 38.4). Check institutional policy for specific guidelines for protecting yourself against exposure.

To administer chemotherapeutic medications and to obtain blood specimens, central lines are typically placed in children with cancer. Provide meticulous care to a surgically implanted central line to avoid a serious infection in a child who is already immunocompromised (see Fig. 23.7).

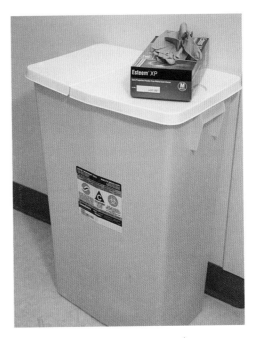

FIGURE 38.4 Chemotherapy waste receptacle.

Leukemia

Leukemia is the most common form of cancer found across childhood, accounting for at least 28% of all cancer diagnoses (Cancer.net, 2023). Leukemia is either lymphocytic or nonlymphocytic in nature. Acute lymphocytic leukemia (ALL) is the most commonly diagnosed leukemia in childhood (75% of all leukemias; St. Jude Children's Research Hospital, 2023c). An excessive number of abnormal immature leukocytes are produced in the bone marrow and then invade the blood and various organs of the child's body. Normal cells in the bone marrow are displaced by these abnormal cells, and therefore insufficient numbers of RBCs, other WBC types, and platelets are formed. The child is at risk for bleeding and infections.

The group at highest risk for a diagnosis of ALL is children between 3 and 5 years of age. The poorest responses to treatment and poorest overall prognoses occur when the child is younger than 1 year, is older than 10, has a total WBC count over $100,000/mm^3$ at diagnosis, or is male.

Diagnosing Leukemia

A child with a potential diagnosis of leukemia may have signs and symptoms including the following:

- Fever
- Fatigue
- Evidence of bleeding, such as petechiae or hemorrhage
- Bone pain
- Weight loss
- Anorexia

Laboratory tests for leukemia include the following:

- CBC with cellular differentiation
- Bone marrow aspiration for blast cell confirmation

- Lumbar puncture to determine CNS involvement/metastasis
- Chest x-ray to detect lung and mediastinal involvement
- Kidney, liver, and spleen scans to detect leukemic cell infiltration
- Bone scans and skeletal surveys to identify the presence of metastasis

Interventions for Leukemia

Leukemia requires medical management through the administration of a chemotherapy medication regimen to prevent abnormal cells from dividing and metastasizing. Treatment is divided into progressive phases:

- *Induction phase*, in which treatment focuses on eradicating the disease or inducing a remission, occurs in the first few weeks from the diagnosis. Induction requires that a child experience the administration of multiple medications in high doses.
- *Intensification phase*, in which the goal of treatment is to combat any involvement of the CNS or any other vital organ.
- *Maintenance therapy* is the last phase, during which the child receives several months to a year of chemotherapy to sustain the remission.

Box 38.5 provides a case study of a child with a new diagnosis of ALL.

Nursing Considerations for Leukemia

Nursing care for a child receiving chemotherapy includes both administering the treatments themselves as well as documenting the child's responses to treatments. Nurses who administer chemotherapy should be certified to give these medications via any route. (Many states require this certification.) Common care concerns include the following:

- Monitor for signs of infection. A fever must be reported immediately to the pediatric oncologist so that antibiotics can be started to prevent sepsis. In general, a fever for an immune compromised child receiving chemotherapy is considered at or above 38.0°C (100.4° F). Always follow institutional policy carefully because a fever can be a clinical sign of a life-threatening infection. The definition of "fever" in immunocompromised children may vary per institution.
- Monitor for reactions to the chemotherapy medications.
- Monitor the child's peripheral and/or central IV site for signs of infiltration. Some chemotherapy medications are vesicants and will cause severe tissue damage and potential cellular death if the medication infiltrates surrounding tissues.
- Offer nutrition only when the child can tolerate eating. Stomatitis or mucositis is a common side effect of chemotherapy and may make the oral consumption of food or fluids difficult.
- Teach the family how to care for the child's central line, including evaluations, flushing, and sterile dressing changes.

Box 38.5

Case Study: Child With a New Diagnosis of Acute Lymphocytic Leukemia

A 10-month-old infant has been seen in the public health clinic of a large urban health center for ongoing fevers, fussiness, poor nutritional intake, weight loss, and pallor. The child had been seen by clinic pediatricians and treated with antibiotics for bilateral otitis media not responsive to the first course of medication. The mother, a Chinese immigrant, needed to bring two older siblings and use public transportation to attend doctor's visits for the infant. The mother, distressed that her infant was still displaying severe symptoms not seen in her other children, finally brought the infant to an emergency department (ED) of a large teaching hospital. Upon evaluation in the ED, the health-care team recognized an abnormally elevated WBC and called a pediatric hematologist/oncologist to consult on the case. Further evaluation was performed on a slide of the child's blood. The child was identified as having suspected leukemia and was admitted into the hospital for further diagnostic workup and central line placement. Using a translator, the family was told that the child had high-risk ALL and required extensive induction chemotherapy followed by at least a 2-year course of treatment. The family responded to the news with shock, and the adults required support and education by several members of the health-care team to adapt to the diagnosis of childhood cancer. The health-care team called in a pediatric social worker, asked the hospital chaplain to provide support, and asked the hospital-based psychologist and members of the oncology team to rapidly become involved in the case. Members of the child life department were asked to work with the infant's siblings to improve their understanding of the crisis of the new diagnosis.

The hospitalized infant had a Broviac central venous catheter line placed and was started on an alkalizing hydration fluid in anticipation of chemotherapy starting as soon as the diagnosis was confirmed. The child stayed in the hospital for over a month for the first cycle of induction chemotherapy and continued to receive supportive care to adapt to the new diagnosis. Multiple family members brought home-cooked meals to the family while the child was hospitalized, and the siblings were allowed to visit provided they had no symptoms of colds, flu, or any infections.

- Address family members' anxiety and concerns. The diagnosis of childhood cancer provokes powerful emotions, and the family will need professional support to maintain a level of functioning that will provide support to the child. Social services and other professionals will need to be involved in the child's care. Spiritual care is important and should be offered to all family members. All family members should be allowed 24-hour visitation privileges.
- Use caution when around children receiving chemotherapy. Wear the appropriate safety gear, know how to clean up a chemotherapy spill, and know in which waste container to place contaminated materials and objects. Follow institutional policy on chemotherapy administration and accidental spill cleanup procedures.

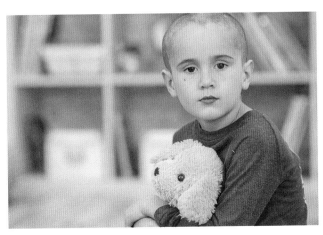

FIGURE 38.5 A child with alopecia. Alopecia is a negative effect associated with cancer treatment that can make the child feel very self-conscious.

- Understand the physical changes that may occur because of cancer treatments. Some children are very sensitive to these changes. Alopecia, or hair loss, from chemotherapy can cause great distress to a child, especially older school-aged children, and teens (Fig. 38.5).

Interventions for Complications Associated With Leukemia

Treatments for leukemia include caring for the complications of bone marrow dysfunction. Dysfunction can be caused by both the cancer within bone marrow as well as the chemotherapy suppressing the bone marrow. The complications include neutropenia, anemia, and thrombocytopenia.

NEUTROPENIA. A reduction of circulating neutrophils, **neutropenia**, is measured by calculating the child's absolute neutrophil count (ANC). The child is considered neutropenic when the calculated value is lower than 1,000/microL. When a child is neutropenic, they are at risk for a serious bacterial infection.

Neutropenia requires the implementation and strict adherence of neutropenic precautions. If a neutropenic child presents with a fever, they must be seen urgently and have a blood culture, urinalysis, and appropriate wide-spectrum antibiotics started STAT until the results of the cultures come back.

Safe and Effective Nursing Care

Ten Tips to Prevent Sepsis in a Neutropenic Child While Hospitalized

1. Implement strict hand washing techniques and hang signs to remind caregivers and family members to perform meticulous hand washing.

2. Prevent the child from being exposed to ill persons.
   - Screen visitors for symptoms of illness and prevent caregivers with any mild illnesses or infections from giving care to the child with neutropenia.
3. Calculate the child's neutropenic state daily (Box 38.6) and plan care according to the severity of the child's myelosuppression.
4. Provide adequate nutrition, calories, fluids, and rest to promote bone marrow recovery after chemotherapy.
5. Avoid fresh fruits, vegetables, and flowers in the child's room because they contain bacteria or fungi.
6. Provide a mask for the child whenever the child must leave their hospital room for diagnostic examinations.
7. Promptly report any evidence of infection, including any fevers, no matter how high.
8. Avoid any trauma to the rectal mucosa by avoiding rectal examinations, rectal suppositories, and rectal temperatures.
9. Provide the child with their own VS evaluation equipment to prevent sharing among children who may pass infection to the child with cancer.
10. Evaluate the child frequently for any breaks in the skin or mucous membranes, such as rashes, cuts, sores, mucositis, hemorrhoids, or any loss of skin integrity.

Box 38.6
Calculating the Absolute Neutrophil Count

The ANC is calculated by multiplying the total WBC count by the combined percentage of neutrophils and bands found in the differential.
Example:
Total WBC is 3,500.
Segmented neutrophils are 21%.
Bands are 2%.
Convert percentages to decimals: 21% = 0.21 and 2% = 0.02.
Add these together: 0.21 + 0.02 = 0.23
(3,500) (0.23) = 805.
An ANC of 805 indicates that the child is neutropenic.

Medication Facts

Treatment for neutropenia includes administering colony-stimulating factors (CSF) starting 1 to 5 days after the child receives chemotherapy. Doses are 5 to 10 mcg/kg, given subcutaneously. Team members should discuss the need for CSF in relation to the expected periods of chemotherapy-induced neutropenia.

· **WORD · BUILDING ·**
neutropenia: neutro–neutrophil + pen–lack + ia–condition

Box 38.7

Neutropenic Precautions

- Check frequently for a fever and immediately report fever to enable the health-care team to implement STAT antibiotic therapy to prevent life-threatening sepsis. Blood cultures should be drawn as ordered, such as every 24 hours. Obtain blood cultures before implementing antibiotic therapy.
- Monitor regularly for any signs and symptoms of infection, such as erythema at central line catheter insertion sites and infections at wound or incision sites. Also monitor any other symptoms of impending or actual infection, including diarrhea, mouth pain, anal pain or perirectal irritation, cough, and rhinorrhea. Neutropenic patients may not produce pus because their total WBC count is low. It is imperative to evaluate for pain, irritation, and redness and to rapidly report any indication of infection, which can be life-saving.
- Maintain a meticulous environment to reduce the possibility of infection. This includes frequent hand washing for the child

and family and preventing exposure to crowds when the child's ANC is lower than 500/microL.
- Prevent nosocomial infections by keeping the child in their hospital room and not allowing the child to play in the playroom unless the institution has clean "neutropenia" play time only for children with neutropenia.
- To reduce the chance of bleeding and infection, do not use rectal thermometers, conduct rectal examinations, or administer rectal suppositories. Children should use only soft toothbrushes to prevent bleeding.
- Perform meticulous hygiene practices, including daily bathing as tolerated and strict mouth care to prevent mucositis.
- Teach the family about neutropenia so that they can be directly involved with the care of protecting their child and monitoring for signs and symptoms of infection.

To provide safety to a child with an oncology disorder such as leukemia, the health-care team must prevent the child from acquiring an infection. Neutropenic precautions are required. See Box 38.7 for a list of neutropenic precautions.

ANEMIA. Children receiving cancer treatment are at risk for developing anemia because of bone marrow suppression. The child will have daily CBC counts with cellular differentiation to monitor the need for a transfusion of RBCs. Typically, when a child becomes symptomatic from their level of

anemia, or the hemoglobin count falls below 7 to 8 g/dL, the child will require a PRBC transfusion.

THROMBOCYTOPENIA. Children receiving cancer treatment are also at risk for developing serious bleeding episodes related to the toxicity of the bone marrow and the reduction of circulating thrombocytes. The child may need to have platelet transfusions to prevent spontaneous bleeds or bleeding episodes related to invasive procedures such as bone marrow aspirations.

Key Points

- Nursing care of children who have an oncological (cancer) or hematological (blood) disease requires specific knowledge and skills. The diagnosis of a hematological/oncological condition can cause great emotional distress for each member of the family, and yet the majority of childhood cancers are curable.
- Blood-product support is often a cornerstone of hematology and oncology therapy. Many treatments to cure cancer produce periods of severe anemia. Children with SCA require blood-product support to optimize the recovery of a sickle cell crisis.
- Iron-deficiency anemia is the most common form of anemia affecting children in the United States. After depletion of maternal iron stores at 6 months of age, the infant must have sufficient iron intake from their nutrition. Risk factors for iron-deficiency anemia include the introduction of solid foods to an infant before the recommended age of 6 months, the introduction of cow's milk before the child's first birthday, or the excessive consumption of cow's milk during the toddler/early childhood period.
- SCA is a type of sickle cell disease that leads the child to have abnormal, sickle-shaped RBCs. Occurring in one out of every 500 live births of African American babies, this condition is marked by chronic hemolytic anemia and vaso-occlusion.

- Hyperbilirubinemia of the newborn most often occurs when there is a physiological immaturity of liver functions or when there is an increased destruction of the RBCs. Typical onset is by 3 days of age.
- ITP is an acquired hemorrhagic disorder in which the child's total number of circulating platelets is severely reduced. The child will present with bruising, bleeding, or injury, most commonly presenting between 2 and 6 years.
- Hemophilia A and B are both X-linked recessive genetic disorders in which the child has an impaired ability to control bleeding.
- Thalassemia major is one of a group of heritable hypochromic (pale) and microcytotic anemias.
- Leukemia is the most common form of malignant cancer found in children.
- The three most common side effects of cancer treatment that are life-threatening are neutropenia, anemia, and thrombocytopenia. Neutropenia is a reduction of circulating neutrophils and is measured by a calculation of the child's ANC. The child is considered neutropenic when the calculated value is lower than 1,000/microL. When a child is neutropenic, they are at risk for a serious bacterial infection.

Review Questions

1. What medications should you plan to have on hand to respond to a blood transfusion reaction?
   1. Acetaminophen and diphenhydramine
   2. Morphine and acetaminophen
   3. Steroidal anti-inflammatory medications and morphine
   4. Diphenhydramine and epinephrine

2. Which developmental stage would be most affected by periods of alopecia associated with chemotherapy treatments?
   1. Late school-aged
   2. Adolescence
   3. Early school-aged
   4. Preschool-aged

3. An RN will instruct a licensed practical nurse (LPN) to report which behavior of a preschool child undergoing chemotherapy treatments?
   1. Brushing teeth regularly with a hard toothbrush
   2. Rinsing the mouth out with salt and soda mouthwash three times daily
   3. Allowing you to check for mouth sores daily
   4. Requesting plain yogurt and oatmeal for breakfast

4. Neutropenic precautions protect an immunosuppressed child during chemotherapy treatments. Which precautions are specifically for patients with neutropenia? **(Select all that apply.)**
   1. Positive air pressure isolation room
   2. No fresh flowers or standing water in room
   3. No acetaminophen-containing pain medications unless approved by physician
   4. A diet rich in raw fruits and vegetables
   5. Strict hand washing techniques for visitors and caregivers
   6. Mask on child when required to leave room
   7. Daily bathing and complete oral hygiene

5. Which developmental stage is most at risk for the development of anemia associated with consuming too much milk?
   1. Early infancy
   2. Adolescence
   3. Early school-aged
   4. Toddlerhood

6. You are caring for a preschool-aged child with a sickle cell vaso-occlusive crisis. Which physician order should you question?
   1. Apply oxygen via nasal cannula for 24 hours after all surgical procedures.
   2. Offer warm packs to place on painful joints.
   3. Give pain medication around the clock (ATC) as needed based on the pain-scale score.
   4. Restrict oral fluids.

7. You have just taught the family of a child with ALL about the potential complications of chemotherapy treatment. You then ask the family to give some examples of these complications. Which response by the family indicates the need for clarification?
   1. Anemia
   2. Elevated liver enzymes
   3. Thrombocytopenia
   4. Neutropenia

8. Which test would be performed to demonstrate a definitive diagnosis of childhood leukemia?
   1. A CBC with differential
   2. Serum titer levels
   3. Serum IgG levels
   4. A bone marrow aspiration

9. Which of the following activities would you recommend to the family of a young child with hemophilia? **(Select all that apply.)**
   1. Soccer
   2. Baseball
   3. Swimming
   4. Fishing
   5. Golfing
   6. Hiking

10. To minimize the effect of chemotherapy-induced nausea for a young child being treated for cancer, what should you recommend?
    1. NPO (nothing by mouth) status
    2. Clear liquid diet
    3. No eating pressures
    4. Full liquid diet

ANSWERS 1. 4; 2. 3; 3. 1; 4. 1, 2, 3, 5, 6; 5. 4; 6. 4; 7. 2; 8. 4; 9. 3, 4, 5, 6; 10. 3

CRITICAL THINKING QUESTIONS

1. Research the resources a family of a school-aged child with a cancer diagnosis would require to support the child's academic progress and success if the child requires 2 years of chemotherapy treatments.

2. How would a parent best tell friends, family, and neighbors about a cancer diagnosis of testicular cancer for an adolescent boy? Keeping in mind the developmental stage of a teenager, how do you think the child would want his diagnosis shared with others?

Resources

For additional resources and information, including Postconference Questions and Activities, Answers, and References, visit www.FADavis.com.

 Student Study Guide

APPENDIX A
Best Practices for Medication Administration for Pediatric Patients

One of the greatest challenges in caring for children is the administration of medications. Regardless of the route (oral, sublingual, intramuscular [IM], intravenous [IV], transdermal, rectal, inhalation, etc.), young children often have strong reactions to medication administration. Whether you are administering the medication or teaching the caregiver to give a medication, children pose unique challenges in accurate medication administration. One must reflect on the child's developmental stage (understanding and ability) and proceed with kindness but firmness.

School-aged children and teens can learn what a medication is indicated for and therefore have a basic understanding of the need for and importance of taking a medication. Infants can be held gently and safely in order to have medications administered without their understanding, but toddlers and preschool children pose special considerations. Toddlers who want to show autonomy, and preschoolers with their magical thinking, are two age groups that need special planning and consideration.

As stated by Gardiner and Dvorkin (2006), "The problem of getting children to follow a treatment regimen is widespread and is frustrating for physicians. The extent to which any patient adheres to a medical regimen is an essential determinant of clinical success" (para. 1). Suggestions made include once a day dosing, clearly written instructions in the family's primary language, and regular communication with the caregivers to ensure knowledge and adherence.

Several of the challenges to consider when administering medications to children include:

- Make sure the child swallows the medication without spitting it up.
- Give the medication in small portions to prevent aversions; don't make them "swig" the medicine down (Children's Hospital Los Angeles, 2022).
- Prevent gagging and vomiting caused by the medication's taste or texture.
- Confirm that the entire dose was administered for the desired effect.
- Know common side effects and learn to observe for these concerns.
- Understand if there are any harmful interactions to be aware of relating to other medications or foods.
- Use the easiest means or mechanisms to get oral medications into a young child (oral medicine droppers, dosing spoons or syringes, medication cups, flavored syrups, and medication "chasers" such as a sweet drink after the medication is in). Swallowing capsules or tablets may be challenging, but some kids prefer this to liquid medications with unpleasant tastes (Medicines for Children, 2023).
- Note that children may feel as if the caregiver or nurse does not understand their distress in taking medications; it is good to provide honest empathetic statements but firmly and without negotiating.
- When a medication is successfully consumed, give the child praise.
- When able, talk to the child and offer them two or three choices on how they want their medication administered.
- If the medication is suspended in sugar solutions, make sure the child's teeth are brushed afterwards.

Overall guidelines for safety:

- Do not administer medications to a crying child as there is a risk for aspiration.
- When administering medications to an infant, give only small amounts at a time via oral syringe to prevent gagging and choking; allow swallowing with each small amount given.
- Never refer to medications as candy. Do not hide medicine in food (Children's Hospital Los Angeles, 2022).
- Do not mix medications or crushed pills in large amounts of fluid as the child may not be able or willing to consume the entire amount.
- Use small amounts of foods with the consistency of applesauce, pudding, or ice cream to help convince a child to take the medication. Cold foods may help.
- Talk to a pediatric pharmacist regarding ideas for safe delivery of medications.
- Never crush time-released medications and never crush medications dispensed as small "beads" as this will potentially create an inconsistent or too rapid medication dose.
- Discuss with caregivers the need for safe storage out of sight and mind of a child.
- Make certain that caregivers understand that adult medications should not be given to children; specific concentrations made for infants and children should be used exclusively. Under no circumstances should adult medications, even routine cold medications, be given to a child.
- Make every attempt to incorporate medication administration into the daily routine, which provides consistency for the family and child and promotes adherence.
- Inquire about concerns with cost of medications. Some families cannot afford insurance or copayments, and this may cause poor adherence. With kindness, you should

inquire about financial concerns for filling prescriptions. This may feel awkward, but it is quite common.

- Understand that caregivers may not be familiar with administering medications and often find it daunting and need specific support, education, and guidelines.

DEVELOPMENTAL GUIDELINES

Infants:

- Hold the infant upright and do not give medications while crying to prevent aspiration or choking.
- Give the medicine in small amounts via a syringe or dropper toward their cheek.
- If you need to mix the medication in a solution, use the smallest amount of breast milk or solution as possible. Do not give free water to newborns or young infants.
- Administer right before a feeding when the infant shows hunger signs and may more readily swallow the medication; promptly follow with breast milk, formula, or, if over 6 months, a small spoon of safe consistency food.
- Ask the caregivers if they have ideas or family practices that have been successful in the past.

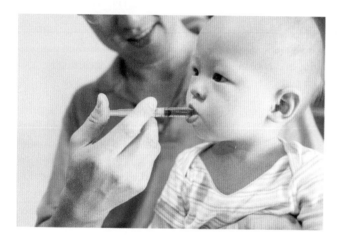

Toddlers:

- Try to give two choices to a toddler by telling the child the medication must be taken, but it can be taken with cherry syrup, chocolate syrup or pancake syrup, or it can be taken now or in 2 minutes, for example.
- Make sure the toddler is as quiet as possible to prevent choking or spitting the medication out.
- If there is a possibility that the toddler will spit or vomit the medication out, talk to the pharmacist about next steps, as it will need to be determined if the medication is repeated or a second reduced dose is given.

Preschoolers:

- Preschoolers should be given a warning that the time for medication administration is impending.

- They also benefit from offering two choices in flavors of syrup, and they benefit from being offered to take their own medication once it has been prepared (offering them the spoon, medical syringe, or med cup).
- Many preschool children benefit from role-playing with a doll or a teddy bear; pretending their favorite toy has to take the medicine first may work.

School-aged children:

- School-aged children want to understand about their medication, including what it is for, how long the prescription will last (number of doses), and how it benefits them.
- School-aged children should be able to take their own medication after it is prepared.

Teens:

- Most teens want independence in medication administration. They should be taught how to take the medication and how to store it.
- Teens should always keep the medication in the original container in case an issue arises.
- For safety, the teen should be taught the importance of the medication, how it will benefit them, consequences of not taking the medication, and side effects.
- Teens benefit from periodic discussions of their medications and checks for adherence.

Further tips for caregivers:

- Set an alarm every day for each dose and work with the child's daily routine (Grambley, 2023).
- Use visual reminders such as notes in common areas.
- Understand that pediatric liquid doses can result in underdosing or overdosing as they need to be measured accurately.
- Do not use everyday kitchen utensils (teaspoons or tablespoons) to measure medications as they may not be accurate. Use pharmacy-provided accurate dispensing devices (Nationwide Children's, 2023).
- Never give children adult medications, especially over-the-counter medications that may be many times more concentrated than medications specifically for children.
- Acetaminophen (paracetamol or Tylenol) comes in various concentrations (24 mg/mL, 48 mg/mL, 50 mg/mL, and 100 mg/mL) and poses a risk of inaccurate dosing (Smith et al., 2022).
- The caregiver should call the health-care provider for guidelines if any doses are missed.
- Do not stop the medication if the child feels better; make sure all doses are taken, such as with antibiotics to fight infection.
- Try cold treats such as frozen juice, ice cubes, or popsicles to attempt to numb a child's taste buds (Smith et al., 2022).
- Do not mix infant medications with honey as there is a risk of acquiring botulism from raw honey.
- To improve adherence, many children benefit from sipping a small amount of medicine/sweet solution from a straw.

References

Children's Hospital Los Angeles. (2022). *6 Tips that will take the strain out of giving your child medication.* https://www.chla.org/blog/health-and-safety-tips/6-tips-will-take-the-strain-out-giving-your-child-medication

Gardiner, P., & Dvorkin, L. (2006). *Promoting medication adherence in children. American Family Physician, 74*(5), 793–798.

Grambley, W. (2023). *Maximizing pediatric medication adherence.* https://allazohealth.com/resources/5-ways-to-improve-medication-adherence-in-children/#:~:text=Incorporate%20the%20Prescribed%20Medicine%20into,the%20likelihood%20of%20medication%20adherence

Medicines for Children. (2023). *Helping your child to swallow tablets.* https://www.medicinesforchildren.org.uk/advice-guides/general-advice-for-medicines/helping-your-child-to-swallow-tablets

Nationwide Children's. (2023). *Medicine; how to give by mouth.* https://www.nationwidechildrens.org/family-resources-education/health-wellness-and-safety-resources/helping-hands/medicine-how-to-give-by-mouth#:~:text=Mixing%20with%20sweet%20or%20cold,let%20your%20child%20drink%20it

Smith, L., Leggett, C., & Borg, C. (2022). Administration of medicines to children: A practical guide. *Australian Prescriber, 45*(6), 188–192. https://doi.org/10.18773/austprescr.2022.067

APPENDIX B

Thirty-Five Types of Medical Errors and Tips for Preventing Harm: Quality and Safety Imperatives for Nurses Caring for Patients Across the Developmental Period

Nurses who care for children must consider safety the primary concern. Medical errors continue to harm or cause death to patients across clinical settings and across the life span at alarming rates. In the United States, previous estimates of approximately 251,000 to 400,000 people dying each year from medical errors may be exaggerated (Anderson & Abrahamson, 2017; Hathaway, 2020; Juneja & Mishra, 2022; Rodziewicz, Houseman, Vaqar, et al., 2024), but continue to be very concerning. Nurses are instrumental in identifying error-prone situations, especially in high-risk intensive care units, and can prevent many errors from occurring. The following list provides a summary of the most common types of medical errors that occur in the United States:

1. *Surgery on the wrong body part:* Participate with the surgical team to ensure that the correct body part has been identified before the patient undergoes anesthesia. Ask patients to mark the correct body part with a felt-tip pen before surgery.

2. *Surgery on the wrong patient:* The procedural or surgical team must call a "time out" before any procedure, minor or major, to ensure that the correct patient is undergoing the correct procedure. Use two forms of patient identification and have them double-checked by another licensed health-care professional.

3. *Wrong surgical procedure performed on a patient:* Participate in a "time out" double-check before any medical procedure. During the "time out," the name of the surgical procedure is said out loud and double-checked with the patient and the patient's medical record.

4. *Object left in patient after surgery:* Strictly follow institutional policy and double-check the count of each dressing, sponge, and medical instrument to reduce the probability of leaving a surgical object in the patient after a surgical procedure is performed. Leaving an instrument, dressing, or sponge in the patient can lead to pain, infection, and the need for a second surgery to remove the object.

5. *Death of a patient, who had been generally healthy, during or immediately after surgery for a localized problem:* Assist in the investigation of all unexpected deaths related to unintentional errors, medication side effects, allergic reactions, or any contributing factors to the death.

6. *Patient death or serious disability associated with the use of contaminated medications, devices, or biologics:* Visually double-check all medications for obvious contaminants, check all expiration dates for multidose containers, and immediately report any concerns to pharmacy. Strictly follow standardized protocols for cleaning instruments.

7. *Patient death or disability associated with the misuse or malfunction of a medical instrument or device:* Double-check all equipment for malfunctions. Label questionable or malfunctioning equipment and notify the appropriate supervisor of the department that oversees medical equipment. Label the faulty equipment clearly and then remove it from patient-care areas so that no other nurse or health-care professional can mistakenly use the device.

8. *Patient death or serious disability associated with intravascular air embolism:* Whenever assisting with the care of a patient with a central line, do not allow air to enter the IV tubing. Take precautions when changing tubing, flushing, drawing blood, or administering medication so that no air can enter the central line system. Intravenous (IV) pumps prevent air from entering the lines by providing a closed-valve system or an immediate clamping of IV tubing when the door is open and the tubing is removed from the pump. This also prevents rapid infusion of IV medications at incorrect rates.

9. *Infant discharged to the wrong person:* Ensure that the correct newborn or infant is discharged to the correct family by double-checking the infant's medical identification. This safety check should include at least two forms of personal identification for the infant and identification of the parent/guardian. Most institutions require that parents wear identification bands at all times.

10. *Patient death or serious disability associated with the patient disappearing for more than 4 hours:* Know where your patients are at all times. In pediatrics, no child is allowed to leave the unit for any reason without an accompanying parent, family member, health-care professional, or hospital transport team member. Stairwells and elevators pose unique risks on a pediatric floor and should be monitored when children are ambulatory. Explain hospital safety policies to adolescents.

11. *Patient suicide or attempted suicide resulting in serious disability:* Participate in a team effort to identify patients, regardless of age, who are at risk for suicide. Hospital policies allow the presence of a 24-hour attendant, such as a certified nursing assistant, to constantly monitor a patient at risk.

12. *Patient death or serious disability associated with a medication error:* Use all medication safety precautions to prevent medication errors. Errors can be acts of commission, acts of omission, scheduling misconceptions, or scheduling noncompliance. Use two patient identifiers before administering medication, and triple-check each medication being prepared.

13. *Patient death or serious disability associated with transfusion of blood or blood products of the wrong type:* Participate in strict patient safety procedures when drawing blood, administering blood, or administering any form of blood products. Two licensed nurses must double-check the patient name, medical record, and date of birth with all blood products.

14. *Maternal death or serious disability associated with labor or delivery in a low-risk pregnancy:* Participate in the investigation of any serious problems associated with labor or delivery.

15. *Patient death or serious disability associated with the onset of hypoglycemia (low blood sugar):* Changes in blood sugar are common in hospital settings where illness causes fluctuations or patients are NPO (nothing by mouth). Knowing the signs and symptoms of both hypoglycemia and hyperglycemia will assist in the early identification of dangerous blood sugar fluctuations.

16. *Patient death or serious disability associated with failure to identify and treat hyperbilirubinemia, a blood abnormality, in newborns:* Participate in the assessment of hyperbilirubinemia in newborns who are at risk for jaundice or who appear to be developing jaundice. Early initiation of bili light therapy assists with the medical complications of rising bilirubin levels in high-risk infants.

17. *Patient death or serious disability caused by spinal manipulative therapy:* Work carefully with members of occupational therapy and physical therapy to follow treatment protocols for patients with spinal injuries or those who are in the postspinal surgical period to ensure safe turning, transfer, and mobility.

18. *Patient death or serious disability associated with an electric shock:* Be diligent in inspecting all electrical wires and lines for frayed materials, sparks, or any concern associated with a piece of electrical equipment.

19. *Any incident in which a line designated for oxygen or other gas to be delivered to a patient contains the wrong gas or is contaminated by toxic substances:* Whenever attaching oxygen to a patient's delivery device, double-check that the line is directly connected to the oxygen tank or wall delivery system. Report immediately any suspected or actual complication from the administration of a gas.

20. *Patient death or serious disability associated with a burn incurred in the hospital:* Be acutely aware of all medical equipment that has the potential to cause a burn. Formula or frozen breast milk must be warmed in a hot water bath or approved bottle warming device rather than in the microwave oven. Do not create a warm or hot pack by heating wet washcloths or other materials in the microwave because serious burns have been documented.

21. *Patient death or injury associated with a fall suffered in the hospital:* Assist with the investigation of all falls leading to the injury, harm, or death of a patient. Infants or toddlers falling from cribs onto hard wood or linoleum floors and suffering skull fractures have been documented.

22. *Patient death or serious injury associated with the use of restraints or bedrails:* Restraints have been documented to cause serious injury, harm, and death to patients. Ensure patient safety before restraints are used. Refer to and follow the institutional policies and procedures for restraint use before applying a restraint. Be sure to have an order for use of restraints and to have the order renewed at least every 24 hours.

23. *Any instance of care ordered by or provided by someone impersonating a physician, medical student, resident, nurse practitioner, nurse, or pharmacist/other licensed health-care provider:* Request identification from any health-care professional who is not familiar to you. Hospitals have lists of approved health-care providers that can be checked for security purposes. Always ask to see a name badge for anyone who is not familiar in the workplace. Call security immediately if there is someone on the maternity or pediatric ward who does not belong.

24. *Abduction of a patient:* Be diligent in determining circumstances where a patient is at risk for abduction. Infants are at particular risk for abduction. Notify security immediately if any suspicious behaviors, abduction attempts, or actual removal of a patient occurs. Institutions have policies and practices for securing exits and stairwells should an abduction occur. Most pediatric units have security doors to screen visitors before entering.

25. *Sexual assault on a patient:* Patients are in a vulnerable position when they are in a hospital environment. Facilities must institute safety precautions to prevent any type of sexual assault.

26. *Death or significant injury of a patient or staff member resulting from a physical assault or violence in the hospital:* Participate in ongoing training programs to learn how to help diffuse dangerous situations that lead to physical assault. Call hospital security immediately to assist in situations where the potential of an assault exists. Ensure that you have direct access to a door if a patient or visitor becomes verbally abusive or threatens violent behavior.

27. *Hospital falls:* Numerous procedures are available to reduce the potential of falls across the life span. Infants are vulnerable to fall from cribs, just as older patients are at risk to fall from beds, wheelchairs, or gurneys. Falls are more likely during transportation, moving from surface to surface, or when ambulating after taking medications that alter neurological, musculoskeletal, or cognitive function. Follow institutional policy carefully and institute all precautions needed to prevent falls, regardless of the age of the patient.

28. *Hospital-acquired central line infections:* Use aseptic technique for all handling of central lines. Use sterile technique for opening lines or changing tubing if the patient is at higher risk for infection, such as pediatric patients who are immunocompromised from chemotherapy.

29. *Hospital-acquired pressure injuries:* Patients with decreased circulation, reduced mobility, incontinence, and other factors can lead to a high risk of skin breakdown or pressure injuries. Regardless of age, place patients on a strict turning schedule with frequent evaluations of skin integrity.

30. *Near misses:* Be confident about reporting near-miss medication errors. Even though an error did not take place and the error was caught before it happened, some set of circumstances led to the potential error. Report these near misses so that steps can be taken to improve processes and prevent near misses from reoccurring.

31. *Failure to use indicated diagnostic or laboratory test results:* Follow-up on the results of tests in order to report them to the appropriate health-care provider or to the person who ordered the test. Report critical values within 60 minutes.

32. *Avoidable delay in providing treatment:* Be aware of the time frame between a diagnosis and the onset of treatment. Foster an appropriate time frame by communicating effectively with other team members and by assisting in the coordination of care.

33. *Inadequate preparation of the child and family before treatment:* Provide education concerning a diagnostic test, laboratory test, or surgical procedure to prevent complications or lack of adequate preparation. Use preprocedural checklists and patient/family education checklists to reduce errors.

34. *Inadequate monitoring of a child after a procedure:* Adhere to safe standards of practice after a patient has undergone a diagnostic test or procedure to make sure that the patient is achieving homeostasis and stability. This includes monitoring vital signs and reactions to dyes and medications, monitoring for a safe airway, and rapidly communicating to the health-care team concerning a change in condition.

35. *Not using automated medication dispensing equipment:* It is imperative to use safe medication dispensing equipment and not workarounds that can lead to dispensing errors.

References

Anderson, J. G., & Abrahamson, K. (2017). Your health care may kill you: Medical errors. *Studies in Health Technology and Informatics, 234,* 13–17. PMID: 28186008

Hathaway, J. (2020). *Estimates of preventable deaths are too high, new study shows.* https://news.yale.edu/2020/01/28/estimates-preventable-hospital-deaths-are-too-high-new-study-shows

Juneja, D., & Mishra, A. (2022). Medication prescription errors in intensive care unit: An avoidable menace. *Indian Journal of Critical Care Medicine, 26*(5), 541–542. https://doi.org/10.5005/jp-journals-10071-24215

National Quality Forum. (2011). *Serious Reportable Events in Healthcare 2011.* https://www.qualityforum.org/Publications/2011/12/Serious_Reportable_Events_in_Healthcare_2011.aspx

Rodziewicz, T. L., Houseman, B., Vaqar, S., & Hipskind, J. E. (2024). *Medical error reduction and prevention.* StatPearls Publishing. https://www.ncbi.nlm.nih.gov/books/NBK499956

APPENDIX C
Conversion Factors

1. Degrees Centigrade to Fahrenheit

Celsius	Fahrenheit
0	32 (freezing point)
32.1	90
32.8	91
33.3	92
34	93
34.4	94
35	95
35.6	96
36.1	97
36.7	98
37	98.6
37.2	99
37.8	100
38.3	101
38.9	102
39.4	103
40	104
40.6	105
41.6	106
42.2	107
100	212 (i.e., boiling point)

From Litwack, K. (2009). Clinical coach for effective nursing care.
In J. Nagtalon-Ramos, *Maternal-newborn nursing care* (Table 12-1,
pp. 261–262). F. A. Davis.

2. Body Mass Index
   Calculated by:
   [(Weight in pounds divided by Height in inches) divided by Height in inches] multiplied by 703
3. Pounds to Kilograms
   Divide the child's weight in pounds by 2.2 to calculate kilograms.
4. Kilograms to Pounds
   Multiply the child's weight in kilograms by 2.2 to calculate pounds.
5. Inches to centimeters
   Multiply the child's height in inches by 2.5 to calculate centimeters.
6. Centimeters to inches
   Divide the child's height in centimeters by 2.5 to calculate inches.

APPENDIX D
Common Medication Administration Calculations in Pediatrics

 EXAMPLES OF MATH/CONVERSIONS

- The majority of medications administered to children are prescribed in milligrams (mg) per the child's weight in kilograms (kg).
- Other calculations include mg of medication per body surface area (BSA), described as mg/m^2.
- All orders in pediatric care require the health-care provider to write the final dose as either mg or mg/m^2. If an order only states milliliters (mL) as the final unit, it must be clarified so that you know exactly how many mg of medication to give the child. This way the nurse can confidently and safely know how many milligrams are being ordered in the milliters ordered.
- Remember to always double-check the "rights" of medication administration! The following include the basic five "rights" often referred to in nursing practice, plus additional "rights" for safe practice.
  - Right patient
  - Right medication
  - Right dose
  - Right route
  - Right time
  - Right assessment before administration
  - Right assessment after administration
  - Right education
  - Right documentation
  - Right to refuse (if over 18 years of age or medically emancipated from parents or legal guardians)

Example #1:
Calculate a dose of oral amoxicillin (Amoxil) suspension in mL for a child with recurring bilateral otitis media with infusion. The child weighs 36 pounds. The order from the pediatrician is for 400 mg per dose bid for 5 days. The safe dose range for this medication is listed in the clinic formulary as 40 to 50 mg/kg/day divided into two doses.

You have on hand 400 mg/5 mL.

1. Convert the child's weight from pounds to kilograms by dividing the weight in pounds by 2.2: 16.4 kg.
2. Calculate the child's required doses per day, taking into account the safe dose range published on this medication: 16.4 kg × 40 = 656 mg per day. The high range of this medication is 16.4 kg × 50 = 820 mg per day. The safe dose range of total medication per day is between 656 and 820 mg.

3. Calculate the frequency of the medication as ordered. The medication is divided into two doses, so the range should be 328 mg per dose up to 410 mg per dose: 656 mg/day divided by 2 × 328 mg/dose; and 820 mg/day divided by 2 × 410 mg/dose.
4. Double-check what the order is now that a safe dose daily range has been determined as well as a safe dose range per dose (bid).
5. Now calculate the mL needed from the concentration available. You have on hand 400 mg/5 mL and you need 400 mg. 400 mg/day divided by 400 mg/5 mL × 5 mL of amoxicillin per dose.
6. The child should have 5 mL per dose.

Example #2:
Calculate a dose of liquid Tylenol suspension in mL for a child with a fever from influenza. The child weighs 22.8 pounds. The order from the pediatrician is for 155 mg per dose, every 4 to 6 hours, up to four doses per day, maximum. The safe dose range for this medication is listed in the clinic formulary as 10 to 15 mg/kg/dose.

You know that pediatric Tylenol comes in two strengths: either Tylenol 160 mg/5 mL for toddlers and older, or Tylenol 80 mg/1 mL for infants. You have on hand the 160 mg/5 mL strength.

1. Convert the child's weight from pounds to kilograms by dividing the weight in pounds by 2.2: 10.4 kg.
2. Calculate the child's required doses per day, taking into account the safe dose range published on this medication: 10.4 kg × 10 = 104 mg per day. Calculate the high range of this medication: 10.4 kg × 15 = 156 mg per day. The safe dose range of total medication per day is between 104 and 156 mg.
3. Double-check what the order is now that a safe dose range has been determined. The dose of 155 mg of Tylenol falls in the safe dose range of 104 to 156 mg.
4. Now calculate the mL needed from the concentration available. You have on hand 160 mg/5 mL and you need 155 mg. 155 mg/X mL divided by 160 mg/5 mL × 4.8 mL of Tylenol per dose.
5. The child should have Tylenol 4.8 mL per dose. The child may have four doses per day, maximum.

Example #3:
A child with leukemia is in the phase of treatment called maintenance. Here the child is to receive 1.5 units of vincristine

(Oncovin) per BSA (m²). The child weighs 92 pounds and is 150 cm tall. The chemotherapy medication vincristine comes already prepared by the pharmacy in a protective "hood" with a final concentration of 1 mg per mL. What is the final dose of the medication for this child?

1. Convert the child's weight from pounds to kilograms: 92 pounds divided by 2.2 × 41.8 kg.
2. Calculate the BSA by multiplying the child's weight in kg by the height in cm, then divide by 3,600, then find the square root of this amount (press square root on the calculator). The square root of (41.8 × 150) divided by 3,600 × 1.32 m².
3. The child is to receive 1.5 units of the medication per BSA. 1.5 units × 1.32 m² × 1.98 units.
4. The final concentration is then determined: 1.98 units of vincristine per dose with a medication concentration of 1 mg of vincristine per mL would be: 1.98 units × 1 = 1.98 units per dose.

Glossary

Abortion: A term used to describe a pregnancy loss or termination before the fetus is viable.

Abuse: A form of potential or actual injury or harm inflicted upon a child that may be physical, emotional, or neglectful in nature.

Acanthosis nigricans: A skin disorder in which dark brown or gray plaques appear on the skin, typically on the neck, groin, upper thighs, and under the arms, in patients with insulin excess, such as obesity or type 2 diabetes mellitus (DM).

Acceleration: An abrupt increase in fetal heart rate above the baseline.

Accidental poisoning: The ingestion of toxic substances or medications by young children who obtain unsafe access to them.

Acidosis: A relative or actual increase in blood acidity because of the accumulation of acids (e.g., renal disease or diabetic acidosis) or an excessive loss of bicarbonates (e.g., renal disease).

Acme: The peak of the contraction.

Acne neonatorum: Clogged hair follicles or pores in the skin present at birth.

Acne vulgaris: A variation of acne, an inflammatory disease of the sebaceous follicles marked by comedones, papules, and pustules, in which there is the presence of cysts, nodules, and scarring.

Acquired immunity: Immunity or resistance to infection or toxicity by the child's natural immune system. Often referred to when a child has experienced an infection and developed antibodies against the infection source or organism.

Acrocyanosis: A blue or purplish discoloration of the hands and feet of the newborn.

Acromegaly: A chronic syndrome of excessive growth hormone, caused by pituitary malfunction, which produces bony enlargement. Acromegaly is diagnosed by an excessive blood level of serum insulinlike growth factor 1 (IGF-1).

Active immunity: Protection from disease that develops when antibodies are formed against specific antigens or foreign substances such as bacteria, viruses, and toxins.

Acts of commission: Child abuse situations in which the responsible person, often the parent, intentionally harms the child via physical, emotional, or sexual abuse.

Acts of omission: Child abuse situations in which a parent or caregiver, to the best of abilities and often inadvertently, cannot provide adequate nutrition, shelter, warmth, appropriate seasonal clothing (winter coats), safety, and/or education for their child.

Acute distress disorder: A disorder that precedes posttraumatic stress disorder (PTSD), manifested as anxiety; considered a predictor for PTSD.

Addiction: An abnormal dependence and compulsive behavior toward a substance such as alcohol, cocaine, opiates, or tobacco that has adverse emotional, psychological, physical, economic, social, and legal ramifications.

Adventitious breath sounds: Abnormal, acquired, or accidental breath sounds.

Afterpains: The contractions of the uterus for the first few days after childbirth.

Alcohol abuse: An abusive state of alcohol consumption associated with the chronic, frequently progressive, and sometimes fatal disease of impaired control of alcohol consumption.

Alkalosis: A relative or actual increase in blood alkalinity because of the accumulation of alkaloids or because of the reduction of acids.

Alveoli/alveolar sacs: The small air sacs of the lungs where gas exchange takes place.

Amblyopia: Unilateral or bilateral decrease of best-corrected vision in an otherwise healthy eye, often because of asymmetric refractive error (i.e., deflection from a straight path or change in direction of light) or the presence of strabismus.

Amenorrhea: Absence of the menstrual period.

Amniocentesis: A procedure in which a thin needle is used to remove amniotic fluid and cells from the amniotic sac surrounding the fetus for testing.

Amnioinfusion: A procedure in which room temperature normal saline is infused into the uterus through an intrauterine pressure catheter to increase the volume of fluid in the uterus. The increase in fluid may relieve the compression of the fetal body on the umbilical cord.

Amniotic band syndrome: A condition in which adhesions between the amnion and fetus occur, causing deformities, such as limb amputation.

Amniotic fluid: Also known as the *bag of waters (BOW),* a fluidlike mixture that provides buoyancy, movement, and protection for the fetus in the uterus.

Amniotic membrane: A thin membrane formed from the ectoderm layer that surrounds the fetus and amniotic fluid.

Amniotomy: Artificial rupture of the uterine membranes with an amniohook.

Analgesia: The absence of a normal sense of pain that is achieved by the administration of pain relievers or anesthetics.

Anaphylaxis: A very serious allergic reaction with symptoms including hypotension, severe airway edema, lightheadedness, and bronchospasms.

Anemia: A reduction in circulating red blood cells.

Anesthesia: A medication delivered by gas or injection that causes partial or complete loss of sensation to an area of the body.

Anhedonia: Lack of pleasure in acts that are normally pleasurable.

Animism: A belief that inanimate objects are alive.

Anorexia nervosa: An eating disorder marked by weight loss, disturbance of body image, and eventual emaciation by consciously withholding calorie consumption.

Anoxia: A condition in which no oxygen reaches cells.

Antepartum: The period of pregnancy between conception and onset of labor.

Anthropometric measurements: The measurements of the body, including weight, height, head circumference, and other measurements.

Antigen: Foreign substances such as bacteria, viruses, toxins, and foreign proteins that stimulate the formation of antibodies.

Apgar score: A systematic method of assessing the newborn's heart rate, muscle tone, response to stimuli, and color at 1 minute after birth and again at 5 minutes after birth.

Apnea: A cessation of breathing.

Apparent life-threatening event (ALTE): Also called an *acute life-threatening event,* an ALTE is a sudden, acute, and unexpected change in a young infant's breathing pattern, which leads to a color change, apnea, limpness, and, often, choking or gagging.

Areola: The dark area around the nipple.

Artificialism: A belief that everything is made by humans.

Ascites: Edema marked by excess serous fluid accumulating in the peritoneal cavity.

Asphyxiation: A state of insufficient oxygen intake related to choking, poisoning, shock, trauma, crushing or compression injuries to the chest, drowning, near drowning, or any source of diminished environmental oxygen.

Assent: The inclusion of the school-aged child in the developmentally appropriate discussions of their health-care treatments. This is not a legal form of consent but a respectful inclusion of the child's thoughts, feelings, and desires.

Astigmatism: A visual disorder where the refraction of a ray of light is spread over a diffuse area rather than sharply focused on the retina. This is because of a difference in the curvature of the cornea and lens of the eye.

Atelectasis: A collapsed or airless condition of the lung often caused by an obstruction by mucous plugs.

Atony: Lack of normal uterine muscle tone.

Attachment: The incorporation of the new baby into the family unit.

Attitude: Referring to the positioning of the fetus. The most common fetal attitude and the most successful for a vaginal delivery is when the fetus is in a fully flexed position.

Augmentation: The stimulation of hypotonic uterine contractions once labor has begun but the contractions are ineffective in producing dilation and labor progression.

Autonomy: The sense that one is separate from others and that one has some control over one's environment and interactions; the actual or desired state of independence. May be considered a state of separation from the child's primary caregiver.

Ballottement: A diagnostic maneuver in pregnancy. The fetal part rebounds when touched by an examiner's finger through the vagina.

Battered: A child who has been physically abused by another; often has lasting marks, erythema, bruises, fractures, or other forms of physical or emotional evidence.

Beneficence: Acting from a spirit of compassion and kindness to benefit others.

Bilirubin: A product of the breakdown of the heme portion of a red blood cell.

Bimanual examination: To determine uterine size and position, the health-care provider places the gloved middle and index fingers into the vagina to identify the cervix. The other hand is placed midway between the umbilicus and the symphysis pubis and presses downward toward the pelvic hand.

Bishop score: A tool used to evaluate cervical ripening that is predictive of readiness for labor.

Blastocyst: A maturing embryo in which some cell differentiation has occurred.

Bonding: The emotional and physical attachment between a mother and her newborn that is initiated in the first hour or two after the birth.

Brachial plexus: A network of nerves that originates in the neck area and branches off to form the nerves that control movement and sensation in the shoulders, arms, and hands.

Brachycephalic: Having a cephalic index of greater than 80%, which demonstrates a short and broad head; considered a short head but not abnormal.

Braxton Hicks contractions: Irregular, mild contractions that occur in late pregnancy and do not produce cervical effacement and dilation.

Bronchodilation: A method of opening the airway to ease respiratory distress; often accomplished through the use of bronchodilating medications.

Broselow tape: Also known as *Broselow pediatric emergency tape;* a color-coded, length-based system for emergency response based on a child's actual or estimated weight that is used in a variety of settings, including emergency departments, acute and critical care units, and outpatient settings. The system covers both equipment for weight and medications precalculated for weight.

Brown fat: A type of fat found in term newborns in the scapular area, the thorax, and behind the kidneys. It can be used by the newborn to produce body heat.

Bulimia: An eating disorder marked by episodes of binge eating followed by intense emotional distress, including guilt and shame, resulting in self-induced vomiting and diarrhea as well as excessive exercise and fasting to reverse the effects of the binge eating.

Bullying: Aggressive behavior among children that is unwanted and demonstrates a feeling of perceived or real power imbalance (Stopbullying.gov, 2019).

Caput succedaneum: A swelling of the scalp of the newborn caused by pressure from the uterus or vaginal wall during delivery.

Carbon monoxide: A colorless, odorless, and tasteless poisonous gas often associated with car engine exhaust, broken heaters, sewers, cellars, and mines. Poisoning can result from burning organic fuels in the home or car exhaust without proper ventilation.

Cardiopulmonary: Relating to both the heart and the lungs.

Cardiovascular: Relating to the heart and entire blood vessel system.

Cataract: An opacity (i.e., cloudy appearance) of the lens of the eye often caused by trauma, aging, metabolic or endocrine disease, or the side effects of certain medications such as steroids.

Catecholamines: Hormones produced by the adrenal glands, such as dopamine, norepinephrine, and epinephrine.

Centers for Disease Control and Prevention (CDC): Located just outside of Atlanta, Georgia, the CDC operates under the Department of Health & Human Services and is the leading agency for protecting the health of U.S. residents.

Central cyanosis: Discoloration because of reduced hemoglobin; associated with reduced oxygen saturation measurements.

Cephalic: A medical term of Latin origin referring to the head.

Cephalohematoma: A swelling on the head that does not cross the suture line. It is caused by birth trauma that causes a rupture of blood vessels between the skull and periosteum.

Cephalopelvic disproportion (CPD): A disproportion or mismatch between the maternal pelvis size and the size or position of the fetal head. This condition occurs when the maternal pelvis is too small for the fetal head.

Cerclage: The use of sutures around the cervix to prevent the opening of the cervix.

Certified nurse midwife (CNM): An advanced-practice registered nurse who has graduated from an accredited school of midwifery and passed a national certification examination that allows the nurse midwife to provide health care during the preconception, prenatal, labor, delivery, and postpartum periods.

Cerumen: A substance secreted by glands at the outer third of the ear canal. Although it typically does not accumulate in the ear canal, it may clog the channel.

Cervical incompetence: The inability of the uterine cervix to retain a pregnancy in the second trimester in the absence of uterine contractions.

Cervix: The lower portion of the uterus that projects into the vagina.

Chadwick sign: A deep blue color of the vagina and cervix because of increased vascularity.

Chain of custody: Labeling and securing of evidence of abuse during processing, holding, and handing over to officials.

Child Protective Services (CPS): In most states, this is a state-run organization that is a designated social services agency that provides assessment, interventions, and treatment for families who have been identified to have child maltreatment, including various forms of abuse and/or neglect.

Chorioamnionitis: Infection of the fetal amnion and chorion membranes.

Choriocarcinoma: A fast-growing cancer that can develop in the uterus following a molar pregnancy.

Chorion: A thick membrane that develops from the trophoblast and becomes part of the placenta villi.

Chorioretinitis: Inflammation of the choroid and retina of the eye.

Chromosomes: A linear strand of protein DNA that carries genetic material.

Chronic illness: An illness that lasts a long period and significantly affects a person's functioning for at least 3 months out of each year.

Chronicity: Pertaining to a condition lasting a long time.

Circumcision: The surgical removal of the end of the foreskin of the penis.

Clinical status: A term used to denote the clinical well-being of a child.

Clostridioides difficile (C. difficile): A gram-positive, anaerobic, spore-forming bacillus that causes watery diarrhea, abdominal pain, fever, and anorexia, and that may produce a pseudomembranous colitis.

Code blue: A phrase used to describe an actual or pending cardiopulmonary arrest.

Collaboration: A process of working together.

Color blindness: An inability to distinguish certain colors or any colors at all.

Colostrum: A fluid rich with antibodies that may be secreted in small amounts during the pregnancy and before milk production. It contains carbohydrates, antibodies, and a small amount of fat.

Communicable: Capable of being transmitted from one individual to another.

Compartment syndrome: A situation in which a traumatic injury causes pressure to build up in a confined space, such as in the rigid fascia surrounding the muscles. If a bleed occurs or there is a buildup of inflammatory fluids, pressure builds up within the muscles, leading to ischemia and necrosis and causing severe tissue damage.

Concrete operations: Created by Dr. Jean Piaget, a Swiss philosopher and psychologist (1896–1980), *concrete operations* refers to the thought processes of the school-aged child who can use and understand logical thinking to interpret their world and understand simple and complex phenomena.

Conduction: The transfer of body heat to a cooler surface.

Conductive hearing loss: Form of hearing impairment where the outer ear has been affected or damaged, such as with repeated otitis media, causing scarring on the tympanic membrane.

Congenital: Inherited, or genetic, disorders that are present at birth.

Contactant: A substance that causes an allergic or sensitivity response when the substance is exposed to the skin.

Contraceptive: A method or device serving to prevent pregnancy.

Convection: The transfer of body heat to the surrounding cool air.

Coping: Adapting to and managing significant change, illness, work, relocation, pain, death, changes in family structure, or chronic illness.

Corpus luteum: A structure that develops from a ruptured ovarian follicle and that secretes the hormone progesterone.

Couvade syndrome: A syndrome in which the father may experience psychosomatic, pregnancy-simulating symptoms of nausea, fatigue, and backache.

Cranial nerves: Twelve pairs of nerves, numbered by the order in which they contact the brain, that originate in the cranial cavity and innervate the head.

Crepitus: A crackling sound heard while auscultating the lungs, such as with pneumonia.

Crohn disease: An inflammatory disease marked by patchy areas of full-thickness inflammation anywhere along the gastrointestinal tract. The condition causes pain, malabsorption, fistulas, and bloody stools.

Cultural awareness: Developing sensitivity and awareness of another ethnic group (Adams, 1995).

Cultural competence: Ability of an individual or organization to function effectively within the cultural context of beliefs, behaviors, and needs of the person or community that they serve (Ritter & Hoffman, 2010).

Cultural sensitivity: The use of neutral language, both verbal and nonverbal, in a way that reflects sensitivity and appreciation for the diversity of another. Cultural sensitivity may be conveyed through words, phrases, and categorizations that are intentionally avoided, especially when referring to any individual who may interpret certain language as impolite or offensive (American Academy of Nursing Expert Panel on Cultural Competence, 2007).

Culture: Learned behavior shared among members of a group; system of shared ideas, concepts, rules, and meanings that underlie and are manifested in ways of life; includes knowledge, beliefs, art, morals, law, customs, and any other capabilities and habits acquired by members of a society (Bird & Osland, 2006; Douglas & Pacquiao, 2010; Soderberg & Holden, 2002).

Cushing syndrome: Also called *hyperadrenocorticism,* this disorder is related to exposure to excessive glucocorticoid hormones. Cushing syndrome is a side effect of pharmacological use of steroids in the management of inflammatory illnesses. Symptoms include muscular weakness, thinning of the skin, easy bruising, rounding facial features, and weight gain.

Cyanosis: A blue, gray, slate-colored, or dark purple discoloration of the skin or mucous membranes when deoxygenated or reduced hemoglobin is in the blood. Cyanosis is associated with severe respiratory distress and poor gas exchange. It may start as subtle cyanosis in the lips (i.e., circumoral), progressing to the nipples and nailbeds, and can be seen on the entire body when severe deoxygenation is present.

Cyberbullying: The use of computer technology and the internet to bully another. Cyberbullying may be in the form of defamation, ridicule, intimidation, or threats of violence.

Cyber threat: A threat made by a person over the internet. Such threats are prevalent and pose a very real danger to an unsuspecting child.

Cystocele: A condition in which the bladder drops down and protrudes through the vagina.

Deafness: Inability to process any acoustic sound with or without hearing devices.

Deceleration: A decrease in fetal heart rate from the baseline.

Decibel: A unit of measure of sound.

Deciduous teeth: Primary (i.e., baby) teeth that are shed to make room for adult or permanent teeth. Deciduous refers to the "falling out" or shedding of the primary teeth.

Decrement: The subsiding of a contraction.

Decubitus: Term used for skin and underlying structures damaged from compression and inadequate perfusion; used synonymously with the term *pressure sore.*

Depression: A mood disorder marked by a loss of interest or pleasure in living, which presents with many symptoms, including poor academic performance, persistent sadness, poor appetite, tearfulness, hopelessness, and loss of energy. Depression is also called *clinical depression, major depressive disorder, dysthymic disorder,* and *unipolar depression.*

Dermal melanosis: Also known as a *Mongolian spot,* this congenital birthmark is caused by melanocytes trapped deep in the skin; it appears flat and bluish-gray or brown, and is located on the back or buttocks.

Dermatological: Pertaining to the skin, or study or science of the skin.

Developmental dysplasia/dislocation of the hip: A spectrum of anatomical abnormalities of the hip joint.

Diabetes insipidus (DI): In this disorder, the opposite of syndrome of inappropriate antidiuretic hormone (SIADH) occurs. In DI, there is a reduced production of posterior pituitary secretion of SIADH and the child's urine has a very low specific gravity. DI causes the child to produce copious urine (i.e., uncontrolled diuresis).

Diabetes mellitus (DM): A chronic metabolic disorder marked by hyperglycemia that results from either failure to produce insulin (i.e., type 1) or insulin resistance with inadequate insulin secretion to sustain metabolism (i.e., type 2).

Diabetic ketoacidosis (DKA): An acidotic state caused by an excess of ketone bodies in patients who do not produce adequate insulin.

Diagonal conjugate: The distance from the lower posterior border of the symphysis pubis to the sacral promontory.

Diaphoresis: Profuse sweating.

Diastasis recti: Separation of the abdominal muscles.

Dilation: The opening of the closed cervix to approximately 10 cm.

Dilation and curettage (D&C): A surgical procedure in which the cervix is dilated and the physician scrapes the lining of the uterus to remove the contents of pregnancy.

Direct or conjugated bilirubin: Bilirubin that is broken down into a water-soluble form for excretion.

Disseminated intravascular coagulation (DIC): A coagulation disorder in which the body responds to hemorrhage by overproducing clotting factors that can cause clots that cut off the blood supply to major organs.

Diuresis: The secretion and passage of large amounts of urine.

Diurnal incontinence: Incontinence of urine occurring every day; when it occurs during the day, it usually has a pathological cause.

Diversity (cultural competency): Differences in race, ethnicity, national origin, religion, age, gender, sexual orientation, ability or disability, social and economic status or class, education, and related attributes of groups of people in society (Andrews & Boyle, 2008).

Dizygotic twins: Fraternal twins who develop from two separate sperm and ova.

Doula: A professional who provides physical, emotional, and informational support to the laboring woman.

Down syndrome: Present in 1 of 700 births in the United States, the clinical consequence of having three #21 chromosomes (i.e., trisomy 21), which results in mild to moderate cognitive impairment and specific physical characteristics, including low-set ears, sloping forehead, single palmar crease, and a tendency to have cardiac disease.

Ductus arteriosus: A blood vessel in the fetus that permits most blood to bypass the lungs.

Ductus venosus: A small blood vessel that allows fetal blood to bypass the liver.

Duration: The actual time that a contraction lasts from beginning to end.

Dysmenorrhea: Painful menstrual periods.

Dyspareunia: Painful sexual intercourse.

Dyspnea: Labored or difficult breathing.

Dysuria: Painful or difficult urination.

Early decelerations: A gradual decrease in fetal heart rate with the onset of deceleration caused by head compression as the fetus moves through the pelvis.

Echocardiography: A test that looks at how blood flows through the heart vessels, valves, and chambers.

Eclampsia: The onset of seizure activity with all the symptoms of severe preeclampsia.

Ectopic pregnancy: A situation in which a fertilized ovum implants outside the uterus.

Effacement: The process of thinning of the cervix.

Elective abortion: A term used to describe a situation in which a woman chooses to terminate a pregnancy.

Emancipation: The granting of legal control over one's decisions or lifestyle. For adolescents who are not yet 18 years of age, emancipation can be the granting of financial independence or related to the granting of rights over health-care decisions.

Embryo: The stage of development between the fertilized ovum and the fetus.

Emesis: Defined as the forceful expulsion or emptying of stomach content caused by either a gastrointestinal disorder or by a nongastrointestinal disorder.

Empowerment: A concept within family-centered care principles that describes assisting a family to feel as though they are supported, listened to, and competent.

Enabling: A concept within family-centered care principles that describes the teaching, supporting, and enabling that allows a family to care for their child.

Encephalopathy: A generalized brain dysfunction of varying degrees that causes an impairment of arousal, orientation, speech, and cognitive processing. It is caused by exposure to toxins, hypoxia, or an infectious process.

Encopresis: Uncontrolled soiling during the day in a child who is 4 years of age or older who had previously mastered toilet training. This condition is associated with stool retention and holding.

Endemic: A condition or a disease that is found regularly among those in a certain area.

Endometrial ablation: A procedure in which the tissues lining the uterus are destroyed.

Endometriosis: A condition in which uterine tissue is growing outside the uterus.

Endometritis: An infection of the endometrium, which is the lining of the uterus.

Endometrium: The mucous membrane that lines the cavity of the uterus. It is the site where the embryo implants after arriving in the uterus.

Engagement: The entrance of the widest diameter of the presenting part of the fetus into the mother's pelvis.

Engorgement: An overfull breast that occurs at times with breastfeeding.

Engrossment: An attitude of total focus on something.

Enucleation: Surgical removal of an eye from the eye socket.

Enuresis: Involuntary elimination of urine after the age in which the child should have or has had bladder control but now has lost it. Control is usually secured by 5 years of age. Enuresis is multifactorial.

Epidemic: The presence, or prevalence, of a disease within a widespread geographical area. Typically refers to a rapid spread or an increased occurrence of a disease within a widespread geographical area.

Epidural: Anesthesia infused through a catheter between the fourth and fifth vertebrae into the epidural space to decrease pain and perception.

Epiglottitis: A medical emergency in which the child's epiglottis becomes inflamed, mostly caused by a viral infection, and in which the child's airway may become completely closed.

Epimetrium: Smooth, transparent membrane that lines most of the external surface of the uterus.

Epiphyseal plate: The center of ossification at the extremity of each of the long bones. Considered the "growth plate" of long bones where new bone growth occurs.

Episiotomy: An incision into the perineum to enlarge the vaginal opening.

Episodic decelerations: Decelerations of fetal heart rate that are not associated with uterine contractions.

Epispadias: A congenital condition in which the meatus, the opening of the urethra, is located on the dorsum of the penis.

Erythema toxicum neonatorum: Also known as a *newborn rash,* this rash may appear as macules, papules, or vesicles and may appear on any part of the body except the palms and soles of the feet.

Esotropia: Inward deviation of the eye laterally.

Estriol: One of three types of estrogens that occur naturally in the body.

Estrogen: A female hormone secreted by the ovaries.

Ethics: Moral principles that guide a person's behavior.

Ethnicity: The perception of oneself and a sense of belonging to a particular ethnic group or to more than one group. Ethnicity includes commitment to cultural customs and rituals. It is not the same as physical traits associated with race (e.g., skin or eye color, hair) related to a geographical origin.

Ethnographic: The scientific description of individual cultures.

Eustachian tubes: Anatomical auditory tubes lined with mucous membranes and located from the middle ear to the nasopharynx. Occlusion can lead to otitis media, an infectious process.

Evaporation: The loss of heat as fluid evaporates.

Exanthem: Any type of a reaction or eruption that appears on the skin as opposed to a reaction or eruption that forms on mucous membranes; often used to describe pediatric rashes.

Exfoliation: The shedding or casting off of a body surface.

Exophthalmos: An abnormal protrusion of the eyeball often because of thyrotoxicosis (i.e., hyperthyroidism).

Exotropia: Outward deviation of the eye laterally.

External cephalic version: An attempt by the health-care provider to move a malpositioned fetus, such as a breech or transverse lie, into a vertex cephalic presentation.

External version: A procedure in which the health-care provider attempts to change the fetal position externally.

Factitious disorder imposed on another: (formally known as Munchausen syndrome by proxy) A mental illness in which one has an inner need for another person (their child) to be seen as injured or ill, and produces this by false claims (Mayo Clinic, 2022).

Failure to thrive (FTT): A term used to denote an infant's or child's growth measurements that are below what is expected; may be associated with pathology, neglect, or poor parenting skills.

Family-centered care: A philosophy of family-focused care in which the family is considered the child's constant. Family is given the opportunity to be included in all medical decision-making, is empowered to make informed decisions for their child, and is enabled to provide all care for their child.

Fetal: Pertaining to a fetus.

Fetal demise: The death of a fetus at any stage of the pregnancy.

Fetal fibronectin (fFN): A protein that helps the amniotic sac to adhere to the uterine wall. It is detected before 22 weeks' gestation and after 37 weeks' gestation.

Fetal lie: The alignment of the fetus with the mother.

Fetal presentation: The part of the fetus that is first to enter the pelvis.

Fetal station: The measurement in centimeters of the fetal presenting part in relationship to the maternal ischial spine in the pelvis.

Fibroids: Benign tumors in the uterus.

Fibromyomas: Benign uterine tumors.

Fistula: An abnormal opening between anatomical structures that should not be there, such as between the rectum and the vagina, or between the trachea and the esophagus.

Fluid maintenance calculation: A standard calculation used in pediatrics to determine the daily maintenance of fluids that should be consumed or administered. Based on the child's weight in kilograms, this is not considered as resuscitative fluids but what should be taken in daily to maintain a balanced fluid status.

Follicle-stimulating hormone (FSH): A hormone that stimulates the development of a follicle in the ovary before ovulation.

Fontanel: Often referred to as the "soft spot" on the baby's head, this fibrous membrane lies between the bones of the cranium.

Food lags and jags: A phrase used to describe how a young child goes through phases of not experiencing hunger and therefore refusing to eat or taking in a reduced number of calories.

Foramen ovale: The opening in the atria of the fetal heart that allows blood to bypass the lungs.

Forceps: A metal instrument that has two curved spoonlike blades with locking handles that fit on either side of the fetal head and assist with delivery of the baby.

Foremilk: The milk produced and stored between feedings.

Frequency: The time between contractions, which is measured from the beginning of one contraction to the beginning of the next contraction.

Fundus: The upper large part of the uterus.

Galactorrhea: Inappropriate or excessive production of milk.

Galactosemia: A rare genetic metabolic disorder that makes it difficult for the infant to metabolize milk sugar, which can damage organs.

Gastroenteritis: An inflammatory process that occurs in the stomach, small intestine, or large intestine.

Gender dysphoria: Discomfort or lack of identification with one's sex assigned at birth.

General anesthesia: Medication given IV to cause the patient to lose consciousness and the subsequent placement of an endotracheal tube in the trachea to allow the administration of oxygen and gas to keep the patient unconscious during a procedure.

Genetics: The study of how genes, chromosomes, and genotypes, or sequencing and combinations of genes, are expressed and responsible for health or disorders.

Genomics: The study of how genetics influence disease.

Gigantism: The excessive development of the body or of a body part.

Glaucoma: A group of eye diseases that leads to increased intraocular pressure and eventually leads to the atrophy of the optic nerve.

Glomerulonephritis: A condition of inflamed glomerular tissue, nephritis, in which the lesions involve the glomeruli. Also called *acute nephritic syndrome*, this condition frequently follows an infection with particular strains of streptococci.

Glucagon: A polypeptide hormone secreted by the α cells of the pancreas. This hormone stimulates the liver to change stored glycogen to glucose.

Gluten intolerance: The inability to tolerate the consumption of foods with gluten, including wheat, oats, barley, and rye. Consumption of glutens in a child with intolerance can cause inflammation, flatus, cramping, fatigue, and diarrhea. In severe cases, it can cause a failure to thrive (FTT) trajectory.

Glycogen: Glucose stored in the liver until needed for energy.

Goiter: An enlargement of the thyroid gland caused by a variety of reasons, including iodine deficiency, thyroiditis, nodules, or any hyperfunction or hypofunction of the thyroid.

Goodell sign: Softening of the cervix caused by the increased vascularity of pregnancy.

Grand mal seizure: A type of seizure activity that crosses over the brain's hemispheres and causes full-body neuromuscular seizure activity. It is associated with a loss of consciousness, tonic/clonic movements, urinary and fecal incontinence, amnesia of the event, and an icteric (i.e., sleepy) state afterward.

Graves disease: A form of hyperthyroidism in which an autoimmune destruction of the thyroid gland takes place. The condition increases production of thyroxine and causes an enlargement of the thyroid gland.

Gravida: The number of times a woman has been pregnant.

Gynecomastia: Enlarged breasts in the newborn caused by maternal hormones.

Hard of hearing: Phrase used to denote the reduced ability to hear but the continued ability to hear and process acoustic sounds at some level.

Health-care disparity: Lack of similarity in access to health care. Many residents of the United States have no access to health care.

Health literacy: The degree to which individuals have the capacity to obtain, process, and understand basic health information and services needed to make appropriate health-related decisions (Institute of Medicine, 2004).

Healthy People 2020: An initiative created by the Surgeon General's office in 1979 that states major health goals for U.S. residents in the upcoming decade.

Hegar sign: A sign of pregnancy; softening of the lower uterine segment.

Hemangioma: Also known as *nevus vascularis,* this growth consists of newly formed and dilated capillaries in the dermal and subdermal layers of the skin.

Hematochezia: The passage of bright-red, fresh blood in the stool.

Hematoma: A collection of blood in the tissues outside a blood vessel.

Hematuria: Blood in the urine.

Hemolytic uremic syndrome (HUS): An acute condition in which microangiopathic hemolytic anemia, thrombocytopenia, and acute nephropathy are present. *Escherichia coli* O157:H7 and *E. coli* O111 are frequently the causative agents, which are acquired from eating contaminated foods or raw meat.

Hemophilia: A group of hereditary bleeding disorders noted by a deficient level of blood clotting proteins. The two major types are hemophilia A (1 in 10,000 males) and hemophilia B (1 in 30,000 males).

Hemoptysis: The presence of blood in respiratory secretions or mucus.

Hemorrhoids: Enlarged veins in the anus and rectal area.

Hereditary: The transmission of genetic characteristics from the parent to the offspring.

Higher level of care: A phrase used to denote the transfer of a child from a lower level of care, such as a hospital pediatric unit bed, to the pediatric intensive care unit.

Hindmilk: Milk that is produced during the breastfeeding session.

Hirsutism: An excessive growth of hair or the presence of hair in unusual places, particularly in women; can be associated with the side effects of certain anticonvulsant medications and hormonal imbalances.

Human chorionic gonadotropin (hCG): A hormone that is produced by the fertilized egg that supports the development of the embryo.

Human papillomavirus (HPV): A papillomavirus found in humans that is considered a common sexually transmitted infection. The virus causes genital warts and can develop into cervical cancer.

Human placental lactogen: A hormone that assists with milk production and increases the mother's metabolism during pregnancy.

Human trafficking: The recruitment, transportation, transfer, harboring, and exploitation of persons by the means of threat, force, or abduction for the use of prostitution, forced labor, slavery, servitude, or the removal of organs for sale (Article 3, paragraph [b]; Migrationdataportal.org, 2019).

Hydatidiform mole: A genetic abnormality that occurs during early placental attachment and fetal development in which the trophoblast cells that would normally attach the ovum to the uterine wall develop abnormally.

Hydrocephalus: An accumulation of excessive quantities of cerebral spinal fluid (CSF) within the ventricles of the brain, which can cause blocking of normal CSF drainage systems and an increasing head circumference.

Hypercapnia: Excessive carbon dioxide in the bloodstream.

Hyperemesis gravidarum: Nausea and vomiting that interferes with adequate intake of fluid and food and/or that persists past 20 weeks' gestation.

Hyperinsulinemia: A condition of excess insulin circulating in the blood.

Hyperinsulinism: A condition in which the amount of insulin in the blood is higher than normal.

Hyperopia: A defect of vision called *farsightedness* caused by a flattening of the globe of the eye where parallel rays of light come to focus behind the retina.

Hyperthermia: A state in which the body temperature is above the normal range.

Hyperventilation: A state that results from an individual's breathing too fast and too deep, which causes a decrease in carbon dioxide in the blood.

Hypocalcemia: Low levels of calcium in the blood.

Hypofibrinogenemia: Lack of fibrin in the blood.

Hypoglycemia: A plasma glucose level of less than 30 mg/dL in the first 24 hours of life and less than 45 mg/dL thereafter.

Hypomagnesemia: Low levels of magnesium in the blood.

Hyponatremia: A decreased concentration of sodium in the bloodstream.

Hypoparathyroidism: Decreased level of parathyroid hormone, which can cause deficiencies of calcium and phosphorus in the blood.

Hypospadias: A congenital condition in which there is an abnormal opening of the meatus on the underside of the penis. This term is also used to describe the condition in which the urethral opening is within the vagina.

Hypothermia: A body temperature below normal.

Hypoxemia: An abnormally low level of oxygen in the blood resulting from respiratory compromise that prevents the lungs from adequately performing gas exchange.

Hypoxia: A decrease in oxygen supply to the tissues.

Hypoxic-ischemic encephalopathy: Acute brain injury caused by asphyxia.

Hysterectomy: A surgical procedure to remove the uterus.

Hysterosalpingography: A diagnostic test that uses dye to visualize the fallopian tubes and uterus.

Hysteroscopy: Procedure in which a lighted scope is placed through the cervix into the uterus to visualize the uterine cavity.

Hysterosonography: Procedure in which a saline infusion ultrasound is used to view the uterus.

Imminent justice: A belief that everything has a determined universal code of law and order.

Immunity: A term that refers to the body's response of developing antibodies against specific bacteria, viruses, and toxins that, once developed, can prevent illness from future exposure to the organism.

Immunizations: The protection of an individual or of groups by the administration of a vaccine or an injection of specific immunoglobulins for a specific disease or infectious material.

Immunoglobulin: A protein that functions as an antibody.

Impaired nurse: A nurse who is not behaving or functioning appropriately because of illness or addiction or who is incapable of carrying out their professional duties.

Incident report: A legal document used in health care to launch a communication sequence related to a near-miss medical or medication error or an actual medication or medical error. An incidence report can be used to document and inform hospital administration of an unusual occurrence that could have led or that did lead to harm.

Increased intracranial pressure: Increased pressure within the brain's ventricles that is caused by either an overproduction or a lack of absorption of cerebral spinal fluid (CSF).

Increment: The onset and buildup of intensity of a contraction.

Incubation period: The interval of time between exposure to a communicable disease or infection and the presentation of the first symptoms.

Indirect or unconjugated bilirubin: Bilirubin that travels through the bloodstream to the liver.

Induction: A phase of chemotherapy administration often used in pediatric oncology practice that is the first phase in the treatment of many cancers. Induction usually includes one or more medications administered with the intent of inducing a remission or having no identifiable (i.e., minimal) residual disease (i.e., evidence of cancer cells).

Inhaler: A device used to breathe inhaled medications into the lungs. Usually a handheld device that can have a mask attached for easier use with children younger than 5.

Insulin resistance: A condition in which the muscle, fat, and liver cells do not respond to insulin and cannot absorb glucose from the bloodstream.

Intensity: The strength of the contraction at the peak, or acme, of the contraction.

Intentional injury: Considered a possible form of physical child abuse, this type of injury is considered an injury that is caused by another person during such activities as discipline. It can include hitting; slapping; pushing; and causing fractures, burns, or severe harm.

Intersex conditions: A variety of conditions that contribute to the development of physical sex characteristics that are atypical.

Intrathecal space: Something that exists within the spinal canal.

Intrauterine growth restriction (IGR): Decreased fetal growth because of a decrease in placenta perfusion during gestation.

Intrauterine pressure catheter (IUPC): A small flexible tube inserted into the uterus along the uterine wall that provides an exact measurement of contraction length and intensity.

Intuitive thinking: The ability to classify information while becoming more aware of cause-and-effect relationships.

Intussusception: The invagination, or folding, of one section of the bowel into the other, which causes acute bowel obstruction, inflammation, and necrosis if not rapidly treated by low-pressure contrast or water enema.

Inverted nipples: Nipples that do not protrude or stand out from the breast.

Involution: The reduction in size of the uterus after childbirth.

Ipecac syrup: An over-the-counter medication known to induce vomiting related to toxic ingestion; it is no longer used in health-care settings because it has been replaced with activated charcoal and whole bowel irrigation.

Iron-deficiency anemia: A reduction in the mass of circulating red blood cells caused by a deficiency of dietary iron.

Ischial tuberosity diameter: The smallest dimension of the pelvis. It should be at least 10 cm to allow the head to pass through the ischial spines of the pelvis.

Isoimmunization: The creation of antibodies against Rh-positive blood that occurs in the mother's body after exposure to fetal Rh-positive blood.

Jaundice: A yellow discoloration of the skin caused by the breakdown of red blood cells that are not cleared by the liver.

Justice: The ethical principle of acting out of fairness for individuals, groups, organizations, and communities.

Juvenile idiopathic arthritis: A group of idiopathic chronic inflammatory joint diseases that first manifest during the early childhood period.

Kegel exercise: An exercise for strengthening the muscles of the perineum and vagina. The patient should repeatedly and rapidly contract and relax the muscles of the perineum and vagina for 10 seconds then relax for 20 seconds, and then repeat the routine. The number of repetitions should be increased gradually to between 50 and 150 per day.

Ketogenic diet: A special high-fat, low-carbohydrate diet that is thought to help control seizures in some people who have a documented history of epilepsy.

Ketones: Acids made when the body uses fat instead of carbohydrates for energy.

Kussmaul's respirations: A deep, gasping, repetitive breathing pattern associated specifically with acidosis.

Kyphosis: A condition of exaggerated angulation of the posterior curvature of the thoracic (i.e., upper) spine. In lay language, kyphosis is also referred to as "humpback" or "hunchback."

Labor induction: The use of mechanical or chemical methods to start cervical effacement, dilation, and contractions.

Lactoferrin: A protein that has bactericidal and iron-binding properties found in breast milk.

Lactogenesis: Production of milk.

Lanugo: A fine hair that covers the forehead, ears, and body of the newborn.

Large-for-gestational age (LGA): Newborn whose weight is greater than 90% for gestational age.

Laryngitis: Inflammation of the larynx or laryngeal mucosa and the vocal cords; characterized by hoarseness and aphonia (i.e., lost voice).

Late decelerations: Deceleration of fetal heart rate that occurs after the uterine contraction begins; the nadir is noted after the peak of the contraction.

Leading Health Indicators: A list of some of the *Healthy People* objectives that were selected because they are high-priority health issues.

Left-to-right blood flow shunt: A cardiovascular conduit through which blood flows from the left side of the heart, which usually perfuses the systemic circulation, to the right side of the heart, which usually perfuses the pulmonary circulation. This may result in pulmonary congestion and eventual heart failure.

Legal blindness: A term used to note that a child's visual acuity is measured or approximated to be below 20/200.

Leiomyoma: A benign tumor of smooth muscle.

Leopold maneuvers: A pattern of maneuvers that can be performed to determine the fetal position in the uterus.

Lethality of attempt: Refers to the determination of the potential threat of suicidal death per the patient's description of plans, methods, reasons, and availability of rescue.

Leukemia: Any class of hematological malignancies (i.e., cancer) of bone marrow cells in which immortal clones of immature blood cells multiply, causing a depletion of normal blood cells. Leukemias are categorized as chronic or acute; by the cell type they originated from; and by the genetic, chromosomal, or growth factor aberration present in the malignant cell.

Leukocoria: Also called "cat's eye reflex," it is a white to yellow glow to the retina seen when light hits the retina; a tumor of the eye, retinoblastoma, is present.

Leukorrhea: A white vaginal discharge that is usually increased in pregnancy.

LGBTQIA: Lesbian, gay, bisexual, transgender, queer/questioning, intersex, asexual, + (all other gender identities and sexual orientations not yet defined).

Lightening: The "dropping" of the fetus descending into the mother's pelvis.

Linea nigra: A dark line that runs from the umbilicus to the pubis in pregnant women; caused by hormonal changes.

Lipodystrophy: A disturbance of fat metabolism with a common finding of localized accumulation of fat under the skin, especially over the trunk.

Lithotomy position: A position in which the patient lies on the back, thighs flexed on the abdomen, legs on thighs, and thighs abducted.

Local anesthesia: Medication injected to numb an area of the body that is infused by the needle.

Lochia: The postpartum discharge of blood, mucus, and uterine tissue from the uterus after childbirth.

Lochia alba: The final stage of uterine sloughing. The discharge is yellow-white and may continue up to 6 weeks after delivery.

Lochia rubra: Postpartum, bright-red uterine discharge that usually lasts for 1 to 3 days after childbirth.

Lochia serosa: Postpartum, pink or brown uterine discharge that lasts for 4 to 9 days after childbirth.

Lordosis: A condition of anterior convexity of the lumbar spine.

Lund-Browder classification tool: A tool that is used to estimate the extent of a burn, allowing for varying proportion of the body surface; used instead of the "rule of nines" in children because of their larger head.

Luteinizing hormone (LH): A hormone causing ovulation that converts the ruptured follicle into the corpus luteum.

Macrosomia: A newborn with a birth weight greater than 4,000 to 4,500 g.

Macular rash: A rash that has flat spots on the skin; a macule is a flat, nonpalpable lesion less than 1 cm in diameter. Examples are freckles and petechiae.

Magical thinking: The invention of stories and fantasies to process a young child's reality.

Maintenance therapy: A phase of chemotherapy administration often used in pediatric oncology practice that is the end phase of treatment. Maintenance therapy has a goal of keeping the child in remission with no evidence of residual disease.

Maladaptive behaviors: Responses to stress that are considered unhealthy, such as the consumption of alcohol, illicit drug use, smoking, not sleeping, not eating well, self-harm, and fighting between family members.

Malpractice: An injury to a patient caused by an action taken by a health-care professional. The action is deemed a failure to meet a reasonable standard of practice.

Mandatory reporters of child abuse and neglect: People who, because of their positions, are legally responsible to report actual or suspected child abuse to authorities. All health-care providers are considered mandatory reporters. Commercial film developers, childcare custodians, and all branches of the law are considered mandatory reporters. Each of these four categories of mandatory reporters has the potential to identify actual or suspected abuse.

Mastitis: An infection in the breast tissue.

Meconium: A newborn's first stool that is composed of secretions from the intestines, bile pigments, mucus, lanugo, epithelial cells, and blood; it is greenish to black in color.

Mediating process: The process when one consciously or unconsciously reacts to manage a stressful situation.

Medical play: Structured play provided by the child life specialist or the nursing staff that provides the opportunity for a child to learn about their diagnosis; procedures; surgery; and diagnostic or medical equipment, including lines, tubes, and devices through the use of anatomically correct dolls or other play equipment used for teaching and demonstration.

Melanocytic nevi: Also known as *moles,* a nevus may be flat or raised. The congenital melanocytic nevus is usually evenly pigmented and brown or black in color.

Melasma: Brown facial skin discoloration. It appears on the upper cheeks, upper lip, forehead, and chin. It is related to sun exposure, hormones such as birth control pills, and hormonal changes in pregnancy.

Meningitis: Inflammation of the membranes of the brain or spinal cord, often caused by an infectious process.

Mental illness: A condition that affects behaviors or mood, such as personality disorders, depression, or schizophrenia.

Mesoderm: Lying between the ectoderm and the endoderm, the mesoderm is the middle embryonic germ layer from which the urogenital and circulatory systems develop.

Microencephaly: The state of having a small brain and head.

Milia: Sebaceous glands occluded with keratin that appear as tiny white papules about 1 mm in size located on the nose, chin, cheeks, and forehead.

Mittelschmerz: A term for the pain that is noticed by a woman during the middle of the menstrual cycle when ovulation occurs.

Monozygotic twins: Identical twins that develop from one fertilized egg.

Morbidity: A disease state.

Mortality: Death.

Multiple pregnancy: A pregnancy in which the woman has two or more embryos in her uterus.

Myelination: The process of growth of a myelin sheath around nerve fibers. This sheath, which acts as an electrical insulator, represents maturity of the nerve body and allows for increased velocity of the impulse.

Myoclonic: Clonic spasms or severe twitching of a muscle or group of muscles.

Myomas: Tumors that contain muscle tissue.

Myometrium: The middle layer of uterine muscle. The function of this layer is to contract and expel the fetus during childbirth.

Myopia: A defect of vision called *nearsightedness* caused by an error of refraction where parallel rays of light come to focus in front of the retina.

Nadir: The lowest point of the fetal heart rate deceleration.

Naegele's rule: The formula used to determine the estimated due date. Subtract 3 months from the first day of the last menstrual period and then add 7 days.

Nasopharyngeal: Relating to the area of the nasopharynx or the area situated above the soft palate.

National Standards for Culturally and Linguistically Appropriate Services in Health Care (CLAS): The collective set of CLAS mandates, guidelines, and recommendations issued by the Health & Human Services (HHS) Office of Minority Health intended to inform, guide, and facilitate required and recommended practices related to culturally and linguistically appropriate health services (Office of Minority Health, Department of Health & Human Services).

Near drowning: A phrase used to denote a level of survival after an immersion in water. This phrase has often been replaced with the phrase *submersion injury.*

Nebulizer: A device that aerates respiratory medications via a machine used for the ease and effectiveness of instilling medications throughout the lung fields. Considered very effective for the administration and distribution of asthma medications, such as nebulized albuterol or levosalbutamol.

Necrosis: The death of cells, tissues, or organs.

Necrotizing enterocolitis: A serious disease of premature infants characterized by damage to the intestinal tract mucosa.

Negativism: The tendency of being negative in attitude, including resisting suggestions, requests, or commands from others. This behavior of a young child is marked by resistance or retreat and is often associated with tantrums.

Neglect: The failure of another to provide for a child's most basic needs. Neglect can be emotional, physical, or educational.

Negligence: The failure of a health-care team member, or the team itself, to provide care according to their professional responsibility. There are four elements of negligence: breach of duty, duty owed, proximate cause, and damages/harm/injuries.

Neonatal sepsis: A blood infection that presents within the first 7 days of life but may occur up to 90 days after birth.

Nephrotic syndrome: A condition marked by an abnormal increase in renal glomerular permeability to serum proteins with subsequent hyperalbuminuria, hypoalbuminemia, and hyperlipidemia.

Neural tube defects: Defects of the spinal cord, spine, or brain.

Neuroleptic: Refers to any medication that is taken to treat psychotic behavior, usually by blocking dopamine receptors in the brain (e.g., chlorpromazine, haloperidol, or clozapine).

Neurotransmitter: A chemical molecule released by the axon terminals of a nerve cell that triggers a reaction that excites or inhibits the activity of the target cell. Serotonin, dopamine, and norepinephrine are examples of neurotransmitters.

Neutropenia: The presence of an abnormally small number of circulating neutrophils in the blood, usually less than 1,500 per microliter.

Nevus flammeus: Also known as a *port wine stain,* this reddish purple skin deformity is made up of dilated skin capillaries.

Nevus simplex: Also known as *stork bite, angel kiss,* or *salmon patch,* this type of benign birthmark is a capillary malformation that fades over time.

New morbidity: A phrase used to describe contemporary issues that affect a given population, such as children, and that is related to illness, injury, disease, and death.

Nightmares: Nighttime dreams that have the potential to, or actually, frighten a child.

Night terrors: Waking up at night with a strong emotional reaction to a nightmare.

Nocturia: Excessive urination during the night, which can be a symptom of renal or bladder problems.

Nocturnal incontinence: Incontinence of urine that occurs during the night, usually with a pathological cause.

Nonaccidental poisoning: When a child takes a toxic substance or medication for abuse, suicide gestures/attempts, or successful self-inflicted death.

Nonmaleficence: The ethical principle of "do no harm" or inflict the least possible harm to reach a beneficial outcome.

Nonsuicidal self-injury: Injury not accompanied by suicidal ideation or intent but rather is a way of coping with anxiety.

Normalcy: The movement toward being normal in one's life; pertains to attaining normal standards in one's life when faced with chronic illness, disability, or impairment.

Nuchal cord: The umbilical cord around the neck of the fetus.

Nystagmus: Involuntary back-and-forth movements of the eyes, most often noticeable when the patient gazes at objects moving by rapidly or at fixed objects.

Obesity: Considered a body mass index of greater than 30 kg/m². It is an unhealthy accumulation of body fat and is the most common metabolic/nutritional disease in the United States, leading to health consequences including diabetes, heart disease, hypertension, stroke, and fatal cancers.

Obstetric conjugate: The diameter from the sacral promontory to the upper inner border of the symphysis pubis; it measures approximately 11 cm.

Oligohydramnios: An abnormally small amount of amniotic fluid.

Ophthalmia neonatorum: An eye infection the newborn receives from exposure to vaginal secretions from untreated sexually transmitted infections.

Orthostatic hypotension: A drop in the blood pressure when a patient stands; caused by low blood volume or low blood pressure.

Osteomyelitis: Inflammation of the bone tissue and the marrow caused by an infection (or other less common sources, such as radiation) that most often occurs in the long bones.

Osteoporosis: A condition in which the bones become thin and fragile.

Otitis media: A viral or bacterial infection that causes the buildup of inflammatory fluids or pus behind the tympanic membrane.

Overflow incontinence: A condition in which an individual is unable to hold urine and then passes urine when the bladder is too full.

Overweight: Having weight in excess of what would be considered normal for a person's height, age, and overall build; person having a body mass index higher than expected for age and height and at the 95th percentile for others of the same age, height, and body mass.

Oxygenation: The exchange of gases in the lungs that allows oxygen to move into the blood.

Oxytocin: A hormone that is produced in the pituitary gland and secreted into the bloodstream.

Papanicolaou (Pap) smear: A test for cervical cancer.

Papular rash: A rash that has raised bumps or pimples rising above the skin and found of various colors; a papule is an elevated, firm, palpable lesion that is less than 1 cm in diameter. Examples include psoriasis and eczema.

Para: A woman who has produced a viable infant (weighing at least 500 g or more than 20 weeks' gestation) regardless of whether the fetus is alive at birth.

Parallel play: A form of play associated with the toddler developmental stage in which the child does not play with another toddler but plays close by, often back to back, with separate toys that they do not have to share.

Passive immunity: Temporary immunity acquired by transfusing immune globulins or antitoxins either artificially from another human or from an animal that has been actively immunized against an antigen or naturally from the mother to the fetus via the placenta.

Pediatric medical traumatic stress (PMTS): Set of psychological and physiological responses of children and their families to injury, pain, serious illness, medical procedures, and invasive or frightening treatment interventions.

Perfusion: The body's ability to circulate blood through the body to oxygenate tissues.

Perimetrium: A serous membrane that lines the external surface of the uterus.

Periodic decelerations: Decelerations of fetal heart rate associated with uterine contractions.

Peripheral cyanosis: Decreased cardiac output with an accompanying decrease in the peripheral blood flow; peripheral cyanosis may not demonstrate a reduced oxygen saturation measurement.

Personal protective equipment (PPE): Equipment that is made available to health-care professionals to prevent the spread of infections or diseases. This equipment includes gloves, gowns, eye shield/glasses, masks, shoe protectors, hair protective coverings, and disposable equipment such as stethoscopes.

Personality disorder: A pathological disturbance that affects communication, thinking, and perception and can manifest in different types such as antisocial and borderline categories.

Petechiae: Very small hemorrhagic purplish spots found on the child's skin when there is a significant reduction in circulating platelets.

Pfannenstiel incision: A "bikini cut" incision above the symphysis pubis.

Pica: The practice of eating nonnutritive foods.

Placenta: An organ that provides the fetus with oxygen and nourishment.

Placenta abruptio: The premature separation of the placenta from the wall of the uterus.

Placenta accreta: A situation in which the placenta is attached too deeply into the wall of the uterus, causing complications with removal.

Placenta previa: A complication of pregnancy in which the placenta implants in the lower uterus and completely or partially covers the cervix.

Pneumonitis: Inflammation of the lungs, usually affecting the bronchioles and alveoli.

Pneumothorax: A collection of air or gas in the pleural cavity. Often follows a perforation through the chest wall; a pneumothorax is sudden in onset with severe, sharp pains in the side of the chest and accompanying dyspnea.

Polycythemia: An excess of red blood cells.

Polydipsia: An experience of excessive thirst, often associated with dehydration, hypovolemia, and hyperglycemia.

Polyhydramnios: Excessive amniotic fluid.

Polyphagia: An experience of excessive hunger and eating abnormally large amounts of food.

Polyuria: An excessive secretion and discharge of urine, defined as more than 50 mL of urine per kg of body weight per day.

Postterm: An infant born after 42 weeks' gestation.

Posttraumatic stress disorder (PTSD): Considered a mental health condition following a traumatic or terrifying event; can be actually experienced or an event that was witnessed. PTSD can last for months to years.

Posttraumatic stress syndrome (PTSS): Set of symptoms experienced by children and adults after an event that is perceived as being traumatic.

Precipitous delivery: An unusually rapid labor of less than 3 hours and ending with a rapid spontaneous delivery of the infant.

Precocious puberty: The appearance of secondary sex characteristics before 8 years in girls and 9 years in boys. The cause of this condition may be premature secretion of sex hormones not caused by pituitary or hypothalamic action.

Preconceptual thinking: A young child's judgment of their environment by visual experiences.

Preeclampsia: Hypertension and proteinuria that is present after 20 weeks' gestation.

Premature rupture of membranes (PROM): Ruptured membranes within the patient that are at least 37 weeks' gestation before the onset of labor.

Prepubescence: The period of growth right before the onset of puberty that is marked by physical changes that denote sexual and reproductive maturation.

Pressure injury: A skin wound that results from impaired circulation or inadequate perfusion from pressure. It often develops from bedrest without consistent turning. It can vary from a superficial depth, appearing as nonblanching redness, to a deep crater that extends into bone tissue. Hospitalized patients with mobility deficits are at high risk.

Preterm: An infant born before 37 weeks' gestation.

Preterm premature rupture of membranes (PPROM): The rupture of membranes before 37 weeks' gestation.

Probiotics: Intestinal bacteria that aid in breaking down food for digestion.

Progesterone: A hormone that is produced by the corpus luteum and the placenta.

Prolactin: The hormone responsible for milk production.

Prolapse: To drop down out of place.

Prostaglandins: Hormonelike substances with a variety of effects on tissues, including the contraction and relaxation of smooth muscle.

Pruritic urticarial papules and plaque of pregnancy (PUPP): A dermatitis of itchy plaques and papules with erythematous patches of papules and vesicles.

Pruritus: Intense itching of the skin.

Pseudomenstruation: A mucus- and blood-tinged vaginal discharge that may be present in the newborn female for a few days until the maternal hormone level decreases.

Psychosis: A state in which a person experiences an impairment of reality testing. They inaccurately evaluate perceptions and thoughts.

Puberty: The time period or stage in a child's life when they become sexually mature and able to reproduce. Typically, this occurs during a rapid period between 13 and 15 years for boys and 9 and 16 years for girls.

Pudendal block: An anesthetic injected into the pudendal nerve to anesthetize the vulva and perineum.

Puerperium: The postpartum period after childbirth that lasts approximately 6 weeks as the reproductive system returns to the prepregnancy state.

Purpura: Any rash in which blood cells leak into the skin or mucous membranes, usually at multiple sites. Purpuric rashes are often associated with disorders of thrombosis or coagulation.

Pustule: A small raised skin lesion protruding above the skin line and filled with pus (i.e., white blood cells); found in many skin disorders, including medication rashes and acne.

Quickening: Fetal movement felt by the mother after 18 to 20 weeks' gestation.

Race: Genetic physical characteristics that are similar among members of a group, such as skin, hair, and eye color (Purnell & Paulanka, 2008).

Radiation: The transfer of body heat to a cooler object, such as a window.

Rales: Also known as *crackles,* adventitious breath sounds associated with fluid collection in the base of the lungs.

Rapid response team: A designated team designed to rapidly assemble at a child's bedside or clinic room to provide emergency response skills and resuscitation if needed.

Reactivity: A set of traits that influences behaviors, also called temperament.

Rectocele: A condition in which the rectum drops down and protrudes into the back wall of the vagina.

Refractory error: A common eye disorder where the eye bends light and is unable to focus because of its abnormal shape.

Regression: Demonstration of behaviors associated with a previous developmental stage. Usually associated with stress and anxiety; a child will regress to earlier behaviors such as bed wetting, use of diapers, wanting to be fed, or tantrums.

Relaxin: A hormone that works with progesterone to maintain the pregnancy and that causes relaxation of pelvis ligaments to aid in birthing.

Respiratory distress syndrome: A severe impairment of the respiratory function of a preterm newborn caused by immature lungs and lack of surfactant.

Respiratory syncytial virus (RSV): A viral infection associated with winter months that sequesters in the lung and causes severe symptoms of respiratory distress in infants. Children younger than 6 months are often hospitalized for supportive treatment.

Restraints: Devices that prevent patients from hurting themselves or others; may infrequently be warranted, although their use is highly discouraged and left for extreme safety issues. Adhering to strict hospital policy concerning the application for restraints is an imperative. All other forms of care and control should be used, such as family members or sitters being present, or child life interventions applied, before the decision to use restraints.

Retained placenta: A placenta that does not detach from the wall of the uterus, or, as the placenta separates from the uterus, small pieces or fragments of the placenta may be left attached to the uterus.

Retinoblastoma: A malignant glioma of the retina, usually unilateral, found in young children and associated with heredity.

Retinopathy of prematurity (ROP): A bilateral disease of the retinal vessels in premature infants leading to neovascularization and retinal detachment in the first few weeks of life. Although the etiology is unknown, ROP is associated with oxygen levels and environmental factors.

Retractions: A pulling in of the skin around the ribs and sternum when inhaling that is observed during respiratory distress.

Reye syndrome: Acute encephalopathy with brain swelling and fatty infiltration of the liver, spleen, kidney, pancreas, and lymph that is associated with the use of salicylates (i.e., aspirin) following a viral infection such as varicella.

Rhonchi: A low-pitched adventitious breath sound when a mucous plug is within a large airway structure; a rattling sound that moves with coughing.

Right-to-left blood flow shunt: A cardiovascular conduit through which blood flows from the right side of the heart, which usually perfuses the pulmonary circulation, to the left side of the heart, which usually perfuses the systemic circulation. This may result in underperfusion of pulmonary circulation and worsening cyanotic changes.

Rugae: The folds in the wall of the vagina.

Rule of nines: An assessment tool used to estimate the extent of a burn; used in late adolescence and adulthood.

Safety precautions: The use of multiple safety measures to keep children safe, including locking the wheels on the crib or bed; keeping the rails up; using high-top cribs for standing young children; keeping appropriately sized emergency equipment at the bedside, such as suction, oxygen, and a resuscitative bag/mask/valve; preventing aspiration; preventing strangulation with IV tubing or any wires in the crib; preventing burns and electrocution; and teaching parents how to use the rapid response team.

Salmonella **food poisoning:** Pathogenic bacilli that produce a range of reactions from mild gastroenteritis to fatal food poisoning. There are more than 1,400 species.

Salpingectomy: Removal of the fallopian tube.

Salpingostomy: A small, linear incision made into a fallopian tube that has become occluded or for drainage purposes.

SBAR: A method of organizing oneself for an oral report or telephone call with a primary health-care provider using four components: **S**ituation, **B**ackground, **A**ssessment, and **R**ecommendation.

Schizophrenia: A thought disorder marked by hallucinations, disorganized speech and behavior, and delusions. The child may be withdrawn, socially isolated, and present with a flat affect.

School vision: When a child is considered to be partially sighted with a measured or approximate visual acuity of 20/70 to 20/200.

Scoliosis: A lateral or *S*-shaped curvature of the spine that often presents with two curves: the abnormal curve and a compensatory curve on the opposite side.

Scope of practice: The boundaries in which a health-care provider can practice as described by the associated professional organization or licensure body; the legal outline of what a nurse can do according to the law of that state.

Selective attention: A demonstration during play, such as reading a book or playing a game, that the child does not hear the voice of a parent or teacher.

Sentinel events: Unexpected occurrences that cause injury or death of a patient.

Separation anxiety: An emotional reaction experienced by an older infant that starts at approximately 8 to 10 months, in which the child expresses anxiety when parents leave or the child is taken from the parents.

Sexual abuse: Inappropriate sexual behavior by an adolescent or adults with a child. This includes fondling the child's genitals, making the child fondle the adult's genitals, incest, intercourse, rape, sodomy, exploitation, exhibitionism, inappropriate sexually oriented photographing of a child, and exposure to pornography.

Sexual latency: A term used to describe the disinterest in the school-aged child's sexuality. This developmental period comes after the phases in infancy and young childhood of "oral" and "anal." The concept was proposed by Dr. Sigmund Freud, an Austrian neurologist and psychoanalyst (1856–1939).

Shock: A clinical syndrome marked by inadequate oxygenation and perfusion of tissues and organs at the cellular level because of markedly low systemic blood pressure; it can be caused by several factors, including sepsis, hemorrhage, severe dehydration, heart disease, burns, spinal cord injury, or trauma.

Shoulder dystocia: A situation during birth that occurs when one or both shoulders become wedged in the maternal pelvis after the head has been delivered.

Sickle cell anemia: An autosomal recessive disorder causing an abnormality of the globin genes in hemoglobin, leading to a chronic anemia disorder with a higher incidence in African Americans, Native Africans, and Mediterranean people. If the child is exposed to low levels of oxygen, the hemoglobin S becomes viscous and causes the red blood cell to become rigid, fragile, sickle-shaped, and sticky, all of which leads to an increase in destruction called *hemolysis*.

Sitz bath: A warm bath for the perineal area to provide comfort and promote healing.

Small-for-gestational age (SGA): An infant whose weight is less than the 10th percentile for their gestational age.

Social determinants of health: Physical conditions and social situations in environments where people are born, live, play, learn, work, worship, and age (*Healthy People 2030*).

Somatic pain: Pain caused by activation of pain receptors in the body surface or musculoskeletal tissues.

Spina bifida: A congenital defect of the spine in which part of the spinal cord and meninges are exposed through an opening in the vertebrae.

Spinal anesthesia: The placement of a needle into the intrathecal space to inject anesthetic medication.

Spiritual distress: A state of disruption in a person's emotional and psychological well-being. An impaired ability to feel connected with self, others, nature, and/or a power greater than oneself.

Spirituality: An awareness of the metaphysical, sublime, or religious. A practice of spirituality typically includes participation in an organized religion and/or meditation, prayer, contemplation, reflection, and/or other activities that foster self-growth.

Standards of care: A model of established practice that is accepted as the correct way to provide care for a patient.

Status epilepticus (SE): Continued seizure activity (i.e., seizures back-to-back) that can rapidly progress to being life-threatening and that require aggressive interventions and medications to prevent injury and death.

Stereotyping: A conception, opinion, or belief about some aspect of an individual or group (Purnell & Paulanka, 2008).

Stomatitis: A painful inflammation of the mouth that can affect the tongue, mucous membranes, and lips.

Strabismus: Disorder of the eye in which optic axes cannot be directed to the same object; found in approximately 4% of children. The child may squint to deviate the alternative eye to the same extent as the eyes are carried in different directions. Lay term for strabismus is "wall eye."

Stranger anxiety: Anxiety experienced by an older infant or young child when they encounter a new person in their environment.

Stress: A state produced by a change in the environment that is perceived as threatening, challenging, or damaging to an individual's dynamic balance or equilibrium.

Stress incontinence: Leaking of urine when coughing or laughing.

Striae gravidarum: Stretch marks located on the abdomen and thighs because of weight gain of pregnancy.

Stridor: A high-pitched harsh sound that occurs during inspiration (often heard without the aid of a stethoscope), which denotes the presence of an obstruction in the upper airway.

Subinvolution: A state in which the uterus fails to complete the involution process after giving birth.

Suicidal ideation: The thought process of considering suicide but without any physical attempts to do so. Many people who contemplate killing themselves have seen a health-care professional in the months before an attempt or successful suicide, showing the importance of early screening, identification, and intervention.

Suicidal thinking: When a child or teen is thinking about suicide but has no plan. This is not uncommon with approximately 3% of the general teen population reporting suicidal thinking at one point of their development.

Suicide: Death associated with taking one's own life via a variety of methods.

Suicide attempt: A situation in which a person attempts to take their life via a variety of means but is unsuccessful.

Surfactant: A mixture of phospholipids and lipoproteins secreted by the lung cells that assists the alveoli to stay open when the newborn begins breathing.

Symbolic functioning: The creation of an image in the mind that represents something as other than it is (e.g., a horse for a pillow or a sheet for a tent).

Tachypnea: Rapid breathing.

Tachysystole: The term for contractions occurring more often than five or more contractions in a 10-minute window averaged over 30 minutes. This can be caused by overstimulation from oxytocin or it may be a spontaneous occurrence.

Tardive dyskinesia: Considered a neurological syndrome of slow, stereotyped rhythmical movements, generalized or focal, of muscle groups. Associated with psychotropic medications, it is an unwanted side effect of therapy requiring medical intervention.

Technology dependent: The dependence on a medical device and/or skill to maintain health and wellness.

Temperament: The combination of the mental, physical, and emotional traits of a person; in toddlerhood, it marks the toddler's predisposition to how they interact with others and their unique environment.

Teratogen: Any substance that may cause a birth defect.

Testosterone: A male hormone produced in the testes.

Therapeutic hugging: The use of a parent's or a caregiver's hugs to hold a child during a procedure such as injections, IV line placement, wound care, or a dressing change. Not considered a restraint but a means to protect and comfort a child during an uncomfortable, painful, or frightening procedure.

Thermoregulation: An intrinsic or extrinsic process of maintaining a normal core body temperature.

Threatened abortion: When vaginal bleeding occurs during the first 20 weeks of pregnancy.

Thrombocytopenia: The presence of an abnormally small number of circulating platelets in the blood. A platelet count of less than per $50,000/mm^3$ may increase the risk of a child bleeding.

Thromboembolism: A condition of an inflammation of a vein in conjunction with a thrombus.

Thrombosis: Formation of a blood clot.

Thrombus: A blood clot.

Tocolytic medications: Medications used to decrease uterine activity and stop preterm labor.

Tonic-clonic seizure: Muscle activity associated with grand mal seizures that is marked by rapid contraction and then relaxation of large muscle groups.

Tort: A wrongful act or injury committed against another that can be pursued in civil court by the party that was injured.

Toxicology: The study of harmful or poisonous levels of chemicals in the body, including their detection, avoidance, chemistry, pharmacological actions, antidotes, and treatments.

Toxoid: A substance that is chemically modified to retain its antigen properties but is no longer considered poisonous; used to make immunizations.

Traction: A therapy used to help in the healing process of a fracture; it often uses two lines of pull for extension and stabilization.

Trial of labor after cesarean (TOLAC): Allowing a woman who desires a vaginal birth after a cesarean birth to begin labor while being closely monitored for progress and complications.

Umbilical cord: The attachment between the fetus and the placenta.

Unintentional abuse or injury: An injury to a child that was unintentionally inflicted. Not considered a form of child abuse, unintentional injury occurs when a child is injured but it was not caused by abuse or neglect.

Urinary retention: A condition in which the bladder cannot empty completely.

Urticaria: A condition associated with allergic reactions and marked by multiple discrete areas of swelling on the skin (also known as *wheals*); can cause severe itching because of the associated secretion of vasoactive mediators from mast cells.

Uterine inversion: A situation in which the uterus inverts and the uterine fundus prolapses to or through the dilated cervix. The inverted uterine wall may extend to or through the cervix. In severe cases, the entire uterus and vagina may invert and prolapse out of the patient's body.

Uterine rupture: A nonsurgical opening of the uterus that can allow the uterine contents to move into the abdomen.

Vacuum extraction: The use of a cuplike device that attaches to the fetal head with suction, which allows the healthcare provider to assist with the birth.

Vaginal birth after cesarean (VBAC): Allowing a woman to attempt a vaginal birth after a previous cesarean birth.

Variability: Fluctuations in the baseline that are irregular in frequency and amplitude because of interactions between the sympathetic and parasympathetic nervous systems.

Variable decelerations: An abrupt decrease in fetal heart rate of 15 beats per minute or more caused by cord compression, which disrupts the oxygenation of the fetus.

Varicose veins: Distended, swollen veins.

Vaso-occlusive episode: During a sickle cell anemia exacerbation, a vaso-occlusive episode (called a *vaso-occlusive crisis* in the past) is when a large number of rigid, sickle-shaped red blood cells infiltrate organs, joints, lung tissue, and the retina, causing hypoxia and damage to the affected tissues. Vaso-occlusive episodes are associated with pain and can be life-threatening if severe.

Vena caval syndrome: Condition when the weight of the uterus on the vena cava causes compression and the reduced blood flow causes hypotension and lightheadedness.

Vernix caseosa: A white protective coating on the skin of the newborn.

Vesicle: A small elevation on the skin that is blisterlike and contains serous fluid; varies in diameter and color.

Viability: A newborn weighing at least 500 g at more than 20 weeks' gestation.

Viable: A term used to describe a fetus that is able to live outside the uterus.

Villi: Fingerlike projections in the placenta that are surrounded by the mother's blood.

Visceral pain: Pain in internal organs caused by the activation of receptors in the chest, abdomen, or pelvic area that send signals to the spinal cord and on to the brain.

Vitiligo: A condition of depigmentation, or loss of natural skin color, that has no known cause.

Vulvovaginitis: Infection of the vagina and vulva.

Wharton jelly: A gelatinous substance that provides support and protection for the vessels inside the umbilical cord.

Wheal: A round and elevated lesion, often temporary, that is white in the center and surrounded by red inflammation; often seen with insect bites and urticaria.

Worldview: A set of explanations used by a group of people to explain life's events and to offer solutions to life's mysteries; also defined as a major thought process of shared cultural backgrounds (Andrews & Boyle, 2008).

Credits

Figure 1.1: Courtesy of the National Institutes of Health, www.nih.gov.

Figure 2.1: monkeybusinessimages/iStock/Thinkstock.

Figure 2.2: BananaStock/BananaStock/Thinkstock.

Figure 2.5: Ryan McVay/Photodisc/Thinkstock.

Figure 3.1: American College of Obstetricians and Gynecologists. (2021). *Effectiveness of contraceptive methods.* https://www.acog.org/womens-health/infographics/effectiveness-of-birth-control-methods

Chapter 4: American College of Obstetricians and Gynecologists. (2017). *Five As Model: Smoking cessation during pregnancy.* ACOG Committee Opinion, number 721. https://www.acog.org/-/media/Committee-Opinions/Committee-on-Obstetric-Practice/co721.pdf?dmc=1&ts=20180201T1832413356; Section 2: Recommendations for Adults (continued). Content last reviewed June 2014. Adapted from Agency for Healthcare Research and Quality, Rockville, MD. https://www.ahrq.gov/prevention/guidelines/guide/section2d.html#Tobacco

Figure 7.1: szeyuen/iStock/Thinkstock.

Figure 7.3: Purestock/Thinkstock.

Figure 9.7: Adapted with permission from Wong, D. L., Perry, S. E., & Hockenberry, M. J. (2002). *Maternal child nursing care* (2nd ed.). Mosby. Copyright 2002.

Figures 9.15, 9.16, and 12.3: Adapted with permission from Lowdermilk, D. L., & Perry, S. E. (2004). *Maternity and women's healthcare* (8th ed.). Mosby. Copyright 2004.

Figure 12.7: Glenda Powers/iStock/Thinkstock.

Figure 15.14: Reprinted from Ballard, J. L., Khoury, J. C., Wedig, K., Wang, L., Eilers-Walsman, B. L., & Lipp, R. (1991). New Ballard Score, expanded to include extremely premature infants. *The Journal of Pediatrics, 119,* 3. https://doi.org/10.1016/s0022-3476(05)82056-6. Copyright 1991, with permission from Elsevier.

Figure 16.3: All images are Copyright ©2015 Medela, Inc.

Figure 17.2: Courtesy of McLeod Regional Medical Center, Florence, SC.

Figures 17.3, 17.4, and 17.6: Courtesy of St. Luke's Hospital, Bethlehem, PA.

Figure 18.1: DragonImages/iStock/Thinkstock.

Figure 19.2: yaoinlove/iStock/Thinkstock.

Figure 20.3: kate_sept2004/iStock/Thinkstock.

Figure 21.1: Ridofranz/iStock/Thinkstock.

Figures 21.2, 21.3, and 24.7: From the Centers for Disease Control and Prevention Public Health Library. http://phil.cdc.gov

Figure 22.4: From *Healthy People 2020.*

Chapter 23: Safe and Effective Nursing Care, QUESTT Tool: Adapted with permission from Wong, D. L., & Wilson, D.

(Eds.). (1999). *Whaley & Wong's nursing care of infants and children* (6th ed.). Copyright Elsevier 1999.

Unnumbered Figure 23.3: Used with permission of OUCHER!.org; ©The African-American version was developed and copyrighted by Mary J. Denyes, PhD, RN, and Antonia M. Villarruel, PhD, RN, USA, 1990. Cornelia Porter, PhD, RN, and Charlotta Marshall, RN, MSN, contributed to the development of the scale.

Figure 25.6: Jupiterimages/Stockbyte/Thinkstock.

Figure 28.1: Gylys, B. A., & Wedding, M. E. (2009). *Medical terminology systems: A body systems approach* (6th ed.). F. A. Davis.

Figure 28.5: Courtesy of D. M. Kocisko.

Figure 29.4: SDI Productions/iStock/Thinkstock.

Figure 32.4: From the Centers for Disease Control and Prevention, Department of Health and Human Services.

Figure 35.3: Adapted from the National Institutes of Health. Retrieved from http://kidney.niddk.nih.gov/kudiseases/pubs/nephrotic.

Figures 36.3, 37.7, 37.8, 39.9, and Unnumbered Figure 37.1: Courtesy of the Centers for Disease Control and Prevention.

Figure 36.7: Courtesy of Dr. Loretta Fiorillo.

Figure 36.12: From Goldsmith, L. A., Lazarus, G. S., & Tharp, M. D. (1997). *Adult and pediatric dermatology.* F. A. Davis Company, p. 121. Vitiligo.

Figure 37.1: From the Centers for Disease Control and Prevention, Department of Health & Human Services, Dr. Heinz F. Eichenwald, 1958. Retrieved March 2012 from http://phil.cdc.gov/phil/details.asp?pid=3187, ID #3187.

Figure 37.2: From the Centers for Disease Control and Prevention, Department of Health & Human Services, Dr. Heinz F. Eichenwald, 1958. Retrieved March 2012 from http://phil.cdc.gov/Phil/details.asp, ID #3168.

Figure 37.3: From the Centers for Disease Control and Prevention, Department of Health & Human Services, NIP/Barbara Rice. Retrieved March 2012 from http://phil.cdc.gov/phil/details.asp?pid=130

Figure 37.4: From the Centers for Disease Control and Prevention, Department of Health & Human Services, 1975. Retrieved March 2012 from http://phil.cdc.gov/Phil/details.asp, ID #4514.

Figure 37.5: From the Centers for Disease Control and Prevention, Department of Health & Human Services, 1969. Retrieved from http://phil.cdc.gov/Phil/details.asp,ID #3318.

Figure 37.6: From the Centers for Disease Control and Prevention, Department of Health & Human Services, 1995. Retrieved March 2012 from http://phil.cdc.gov/phil/details.asp, ID #6121.

Figure 37.10: From the Centers for Disease Control and Prevention, Department of Health & Human Services, 2007. Retrieved from http://phil.cdc.gov/Phil/details.asp, ID #9875.

Figure 38.2: FangXiaNuo/iStock/Thinkstock.

Figure 38.5: FatCamera/iStock/Thinkstock.

Index

References followed by the letter "f" are for figures, "t" are tables, and "b" are boxes.

Granulocyte transfusion, 694
Graves disease, 567
Gravida, 76–77
Greenstick fractures, 582, 582b, 582f
Grief, perinatal loss and, 183–184
Gross motor development, 303b, 340, 340t, 341f
Group B streptococci test (GBS), 81, 146
Group B streptococcus screen, 101t, 102
Growth, concept of, 76
Growth and development
    of adolescents
        acne and, 385–386, 385f, 650–651, 651f
        anticipatory guidance for, 382–383
        challenges in, 385–387
        cognitive development and, 378–379
        depression and, 386
        emotional development and, 381
        hormones and, 375–376
        injury prevention and, 384–385
        legal issues and, 382
        LGBTQIA+, 380
        nutrition and, 376–377
        overweight and obesity in, 377
        physical, 376–378, 376b, 376t
        psychological growth and development of, 381–382, 382f
        screening and, 384
        self-harm and, 386–387, 387f
        sexual development and, 379–380, 379f, 380f
        sleep and, 377–378
        socialization of, 382, 382f
        spiritual development and, 381–382
        suicide and, 386
        violence and, 386
    cardiac conditions and, 547
    development theories, 304t
    of infants (birth to one year)
        anticipatory guidance for, 305–306, 305b, 306f
        cognitive development and, 300, 303
        communication in, 304, 304f
        disease and injury prevention for, 311
        disorders of, 312, 312t–314t, 315, 315b
        growth charts for, 300, 301f, 302f
        hereditary and genetic influences in, 294
        hospitalized infant safety, 308–311, 308t–310t, 310f
        medication administration guidelines for, 706
        milestones of, 293
        physical growth and development in, 294–300, 296t, 298t, 299t, 301f–304f, 303–304, 303b, 304t
        psychosocial needs and bonding in, 304–305
        safety for, 293, 306
        screenings for, 306–308, 307t, 308t
        visual impairment or blindness in, 500

    of preschoolers
        allergies and, 341
        anticipatory guidance for, 349–352, 350b, 352b, 352f
        body image of, 349
        cheating and, 348
        cognitive development and, 342–344, 343b, 343f, 344t
        concept of time, 343
        dentition and, 351
        discipline and, 346
        encopresis and, 353, 356–357
        enuresis and, 346
        family meals and, 341
        family relationships and, 346
        germ avoidance for, 353
        gross motor development and, 340, 340t, 341f
        hand washing and, 353
        hospitalized preschoolers, 347, 352
        imaginary friends and, 347–348
        imagination, magical thinking and, 343
        immunizations for, 339–340
        infectious disease and, 353, 354t–355t
        injury prevention for, 353
        language development and, 343–344, 344t
        medical concerns and, 350
        medical play and, 351–352, 352b, 352f
        medical terminology and, 351
        medication administration guidelines for, 706
        medication safety for, 350–351
        moral and spiritual development of, 345, 345b, 345f
        MyPlate for, 341, 342f
        numbers, colors, letters and, 344
        nutrition and, 340–341, 342f
        obesity and, 341
        physical development and, 339
        play and, 347–349, 348b
        preschool readiness and, 349
        protective equipment for, 349
        psychological growth and development and, 344–346, 345b, 345f
        screenings for, 352
        selective attention and, 343, 343f
        sexual development and, 349
        sleep and, 341–342
        socialization and, 344–345
        technology and, 348
        temperament and, 345
        thumb sucking and, 351
        toys, crafts, arts and games for, 348–349, 348b
    of school-aged child
        anticipatory guidelines for, 366
        bullying and, 367, 368t, 369
        cognitive development and, 362–363, 362b
        concerns for, 366–369, 367t, 368t
        family dynamics and, 365, 365b
        friendship and, 366

        hospitalized school-aged child safety, 372
        injury prevention for, 369–371, 369b, 369f, 370b
        medication administration guidelines for, 706
        moral development and, 364
        musculoskeletal health of, 361
        nutrition and, 361–362
        obesity and, 366–368, 367t
        physical growth and development and, 360–362, 360f, 361b, 362b, 362f
        play and, 366
        psychological growth and development and, 363–366, 363b, 364t, 365b
        screenings and, 371–372, 371f, 496–497
        sleep and, 362, 362f
        socialization and, 363–364, 363b, 364t
        spirituality and, 364–365
        temperament and, 365
    sensory impairments and, 496
    skin conditions and, 638
    of toddlers
        anticipatory guidance for, 327–331, 328f, 329b
        auditory acuity and, 328
        autism spectrum disorder and, 334
        autonomy in, 318
        car seat safety and, 330–332
        causality and, 321
        child abuse and, 332, 334
        cognitive development and, 321–322, 322t
        communication development and, 322–323, 322t
        dentition and, 327–328, 328f
        discipline and, 325–326, 326b
        disorders of, 332, 334–335
        environmental exploration and, 321
        exploratory play and, 319, 319f
        home safety for, 328–329, 329b
        infectious diseases and, 335
        injury prevention for, 332, 333t
        iron-deficiency anemia and, 334
        medication administration guidelines for, 706
        medication safety and, 330
        moral development of, 324
        nutrition and, 320
        object permanence and, 321
        parallel play and, 326, 326f
        pet safety for, 329
        physical development and, 319–321, 319f
        poisoning and, 329–330
        psychosocial development and, 323–324
        safety in, 318
        screenings for, 331–332, 331t–332t
        separation anxiety and, 324
        sleep patterns in, 321
        socialization of, 320, 323
        spatial relationships and, 321